One Health Reviews: 2019–2025

One Health Reviews: 2019–2025

Edited by

David Hemming

CABI

CABI is a trading name of CAB International

CABI
Nosworthy Way
Wallingford
Oxfordshire OX10 8DE
UK

Tel: +44 (0)1491 832111
E-mail: info@cabi.org
Website: www.cabi.org

CABI
200 Portland Street
Boston
MA 02114
USA

T: +1 (617)682-9015
E-mail: cabi-nao@cabi.org

A catalogue record for this book is available from the British Library, London, UK.

ISBN-13: 9781836991458 (hardback)
9781836991465 (ePDF)
9781836991472 (ePub)

DOI: 10.1079/9781836991472.0000

Commissioning Editor: David Hemming
Editorial Assistant: Theresa Regueira
Production Editor: Helen Elliott

Typeset by Exeter Premedia Services Pvt Ltd, Chennai, India
Printed and bound in the UK by CPI Group (UK) Ltd, Croydon, CR0 4YY

Contents

Supplementary Content

https://www.cabidigitallibrary.org/doi/book/10.1079/9781836991472.0000

Chapter 1 includes supplementary material:

S1.1 Electronic Boolean Search

S1.2 Table of Data Extraction

Original Publication Details

1 **Design characteristics of integrated surveillance of antimicrobial resistance at the human, animal, and environment interfaces**
Erda Eni Rame Hau, Peter D. Sly, Deirdre Mikkelsen, Neelam Taneja, Kinley Penjor, Sukhyun Ryu, Erica Donner, Joanne Mollinger, Jorge Pinto Ferreira, Mark Schipp and Ricardo J. Soares Magalhaes
Previously published in CABI Reviews (2024)
https://doi/10.1079/cabireviews.2024.0047

2 **An insight on the last two decades of global research on animal tuberculosis: Bibliometric analysis**
Latifah Abdullah Alhusayni, Mohamed Marzok, Yamen Hegazy, Fatma A. El-Gohary and Sabry El-Khodery
Previously published in CABI Reviews (2024)
https://doi.org/10.1079/cabireviews.2024.0035

3 **Local food systems as a resilient strategy to ensure sustainable food security in crisis: Lessons from COVID-19 pandemic and perspectives for the post-pandemic world**
Anju Thattantavide and Ajay Kumar
Previously published in CABI Reviews (2024)
https://doi.org/10.1079/cabireviews.2024.0020

4 **Multiple approaches in the study of ancient human microbiome**
Santiago Rosas-Plaza, Ximena Rosas-Plaza and Rene Cerritos
Previously published in CABI Reviews (2024)
https://doi.org/10.1079/cabireviews.2024.0011

5 **More than food: Why restoring the cycle of organic matter in sustainable plant production is essential for the One Health nexus**
Cindy E. Morris, Andrea Radici, Christine N. Meynard, Nicolas Sauvion, Claire Nedellec, Ghislain Geniaux and Samuel Soubeyrand
Previously published in CABI Reviews (2024)
https://doi.org/10.1079/cabireviews.2024.0008

6 Foodborne pathogens and their association with well-known enteric infections and emerging non-communicable disorders
Asma Afshari, Ramin Rezaee and Golshan Shakeri
Previously published in CABI Reviews (2024)
https://doi.org/10.1079/cabireviews.2024.0009

7 Current perspectives for the use of medical ozone in veterinary medicine
Haytham Aamer, Eman Nour, Ayman Refaie, Mohamed Youssef and Maged El-Ashker
Previously published in CABI Reviews (2023)
https://doi.org/10.1079/cabireviews.2023.0043

8 Dengue a global threat: An insight into management and control
Muhammad Jamil, Ashiq Saleem, Rida Naz, Sajad Ahmad, Faiqah Ramzan, Mubarik Ali and Norina Jabeen
Previously published in CABI Reviews (2023)
https://doi.org/10.1079/cabireviews.2023.0040

9 Impacts of climate change on animal welfare
Joe Joseph, Renae Charalambous, Harsh Pahuja, Dylan Fox, Jiwoo Jeon, Ning-Yuan Ko, Nishit Rao, Zhiheng Wang, Sneh Kashinath Nerurkar, Sharvari Avinash Sherekar, Yifei Yang, Kate Dutton-Regester and Edward Narayan
Previously published in CABI Reviews (2023)
https://doi.org/10.1079/cabireviews.2023.0020

10 Tuberculosis vaccines for cattle
Federico Blanco, Julia Sabio y Garcia and Fabiana Bigi
Previously published in CABI Reviews (2023)
https://doi.org/10.1079/cabireviews.2023.0010

11 How agricultural practices affect the risk of human contamination by infectious pathogens: the need for a 'One Health' perspective
Alain Ratnadass and Samira Sarter
Previously published in CABI Reviews (2023)
https://doi.org/10.1079/cabireviews.2023.0003

12 The role of agriculture in human infectious disease outbreaks
Serge Morand
Previously published in CABI Reviews (2022)
https://doi.org/10.1079/cabireviews202217060

13 Man's best friend and our shared infectious diseases
Maxine L.A. Macpherson, Rhonda Pinckney, Wayne Sylvester, Satesh Bidaisee and Calum N.L. Macpherson
Previously published in CABI Reviews (2022)
https://doi.org/10.1079/cabireviews202217052

14 Food systems during the COVID-19 pandemic: vulnerabilities, adaptations, and resilience
Jill E. Hobbs
Previously published in CABI Reviews (2022)
https://10.1079/cabireviews202217014

15 Constraints to using livestock to meet dietary needs in developing countries: role of vaccines
Cynthia L. Baldwin and Samuel J. Black
Previously published in CABI Reviews (2021)
https://doi.org/10.1079/PAVSNNR202116058

16 Cattle tick control in Africa: potential of ethnoveterinary plants
Brighton M. Mvumi, Emmanuel T. Nyahangare, Jacobus N. Eloff, Steven R. Belmain and Philip C. Stevenson
Previously published in CABI Reviews (2021)
https://doi.org/10.1079/PAVSNNR202116042

17 Zoonotic diseases: a One Health perspective
Assadullah Samadi and Nabil Hailat
Previously published in CABI Reviews (2021)
https://doi.org/10.1079/PAVSNNR202116027

18 Pursuing effective vaccines against cattle diseases caused by apicomplexan protozoa
Monica Florin-Christensen, Leonhard Schnittger, Reginaldo G. Bastos, Vignesh A. Rathinasamy, Brian M. Cooke, Heba F. Alzan and Carlos E. Suarez
Previously published in CABI Reviews (2021)
https://doi.org/10.1079/PAVSNNR202116024

19 Impacts of COVID-19 on agriculture and food security in developing countries: potential mitigation strategies
Kehinde O. Erinle, Matthew C. Ogwu, Smith E. Evivie, Muhammad S. Zaheer, Solabomi O. Ogunyemi and Samson O. Adeniran
Previously published in CABI Reviews (2021)
https://doi.org/10.1079/PAVSNNR202116016

20 Emotional contagion and its implications for animal welfare
Sandra Düpjan, Annika Krause, Liza R. Moscovice and Christian Nawroth
Previously published in CABI Reviews (2020)
https://doi.org/10.1079/PAVSNNR202015046

21 Direct and indirect threats imposed by plant pathogenic and saprophytic fungi on humans and animals
Elham Ahmed Kazerooni, Rethinasamy Velazhahan, Musthafa Mohamed Essa and Abdullah Mohammed Al-Sadi
Previously published in CABI Reviews (2020)
https://doi.org/10.1079/PAVSNNR202015036

22 *Toxocara* and its species
Molly A. Ziegler and Calum N.L. Macpherson
Previously published in CABI Reviews (2019)
https://doi.org/10.1079/PAVSNNR201914053

23 Feline obesity and diabetes: a One Health perspective
Moira S. Lewitt
Previously published in CABI Reviews (2019)
https://doi.org/10.1079/PAVSNNR201914017

24 Integrative view of diseases in ruminants: towards a holistic model
Ricardo Piña-Martínez, Cintli Martínez-Ortiz-de-Montellano, Claudia Cecilia Márquez-Mota and Edgar Dantán-González
Previously published in CABI Reviews (2025)
https://doi.org/10.1079/cabireviews.2025.0015

Contributors

Haytham Aamer: Faculty of Medicine, Urology & Nephrology Centre, Animal Research Facility, Mansoura University, Mansoura, Egypt

Latifah Abdullah Alhusayni: Department of Clinical Sciences, College of Veterinary Medicine, King Faisal University, Al-Ahsa, Saudi Arabia

Samson O. Adeniran: Department of Animal Genetics, Breeding and Reproduction, College of Animal Science and Technology, Northeast Agricultural University, Harbin, 150030, China

Asma Afshari: Department of Nutrition, Faculty of Medicine, Mashhad University of Medical Sciences, Mashhad, Iran

Sajad Ahmad: Regional Blood Centre, Dera Ismail Khan, 29050, Pakistan

Mubarik Ali: Animal Science Institute, National Agricultural Research Center, Islamabad, 54000, Pakistan

Abdullah Mohammed Al-Sadi: Department of Crop Sciences, College of Agricultural and Marine Sciences, Sultan Qaboos University, Muscat, 123, Sultanate of Oman

Heba F. Alzan: Department of Veterinary Microbiology and Pathology, Washington State University, P.O. Box 647040, Pullman, WA, 991664-7040, United States; Parasitology and Animal Diseases Department, National Research Center, Giza, 12622, Egypt

Cynthia L. Baldwin: Department of Veterinary & Animal Sciences, 661 North Pleasant Street, University of Massachusetts, Amherst, MA 01003, United States; Program in Molecular & Cellular Biology, University of Massachusetts, Amherst, MA 01003, United States

Reginaldo G. Bastos: Department of Veterinary Microbiology and Pathology, Washington State University, P.O. Box 647040, Pullman, WA, 991664-7040, United States

Steven R. Belmain: Natural Resources Institute, University of Greenwich, Chatham Maritime, Chatham, Kent ME4 4TB, United Kingdom

Satesh Bidaisee: School of Graduate Studies, St. George's University, Grenada, West Indies; Windward Islands Research and Education Foundation, St. George's University, Grenada, West Indies; School of Medicine, St. George's University, True Blue, Grenada, West Indies

Fabiana Bigi: Instituto de Biotecnologia, CICVyA, Instituto Nacional de Tecnologia Agropecuaria, Argentina (INTA) and Instituto de Agrobiotecnologia y Biologia Molecular, (IABIMO) INTA-CONICET, Hurlingham CP1686, Buenos Aires, Argentina

Samuel J. Black: Department of Veterinary & Animal Sciences, 661 North Pleasant Street, University of Massachusetts, Amherst, MA 01003, United States; Program in Molecular & Cellular Biology, University of Massachusetts, Amherst, MA 01003, United States

Federico Blanco: Instituto de Biotecnologia, CICVyA, Instituto Nacional de Tecnologia Agropecuaria, Argentina (INTA) and Instituto de Agrobiotecnologia y Biologia Molecular, (IABIMO) INTA-CONICET, Hurlingham CP1686, Buenos Aires, Argentina

Rene Cerritos: Centro de Investigacion en Politicas, Poblacion y Salud, Universidad Nacional Autonoma de Mexico, Mexico City, Mexico; CONACHYT, Cibiogem (Comision Intersecretarial de Bioseguridad y Organismos Geneticamente Modificados), Mexico City, Mexico

Renae Charalambous: School of Agriculture and Food Sustainability, The University of Queensland, Gatton Campus, QLD 4343, Australia

Brian M. Cooke: Australian Institute of Tropical Health and Medicine, James Cook University, Cairns, Queensland, 4870, Australia

Edgar Dantán-González: Centro de Investigación en Biotecnología, Universidad Autónoma del Estado de Morelos, Av. Universidad 1001, Colonia Chamilpa, Cuernavaca, Morelos, 62209, México

Erica Donner: Future Industries Institute, University of South Australia, Adelaide, South Australia, Australia

Sandra Düpjan: Institute of Behavioural Physiology, Leibniz Institute for Farm Animal Biology (FBN), 18196 Dummerstorf, Germany

Kate Dutton-Regester: School of Agriculture and Food Sustainability, The University of Queensland, Gatton Campus, QLD 4343, Australia

Maged El Ashkcr: Faculty of Veterinary Medicine, Department of Internal Medicine and Infectious Diseases, Mansoura University, Mansoura, 35516, Egypt

Fatma A. El-Gohary: Department of Hygiene and Zoonoses, Faculty of Veterinary Medicine, Mansoura University, Mansoura, 35516, Egypt

Sabry El-Khodery: Department of Internal Medicine and Infectious Diseases, Faculty of Veterinary Medicine, Mansoura University, Mansoura, 35516, Egypt

Jacobus N. Eloff: Phytomedicine Programme, Faculty of Veterinary Science, University of Pretoria, Private Bag X04, Onderstepoort 0110, Pretoria, South Africa

Erda Eni Rame Hau: Queensland Alliance for One Health Sciences, School of Veterinary Science, The University of Queensland, Gatton, Queensland, Australia

Kehinde O. Erinle: School of Agriculture, Food and Wine, The University of Adelaide, South Australia, Urrbrae SA 5064, Australia

Musthafa Mohamed Essa: Department of Food Science and Nutrition, Sultan Qaboos University, Muscat, 123, Sultanate of Oman

Smith E. Evivie: Key Laboratory of Dairy Science, Ministry of Education, College of Food Science, Northeast Agricultural University, Harbin, 150030, China; Department of Animal Science, Faculty of Agriculture, University of Benin, Benin City, 300001, Nigeria; Department of Food

Science and Human Nutrition, Faculty of Agriculture, University of Benin, Benin City, 300001, Edo State, Nigeria

Monica Florin-Christensen: Instituto de Patobiologia Veterinaria, Centro de Investigaciones en Ciencias Veterinarias y Agronomicas (CICVyA), Instituto Nacional de Tecnologia Agropecuaria (INTA), Hurlingham 1686, Argentina; Consejo Nacional de Investigaciones Cientificas y Tecnologicas (CONICET), C1425FQB Buenos Aires, Argentina

Dylan Fox: School of Agriculture and Food Sustainability, The University of Queensland, Gatton Campus, QLD 4343, Australia

Ghislain Geniaux: INRAE, Ecodeveloppement UR 767, F-84914, Avignon, France

Nabil Hailat: Pathology and Public Health Department, Faculty of Veterinary Medicine, Jordan University of Science and Technology (JUST), P.O. Box 3030, Irbid, Irbid 22110, Jordan

Yamen Hegazy: Department of Clinical Sciences, College of Veterinary Medicine, King Faisal University, Al-Ahsa, Saudi Arabia

Jill E. Hobbs: Department of Agricultural and Resource Economics, University of Saskatchewan, 51 Campus Drive (3D34.1), Saskatoon, S7N 5A8, Canada

Norina Jabeen: Department of Rural Sociology, University of Agriculture Faisalabad, 37000, Pakistan

Muhammad Jamil: PARC Arid Zone Research Centre, Dera Ismail Khan, 29050, Pakistan

Jiwoo Jeon: School of Agriculture and Food Sustainability, The University of Queensland, Gatton Campus, QLD 4343, Australia

Joe Joseph: School of Agriculture and Food Sustainability, The University of Queensland, Gatton Campus, QLD 4343, Australia

Elham Ahmed Kazerooni: Department of Crop Sciences, College of Agricultural and Marine Sciences, Sultan Qaboos University, Muscat, 123, Sultanate of Oman

Ning-Yuan Ko: School of Agriculture and Food Sustainability, The University of Queensland, Gatton Campus, QLD 4343, Australia

Annika Krause: Institute of Behavioural Physiology, Leibniz Institute for Farm Animal Biology (FBN), 18196 Dummerstorf, Germany

Ajay Kumar: Department of Plant Science, School of Biological Sciences, Central University of Kerala, Kasaragod, 671316, Kerala, India

Moira S. Lewitt: School of Health and Life Sciences, University of the West of Scotland, PA1 2BE, UK

Calum N.L. Macpherson: School of Graduate Studies, St. George's University, Grenada, West Indies; Windward Islands Research and Education Foundation, St. George's University, Grenada, West Indies; School of Medicine, St. George's University, True Blue, Grenada, West Indies

Maxine L.A. Macpherson: School of Graduate Studies, St. George's University, Grenada, West Indies; School of Veterinary Medicine, St. George's University, Grenada, West Indies; Windward Islands Research and Education Foundation, St. George's University, Grenada, West Indies

Claudia Cecilia Márquez-Mota: Departamento de Nutrición Animal y Bioquímica, Facultad de Medicina Veterinaria y Zootecnia, Universidad Nacional Autónoma de México, Colonia UNAM, CU, Delegación Coyoacán, C.P. 04510, Ciudad de México, México

Cintli Martínez-Ortiz-de-Montellano: Departamento de Parasitología, Facultad de Medicina Veterinaria y Zootecnia, Universidad Nacional Autónoma de México, Colonia UNAM, CU, Delegación Coyoacán, C.P. 04510, Ciudad de México, México

Mohamed Marzok: Department of Clinical Sciences, College of Veterinary Medicine, King Faisal University, Al-Ahsa, Saudi Arabia; Department of Surgery, Faculty of Veterinary Medicine, Kafrelsheikh University, Kafrelsheikh, Egypt

Christine N. Meynard: CBGP, INRAE, CIRAD, IRD, Montpellier SupAgro, Univ Montpellier, Montpellier, France

Deirdre Mikkelsen: School of Agriculture and Food Science, The University of Queensland, Queensland, Australia

Joanne Mollinger: Department of Agriculture and Fisheries, Biosecurity Queensland, Brisbane, Queensland, Australia

Serge Morand: MIVEGEC, CNRS-IRD, Montpellier University, Montpellier, France; Faculty of Veterinary Technology, Kasetsart University, Bangkok, Thailand; Faculty of Tropical Medicine, Mahidol University, Bangkok, Thailand

Cindy E. Morris: INRAE, Pathologie Vegetale, F-84140, Montfavet, France

Liza R. Moscovice: Institute of Behavioural Physiology, Leibniz Institute for Farm Animal Biology (FBN), 18196 Dummerstorf, Germany

Brighton M. Mvumi: Department of Agricultural and Biosystems Engineering, Faculty of Agriculture, Environment and Food Systems, University of Zimbabwe, P.O. Box MP167, Mt. Pleasant, Harare, Zimbabwe

Edward Narayan: School of Agriculture and Food Sustainability, The University of Queensland, Gatton Campus, QLD 4343, Australia; Queensland Alliance for Agriculture and Food Innovation, The University of Queensland, St Lucia, QLD 4072, Australia

Christian Nawroth: Institute of Behavioural Physiology, Leibniz Institute for Farm Animal Biology (FBN), 18196 Dummerstorf, Germany

Rida Naz: Regional Blood Centre, Dera Ismail Khan, 29050, Pakistan

Claire Nedellec: Universite Paris-Sacl, INRAE, MaIAGE, F-78352 Jouy-en-Josas, France

Sneh Kashinath Nerurkar: School of Agriculture and Food Sustainability, The University of Queensland, Gatton Campus, QLD 4343, Australia

Eman Nour: Faculty of Medicine, Urology & Nephrology Centre, Animal Research Facility, Mansoura University, Mansoura, Egypt

Emmanuel T. Nyahangare: Department of Livestock Sciences, Faculty of Agriculture, Environment and Food Systems, University of Zimbabwe, P.O. Box MP167, Mt. Pleasant, Harare, Zimbabwe

Solabomi O. Ogunyemi: State Key Laboratory of Rice Biology, Ministry of Agriculture Key Lab of Molecular Biology of Crop Pathogens and Insects, Institute of Biotechnology, Zhejiang University, Hangzhou, 310058, China

Matthew C. Ogwu: Department of Plant Biology and Biotechnology, Faculty of Life Sciences, University of Benin, Ugbowo, Benin City, PMB 1154, Edo State, Nigeria; School of Biosciences and Veterinary Medicine, University of Camerino – Center for Floristic Research of the Apennine, 67021, L'Aquila, Italy

Harsh Pahuja: School of Agriculture and Food Sustainability, The University of Queensland, Gatton Campus, QLD 4343, Australia

Kinley Penjor: Bhutan Agriculture and Food Regulatory Authority, Ministry of Agriculture and Forests, Bhutan

Ricardo Piña-Martínez: Departamento de Parasitología, Facultad de Medicina Veterinaria y Zootecnia, Universidad Nacional Autónoma de México, Colonia UNAM, CU, Delegación Coyoacán, C.P. 04510, Ciudad de México, México

Rhonda Pinckney: School of Graduate Studies, St. George's University, Grenada, West Indies; School of Veterinary Medicine, St. George's University, Grenada, West Indies

Jorge Pinto Ferreira: Food and Agriculture Organization of the United Nations (FAO), 00153 Rome, Italy

Andrea Radici: INRAE, BioSP, F-84914 Avignon, France

Faiqah Ramzan: Faculty of Veterinary and Animal Sciences, Gomal University Dera Ismail Khan, 29050, Pakistan

Nishit Rao: School of Agriculture and Food Sustainability, The University of Queensland, Gatton Campus, QLD 4343, Australia

Vignesh A. Rathinasamy: Australian Institute of Tropical Health and Medicine, James Cook University, Cairns, Queensland, 4870, Australia

Alain Ratnadass: CIRAD, UPR Aida, F-97410 Saint-Pierre, Réunion, France; Aida, Univ Montpellier, CIRAD, Montpellier, France

Ayman Refaie: Nephrology and Transplantation Unit, Urology and Nephrology Center, Mansoura University, Mansoura, Egypt

Ramin Rezaee: Clinical Research Development Unit, Imam Reza Hospital, Faculty of Medicine, Mashhad University of Medical Sciences, Mashhad, Iran; Applied Biomedical Research Center, Mashhad University of Medical Sciences, Mashhad, Iran

Santiago Rosas-Plaza: Centro de Investigacion en Politicas, Poblacion y Salud, Universidad Nacional Autonoma de Mexico, Mexico City, Mexico

Ximena Rosas-Plaza: Facultad de Medicina Veterinaria y Zootecnia, Universidad Nacional Autonoma de Mexico, Mexico City, Mexico

Sukhyun Ryu: Department of Preventive Medicine, College of Medicine, The Catholic University of Korea, Republic of Korea

Julia Sabio y Garcia: Instituto de Biotecnologia, CICVyA, Instituto Nacional de Tecnologia Agropecuaria, Argentina (INTA) and Instituto de Agrobiotecnologia y Biologia Molecular, (IABIMO) INTA-CONICET, Hurlingham CP1686, Buenos Aires, Argentina

Ashiq Saleem: PARC Arid Zone Research Centre, Dera Ismail Khan, 29050, Pakistan

Assadullah Samadi: Paraclinic Department, Faculty of Veterinary Science, Kabul University, Jamal Mina, Kabul, Kabul 1006, Afghanistan

Samira Sarter: CIRAD, UMR ISEM, F-34398 Montpellier, France; ISEM, Univ Montpellier, CNRS, EPHE, IRD, Montpellier, France

Nicolas Sauvion: PHIM, Univ Montpellier, INRAE, CIRAD, IRD, Institut Agro, Montpellier, France

Mark Schipp: The Australian Veterinary Association Member Board of Directors, Canberra, Australian Capital Territory, Australia

Leonhard Schnittger: Instituto de Patobiologia Veterinaria, Centro de Investigaciones en Ciencias Veterinarias y Agronomicas (CICVyA), Instituto Nacional de Tecnologia Agropecuaria (INTA),

Hurlingham 1686, Argentina; Consejo Nacional de Investigaciones Cientificas y Tecnologicas (CONICET), C1425FQB Buenos Aires, Argentina

Golshan Shakeri: Department of Nutrition, Faculty of Medicine, Mashhad University of Medical Sciences, Mashhad, Iran; The German Federal Institute for Risk Assessment, Diedersdorfer Weg 1, D-12277 Berlin, Germany

Sharvari Avinash Sherekar: School of Agriculture and Food Sustainability, The University of Queensland, Gatton Campus, QLD 4343, Australia

Peter D. Sly: Children's Health and Environment Program, Children Health Research Centre, The University of Queensland, Brisbane, Queensland, Australia

Ricardo J. Soares Magalhaes: Queensland Alliance for One Health Sciences, School of Veterinary Science, The University of Queensland, Gatton, Queensland, Australia; Children's Health and Environment Program, Children Health Research Centre, The University of Queensland, Brisbane, Queensland, Australia

Samuel Soubeyrand: INRAE, BioSP, F-84914 Avignon, France

Philip C. Stevenson: Natural Resources Institute, University of Greenwich, Chatham Maritime, Chatham, Kent ME4 4TB, United Kingdom; Royal Botanic Gardens, Kew, Surrey TW9 3AB, United Kingdom

Carlos E. Suarez: Department of Veterinary Microbiology and Pathology, Washington State University, P.O. Box 647040, Pullman, WA, 991664-7040, United States; Animal Disease Research Unit, Agricultural Research Service, USDA, WSU, P.O. Box 646630, Pullman, WA, 99164-6630, United States

Wayne Sylvester: School of Graduate Studies, St. George's University, Grenada, West Indies; School of Veterinary Medicine, St. George's University, Grenada, West Indies

Neelam Taneja: Department of Medical Microbiology, Postgraduate Institute of Medical Education & Research, Chandigarh, India

Anju Thattantavide: Department of Plant Science, School of Biological Sciences, Central University of Kerala, Kasaragod, 671316, Kerala, India

Rethinasamy Velazhahan: Department of Crop Sciences, College of Agricultural and Marine Sciences, Sultan Qaboos University, Muscat, 123, Sultanate of Oman

Zhiheng Wang: School of Agriculture and Food Sustainability, The University of Queensland, Gatton Campus, QLD 4343, Australia

Yifei Yang: School of Veterinary Sciences, The University of Queensland, Gatton Campus, QLD 4343, Australia

Mohamed Youssef: Faculty of Veterinary Medicine, Department of Internal Medicine and Infectious Diseases, Mansoura University, Mansoura, 35516, Egypt

Muhammad S. Zaheer: Department of Agricultural Engineering, Khwaja Fareed University of Engineering and Information Technology, Rahim Yar Khan, 64200, Pakistan; Department of Agronomy, University College of Agriculture and Environmental Sciences, Islamia University of Bahawalpur, 63100, Pakistan

Molly A. Ziegler: School of Graduate Studies, St. George's University, Windward Islands Research and Education Foundation, True Blue Campus, Grenada, West Indies

Introduction

As described by the World Health Organization, 'One Health is an integrated, unifying approach that aims to sustainably balance and optimize the health of people, animals and ecosystems.' They note that it recognizes that the health of humans, domestic and wild animals, plants, and the wider environment (including ecosystems) are closely linked and interdependent. Research in this area is cross-cutting, utilizing evidence and expertise from researchers in human and veterinary medicine, and plant science and ecology.

This specially selected collection of articles from CABI Reviews brings together topics relating to One Health, and related papers on zoonotic diseases and integrated approaches in agriculture, veterinary and human health. This includes major diseases such as COVID-19, tuberculosis, *Toxocara* and dengue fever, and research addressing the role of organic agriculture, antimicrobial resistance and climate change.

1 Design Characteristics of Integrated Surveillance of Antimicrobial Resistance at the Human, Animal, and Environment Interfaces

Erda Eni Rame Hau[1]*, Peter D. Sly[2], Deirdre Mikkelsen[3], Neelam Taneja[4], Kinley Penjor[5], Sukhyun Ryu[6], Erica Donner[7], Joanne Mollinger[8], Jorge Pinto Ferreira[9], Mark Schipp[10] and Ricardo J. Soares Magalhaes[1,2]

[1]Queensland Alliance for One Health Sciences, School of Veterinary Science, The University of Queensland, Gatton, Queensland, Australia; [2]Children's Health and Environment Program, Children Health Research Centre, The University of Queensland, Brisbane, Queensland, Australia; [3]School of Agriculture and Food Science, The University of Queensland, Queensland, Australia; [4]Department of Medical Microbiology, Postgraduate Institute of Medical Education & Research, Chandigarh, India; [5]Bhutan Agriculture and Food Regulatory Authority, Ministry of Agriculture and Forests, Bhutan; [6]Department of Preventive Medicine, College of Medicine, The Catholic University of Korea, Republic of Korea; [7]Future Industries Institute, University of South Australia, Adelaide, South Australia, Australia; [8]Department of Agriculture and Fisheries, Biosecurity Queensland, Brisbane, Queensland, Australia; [9]Food and Agriculture Organization of the United Nations (FAO), Rome, Italy; [10]The Australian Veterinary Association Member Board of Directors, Canberra, Australian Capital Territory, Australia

Abstract

Efforts have been made to strengthen national and global antimicrobial resistance (AMR) surveillance programs by integrating data collection across the human, animal, and environmental sectors. We searched the literature to review published studies reporting the implementation of integrated AMR surveillance approaches, and we identified a total of 96 articles from 36 countries published from 2000 to 2022, which met our inclusion criteria. Standard review protocols were applied in our study. Out of 96 studies, 47 (49%) articles integrated AMR analysis from human and animal (HA) populations, 24 (25%) considered human, animal, and environmental (HAE) samples together, 11 (12%) studies included animal and environment (AE) samples, and 12 (13%) integrated human and environmental (HE) surveillance. Human isolate-based and animal isolate-based surveillance were the most common study designs (38, 52.8%), with the remainder applying human case-based and isolate-based for animal populations (32, 44.4%). Finally, our results demonstrate that AMR studies on *E. coli* revealed a lower correlation between human and animal AMR prevalence compared to *Salmonella* spp. and *Campylobacter* spp.

*Corresponding author: e.ramehau@student.uq.edu.au

studies. Different aspects of surveillance design were associated with the level of correlation of AMR prevalence between sectors. Our study found that while global efforts for integrated AMR surveillance have increased in the past 10 years, significant variation exists between studies with regard to the epidemiological and laboratory aspects of their surveillance designs. Our findings indicate that to enable the generation of comparable epidemiological data across countries and sectors, there is a need for the development of a global protocol to support the design of surveillance programs that aim to conduct integrated surveillance of AMR.

Keywords: antimicrobial resistance, integrated surveillance, epidemiology, human, animals, environment

Introduction

Antimicrobial resistance (AMR) is a significant global public health threat that impacts human and animal health and welfare by limiting antimicrobial therapy choices for the treatment of infectious diseases. A study of Antimicrobial Resistance Collaborators estimated that the death of about 4.95 million (3.62–6.57) people in 2019 is correlated with bacterial AMR, and among these are 1.27 million deaths directly due to bacterial AMR (Murray *et al.*, 2022). This number is already half of the UK government's prediction in 2014, estimating that by 2050, around 10 million people will die annually related to AMR, more than 10 times higher than the death rate in 2014 (O'Neill, 2014).

AMR is a complex public health problem due to the possibility for bacterial resistance to emerge in the human, animal, and environmental sectors. However, the main driver of AMR emergence is a lack of stewardship in antimicrobial use (AMU) when treating human and animal infections, including misuse and/or overuse of antibiotics (Castro-Sánchez *et al.*, 2016). Between 2000 and 2015, a 65% growth (21.1–34.8 billion defined daily doses, DDDs) of worldwide human antibiotic consumption was reported corresponding to a 39% rise in antibiotic consumption rate (11.3–15.7 DDDs per 1000 inhabitants per day) (WHO, 2017a). DDD is defined as the assumed average maintenance dose per day for a drug used for its main indication in adults. Drug utilization figures expressed in DDDs are generally reported in units that control for population size differences (such as 1000 persons). This provides a measure of exposure or therapeutic intensity in a defined population, allowing comparison across various time periods and population groups (WHO Collaborating Centre for Drug Statistics Methodology, 2023). The reported increase was attributed to low- and middle-income countries (LMICs) and associated with growth in gross domestic product per capita (GDPPC). In the absence of regulatory change, global antibiotic consumption in humans is projected to increase by 200% from 2015 to 2030, reaching an estimated total consumption of 42 billion DDDs (Klein *et al.*, 2018).

AMU in food production is also predicted to increase. For example, reports anticipate that between 2010 and 2030 AMU in food animals will increase by 67%, from 63,151 to 105,596 tons (Van Boeckel *et al.*, 2015). This projected increase is due to the global rise in demand for animal food products and the shifting trend from extensive to more intensive farming systems in LMICs, where antimicrobials are often used routinely with little regulatory guidance (Van Boeckel *et al.*, 2017). In addition to therapeutic use, antimicrobials are also used in animal production as prophylactics and metaphylactics for disease prevention and control. In addition, the World Organization for Animal Health (WOAH, founded as OIE) 2017 Annual Report on Antimicrobial Agents Intended for Use in Animals reported that 25% of countries (40 out of 157) use antimicrobials for growth promotion (OIE, World Organization for Animal Health, 2017).

In this context, the lived environment acts both as a source of AMR bacteria and a reservoir for several AMR inputs from the human and animal sectors. Rapid selection and proliferation of mobile resistance and multi-drug resistance are driven by human and animal activities through contact with resistant bacteria, antibiotics and their residues, and chemical agents, including released heavy metals (Baker *et al.*, 2018). Transfer of resulting AMR bacteria in the environment to people and livestock can result from direct exposure to more resistant bacteria or food and water consumption.

Several initiatives at the global and national level have been undertaken to advocate for a unified approach to tackling AMR. The World Health Organization (WHO), the Food and Agricultural Organization (FAO), and the World Organization for Animal Health (WOAH) Tripartite, which became Quadripartite with the inclusion of UN Environment Programme (UNEP), produced a manual on developing National Action Plans (NAPs) to assist countries in the initial phase of developing new or refining existing national action plans in line with the strategic objectives of the Global Action Plan (GAP). The initiative of the Tripartite alliance has been instrumental in ensuring advocacy for comprehensive surveillance, monitoring, data sharing, and policy implementation across the three sectors (Jinks *et al.*, 2016).

Many countries have followed the guidance in the manual for developing NAPs and taken steps toward implementing them through multisectoral collaboration across the human, animal, and environmental domains (Ogyu *et al.*, 2020; WHO, 2021). However, examples of truly integrated AMR surveillance remain relatively rare, requiring coordination of activities across AMR programs across sectors with surveillance resources being shared across departments, increasing efficiencies. The WHO report 'Antimicrobial Resistance: Global Report on Surveillance' (WHO, 2014) highlighted significant gaps in surveillance, lack of standards for methodology, data sharing, and coordination, all of which were considered barriers to effective global surveillance, reinforcing the importance of harmonized, integrated surveillance of AMR in humans, food-producing animals, and food (WHO, 2014). Indeed, several high-income countries such as Denmark (DANMAP program), the Netherlands (MARAN and NethMap programs), the United States of America (NARMS), and Canada (CIPARS) have paved the way, demonstrating the feasibility of the approach, but most, if not all, are lacking the environment sector. Although DANMAP, MARAN, and NARMS are One Health Reports, the AMR data of humans and animals are usually displayed in separate chapters, with limited integrated data analysis, while CIPARS is an example of a program implementing integrated analysis across sectors. Finally, one of the major attempts worldwide to jointly analyze AMR and AMU data in humans and animals in Europe is the third joint inter-agency report on integrated analysis of antimicrobial agent consumption and occurrence of AMR in bacteria from humans and food-producing animals (JIACRA), prepared by the three agencies, the European Centre for Disease Prevention and Control (ECDC), the European Food Safety Authority (EFSA), and the European Medicines Agency (EMA), at the request of the European Commission (EC) (ECDC, EFSA, and EMA, 2021). The report highlighted that despite the different purposes of various AMU and AMR surveillance and monitoring systems, the agencies continue working on improving surveillance harmonization and integration across sectors to better understand AMU and AMR (Klees *et al.*, 2020). A recent study reviewing the French antimicrobial surveillance system reported that it is highly fragmented, has overlaps between programs, and has some gaps, emphasized by the insufficient coverage of the environmental sector (Collineau *et al.*, 2023). Questions remain concerning the heterogeneity of results across jurisdictions and the feasibility and opportunities for scaling these approaches to LMICs. This latter issue is crucial as while AMR in some high-income countries has leveled off, AMR and AMU continue in an upward trend in many LMICs (Laxminarayan *et al.*, 2020).

Since the recognition that AMR surveillance that combines data from humans, animals, and the environment is the most appropriate approach for studying and guiding AMR prevention and control interventions (WHO, 2017b), the implementation of integrated AMR surveillance is gaining popularity. As a result, an increasing number of studies have recently shown evidence of the relationships between AMR in humans, animals, and the environment (Tang *et al.*, 2017; ECDC, EFSA, and EMA, 2021). Important aspects that need to be considered for the design of a truly integrated AMR surveillance system are the surveillance objective, the selection of the sample type within each sector, the locations for samples for each sector, the selection of the bacterial species to be included, the selection of antimicrobials against bacterial species, and the antimicrobial susceptibility methodology for the susceptibility test (WHO, 2017b; OIE, 2018). The absence of high-quality data yielded by integrated AMR programs on the prevalence and epidemiological relationships between resistant bacteria and associated resistance genes in humans, animals, and the environment limits countries' ability to measure the actual burden of AMR, evolutionary and transmission pathways and meet the goals of the NAPs (Tacconelli *et al.*, 2018).

This review aims to highlight the surveillance design characteristics across studies or programs that attempted some kind of integrated AMR surveillance reported worldwide, which considered biological samples from humans, animals, and the environment or a combination of those. In doing so, we critically appraise the surveillance design aspects that could partially explain correlations between AMR prevalence in each sector and surveillance design.

Materials and Methods

Review methodology

We searched databases including Scopus, Web of Science, PubMed, and EMBASE. Combination search terms used to find relevant articles are 'integrated surveillance,' 'antimicrobial resistance,' 'human,' 'animal,' and 'environment.' No restrictions on language or publication date applied. We used reference lists from the included articles to check for other additional relevant publications that were not identified by the original search. EndNoteTM was used as a reference manager for storage and duplication checks of all retrieved articles.

Joanna Briggs Institute methodology guidelines were used as a guideline in conducting this review (Peters *et al.*, 2015) and Preferred Reporting Items for Systematic Reviews and Meta-Analyses Extension for Reviews (PRISMA-ScR) was used for reporting (Tricco, 2018). Arskey and O'Malley framework describes the methodology as followed: (1) research question identification; (2) relevant studies identification; (3) study selection; (4) data charting; and (5) results organizing, summarizing, and reporting (Arksey and O'Malley, 2005). Details of the protocol for this review were specified and registered in Figshare with DOI 10.6084/m9.figshare.24658395. The protocol is available in full and can be accessed on the Figshare website (Available at: https://figshare.com/account/items/24658395, accessed 29 November 2023). Relevant articles meeting inclusion criteria were screened based on the titles and abstracts by one reviewer (ERH). All articles available with full text were then thoroughly reviewed for eligibility by two authors (ERH and RJSM).

Inclusion and exclusion criteria

Studies were eligible for inclusion if they applied integration of human, animal, and/or environment as part of their AMR surveillance. AMR integrated surveillance included studies integrating human and animal surveillance (i.e. classified as HA studies), animal, and environmental surveillance (i.e. classified as AE studies), or integrating these three sectors (i.e. classified as HAE studies). For the purpose of our data extraction tool, environmental samples included water, soil, effluent, rivers, and ponds. Other than these three main groups of integrated surveillance, some other integrated approaches have been implemented, human and environment populations (i.e. classified as HE studies), and also these populations combined with others such as horticulture produce (e.g. fruits and vegetables), which were then grouped as 'others' in this review (i.e. classified O), such as human and food, or animal and food (Supplementary File S1.2).

Papers were excluded if: (a) abstract or full paper was not available; (b) they were experimental design studies, case series, or case reports of AMR without involving the integration of HA, HE, AE, or HAE; or (c) they were short communications, conference proceedings, commentaries, review articles, books or book sections.

Data extraction

For each eligible article, we extracted and summarized data on study location, year of publication, target population (HA, HE, AE, or HAE), study design (cross-sectional, case-control, cohort), type of surveillance (case-based, sample-based, isolate-based), target human population (patients/ healthy people/ community), target animal sites (farms, slaughterhouses, markets, hospitals/ clinics, households), environmental sample type (water, soil), geographical and temporal study design (whether human, animal, and environment samples are geographically collocated [setting based collocated (SC) or regional-based collocated (RC) or random (R)], and temporally dependent, mixed or independent), the sample size of each human, animal, and environment population, bacteriological methods for each human, animal, and environment sample, resistance patterns, and prevalence of AMR within each sector and bacteria under surveillance. Geographical settings describe the study design based on the locations of those different population groups (human, animal, and environment), whether they are chosen based on the study settings, whether they are located nearby, or whether they are from random locations. Furthermore, temporally settings show how samples are collected from time perspectives, whether samples of the three different populations are collected in the one-point time frame, mixed of two different times, or the sample collection time is independent between one and others. Reports about descriptive information of studies were conducted in the spreadsheet as well as narrative synthesis of findings from the studies focusing on study design summary of integrated AMR surveillance.

Correlation of AMR prevalence between humans and animal populations of *E. coli*, *Salmonella* spp., and *Campylobacter* spp. was performed using the coefficient of determination R^2. Moreover, comparisons were also performed between different geographical and temporal study settings. All data management and analyses were performed in Microsoft Excel.

Results

General characteristics of studies included in the review

A total of 1315 publications were found during our database search and an additional 28 records were considered from further evaluation of the reference lists of included publications (Fig. 1.1). In the screening process, 314 out of 1315 records were removed due to duplication, and then 673 publications were excluded because they did not meet criteria such as irrelevant titles and abstracts and types of articles (review, letter, proceedings). Following this screening, 232 publications were then excluded because they did not meet inclusion criteria, where they were not integrated surveillance studies. The remaining 96 records were then included in this review synthesis.

Our results show that most integrated AMR surveillance studies are represented by a small set of countries worldwide (Fig. 1.2). Out of 96 studies included in our review, 47 (49%) studies reported integrated surveillance for AMR in human and animal populations (HA studies). Among HA studies, most of

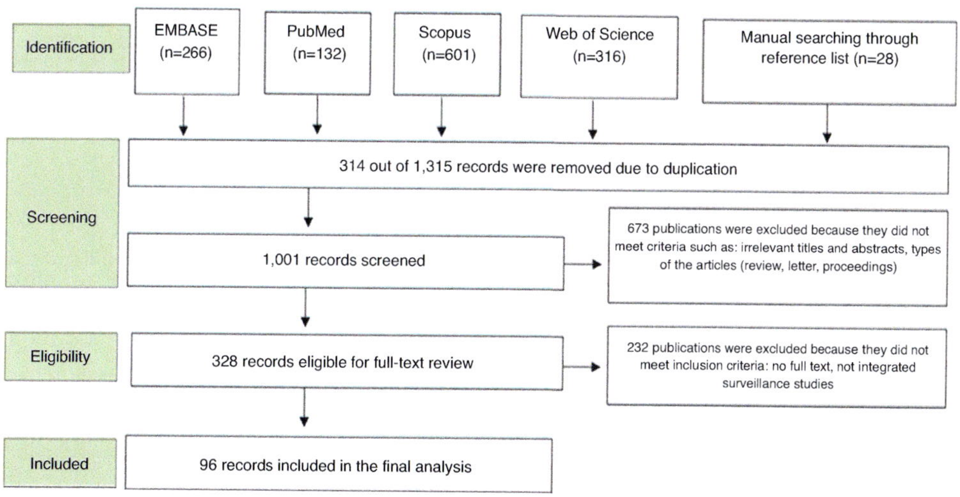

Fig. 1.1. Flow diagram for retrieval of articles.

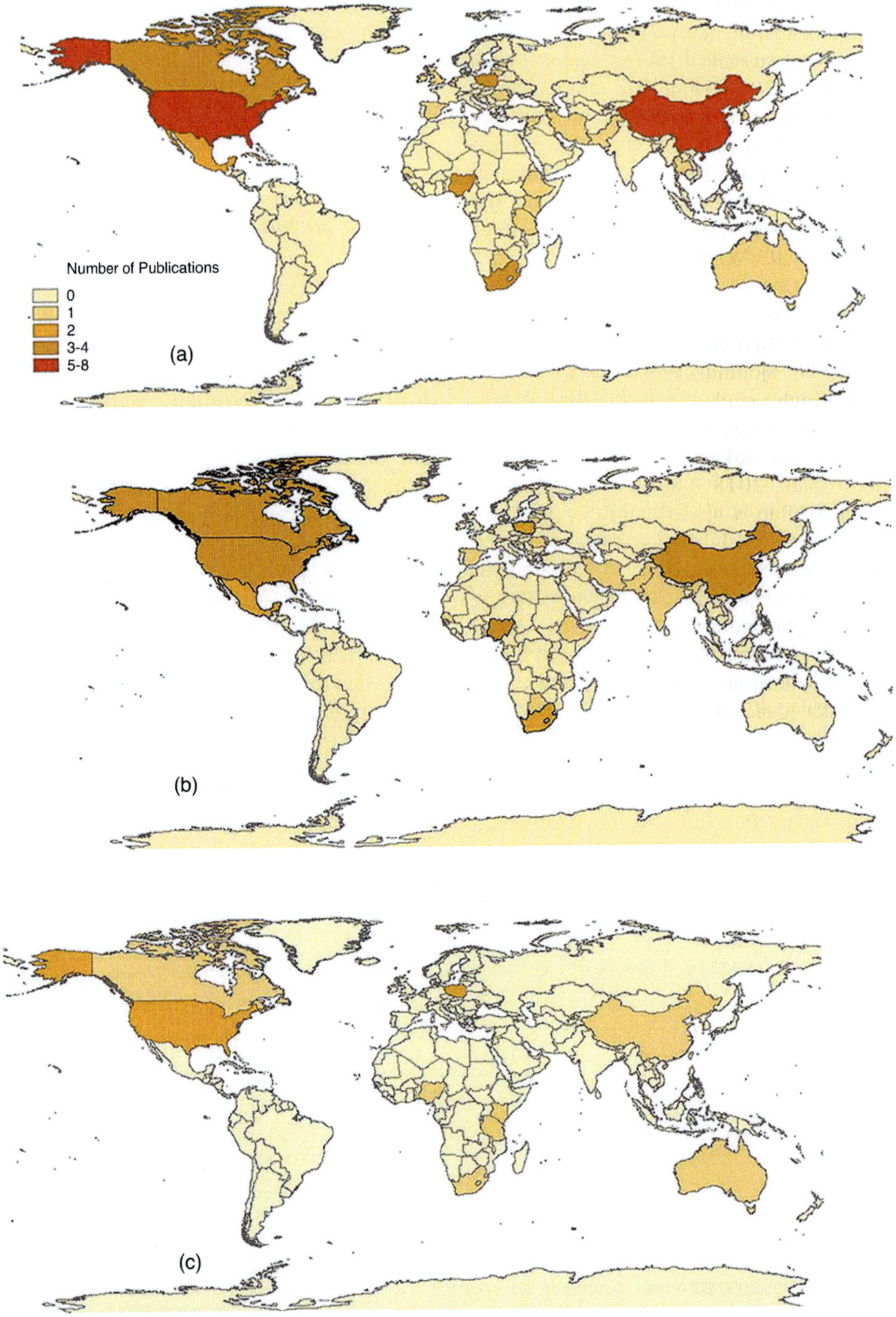

Fig. 1.2. Distribution of all selected papers on antimicrobial surveillance integrated surveillance (a), papers with integrated human and animal (b), papers with integrated human, animal, and environment (c).

them targeted their investigations into 3 main microorganisms including *E. coli* (n=17, 36%) (van den Bogaard *et al.*, 2001; Miles *et al.*, 2006; Johnson *et al.*, 2007; Unno *et al.*, 2010; Sahoo *et al.*, 2012; Boonyasiri *et al.*, 2014; Kazemnia *et al.*, 2014; Maciuca *et al.*, 2015; Dhaka *et al.*, 2016; Purohit *et al.*, 2017; Abbas *et al.*, 2019; Hassell *et al.*, 2019; Kalule *et al.*, 2019; Li *et al.*, 2019; Olowe *et al.*, 2019; Oporto *et al.*, 2019; Dandachi *et al.*, 2020; Lunha *et al.*, 2020; Tamta *et al.*, 2020; Shawa *et al.*, 2021; Badr *et al.*, 2022; Primeau *et al.*, 2023), *Salmonella* spp. (n=11, 23%) (Cardinale *et al.*, 2005; Oloya *et al.*, 2009; Sjölund-Karlsson *et al.*, 2013; Edirmanasinghe *et al.*, 2017; Xu *et al.*, 2017; Eguale *et al.*, 2018; Fashae *et al.*, 2018; Ma *et al.*, 2018; Pornsukarom *et al.*, 2018; Realpe-Quintero *et al.*, 2018; Viana *et al.*, 2019; He *et al.*, 2020; Rao *et al.*, 2020; Talukder *et al.*, 2021; Listorti *et al.*, 2022; Primeau *et al.*, 2023), and *Campylobacter* spp. (n=10, 21%) (Guévremont *et al.*, 2006; Rozynek *et al.*, 2008; Skjot-Rasmussen *et al.*, 2009; Rozynek *et al.*, 2010; Thakur *et al.*, 2010; Zaidi *et al.*, 2012; Maesaar *et al.*, 2016; Cha *et al.*, 2017; Szczepanska *et al.*, 2017; Aksomaitiene *et al.*, 2018; de Vries *et al.*, 2018; Wieczorek *et al.*, 2018). Studies that included human, animal, and environment as their target populations (HAE studies) accounted for 25% of all studies reviewed (n=24/96). Among them, 46% of studies targeted *E. coli* (n=11/24) (Scott *et al.*, 2005; Boonyasiri *et al.*, 2014; Dhaka *et al.*, 2016; Purohit *et al.*, 2017; Hassell *et al.*, 2019; Kalule *et al.*, 2019; Shen *et al.*, 2019; Dandachi *et al.*, 2020; Subbiah *et al.*, 2020; Rousham *et al.*, 2021), and the rest were for *Campylobacter* spp., *Staphylococcus* spp., and *Salmonella* spp.

Since 2016 onwards our results show an increasing trend in the number of studies reporting integrated AMR surveillance, reaching a total of 14 publications in 2019 and 13 publications in 2020, almost five times higher compared to 2015 (Fig. 1.3). From 2016 to 2020, HA studies remained the most predominant study type (49%, n=24/49) followed by HAE studies (31%, n=15/49). *E. coli* remained the predominant bacteria among integrated surveillance of AMR conducted in the period of 2016–2020 (42%, n=21/49), followed by *Salmonella* spp. (23%, n=11/49).

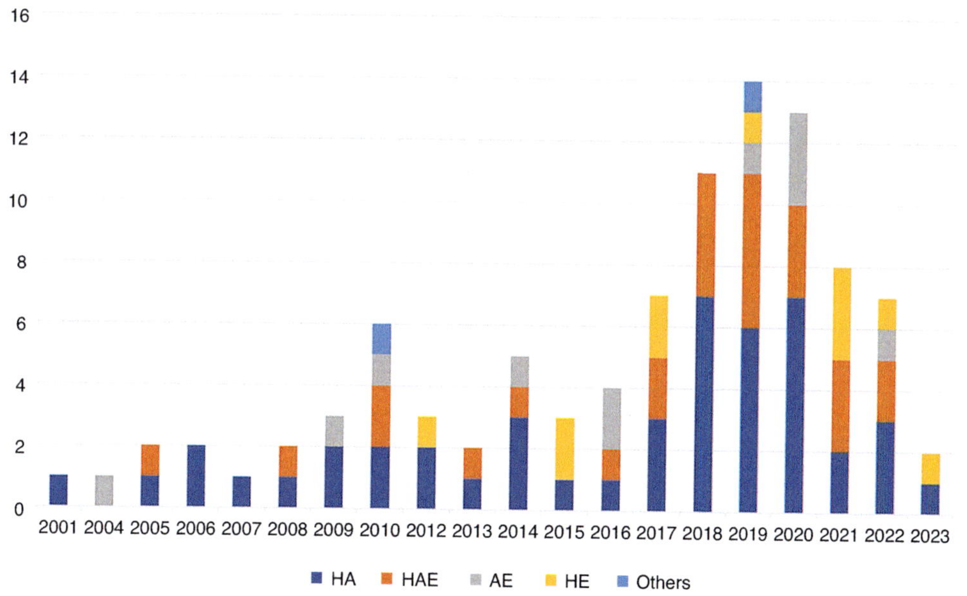

Fig. 1.3. Number of included articles in the review classified by time period (HA: Studies of Human and Animal; HAE: Studies of Human, Animal, and Environment; AE: Studies of Animal and Environment; HE: Studies of Human and Environment; Others: Other Integrated Studies).

Types of sampling strategies of integrated antimicrobial resistance surveillance

Our results showed that studies under review employed different sampling strategies in different target populations (Table 1.1). Findings indicate that a little more than half (53%, *n*=38/72) of integrated AMR surveillance studies where human samples were collected were conducted taking an isolate-based approach, and most integrated AMR studies using animal samples used an isolate-based approach (97%, *n*=70/72). The most common type of sampling strategy of HA studies was studies combining human isolate-based and animal isolate-based surveillance (53%, *n*=38/72), in which the samples were collected from representative populations, and then antimicrobial susceptibility was tested from the recovered isolates of interest. This approach was closely followed by 44% (*n*=25/57) of HA studies applying case-based surveillance in human populations, in which isolates were recovered from samples of patients with specific suspected diseases and isolate-based for animal target populations. Case-based surveillance is defined as prospective surveillance using defined patient groups as the population of interest, such as patients with specific clinical characteristics, including urinary tract infections, diarrhea, and other infections (Ryu *et al.*, 2019). Only two studies were identified in our literature search that employed case-based surveillance.

Of the 32 studies combining human case-based and animal isolate-based approaches, *Campylobacter* spp. [41% (*n*=13/32)] and *Salmonella* spp. [31%, (*n*=10/32)] were the most commonly targeted bacteria. From the total of 29 publications focusing on *E. coli* as the target pathogen, the majority (76%, *n*=22/29) of studies conducted an isolate-based approach for both human and animal samples, and only six studies performed a case-based approach for human samples and isolate-based approach for animal samples. Similarly, all six studies focusing on *Staphylococcus* spp. were performed using an isolate-based approach for both human and animal samples. For studies including environmental samples (HAE and AE studies), the majority (92%, *n*=12/13) were conducted using an isolate-based approach for all the samples, only 1 study was case-based for human samples and isolate-based for other samples.

From a geographical and temporal study design perspective, the majority of studies were geographically setting-based collocated and temporally dependent (SC-D) (32%, *n*=31/96), followed by geographically regional-based collocated and temporally dependent (29%, *n*=28/96). These were then followed by geographically regional-based, collocated, and temporally mixed (15%, *n*=14/96) and geographically random and temporally independent (11%, *n*=11/96) studies (Table 1.2).

Table 1.1. Number of publications with different surveillance type combinations in humans and animals for different pathogens.

	IBH[a]-IBA[b] (%)	CBH[c]-IBA (%)	CBH-CBA[d] (%)	Total (%)
Escherichia coli	22 (30. 6)	6 (8.3)	1 (1.4)	29 (40.3)
Campylobacter spp.	–	13 (18.1)	1 (1.4)	14 (19.4)
Salmonella spp.	7 (9.7)	10 (13.9)	–	17 (23.6)
Staphylococcus spp.	7(9.7)	–	–	7 (7.7)
Aeromonas spp.	–	1 (1.4)	–	1 (1.4)
Enterococcus spp.	–	2 (2.8)	–	2 (2.8)
Enterobacteriaceae	2 (2.8)	–	–	2 (2.8)
Total	38 (52.8)	32 (44.4)	2 (2.8)	72 (100)

[a]IBH: isolate-based human.
[b]IBA: isolate-based animal.
[c]CBH: case-based human.
[d]CBA: case-based animal.

Table 1.2. Number of integrated AMR studies implemented different study designs temporally and geographically.

	Temporally			
Geographically	Dependent (D) (%)	Mix (M) (%)	Independent (I) (%)	Total (%)
Setting-based collocated (SC)	31 (32.3)	–	–	31 (32.3)
Regional-based collocated (RC)	28 (29.3)	14 (14.6)	3 (3.1)	45 (46.9)
Random (R)	1 (1.0)	8 (8.3)	11 (11.5)	20 (20.8)
Total	60 (632.5)	22 (22.9)	14 (14.6)	96

Correlation between AMR prevalence in different study populations and different surveillance design characteristics

Our results indicate that the correlation between *E. coli* AMR prevalence in humans and animal populations based on phenotypic results was lower than *Salmonella* spp. and *Campylobacter* spp (Fig. 1.4). The highest correlation in AMR prevalence between human and animal isolates was found in studies that targeted *Campylobacter* spp. ($R^2 = 0.86$) (Fig. 1.4e).

Within all *Campylobacter* spp. in AMR studies, the highest AMR prevalence correlation between human and animal samples was seen among studies that employed a case-based approach in the human sector. Within *E. coli* studies, the highest correlation between AMR prevalence in different populations was in AE studies ($R^2 = 0.77$) followed by HA ($R^2 = 0.62$) and HE studies ($R^2 = 0.23$) (Fig. 1.4).

Our results also indicate that the level of correlation between the prevalence of AMR in human and animal populations was highest in studies that employed a setting-based collocated, in which the samples of humans and animals were set to be taken from the same location settings, and temporally dependent sampling design, which samples of both populations were taken in the same time frame ($R^2 = 0.89$) (Fig. 1.5a). This is followed by regionally-based collocated, in which samples of both populations were taken from the same regional area, and temporally dependent studies ($R^2 = 0.77$) (Fig. 1.5b), and then regionally-based collocated and temporally mixed studies, in which the samples of human populations were not taken in the same time frame as animal samples ($R^2 = 0.75$) (Fig. 1.5c). Among these major studies, the weakest correlation between the prevalence of AMR in human and animal populations was found in geographically random temporally independent study designs, in which samples of both human and animal populations were taken from random unrelated locations and different time frames ($R^2 = 0.01$) (Fig. 1.5d).

Discussion

General characteristics of studies included in the review

This review has shown that a growing number of studies worldwide are pursuing integrated AMR surveillance using biological samples from human subjects, animal species, and their shared environments. These studies have been designed to gather knowledge on AMR prevalence, understand the relationship between isolates, and elucidate transmission mechanisms.

Global efforts to tackle AMR require integrated One Health surveillance programs that provide information on the resistance profiles of pathogens of public health interest. Our results indicate that this has become an area of growing interest, with 96 studies meeting the inclusion criteria for this review. Among these, the most common combination was integrated human and animal-derived AMR sampling (HA studies). This reflects the understanding that AMU in animals is correlated with the occurrence of resistant bacterial strains and can result in resistance transferring to human microbiomes via colonizing organisms or genetic elements (Holmes *et al.*, 2016). Previous studies have shown that lakes, rivers, sewage, and drinking water can be contaminated with antimicrobial-resistant bacteria, antimicrobial

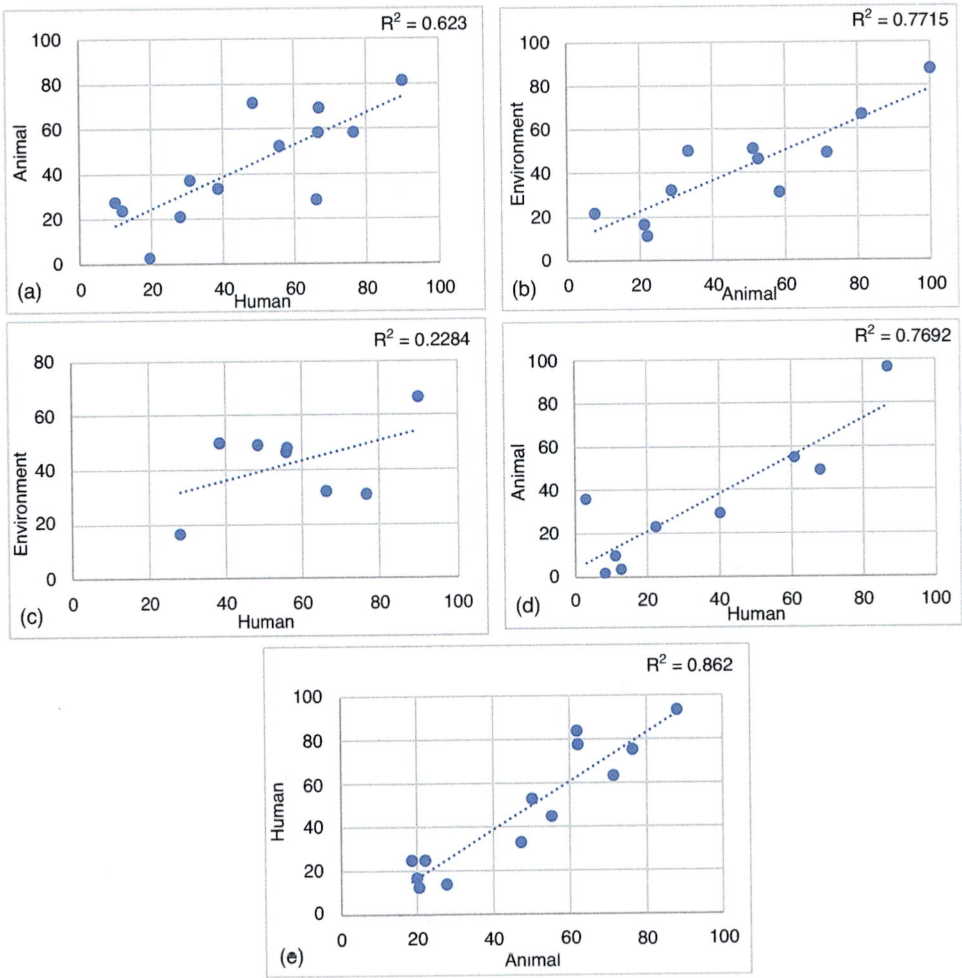

Fig. 1.4. Correlation of *Escherichia coli* antimicrobial AST resistance prevalence between humans and animals (a), animals and environment (b), and humans and environment (c), correlation of *Salmonella* spp. antimicrobial resistance prevalence between humans and animals (d), correlation of *Campylobacter* spp. antimicrobial resistance prevalence between humans and animals (e). Each dot represents one study.

residues, and AMR drivers such as heavy metals (Pehrsson *et al.*, 2016). However, although the environment has been recognized as both a 'source' and a 'sink' for AMR genes for some time, environmental sampling has only recently been added to integrated AMR surveillance efforts (HAE studies) (Rousham *et al.*, 2018). Most of the HAE studies examined here aimed to investigate AMR across humans, animals, and the environment to understand the phenotypic and genetic relationships (Hutinel *et al.*, 2019). Under the search terms investigated, the first integrated AMR study was published in 2001, targeting food production animal species (poultry farms) and their associated farmers and poultry slaughterers (van den Bogaard *et al.*, 2001). The year 2005 was the landmark year for the first publication of integrated human, animal, and environment (HAE) surveillance (Scott *et al.*, 2005). These first publications coincided with global expert discussions that led to the establishment of the WHO Advisory Group

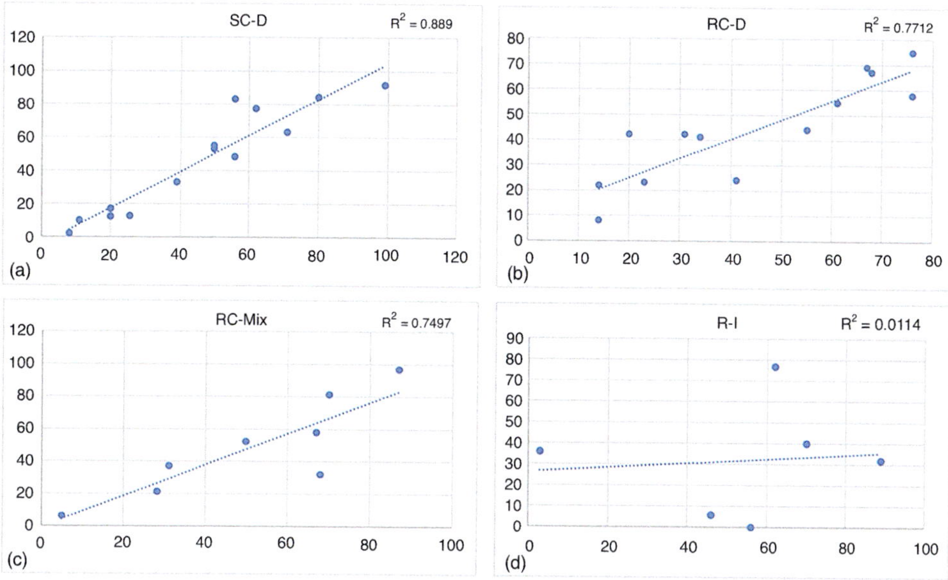

Fig. 1.5. Correlation of antimicrobial AST resistance prevalence between humans and animals between different study design settings: Geographically setting based collocated and temporally dependent (samples of both populations were taken in the same time frame) (SC-D) (a); Geographically regional based collocated and temporally dependent (RC-D) (b); Geographically regional based collocated and temporally mixed (RC-Mix) (c); and Geographically random and temporally independent (R-I) (d).

on Integrated Surveillance of Antimicrobial Resistance (AGISAR) in 2008 aiming to support WHO in reducing the impact of AMR on public health. Since then, the number of HA and HAE studies has steadily increased, particularly from 2016 onwards. This is likely in response to the release of the WHO Global Action Plan on Antimicrobial Resistance in 2015. One of the critical knowledge gaps identified in the Global Action Plan is the lack of understanding of how AMR evolves and spreads, including the circulation within and between humans, animals, and environment. These gaps need to be filled, along with the provision of new tools, policies, and regulatory developments.

Although integrated AMR surveillance is a critical approach to providing actionable data, studies and/or programs in this area have not been implemented or reported in many countries. Geographically, 30% of the studies that have published integrated AMR surveillance data covered in this review were derived from Canada, the USA, and China. Relatively few of the integrated surveillance studies reviewed were derived from LMICs; these need to be supported with upskilling for surveillance, data management, and stakeholder collaboration for integrated surveillance and response. We note, however, that the geographic distribution observed only pertains to published journal articles and thus omits sources such as national AMR program reports. Some well-known national programs, e.g. The Monitoring of Antimicrobial Resistance and Antimicrobial Usage in Animals in the Netherlands (MARAN), and the Danish Integrated Antimicrobial Resistance Monitoring and Research Programme (DANMAP), have not yet published their findings in scientific journals.

Among all studies reviewed, *E. coli* was the predominant bacterium targeted for investigation, followed by *Campylobacter* spp. and *Salmonella* spp. This emerging trend reflects the importance of *E. coli* in human, animal, and environmental health, and encourages (e.g. through GLASS) adoption of a single indicator that can be standardized for cost-effective surveillance across nations of varying lab capacity. Infections with Extended-Spectrum-β-Lactamase producing *Escherichia coli* (ESBL-Ec) result in severe morbidity and mortality in humans, with substantial health costs and disease burdens. As a commensal, opportunistic bacteria, *E. coli* is always present in human and animal digestive tracts and in their waste. *E. coli* survival in the environment is strain-dependent, with those closely linked to fecal pollution typically dying off once in the external environment, and others naturalized and persisting in the environment (Flint, 1987; Van Elsas *et al.*, 2011). *E. coli* may function as reservoirs of resistance genes, potentially transferring these to human pathogens transiting the intestinal tract. Thus, it may provide important information on the potential flow of bacterial resistance traits in the food chain.

Type of integrated antimicrobial resistance surveillance design

The results show that if the surveillance objective is to compare across sectors, there has been significant heterogeneity in surveillance design with regard to sampling frames, target populations, and how these were approached for sampling. Sampling design is a crucial element of surveillance as it determines the quality of data available for meeting surveillance objectives, which may include quantifying trends and profiling risk factors for any observed differences in disease frequency between populations. The decision making processes in surveillance sampling design are challenging in integrated AMR surveillance due to the need to maximize precision across multiple sectors. Our findings show that almost half of the studies combined case-based sampling for human-derived samples with isolate-based sampling for animal-derived samples, and the rest implemented isolate-based approaches for both sources. A case-based approach to surveillance has been noted to have advantages compared to isolate- or sample-based designs, due to the availability of clinical data to supplement isolate information for risk factor analysis (Ryu *et al.*, 2019). Nevertheless, the collection of isolate-based animal data is also of value. Although it is generally obtained from healthy animals in the food chain and thus lacks accompanying clinical data, it is potentially more relevant for understanding food chain risks as humans will most often be eating healthy animals.

Our results also indicate that the type of study design is likely to contribute to the level of correlation in AMR prevalence between human, animal, and environmental samples. Our results show that whether studies had a case-based or isolate-based approach to sample selection significantly impacted the AMR prevalence correlation between humans and animals. In general, it can be concluded that the group of studies that employed a case-based sampling design resulted in a higher correlation between human and animal AMR compared to those with an isolate-based design. This is intuitive given that case-based studies took samples from specific groups of patients with similar infections and specific pathogens and checked for those specific pathogens' antimicrobial susceptibility (Ryu *et al.*, 2019). The fundamental concept of case-based surveillance is prospective surveillance for a specific, defined patient group that is infected by particular pathogens. Therefore, the denominator of this surveillance is those specific patients with specific infection conditions (Ryu *et al.*, 2019). This setting will possibly give a higher correlation of these specific conditions sampling AMR prevalence to the AMR prevalence of the specific isolates from the animal population.

Sampling should be done continuously or regularly using consistent methods to permit analysis of AMR trends (WHO, 2017b). In the studies examined here, the most common design was a cross-sectional design with a single evaluation time point, and only two longitudinal studies were conducted (Bondo *et al.*, 2016; Hutinel *et al.*, 2019). This may be partly due to the studies' aim to obtain snapshot surveillance of AMR in target populations and partly due to funding constraints. This could potentially be the impact of the exclusion criteria, where surveillance reports are excluded. The two longitudinal designs involved multiple sampling observations, with eight sampling events in one study (Tamta *et al.*, 2020) and weekly sampling in another (Bondo *et al.*, 2016; Hutinel *et al.*, 2019). By observing the same population multiple times, AMR trends can be tracked over time across sectors, not just in terms of prevalence but also for the incidence of AMR acquisition and investigation of AMR transmission and evolutionary trajectories between sectors.

Another important aspect of integrated surveillance design is site selection, and interdependencies between sites may need to be factored into site selection protocols. A study by Mughini-Gras *et al.* about ESBL and pAmpC *E. coli* revealed that although human-to-human transmission is the community-acquired carriage followed by food, animal, and environmental sources, this transmission within the community is not feasible without transmission to and from non-human sources as they require large reservoirs of infection, contamination, and dissemination, to which humans remain continuously exposed and subsequently contribute to further spread among individuals (Mughini-Gras *et al.*, 2019). This issue is particularly pertinent when the surveillance objective is source attribution, i.e., by accurately measuring the clonal relationships between isolates from the three different domains: human, animal, and environment, to ascertain the source (Bolukaoto *et al.*, 2019). Ideally, the sampling design of integrated surveillance needs to be geographically and temporally correlated so the correlation will be represented in the results. Potential drivers of AMR persistence, evolution, and the opportunity for a more refined microbial risk analysis based on the association of resistance traits with specific sources can also be discovered by this type of surveillance (Hendriksen *et al.*, 2019). With this regard, our study demonstrated that geographical and temporal decisions regarding sampling design were also observed to affect the correlation between AMR prevalence in human and animal samples. Not surprisingly, studies with geographically random and temporally independent designs showed the weakest correlation between human and animal AMR prevalence.

Based on the results found, the features of an AMR surveillance system are fundamentally dependent on the objective of the system. In the context of AMR surveillance that aims to compare data across sectors a case-based sampling design targeting the human population offers efficiencies for the collection of adequate data to achieve that objective. Utilizing existing sentinel surveillance in hospitals and other healthcare settings, the case-based approach allows systematic collection of a minimum dataset across a range of pathogens, as well as providing comprehensive metadata on patients' characteristics (Ryu *et al.*, 2019). Moreover, longitudinal studies are recommended due to advantages of detecting development or changes in characteristics of the target population at a group or individual level as they extend beyond a single moment and establish sequences of events (Rindfleisch *et al.*, 2008). Lastly, geographically and temporally correlated surveillance designs are important to be considered in the context of integrated AMR surveillance as this design allows us to see clearly how human, animal, and environment AMR patterns are geospatially associated. In the livestock context, FAO has released detailed guidelines for surveillance, which form the basis of surveillance system requirements for sampling, sample collection storage, and processing (FAO, 2019; FAO and WOAH, 2023; FAO, NParks, and SFA, 2023).

Limitations

Although we conducted an extensive literature search, including a wide range of electronic databases, the studies under review included only those reported in English. Furthermore, this study only included published articles, and additional integrated AMR surveillance systems, such as the ones mentioned above, were only available as part of annual AMR surveillance reports and thus not included in the present study (Supplementary File S1.1).

Conclusions

The results of this review show the importance of approaching AMR surveillance through an integrated lens, where data collection across the human, animal, and environmental sectors is coordinated. Furthermore, a number of studies provide excellent examples to be considered when developing national AMR action plans that incorporate integrated AMR surveillance. The results also highlight some important points of the approaches implemented to date, including variation between studies with regard to the type of integration implemented, sampling designs, and AMR profiling methods. The study highlights the need for the development of standard guidance for integrated AMR surveillance on par with the AMR surveillance guidelines that the Food and Agriculture Organization has been releasing in the context of AMR surveillance in livestock industries. Harmonization of integrated surveillance designs needs to be addressed if such an approach is to be scaled globally to produce comparable data.

Funding

This work was supported by the Lembaga Pengelola Dana Pendidikan (LPDP) Scholarship, Ministry of Finance, Government of Indonesia (grant number 201911220315663).

Conflict of Interest

The authors have no conflicts of interest to declare.

Supplementary Content

Refer to supplementary material on the CABI Digital Library: https://www.cabidigitallibrary.org/doi/book/10.1079/9781836991472.0000

References

Abbas, G. *et al.* (2019) High rates of CTX-M group-1 extended-spectrum β-lactamases producing *Escherichia coli* from pets and their owners in Faisalabad, Pakistan. *Infection and Drug Resistance* 12, 571–578.

Aksomaitiene, J. *et al.* (2018) Prevalence of genetic determinants and phenotypic resistance to ciprofloxacin in *Campylobacter jejuni* from Lithuania. *Frontiers in Microbiology* 9, 203.

Arksey, H. and O'Malley, L. (2005) Scoping studies: Towards a methodological framework. *International Journal of Social Research Methodology* 8(1), 19–32.

Badr, H. *et al.* (2022) Multidrug-resistant and genetic characterization of extended-spectrum beta-lactamase-producing *E. coli* recovered from chickens and humans in Egypt. *Animals* 12(3), 346.

Baker, S. *et al.* (2018) Genomic insights into the emergence and spread of antimicrobial-resistant bacterial pathogens. *Science* 360(6390), 733–738.

Bolukaoto, J.Y. *et al.* (2019) Molecular characteristics and genotypic diversity of enterohaemorrhagic *Escherichia coli* O157:H7 isolates in Gauteng region, South Africa. *Science of the Total Environment* 692, 297–304.

Bondo, K.J. *et al.* (2016) Epidemiology of antimicrobial resistance in *Escherichia coli* isolates from raccoons (*Procyon lotor*) and the environment on swine farms and conservation areas in Southern Ontario. *PLoS ONE* 11(11), e0165303.

Boonyasiri, A. *et al.* (2014) Prevalence of antibiotic resistant bacteria in healthy adults, foods, food animals, and the environment in selected areas in Thailand. *Pathogens and Global Health* 108(5), 235–245.

Cardinale, E. *et al.* (2005) Epidemiological analysis of *Salmonella enterica* ssp. enterica serovars Hadar, Brancaster and Enteritidis from humans and broiler chickens in Senegal using pulsed-field gel electrophoresis and antibiotic susceptibility. *Journal of Applied Microbiology* 99(4), 968–977.

Castro-Sánchez, E. *et al.* (2016) What are the factors driving antimicrobial resistance? Perspectives from a public event in London, England. *BMC Infectious Diseases* 16(1), 465–465.

Cha, W. *et al.* (2017) Comparing the genetic diversity and antimicrobial resistance profiles of *Campylobacter jejuni* recovered from cattle and humans. *Frontiers in Microbiology* 8(May), 818.

Collineau, L. *et al.* (2023) Towards one health surveillance of antibiotic resistance: Characterisation and mapping of existing programmes in humans, animals, food and the environment in France, 2021. *Eurosurveillance* 28, 22.

Dandachi, I. *et al.* (2020) Dissemination of multidrug-resistant and mcr-1 gram-negative bacilli in broilers, farm workers, and the surrounding environment in Lebanon. *Microbial Drug Resistance* 26(4), 368–377.

de Vries, S.P.W. *et al.* (2018) Phylogenetic analyses and antimicrobial resistance profiles of *Campylobacter* spp. from diarrhoeal patients and chickens in Botswana. *PLoS One* 13(3), e0194481.

Dhaka, P. *et al.* (2016) Genetic diversity and antibiogram profile of diarrhoeagenic *Escherichia coli* pathotypes isolated from human, animal, foods and associated environmental sources. *Infection Ecology & Epidemiology* 6, 31055.

ECDC, EFSA, and EMA (2021) *Third Joint Inter-Agency Report on Integrated Analysis of Consumption of Antimicrobial Agents and Occurrence of Antimicrobial Resistance in Bacteria from Humans and Food-Producing Animals in the EU/EEA, JIACRA III*. European Centre for Disease Prevention and Control (ECDC), European Food Safety Authority (EFSA) and European Medicines Agency (EMA), Stockholm, Parma, Amsterdam.

Edirmanasinghe, R. *et al.* (2017) A whole-genome sequencing approach to study cefoxitin-resistant *Salmonella* enterica serovar Heidelberg isolates from various sources. *Antimicrobial Agents and Chemotherapy* 61(4), e01919–16.

Eguale, T. *et al.* (2018) Phenotypic and genotypic characterization of temporally related nontyphoidal *Salmonella* strains isolated from humans and food animals in central Ethiopia. *Zoonoses and Public Health* 65(7), 766–776.

FAO (2019) Monitoring and surveillance of antimicrobial resistance in bacteria from healthy food animals intended for consumption. In: *Regional Antimicrobial Resistance Monitoring and Surveillance Guidelines – Volume 1*. FAO, Bangkok.

FAO and WOAH (2023) *Guidelines on Monitoring Antimicrobial Use at the Farm Level, in Regional Guidelines for the Monitoring and Surveillance of Antimicrobial Resistance, Use and Residues in Food and Agriculture. Volume 5*. Bangkok.

FAO, NParks, and SFA (2023) Monitoring and surveillance of antimicrobial resistance in bacterial pathogens from aquaculture. In: *Regional Guidelines for The Monitoring and Surveillance of Antimicrobial Resistance, Use and Residues in Food and Agriculture Volume 3*. Bangkok.

Fashae, K., Leekitcharoenphon, P. and Hendriksen, R.S. (2018) Phenotypic and genotypic comparison of *salmonellae* from diarrhoeic and healthy humans and cattle, Nigeria. *Zoonoses and Public Health* 65(1), e185–e195.

Flint, K.P. (1987) The long-term survival of *Escherichia coli* in river water. *Journal of Applied Bacteriology* 63(3), 261–270.

Guévremont, E. *et al.* (2006) Antimicrobial susceptibilities of thermophilic *Campylobacter* from humans, swine, and chicken broilers. *Canadian Journal of Veterinary Research = Revue Canadienne de Recherche Veterinaire* 70(2), 81–86.

Hassell, J.M. *et al.* (2019) Clinically relevant antimicrobial resistance at the wildlife-livestock-human interface in Nairobi: An epidemiological study. *Lancet Planet Health* 3(6), e259–e269.

He, J. *et al.* (2020) Multidrug resistance and prevalence of quinolone resistance genes of *Salmonella* enterica serotypes 4,[5],12:i: – in China. *International Journal of Food Microbiology* 330.

Hendriksen, R.S. *et al.* (2019) Using genomics to track global antimicrobial resistance. *Frontiers in Public Health* 7, 242–242.

Holmes, A.H. *et al.* (2016) Understanding the mechanisms and drivers of antimicrobial resistance. *The Lancet* 387(10014), 176–187.
Hutinel, M. *et al.* (2019) Population-level surveillance of antibiotic resistance in *Escherichia coli* through sewage analysis. *Eurosurveillance* 24(37), 6–16.
Jinks, T. *et al.* (2016) A time for action: Antimicrobial resistance needs global response. *Bulletin of the World Health Organization* 94(8), 558–558a.
Johnson, J.R. *et al.* (2007) Antimicrobial drug-resistant *Escherichia coli* from humans and poultry products, Minnesota and Wisconsin, 2002–2004. *Emerging Infectious Diseases* 13(6), 838–846.
Kalule, J.B. *et al.* (2019) Prevalence and antibiotic susceptibility patterns of enteric bacterial pathogens in human and non-human sources in an urban informal settlement in Cape Town, South Africa. *BMC Microbiology* 19(1), 244.
Kazemnia, A., Ahmadi, M. and Dilmaghani, M. (2014) Antibiotic resistance pattern of different *Escherichia coli* phylogenetic groups isolated from human urinary tract infection and avian colibacillosis. *Iranian Biomedical Journal* 18(4), 219.
Klees, S. *et al.* (2020) Prevalence and epidemiology of multidrug-resistant pathogens in the food chain and the urban environment in Northwestern Germany. *Antibiotics-Basel* 9(10), 14.
Klein, E.Y. *et al.* (2018) Global increase and geographic convergence in antibiotic consumption between 2000 and 2015. *Proceedings of the National Academy of Sciences* 115(15), E3463.
Laxminarayan, R. *et al.* (2020) The lancet infectious diseases commission on antimicrobial resistance: 6 years later. *The Lancet Infectious Diseases* 20(4), e51–e60.
Li, J. *et al.* (2019) Inter-host transmission of carbapenemase-producing *Escherichia coli* among humans and backyard animals. *Environmental Health Perspectives* 127(10), 107009.
Listorti, V. *et al.* (2022) Antimicrobial resistance of *Salmonella* strains isolated from human, wild boar, and environmental samples in 2018–2020 in the Northwest of Italy. *Pathogens* 11(12), 1446.
Lunha, K. *et al.* (2020) Antimicrobial resistance in fecal *Escherichia coli* from humans and pigs at farms at different levels of intensification. *Antibiotics* 9(10), 1–11.
Ma, Y. *et al.* (2018) High-levels of resistance to quinolone and cephalosporin antibiotics in MDR-ACSSuT *Salmonella* enterica serovar enteritidis mainly isolated from patients and foods in Shanghai, China. *International Journal of Food Microbiology* 286, 190–196.
Maciuca, I.E. *et al.* (2015) High prevalence of *Escherichia coli*-producing CTX-M-15 extended-spectrum beta-lactamases in poultry and human clinical isolates in Romania. *Microbial Drug Resistance* 21(6), 651–662.
Maesaar, M. *et al.* (2016) Antimicrobial resistance profiles of *Campylobacter* spp. isolated from broiler chicken meat of Estonian, Latvian and Lithuanian origin at Estonian retail level and from patients with severe enteric infections in Estonia. *Zoonoses Public Health* 63(2), 89–96.
Miles, T.D., McLaughlin, W. and Brown, P.D. (2006) Antimicrobial resistance of *Escherichia coli* isolates from broiler chickens and humans. *BMC Veterinary Research* 2, 7.
Mughini-Gras, L. *et al.* (2019) Attributable sources of community-acquired carriage of *Escherichia coli* containing β-lactam antibiotic resistance genes: A population-based modelling study. *Lancet Planet Health* 3(8), e357–e369.
Murray, C.J. *et al.* (2022) Global burden of bacterial antimicrobial resistance in 2019: A systematic analysis. *The Lancet* 399(10325), 629–655.
O'Neill, J. (2014) Antimicrobial resistance: Tackling a crisis for the health and wealth of nations. *Review on Antimicrobial Resistance. Review on Antimicrobial Resistance*. Available at: https://amr-review.org/sites/default/files/AMR%20Review%20Paper (accessed 16 September 2021).
Ogyu, A. *et al.* (2020) National action to combat AMR: A one-health approach to assess policy priorities in action plans. *BMJ Global Health* 5(7), 10.
OIE (2018) *Harmonisation of National Antimicrobial Resistance Surveillance and Monitoring Programmes*. Terrestrial Animal Health Code, Paris, France.
OIE, World Organization for Animal Health (2017) *OIE Annual Report on Antimicrobial Agents Intended for Use in Animals; Better Understanding of the Global Situation, in Second Report*. World Organization for Animal Health, Paris, France.
Olowe, O.A. *et al.* (2019) Phylogenetic grouping and biofilm formation of multidrug resistant *Escherichia coli* isolates from humans, animals and food products in South-West Nigeria. *Scientific African* 6, e00158.

Oloya, J., Doetkott, D. and Khaitsa, M.L. (2009) Antimicrobial drug resistance and molecular characterization of *Salmonella* isolated from domestic animals, humans, and meat products. *Foodborne Pathogens and Disease* 6(3), 273–284.

Oporto, B. *et al.* (2019) Zoonotic approach to Shiga toxin-producing *Escherichia coli*: Integrated analysis of virulence and antimicrobial resistance in ruminants and humans. *Epidemiology and Infection* 147, e164.

Pehrsson, E.C. *et al.* (2016) Interconnected microbiomes and resistomes in low-income human habitats. *Nature* 533(7602), 212–216.

Peters, M. *et al.* (2015) *Joanna Briggs Institute Reviewer's Manual 2015: Methodology for JBI Scoping Reviews. UniSA Clinical and Health Sciences*. JBI, Australia.

Pornsukarom, S., Vliet, A.H.M. and Thakur, S. (2018) Whole genome sequencing analysis of multiple *Salmonella* serovars provides insights into phylogenetic relatedness, antimicrobial resistance, and virulence markers across humans, food animals and agriculture environmental sources. *BMC Genomics* 19, 801.

Primeau, C.A. *et al.* (2023) Integrated surveillance of extended-spectrum beta-lactamase (ESBL)-producing *Salmonella* and *Escherichia coli* from humans and animal species raised for human consumption in Canada from 2012 to 2017. *Epidemiology & Infection* 151, e14.

Purohit, M.R. *et al.* (2017) Antibiotic resistance in an indian rural community: A 'One-Health' observational study on commensal coliform from humans, animals, and water. *International Journal of Environmental Research and Public Health* 14(4), 386.

Rao, S. *et al.* (2020) Genomic diversity of class I integrons from antimicrobial resistant strains of *Salmonella* Typhimurium isolated from livestock, poultry and humans. *PLoS ONE* 15, 12 December.

Realpe-Quintero, M. *et al.* (2018) Genetic diversity and antimicrobial resistance of *Salmonella* serotypes recovered throughout the beef production chain and from patients with salmonellosis. *PeerJ* 2018(8), e5482.

Rindfleisch, A. *et al.* (2008) Cross-sectional versus longitudinal survey research. *Journal of Marketing Research – Chicago* 45, 261–279.

Rousham, E.K., Unicomb, L. and Islam, M.A. (2018) Human, animal and environmental contributors to antibiotic resistance in low-resource settings: Integrating behavioural, epidemiological and One Health approaches. *Proceedings of the Royal Society B: Biological Sciences* 285(1876), 20180332.

Rousham, E.K. *et al.* (2021) Human colonization with extended-spectrum beta-lactamase-producing *E. coli* in relation to animal and environmental exposures in Bangladesh: An observational one health study. *Environmental Health Perspectives* 129(3).

Rozynek, E. *et al.* (2008) Comparison of antimicrobial resistance of *Campylobacter jejuni* and *Campylobacter coli* isolated from humans and chicken carcasses in Poland. *Journal of Food Protection* 71(3), 602–607.

Rozynek, E. *et al.* (2010) Genetic similarity of *Campylobacter* isolates in humans, food, and water sources in Central Poland. *Foodborne Pathogens and Disease* 7(5), 597–600.

Ryu, S. *et al.* (2019) Case-based surveillance of antimicrobial resistance with full susceptibility profiles. *JAC-Antimicrobial Resistance* 1(3), dlz070.

Sahoo, K.C. *et al.* (2012) Geographical variation in antibiotic-resistant *Escherichia coli* isolates from stool, cow-dung and drinking water. *International Journal of Environmental Research and Public Health* 9(3), 746–759.

Scott, H.M. *et al.* (2005) Patterns of antimicrobial resistance among commensal *Escherichia coli* isolated from integrated multi-site housing and worker cohorts of humans and swine. *Foodborne Pathogens and Disease* 2(1), 24–37.

Shawa, M. *et al.* (2021) Clonal relationship between multidrug-resistant *Escherichia coli* ST69 from poultry and humans in Lusaka, Zambia. *FEMS Microbiology Letters* 368, 21–24.

Shen, Y. *et al.* (2019) Integrated aquaculture contributes to the transfer of mcr-1 between animals and humans via the aquaculture supply chain. *Environment International* 130, 104708.

Sjölund-Karlsson, M. *et al.* (2013) Occurrence of β-lactamase genes among non-Typhi *Salmonella* enterica isolated from humans, food animals, and retail meats in the United States and Canada. *Microbial Drug Resistance* 19(3), 191–197.

Skjot-Rasmussen, L. *et al.* (2009) Trends in occurrence of antimicrobial resistance in *Campylobacter jejuni* isolates from broiler chickens, broiler chicken meat, and human domestically acquired cases and travel associated cases in Denmark. *International Journal of Food Microbiology* 131(2–3), 277–279.

Subbiah, M. *et al.* (2020) Antimicrobial resistant enteric bacteria are widely distributed amongst people, animals and the environment in Tanzania. *Nature Communications* 11(1), 228.

Szczepanska, B. *et al.* (2017) Prevalence and antimicrobial resistance of *Campylobacter jejuni* and *Campylobacter coli* isolated from children and environmental sources in urban and suburban areas. *BMC Microbiology* 17(1), 80.

Tacconelli, E. *et al.* (2018) Discovery, research, and development of new antibiotics: The WHO priority list of antibiotic-resistant bacteria and tuberculosis. *The Lancet Infectious Diseases* 18(3), 318–327.

Talukder, S. *et al.* (2021) Epidemiology and antimicrobial resistance profiles of *Salmonella* in chickens, sewage, and workers of broiler farms in selected areas of Bangladesh. *Journal of Infection in Developing Countries* 15(8), 1155–1166.

Tamta, S. *et al.* (2020) Faecal carriage of extended spectrum beta-lactamase (ESBL) and New Delhi metallo beta-lactamase(NDM) producing *Escherichia coli* between piglets and pig farmworkers. *Comparative Immunology, Microbiology and Infectious Diseases* 73, 101564.

Tang, K.L. *et al.* (2017) Restricting the use of antibiotics in food-producing animals and its associations with antibiotic resistance in food-producing animals and human beings: A systematic review and meta-analysis. *Lancet Planet Health* 1(8), e316–e327.

Thakur, S. *et al.* (2010) Antimicrobial resistance, virulence, and genotypic profile comparison of *Campylobacter jejuni* and *Campylobacter coli* isolated from humans and retail meats. *Foodborne Pathogens and Disease* 7(7), 835–844.

Tricco, A.C. *et al.* (2018) PRISMA extension for scoping reviews (PRISMA-ScR): Checklist and explanation. *Annals of Internal Medicine* 169(7), 467–473.

Unno, T. *et al.* (2010) High diversity and abundance of antibiotic-resistant *Escherichia coli* isolated from humans and farm animal hosts in Jeonnam Province, South Korea. *Science of the Total Environment* 408(17), 3499–3506.

Van Boeckel, T.P. *et al.* (2015) Global trends in antimicrobial use in food animals. *Proceedings of the National Academy of Sciences* 112(18), 5649.

Van Boeckel, T.P. *et al.* (2017) Reducing antimicrobial use in food animals. *Science* 357(6358), 1350–1352.

van den Bogaard, A.E. *et al.* (2001) Antibiotic resistance of faecal *Escherichia coli* in poultry, poultry farmers and poultry slaughterers. *Journal of Antimicrobial Chemotherapy* 47(6), 763–771.

Van Elsas, J.D. *et al.* (2011) Survival of *Escherichia coli* in the environment: Fundamental and public health aspects. *Isme j* 5(2), 173–183.

Viana, C. *et al.* (2019) Distribution, diversity, virulence genotypes and antibiotic resistance for *Salmonella* isolated from a Brazilian pork production chain. *International Journal of Food Microbiology* 310, 108310.

WHO (2014) *Antimicrobial Resistance: Global Report on Surveillance*. World Health Organization, Geneva.

WHO (2017a) *Critically Important Antimicrobials for Human Medicine: Ranking of Antimicrobial Agents for Risk Management of Antimicrobial Resistance Due to Non-Human Use*. WHO, Geneva.

WHO (2017b) *Integrated Surveillance of Antimicrobial Resistance in Foodborne Bacteria: Application of a One Health Approach: Guidance from the WHO Advisory Group on Integrated Surveillanec of Antimicrobial Resistance (AGISAR)*. WHO, Geneva.

WHO (2021) *WHO Integrated Global Surveillance on ESBL-Producing E. coli using a "One Health" Approach: Implementation and Opportunities*. WHO, Geneva.

WHO Collaborating Centre for Drug Statistics Methodology (2023) *Guidelines for ATC Classification and DDD Assignment 2024*. Norwegian Institute of Public Health, Oslo, Norway.

Wieczorek, K., Wołkowicz, T. and Osek, J. (2018) Antimicrobial resistance and virulence-associated traits of *Campylobacter jejuni* isolated from poultry food chain and humans with diarrhea. *Frontiers in Microbiology* 9, 1508.

Xu, C. *et al.* (2017) Phenotypic characteristics and genetic diversity of *Salmonella* enterica serotype derby isolated from human patients and foods of animal origin. *Foodborne Pathogens and Disease* 14(10), 593–599.

Zaidi, M.B. *et al.* (2012) Antimicrobial-resistant *Campylobacter* in the food chain in Mexico. *Foodborne Pathogens and Disease* 9(9), 841–847.

2 An Insight on the Last Two Decades of Global Research on Animal Tuberculosis: Bibliometric analysis

Latifah Abdullah Alhusayni[1], Mohamed Marzok[1,2]*, Yamen Hegazy[1], Fatma A. El-Gohary[3] and Sabry El-Khodery[4]

[1]Department of Clinical Sciences, College of Veterinary Medicine, King Faisal University, Al-Ahsa, Saudi Arabia; [2]Department of Surgery, Faculty of Veterinary Medicine, Kafrelsheikh University, Kafrelsheikh, Egypt; [3]Department of Hygiene and Zoonoses, Faculty of Veterinary Medicine, Mansoura University, Mansoura, Egypt; [4]Department of Internal Medicine and Infectious Diseases, Faculty of Veterinary Medicine, Mansoura University, Mansoura, Egypt

Abstract

Animal tuberculosis is of global concern because of its economic and zoonotic importance. Bibliometric analysis is an important methodology used to analyze articles and other publications in literature. In this study, we performed quantitative studies on animal tuberculosis for the last two decades to March 2024. The data were retrieved from the Web of Science (WOS) database. Statistical data were set for each studied item using the VOSviewer software, with a focus on the top ten results for each item. A total of 11,155 documents were finally included in the evaluation. Results revealed that author Vordermeier H.M. had the highest number of published papers (151, 1.35%), and the publications in 2021 (693, 6.21%) were at the forefront. The United States Department of Health and Human Services was the top funding agency (1093, 9.79%), and the USA was the top nation in publications (3137, 28.12%). The most publications were in English (10898, 97.69%) and the highest publications in WOS categories were collected from Veterinary Sciences (2588, 23.2%). Research articles were the most abundant form (9271, 83.11%). Citation meso indicated that tuberculosis and leprosy (6628, 59.4%) were the top and Elsevier was the main publisher (2577, 23.1%). The results of this bibliometric analysis indicate a growing number of studies on tuberculosis in animals, which reflects the re-emergence of the disease to an alarming degree. The results can help to establish the possible forthcoming plans for its prevention and control.

Keywords: cattle, *Mycobacterium bovis*, *Mycobacterium caprae*, bibliometric analysis, publications

Introduction

Mycobacterium tuberculosis complex is a group of *Mycobacterium* species that can induce tuberculosis in both animals and humans (Costa *et al.*, 2014; Siala *et al.*, 2017; Elsayed and Amer, 2019; Goosen *et al.*, 2020). Bovine tuberculosis (BTB) is an economically important disease with zoonotic potential, particularly in developing countries (Vordermeier *et al.*, 2012). Caprine tuberculosis

*Corresponding author: mmarzok@kfu.edu.sa

has also the same economic and zoonotic importance (Ayana, 2020; Njoga *et al.*, 2023). The cost of surveillance is a major challenge, especially in low-income countries (Schwoebel, 2020). Although the disease presents a serious challenge in developing countries, regional disease foci that are not considered free of BTB continue to exist in several European countries and the USA (Murai *et al.*, 2019). Moreover, BTB is a major concern for the cattle industry in the United Kingdom (Fielding *et al.*, 2021).

The transmission of *Mycobacterium bovis* (*M. bovis*) from animals to humans is a major public health concern worldwide (Ayele *et al.*, 2004; Olea-Popelka *et al.*, 2017; Singh *et al.*, 2022). Mycobacterium tuberculosis can survive in the host under adverse conditions (Hade *et al.*, 2020). *M. bovis* infects nearly one-third of the human population (Zumla *et al.*, 2011). Moreover, human patients with *M. bovis* infection are more likely to receive less efficient treatment because *M. bovis* is resistant to pyrazinamide (Ayalew *et al.*, 2023). Globally, by 2022, the reported number of people newly diagnosed with tuberculosis was 7.5 million. This is the highest number since the World Health Organization (WHO) started global tuberculosis monitoring in 1995 and is responsible for approximately 1.6 million deaths per year (Bagcchi, 2023). In addition to the economic and zoonotic importance of BTB, studies on the disease in cattle are essential because cattle have been found to be a suitable model for the development of vaccines against human tuberculosis, as it is comparatively easy to collect large volumes of blood from calves at intervals following vaccination (Buddle *et al.*, 2005).

Analysis of the status and anticipation of emerging studies on BTB necessitates evaluating the publication's coherence and quality. Recently, several review articles and meta-analyses on BTB have been conducted regionally (Sibhat *et al.*, 2017; Ferluga *et al.*, 2020; Refaya *et al.*, 2020; Fielding *et al.*, 2021; Byrne *et al.*, 2022). However, few meta-analytical studies have been conducted on these diseases. In contrast to traditional literature reviews, such as systematic literature reviews or meta-synthesis, which may show analysis bias or even publication bias, bibliometric analysis provides a more objective evaluation of specific literature. Additionally, bibliometric analysis offers considerable issues for researchers that guide the most effective studies before they start reading, helping them find the current gaps in a specific field of research and inspiring new ideas to study, identify, and map research trends to appreciate the conceptual, social, or cognitive structure of their future studies (Zupic and Čater, 2015; Donthu *et al.*, 2021).

Bibliometric analysis is an analytical approach that utilizes statistics to quantitatively evaluate research productivity for a certain scientific trend (Drijvers *et al.*, 2020). The term 'bibliometrics' can be defined as an expression substitution for the term 'statistical bibliography' (Pritchard, 1969). Bibliometric analysis was employed to establish descriptive guidelines for scientific literature concerning core research publications in a specific field worldwide. It includes a wide range of evaluation bases, providing insight into the current situation, possible prospective output, and the effects of the studied fields (Hsu *et al.*, 2020). Focusing on these words, it could be helpful to flare up to the point where a research field is present. At the literature level, various descriptive items are categorized and analyzed, such as handling specific research fields, authors and co-authors contributions, specific veterinary journals (Pelzer and Wiese, 2003; Crawley-Low, 2006; Krauskopf *et al.*, 2017; Schoenfeld-Tacher and Alpi, 2021) collaborative and interdisciplinary publications, and universities.

Several types of bibliometric analysis are typically used in scientific research. Citation, co-citation, co-occurrence, bibliographic coupling, and co authorship analyses are the most commonly used methods (van Eck and Waltman, 2014). Although BTB has received global attention, there has been no bibliometric analysis describing the dynamics and distribution of this disease in the last period. Therefore, the aim of the present investigation was to present a bibliometric analysis of research studies on animal tuberculosis in the last two decades to highlight the veterinary and zoonotic importance of this disease.

Review Methodology

Searching plan and data source

First, the data were collected by identifying the databases and choosing appropriate search strategy methods, data retrieval, and cleaning the data before the analysis and visualization process. In the present bibliometric analysis, publications on animal tuberculosis research up to March 1, 2024, were retrieved from the Web of Science (WoS) database. The search was done by using the main terms of animal tuberculosis identified in the literature as follows: ('ANIMAL' and 'TUBERCULOSIS'). Additional keywords '*Mycobacterium bovis*' and '*Mycobacterium caprae*' were used. The search was performed using the WoS topic field, which included the title, abstract, and author keywords. Moreover, the search was completed in a single day to avoid bias caused by a daily database update.

Raw data were extracted in BibTeX and Txt formats using the WoS extraction tool. Information fields related to authors, affiliations, countries of publication, citation topics, WOS categories, article types, languages, research areas, funding agencies, publishers, journals, and years of publication were included in the extraction process.

Eligible criteria

In the bibliometric analysis, only original articles and reviews published in field research on animal tuberculosis were implicated. Retracted publications, corrections, and biographies were excluded.

Data analysis

The search results included authors, affiliations, countries of publication, citation topics, WOS categories, publication type, languages, research areas, funding agencies, publishers, journals, and publishing year. The relationships among the most highly productive countries, research institutions, and frequently used keywords were analyzed using specific software (VOSviewer, version 1.6.14), co-citation, coupling document, and coupling institution. Cluster analysis and social network maps (consisting of nodes and links) for countries, institutions, and keywords were also generated (Mulet-Forteza *et al.*, 2019). Two or four times the minimum frequency of keyword occurrence in the publications, reflecting the number of included studies (11,155) and the consequent analysis results, respectively, were set. Different nodes in a map represent elements including a country, institution, or keywords. The size of the nodes reflects the number of publications or frequencies; the larger the node, the greater the number of publications or frequencies (Liang *et al.*, 2017). Furthermore, the link between nodes represents the relationships among collaboration, co-occurrence, and co-citation. The colors of the nodes and lines represent different clusters (Gao *et al.*, 2019).

Results

The terms 'Tuberculosis' and 'Animal' in the title, abstract, and keywords were searched in the WOS database and a total of 11,155 documents were extracted in the last decade until March 1, 2024.

Authors

A total of 11,155 publications related to animal tuberculosis have been published. The top ten authors are as follows: Vordermeier HM had the highest number of published papers (151, 1.35%), followed by Hewinson RG (147, 1.318%), Waters WR (127, 1.139%), Palmer MV (115, 1.031%), Gortázar C (108, 0.96%), Delahay RJ (100, 0.89%), Buddle BM (98, 0.87%), Romero B (93, 0.83%), Vicente J (89, 0.79%), and Bezos J (87, 0.78%). The co-authorship networks at the author's level and organization by VOSviewer of 3526 publications related to animal tuberculosis and their implications in global studies are shown in Figs. 2.1 and 2.2.

Publication year

Regarding the publication year, the last decade showed a significant increase in research on animal tuberculosis. A total of of 693 publications were published in 2021 (6.21%), followed by 662 articles in 2016 (5.93%), 653 articles in 2017 (5.85%), 638 articles in 2014 (5.71%), 635 articles in 2020 (5.69%), 633 articles in

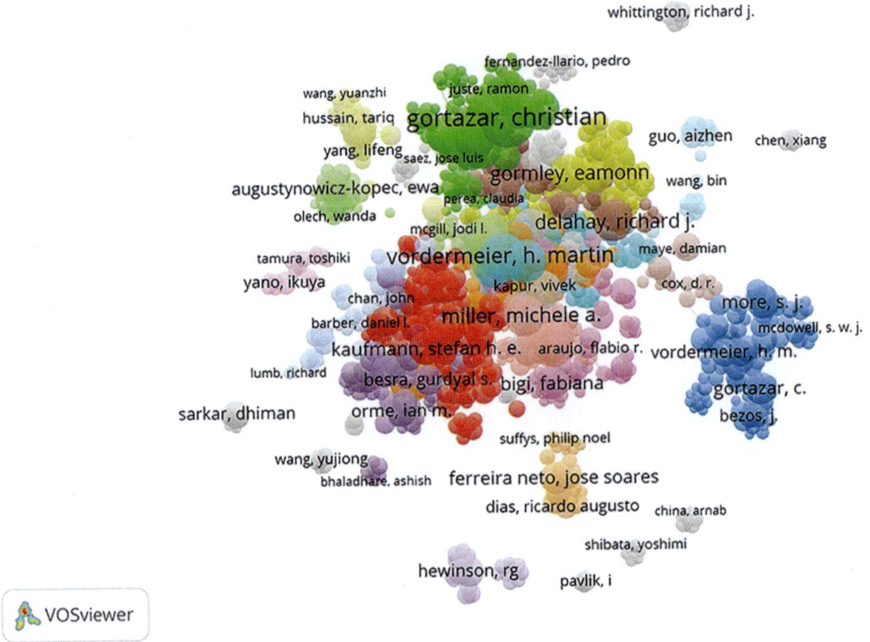

Fig. 2.1. VOSviewer diagram on authors contributing research on animal tuberculosis.

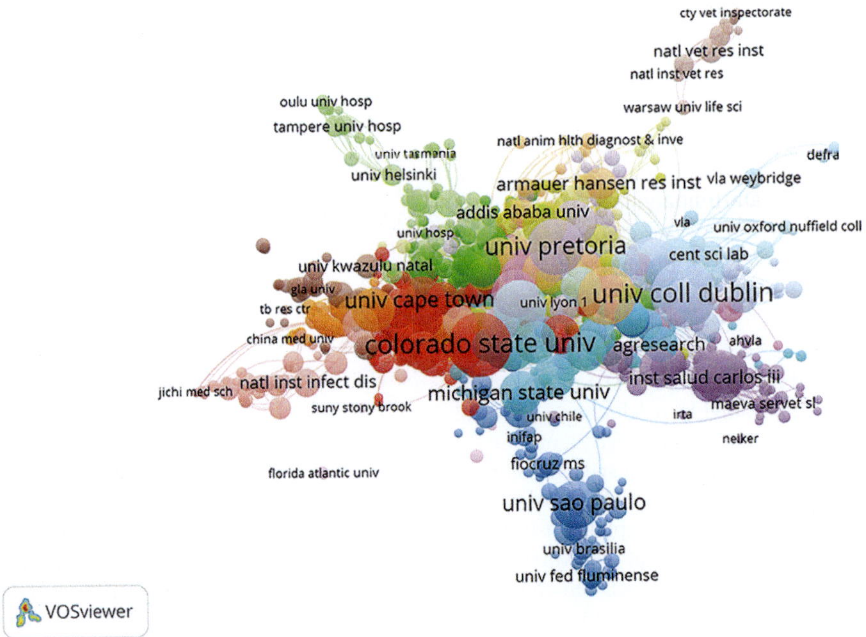

Fig. 2.2. VOSviewer diagram on co-author organization contributing research on animal tuberculosis.

2015 (5.67%), 614 articles in 2018 (5.5%), 607 papers in 2019 (5.44%), 599 papers in 2011 (5.37%), 588 papers in 2012 (5.27%), and 587 papers in 2013 (5.26%).

Institutions

The United States Department of Agriculture USDA had the highest number of publications (355, 3.18%), followed by the University of London (332, 2.97%), University College Dublin (288, 2.58%), Consejo Superior De Investigaciones Cientificas CSIC (271, 2.41%), Stellenbosch University (249, 2.23%), Colorado State University (247, 2.21%), Centre National De La Recherche Scientifique CNRS (241, 2.16%), University of California System (240, 2.16%), Veterinary Laboratories Agency (237, 2.1%), and Animal Plant Health Agency UK (233, 2.08%).

Funding agencies

Regarding funding agencies, the highest number of publications received funding from the United States Department of Health and Human Services (1093, 9.79%), followed by the National Institutes of Health (NIH) USA (1063, 9.52%), UK Research Innovation (UKRI) (677, 6.06%), European Union (EU) (447, 4.0%), National Institute of Allergy Infectious Diseases (NIAID) (436, 3.9%), National Natural Science Foundation of China (NSFC) (333, 2.98%), Medical Research Council (MRC) UK (331, 2.96%), Wellcome Trust (303, 2.71%), Spanish Government (295, 2.64%), and Biotechnology and Biological Sciences Research Council (BBSRC) (264, 2.63%).

Countries of publication

The top ten nations regarding the total number of publications on animal tuberculosis are presented in Table 2.1. The USA recorded the highest number of publications (3137, 28.12%).

Table 2.1. Countries contribution on research regarding animal tuberculosis in the last two decades.

Countries/regions	Record count	% of 11,155
USA	3137	28.122
England	1787	16.020
Spain	764	6.849
France	719	6.446
People's Republic of China	715	6.410
India	649	5.818
South Africa	637	5.710
Germany	536	4.805
Brazil	523	4.688
Canada	415	3.720

Language

Most publications were in English (10898, 97.69%). The other publications were in Spanish (65, 0.58%), French (47, 0.42%), Portuguese (42, 0.37%), German (24, 0.27%), Turkish (17, 0.15%), Polish (11, 0.10%), Hungarian (10, 0.09%), Korean (8, 0.07%), and Italian (6, 0.06%).

WOS categories

The top ten WOS categories for all 11,155 publications were Veterinary Sciences (2588, 23.2%), followed by Immunology (2541, 22.77%), Microbiology (2188, 19.61%), Infectious diseases (1484, 13.3%), Multidisciplinary Sciences (744, 6.6%), Medicine Research Experimental (612, 5.4%), Biochemistry Molecular Biology (573, 5.13%), Pharmacology Pharmacy (481, 4.31%), Respiratory System (463, 4.15%), and Ecology (390, 3.49%).

Citation topics

According to the citation topics meso, the ten most highly cited publications are presented in Table 2.2. The VOSviewer network for citation source, citation authors, and citation organization are presented in Figs. 2.3–2.6.

Publication type

Regarding publication type, research articles were the prevalent (9271, 83.11%), followed by book chapters (266, 2.38%), meeting abstracts (184, 1.64%), editorial material (156, 1.39%), letters (124, 1.11%), books (5, 0.04%), book reviews (5, 0.04%) and data papers (4, 0.036%).

Table 2.2. Citation topics meso of articles on animal tuberculosis in the last two decades.

Citation topics meso	Record count	% of 11,155
Tuberculosis & Leprosy	6628	59.417
Immunology	433	3.882
Zoology & Animal Ecology	339	3.039
Pelvic & Renal Disorders	334	2.994
Bacteriology	213	1.909
Virology–General	208	1.865
Zoonotic Diseases	185	1.658
Parasitology–General	116	1.040
Virology–Tropical Diseases	108	0.968
Antibiotics & Antimicrobials	93	0.834

Publishers

The main publishers of documents on animal tuberculosis were Elsevier (2577, 23.1%), Springer Nature (1072, 9.61%), Wiley (1071, 9.6%), American Society of Microbiology (756, 6.77%), Public Library Science (522, 4.68%), Frontiers Media SA (508, 4.55%), MDPI (357, 3.2%), Oxford University Press (287, 2.57%), Taylor & Francis (247, 2.21%), and Nature Portfolio (200, 1.79%).

Publication titles (Journals)

The top ten journals which published research on animal tuberculosis were PloS One (393, 3.52%), followed by Preventive Veterinary Medicine (246, 2.20%), Tuberculosis (238, 2.13%), Vaccine (233, 2.08%), Infection and Immunity (185, 1.65%), Frontiers in Veterinary Science (161, 1.44%), Veterinary Immunology and Immunopathology (160, 1.43%), Veterinary Microbiology (157, 1.4%), Clinical

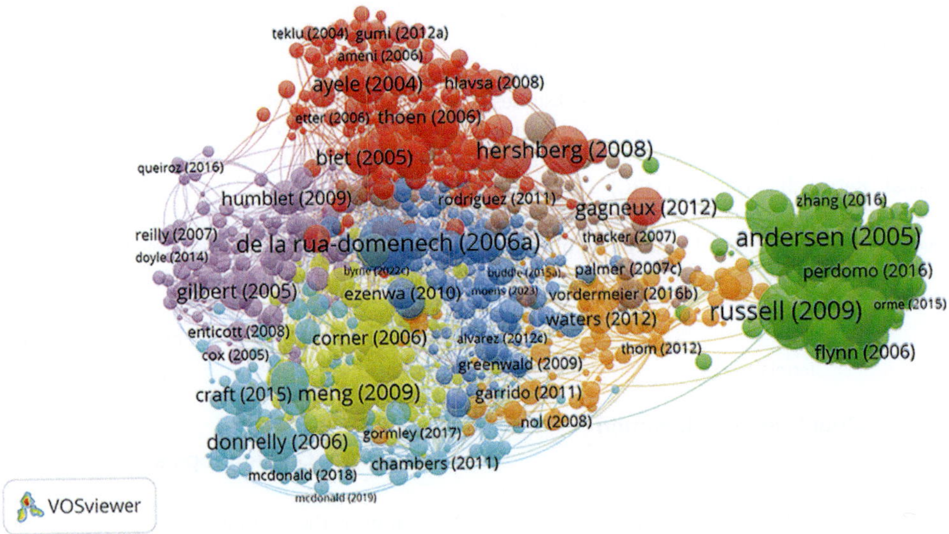

Fig. 2.3. VOSviewer diagram on citation-document regarding animal tuberculosis.

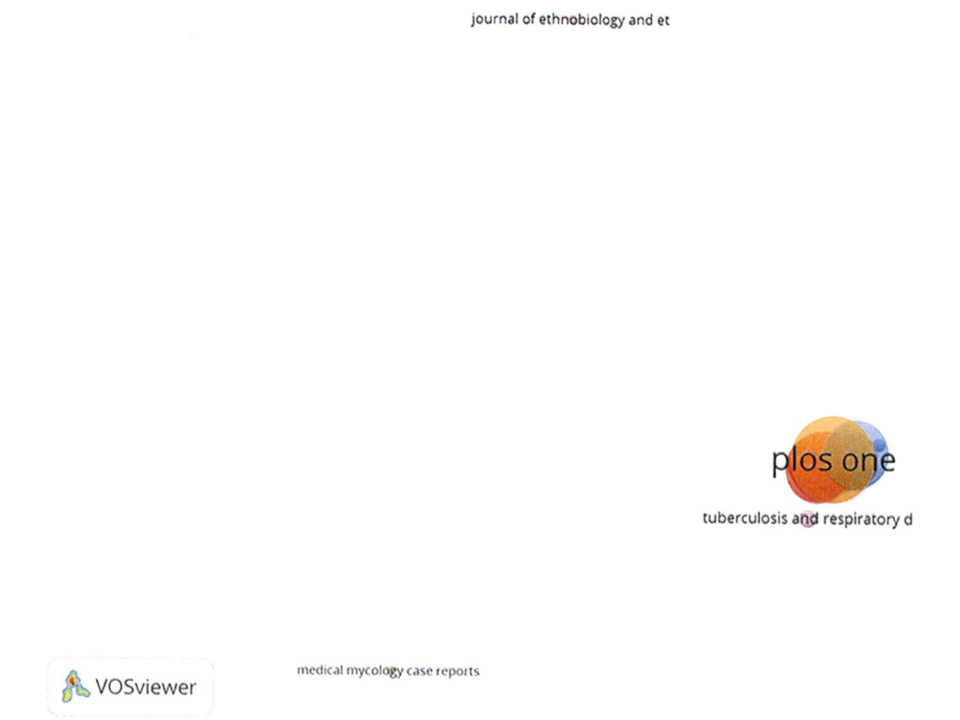

Fig. 2.4. VOSviewer diagram on citation-source regarding animal tuberculosis.

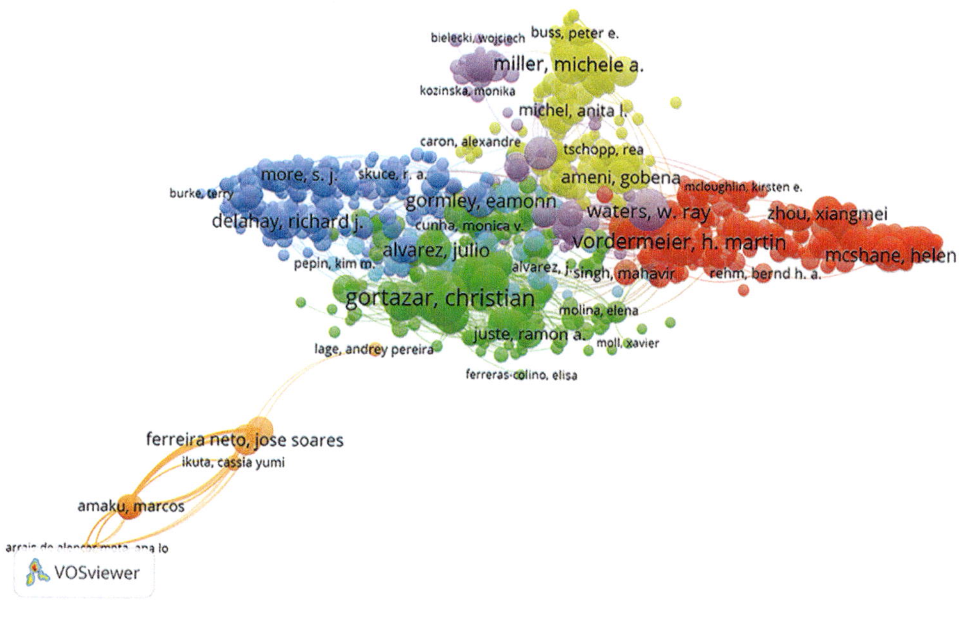

Fig. 2.5. VOSviewer diagram on citation-author regarding animal tuberculosis.

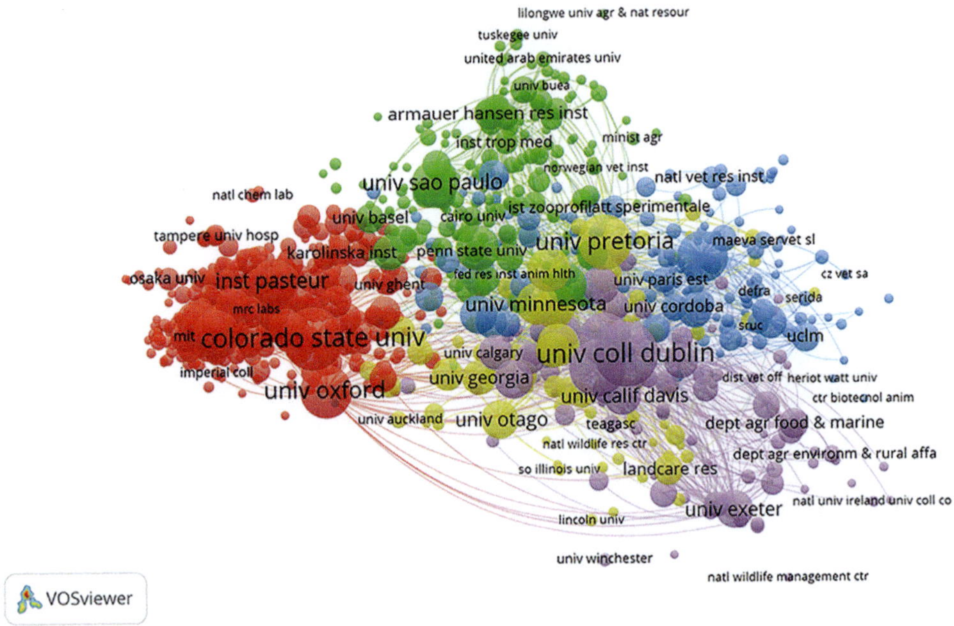

Fig. 2.6. VOSviewer diagram on citation-organization regarding animal tuberculosis.

and Vaccine Immunology (152, 1.36%), and Scientific Reports (149, 1.33%).

Co-occurrence analysis

We conducted a co-occurrence analysis to identify the most focused and accentuated content, topics, or keywords on the topic of animal tuberculosis. The minimum number of occurrences of a keyword was selected as five. Figure 2.7 shows the VOSviewer network of keywords that frequently occur in animal tuberculosis. The size of each node indicates the number of keyword occurrences across different studies. However, if the lines among nodes indicate that the two connected keywords co-occurred in a research study, the thickness of the line represents the number of co-occurrences.

Bibliographic coupling

The bibliographic coupling document, source, authors, and organizations are presented in Figs 2.8–2.11.

Discussion

Epidemiological longitudinal herd-level surveillance of tuberculosis provides information on the changes in pathogen genotype abundance over time (Skuce *et al.*, 2020). However, bibliometric analysis allows for the interpretation of minute differences by analyzing a huge input of data over a long period of time (Zan, 2012; Zheng *et al.*, 2022). The application of bibliometric analysis in veterinary research is relatively limited and considerable effort is required to accomplish it. In this study, we present an overview of the global rush point concerning research on animal tuberculosis, following the standard pathway of bibliometric analysis.

At the authors' level, Vordermeier H.M. had the highest number of published papers (151, 1.35%). Vordermeier focused on animal tuberculosis, with a total publication of 249. A highly cited paper by Vordermeier was published in Research in Veterinary Science 529. The co-authorship networks at the author level showed that Glyn Hewinson was the top co-author (119 articles). However, this type of metric analysis was applied to discover the social structure

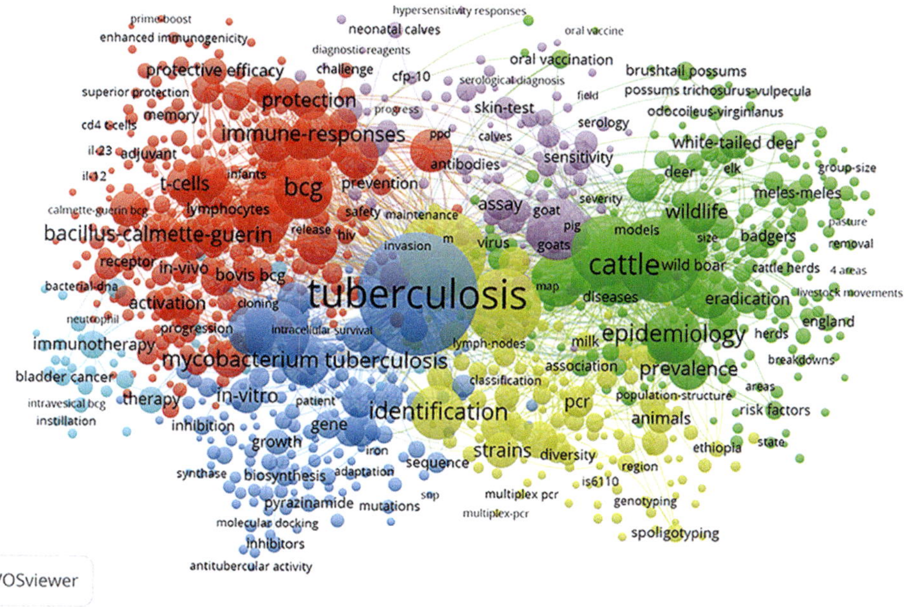

Fig. 2.7. VOSviewer diagram on co-occurrence (all keywords) regarding animal tuberculosis.

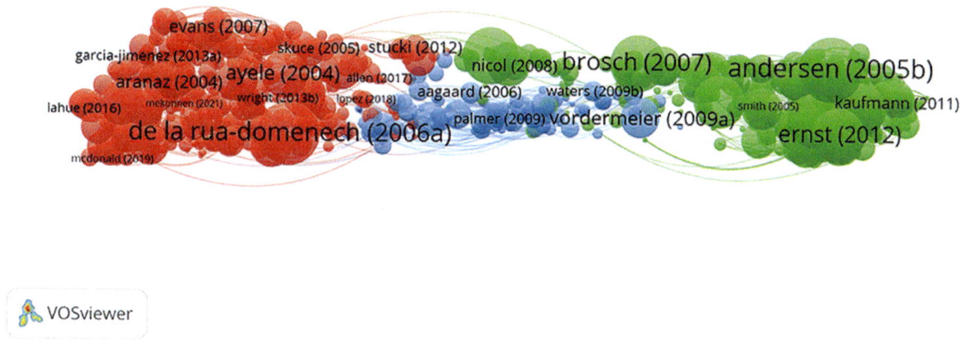

Fig. 2.8. VOSviewer diagram shows the bibliographic coupling-document regarding research on animal tuberculosis.

instead of the authors' intellectual structure (Lu and Wolfram, 2012). On the other hand, co-citation analysis visualizes the co-citied publications in the form of thematic clusters, where the common references between two publications do not change over time and remain identical (Jarneving, 2005; Lu and Wolfram, 2012).

Regarding the publication time analysis, the results show a steady increase in the output since 2004, with the highest number of publications emitted in 2021 (693, 6.21%). This finding may reflect global attention toward this disease. As a general concept, over time, the attitudes towards animal sciences and diseases have augmented worldwide (Pifer *et al.*, 1994). It could be that any research gate provides an opportunity for new horizons for other gates as continuousness for assumed research ideas. The topic here is no different, where research on animal tuberculosis continues to be emphasized based on economic and public health importance. Several factors may motivate such

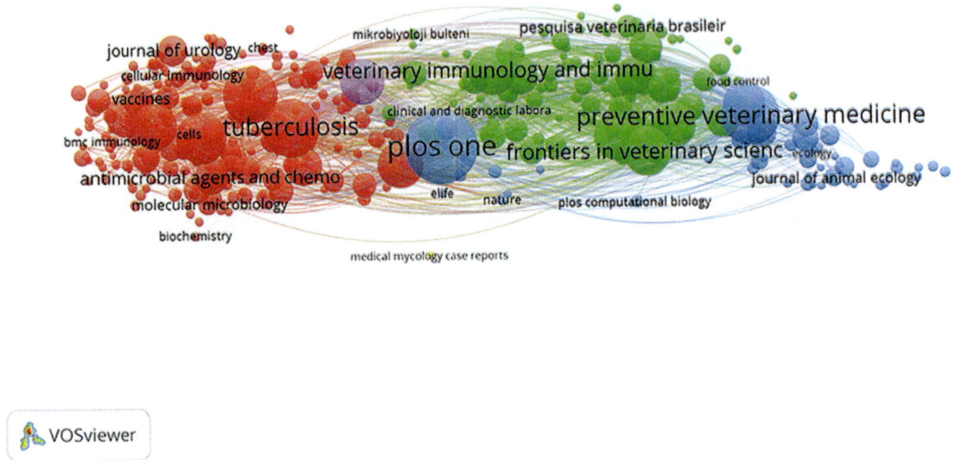

Fig. 2.9. VOSviewer diagram shows the bibliographic coupling-source regarding research on animal tuberculosis.

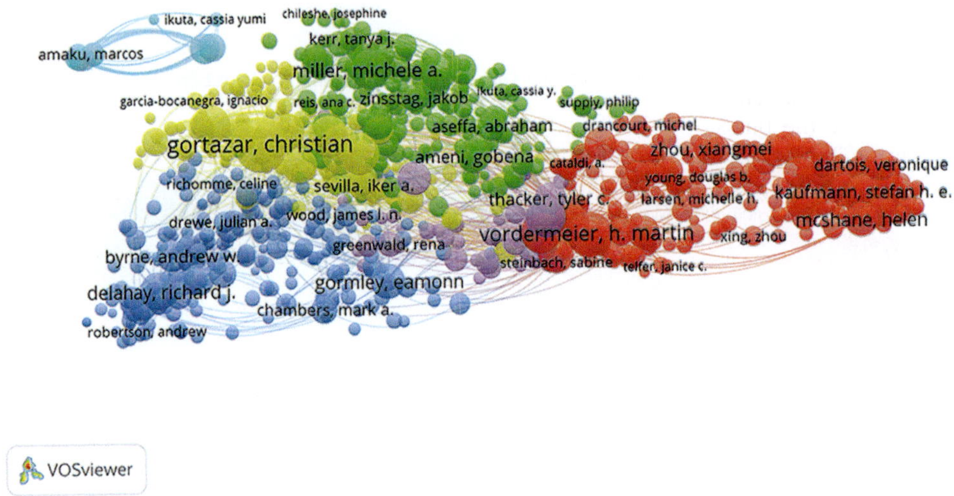

Fig. 2.10. VOSviewer diagram shows the bibliographic coupling-author regarding research on animal tuberculosis.

attention, such as environmental changes that are parallel to the flaring of animal tuberculosis. Therefore, temporal evaluation of animal tuberculosis has recently received more attention globally (Acevedo *et al.*, 2019; Aranha *et al.*, 2021; Blanco Vázquez *et al.*, 2021; Schwarz *et al.*, 2021; Herraiz *et al.*, 2023).

Institutions play an important role in most available publications. In the current study, the United States Department of Agriculture and Research Institutes in the United Kingdom were the major institutes contributing to research on animal tuberculosis. These findings may reflect the increased need to conduct further studies on these diseases. Interestingly, funding agencies provide support for research projects (Gläser and Velarde, 2018). The UK Research Innovation UKRI is the top funding agency, which explains why institutes in this country are highly affiliated.

Continuing the overall characterization of the research input on animal tuberculosis, the

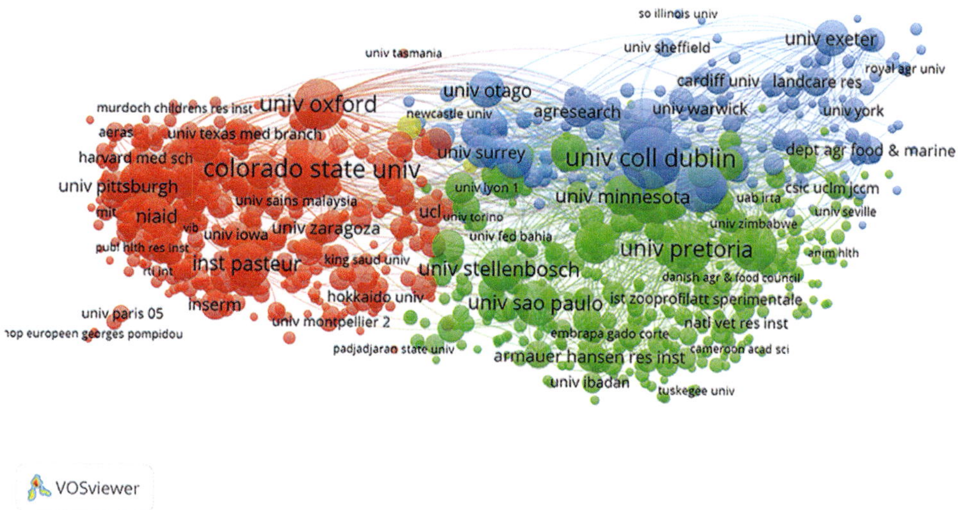

Fig. 2.11. VOSviewer diagram shows the bibliographic coupling-organization regarding research on animal tuberculosis.

top countries regarding the total publication number were the United Kingdom, the USA, and Spain. This finding may reflect the interest of funding agencies and institutes in conducting research on such topics to answer several questions regarding this issue. In the UK, more tests for BTB are performed on cattle herds, and each positive herd test triggers more testing, which may contribute to the final number of articles on tuberculosis (van Dijk, 2013).

In this study, the WoS Core collection was used because of the definite collection and evaluation process of academic articles, which is commonly considered ideal for detailed bibliometric analysis. This analysis enables scholars to objectively determine the performance of papers related to scope and citation features. WoS incorporates more than 252 subject categories in science, social sciences, arts, and humanities. In the present investigation, the highest number of publications were registered in Veterinary Sciences category (2588, 23.2%). This scheme is implemented by assigning each journal to one or more topic groups. However, because it is often difficult to assign a journal to a single category, overlapping coverage of the categories may occur. Each published item inherits all the subject categories assigned to the parent journal (Birkle *et al.*, 2020).

Referring to citation topics, the results revealed that the main topics focused on tuberculosis and leprosy, which may reflect the zoonotic potential of animal tuberculosis. The second topic was immunology, which may indicate the increased studies on the antibiotic resistance and vaccine development. However, animal health and production sciences are of great interest globally, as there is an expected significant increase in the world population (Hernández-Castellano *et al.*, 2019). Citation analysis aims to measure the effects of relevant research units in the scientific field, such as authors, journals, and institutions (Hallinger and Kovačević, 2021). These research units are expected to receive more citations, which are considered the most significant, indicating greater effectiveness, rank, and quality (Donthu *et al.*, 2021). Henry Small was the first to use co-citation analysis to detect the strengths and weaknesses of an institution (Surwase *et al.*, 2011). Furthermore, co-citation analysis shows whether the two research units appear together in the bibliography, indicating a strong co-citation relationship (van Eck and Waltman, 2014). Moreover, co-occurrence analysis clarifies the ideas that are often shared in abstracts, titles, or even keywords of publications based on thematic clusters created by the relationships between these concepts and visualizes them as a network (Donthu *et al.*, 2021). Additionally, co-authorship analysis was used to display social partnerships in a field study (Rousseau *et al.*, 2018).

Concerning the publication type, the form of research articles was the most prevalent. This seems quite similar to what is commonly known by researchers in other fields of study. Research papers are usually more detailed and thorough than reviews. A research paper is usually peer-reviewed, but a review paper is not always available. Generally, research articles are usually more formal than review articles (Booth *et al.*, 2003; Ömer Gülpınar, 2013). Regarding the publishers, Elsevier had the highest number of publications (2577, 23.1%). Elsevier is a leading publisher of the most well-respected science journals worldwide. Therefore, publishing research in Elsevier is expected to be widely disseminated. Elsevier journals are a smart choice for scientific authors, including those interested in farm animal practices, microbiology, and emerging diseases. In the aspect concerning the most publication titles (Journals) interested in animal tuberculosis, the highest publication title was PloS One, which publishes evidence of improvements and the expansion of scientific knowledge supporting infectious diseases (Silver *et al.*, 2011). It has been reported that, indisputably, specialist journals have a higher attraction for papers than less highly specialist journals in practice.

In the present study, using VOSviewer, we obtained a co-occurrence analysis to recognize the most focused and accentuated content, topics, and keywords in the animal tuberculosis research field. Co-occurrence analysis has been found to offer perceptions of the most common ideas, trends, topics, and patterns that may be considered in future planning of scientific research (Wang and Chai, 2018). One of the most important variables for the analysis of publications is the bibliographic coupling of documents and organization. In this analysis, two documents from two organizations were coupled to cite the third document. Bibliographic coupling can be evaluated using bibliographic coupling strength (Moed, 2006). It also considers recently published research articles with fewer citations. Bibliographic coupling displays all current studies, and old and seminal studies appear in co-citation analysis. It depicts the current situation of intellectual structure in a certain scientific trend (Boyack and Klavans, 2010). Coupling analysis has been reported to be stronger than co-citation analysis (Zhao and Strotmann, 2015).

Conclusion

In this work, for the first time, using bibliometric analysis, we provide insight into studies conducted on animal tuberculosis in the last two decades. The results indicate a growing number of studies on tuberculosis in animals, which reflects the re-emergence of the disease to an alarming degree. The results can help to establish the possible forthcoming plans for its prevention and control.

Conflict of Interest

The authors declare that there is no conflict of interest.

Funding

This work was supported through the Annual Funding track by the Deanship of Scientific Research, Vice Presidency for Graduate Studies and Scientific Research, King Faisal University, Saudi Arabia (Grant A317).

Data Availability

Data are available on request.

References

Acevedo, P., Prieto, M., Quirós, P., Merediz, I., Juan, L. *et al.* (2019) Tuberculosis epidemiology and badger (meles meles) spatial ecology in a hot-spot area in Atlantic Spain. *Pathogens* 8, 292–309.

Aranha, J., Abrantes, A.C., Gonçalves, R., Miranda, R., Serejo, J. *et al.* (2021) GIS as an epidemiological tool to monitor the spatial-temporal distribution of tuberculosis in large game in a high-risk area in Portugal. *Animals (Basel)* 11.

Ayalew, S., Habtamu, G., Melese, F., Tessema, B., Ashford, R.T. *et al.* (2023) Zoonotic tuberculosis in a high bovine tuberculosis burden area of Ethiopia. *Frontiers in Public Health* 11, 1204525.

Ayana, D.Z. (2020) Review on epidemiology and public health importance of goat tuberculosis in Ethiopia. *Veterinary Medicine International* 8898874.

Ayele, W.Y., Neill, S.D., Zinsstag, J., Weiss, M.G. and Pavlik, I. (2004) Bovine tuberculosis: An old disease but a new threat to Africa. *The International Journal of Tuberculosis and Lung Disease* 8, 924–937.

Bagcchi, S. (2023) WHO's global tuberculosis report 2022. *The Lancet Microbe* 4, e20.

Birkle, C., Pendlebury, D.A., Schnell, J. and Adams, J. (2020) Web of science as a data source for research on scientific and scholarly activity. *Quantitative Science Studies* 1, 363–376.

Blanco Vázquez, C., Barral, T.D., Romero, B., Queipo, M., Merediz, I. *et al.* (2021) Spatial and temporal distribution of mycobacterium tuberculosis complex infection in eurasian badger (meles meles) and cattle in Asturias, Spain. *Animals (Basel)* 11.

Booth, W.C., Colomb, G.G. and Williams, J.M. (2003) *The Craft of Research*. University of Chicago Press, Chicago, IL.

Boyack, K.W. and Klavans, R. (2010) Co-citation analysis, bibliographic coupling, and direct citation: Which citation approach represents the research front most accurately? *Journal of the American Society for Information Science and Technology* 61, 2389–2404.

Buddle, B.M., Skinner, M.A., Wedlock, D.N., Lisle, G.W., Vordermeier, H.M. *et al.* (2005) Cattle as a model for development of vaccines against human tuberculosis. *Tuberculosis (Edinburgh, Scotland)* 85, 19–24.

Byrne, A.W., Barrett, D., Breslin, P., Fanning, J., Casey, M. *et al.* (2022) Bovine tuberculosis in youngstock cattle: A narrative review. *Frontiers in Veterinary Science* 9, 1000124.

Costa, P., Amaro, A., Ferreira, A.S., Machado, D., Albuquerque, T. *et al.* (2014) Rapid identification of veterinary-relevant *Mycobacterium tuberculosis* complex species using 16S rDNA, IS6110 and regions of difference-targeted dual-labelled hydrolysis probes. *Journal of Microbiological Methods* 107, 13–22.

Crawley-Low, J. (2006) Bibliometric analysis of the American Journal of Veterinary Research to produce a list of core veterinary medicine journals. *Journal of the Medical Library Association* 94, 430.

Donthu, N., Kumar, S., Mukherjee, D., Pandey, N. and Lim, W.M. (2021) How to conduct a bibliometric analysis: An overview and guidelines. *Journal of Business Research* 133, 285–296.

Drijvers, P., Grauwin, S. and Trouche, L. (2020) When bibliometrics met mathematics education research: The case of instrumental orchestration. *ZDM* 1–15.

Elsayed, M. and Amer, A. (2019) The rapid detection and differentiation of Mycobacterium tuberculosis complex members from cattle and water buffaloes in the delta area of Egypt, using a combination of real-time and conventional PCR. *Molecular Biology Reports* 46, 3909–3919.

Ferluga, J., Yasmin, H., Al-Ahdal, M.N., Bhakta, S. and Kishore, U. (2020) Natural and trained innate immunity against Mycobacterium tuberculosis. *Immunobiology* 225, 151951.

Fielding, H.R., McKinley, T.J., Delahay, R.J., Silk, M.J. and McDonald, R.A. (2021) Characterization of potential superspreader farms for bovine tuberculosis: A review. *Veterinary Medicine and Science* 7, 310–321.

Gao, Y., Ge, L., Shi, S., Sun, Y., Liu, M. *et al.* (2019) Global trends and future prospects of e-waste research: A bibliometric analysis. *Environmental Science and Pollution Research* 26, 17809–17820.

Gläser, J. and Velarde, K.S. (2018) Changing funding arrangements and the production of scientific knowledge: Introduction to the special issue. *Minerva* 56, 1–10.

Goosen, W.J., Kerr, T.J., Kleynhans, L., Buss, P., Cooper, D. *et al.* (2020) The VetMAX™ M. tuberculosis complex PCR kit detects MTBC DNA in antemortem and postmortem samples from white rhinoceros (*Ceratotherium simum*), African elephants (*Loxodonta africana*) and African buffaloes (*Syncerus caffer*). *BMC Veterinary Research* 16, 220.

Hade, M.D., Sethi, D., Datta, H., Singh, S., Thakur, N. *et al.* (2020) Truncated hemoglobin O carries an autokinase activity and facilitates adaptation of *Mycobacterium tuberculosis* under hypoxia. *Antioxidants & Redox Signaling* 32, 351–362.

Hallinger, P. and Kovačević, J. (2021) Science mapping the knowledge base in educational leadership and management: A longitudinal bibliometric analysis, 1960 to 2018. *Educational Management Administration & Leadership* 49, 5–30.

Hernández-Castellano, L.E., Nally, J.E., Lindahl, J., Wanapat, M., Alhidary, I.A. *et al.* (2019) Dairy science and health in the tropics: Challenges and opportunities for the next decades. *Tropical Animal Health and Production* 51, 1009–1017.

Herraiz, C., Vicente, J., Gortázar, C. and Acevedo, P. (2023) Large scale spatio-temporal modelling of risk factors associated with tuberculosis exposure at the wildlife-livestock interface. *Preventive Veterinary Medicine* 220, 106049.

Hsu, Y.-H.E., Yang, Y.-T., Wang, M.-H. and Ho, Y.-S. (2020) Bibliometric analysis of highly cited publications in health policy and services. *COLLNET Journal of Scientometrics and Information Management* 14, 177–202.

Jarneving, B. (2005) A comparison of two bibliometric methods for mapping of the research front. *Scientometrics* 65, 245–263.

Krauskopf, E., Garcia, F. and Funk, R. (2017) Bibliometric analysis of multi-language veterinary journals. *Transinformação* 29, 343–353.

Liang, Y.-D., Li, Y., Zhao, J., Wang, X.-Y., Zhu, H.-Z. *et al.* (2017) Study of acupuncture for low back pain in recent 20 years: A bibliometric analysis via CiteSpace. *Journal of Pain Research* 951–964.

Lu, K. and Wolfram, D. (2012) Measuring author research relatedness: A comparison of word-based, topic-based, and author cocitation approaches. *Journal of the American Society for Information Science and Technology* 63, 1973–1986.

Moed, H.F. (2006) *Citation Analysis in Research Evaluation*. Springer Science & Business Media, Dordrecht, The Netherlands.

Mulet-Forteza, C., Genovart-Balaguer, J., Merigó, J.M. and Mauleon-Mendez, E. (2019) Bibliometric structure of IJCHM in its 30 years. *International Journal of Contemporary Hospitality Management* 31, 4574–4604.

Murai, K., Tizzani, P., Awada, L., Mur, L., Mapitse, N. *et al.* (2019) Panorama 2019-1: Bovine tuberculosis: Global distribution and implementation status of prevention and control measures according to WAHIS data. *Bulletin de l'OIE* 1–3.

Njoga, E.O., Ilo, S.U., Nwobi, O.C., Onwumere-Idolor, O.S., Ajibo, F.E. *et al.* (2023) Pre-slaughter, slaughter and post-slaughter practices of slaughterhouse workers in Southeast, Nigeria: Animal welfare, meat quality, food safety and public health implications. *PLoS One* 18, e0282418.

Olea-Popelka, F., Muwonge, A., Perera, A., Dean, A.S., Mumford, E. *et al.* (2017) Zoonotic tuberculosis in human beings caused by *Mycobacterium bovis* – A call for action. *The Lancet Infectious Diseases* 17, e21–e25.

Ömer Gülpınar, A.G.G. (2013) How to write a review article? *Turkish Journal of Urology* 39(Supplement 1), 44–48.

Pelzer, N.L. and Wiese, W.H. (2003) Bibliometric study of grey literature in core veterinary medical journals. *Journal of the Medical Library Association* 91, 434.

Pifer, R., Shimizu, K. and Pifer, L. (1994) Public attitudes toward animal research: Some international comparisons. *Society and Animals* 2, 95–113.

Pritchard, A. (1969) Statistical bibliography or bibliometrics. *Journal of Documentation* 25, 348.

Refaya, A.K., Bhargavi, G., Mathew, N.C., Rajendran, A., Krishnamoorthy, R. *et al.* (2020) A review on bovine tuberculosis in India 122, 101923.

Rousseau, R., Egghe, L. and Guns, R. (2018) *Becoming Metric-Wise: A Bibliometric Guide for Researchers*. Chandos Publishing, Witney, UK.

Schoenfeld-Tacher, R.M. and Alpi, K. (2021) A 45-year retrospective content analysis of JVME articles. *Journal of Veterinary Medical Education* 48, 729–746.

Schwarz, D.G.G., Sousa Júnior, P.F., Silva, L., Polveiro, R.C., Oliveira, J.F. *et al.* (2021) Spatiotemporal distribution and temporal trends of brucellosis and tuberculosis in water buffalo (*Bubalus bubalis*) in Brazil. *Preventive Veterinary Medicine* 193, 105417.

Schwoebel, V. (2020) Surveillance of tuberculosis. *The Indian Journal of Tuberculosis* 67, S33–s42.

Siala, M., Smaoui, S., Taktak, W., Hachicha, S., Ghorbel, A. *et al.* (2017) First-time detection and identification of the *Mycobacterium tuberculosis* complex members in extrapulmonary tuberculosis clinical samples in south Tunisia by a single tube tetraplex real-time PCR assay. *PLoS Neglected Tropical Diseases* 11, e0005572.

Sibhat, B., Asmare, K., Demissie, K., Ayelet, G., Mamo, G. *et al.* (2017) Bovine tuberculosis in Ethiopia: A systematic review and meta-analysis. *Preventive Veterinary Medicine* 147, 149–157.

Silver, I., Jeffcott, L. and Rossdale, P. (2011) Fifty years of the British Equine Veterinary Association as a facilitator of progress in equine clinical science. *Equine Veterinary Journal* 43, 618–631.

Singh, A.V., Yadav, V.S., Chauhan, D.S. and Singh, S.V. (2022) *Mycobacterium bovis* induced human tuberculosis in India: Current status, challenges & opportunities. *The Indian Journal of Medical Research* 156, 21–30.

Skuce, R., Breadon, E., Allen, A., Milne, G., McCormick, C. *et al.* (2020) Longitudinal dynamics of herd-level *Mycobacterium bovis* MLVA type surveillance in cattle in Northern Ireland 2003–2016. *Infection, Genetics and Evolution* 79, 104131.

Surwase, G., Sagar, A., Kademani, B. and Bhanumurthy, K. (2011) Co-citation analysis: An overview. In: *Beyond Librarianship: Creativity, Innovation and Discovery*. Mumbai (India).

van Dijk, J. (2013) Towards risk-based test protocols: Estimating the contribution of intensive testing to the UK bovine tuberculosis problem. *PLoS One* 8, e63961.

van Eck, N.J. and Waltman, L. (2014) Visualizing bibliometric networks. In: *Measuring Scholarly Impact: Methods and Practice*. Springer, Cham, Heidelberg, New York, Dordrecht, London, pp. 285–320.

Vordermeier, M., Ameni, G., Berg, S., Bishop, R., Robertson, B.D. *et al.* (2012) The influence of cattle breed on susceptibility to bovine tuberculosis in Ethiopia. *Comparative Immunology, Microbiology and Infectious Diseases* 35, 227–232.

Wang, M. and Chai, L. (2018) Three new bibliometric indicators/ approaches derived from keyword analysis. *Scientometrics* 116, 721–750.

Zan, B. (2012) *A Comparative Bibliometric Analysis Study in Scinentific Disciplines at Turkey*. Ankara University, Ankara.

Zhao, D. and Strotmann, A. (2015) *Analysis and Visualization of Citation Networks*. Morgan & Claypool Publishers, New England, Northeastern US.

Zheng, M.Q., Li, X.X., Xu, R., Liu, S., Rui, Z.Y. *et al.* (2022) Bibliometric analysis of tuberculosis molecular epidemiology based on CiteSpace. *Frontiers in Public Health* 10, 1040176.

Zumla, A., Atun, R., Maeurer, M., Mwaba, P., Ma, Z. *et al.* (2011) Viewpoint: Scientific dogmas, paradoxes and mysteries of latent *Mycobacterium tuberculosis* infection. *Tropical Medicine & International Health* 16, 79–83.

Zupic, I. and Čater, T. (2015) Bibliometric methods in management and organization. *Organizational Research Methods* 18, 429–472.

3 Local Food Systems as a Resilient Strategy to Ensure Sustainable Food Security in Crisis: Lessons From COVID-19 Pandemic and Perspectives for the Post-Pandemic World

Anju Thattantavide and Ajay Kumar*

Department of Plant Science, School of Biological Sciences, Central University of Kerala, Kasaragod, 671316, Kerala, India

Abstract

The COVID-19 pandemic adversely affected food supply chains and threatened global food security. The nations excessively relying on the import of food were severely affected. The food shortages in various countries worldwide were due to multiple reasons, such as unavailability of land, infertility of the available land, and excessive reliance on the import of foods. The excessive dependence on a few mainstream crops increases the vulnerabilities of the communities. However, several plants, known as traditional or indigenous food plants, are consumed by local populations and form the basis of robust local food systems. They are not cultivated at a large scale in a large area, but local communities have access to the locally available plants that grow near their settlements. Local foods are particularly vital during situations similar to pandemics and wars when the global supply chains are disrupted. This article emphasises the potential of local food system supply chains as a resilient strategy for food security in emergencies such as COVID-19. It further attempts to provide important insights into the vulnerabilities associated with mainstream foods, their impact on food insecurity, and the forthcoming roles of alternative local food systems based on local indigenous plants.

Keywords: local foods, traditional food plants, traditional food systems, poverty, COVID-19, sustainable development goals, food security

Introduction

The world population is expected to reach nine billion by 2050 (Béné *et al.*, 2015). An increased population means increased demand for food for their food security. Food production is already battling many issues due to climate change, shrinkage of agricultural land, and increased incidences of disease outbreaks and stresses (Masters *et al.*, 2010). The current agricultural production systems are environmentally not very sustainable as they contribute

*Corresponding author: botanistajay@gmail.com
Both authors contributed equally to this work.

to environmental degradation, biodiversity loss, and depletion of soil and water (Foley *et al.*, 2011; Bakalis *et al.*, 2020). Additionally, the COVID-19 pandemic disturbed the whole food system, from production to consumption (Belik, 2020; Haron and Jalil, 2023). The food-producing and exporting regions lost employment, whereas the food-importing regions faced food shortages (Belik, 2020). Besides the massive death of humans, it created losses for economic sectors, goods manufacturing, supply chains, and logistics (Barman *et al.*, 2021; Kazancoglu *et al.*, 2023; Verma *et al.*, 2023). This planet has experienced several pandemics in the past as well (Kilbourne, 2006), but unlike the past pandemics, COVID-19 forced the cessation of all commercial activities and disrupted daily activities, including employment and education (Zhou and Kan, 2021).

The COVID-19 pandemic has revealed the negative side of the current food production systems (Kubatko *et al.*, 2023). Mainstream food crops are commonly consumed food plants that are widely available and popular among the general population. They play a pivotal role in the global food system, as they are widely consumed by people across different regions and cultures. COVID-19 affected mainstream agriculture in various dimensions. The decreased availability of workers or workforce for agriculture resulted in a temporary reduction in productivity (Devereux *et al.*, 2020; Purwantini, 2023). Agricultural inputs such as manures, fertilisers and pesticides were also less available and more expensive during the pandemic, resulting in decreased crop yields (Lamichhane and Reay-Jones, 2021). The limited availability of inputs due to movement restrictions impacted agricultural productivity (OCED, 2020). Southeast Asia's agricultural labour force (ALF) decreased by 1.4% in 2020 compared to 2019 (Gregorio and Ancog, 2020). Due to an overreliance on a couple of major crops, the severity of the problem increased. Despite diverse flowering plants on this planet, we currently cultivate only a few plants for the dietary requirements, including rice, maize, wheat, potato, sorghum, soybean, and plantains (Hammer *et al.*, 2003; Dulloo *et al.*, 2014). The vulnerability of mainstream crops to stresses and other innate limitations highlights the necessity of diversifying our food systems. The homogenised food systems involving long-distance transportation are vulnerable to various challenges. These include natural disasters, rising fuel prices, disease outbreaks, and the impacts of climate change (Breiling and Anbumozhi, 2020). The COVID-19 pandemic revealed the limitations of homogenised global food systems based on mainstream crops (Hamilton *et al.*, 2020). Due to the limitations of mainstream crops, local food crops that are regionally adapted gain greater importance (Enthoven and Van den Broeck, 2021).

Besides affecting agricultural productivity and crop yields, the COVID-19 pandemic disrupted global food supply chains and disconnected the links between food producers and consumers (Belik, 2020). Typically, food covers extensive distances before it reaches consumers (Lamine and Dawson, 2018; Bakalis *et al.*, 2020; Belik, 2020; McKeon, 2021). A breakdown in the food supply chains led to food shortages in many regions (Esfahani *et al.*, 2022). Food security was severely affected in underdeveloped countries heavily dependent on food imports and donations (FAO and WFP, 2020). Food supply chains have faced disruptions long before COVID-19. Several countries have encountered challenges in their food supply chains due to conflicts, natural disasters, and pest outbreaks (Leat and Revoredo-Giha, 2013). However, the COVID-19 pandemic was rapid, and it crippled even the most developed and advanced economies in the world (Marti and Puertas, 2021). The Global Report on Food Crisis 2020 states that acute food insecurity affected 155 million people worldwide in 2020, an increase of 20 million from the figures of 2019 (FSIN, 2021). This indicates that the COVID-19 pandemic caused nearly 20 million people to experience acute food insecurity (FSIN, 2021). The pandemic led to a realisation that long-distance food supply chains have undesirable effects, especially during untoward situations such as wars, pandemics, and natural disasters. Sovereign states must have locally available resilient food systems not only to tide over pandemic-like situations but also for untoward situations in the future. It is also necessary to strengthen short-food supply chains and regional food systems to prevent food insecurity (Cappelli and Cini, 2020). In this background, the paper discusses the significance of local food systems and local supply chains in maintaining food security as a robust and sustainable production strategy. Local food systems are also deeply rooted in regional cultures, making them more resilient in unpredictable situations and emergencies.

Review Methodology

To investigate the impact of the COVID-19 pandemic on food security and supply chains, the study analysed scholarly articles addressing key themes related to the effect of the pandemic on food systems. The three major databases, Scopus, PubMed, and Google Scholar, were used to search for scholarly articles. The keywords used in the search query include COVID-19, food security, global food supply chain, local supply chain, local food plants, sustainable production, post-pandemic transition, sustainable development goals, technologies for reviving local food systems and resilience. We retrieved articles related to the impact of COVID-19 on food security, supply chains, and post-pandemic food system transitions. The analysis centred on understanding how the pandemic affected food security, supply chains and the resilience of food systems. The study also explored strategies for sustainable production and including local food systems in recovery efforts. Based on the reviewed literature, we developed insights into actionable recommendations for policymakers, practitioners, and researchers. The goal was to understand the challenges posed by over-reliance on major crops during crises like COVID-19 and the role of local food systems in building better strategies.

Mainstream Food Systems, COVID-19, and Food Security

Mainstream food systems during the COVID-19 pandemic

Mainstream food crops refer to commonly consumed food items that are widely available and popular among the general population. Mainstream food crops play a pivotal role in the global food system as they are widely consumed by people across different regions and cultures (Erenstein *et al.*, 2022). Global food systems, especially global food trade networks, are highly interconnected, and any adverse effects on any component within the system can affect the entire system (Ji *et al.*, 2024). The globalisation of the food systems has resulted in an increased distance between consumers and producers, damaging the people's agri-food culture (Iga, 2014). The control of industrial food production is neither in the hands of producers nor consumers (Donkers, 2014). Unlike our ancestors, who used to grow their own foods for their consumption, we import them from long distances. The food produced in one area travels long distances before reaching consumers (Pretty *et al.*, 2005). Globalisation has led to an excessive homogenisation of food systems worldwide. Similar diets are recommended for different geographically distant regions of the world. As a result, locally and regionally available foods have reduced in size and have been supplanted by industrial and processed foods (Hamilton *et al.*, 2020). It has been found that industrial food production systems are unsustainable and highly vulnerable to pests, insect attacks, diseases and climate change (Altieri and Nicholls, 2020). Many of the current diseases that affect humans are basically due to the type of diet we eat. An evolutionary health promotion perspective also suggests that ancestral palaeolithic diets (PD) might be beneficial against lifestyle-related diseases (Eaton *et al.*, 2002). A meta-analysis of the effect of PDs on chronic vascular diseases (CVDs) suggests its positive impact on lowering CVDs (Ghaedi *et al.*, 2019). Current mainstream food systems are highly expensive economically and compromise the planet's health. They destroy the water, land, climate and biodiversity globally (Foley *et al.*, 2011). A comparison between mainstream and local foods is given in Table 3.1.

Impact of the COVID-19 pandemic on global food supply chains

The development of a nation is ultimately linked to its economic growth. Agricultural

Table 3.1. The comparison between mainstream and local foods.

Mainstream foods	Local foods	References
Disconnection between the consumers and producers	Consumers and producers are connected	O'Hara and Stagl (2001)
Long-distance transportation	Short-distance transportation	O'Hara and Stagl (2001)
Requirement of extra fuel, transport, logistics – hike in prices	Less cost than imported food products from other regions	Atallah *et al*. (2014); McCarthy *et al*. (2018)
Loss of freshness and nutrients	Fresh and nutrient-rich	Maherani *et al*. (2016); Vargas *et al*. (2021)
Supply-chain disruptions (due to wars, disasters and pandemics)	Fewer chances of supply-chain disruptions	Zollet *et al*. (2021); Khan *et al*. (2022)
Unsustainable	Sustainable during disruptions	La Trobe and Acott (2000); Donkers (2014)
Disruption between production and consumption increases vulnerabilities. Less resilient	Resilient during times of crisis	Uščа and Tisenkopfs (2023); Ujjwal *et al*. (2024)
Uniform foods are not suitable for everyone	Locally available foods are more suited to the climate and genetic makeup	Rotz and Fraser (2015); Borelli *et al*. (2020)
More chemical inputs	Reduced use of pesticides and fertilisers	Martinez *et al*. (2010); Thomson *et al*. (2012)
Same food during all seasons	Seasonal food availability is suitable for the body	Cruz-Garcia and Struik (2015); The Food Systems Dashboard (2023)
Homogenous foods for everyone	More diversity	Johns *et al*. (2013); Khoury *et al*. (2014)
High greenhouse gas emission causes global warming and environmental pollution	Low greenhouse gas emissions since transportation involves short distances	Li *et al*. (2022); Stein and Santini (2022)
More energy consumption	Energy efficient	Jones (2002); Usubiaga-Liaño *et al*. (2020)

productivity is a significant source of a country's income, savings, and investment (Noort *et al.*, 2022). However, primary agricultural productivity is insufficient to provide added value to the economy. The marketing supply chain with upstream processing of food and consumer distribution offers more value to economic development (Noort *et al.*, 2022). In high-income-generating countries, the major source of economic profits is branded food products. Therefore, food processing and supply chains are crucial in determining the development of a country (IFPRI, 2020). Supply systems act as a link between consumers and producers (Weber *et al.*, 2021). The supply system is related to food production, distribution, and usage activities. It encompasses production, preservation, transportation, marketing, processing, consumption, and waste disposal. It is strongly influenced by labour, capital, government policies, market structure, and legislation (van Berkum *et al.*, 2018). The spread of the COVID-19 pandemic collapsed the global food supply chains. The breakage of supply chains destroyed agricultural products from the field itself (Aday and Aday, 2020). The movement of food was hindered in various corners of the world. The supply chain disruption also resulted in rising food demand. For instance, the demand increased in European nations by about 52% for vegetables and 76% for bread (Barman *et al.*, 2021; GoCrisp, 2022). The restriction on moving outside hugely changed the food consumption pattern of consumers (Janssen *et al.*, 2021). Homely food was preferred because of difficult-to-access restaurants and markets (Stephens *et al.*, 2020). The fear of virus infection through the market and exposure to crowded areas also caused the consumers' aversion towards market-available food. Consumers' choices have changed to the home delivery system and food products with a long shelf life (Sgroi and Modica, 2022). The non-availability of labourers also severely affected the supply system (Stephens *et al.*, 2020).

The COVID-19 pandemic has highlighted the risks associated with the globalised food systems. This excessive reliance on food imports compromises food security's sustainability and resilience dimensions (HLPE, 2020). One of today's most pressing concerns is the disruption of supply chains, which jeopardises food security in food-importing regions (Altieri and Nicholls, 2020). The situation has been recently exposed due to recurrent lockdowns in almost all countries. The aquatic food supply chains in various countries such as Bangladesh, Egypt, India, Myanmar, and Nigeria were found to be highly disrupted during the pandemic (Belton *et al.*, 2021). It affected the production of aquatic foods, their supply, and the labour force. In Bangladesh, an analysis of the effects of the pandemic on small-scale fishermen found a decline in the demand for fish resulting from supply chain disruptions. The decline in demand led to reduced sales and a loss of income for the fishermen (Hoque *et al.*, 2021). A study shows that, during COVID-19, people adapted to the crisis and turned to local and regional systems for the supply and distribution of seafood due to the disruptions in the supply of aquatic foods (Bassett *et al.*, 2021). At the same time, COVID-19 exposed the disparities between global and local farmers in the use of technology for supply and distribution systems. Even though the technology is crucial for repurposing distribution networks, small-scale farmers did not have equal access to those technologies, severely limiting the supply of local aquatic seafood (Bassett *et al.*, 2021). This shows the risks of over-dependence on global trade networks. Therefore, it is suggested that domestic supply chains be strengthened to prevent and lessen the effects of upcoming significant disruptions. We require resilient food production systems that can withstand macroeconomic shocks and keep the population alive even if we encounter such shocks in the future (Bassett *et al.*, 2021).

During the pandemic, the middlemen raised their market prices to stay profitable and cover cost increases. Farmers decreased labour costs by reducing the number of employees and their wages to offset rising operational costs and decreased income (Hasan *et al.*, 2021). In the global food market, product prices are determined by fuel prices, climate change, government subsidies, and stockpiles (Amedeo and Eztevez, 2022). The hike in food prices is already an issue of concern for many people, especially in North Africa and Asia, as their purchasing power is very low (Barua, 2022). In low and middle-income countries, local food systems are prevalent and strengthening local food supply chains can solve the issue (Béné, 2020).

Various countries adopted measures to tackle supply chain disruptions (Veselovská, 2020). More robust and resilient food supply chains are essential to stabilise the economy and growth of the country (Singh *et al.*, 2021). As discussed above, local or regional food supply chains gained more attention from consumers, producers, policymakers, and governments during the pandemic. Since local food systems are more accessible and obvious to consumers and producers, they were promoted during the pandemic. In a local food system, food products can be purchased from farmers directly, on-field, at farmer's markets, local stores, and restaurants (Martinez *et al.*, 2010). However, some studies reported that, as an effect of continuous lockdown, the local markets were also closed, resulting in income loss in some regions. For instance, among Ho tribal communities of India, during the second wave, food procurement faced challenges in local markets due to lockdowns, transport restrictions, and reduced availability of certain seasonal vegetables. The reduced production of vegetables or household consumption also contributed to this situation (Ghosh-Jerath *et al.*, 2024). Simultaneously, online markets flourished during the period. However, local food supply chains remained resilient in several other corners of the world to mitigate the food security challenges during the pandemic. Through quantitative and qualitative surveys, a study reported that, in the urban areas of Italy, grassroots alternative food networks (AFN) or small-scale local supply chains and food production helped access and distribute food during the pandemic (Zollet *et al.*, 2021).

Effect of the COVID-19 pandemic on food security

Given the increasing prevalence of food insecurity on a global scale, sustainable development goals 1 and 2 are unlikely to be achieved by 2030, which envisage ending poverty and hunger by 2030, respectively, in all forms everywhere. It has been reported that nearly three billion people around the world lack access to wholesome, natural foods that are fresh and unprocessed (FAO *et al.*, 2021). Food insecurity directly impacts health and wellness (Smith and Wesselbaum, 2020). Food security encompasses four essential dimensions: availability, which refers to having an adequate supply of food; access, which involves economic, physical, and social means to obtain food; utilisation, which focuses on consuming nutritious and safe food according to dietary requirements; and stability, which ensures consistency across these dimensions over time (CELAC, 2024). Besides, the High-Level Panel of Experts on Food Security and Nutrition added 'agency' and 'sustainability' as additional pillars of food security (HLPE, 2020). Agency refers to the capability of the individual or community to decide on its food systems (policies), and sustainability refers to the system's long-term viability (Clapp *et al.*, 2022). Food security must be ensured for all individuals in urban and rural areas. COVID-19 has significantly affected food security in both rural and urban regions worldwide. For example, 88% of households reported food insecurity in Nairobi, Kenya, during the pandemic (Shupler *et al.*, 2021). Many Mexican households also faced food insecurity during COVID-19 (Monroy-Torres *et al.*, 2021). The Global Report on Food Crisis (GRFC) reported that, due to COVID-19, 55 countries around the globe, including Ethiopia, Yemen, Nigeria, South Sudan, Haiti, Zimbabwe, and Afghanistan, suffered severe hunger and malnutrition issues (FSIN, 2021). COVID-19-induced restrictions affected Liberia's food and nutritional security (Pewee and Mulbah, 2021). The COVID-19 outbreak coincided with a locust infestation that threatened food security in Central and East Africa, diminishing food resources and pushing 20.2 million people from eight nations (Iran, Saudi Arabia, Sudan, Yemen, South Sudan, Kenya, Ethiopia, and Somalia) into drastic food insecurity (FAO *et al.*, 2020; Ma *et al.*, 2021). In Lebanon, the lockdowns worsened the challenges faced by its population due to the existing economic crisis. There was a price increase in foods, a reduction in revenue, and people had no access to food (Hammad *et al.*, 2023). Conflict-ridden states such as Yemen, Syria, and Sudan were worse hit by the pandemic (Ma *et al.*, 2021). Therefore, it is clear that the pandemic caused acute problems for food security around the globe. A survey conducted in Nigeria revealed that personal savings and income experienced a decline in households (Akinleye *et al.*, 2023). Simultaneously, the importance of a robust local support system increased the number of households (Akinleye *et al.*, 2023). In Eastern European countries, especially Ukraine and Azerbaijan, the local markets named '*Babushka*' are predominant, which act as a survival strategy for them during emergencies (Sõukand *et al.*, 2020). A study regarding the food insecurity issues of Ukraine during the Russo-Ukraine war suggested that introducing more regionally adapted local food crops in the supply chain can prevent food insecurity issues in conflict areas (Ben Hassen and El Bilali, 2022). A study documented that when Ukraine's neoliberal agricultural system was shattered during the war, the Ukrainians cultivated their own food (as Victory Gardens) and promoted small-scale agriculture and short supply chains for survival (Mamonova, 2023).

Several studies reported that the local food system supply chains were very strong and efficiently functioning during the pandemic, which helped them achieve food security. For example, the re-emergence of local food systems in

Canada, Argentina, the United Kingdom, Italy, France, Spain, Norway, and Australia during COVID-19 was reported (Nemes *et al.*, 2021). The study discussed that the short supply chains with supermarkets, canteens, groceries, mobile stalls, roadside selling points, on-farm markets, farm-gate shops, and home delivery systems were more active during the pandemic. Another study reported that, during the pandemic, the challenges such as a rise in cost and demand, changes in the mode of sale and requirement of online literacy, the Canadian Antigonish Farmer's market showed a higher degree of adaptability (Weinkauf and Everitt, 2023). This shows the importance of local farmers. Similarly, a report from Peru suggested that, during the pandemic period, the focus on the local community's production system helped them to incline the availability and affordability of a wide diversity of food items such as indigenous potato cultivars, kiwicha, quinoa, and other tubers which were cultivated with the aid of traditional agro-ecological practices (Valdivia, 2020). In the Netherlands, local initiatives with producers such as food banks and community-based food organisations also helped to fight against the COVID-19 crisis (Dekkinga *et al.*, 2022). Consumers in Romania during the pandemic period preferred more local foods over other staple foods when shopping online (Petrescu-Mag *et al.*, 2020). During the COVID-19 period, consumers in Greece expressed greater satisfaction with locally produced and processed food in terms of quality and cost (Skalkos *et al.*, 2021). By interviewing 34 farmers from Austria, Meixner reported that the pandemic resulted in a rise in the importance of local or regional food production and short food value chains (Meixner *et al.*, 2022). Similar to other countries, due to lack of labour, breakage of transportation, and maintaining crop balance, the local food system and short supply chains were also prevalent in Finland and China (Fei *et al.*, 2020; Sözer *et al.*, 2021). The Ministry of Agriculture in Thailand introduced a programme entitled 'Eat Thai First' to promote the consumption of local Thai fruits, and the government encouraged domestic agriculture on a large scale during COVID-19 (Neo, 2020). During the crisis period, a strong local network for food production and distribution was developed between the farmers and communities of Japan. Local food systems in Japan with small-scale systems were more resilient during COVID-19 (Kondo and Lichten, 2020). A transition in the food behaviour of Russians was also observed (Zhuravleva *et al.*, 2022). The study noted an increased preference for local foods and local food markets. In South Korea, consumers preferred safe, healthy, fresh, and nutritious food after COVID-19 (Rha *et al.*, 2021). In the case of the Philippines, Myanmar, and Cambodia, as in other countries, traditional agricultural systems continued to operate with minimal restrictions during the limitations imposed by COVID-19 (Espino *et al.*, 2021). Various kinds of regional tubers, vegetables, cereals, and pulses diversified the diet of consumers during the pandemic period in these three countries (Espino *et al.*, 2021).

Local Foods as a Sustainable and Resilient Strategy

Besides biodiversity loss, climate change, accumulation of waste, and natural resource depletion are the major issues caused by anthropogenic activities (Mahmoud and Gan, 2018). Industrial activities are the major causes of pollution and natural resource exploitation. The food production system causes 26% of the world's GHG emissions (Ritchie *et al.*, 2022). Besides that, the agriculture industry is responsible for soil degradation, groundwater source exploitation, and loss of biodiversity (Kanianska, 2016). Global food production consumes huge amounts of freshwater and expels significant food as waste (UNESCO World Water Assessment Programme, 2012). These issues threaten planet Earth and pose significant challenges to achieving sustainable development goals. For the existence of a healthy planet and a human population, it is necessary to adopt novel, sustainable, and environmentally friendly strategies. The major environmental consequences of the global food production system arise from raw material accumulation, processing, packaging, distribution, and waste disposal (Andersson *et al.*, 1994). At each stage of the food chain, there is a significant environmental footprint, which adversely impacts the ecosystem. To minimise the environmental impact of food production, it is essential to reduce raw material loss and atmospheric emissions (Ritchie *et al.*, 2022; Shabir *et al.*, 2023). It is crucial to efficiently utilise energy, raw materials, and water during the initial production stage. However, in pursuing cleaner food production, we must ensure that taste, quality, cultural preferences, price, cost, and safety remain uncompromised (Ramos *et al.*, 2020).

Considering the fragility of the current mainstream food systems, finding alternative systems of sustainable food production strategies is necessary. To this end, there are pertinent questions, such as whether we need a complete turnaround in the food production systems to achieve this or is there any evidence of sustainable and resilient food systems capable of feeding communities with the least environmental impact during supply chain disruptions and global economic slowdowns? Answers to these questions involve strengthening and revamping local food systems because regionally available local food systems are geographically restricted and regionally important (Feenstra, 1997). The local food systems include locally produced, sourced, or procured items. It also includes local markets where small-scale farmers sell lesser-known food items grown on small plots of land or harvested directly from the wild (Feenstra, 1997; Anju and Kumar, 2022). The global food supply chains account for approximately 20% of total food system emissions. The transportation of vegetables and fruits globally accounts for 36% of food miles emissions, nearly double the greenhouse gases emitted during their production (Li *et al.*, 2022). This study suggested a transition towards plant-based local foods to minimise greenhouse gases, particularly in wealthier nations. A case study based on dessert apples reported that local food sourcing reduces energy consumption and transportation-related carbon dioxide emissions (Jones, 2002). In contrast to nationally and globally sourced products, the environmental impact of transportation can be reduced by using local supply chains (Jones, 2002). Due to the addition of fertilisers and pesticides to the soil, industrial agriculture causes the excessive emission of nitric oxide into the atmosphere through microbial activity (Thomson *et al.*, 2012). However, local food crops, having adapted to their native land, exhibit varying degrees of resilience, adaptability, and sometimes even a weedy nature, which indicates their reduced need for maintenance (Kumar *et al.*, 2021c). Local food crops possess the disease-resistance potential and pathogen resistance, enabling them to thrive and flourish with minimal agricultural inputs (Kumar *et al.*, 2021a). The requirement of minimal inputs benefits the local food plants for their own growth and also has a positive impact on the health and fertility of the soil. For consumers, consuming food with pesticide residues poses potential health risks. Certain pesticides have been linked to adverse effects on the nervous system, reproductive system, and overall well-being. Minimising the use of insecticides and fertilisers can reduce the toxicological effects associated with food production (Carvalho, 2017). Many local food crops are available in different seasons and can be freshly harvested (Shelef *et al.*, 2017). But mainstream foods are kept in storage for a long time, and hence, they are preserved. They demand more energy, preservatives, and refrigeration facilities, increasing their environmental impact (Garnett, 2011; Nayak and Waterson, 2019).

Local food systems have recently demonstrated reliability, resilience, and sustainability – particularly during blockades or import restrictions caused by the COVID-19 pandemic (Nemes *et al.*, 2021). Within this context, resilience emerges as a fundamental attribute of food systems. Resilience encompasses the capacity to adapt to change, withstand shocks, and recover swiftly from crises (Walker *et al.*, 2004; Biggs *et al.*, 2015; Tendall *et al.*, 2015). The food system's resilience can be improved by adopting cleaner production practices. Cleaner production practices are preventive and aim to minimise waste and maximise product output. It emphasises resource efficiency, energy optimisation, and reduction of environmental impact (Tschiggerl and Topic, 2019). Adopting cleaner production practices within food systems enhances environmental sustainability and fortifies their resilience by minimising risks, optimising resource use, and fostering adaptability. The cleaner production practices and resilient properties of the food system contribute to sustainable development and food security around the globe. The link between the major dimensions of cleaner production, resilient food systems, and food security with sustainable development is given in Fig. 3.1.

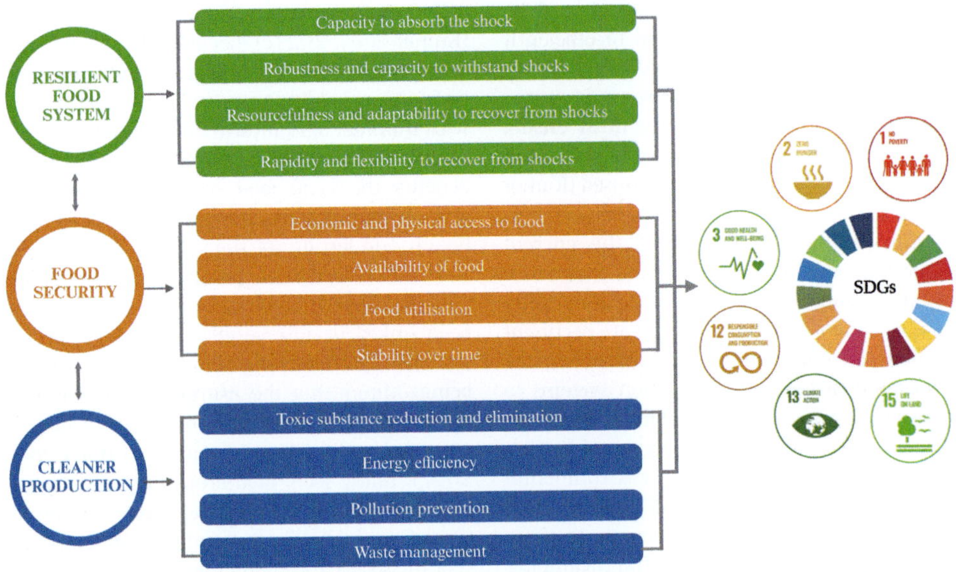

Fig. 3.1. The link between cleaner production, resilient food system, and dimensions of food security with sustainable development goals 1 (no poverty), 2 (zero hunger), 3 (good health and well-being), 12 (responsible consumption and production), 13 (climate action), and 15 (life on land) (Tendall *et al.*, 2015; United Nations, 2015; CELAC, 2024).

Another benefit of local food systems lies in their ability to provide consumers with diverse foods. Many local food plants are consumed in various parts of the world. While local food systems may not be widely known, each region upholds unique local food systems and dietary practices. Crop diversity encompasses more than the mere presence of a varied selection of fruits, vegetables, and grains for consumption – it is a fundamental component that enhances the robustness and adaptability of the food system. The diversity of available crops plays a crucial role in resilience against plant diseases and climate-related challenges like droughts, disease outbreaks, and pest invasions. Since various crops respond differently to stress and disturbances, all crops are less likely to fail simultaneously (Kotschy *et al.*, 2015). Therefore, diversified food systems are widely considered more resilient, and heterogeneity is important for resilience at species, molecular, and habitat levels (Biggs *et al.*, 2015; Kotschy *et al.*, 2015; Staudacher *et al.*, 2018). In contrast, uniform food crops are vulnerable to disease, pest outbreaks, and unexpected weather events since they respond uniformly to these disturbances (Massawe *et al.*, 2016). Historical events such as the Irish potato famine, which devastated Ireland, exemplify this (Powderly, 2019). Notably, locally available food tends to be more nutritious than food transported over long distances. They have freshness, aroma, minimal damage, and overall quality (Vargas *et al.*, 2021). It has been documented that the vitamin and nutrient content of food diminishes when stored for an extended period, even under refrigerated conditions (Spínola *et al.*, 2012; Li *et al.*, 2017). Therefore, locally available food products can ensure more nutritional security than stored commercial ones. Rising fuel prices, natural disasters, and transportation challenges associated with current food production can lead to heightened demand but diminished supply of mainstream foods, resulting in increased costs (FAO, 2021). On the other hand, local food supply chains are partially independent of these factors, and therefore, local foods remain affordable to rural and urban consumers. Shorter distances in the local food system may reduce the impact of fuel price fluctuations and transportation challenges, and they may recover faster from natural calamities than mainstream crops due to their proximity and regional adaptations. The local food systems also offer more opportunities and financial support for small-scale farmers who are pillars of the rural socioeconomic structure (Rahimi and Demirbaş, 2023). Overall, the local food supply chains are a good strategy to enhance the resilience of the food system. Considering the multiple benefits of local foods, efforts are needed to support local food systems, redefine local products in the markets, strengthen local short-supply chains, and promote their marketing. These efforts will help create long-term capacities to improve the local food systems for a sustainable future.

Does Evidence Suggest COVID-19 Triggered Transitions in Food Production and Consumption of Local Foods?

As a result of the COVID-19 spread, transitions in the purchase and consumption patterns of consumers were observed. When COVID-19-related restrictions were announced in various parts of the world, people resorted to home delivery of groceries and food items to avoid the risk of virus exposure (Fardkhales and Lincoln, 2021). The behavioural changes among consumers in various countries were observed during COVID-19. For instance, the desert country Jordan depended heavily on food imports to meet its dietary needs. However, during repeated lockdowns of COVID-19, imports from other countries stopped, prompting Jordan farmers to shift their focus towards less water-intensive crops well-suited to local conditions (Al-Saidi and Hussein, 2021). Likewise, there are additional instances where local food plants were encouraged during the pandemic, which are discussed in the following sections.

Home gardens and home food procurement

Home food procurement (HFP) involves various activities such as fishing, hunting, foraging, gardening, keeping livestock in the backyard, and canning (Niles *et al.*, 2021). HFPs, or homegrown foods, have been a significant part of sustainable human diets for improving food security (Kortright and Wakefield, 2011; Palar *et al.*, 2019; Abdoellah *et al.*, 2020; Nova *et al.*, 2020; Niles *et al.*, 2021). Several studies show that the increase in HFP activity following the onset of the pandemic offers a crucial safety net for those severely affected by COVID-19. Individuals who lost their jobs might face difficulty accessing affordable market foods. In such circumstances, the availability of HFP can provide them with temporary relief (Niles *et al.*, 2021). Home gardens are reported to impact household finances positively (Algert *et al.*, 2014; Gray *et al.*, 2014). These home gardens also impart a sense of community engagement, sharing of horticultural knowledge, and providing access to fresh produce (Gray *et al.*, 2014). During COVID-19, more households started practising home food procurement (D'Amelio, 2020; Rao, 2020; Niles *et al.*, 2021). These examples suggest that COVID-19 revitalised home and community gardens, leading to increased production of homegrown foods worldwide. When large-scale disruption of bean production was reported during the COVID-19 pandemic, villagers in peri-urban and urban areas of Eastern and Southern Africa survived by relying on home gardens (Nchanji and Lutomia, 2021). The production of locally available foods has also been historically important. For example, during World War II, the production of local foods was encouraged as a patriotic act to reduce the burden on the government (Howard, 2020). Emerging evidence suggests that changes in food consumption and production patterns and the revival or reinforcement of local food systems during challenging times like the COVID-19 pandemic enhance food security.

Innovations emerging out of COVID-19

Human beings fought against the COVID-19 pandemic with novel and rapidly developed efficient innovations by researchers, government authorities, policymakers, and communities (Bongini *et al.*, 2020; Ding and Li, 2021;

Tsai *et al.*, 2021). To maintain food security, the established link between food sources and institutions proved highly beneficial (Heck *et al.*, 2020). The development of small food hubs was also a milestone in innovations that emerged during COVID-19. During the pandemic, local farmers encountered difficulties selling their products directly to upscale restaurants. The closure of these restaurants due to COVID-19 resulted in financial setbacks for the farmers. However, food hubs, essential for distributing local foods, experienced heightened demand. Estimates suggest that food hubs delivered more local foods in 2020 than 2019 (Fardkhales and Lincoln, 2021). For instance, the colonisation of Hawaii led to a shift from local foods to industrial plantation crops, resulting in the decline of local food systems. However, during the COVID-19 pandemic, food hubs were crucial to Hawaii's food security. Their local food systems supported 400,000 to 800,000 people (Fardkhales and Lincoln, 2021). Several innovations emerged during the pandemic period in the food supply chain. For example, restaurants rapidly switched to a home delivery system during lockdowns. Software engineers and entrepreneurs developed regional mobile applications to deliver groceries and food items. For instance, restaurants swiftly transitioned to home delivery systems when faced with lockdowns. Software engineers and entrepreneurs also developed regional mobile applications to deliver groceries and food items (Zanetta *et al.*, 2021). These pandemic-driven innovations played a crucial role in supporting rural communities by safeguarding their economic and physical well-being.

Envisioning Post-Pandemic Transitions in Food Production and Consumption Patterns

Role of local food systems for sustainable food security, human health and well-being

A food system involves all the activities connected with the consumption of food, such as manpower, the environment, agricultural inputs, processing, distribution, and infrastructure (Béné, 2020). A food system dependent on natural resources and where consumption is associated with sociocultural aspects is considered a local food system. It is more reliable and robust than the globalised food system, and local resources are the foundation of the local food systems (Domingo *et al.*, 2021). The production of local foods is rooted in the culture, and consumers are more connected to the producers. It provides more opportunities for decision-making regarding food consumption both regionally and nationally (Donkers, 2014). The short food production and supply chain surveillance is less complex than the globalised food system. It allows proper monitoring of food security parameters regionally. Promoting the local food system allows the cultivation and consumption of plants suitable for the regional climate and soil conditions (Donkers, 2014). It is possible to produce food products proportional to the population in the region, which minimises the wastage of products (Donkers, 2014). Hence, local food systems have the potential to improve social, economic, and environmental outcomes significantly. It benefits local development, farmer welfare, and community well-being in general. It also leads to job creation and skill development (Mundler and Laughrea, 2016).

The homogenisation of the products in the markets can be prevented by promoting the local food system (Berti and Mulligan, 2016). Regionally adapted food crops are ideal for sustainable agricultural production since they efficiently utilise natural resources such as soil and water (Çakmakçı *et al.*, 2023). A comparative analysis of pasta production using traditional and industrial methods shows that the production of pasta through traditional methods has far less impact on the environment and is more sustainable (Recchia *et al.*, 2019). The results suggest that the local systems have less effect on natural resource consumption, soil degradation, and agrobiodiversity losses. The food system with local food plants can provide consumers with nutritional, environmental, sociocultural, and economic benefits (Akinola *et al.*, 2020). Consequently, local foods and supply chains can create a sustainable, robust, and nutritious food system.

Sustainable production-consumption-challenges to local food systems

Besides several benefits, various challenges are associated with local food systems. To promote the local food market, it is essential to consider dimensions such as safety, quality, healthiness, sustainability, and locality (Berti and Mulligan, 2016). The link between already established local markets, exclusive control over existing markets without interference from outside authorities, and the development of new markets are also necessary to popularise the local food systems (van der Ploeg *et al.*, 2012). It is also essential to maintain transparency in food production (Payne, 2022). Competition with the global food system is also a significant obstacle for the local food system (Willis, 2012). The conditions are not different in other countries. As a result, to meet food demand and ensure sustainability, local food should be produced on a large scale (Stein and Santini, 2022). Similarly, the number of local food sellers and outlets should be scaled up. The development of good infrastructure is required to increase the local agricultural output. The sustainability of the local food system depends on coordination and cooperation between local food suppliers and other actors (Anggraeni *et al.*, 2022). While scaling up production and distribution, its quality and quantity should not be compromised. Stability in distribution should be maintained for small-scale purchasers (household purchases) and large-scale purchasers (functions, restaurants) (UNIDO, 2020). A diversity of products should be provided for various needs according to the consumers' choices. Food affordability is also a main concern from the consumer's perspective (Ward *et al.*, 2013). However, locally-produced food products have the potential to meet these conditions since they are regionally adapted and suitable for that environment (Akinola *et al.*, 2020). The local food plants have minimum requirements for agricultural inputs such as manure and fertiliser, and consistent maintenance of crops is not mandatory. Besides that, the familiarity of the farmers with the local plants makes the production procedure easier. Other challenges are also associated with local food systems; for example, the local food markets of Uttarakhand, India (Northwestern Himalaya), still remain poorly developed (Bisht *et al.*, 2018). The local people occasionally use the barter system to trade their produce. The decisions are mainly based on their consumption and cultural preferences, and farmers are least aware of profit maximisation and market prices. Therefore, providing commercial potential and strategies for local foods among communities is essential (Bisht *et al.*, 2018). The important factor is that only the local communities are predominantly capable of developing community-based food hubs in rural regions that require modern thinking and innovation. Community-based grassroots innovations efficiently promote local foods regionally (Seyfang and Haxeltine, 2012).

The apathy of the younger generation towards local foods is another challenge (Pereira *et al.*, 2022). The younger generation is unwilling to cultivate and consume local foods and shows poor interest in farming. Global marketing campaigns and trends have drawn the attention of the new generation towards branded processed food products, leading to a decline in awareness about local food crops (Pereira *et al.*, 2022). The proper documentation of cultivation seasons, farming practices, processing, cooking, and consumption patterns of local food plants is crucial in the current scenario (Kuhnlein *et al.*, 2006). If not, the local food systems will remain unviable and unsustainable. Restaurant supplies of local food also face several challenges. Qualitative and quantitative data collected from 71 restaurants in the state of Ohio found that the chefs tried to promote local foods by conducting cooking classes and other activities (Inwood *et al.*, 2009). However, major barriers include the lack of network association between producers and restaurants, distribution issues, and difficulty convincing consumers (Inwood *et al.*, 2009). Therefore, global awareness programmes should be conducted to popularise the significance of local foods.

Sustainable development goals and the future of food production systems

The UN Agenda 2015 seeks to achieve 17 sustainable development goals (SDGs) by 2030 (United Nations, 2015). However, given the circumstances, it is difficult to achieve the goals by 2030 (Kumar *et al.*, 2021b). Attaining food security via a sustainable food system contributes to a more efficient fulfilment of the SDGs. Providing nutritious and sufficient food to the global population while simultaneously minimising environmental harm poses a substantial challenge in pursuing sustainable development goals (Herrero *et al.*, 2021), because the supply of sufficient nutritious food to the consumers alone will not meet the SDGs. Addressing climate change requires considering other factors, including social incorporation of people, ecosystem conservation, environmental protection, and climate change mitigation (UN, 2015). The 17 SDGs are interlinked and connected with food system sustainability (Herrero *et al.*, 2021). Even though the second goal, i.e. ending global malnutrition and hidden hunger by 2030, is more related to food systems, other goals are also interconnected with agriculture and the food system.

The prevention of agricultural losses and the recycling of agri-waste are the primary concerns of the sustainable food system, but the present food supply chains are inefficient in dealing with global food loss and wastage (Bombelli *et al.*, 2019). Alterations in consumption patterns, improved food diversity, waste management, sufficient food access, and preservation of culturally significant local foods are essential to food security. (Bombelli *et al.*, 2019). Similarly, the producers and farmers willing to do sustainable food production require more support for entrepreneurship, novel market access, advanced extension services, and professional technical support (Kahan, 2012). The current industrial food production system causes water source depletion, aquatic pollution, loss of agrobiodiversity, soil depletion, and deforestation, which can be considered unsustainable (IPES-Food, 2016). For every nation, the central challenge lies in attaining food security within the existing global food systems, which are currently unsustainable. However, changes in consumption patterns, food production, and supply systems can lead to a transition from an unsustainable food system to a sustainable, nutritious diet (Rocha and Spagnuolo, 2019). For instance, the increased popularity of wheat bread over traditional cassava, pulses, and sorghum varieties in sub-Saharan Africa resulted in major nutritional and food insecurity issues (Noort *et al.*, 2022). These facts demonstrate the value of a diverse diet and local food system in ensuring food security for consumers. Therefore, strengthening the local food system can contribute significantly to achieving sustainable food security.

Innovative systems for the production of local foods

An effective, innovative system for local foods requires the participation of policymakers, government employees, producers, organisations, and individuals who are ultimately focused on developing new items, concepts, procedures, and formats for promoting economic development and social change (Pound and Conroy, 2017). The implementation of innovative agricultural systems has the potential to support transformative changes in our food systems (Klerkx and Begemann, 2020). The present conditions of global food system insecurity demand a transformation to a more environmentally friendly, economical, regenerative, circular, and democratic food system that ensures sustainability (FAO, 2018). Government, non-governmental organisations, research institutions, and civil society must participate equally in a successful transformation (Herens *et al.*, 2022). The major focus of future food system innovations includes advanced farming systems such as precision agriculture, bio-saline agriculture, hydroponics, terrace gardening, and home kitchens (Hemathilake and Gunathilake, 2022). The innovations in agriculture are linked to the blending of information technology, biotechnology, satellite technology, and artificial intelligence (Ayed *et al.*, 2022). Achieving efficient food transformations should be aimed at economic development, clean earth conditions, biodiversity protection, social welfare, and animal well-being (Çakmakçı *et al.*, 2023).

Regarding the regional food supply system, chefs play a considerable role in promoting local

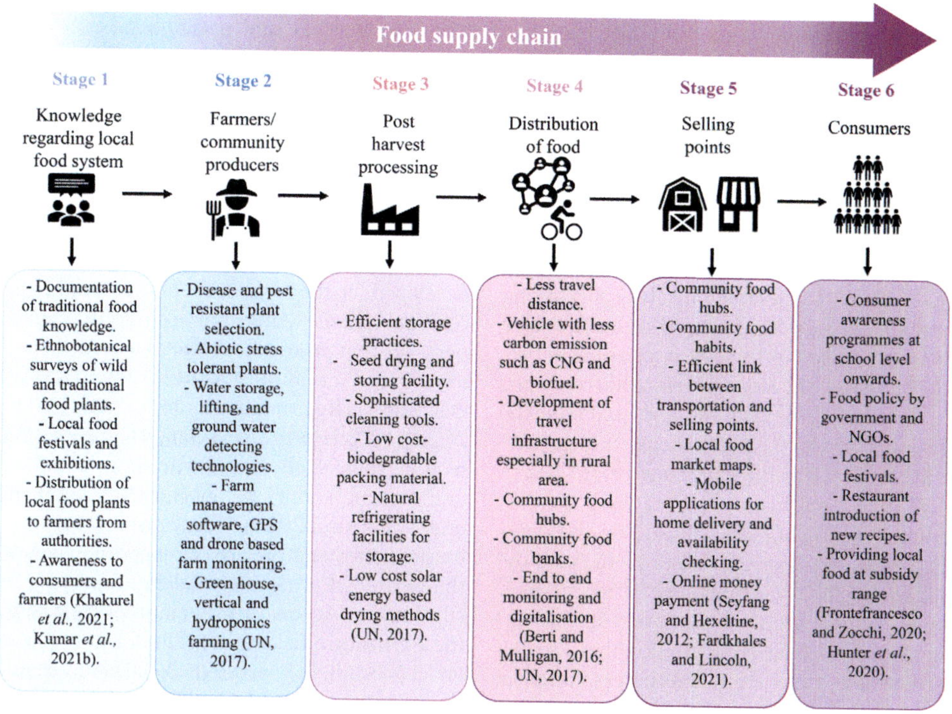

Fig. 3.2. The technological innovations necessary for promoting local food systems and supply chain sustainability (Seyfang and Haxeltine, 2012; Berti and Mulligan, 2016; United Nations, 2017; Fontefrancesco and Zocchi, 2020; Hunter *et al.*, 2020; Fardkhales and Lincoln, 2021; Khakurel *et al.*, 2021; Kumar *et al.*, 2021b).

foods in restaurants (Inwood *et al.*, 2009). The introduction of new local food recipes and the attractive presentation of the food to consumers can increase the popularity of food at the restaurant level. The large-scale production of local foods also needs government and institute-funded innovative programmes. For example, in England, the Royal Society of Wildlife Trusts launched the Big Lottery's 'Changing Spaces' programme to provide funding for various food-related projects to increase the availability, affordability, and accessibility of local food to nearby communities (Kirwan *et al.*, 2013). Such innovative programmes are also required to promote local food systems on a large scale (Kirwan *et al.*, 2013). Innovations facilitating the delivery system from producers to consumers are also necessary (Fardkhales and Lincoln, 2021). Telecommunication and social media campaigns can also be explored for the large-scale commercialisation of local foods. The necessary agricultural innovations to strengthen the local food systems and supply chains are described in Fig. 3.2.

Financing and use of enabling technologies for the revival of local food systems

The popularisation/adoption of local food systems demands market and transport facilities, legal frameworks, and financial support for the producers (Poulton *et al.*, 2010). Federal, state, and local government policies must improve and popularise the local food system (Martinez *et al.*, 2010). In the US, the government developed several programmes to support the local food system financially to empower the producers and consumers, such as the National Farmer's

Market Promotion Programme, Crop Block Grant Programme, Community Food Project Grant Programme, and Federal State Marketing Improvement Programme (Martinez *et al.*, 2010). In the post-pandemic period, it is essential to implement such programs that promote and support the local food systems. Community farming can also offer financial support to the local food production system. The concept originated in Switzerland and Japan during the 1960s, and it traditionally involves purchasing shares of the expected harvest on the farm by a group of people. In the system, consumers take risks by paying the amount before harvest (they are unaware of the quantity and quality of the harvested product), which helps the sustainability of local farming (Anggraeni *et al.*, 2022). Local-level coordination is required for this system (Anggraeni *et al.*, 2022). The producers themselves can develop companies to retail the products regionally. Around 263 producer companies in India are growing rapidly and profiting from local food products (Trebbin, 2014). Furthermore, rural areas can increase internal funding schemes to ensure the long-term viability of their local food systems (Kneafsey *et al.*, 2013). For instance, in European countries, schemes such as Voedselteams, Community Farm Chew Magna, Aarstiderne, and Einkaufen Auf dem Bauernhof are important (Kneafsey *et al.*, 2013). Under these schemes, consumers pay a fee at an interval of a week, a month, or annual (during harvest) to maintain the running of the local food stores. External funding, such as rural development funds and other sources, can support reviving the local food system (Kneafsey *et al.*, 2013).

Local, national, and international supporters can introduce various technologies to strengthen and revive traditional food knowledge and local food systems (Guell *et al.*, 2022). Advancements in technology should be made for economic profit, efficiency, and sustainability of the country's development (Trolio *et al.*, 2016). Technological inventions should be applied to various biotechnological improvements of plants, harvest and post-harvest processing, market infrastructure, and supply chains (Trolio *et al.*, 2016). Long-term preservation techniques such as canning can protect the food during supply, while other advanced technologies can increase local food plants' yield and agricultural efficiency (Adeyeye, 2017). The production efficiency of the plants can be improved by using resilient smart plants, sophisticated planting tools, and small-scale production units with high efficiencies, such as hydroponics, vertical farming, and greenhouses (Avgoustaki and Xydis, 2020). The latest technology, bounded seed dispersal units and propagule planting units should be developed for the large-scale production of the regional plants. After harvesting, the freshness of the products should be maintained for a long time to meet marketing and selling demands (Ngairangbam and Athokpam, 2023). Therefore, post-harvest processing technologies such as dehydrating, canning, and freezing should be applied (Ngairangbam and Athokpam, 2023). The transportation and market infrastructure are the expensive sides of the local food production system, especially in rural areas. Access to water and electricity in the agriculture field at subsidised rates for the farmers can help improve the local food system. These initiatives and financial support can help strengthen and empower the local food systems. All governments, NGOs, policymakers, institutions, and communities should take similar actions to promote the local food systems. A detailed flowchart of measures to popularise the local food systems is given in Fig. 3.3.

Food security within the context of sustainability and resilience

Achieving sustainable food security is a major concern in developed and developing countries. A major barrier to ensuring food security is the inability of the food production and supply systems to recover from various shocks or issues (Panghal *et al.*, 2022). The ability of the food system to continue operating in the face of shocks and disturbances is referred to as resilience (Hoddinott, 2023). The sustainability of food security is crucial for the survival of the human population in times of crisis. The globalised food system was disrupted during the pandemic, and food security was challenged. During the pandemic, all food security

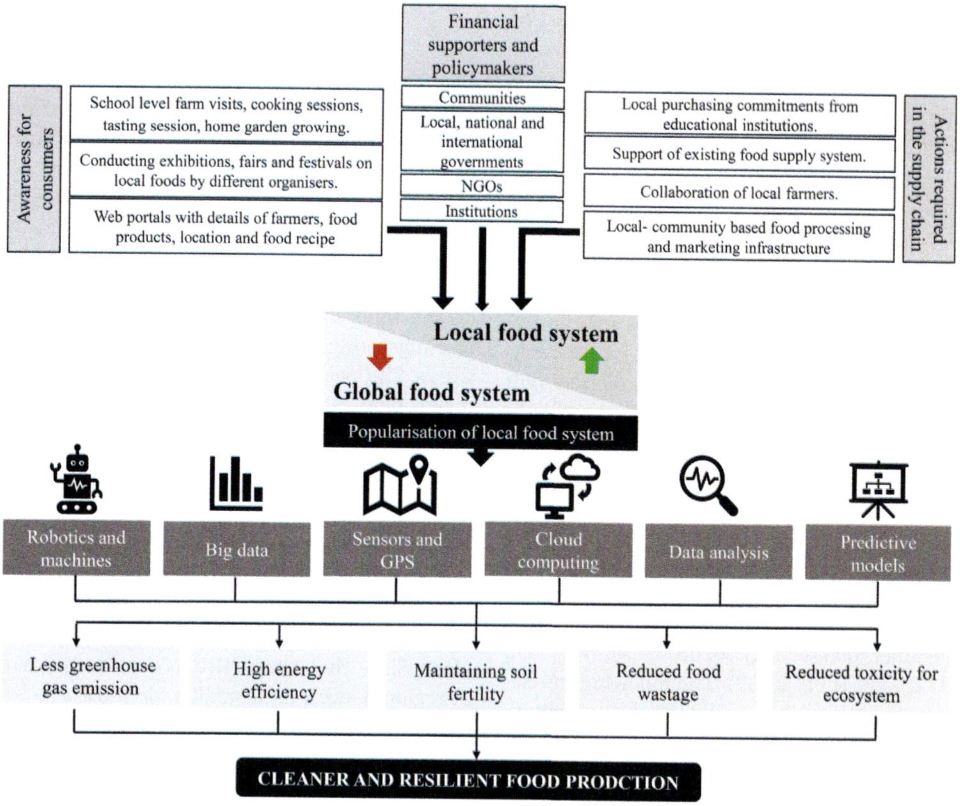

Fig. 3.3. Flowchart of measures required to revive and sustain local food systems (United Nations, 2017; Fontefrancesco and Zocchi, 2020; Ayed *et al.*, 2022; Charatsari *et al.*, 2022; Stein and Santini, 2022).

dimensions – i.e., accessibility, availability, utilisation, and sustainability were compromised. However, reliance on the local food system can help to solve food security issues and ensure sustainability, as previously discussed (Stein and Santini, 2022). Local and regional food systems demonstrated resilience during the pandemic (Ušča and Tisenkopfs, 2023).

Nutrient deficiency, or hidden hunger, represents a significant challenge to achieving global food security. Providing macro and micronutrients during emergencies is crucial for the health and well-being of humans (Bakalis *et al.*, 2020). For instance, during the COVID-19 pandemic, consumers were more likely to experience vitamin D deficiency due to increased indoor confinement. It is essential to provide consumers with affordable and readily accessible foods rich in vitamin D (Bakalis *et al.*, 2020). Therefore, shorter supply chains are considered more resilient in such crisis situations. Innovations can strengthen local food systems in the future to build more resilience (Charatsari *et al.*, 2022). Additionally, food available in local markets tends to be more nutritious than long-distance food. Long-distance foods often lose nutrients over time during transportation (Caixeta-Filho, 1999), and they may also contain toxic preservatives and additives, which can deprive consumers of the freshness found in locally sourced foods (Ng and von Goetz, 2017). Therefore, compared to conventional crops, local foods offer greater nutritional security. Regional foods can better ensure consumer food security, particularly in times of crisis.

Inclusion of local food system as a part of building back better strategy

The post-pandemic world demands complex needs for the survival of the population. COVID-19 has taught mankind several lessons, including the value of food and supply chains. However, recovery strategies need long-term effects, environmental friendliness, and sustainability (Sarkis, 2020). The term 'Build back better strategy' indicates the necessity of improving the quality of the action plan for recovery. The world needs a more resilient food system to deal with pandemics, population growth, and climate change (Bellamy *et al.*, 2021). The resilience of the food system is ultimately influenced by the capacity to anticipate, respond to, and recover from disruptive events (Hecht *et al.*, 2019). During the COVID-19 pandemic, there were several examples globally where the local food system was a resilient strategy for ensuring consumer food security (Béné, 2020; Fan *et al.*, 2021; Kent *et al.*, 2022). The following 10 elements were identified as potential contributors to organisational resilience: formal emergency preparatory work, staff education, pre-event attendance, redundancy of the food supply, food suppliers, location, infrastructure, service providers, insurance, and learning from the experience (Hecht *et al.*, 2019). It is possible to create a resilient food system for long-term food security by incorporating these elements into the local food system. Furthermore, nutritional education for the general public, the establishment of school and college gardens with local plants, institutional initiatives and programs, school-oriented snack distribution made from local food plants, and the introduction of local food recipes in restaurants can all contribute to the rapid incorporation of local food plants into the food system (Hunter *et al.*, 2020). Reviving local food knowledge is also essential for promoting the local food systems (Egeland *et al.*, 2009). The success story of the Pink Asparagus Festival in Mezzago, Italy, reveals the importance of food festivals in refreshing and maintaining knowledge regarding local foods (Fontefrancesco and Zocchi, 2020). By adopting these strategies, it is possible to foster a food system that sustains the physical well-being of consumers and enhances the capacity to withstand future challenges.

Conclusions

The paper discusses the relevance of the local food systems and local food supply chains during the COVID-19 pandemic and provides future perspectives on their future roles. The loss of income, decline of purchasing power, and fear of the spread of viral infection forced consumers to depend on locally available foods based on plants. The local supply chains were also strengthened during the COVID-19 pandemic with the help of e-marketing innovations and connected networks. The local food systems serve as a resilient means of survival for the population in several countries, and they have less environmental impact than the globally interconnected food supply chains. Fig. 3.4 summarises the roles of local food systems in realising food security and sustainable development goals. Many scientists are working to design crops that are more resistant to stresses and can perform well under unfavourable conditions. Globally, scientists also believe that alternative food plants grown at regional levels on a small scale must also be exploited to ensure food security. In the post-COVID-19 world, perspective has shifted away from globalised, interconnected food supply chains. Instead, there is now greater emphasis on regional supply chains and direct connections between producers and local consumers (Elghannam *et al.*, 2019).

Considering the environmental impact of the present food production systems involving long supply chains and the use of fossil fuels, in the future, we must look into other aspects of food production systems, such as shorter food supply chains. Environmental, social, and economic issues also must be integrated into food systems. Resilience and sustainability must be at the heart of food production-consumption supply systems. Local food systems must be robust and reliable, and food security must be ensured even in emergencies. Policymakers, institutes, governments, and communities must support local and regional food system innovations to popularise regionally adapted food plants. Therefore, regional planning in food production systems is very important to ensure people's food security in times of crisis. There should be provision for the local production of foods, which may act as a means to protect people in emergencies like COVID-19.

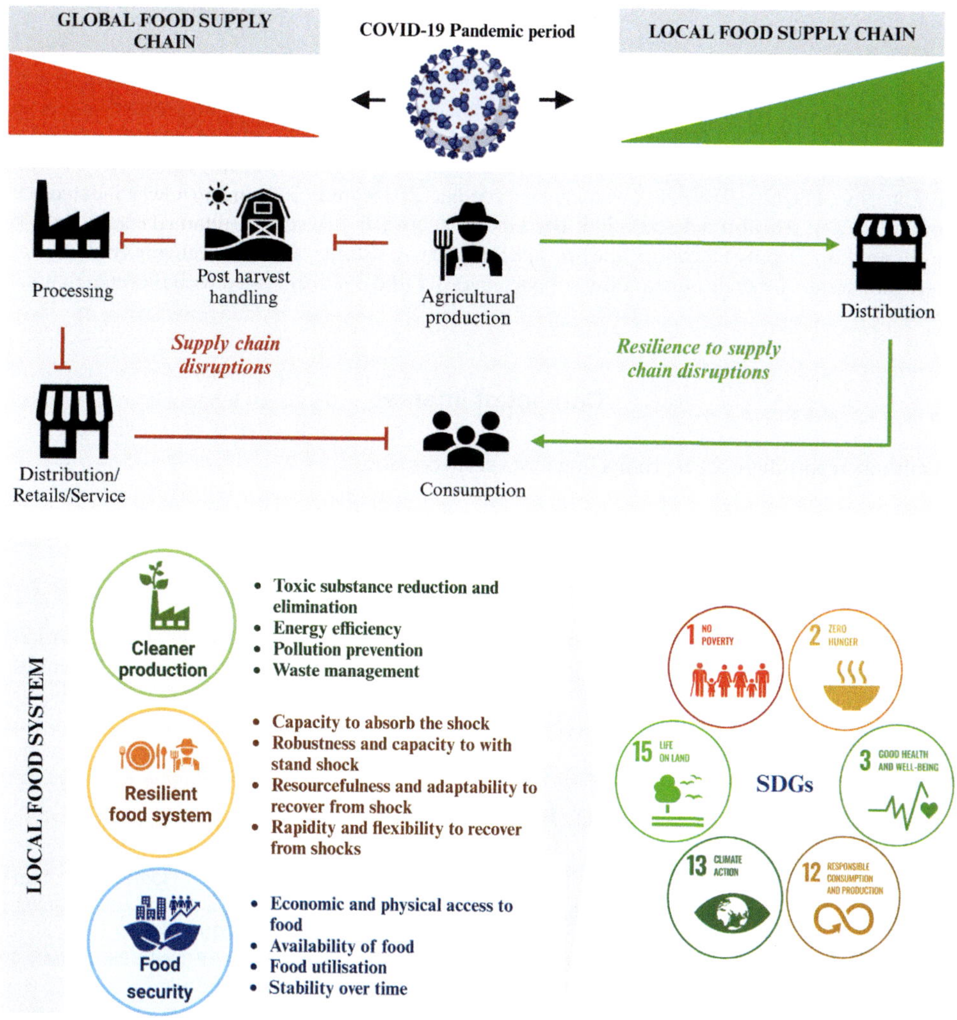

Fig. 3.4. Summary of the role of local food systems in realising food security and sustainable development goals.

Abbreviations

ALF	Agricultural labour force
COVID-19	Coronavirus disease 2019
FAO	Food and Agricultural Organization
GHG	Greenhouse gas
HFP	Home food procurement
SDGs	Sustainable development goals

Acknowledgements

This research received no specific grant from funding agencies in the public, commercial, or not-for-profit sectors. However, the research in AK lab is supported by the Indian Council of Social Science Research (ICSSR; vide File No. 02/124/2022–23/ST/TS/ RP dated 1 September 2023) and Department of Science and Technology-Science and Engineering Research Board (DST-SERB; vide File Nos. EEQ/2019/000441 dated 2 December 2019 and EEQ/2023/000995 dated 19 February 2024). AK also acknowledges the Library team (Dr J. Vivekavardhan, Librarian, Dr P. Senthilkumaran, Deputy Librarian, and Sreeja KP, Library Assistant) of Central University of Kerala, Kasaragod, Kerala, for their outstanding support. Figs 3.1 and 3.4 are created with Biorender.com.

Conflict of Interest

The authors report there are no competing interests to declare.

Author Contributions

AT: investigation, writing – original draft, data curation, visualisation; AK: conceptualization, investigation, validation, writing – original draft, review and editing, visualisation, resources, supervision.

References

Abdoellah, O.S., Schneider, M., Nugraha, L.M., Suparman, Y., Voletta, C.T. *et al.* (2020) Homegarden commercialization: Extent, household characteristics, and effect on food security and food sovereignty in rural Indonesia. *Sustainability Science* 15, 797–815. DOI: 10.1007/s11625-020-00788-9.

Aday, S. and Aday, M.S. (2020) Impact of COVID-19 on the food supply chain. *Food Quality and Safety* 4, 167–180. DOI: 10.1093/fqsafe/fyaa024.

Adeyeye, S.A.O. (2017) The role of food processing and appropriate storage technologies in ensuring food security and food availability in Africa. *Nutrition and Food Science* 47, 122–139. DOI: 10.1108/NFS-03-2016-0037.

Akinleye, S.O., Dauda, R.O.S., Iwegbu, O. and Popogbe, O.O. (2023) Impact of COVID-19 pandemic on financial health and food security in Negeria: A survey-based analysis. *Journal of Public Affairs* 23, e2859. DOI: 10.1002/pa.2859.

Akinola, R., Pereira, L.M., Mabhaudhi, T., Bruin, F.M. and Rusch, L. (2020) A review of indigenous food crops in Africa and the implications for more sustainable and healthy food systems. *Sustainability* 12, 3493. DOI: 10.3390/su12083493.

Algert, S.J., Baameur, A. and Renvall, M.J. (2014) Vegetable output and cost savings of community gardens in San Jose, California. *Journal of the Academy of Nutrition and Dietetics* 114, 1072–1076. DOI: 10.1016/j.jand.2014.02.030.

Al-Saidi, M. and Hussein, H. (2021) The water-energy-food nexus and COVID-19: Towards a systematization of impacts and responses. *Science of The Total Environment* 779, 146529. DOI: 10.1016/j.scitotenv.2021.146529.

Altieri, M.A. and Nicholls, C.I. (2020) Agroecology and the reconstruction of a post-COVID-19 agriculture. *The Journal of Peasant Studies* 47, 881–898. DOI: 10.1080/03066150.2020.1782891.

Amedeo, K. and Eztevez, E. (2022) 5 causes of high food prices. Available at: https://www.thebalance.com/why-are-food-prices-rising-causes-of-food-price-inflation-3306099 (accessed 30 August 2022).

Andersson, K., Ohlsson, T. and Olsson, P. (1994) Life cycle assessment (LCA) of food products and production systems. *Trends in Food Science and Technology* 5, 134–138. DOI: 10.1016/0924-2244(94)90118-X.
Anggraeni, E.W., Handayati, Y. and Novani, S. (2022) Improving local food systems through the coordination of agriculture supply chain actors. *Sustainability* 14, 3281. DOI: 10.3390/su14063281.
Anju, T. and Kumar, A. (2022) Traditional food plants in the face of global change: Past, present, and future. *Annual Plant Reviews Online* 5, 383–454. DOI: 10.1002/9781119312994.apr0796.
Atallah, S.S., Gómez, M.I. and Björkman, T. (2014) Localization effects for a fresh vegetable product supply chain: Broccoli in the eastern United States. *Food Policy* 49, 151–159. DOI: 10.1016/j.foodpol.2014.07.005.
Avgoustaki, D.D. and Xydis, G. (2020) How energy innovation in indoor vertical farming can improve food security, sustainability, and food safety? In: Cohen, M.J. (ed.) *Advances in Food Security and Sustainability*. Elsevier Inc, Amsterdam, Netherlands, pp. 1–51.
Ayed, R.B., Hanana, M., Ercisli, S., Karunakaran, R., Rebai, A. *et al.* (2022) Integration of innovative technologies in the agri-food sector: The fundamentals and practical case of DNA-based traceability of olives from fruit to oil. *Plants* 11, 1230. DOI: 10.3390/plants11091230.
Bakalis, S., Valdramidis, V.P., Argyropoulos, D., Ahrne, L., Chen, J. *et al.* (2020) Perspectives from CO+RE: How COVID-19 changed our food systems and food security paradigms. *Current Research in Food Science* 3, 166–172. DOI: 10.1016/j.crfs.2020.05.003.
Barman, A., Das, R. and De, P.K. (2021) Impact of COVID-19 in food supply chain: Disruptions and recovery strategy. *Current Research in Behavioral Sciences* 2, 100017. DOI: 10.1016/j.crbeha.2021.100017.
Barua, A. (2022) Sizzling Food Prices are Leading to Global Heartburn. Available at: https://www2.deloitte.com/xe/en/insights/economy/global-food-prices-inflation.html (accessed 30 August 2022).
Bassett, H.R., Lau, J., Giordano, C., Suri, S.K., Advani, S. *et al.* (2021) Preliminary lessons from COVID-19 disruptions of small-scale fishery supply chains. *World Development* 143, 105473. DOI: 10.1016/j.worlddev.2021.105473.
Belik, W. (2020) Sustainability and food security after COVID-19: Relocalizing food systems? *Agricultural and Food Economics* 8, 23. DOI: 10.1186/s40100-020-00167-z.
Bellamy, A.S., Furness, E., Nicol, P., Pitt, H. and Taherzadeh, A. (2021) Shaping more resilient and just food systems: Lessons from the COVID-19 pandemic. *Ambio* 50, 782–793. DOI: 10.1007/s13280-021-01532-y.
Belton, B., Rosen, L., Middleton, L., Ghazali, S., Mamun, A.-A. *et al.* (2021) COVID-19 impacts and adaptations in Asia and Africa's aquatic food value chains. *Marine Policy* 129, 104523. DOI: 10.1016/j.marpol.2021.104523.
Ben Hassen, T. and El Bilali, H. (2022) Impacts of the Russia-Ukraine war on global food security: Towards more sustainable and resilient food systems? *Foods* 11, 2301. DOI: 10.3390/foods11152301.
Béné, C. (2020) Resilience of local food systems and links to food security – A review of some important concepts in the context of COVID-19 and other shocks. *Food Security* 12, 805–822. DOI: 10.1007/s12571-020-01076-1.
Béné, C., Barange, M., Subasinghe, R., Pinstrup-Andersen, P., Merino, G. *et al.* (2015) Feeding 9 billion by 2050 – putting fish back on the menu. *Food Security* 7, 261–274. DOI: 10.1007/s12571-015-0427-z.
Berti, G. and Mulligan, C. (2016) Competitiveness of small farms and innovative food supply chains: The role of food hubs in creating sustainable regional and local food systems. *Sustainability* 8, 616. DOI: 10.3390/su8070616.
Biggs, R., Schlüter, M. and Schoon, M.L. (eds) (2015) *Principles for Building Resilience: Sustaining Ecosystem Services in Social-Ecological Systems*, 1st edn. Cambridge University Press, Cambridge, UK.
Bisht, I.S., Mehta, P.S., Negi, K.S., Verma, S.K., Tyagi, R.K. *et al.* (2018) Farmers' rights, local food systems, and sustainable household dietary diversification: A case of Uttarakhand Himalaya in North-Western India. *Agroecology and Sustainable Food Systems* 42, 77–113. DOI: 10.1080/21683565.2017.1363118.
Bombelli, A., Paola, A., Chiriacò, M.V., Perugini, L., Castaldi, S. *et al.* (2019) Climate change, sustainable agriculture and food systems: The world after the Paris agreement. In: Valentini, R., Sievenpiper, J.L., Antonelli, M. and Dembska, K. (eds) *Achieving the Sustainable Development Goals Through Sustainable Food Systems*. Springer International Publishing, Cham, pp. 25–34.
Bongini, P., Trezza, A., Bianchini, M., Spiga, O. and Niccolai, N. (2020) A possible strategy to fight COVID-19: Interfering with spike glycoprotein trimerization. *Biochemical and Biophysical Research Communications* 528, 35–38. DOI: 10.1016/j.bbrc.2020.04.007.

Borelli, T., Hunter, D., Padulosi, S., Amaya, N., Meldrum, G. *et al.* (2020) Local solutions for sustainable food systems: The contribution of orphan crops and wild edible species. *Agronomy* 10, 231. DOI: 10.3390/agronomy10020231.

Breiling, M. and Anbumozhi, V. (2020) *Vulnerability of Agricultural Production Networks and Global Food Value Chains Due to Natural Disasters*. Economic Research Institute for ASEAN and East Asia, Jakarta, Indonesia.

Caixeta-Filho, J.V. (1999) Losses in the transportation of fruits and vegetables: A Brazilian case study. *International Journal of Logistics: Research and Applications* 2, 325–341.

Çakmakçı, R., Salık, M.A. and Çakmakçı, S. (2023) Assessment and principles of environmentally sustainable food and agriculture systems. *Agriculture* 13, 1073. DOI: 10.3390/agriculture13051073.

Cappelli, A. and Cini, E. (2020) Will the COVID-19 pandemic make us reconsider the relevance of short food supply chains and local productions? *Trends in Food Science and Technology* 99, 566–567. DOI: 10.1016/j.tifs.2020.03.041.

Carvalho, F.P. (2017) Pesticides, environment, and food safety. *Food and Energy Security* 6, 48–60. DOI: 10.1002/fes3.108.

CELAC (2024) *CELAC Plan for Food Security, Nutrition and the Eradication of Hunger 2030*. FAO, Santiago.

Charatsari, C., Lioutas, E.D., Rosa, M. and Vecchio, Y. (2022) Technological innovation and agrifood systems resilience: The potential and perils of three different strategies. *Frontiers in Sustainable Food Systems* 6, 872706. DOI: 10.3389/fsufs.2022.872706.

Clapp, J., Moseley, W.G., Burlingame, B. and Termine, P. (2022) Viewpoint: The case for a six-dimensional food security framework. *Food Policy* 106, 102164. DOI: 10.1016/j.foodpol.2021.102164.

Cruz-Garcia, G.S. and Struik, P.C. (2015) Spatial and seasonal diversity of wild food plants in home gardens of Northeast Thailand. *Economic Botany* 69, 99–113. DOI: 10.1007/s12231-015-9309-8.

D'Amelio, J. (2020) "Victory Gardens" for the war against COVID-19. *CBC News*.

Dekkinga, P., Horst, H. and Andriessen, T. (2022) "Too big to fail": The resilience and entrenchment of food aid through food banks in the Netherlands during the COVID-19 pandemic. *Food Security* 14, 781–789. DOI: 10.1007/s12571-022-01260-5.

Devereux, S., Béné, C. and Hoddinott, J. (2020) Conceptualising COVID-19's impacts on household food security. *Food Security* 12, 769–772. DOI: 10.1007/s12571-020-01085-0.

Ding, A.W. and Li, S. (2021) National response strategies and marketing innovations during the COVID-19 pandemic. *Business Horizons* 64, 295–306. DOI: 10.1016/j.bushor.2020.12.005.

Domingo, A., Charles, K.-A., Jacobs, M., Brooker, D. and Hanning, R.M. (2021) Indigenous community perspectives of food security, sustainable food systems and strategies to enhance access to local and traditional healthy food for partnering williams treaties first nations (Ontario, Canada). *International Journal of Environmental Research and Public Health* 18, 4404. DOI: 10.3390/ijerph18094404.

Donkers, H. (2014) Sustainable food security, a paradigm for local and regional food systems. *International Journal of Humanities and Social Science* 4, 89–102.

Dulloo, M.E., Hunter, D. and Leaman, D. (2014) Plant diversity in addressing food, nutrition and medicinal needs. In: Gurib-Fakim, A. (ed.) *Novel Plant Bioresources: Applications in Food, Medicine and Cosmetics*. John Wiley and Sons, Ltd, Hoboken, NJ, pp. 1–21.

Eaton, S.B., Cordain, L. and Lindeberg, S. (2002) Evolutionary health promotion: A consideration of common counterarguments. *Preventive Medicine* 34, 119–123. DOI: 10.1006/pmed.2001.0966.

Egeland, G.M., Charbonneau-Roberts, G., Kuluguqtuq, J., Kilabuk, J., Okalik, L. *et al.* (2009) Back to the future: Using traditional food and knowledge to promote a healthy future among inuit. In: FAO, Alliance of Bioversity International and CIAT, f (ed.) *Indigenous Peoples' Food Systems: The Many Dimensions of Culture, Diversity and Environment for Nutrition and Health*. FAO, Rome, pp. 9–22.

Elghannam, A., Mesias, F.J., Escribano, M., Fouad, L., Horrillo, A. *et al.* (2019) Consumers' perspectives on alternative short food supply chains based on social media: A focus group study in Spain. *Foods* 9, 22. DOI: 10.3390/foods9010022.

Enthoven, L. and van den Broeck, G. (2021) Local food systems: Reviewing two decades of research. *Agricultural Systems* 193, 103226. DOI: 10.1016/j.agsy.2021.103226.

Erenstein, O., Jaleta, M., Sonder, K., Mottaleb, K. and Prasanna, B.M. (2022) Global maize production, consumption and trade: Trends and R&D implications. *Food Security* 14, 1295–1319. DOI: 10.1007/s12571-022-01288-7.

Esfahani, B., Asadaraghi, A. and Moghaddam, S.K. (2022) Analyzing the effects of COVID-19 on food supply chains: A case study on ranking the obstacles with ANP methodology. *IFAC-PapersOnLine* 55, 1876–1881. DOI: 10.1016/j.ifacol.2022.09.672.

Espino, E., Itliong, I., Ruba, C.D., Thy, O., Barbon, W.J. *et al.* (2021) COVID-19 impact on local agri-food systems in Cambodia, Myanmar, and The Philippines. *CCAFS Working Paper No.357*. CGIAR Research Program on Climate Change, Agriculture and Food Security, Wageningen, the Netherlands.

Fan, S., Teng, P., Chew, P., Smith, G. and Copeland, L. (2021) Food system resilience and COVID-19 – Lessons from the Asian experience. *Global Food Security* 28, 100501. DOI: 10.1016/j.gfs.2021.100501.

FAO (2018) *Sustainable Food Systems Concept and Framework*. FAO, Rome.

FAO (2021) *The Impact of Disasters and Crises on Agriculture and Food Security: 2021*. FAO, Rome.

FAO and WFP (2020) *FAO-WFP Early Warning Analysis of Acute Food Insecurity Hotspots. July 2020. Rome*. FAO and WFP, Rome.

FAO, UNICEF, IFAD, WFP, and WHO (2020) *The State of Food Security and Nutrition in the World 2020: Transforming food systems for affordable healthy diets*. FAO, Rome.

FAO, IFAD, UNICEF, WFP, and WHO (2021) *The State of Food Security and Nutrition in the World 2021*. FAO, Rome.

Fardkhales, A.S. and Lincoln, N. (2021) Food hubs play an essential role in the COVID-19 response in Hawai'i. *Journal of Agriculture, Food Systems, and Community Development* 10, 1–18. DOI: 10.5304/jafscd.2021.102.036.

Feenstra, G.W. (1997) Local food systems and sustainable communities. *American Journal of Alternative Agriculture* 12, 28–36. DOI: 10.1017/S0889189300007165.

Fei, S., Ni, J. and Santini, G. (2020) Local food systems and COVID-19: An insight from China. *Resources, Conservation and Recycling* 162, 105022. DOI: 10.1016/j.resconrec.2020.105022.

Foley, J.A., Ramankutty, N., Brauman, K.A., Cassidy, E.S., Gerber, J.S. *et al.* (2011) Solutions for a cultivated planet. *Nature* 478, 337–342. DOI: 10.1038/nature10452.

Fontefrancesco, M.F. and Zocchi, D.M. (2020) Reviving traditional food knowledge through food festivals. The case of the pink asparagus festival in Mezzago, Italy. *Frontiers in Sustainable Food Systems* 4, 596028. DOI: 10.3389/fsufs.2020.596028.

FSIN (2021) Global Report on Food Crises – 2021 | World Food Programme. Available at: https://www.wfp.org/publications/global-report-food-crises-2021 (accessed 21 August 2022).

Garnett, T. (2011) Where are the best opportunities for reducing greenhouse gas emissions in the food system (including the food chain)? *Food Policy* 36, S23–S32. DOI: 10.1016/j.foodpol.2010.10.010.

Ghaedi, E., Mohammadi, M., Mohammadi, H., Ramezani-Jolfaie, N., Malekzadeh, J. *et al.* (2019) Effects of a paleolithic diet on cardiovascular disease risk factors: A systematic review and meta-analysis of randomized controlled trials. *Advances in Nutrition* 10, 634–646. DOI: 10.1093/advances/nmz007.

Ghosh-Jerath, S., Dhasmana, A., Nair, S.C. and Kapoor, R. (2024) Impact of the second wave of COVID-19 pandemic on food security among ho indigenous community of Jharkhand, India. *Agriculture and Food Security* 13, 17. DOI: 10.1186/s40066-024-00469-1.

GoCrisp (2022) Retail Data for the CPG Industry. Available at: https://www.gocrisp.com/ (accessed 16 August 2022).

Gray, L., Guzman, P., Glowa, K.M. and Drevno, A.G. (2014) Can home gardens scale up into movements for social change? The role of home gardens in providing food security and community change in San Jose, California. *Local Environment* 19, 187–203. DOI: 10.1080/13549839.2013.792048.

Gregorio, G. and Ancog, R. (2020) Assessing the impact of the COVID-19 pandemic on agricultural production in Southeast Asia: Toward transformative change in agricultural food system. *Asian Journal of Agriculture and Development* 17, 1–14. DOI: 10.37801/ajad2020.17.1.1.

Guell, C., Brown, C.R., Navunicagi, O.W., Iese, V., Badrie, N. *et al.* (2022) Perspectives on strengthening local food systems in small island developing states. *Food Security* 14, 1227–1240. DOI: 10.1007/s12571-022-01281-0.

Hamilton, H., Henry, R., Rounsevell, M., Moran, D., Cossar, F. *et al.* (2020) Exploring global food system shocks, scenarios and outcomes. *Futures* 123, 102601. DOI: 10.1016/j.futures.2020.102601.

Hammad, H.M., Nauman, H.M.F., Abbas, F., Jawad, R., Farhad, W. *et al.* (2023) Impacts of COVID-19 pandemic on environment, society, and food security. *Environmental Science and Pollution Research* 30, 99261–99272. DOI: 10.1007/s11356-023-25714-1.

Hammer, K., Arrowsmith, N. and Gladis, T. (2003) Agrobiodiversity with emphasis on plant genetic resources. *Naturwissenschaften* 90, 241–250. DOI: 10.1007/s00114-003-0433-4.

Haron, M.Z. and Jalil, R.A. (2023) Food insecurity during COVID-19: A neglected priority? *IIUM Medical Journal Malaysia* 22, 3–11. DOI: 10.31436/imjm.v22i2.1933.

Hasan, N.A., Heal, R.D., Bashar, A., Bablee, A.L. and Haque, M.M. (2021) Impacts of COVID-19 on the finfish aquaculture industry of Bangladesh: A case study. *Marine Policy* 130, 104577. DOI: 10.1016/j.104577/marpol.2021.104577.

Hecht, A.A., Biehl, E., Barnett, D.J. and Neff, R.A. (2019) Urban food supply chain resilience for crises threatening food security: A qualitative study. *Journal of the Academy of Nutrition and Dietetics* 119, 211–224. DOI: 10.1016/j.jand.2018.09.001.

Heck, S., Campos, H., Barker, I., Okello, J.J., Baral, A. *et al.* (2020) Resilient agri-food systems for nutrition amidst COVID-19: Evidence and lessons from food-based approaches to overcome micronutrient deficiency and rebuild livelihoods after crises. *Food Security* 12, 823–830. DOI: 10.1007/s12571-020-01067-2.

Hemathilake, D.M.K.S. and Gunathilake, D.M.C.C. (2022) High-productive agricultural technologies to fulfill future food demands: Hydroponics, aquaponics, and precision/smart agriculture. In: Bhat, R. (ed.) *Future Foods*. Elsevier, Amsterdam, Netherlands, pp. 555–567.

Herens, M.C., Pittore, K.H. and Oosterveer, P.J.M. (2022) Transforming food systems: Multi-stakeholder platforms driven by consumer concerns and public demands. *Global Food Security* 32, 100592. DOI: 10.1016/j.gfs.2021.100592.

Herrero, M., Thornton, P.K., Mason-D'Croz, D., Palmer, J., Bodirsky, B.L. *et al.* (2021) Articulating the effect of food systems innovation on the sustainable development goals. *The Lancet Planetary Health* 5, e50–e62. DOI: 10.1016/S2542-5196(20)30277-1.

HLPE (2020) In: *Impacts of COVID-19 on Food Security and Nutrition: Developing Effective Policy Responses to Address the Hunger and Malnutrition Pandemic*. Food and Agricultural Organisation, Rome.

Hoddinott, J. (2023) Food systems, resilience, and their implications for public action. In: Béné, C. and Devereux, S. (eds) *Resilience and Food Security in a Food Systems Context*. Springer International Publishing, Cham, pp. 185–206.

Hoque, M.S., Bygvraa, D.A., Pike, K., Hasan, M.M., Rahman, M.A. *et al.* (2021) Knowledge, practice, and economic impacts of COVID-19 on small-scale coastal fishing communities in Bangladesh: Policy recommendations for improved livelihoods. *Marine Policy* 131, 104647. DOI: 10.1016/j.marpol.2021.104647.

Howard, E. (2020) Victory gardens: A war-time hobby that's back in fashion. Available at: https://www.bbc.com/travel/article/20200524-victory-gardens-a-war-time-hobby-thats-back-in-fashion (accessed 21 August 2022).

Hunter, D., Monville-Ora, E., Burgos, B., Rogel, C.N., Calub, B. *et al.* (eds) (2020) *Agrobiodiversity, School Gardens and Healthy Diets: Promoting Biodiversity, Food and Sustainable Nutrition*. Routledge, Abingdon, Oxon, New York, NY.

IFPRI, F. (2020) *Global Food Policy Report: Building Inclusive Food Systems*. International Food Policy Research Institute, Washington, DC.

Iga, M. (2014) Changing agri-food systems in the global economy. *Japanese Journal of Human Geography* 66, 552–564. DOI: 10.4200/jjhg.66.6_552.

Inwood, S.M., Sharp, J.S., Moore, R.H. and Stinner, D.H. (2009) Restaurants, chefs and local foods: Insights drawn from application of a diffusion of innovation framework. *Agriculture and Human Values* 26, 177–191. DOI: 10.1007/s10460-008-9165-6.

IPES-Food (2016) *From Uniformity to Diversity: A Paradigm Shift from Industrial Agriculture to Diversified Agroecological Systems*. International Panel of Experts on Sustainable Food Systems, Brussels.

Janssen, M., Chang, B.P.I., Hristov, H., Pravst, I., Profeta, A. *et al.* (2021) Changes in food consumption during the COVID-19 pandemic: Analysis of consumer survey data from the first lockdown period in Denmark, Germany, and Slovenia. *Frontiers in Nutrition* 8, 635859. DOI: 10.3389/fnut.2021.635859.

Ji, G., Zhong, H., Feukam Nzudie, H.L., Wang, P. and Tian, P. (2024) The structure, dynamics, and vulnerability of the global food trade network. *Journal of Cleaner Production* 434, 140439. DOI: 10.1016/j.jclepro.2023.140439.

Johns, T., Powell, B., Maundu, P. and Eyzaguirre, P.B. (2013) Agricultural biodiversity as a link between traditional food systems and contemporary development, social integrity and ecological health: Traditional food systems, agricultural biodiversity and sustainable development. *Journal of the Science of Food and Agriculture* 93, 3433–3442. DOI: 10.1002/jsfa.6351.

Jones, A. (2002) An environmental assessment of food supply chains: A case study on dessert apples. *Environmental Management* 30, 560–576. DOI: 10.1007/s00267-002-2383-6.

Kahan, D. (2012) *Entrepreneurship in Farming*. Food and Agriculture Organization of the United Nations, Rome.

Kanianska, R. (2016) Agriculture and its impact on land use, environment and ecosystem services. In: Almusaed, A. (ed.) *Landscape Ecology: The Influences of Land Use and Anthropogenic Impacts of Landscape Creation*. InTech Open, London, pp. 3–26.

Kazancoglu, Y., Ekinci, E., Mangla, S.K., Sezer, M.D. and Ozbiltekin-Pala, M. (2023) Impact of epidemic outbreaks (COVID-19) on global supply chains: A case of trade between Turkey and China. *Socio-Economic Planning Sciences* 85, 101494. DOI: 10.1016/j.seps.2022.101494.

Kent, K., Gale, F., Penrose, B., Auckland, S., Lester, E. *et al.* (2022) Consumer-driven strategies towards a resilient and sustainable food system following the COVID-19 pandemic in Australia. *BMC Public Health* 22, 1539. DOI: 10.1186/s12889-022-13987-z.

Khakurel, D., Uprety, Y., Łuczaj, Ł. and Rajbhandary, S. (2021) Foods from the wild: Local knowledge, use pattern and distribution in Western Nepal. *PLOS ONE* 16. DOI: 10.1371/journal.pone.0258905.

Khan, S.A.R., Razzaq, A., Yu, Z., Shah, A., Sharif, A. *et al.* (2022) Disruption in food supply chain and undernourishment challenges: An empirical study in the context of Asian countries. *Socio-Economic Planning Sciences* 82, 101033. DOI: 10.1016/j.seps.2021.101033.

Khoury, C.K., Bjorkman, A.D., Dempewolf, H., Ramirez-Villegas, J., Guarino, L. *et al.* (2014) Increasing homogeneity in global food supplies and the implications for food security. *Proceedings of the National Academy of Sciences* 111, 4001–4006. DOI: 10.1073/pnas.1313490111.

Kilbourne, E.D. (2006) Influenza pandemics of the 20th century. *Emerging Infectious Diseases* 12, 9–14. DOI: 10.3201/eid1201.051254.

Kirwan, J., Ilbery, B., Maye, D. and Carey, J. (2013) Grassroots social innovations and food localisation: An investigation of the local food programme in England. *Global Environmental Change* 23, 830–837. DOI: 10.1016/j.gloenvcha.2012.12.004.

Klerkx, L. and Begemann, S. (2020) Supporting food systems transformation: The what, why, who, where and how of mission-oriented agricultural innovation systems. *Agricultural Systems* 184, 102901. DOI: 10.1016/j.agsy.2020.102901.

Kneafsey, M., Venn, L., Schmutz, U., Balázs, B., Trenchard, L. *et al.* (2013) *Short Food Supply Chains and Local Food Systems in the EU. A State of Play of Their Socio-Economic Characteristics*. JRC Scientific and Policy Report, European Commission, Joint Research Centre, Institute for Prospective Technological Studies.

Kondo, C. and Lichten, J. (2020) Resilient Japanese local food systems thrive during covid-19: Ten groups, ten outcomes. *The Asia-Pacific Journal: Japan Focus* 18, 5484.

Kortright, R. and Wakefield, S. (2011) Edible backyards: A qualitative study of household food growing and its contributions to food security. *Agriculture and Human Values* 28, 39–53. DOI: 10.1007/s10460-009-9254-1.

Kotschy, K., Biggs, R., Daw, T., Folke, C. and West, P.C. (2015) Principle 1 – Maintain diversity and redundancy. In: Biggs, R., Schlüter, M. and Schoon, M.L. (eds) *Principles for Building Resilience*, 1st edn. Cambridge University Press, Cambridge, UK, pp. 50–79.

Kubatko, O., Merritt, R., Duane, S. and Piven, V. (2023) The impact of the COVID-19 pandemic on global food system resilience. *Mechanism of an Economic Regulation* 1, 144–148. DOI: 10.32782/mer.2023.99.22.

Kuhnlein, H.V., Smitasiri, S., Yesudas, S., Bhattacharjee, L., Dan, L. *et al.* (2006) *Documenting traditional food systems of indigenous peoples: International case studies*. Centre for Indigenous Peoples' Nutrition and Environment, McGill University, Canada.

Kumar, A., Anju, T., Kumar, S., Chhapekar, S.S., Sreedharan, S. *et al.* (2021a) Integrating omics and gene editing tools for rapid improvement of traditional food plants for diversified and sustainable food security. *International Journal of Molecular Sciences* 22, Article 8093. DOI: 10.3390/ijms22158093.

Kumar, A., Kumar, S., Komal, cs, Ramchiary, N. and Singh, P. (2021b) Role of traditional ethnobotanical knowledge and indigenous communities in achieving sustainable development goals. *Sustainability* 13, 3062. DOI: 10.3390/su13063062.

Kumar, A., Sreedharan, S., Singh, P., Achigan-Dako, E.G. and Ramchiary, N. (2021c) Improvement of a traditional orphan food crop, *Portulaca oleracea* L. (purslane) using genomics for sustainable food security and climate-resilient agriculture. *Frontiers in Sustainable Food Systems* 5, 711820. DOI: 10.3389/fsufs.2021.711820.

Lamichhane, J.R. and Reay-Jones, F.P.F. (2021) Editorial: Impacts of COVID-19 on global plant health and crop protection and the resulting effect on global food security and safety. *Crop Protection* 139, 105383. DOI: 10.1016/j.cropro.2020.105383.

Lamine, C. and Dawson, J. (2018) The agroecology of food systems: Reconnecting agriculture, food, and the environment. *Agroecology and Sustainable Food Systems* 42, 629–636. DOI: 10.1080/21683565.2018.1432517.

La Trobe, H.L. and Acott, T.G. (2000) Localising the global food system. *International Journal of Sustainable Development and World Ecology* 7, 309–320. DOI: 10.1080/13504500009470050.

Leat, P. and Revoredo-Giha, C. (2013) Risk and resilience in agri-food supply chains: The case of the ASDA porklink supply chain in Scotland. *Supply Chain Management: An International Journal* 18, 219–231. DOI: 10.1108/13598541311318845.

Li, L., Pegg, R.B., Eitenmiller, R.R., Chun, J.-Y. and Kerrihard, A.L. (2017) Selected nutrient analyses of fresh, fresh-stored, and frozen fruits and vegetables. *Journal of Food Composition and Analysis* 59, 8–17. DOI: 10.1016/j.jfca.2017.02.002.

Li, M., Jia, N., Lenzen, M., Malik, A., Wei, L. *et al.* (2022) Global food-miles account for nearly 20% of total food-systems emissions. *Nature Food* 3, 445–453. DOI: 10.1038/s43016-022-00531-w.

Ma, N.L., Peng, W., Soon, C.F., Noor Hassim, M.F., Misbah, S. *et al.* (2021) COVID-19 pandemic in the lens of food safety and security. *Environmental Research* 193, 110405. DOI: 10.1016/j.envres.2020.110405.

Maherani, B., Hossain, F., Criado, P., Ben-Fadhel, Y., Salmieri, S. *et al.* (2016) World market development and consumer acceptance of irradiation technology. *Foods* 5, 79. DOI: 10.3390/foods5040079.

Mahmoud, S.H. and Gan, T.Y. (2018) Impact of anthropogenic climate change and human activities on environment and ecosystem services in arid regions. *Science of The Total Environment* 633, 1329–1344. DOI: 10.1016/j.scitotenv.2018.03.290.

Mamonova, N. (2023) Food sovereignty and solidarity initiatives in rural Ukraine during the war. *The Journal of Peasant Studies* 50, 47–66. DOI: 10.1080/03066150.2022.2143351.

Marti, L. and Puertas, R. (2021) European countries' vulnerability to COVID-19: Multicriteria decision-making techniques. *Economic Research-Ekonomska Istraživanja* 34, 3309–3320. DOI: 10.1080/1331677X.2021.1874462.

Martinez, S., Hand, M.S., Pra, M.D., Pollack, S., Ralston, K. *et al.* (2010) *Local Food Systems: Concepts, Impacts, and Issues*. Economic Report, USDA, Washington, DC.

Massawe, F., Mayes, S. and Cheng, A. (2016) Crop diversity: An unexploited treasure trove for food security. *Trends in Plant Science* 21, 365–368. DOI: 10.1016/j.tplants.2016.02.006.

Masters, G., Baker, P. and Flood, J. (2010) Climate change and agricultural commodities. *CABI Working Paper* 2, 1–38.

Mc Carthy, U., Uysal, I., Badia-Melis, R., Mercier, S., O'Donnell, C. *et al.* (2018) Global food security – Issues, challenges and technological solutions. *Trends in Food Science and Technology* 77, 11–20. DOI: 10.1016/j.tifs.2018.05.002.

McKeon, N. (2021) Global food governance. *Development* 64, 48–55. DOI: 10.1057/s41301-021-00299-9.

Meixner, O., Quehl, H.E., Pöchtrager, S. and Haas, R. (2022) Being a farmer in Austria during COVID-19 – A qualitative study on challenges and opportunities. *Agronomy* 12, 1240. DOI: 10.3390/agronomy12051240.

Monroy-Torres, R., Castillo-Chávez, Á., Carcaño-Valencia, E., Hernández-Luna, M., Caldera-Ortega, A. *et al.* (2021) Food security, environmental health, and the economy in Mexico: Lessons learned with the covid-19. *Sustainability* 13, 7470. DOI: 10.3390/su13137470.

Mundler, P. and Laughrea, S. (2016) The contributions of short food supply chains to territorial development: A study of three quebec territories. *Journal of Rural Studies* 45, 218–229. DOI: 10.1016/j.jrurstud.2016.04.001.

Nayak, R. and Waterson, P. (2019) Global food safety as a complex adaptive system: Key concepts and future prospects. *Trends in Food Science and Technology* 91, 409–425. DOI: 10.1016/j.tifs.2019.07.040.

Nchanji, E.B. and Lutomia, C.K. (2021) COVID-19 challenges to sustainable food production and consumption: Future lessons for food systems in eastern and Southern Africa from a gender lens. *Sustainable Production and Consumption* 27, 2208–2220. DOI: 10.1016/j.spc.2021.05.016.

Nemes, G., Chiffoleau, Y., Zollet, S., Collison, M., Benedek, Z. *et al.* (2021) The impact of COVID-19 on alternative and local food systems and the potential for the sustainability transition: Insights from 13 countries. *Sustainable Production and Consumption* 28, 591–599. DOI: 10.1016/j.spc.2021.06.022.

Neo, P. (2020) Thailand's COVID-19 'War': Local food production centre of focus as government guarantees supplies. Available at: https://www.foodnavigator-asia.com/Article/2020/04/06/Thailand-s-COVID-19-war-Local-food-production-centre-of-focus-as-government-guarantees-supplies (accessed 27 August 2022).

Ngairangbam, H. and Athokpam, V. (2023) Post-harvest storage and processing technology of horticultural crops. In: *Current Trends in Agricultural Sciences and Technology*. Vital Biotech Publication, Rajasthan, India, pp. 199–208.

Ng, C.A. and von Goetz, N. (2017) The global food system as a transport pathway for hazardous chemicals: The missing link between emissions and exposure. *Environmental Health Perspectives* 125, 1–7. DOI: 10.1289/EHP168.

Niles, M.T., Wirkkala, K.B., Belarmino, E.H. and Bertmann, F. (2021) Home food procurement impacts food security and diet quality during COVID-19. *BMC Public Health* 21, 945. DOI: 10.1186/s12889-021-10960-0.

Noort, M.W.J., Renzetti, S., Linderhof, V., Rand, G.E., Marx-Pienaar, N.J.M.M. *et al.* (2022) Towards sustainable shifts to healthy diets and food security in sub-saharan Africa with climate-resilient crops in bread-type products: A food system analysis. *Foods* 11, 135. DOI: 10.3390/foods11020135.

Nova, P., Pinto, E., Chaves, B. and Silva, M. (2020) Urban organic community gardening to promote environmental sustainability practices and increase fruit, vegetables and organic food consumption. *Gaceta Sanitaria* 34, 4–9. DOI: 10.1016/j.gaceta.2018.09.001.

OCED (2020) COVID-19 and the Food and Agriculture Sector: Issues and Policy Responses. Available at: https://www.oecd.org/coronavirus/policyresponses/covid-19-and-the-food-andagriculture-sector-issues-andpolicy-responses-a23f764b/ (accessed 12 May 2024).

O'Hara, S.U. and Stagl, S. (2001) Global food markets and their local alternatives: A socio-ecological economic perspective. *Population and Environment* 22, 533–554. DOI: 10.1023/A:1010795305097.

Palar, K., Lemus Hufstedler, E., Hernandez, K., Chang, A., Ferguson, L. *et al.* (2019) Nutrition and health improvements after participation in an urban home garden program. *Journal of Nutrition Education and Behavior* 51, 1037–1046. DOI: 10.1016/j.jneb.2019.06.028.

Panghal, A., Mor, R.S., Kamble, S.S., Khan, S.A.R., Kumar, D. *et al.* (2022) Global food security post COVID-19: Dearth or dwell in the developing world? *Agronomy Journal* 114, 878. DOI: 10.1002/agj2.20932.

Payne, J. (2022) Why farm-to-fork transparency is essential. Available at: https://www.aptean.com/en-EU/insights/blog/farm-to-fork-transparency (accessed 30 August 2022).

Pereira, L.M., Kushitor, S.B., Cramer, C., Drimie, S., Isaacs, M. *et al.* (2022) Leveraging the potential of wild food for healthy, sustainable, and equitable local food systems: Learning from a transformation lab in the Western Cape Region. *Sustainability Science* s11625–022. DOI: 10.1007/s11625-022-01182-3.

Petrescu-Mag, R.M., Vermeir, I., Petrescu, D.C., Crista, F.L. and Banatean-Dunea, I. (2020) Traditional foods at the click of a button: The preference for the online purchase of romanian traditional foods during the COVID-19 pandemic. *Sustainability* 12, 9956. DOI: 10.3390/su12239956.

Pewee, F. and Mulbah, H. (2021) COVID-19, food insecurity and health in Liberia. *Current Journal of Applied Science and Technology* 40, 84–90. DOI: 10.9734/cjast/2021/v40i1731438.

Poulton, C., Dorward, A. and Kydd, J. (2010) The future of small farms: New directions for services, institutions, and intermediation. *World Development* 38, 1413–1428. DOI: 10.1016/j.worlddev.2009.06.009.

Pound, B. and Conroy, C. (2017) The innovation systems approach to agricultural research and development. In: Snapp, S. and Pound, B. (eds) *Agricultural Systems*, 2nd edn. Academic Press, San Diego, pp. 371–405.

Powderly, W.G. (2019) How infection shaped history: Lessons from the Irish famine. *Transactions of the American Clinical and Climatological Association* 130, 127–135.

Pretty, J.N., Ball, A.S., Lang, T. and Morison, J.I.L. (2005) Farm costs and food miles: An assessment of the full cost of the UK weekly food basket. *Food Policy* 30, 1–19. DOI: 10.1016/j.foodpol.2005.02.001.

Purwantini, T.B. (2023) Human capital performance in the agriculture sector during the era of COVID-19. In: *Proceedings of the 1st UMSurabaya Multidisciplinary International Conference 2021 (MICon 2021)*, Atlantis Press. Amsterdam, Netherlands, pp. 649–656.

Rahimi, M. and Demirbaş, N. (2023) Importance of local food markets in terms of sustainable agriculture: Constraints and recommendations. In: *Africa 2nd International conference on new horizons in Sciences*, Academy Global Conferences and Publishing, Cairo, pp. 256–269.

Ramos, S., Etxebarria, S., Cidad, M., Gutierrez, M., San Martin, D. *et al*. (2020) Cleaner production strategies for the food industry. In: Galanakis, C.M. (ed.) *The Interaction of Food Industry and Environment*. Elsevier, Amsterdam, Netherlands, pp. 1–34.

Rao, T. (2020) Food supply anxiety brings back victory gardens. *The New York Times*.

Recchia, L., Cappelli, A., Cini, E., Garbati Pegna, F. and Boncinelli, P. (2019) Environmental sustainability of pasta production chains: An integrated approach for comparing local and global chains. *Resources* 8, 56. DOI: 10.3390/resources8010056.

Rha, J.-Y., Lee, B., Nam, Y. and Yoon, J. (2021) COVID-19 and changes in Korean consumers' dietary attitudes and behaviors. *Nutrition Research and Practice* 15, S94. DOI: 10.4162/nrp.2021.15.S1.S94.

Ritchie, H., Rosado, P. and Roser, M. (2022) Environmental Impacts of Food Production. Available at: https://ourworldindata.org/environmental-impacts-of-food (accessed 11 May 2024).

Rocha, C. and Spagnuolo, D. (2019) Sustainable and healthy diets for achieving the SDGS: The role of consumers. In: Valentini, R., Sievenpiper, J.L., Antonelli, M. and Dembska, K. (eds) *Achieving the Sustainable Development Goals Through Sustainable Food Systems*. Springer International Publishing, Cham, pp. 143–155.

Rotz, S. and Fraser, E.D.G. (2015) Resilience and the industrial food system: Analyzing the impacts of agricultural industrialization on food system vulnerability. *Journal of Environmental Studies and Sciences* 5, 459–473. DOI: 10.1007/s13412-015-0277-1.

Sarkis, J. (2020) Supply chain sustainability: Learning from the COVID-19 pandemic. *International Journal of Operations and Production Management* 41, 63–73. DOI: 10.1108/IJOPM-08-2020-0568.

Seyfang, G. and Haxeltine, A. (2012) Growing grassroots innovations: Exploring the role of community-based initiatives in governing sustainable energy transitions. *Environment and Planning C: Government and Policy* 30, 381–400. DOI: 10.1068/c10222.

Sgroi, F. and Modica, F. (2022) Consumers' eating habits during the covid-19 pandemic: Evidence of an experimental analysis in Italy. *International Journal of Gastronomy and Food Science* 28, 100538. DOI: 10.1016/j.ijgfs.2022.100538.

Shabir, I., Dash, K.K., Dar, A.H., Panddey, V.K., Fayaz, U. *et al*. (2023) Carbon footprints evaluation for sustainable food processing system development: A comprehensive review. *Future Foods* 7, 100215. DOI: 10.1016/j.fufo.2023.100215.

Shelef, O., Weisberg, P.J. and Provenza, F.D. (2017) The value of native plants and local production in an era of global agriculture. *Frontiers in Plant Science* 8, 2069.

Shupler, M., Mwitari, J., Gohole, A., Cuevas, R., Puzzolo, E. *et al*. (2021) COVID-19 impacts on household energy and food security in a Kenyan informal settlement: The need for integrated approaches to the SDGs. *Renewable and Sustainable Energy Reviews* 144, 111018. DOI: 10.1016/j.rser.2021.111018.

Singh, S., Kumar, R., Panchal, R. and Tiwari, M.K. (2021) Impact of COVID-19 on logistics systems and disruptions in food supply chain. *International Journal of Production Research* 59, 1993–2008. DOI: 10.1080/00207543.2020.1792000.

Skalkos, D., Kosma, I.S., Chasioti, E., Skendi, A., Papageorgiou, M. *et al*. (2021) Consumers' attitude and perception toward traditional foods of northwest Greece during the COVID-19 pandemic. *Applied Sciences* 11, 4080. DOI: 10.3390/app11094080.

Smith, M.D. and Wesselbaum, D. (2020) COVID-19, food insecurity, and migration. *The Journal of Nutrition* 150, 2855–2858. DOI: 10.1093/jn/nxaa270.

Sõukand, R., Stryamets, N., Fontefrancesco, M.F. and Pieroni, A. (2020) The importance of tolerating interstices: Babushka markets in Ukraine and Eastern Europe and their role in maintaining local food knowledge and diversity. *Heliyon* 6, e03222. DOI: 10.1016/j.heliyon.2020.e03222.

Sözer, N., Heinonen, M., Kolehmainen, M., Maunuksela, L., Vilkki, J. *et al*. (2021) *A Food Research and Innovation Strategy for Finland 2021–2035*. Finnish Food Research and Innovation, Finland.

Spínola, V., Mendes, B., Câmara, J.S. and Castilho, P.C. (2012) An improved and fast UHPLC-PDA methodology for determination of L-ascorbic and dehydroascorbic acids in fruits and vegetables. evaluation of degradation rate during storage. *Analytical and Bioanalytical Chemistry* 403, 1049–1058. DOI: 10.1007/s00216-011-5668-x.

Staudacher, K., Rennstam Rubbmark, O., Birkhofer, K., Malsher, G., Sint, D. *et al*. (2018) Habitat heterogeneity induces rapid changes in the feeding behaviour of generalist arthropod predators. *Functional Ecology* 32, 809–819. DOI: 10.1111/1365-2435.13028.

Stein, A.J. and Santini, F. (2022) The sustainability of "local" food: A review for policy-makers. *Review of Agricultural, Food and Environmental Studies* 103, 77–89. DOI: 10.1007/s41130-021-00148-w.

Stephens, E.C., Martin, G., Wijk, M., Timsina, J. and Snow, V. (2020) Editorial: Impacts of COVID-19 on agricultural and food systems worldwide and on progress to the sustainable development goals. *Agricultural Systems* 183, 102873. DOI: 10.1016/j.agsy.2020.102873.

Tendall, D.M., Joerin, J., Kopainsky, B., Edwards, P., Shreck, A. *et al.* (2015) Food system resilience: Defining the concept. *Global Food Security* 6, 17–23. DOI: 10.1016/j.gfs.2015.08.001.

The Food Systems Dashboard (2023) *The Global Alliance for Improved Nutrition (GAIN)*. Switzerland, Geneva.

Thomson, A.J., Giannopoulos, G., Pretty, J., Baggs, E.M. and Richardson, D.J. (2012) Biological sources and sinks of nitrous oxide and strategies to mitigate emissions. *Philosophical Transactions of the Royal Society B: Biological Sciences* 367, 1157. DOI: 10.1098/rstb.2011.0415.

Trebbin, A. (2014) Linking small farmers to modern retail through producer organizations – Experiences with producer companies in India. *Food Policy* 45, 35–44. DOI: 10.1016/j.foodpol.2013.12.007.

Trolio, J., Eckman, M. and Mehta, K. (2016) Leveraging globalization to revive traditional foods. *Journal of Sustainable Development* 9, 212–219. DOI: 10.5539/jsd.v9n6p212.

Tsai, S.C., Lu, C.C., Bau, D.T., Chiu, Y.J., Yen, Y.-T. *et al.* (2021) Approaches towards fighting the COVID-19 pandemic. *International Journal of Molecular Medicine* 47, 3–22. DOI: 10.3892/ijmm.2020.4794.

Tschiggerl, K. and Topic, M. (2019) Cleaner production and sustainable development. In: Leal Filho, W. (ed.) *Encyclopedia of Sustainability in Higher Education*. Springer International Publishing, Cham, pp. 204–215.

Ujjwal, K.C., Campbell-Ross, H., Godde, C., Friedman, R., Lim-Camacho, L. *et al.* (2024) A systematic review of the evolution of food system resilience assessment. *Global Food Security* 40, 100744. DOI: 10.1016/j.gfs.2024.100744.

UN (2015) *Eradication of Hunger and Malnutrition, Social Incorporation of All People; Overall Equity, Literacy, Health, Ecosystem Conservation, Environmental Protection, Sustainable Energy and Climate Change Mitigation Are Also Required*. United Nations, New York City, USA.

UNESCO World Water Assessment Programme (2012) United Nations world water development report 4: Managing water under uncertainty and risk. UNESCO, Paris. Thematic report.

UNIDO (2020) *Short Food Supply Chains for Promoting Local Food on Local Markets*. United Nations Industrial Development Organization, Vienna, Austria.

United Nations (2015) THE 17 GOALS | Sustainable Development. Available at: https://sdgs.un.org/goals (accessed 27 February 2023).

United Nations (2017) *The role of Science, Technology and Innovation in Ensuring Food Security by 2030*. In: *United Nations Conference on Trade and Development*, UN.

Ušča, M. and Tisenkopfs, T. (2023) The resilience of short food supply chains during the COVID-19 pandemic: A case study of a direct purchasing network. *Frontiers in Sustainable Food Systems* 7, 1146446. DOI: 10.3389/fsufs.2023.1146446.

Usubiaga-Liaño, A., Behrens, P. and Daioglou, V. (2020) Energy use in the global food system. *Journal of Industrial Ecology* 24, 830–840. DOI: 10.1111/jiec.12982.

Valdivia, M. (2020) In Peru, ancestral values shine during COVID-19 crisis. Available at: https://www.localfutures.org/in-peru-ancestral-values-shine-during-covid-19-crisis (accessed 27 August 2022).

van Berkum, S., Dengerink, J. and Ruben, R. (2018) *The Food Systems Approach: Sustainable Solutions for a Sufficient Supply of Healthy Food*. Wageningen Economic Research, Hague.

van der Ploeg, J.D., Jingzhong, Y. and Schneider, S. (2012) Rural development through the construction of new, nested, markets: Comparative perspectives from China, Brazil and the European Union. *Journal of Peasant Studies* 39, 133–173. DOI: 10.1080/03066150.2011.652619.

Vargas, A.M., Moura, A.P., Deliza, R. and Cunha, L.M. (2021) The role of local seasonal foods in enhancing sustainable food consumption: A systematic literature review. *Foods* 10, 2206. DOI: 10.3390/foods10092206.

Verma, G., Singla, N. and Singh, S. (2023) COVID-19, livestock supply chains and livelihoods in India: A review of impacts and implications. *Journal of Agribusiness in Developing and Emerging Economies*. DOI: 10.1108/JADEE-01-2023-0015.

Veselovská, L. (2020) Supply chain disruptions in the context of early stages of the global COVID-19 outbreak. *Problems and Perspectives in Management* 18, 490–500. DOI: 10.21511/ppm.18(2).2020.40.

Walker, B., Holling, C.S., Carpenter, S. and Kinzig, A. (2004) Resilience, adaptability and transformability in social–ecological systems. *Ecology and Society* 9, 5. DOI: 10.5751/ES-00650-090205.
Ward, P.R., Verity, F., Carter, P., Tsourtos, G., Coveney, J. *et al*. (2013) Food stress in Adelaide: The relationship between low income and the affordability of healthy food. *Journal of Environmental and Public Health* e968078. DOI: 10.1155/2013/968078.
Weber, H., Loschelder, D.D., Lang, D.J. and Wiek, A. (2021) Connecting consumers to producers to foster sustainable consumption in international coffee supply – A marketing intervention study. *Journal of Marketing Management* 37, 1148–1168. DOI: 10.1080/0267257X.2021.1897650.
Weinkauf, K. and Everitt, T. (2023) Food system resilience during COVID-19: The role of local producers in rural Canada. *Canadian Food Studies* 10, 82–101. DOI: 10.15353/cfs-rcea.v10i2.594.
Willis, G. (2012) *From Field to Fork: The Value of England's Local Food Webs*. CPRE, London.
Zanetta, L.D., Hakim, M.P., Gastaldi, G.B., Seabra, L.M.J., Rolim, P.M. *et al*. (2021) The use of food delivery apps during the COVID-19 pandemic in Brazil: The role of solidarity, perceived risk, and regional aspects. *Food Research International* 149, 110671. DOI: 10.1016/j.foodres.2021.110671.
Zhou, M. and Kan, M.-Y. (2021) The varying impacts of COVID-19 and its related measures in the UK: A year in review. *PLOS ONE* 16, e0257286. DOI: 10.1371/journal.pone.0257286.
Zhuravleva, L., Zarubina, E., Kruzhkova, T., Rushitskaya, O. and Ruchkin, A. (2022) Changes in food behavior of Russians in the context of the COVID-19 pandemic. *IOP Conference Series: Earth and Environmental Science* 949, 012083. DOI: 10.1088/1755-1315/949/1/012083.
Zollet, S., Colombo, L., Meo, P., Marino, D., McGreevy, S.R. *et al*. (2021) Towards territorially embedded, equitable and resilient food systems? Insights from grassroots responses to COVID-19 in Italy and the city region of Rome. *Sustainability* 13, 2425. DOI: 10.3390/su13052425.

4 Multiple Approaches in the Study of Ancient Human Microbiome

Santiago Rosas-Plaza[1], Ximena Rosas-Plaza[2] and René Cerritos[1,3*]
[1]Centro de Investigación en Políticas, Población y Salud, Universidad Nacional Autónoma de México, Mexico City, Mexico; [2]Facultad de Medicina Veterinaria y Zootecnia, Universidad Nacional Autónoma de México, Mexico City, Mexico; [3]CONACHYT, Cibiogem (Comisión Intersecretarial de Bioseguridad y Organismos Genéticamente Modificados), Mexico City, Mexico

Abstract

Research related to the analysis of microbial communities in ancient human samples began two decades ago. Since then, new technologies as well as new bioinformatic tools have been developed for the manipulation of massive data. All this together with the theoretical knowledge generated from microbial ecology has expanded our understanding of the human microbiome. Despite the challenge of studying ancient samples and their microbiome, some approaches applied to the contemporary human microbiome have been successfully applied to ancient samples. Most studies in ancient samples have focused on taxonomic profiling at the community level with metagenomic or high-throughput 16S rRNA gene amplicon sequencing data. However, other approaches have emerged in order to get deeper understanding of the ancient human microbiome. Therefore, the aim of this review is to discuss all the approaches and methodologies successfully applied to ancient samples and ancient microbiome as well as the information that can be generated using them, in order to understand the evolution of human microbiome interactions throughout history.

Keywords: ancient DNA, ancient microbiome, metagenomics, microbial diversity, multi-omics, paleogenomics, 16S rRNA gene

Introduction

The constant development of new technologies has been a turning point in the study of ancient DNA (aDNA). This has allowed us to explore new fields of knowledge such as paleogenomics, a discipline based on the reconstruction and analysis of ancient genomes (Lindqvist and Rajora, 2019). While paleogenomic data has offered insights into a portion of human evolutionary history (Kuhlwilm *et al.*, 2016), advances in the study of microbial ecology have shown that humans are the hosts of different symbiotic microorganisms that play a determining role in our body (Selber-Hnativ *et al.*, 2017). Concepts such as the holobiont have been taken up in order to highlight the importance of considering this association as a single biological unit of study (van de Guchte *et al.*, 2018). Since host-microbiome relationship is

*Corresponding author: renecerritos@gmail.com

crucial for the development and survival of its host, it is probable that these interactions have been playing an important role in the evolutionary history of humans. For this reason, it has been proposed that the study of human evolution should implement a line of research focused on the microorganisms that have been involved in development, growth, and health (Warinner *et al.*, 2015). Despite the challenges in the study of ancient microbiome, relevant information has been exposed, mainly related to the taxonomic composition of the ancient oral and gut microbiome through DNA sequencing. However, other approaches that have been applied in current studies of the human microbiome have been rarely applied to understand ancient microbiome. Therefore, this review aims to describe the different approaches and some methodologies (such as functional diversity, intra-species diversity, and the identification of new species with metagenome-assembled genomes) that have been or could be potentially applied in the study of ancient microbiome in order to generate more detailed information about the evolution of human-microbiome interaction.

Review Methodology

For this review, a comprehensive search was conducted across various databases, including Google Scholar, Scopus, PubMed, and ScienceDirect. The search utilized a carefully selected set of keywords to ensure a broad exploration of the subject matter. Terms such as 'coprolites,' 'paleofeces,' 'ancient DNA,' 'ancient microbiome,' 'ancient genomes,' 'ancient bacteria,' 'multi-omics,' 'anthropology genetics,' 'ancient proteomics,' and 'ancient metabolomics' were employed to retrieve relevant literature. Additional materials and references were obtained from downloaded articles. We also consulted key books, such as 'Paleogenomics: Genome-Scale Analysis of Ancient DNA' (Lindqvist and Rajora, 2019). By employing this methodology, we obtained over 130 references, each contributing to the enrichment of this article's review.

Why and How to Study Ancient Human Microbiome?

Several studies have found that the human microbiome is influenced by different factors, including age, geographic location, host genetics, diet, environment, and lifestyle (De Filippo *et al.*, 2010; Yatsunenko *et al.*, 2012; Schnorr *et al.*, 2014; Jha *et al.*, 2018; Ayeni *et al.*, 2018; Hansen *et al.*, 2019). Considering that these factors directly affect the diversity and composition of the human microbiome, it is possible that through the evolution of humans, and the changes that the development of human societies entails, alteration in the human microbiome has been promoted. For example, the transition from hunter-gatherers to modern societies represents major modifications in diet, hygiene practices, health care (including antibiotics), access to resources, and the way humans interact with each other and with the environment (Jha *et al.*, 2018; Hansen *et al.*, 2019). Also, research carried out on the gut microbiome of populations that still practice traditional hunting and gathering has revealed differences compared to modern societies. Furthermore, changes in diversity have been documented across current human populations with different lifestyles (Rosas-Plaza *et al.*, 2022). This implies that local adaptation to different environments, as well as cultural practices, could be promoting differences in the microbiome of populations living within the same time frame. Thus, considering the vast diversification of cultures, local practices, and various environments where humans settled throughout history, along with processes of local adaptation and geographic isolation, we would expect to find differences in the human microbiome at both temporal and regional scales. All this together raises the question whether changes throughout human history could reflect changes in the human microbiome in time and space. Nowadays, thanks to environmental processes that have facilitated the preservation of ancient samples, it is possible to analyze the ancient human microbiome from different sources such as: coprolites, paleofeces, and mummified intestinal tissue for gut microbiome and dental calculus for oral microbiome (Fig. 4.1). These remains

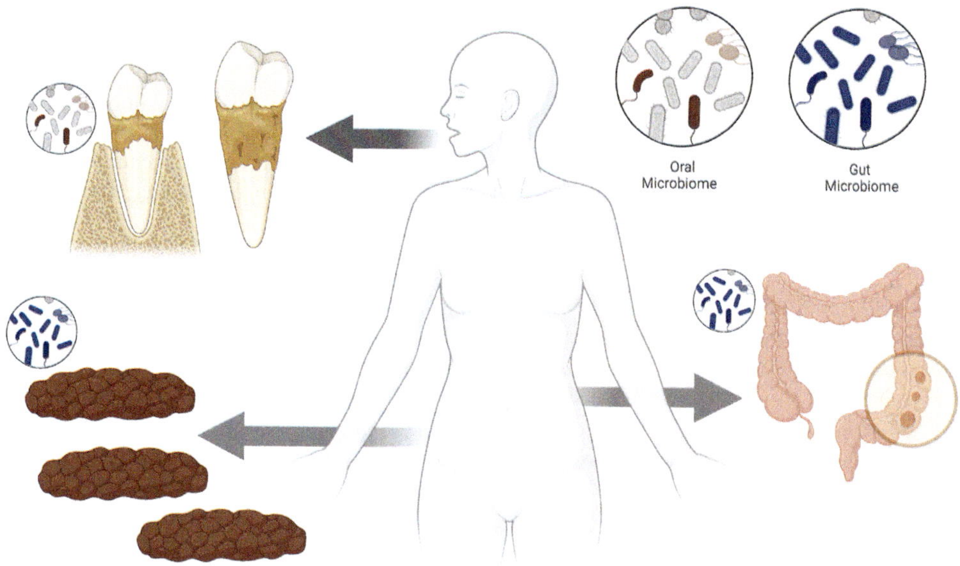

Fig. 4.1. Samples used in the study of ancient human microbiome. Dental calculus, coprolites or paleofeces, and intestinal tissue are fundamental samples in the study of ancient human microbiome. The color of the microorganism in the circles (brown or blue) next to the sample type represents the microbiome (oral or gut microbiome) that can be analyzed. Figure created with BioRender.com.

can be analyzed through different molecules or compounds in order to get insight into ancient human microbiome (DNA, RNA, proteins, and metabolites).

Retrieving Metagenomic Data for Ancient Microbiome Studies

DNA extraction from ancient samples represents a crucial step for the analysis of ancient microbial communities. The selection of extraction methodologies significantly influences the success of retrieving amplicon and metagenomic data, emphasizing the need for careful protocol considerations. The constant refinement of library preparation protocols and the emergence of innovative techniques contribute to advancing our knowledge of the ancient microbial world and its interactions with human populations over time. In this section, we will discuss the main techniques employed for retrieving ancient DNA as well as the sequencing strategies to study ancient human microbiome.

Ancient DNA extraction

Various methodologies have been proposed for the extraction of aDNA from coprolites, paleofeces, and dental calculus (Adler *et al.*, 2013; Hagan *et al.*, 2020). Protocols for aDNA extraction commonly recommend an overnight predigestion step in an EDTA-based lysis buffer, typically containing sodium dodecyl sulfate (SDS) and proteinase K (Adler *et al.*, 2013; Warinner *et al.*, 2014; Huynh *et al.*, 2016). Subsequent DNA extraction can be performed using commercial DNA extraction kits (Tito *et al.*, 2012; Adler *et al.*, 2013; Santiago-Rodriguez *et al.*, 2019), or in-house DNA extraction method (phenol-chloroform or guanidine hydrochloride) (Warinner *et al.*, 2014; Ziesemer *et al.*, 2015; White *et al.*, 2021). This is followed by a purification step with silica-membrane- based methods, often employing a PCR Purification Kit (Warinner *et al.*, 2014; Ziesemer *et al.*, 2015; Jensen *et al.*, 2019). Notably, studies comparing commercial kits with phenol-chloroform protocols have demonstrated that the latter yields higher DNA concentrations in paleofeces (Hagan *et al.*, 2020). This underscores the importance of selecting optimal extraction methods to ensure the successful retrieval of ancient metagenomic data for ancient microbiome analysis. All DNA extraction processes require rigorous contamination control measures, including the use of negative controls and laboratory blanks.

Sequencing methodologies for ancient human microbiome

Various sequencing methods are available for the comprehensive analysis of ancient microbiome, with the selection based on the specific objectives of the investigation, including taxonomic identification, functional analysis, or targeting the genome of a specific bacterial group for evolutionary studies. Among these methods, next-generation amplicon sequencing, primarily focusing on the 16S rRNA gene, is frequently employed for identifying microbial groups in ancient samples (Tito *et al.*, 2012; Adler *et al.*, 2013; Santiago-Rodriguez *et al.*, 2013, 2019). Specifically, the v3 region of 16S rRNA gene has been used in ancient microbiome studies due to its ability to generate a relatively small amplicon size (approximately 190 base pairs) (Adler *et al.*, 2013; Ziesemer *et al.*, 2015), aligning well with the highly fragmented nature of aDNA (Dabney *et al.*, 2013).

The sequences of the 16S rRNA gene generated with next-generation platforms can be processed and classified using bioinformatic tools like QIIME (Table 4.1). Taxonomic assignment is achieved through reference databases such as RDP (Cole *et al.*, 2014), SILVA (Yilmaz *et al.*, 2014), and Greengenes (McDonald *et al.*, 2012). The resulting data can be employed for diverse analyses, including taxonomic abundance screening, alpha and beta diversity assessments, and comparisons with modern human microbiomes for authentication purposes (Box 4.1).

Amplicon-based 16S rRNA gene sequencing serves as an exceptionally cost-effective methodology for conducting a preliminary and broad qualitative characterization of ancient microbiome samples. However, when compared with shotgun metagenomic data, it becomes evident that this method lacks reliability in reconstructing quantitative information about microbial diversity, functional, and taxonomic frequency in ancient microbial communities (Ziesemer *et al.*, 2015). Additionally, the authentication of aDNA through the analysis of cytosine deamination patterns cannot be performed with amplicon sequencing approaches (Box 4.1).

On the other hand, shotgun metagenomic sequencing has been effectively applied to ancient microbiome studies. This approach provides a comprehensive understanding of ancient microbial communities in a more profound manner (Ziesemer *et al.*, 2015). This is because it is not confined to a single, short region of the genome and does not discriminate between bacteria, archaea, eukaryotes, or any other source of DNA present in the sample (Pérez-Cobas *et al.*, 2020). However, the optimization of library preparation protocols for shotgun sequencing represents a crucial step in the analysis of aDNA studies (Henneberger *et al.*, 2019).

Ancient DNA sequencing can be conducted through two primary approaches: (1) utilizing double-stranded DNA or (2) employing single-stranded DNA (Henneberger *et al.*, 2019). In the context of ancient microbiome studies, the double-stranded library preparation protocol has been the most employed sequencing approach, typically using the Illumina platform with single or double indexed libraries (Warinner *et al.*, 2014; Eisenhofer *et al.*, 2020; Rifkin *et al.*, 2020; Granehäll *et al.*, 2021; Wibowo *et al.*, 2021; Quagliariello *et al.*, 2022).

The double-stranded protocol for aDNA involves a preliminary step in library preparation where blunt-ended adapters are ligated to double-stranded DNA, followed by the standard Illumina sequencing protocol (Meyer and Kircher, 2010). Notably, a recently developed single-tube library preparation for degraded DNA has been introduced, promising reduced processing time and lower laboratory costs (Carøe *et al.*, 2018). This protocol has found successful application in ancient human microbiome studies (Jensen *et al.*, 2019; Rampelli *et al.*, 2021; White *et al.*, 2021).

Depending on the intended analysis, uracil-DNA glycosylase (UDG) repairment may be performed before library preparation to remove deaminated nucleotide bases, leaving abasic sites instead of uracils (Briggs *et al.*, 2009).

Table 4.1. Bioinformatics tools for ancient microbiome analysis with amplicon and metagenomic data.

Type of data and analysis	Task	Software	Reference
Taxonomic profiling with amplicon sequence data	Taxonomic classification and microbial community analysis	QIIME	Caporaso *et al.* (2010)
		Mothur	Schloss *et al.* (2009)
Taxonomic and functional profiling with metagenomic sequence data	Taxonomic classification	MetaPhlAn2	Truong *et al.* (2015)
		MALT	Herbig *et al.* (2016)
		Kraken	Wood and Salzberg (2014)
		MegaBLAST	Chen *et al.* (2015)
		ClaMS	Pati *et al.* (2011)
		SPARSE	Zhou *et al.* (2017)
		MIDAS	Zhao *et al.* (2023)
		GTDB-Tk	Chaumeil *et al.* (2020)
	Ancient metagenomic profiling (taxonomic classification and aDNA authentication)	aMeta	Pochon *et al.* (2023)
		HOPS	Hübler *et al.* (2019)
	Functional profiling	HUMAnN 2.0	Franzosa *et al.* (2018)
aDNA and microbiome authentication	Ancient damage analysis	MapDamage2.0	Ginolhac *et al.* (2011)
		AuthentiCT	Peyrégne and Peter (2020)
		DamageProfiler	Neukamm *et al.* (2021)
	Microbiome source authentication	Sourcetracker	Knights *et al.* (2011)
		CoproID	Borry *et al.* (2020)
		FEAST	Shenhav *et al.* (2019)
Ancient genome reconstruction with metagenomic data (MAGS)	*de novo* metagenomic assembly	metaSpades	Nurk *et al.* (2017)
		MEGAHIT	Li *et al.* (2015)
	Metagenome binning for genome reconstruction	MetaBat2	Kang *et al.* (2019)
		MaxBin2	Wu *et al.* (2016b)
	Assessing quality of microbial genomes recovered from metagenomic data	CheckM	Parks *et al.* (2015)
Strain-level analysis with metagenomic data	Strain-level heterogeneity analysis for metagenome assembled genomes	CMseq	Tett *et al.* (2019)
	Metagenomic strain-level population genomics analysis	StrainPhlAn	Truong *et al.* (2017)
Integrated pipelines for aDNA	SNP detection, phylogenomic, and metagenomic analysis	PALEOMIX	Schubert *et al.* (2014)

UDG treatment is crucial when the analysis is focused on within-species evolutionary relationships, as accurate identification of single nucleotide polymorphisms is critical for reliable evolutionary inferences (Spyrou *et al.*, 2019). It is essential to recognize that this step tends to eliminate the signature of postmortem damage, posing challenges in identifying damage patterns in these samples (Renaud *et al.*, 2019) (Box 4.1). To address this, some studies have categorized DNA samples into two groups: those not subjected to UDG treatment for damage pattern analysis and those with treatment for straightforward analysis (Rohland *et al.*, 2015). However, new protocols have been developed that require a single library preparation per sample (partially UDG-treated libraries). This allows the assessment of aDNA damage patterns in the library while enabling straightforward analysis (Rohland *et al.*, 2015).

Several bioinformatic tools have been developed to facilitate the processing and analysis of metagenomic data offering a diverse range of functionalities (Table 4.1). Comparisons between different bioinformatic tools for taxonomic classification of ancient microbiome metagenomic

Box 4.1. Challenges and considerations in the analysis of ancient microbiome

Because ancient samples remain in contact with the environment for thousands of years, they are susceptible to different sources of contamination. Therefore, one of the greatest challenges in paleogenomics is the authentication of endogenous DNA (Peyrégne and Prüfer, 2020). This challenge is even greater when the research is focused in the bacterial composition of ancient microbiome, as the largest source of exogenous DNA contamination comes from bacteria and other microorganisms that accumulate over time (Der Sarkissian *et al.*, 2014). In addition, DNA extraction reagents (both commercial kits and home methods) and sequencing reagents have been reported to contain microbial DNA, contributing to contamination of ancient samples in the extraction and sequencing process (Glassing *et al.*, 2016; Weyrich *et al.*, 2019). All these factors make the authentication of endogenous ancient DNA crucial. Strategies such as identifying DNA damage patterns and comparing microbial composition with similar microbial sources has been complemented in this line of research in order to corroborate the ancient microbiome source. Furthermore, identifying groups of microorganisms reported as possible contaminants in reagents is important in ancient microbiome studies.

DAMAGE PATTERNS IN ANCIENT DNA

Damage such as hydrolytic depurination in aDNA causes its fragmentation (Dabney *et al.* 2013). Typically, the fragment size of aDNA ranges from 100 to 500 bp (Grigorenko *et al.*, 2009). This peculiarity was first studied in this area by corroborating through the visualization and comparison of different PCR product sizes in agarose gels (Grigorenko *et al.*, 2009). Another damage pattern in ancient samples is cytosine (C) deamination. This process converts C to uracil (U), leading to adenine (A) incorporation during DNA replication. Consequently, this results in apparent C to T or G to A substitutions. Deaminated cytosines primarily accumulate at the end of DNA fragments (Dabney *et al.*, 2013). Some bioinformatics tools have been developed to analyze these damage patterns across genomes (e.g. mapDamage) (Ginolhac *et al.*, 2011; Peyrégne and Peter, 2020).

ANALYZING THE PROPORTION OF ANCIENT HUMAN MICROBIOME AND OTHER MICROBIAL COMMUNITIES IN ANCIENT SAMPLES

One way to corroborate that you are working with ancient human microbiome is by comparing it with current human microbiome data and other environmental sources. Programs such as SourceTracker and FEAST analyze the microbial composition associated with a sample in order to estimate the proportion that corresponds to a particular environment (Knights *et al.*, 2011; Shenhav *et al.*, 2019). These tools have been essential in corroborating the presence of human gut microbiome in ancient samples (Tito *et al.*, 2012; Santiago-Rodriguez *et al.*, 2013; Hagan *et al.*, 2020; Sabin *et al.*, 2020). Based on the same principle, a new proposal has recently emerged that combines the analysis of bacterial communities as well as the proportion of potential host DNA (Borry *et al.*, 2020). With this new approach, in addition to ensuring that the bacterial communities found in coprolites correspond to a human gut microbiome, it is intended to predict the probable host. This is important because coprolites of other mammals may be confused with human coprolites (Borry *et al.*, 2020).

data suggest that MIDAS (Zhao *et al.*, 2023) and MetaPhlAn2 (Truong *et al.*, 2015) are reliable options for accurately reconstructing community structures (Velsko *et al.*, 2018). However, new bioinformatic tools focused on ancient metagenomic data have emerged in recent years (Table 4.1).

In summary, the continuous evolution of these methodologies holds the promise of revealing insights into the complex relationships between microbes and their hosts across different historical periods. With persistent technological advancements and meticulous technique refinement, the potential to comprehend the ancient microbial world expands, unveiling new and intriguing avenues for the study of this ever-evolving field.

What We Know About Ancient Human Microbiome: A Brief Story

Ancient gut microbiome

Advancements in the study of the ancient human microbiome align with the evolution of new technologies (Fig. 4.2). The earliest attempts to recover ancient human gut-associated bacteria date back to 1936 with the analysis of cave coprolites found in the Ozark Mountains of Arkansas (Wakefield and Dellinger, 1936). However, the bacteriological culture methods of those years did not allow the growth of the bacterial groups associated with the samples. Subsequently, other groups tried to cultivate bacteria from other coprolites without success (Reinhard and Vaughn, 1992).

With the arrival of PCR, it was possible for the first time to amplify, clone, and sequence the 16S rRNA gene from various ancient human sources, including the colon of mummies (Ubaldi *et al.*, 1998; Cano *et al.*, 2000; Rollo *et al.*, 2007) and coprolites (Luciani *et al.*, 2006). In these studies, although DNA sequences related to environmental bacteria were identified, a significant portion was associated with human gut bacteria. The bacterial groups identified included members of the *Clostridiaceae* (*Clostridium intestinalis*, *C. irregularis*, *C. perfringens*, *C. sordelli*, *C. ghoni*), *Bacteroidaceae* (*Bacteroides spp.*), and *Eubacteriaceae* (*Eubacterium tenue*) families (Ubaldi *et al.*, 1998; Cano *et al.*, 2000). However, it is important to note that these studies identified less than 1% of the 1500 species that have been described as members of the human gut microbiome (Lloyd-Price *et al.*, 2016). Despite these techniques only recovering a small fraction of bacterial groups associated with the human gut, they opened the possibility for retrieving ancient bacterial DNA from coprolites and mummified intestinal tissue dating back up to 5000 years (Tyrolean Iceman) (Cano *et al.*, 2000).

A significant advancement occurred with the advent of Next Generation Sequencing (NGS) techniques and the introduction of new bioinformatic tools specifically designed for the analysis of extensive DNA sequence data. Through the high-throughput sequencing of the 16S rRNA gene and bioinformatic tools focused on the analysis of microbial communities (e.g. QIIME) (Caporaso *et al.*, 2010) (Table 4.1), it was possible to perform a more detailed analysis of the bacterial communities associated with the ancient gut microbiome (Tito *et al.*, 2012). In particular, the analysis carried out with coprolites from Rio Zape (dated 1400 BP) in northern Mexico represented a turning point in this line of research (Tito *et al.*, 2012). This marked a pivotal moment as it became possible, for the first time, to validate through bioinformatic tools that the bacterial composition found in the Rio Zape coprolites corresponded to the human gut microbiome (e.g. Sourcetracker) (Knights *et al.*, 2011) (Table 4.1). Notably, the Rio Zape coprolites exhibited a gut microbiome signature similar to that of children from rural regions of Africa. Additionally, the Rio Zape coprolites were rich in bacterial groups such as *Prevotella*, *Treponema*, and the *Bifidobacterium* genera, which are known to be representative of human populations in regions practicing traditional agriculture and hunting-gathering (Rosas-Plaza *et al.*, 2022). It is important to note that other coprolites analyzed in this study, such as the Caserones and Hinds Cave coprolites, demonstrated limited similarity to a gut microbiome environment. This underscores the significance of ancient sample conservation in preserving the integrity and relevance of microbial data.

Taxonomic microbial profiling using metagenomic data or the 16S rRNA gene has been applied to paleofeces, coprolites, and mummified intestinal tissue from different regions of the world. These studies include ancient samples from Peru (dated between 980–1170

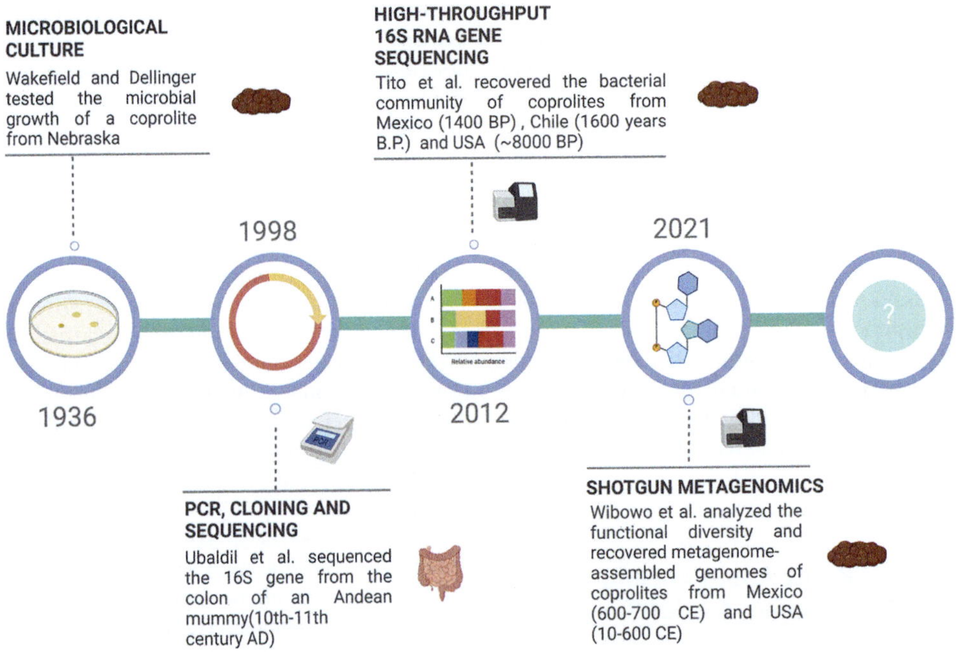

Fig. 4.2. Timeline of ancient human gut microbiome studies. Key points in the study of the ancient human gut microbiome and its relationship with the development of new technologies, from microbiological culturing in 1936, to shotgun sequencing in 2021. The image of a stool (coprolite and paleofeces) or a gut (mummified intestines) represents the type of samples analyzed in each study. Figure created with BioRender.com.

CE) (Santiago-Rodriguez *et al.*, 2015), Puerto Rico (dated between 300–400 CE) (Cano *et al.*, 2014), and Belgium (14th-century) (Appelt *et al.*, 2014). In a Pre-Columbian Andean mummy, amplicon and metagenomic data analysis revealed differences between the microbial composition of mummified tissue and paleofeces. While *Clostridium* spp. constituted up to 96.2% of the mummified tissue, *Turicibacter* spp. accounted for 89.2% of the bacteria identified in the paleofeces (Santiago-Rodriguez *et al.*, 2015). Furthermore, the analysis of the Andean mummy's gut revealed the presence of *Clostridium botulinum*, *Trypanosoma cruzi*, and various antibiotic-resistance genes. This suggests that resistance might have been a natural component of gut microbial communities preceding the emergence of antibiotics (Santiago-Rodriguez *et al.*, 2015). On the other hand, while analyzing Middle Ages coprolites, a variety of members of the mammal gut microbiota were detected, including human gut *Bacteroides* species (*B. finegoldii*, *B. vulgatus*, and *B. coprocola*) (Appelt *et al.*, 2014). Pathogens belonging to *Bartonella* and *Bordetella* were also identified for the first time in the Middle Ages coprolites, expanding our insights into ancient microbial pathogens (Appelt *et al.*, 2014).

While previous investigations have described taxonomic bacterial composition in coprolites and paleofeces, the functional analysis of the ancient gut microbiome has been less explored (Santiago-Rodriguez *et al.*, 2016; Rifkin *et al.*, 2020; Jacobson *et al.*, 2020; Wibowo *et al.*, 2021). Metagenomic analysis on paleofeces from the United States (Boomerang Shelter and Arid West Cave) (10–60 CE) and Mexico (Río Zape) (600–900 CE) has provided valuable insights into the study of the ancient gut microbiome (Wibowo *et al.*, 2021). Paleofeces showed a high abundance of polysaccharide degradation genes, transposase enrichment, and low abundance of antibiotic resistance genes compared to the modern human gut microbiome (Wibowo *et al.*,

2021). Moreover, microbial groups in the paleofeces, such as *Oscillospiraceae*, *Lachnospiraceae*, and *Clostridiaceae*, showed genes associated with chitin degradation, suggesting historical insect consumption (Wibowo *et al.*, 2021). Additionally, different keystone taxa involved in short chain fatty acids (SCFAs) production (*Eubacterium biforme* and *Phascolarctobacterium succinatutens*) were identified in Rio Zape coprolites (Jacobson *et al.*, 2020). Particularly, acetate production was the most abundant SCFA in the Rio Zape samples (Jacobson *et al.*, 2020).

In the same context, the comparison of paleofeces from Middle Iron Age Bantu-speakers with modern gut microbiome has also revealed significant differences in metabolic functions (Rifkin *et al.*, 2020). The paleofeces showed an enrichment of genes related to the biosynthesis of secondary toxic metabolites, indicating a diet rich in natural and unprocessed foods. In contrast, specific genes involved in metabolizing soy, coffee, cacao, citrus, and wine were depleted in the paleofeces but enriched in the modern gut microbiome (Rifkin *et al.*, 2020). The analysis also found an enrichment of xenobiotic degradation pathways associated with toxic environmental pollutants in the modern human microbiome, possibly due to continuous exposure to such compounds in industrialized and urban environments (Rifkin *et al.*, 2020).

Finally, metagenomic and amplicon analyses of ancient gut microbiomes have expanded our understanding of the intricate relationships between historical human populations and their microbial communities. Comparisons with modern populations further highlight the resilience and adaptability of the human gut microbiome across different eras. The marked differences in metabolic functions, dietary habits, and responses to environmental exposures highlight the dynamic nature of the gut microbiome throughout history.

Ancient oral microbiome

In conjunction with the analysis of the ancient gut microbiome, substantial research has been dedicated to exploring the ancient oral microbiome. Initial investigations focused on the 16S rRNA gene in human dental calculus, revealed that ancient samples from the Mesolithic, Neolithic, Bronze Age, and Medieval presented similar bacterial composition compared to modern oral samples (Adler *et al.*, 2013). However, ancient calculus exhibited greater diversity in comparison to the contemporary European oral microbiome (Adler *et al.*, 2013). Notably, the modern European oral microbiome showed a higher abundance of pathogens like *Streptococcus mutans* compared to Mesolithic and Neolithic samples. It has been suggested that the high carbohydrate intake is associated with an increase in the prevalence of periodontal disease in the early Neolithic period and caries in the recent past (Adler *et al.*, 2013). Similarly, the identification of *Actinomyces* in the pre-Columbian oral microbiome from the Caribbean has been linked to periodontal diseases, also attributed to the consumption of fermentable carbohydrates in that culture (Santiago-Rodriguez *et al.*, 2017). Furthermore, with 16S rRNA gene various pathogenic bacteria in the Middle Ages samples have been identified, including some associated with cystic fibrosis (*Burkholderia gladioli* and *Inquilinus limosus*), respiratory tract infections (*Tsukamurella pulmonis*), and nosocomial pathogens (*Methylobacterium mesophilicum*) (Santiago-Rodriguez *et al.*, 2019).

After the validation of the ancient oral microbiome through the utilization of the 16S rRNA gene, other investigations have employed metagenomic data in ancient oral microbiome studies. The analysis of medieval dental calculus (950–1200 CE) revealed that the most abundant bacterial groups are similar to those prevalent in modern human oral microbiome (Warinner *et al.*, 2014). Alongside the metagenomic data, the integration of protein analysis have successfully confirmed the presence of members of the red complex bacteria pathogens, including *Tannerella forsythia*, *Porphyromonas gingivalis*, and *Treponema denticola* (Warinner et *al.*, 2014). In general, the use of metagenomic data has made it possible to identify bacteria from the red complex in various ancient calculus and teeth samples, spanning different periods and cultures around the world. This includes samples from 2000-year- old Egyptian mummified individuals, Roman Iron Age individuals, Medieval individuals, 18th-century Kazakh individuals, and ancient Japanese populations (Eisenhofer *et al.*, 2020; Neukamm *et al.*, 2020; Philips *et al.*,

2020; White *et al.*, 2021). Moreover, members of the red complex have been recognized as a keystone taxa in ancient and historic samples (Jacobson *et al.*, 2020). All this together suggests that this group of bacteria has been associated with humans for thousands of years, despite differences in lifestyle, hygiene, geography, and diet.

Furthermore, the comparative analysis of dental calculus from Palaeolithic hunter-gatherers (31,000–11,000 BC), Neolithic (6200–4000 BC), and Copper Age (3500–2200 BC) farmers revealed specific trends in the taxonomic groups of the oral microbiome that could be associated with the introduction of agriculture (Quagliariello *et al.*, 2022). One trend is the increase in the representation of species at the beginning of the Neolithic period that are poorly represented in Palaeolithic samples. These species include members of the red complex (*P. gingivalis*, *T. forsythia*, and *T. denticola*), orange complex (*Campylobacter gracilis*, *C. rectus*, *C. showae*, and *P. intermedia*), and green complex (*Capnocytophaga endotelialis*, *C. haemolytica*, *C. ochracea*, *C. sputigena*, and *C. corrodens*) (Quagliariello *et al.*, 2022). Notably, the red and orange complexes consist of species recognized as the major etiologic agents of periodontal diseases (Mohanty *et al.*, 2019). Conversely, species that are more prevalent within the Palaeolithic samples decrease over time, reaching the lowest abundance in the late Neolithic and Copper Age. These species are members of the purple complex (*Actinomyces* spp.) and yellow complex (*Streptococcus gordonii*, *S. mitis*, *S. oralis*, and *S. sanguinis*) (Quagliariello *et al.*, 2022). Species from the yellow and purple complexes are early colonizers of the dental biofilm, preceding the proliferation of pathogenic orange and red complexes (Mohanty *et al.*, 2019). Collectively, these findings support the hypothesis that the introduction of agriculture may have influenced the oral human microbiome.

Finally, it is crucial to consider the distinction between dental calculus and dental plaque. Despite the valuable insights gained from the analysis of ancient dental calculus, it has been observed that these two oral features harbor distinct microbial communities (Velsko *et al.*, 2019; Kazarina *et al.*, 2021). Comprehensive investigations using metagenomics and proteomics on both modern and historical samples have revealed that microbial profiles in historic and modern calculus share a high degree of similarity, setting them apart from dental plaque (Velsko *et al.*, 2019; Kazarina *et al.*, 2021). Notably, the abundance of red complex species is significantly higher in dental calculus, both historic and modern, compared to dental plaque (Velsko *et al.*, 2019). This underscores the importance of recognizing the unique characteristics of dental calculus and dental plaque in the study of oral microbiomes.

All the findings from these studies, along with research on the current human microbiome across diverse populations, contribute to the growing evidence that oral and gut microbial communities have evolved alongside humans and societies. Comparing ancient and modern microbiomes highlights a dynamic interplay between microbial communities and human societies, emphasizing how lifestyle changes, dietary habits, and environmental exposures have shaped the structure and function of the gut and oral microbiome over time. As we delve deeper into understanding these complexities, it becomes evident that the microbiome is a dynamic entity intricately linked to human health.

Beyond Taxonomic Composition: Different Approaches in the Study of the Ancient Microbiome

As described above, most research has focused on describing the taxonomic composition of different sources of ancient microbiome (coprolites, mummified tissue, and dental calculus). Although it has been crucial to describe the microbial composition in order to understand the evolution of human-microbiome interactions, new approaches have emerged in recent years that could enrich this line of research, such as: *de novo* genome assembly, multi-omics, the study of intra-species diversity, and the recovery of ancient microbiome from sediments. This section discusses approaches that have been little explored in studies of the ancient microbiome but have great potential to expand our knowledge within this area.

Recovering ancient bacterial species

In early studies of the ancient human microbiome (through high-throughput 16S rRNA sequencing and metagenomics), taxonomic characterizations were carried out with contemporary human microbiome databases (known as reference database-approach). However, this approach has a major bias in identifying only species of the current human microbiome. This compromises the identification of potential microorganisms that were part of the ancient microbiome but are no longer in the current human microbiome. Studies of human gut microbiome from populations with different lifestyles and from ancient populations have shown that some groups such as *Treponema* genus have disappeared from the gut microbiome of modern societies (Wibowo *et al.*, 2021; Rosas-Plaza *et al.*, 2022). However, more information about the loss of other groups and their metabolic functions is crucial in order to understand the evolution of human-microbiome interactions. Therefore, one of the challenges in human ancient microbiome is to identify the species of microorganisms that could potentially belong to ancient populations. For this goal two approaches for the recovery of ancient bacterial species are described: *de novo* metagenomes assembly and high-throughput culture (culturomics) (Fig. 4.3).

Multiple bioinformatic tools and protocols have emerged for *de novo* genome assembly from metagenomic data (Table 4.1) (Li *et al.*, 2015; Nurk *et al.*, 2017; Kang *et al.*, 2019). The recovery of metagenome-assembled genomes (MAGs) has become an important tool in the study of microbial communities. It has been widely used for the identification of new species in different environments (Wilkins *et al.*, 2019; Youngblut *et al.*, 2020; Kim *et al.*, 2021), including the human gut microbiome (Pasolli *et al.*, 2019). As a strategy free of reference databases, it has the potential to be used in the identification of new species and their metabolic roles in the ancient microbiome (Sarhan *et al.*, 2021; Wibowo *et al.*, 2021).

By applying this methodology to coprolites from the United States (dated between 10–600 CE) and Mexico (dated between 600–900 CE), 61 novel species-level genome bins (SGBs) and 18 novel genera were successfully identified (Wibowo *et al.*, 2021). Remarkably, these 61 novel species constitute 39% of the reconstructed SGBs, indicating that a considerable portion of the ancient human gut microbiome remains undescribed. The taxonomic classification of these ancient novel SGBs revealed several genera, including *Eubacterium*, *Prevotella*, *Ruminococcus*, *Solobacterium*, *Bacteroides*, *Catenibacterium*, *Faecalibacterium*, *Faecalicatena*, and *Holdemanella* (Wibowo *et al.*, 2021).

MAGs have been also employed in the study of oral microbiome. Importantly, they allowed the reconstruction of 11 *Methanobrevibacter* genomes from ancient dental calculus (Granehäll *et al.*, 2021). These samples from Trentino-South Tyrol date from the Neolithic (6000–3500 BCE) to the Early Middle Ages (400–1000 CE). The analysis resulted in the identification of two novel *Methanobrevibacter* species named TS-1 and TS-2, alongside the identification of *Methanobrevibacter oralis*. When comparing modern and ancient calculus, a particular pattern emerged regarding the prevalence of *Methanobrevibacter* species based on sample age. Specifically, *M. oralis* exhibited predominance in both modern and younger ancient calculus, while TS-1 was more prevalent in older samples, notably absent in calculus younger than 700 years (Granehäll *et al.*, 2021). Conversely, TS-2 was found in both prehistoric and more recent samples, spanning a timeframe of at least 6000 years (Granehäll *et al.*, 2021). This finding not only remarks on the prevalence of certain bacterial groups over time but also the depletion of other taxa that were once integral parts of the oral microbiome, suggesting that the depletion of oral bacterial groups has been occurring throughout human history and in more recent years.

This advanced understanding of microbial diversity within ancient coprolites and dental calculus provides a significant contribution to the field, offering insights into previously undiscovered species and genera and enhancing our understanding of the ecology of the human oral and gut microbiome during historical periods. In this way, MAGs represent a possibility to overcome the significant bias of using contemporary databases in ancient microbiome studies.

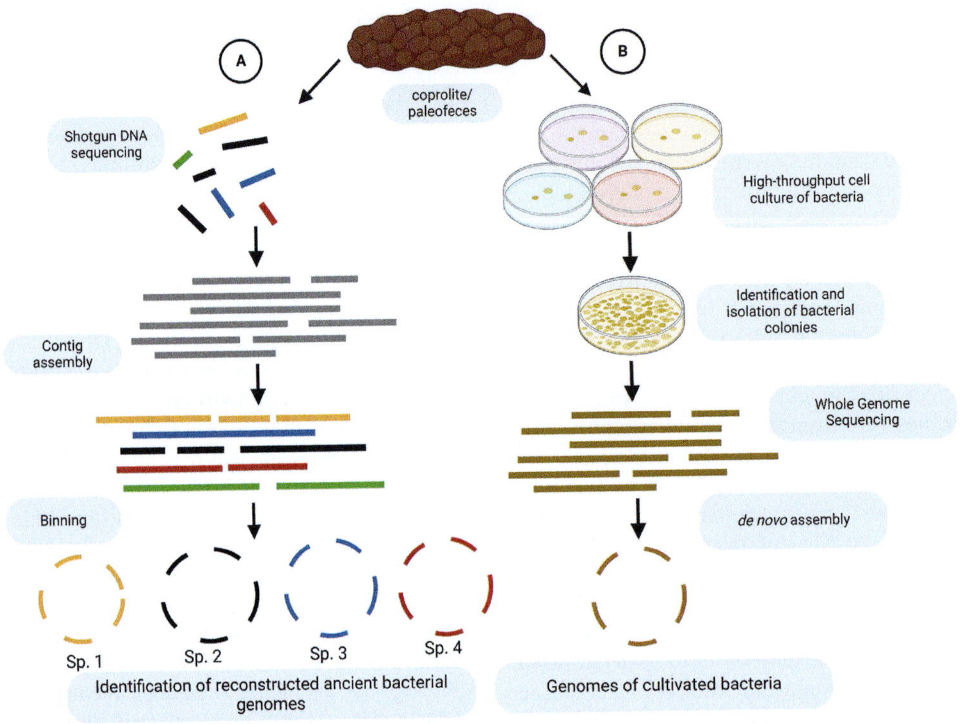

Fig. 4.3. Strategies for the recovery of ancient bacterial species: (A) basic steps for the construction of metagenome-assembled genomes (MAGs). From shotgun sequencing to binning of contigs for the subsequent taxonomic profiling and identification of potential ancient bacterial genomes, and (B) high-throughput culture (culturomics) workflow. The growth and isolation of different colonies, identification with mass spectrometry (MALDI-TOF), and the sequencing of unidentified colonies for the description of potential ancient bacteria. Figure created with BioRender.com.

On the other hand, microbial culture has been essential for the identification of species and their metabolic functions (Browne *et al.*, 2016). In the last decade, there has been progress in high-throughput culturing methods applied in conjunction with metagenomics and mass spectrometry for the analysis of bacterial communities (Lagier *et al.*, 2016). This approach known as culturomics has enabled the growth and identification of bacteria that were thought to be impossible to culture. Through culturomics 77% of the 1525 prokaryotes of the human intestine have been cultivated (Lagier *et al.*, 2016), and potential new species of the gut microbiome have been identified (Browne *et al.*, 2016; Lagier *et al.*, 2016). Furthermore, by using culturomics it was possible to cultivate and sequence 28 ancient bacterial genomes from the permafrost (Afouda *et al.*, 2020). Considering this, culturomics stand as a novel methodology alternative in the ancient microbiome analysis. However, considerations related to the environmental conditions should be made, for example, to take into account where the samples have remained or the phenotypic characteristics of the microorganisms under study. For instance, it has been shown that cold and dry environments favor the preservation of old samples and the survival of ancient microorganisms, while changes in temperature and humidity favor their degradation (Smith *et al.*, 2019; Afouda *et al.*, 2020). On the other hand, microorganisms that are capable of forming resistant structures (e.g. spores) can remain viable for thousands of years (Nicholson *et al.*, 2000). The latter is relevant since it was suggested that at least 60% of the bacterial genera of the intestinal microbiome produce resistant spores (Browne *et al.*, 2016), so the identification of ancient spore-forming bacteria through culturomics could be a viable strategy in the future.

Multi-omics for the analysis of ancient microbiome

With metagenomics it has been possible to analyze the taxonomic composition of microorganisms and their potential metabolic function in the ancient gut microbiome. However these techniques are unable to differentiate between metabolically active and non-viable microorganisms (Daliri *et al.*, 2021). For example, studies have reported that the abundance of some taxonomic groups of the human gut microbiome does not reflect transcriptional activity (Abu-Ali *et al.*, 2018). Techniques such as metatranscriptomics, metaproteomics, and metabolomics provide a more accurate approach to analyze active metabolic functions at a given time. In addition to the above, the rapid advancement of paleoproteomics, ancient transcriptomics and ancient metabolomics opens the possibility that multi-omics can be applied to the study of the ancient microbiome (Fig. 4.4).

Metatranscriptomics consists in the identification and quantification of messenger RNA (mRNA) in a community of microorganisms or a particular environment. This approach enables the investigation of active genes and metabolic pathways in a given sample (Daliri *et al.*, 2021). In ancient samples, RNA has been less explored because its degradation is faster than other molecules such as DNA or proteins (Fordyce *et al.*, 2013b). However, studies focused on ancient transcriptomics have reported the sequencing of RNA from historical samples of animal and plant origin (Fordyce *et al.*, 2013a; Smith *et al.*, 2019), as well as the reconstruction of ancient RNA virus genomes (Smith *et al.*, 2014). The sequencing and identification of mRNA in ancient samples has changed the perception that this molecule is not preserved for thousands of years, opening the possibility that this technique could be applied to the analysis of ancient microbiome in the future. In particular, the presence of antibiotic resistance genes (ARGs) in the ancient gut microbiome has been explored with metagenomics (Wibowo *et al.*, 2021), but metatranscriptomic research of the human gut microbiome has shown that more than 50% of the ARGs in current human gut microbiome are not expressed (Wang *et al.*, 2020). Metatranscriptomic studies involving the expression of ARGs in the ancient human gut microbiome could improve our understanding of ARGs evolution. However, the lack of strategies to detect damage patterns in ancient RNA represents an obstacle in this field of research (Smith *et al.*, 2019).

Contrary to RNA, proteins are better preserved for long periods of time, which has resulted in a more attractive and developed field in the analysis of ancient samples (Wadsworth *et al.*, 2017; Lindqvist and Rajora, 2019). Metaproteomics is an approach that studies the set of proteins of a microbial community. The identification and quantification of proteins allow a better characterization of microbial systems at the functional level (Lin *et al.*, 2019). Nowadays, with bioinformatics tools it is possible to associate the presence of certain peptides with microorganisms (Muth *et al.*, 2015). Although metaproteomic analysis has not been applied to the ancient gut microbiome, a significant number of investigations have delved into dental calculus employing this approach.

In metaproteomics applied to dental calculus from Italy (1st–3rd century CE) and the United Kingdom (2nd–5th century CE), 42–241 proteins have been identified (Mackie *et al.*, 2017). In medieval Danish dental calculus (1100–1450 CE), over 3000 proteins were detected, with more than 85% attributed to bacteria, covering approximately 220 species and 81 genera (Jersie-Christensen *et al.*, 2018). Milk proteins from bovine and caprine sources were also recognized, indicating medieval dairy consumption practices (Jersie-Christensen *et al.*, 2018). This approach has also contributed to the identification of several periodontal pathogens in the ancient samples, including *C. rectus*, *C. showae*, *P. gingivalis*, and *T. forsythia* (Mackie *et al.*, 2017). Additionally, this technique has

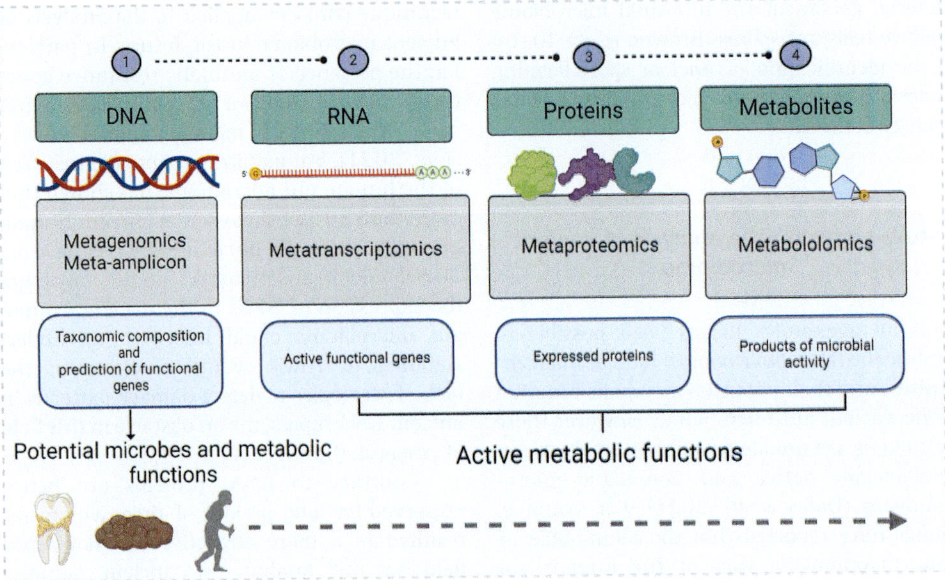

Fig. 4.4. Multi-omics approach for the study of the human ancient microbiome. Different molecules have the potential to be used in the study of ancient microbial communities and their metabolic functions. While DNA (metagenomics and meta-amplicon of 16S rRNA gene) has been widely applied for the characterization of microbial communities and prediction of metabolic functions, other molecules, and compounds such as (1) DNA (metagenomics and meta-amplicon), (2) RNA (metatranscriptomics), (3) proteins (metaproteomics), and (4) metabolites (metabolomics) can be used to directly analyze metabolic functions in ancient microbiome. Figure created with BioRender.com.

proven effective in validating microbial groups previously detected through metagenomic analysis (Warinner *et al.*, 2014; Mackie *et al.*, 2017).

With all the information generated in these studies, dental calculus has been proposed as a stable, long-term reservoir of proteins (Mackie *et al.*, 2017). In addition, it is possible to corroborate the presence of some ancient proteins thanks to the characterization of ancient damage patterns (Hendy, 2021). All this together emphasizes metaproteomics as an important approach for the study of the ancient human microbiome.

Similar to proteins, metabolites are preserved for long periods of time (Velsko *et al.*, 2017). Metabolomics studies all the metabolites in a biological sample (Daliri *et al.*, 2017). Metabolite analyses provide an advantage over the methodologies described above, as they directly reflect the biochemical reactions of cells or the metabolic state of an organism (Xu and Yang, 2021). Nowadays, there are bioinformatics tools that integrate metabolomic and metagenomic data to get a better understanding of ecological communities (Shaffer *et al.*, 2019; Reiman *et al.*, 2021). In ancient samples, metabolomic approaches have primarily concentrated on identifying plant species in artifacts such as ancient smoking pipes and in the study of ancient dental calculus (Brownstein *et al.*, 2020).

A characterization of the human dental calculus metabolome was conducted with modern and historic samples from the United Kingdom, dating back 200 years (Velsko *et al.*, 2017). Analysis involved high-resolution gas chromatography–mass spectrometry (GC–MS) and ultra-performance liquid chromatography–tandem mass spectrometry (UPLC–MS/MS). A total of 285 metabolites were identified, with 185 observed in both historical and modern samples. Notably, historical samples exhibited lower representation in specific metabolite categories, such as amino acids, vitamins, cofactors, carbohydrates, nucleotides, and peptides. In contrast, lipids (unmodified and saturated classes) demonstrated superior preservation in historical calculus, highlighting their stability over time. While the specific identification of bacterial contributions to the calculus metabolome proved challenging (Velsko *et al.*, 2017), this study represents a significant advancement in the analysis of ancient metabolomes.

On the other hand, metabolites such as bile acids and oxo-metabolites have been used for the identification of ancient human feces (coprolites) (Porru *et al.*, 2021). However, no metabolomic analyses have been conducted on ancient gut microbiomes. In particular, it has been proposed that Western modern societies (with vegan and omnivorous diet) have a restrictive gut microbiome that is not capable to produce high levels of SCFAs compared to non-Western traditional populations, even when high levels of fermentable plants are consumed (Wu *et al.*, 2016a). Furthermore, investigations have found that ancient and non-Western populations, in contrast to Western populations, exhibit greater intraspecific functional diversity in *Prevotella copri*, which is associated with active carbohydrate enzymes (CAZymes) (Tett *et al.*, 2019). It is important to highlight that CAZymes are involved in the production of short-chain fatty acids (SCFAs). In this context, the exploration of the ancient human gut microbiome, alongside metabolomics and metagenomics, could enhance our understanding of the evolution of specific gut bacteria that played a crucial role in producing health-relevant metabolites such as SCFAs. The potential of employing the aforementioned techniques in the field of ancient microbiomes has been demonstrated in recent analyses, where patterns of damage in ancient metabolites were reported in dental calculus (Velsko *et al.*, 2017). This opens the possibility of describing ancient damage patterns in other types of sources, such as coprolites and paleofeces.

In summary, despite the fact that the strategies described above have some methodological limitations that compromise their application (Johnson and Gonzalez, 2012; Schubert *et al.*, 2017), multi-omics could be used as an integral approach to obtain more information of the evolution of human-microbiome interaction.

Intra-species diversity in the ancient human microbiome

Most studies on ancient microbiome have focused on taxonomic composition and functional diversity at the species level. However, we know that human gut microbiome is also composed by genomic variants of the same bacterial species (Schloissnig *et al.*, 2013) (Fig. 4.5). This variation comprises single nucleotide variants (SNVs), insertions, inversions, deletions, and structural variants in the bacterial genome (Schloissnig *et al.*, 2013; Truong *et al.*, 2017). Genomic variants are the result of evolutionary forces (mutation and horizontal gene transfer) that lead to new strains within human gut microbiome (Gordo, 2019; Scanlan, 2019). Through these mechanisms microorganisms acquire new traits, such as antibiotic resistance and diversification of metabolic functions (Jernberg *et al.*, 2010; Maurice *et al.*, 2013; Scanlan, 2019). In the particular case of the human microbiome, it has been suggested that intra- species diversity is associated with differences in gene content and metabolic functions that impact the health of the hosts (Ellegaard and Engel, 2016) (Fig. 4.5). For example, different strains of *Blautia wexlerae* and *Ruminococcus gnavus* were recently reported to be involved in different metabolic pathways in the human gut microbiome (Sorbara *et al.*, 2020). Similarly, different strains of *P. copri* exhibit functional differences in carbohydrate metabolism in the human gut (Tett *et al.*, 2019), supporting the hypothesis that intra-species diversity also affects functional diversity.

Particularly, greater intra-species diversity has been observed in the gut microbiome of non-industrialized populations compared to Western modern societies (Pasolli *et al.*, 2019). Moreover, investigation into the intra-species diversity of *P. copri* across modern individuals and ancient samples suggested a recent loss of intraspecific diversity in modern Western societies (Tett *et al.*, 2019). Through the construction of MAGs, researchers identified four distinct clades within *P. copri* (*P. copri* complex) (Tett *et al.*, 2019). Notably, 61% of non-Western individuals exhibited all four clades, while only 4.6% of Western individuals showed the four clades. The presence of the *P. copri* complex was

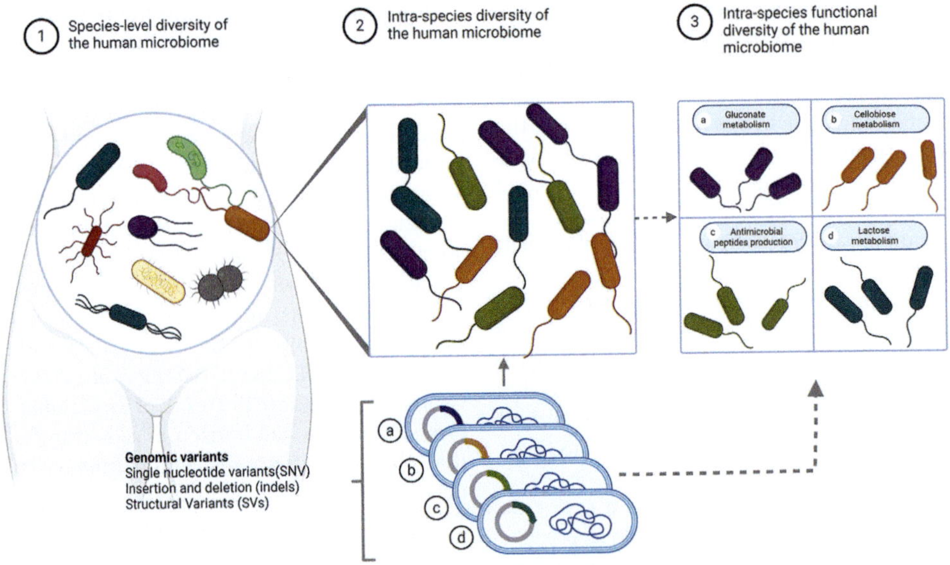

Fig. 4.5. Intraspecies diversity of the human gut microbiome: (1) the human microbiome constitutes different species of bacteria, among others, which contribute to intraspecies diversity, (2) when we delve into the study of a particular bacterial species of the human microbiome, we can find that there are genomic variants that contribute to intra-species diversity, including single nucleotide variants, insertions and deletions, and long structure variants, and (3) in addition to increasing intraspecies diversity, genomic variants may be associated with different metabolic functions, contributing to intraspecies functional diversity. Figure created with BioRender.com.

corroborated in ancient metagenomes (Tett *et al.*, 2019). This study also suggests that the divergence within the *P. copri* complex occurred before the first human migration out of Africa (Tett *et al.*, 2019), indicating that this complex has accompanied human beings for thousands of years.

In summary, modern lifestyle might not only have affected the species diversity in the gut and oral microbiome but also intra-species and functional diversity. In this sense, the analysis of the intra-species diversity of other commensal groups in the ancient human microbiome could provide relevant information on the diversification of strains and metabolic functions throughout human evolution. Particularly, this analysis can target specific microbial groups, such as *Treponema succinifaciens*, which are underrepresented in the microbiome of modern Western populations (Angelakis *et al.*, 2019).

Population structure of ancient human microbiome

The genetic population structure consists in the distribution of the genetic variation within and between populations of the same species. This structure is shaped by various evolutionary processes, including recombination, mutation, genetic drift, demographic history, and natural selection (Andam *et al.*, 2017). All this together in addition to ecological processes, determines the distribution of genes across populations of the same species. In general, few studies have focused on the population structure of the human microbiome. However, it has been proposed that the population structure of some species of the human gut are correlated with the geographic location of the host (Truong *et al.*, 2017). This is the case of *P. copri*, *Eubacterium rectale*, *Bacteroides coprocola*, and *Ruminococcus bromii* (Truong *et al.*, 2017).

In the same context, members of the oral human microbiome have been proposed as a valuable tool for exploring the demographic history of humans. This approach was implemented by analyzing metagenomic data obtained from dental calculus of individuals from two ancient cultural periods in Japan: Jomon period hunter–gatherers (3000 BP) and Edo period agriculturalists (400–150 BP) (Eisenhofer *et al.*, 2020). Whole-genome phylogenetic reconstruction revealed the presence of at least two distinct lineages of *Anaerolineaceae* strains in ancient Japan with a clear separation between Edo-associated *Anaerolineaceae* lineages and Jomon-associated *Anaerolineaceae* lineages. The origin of these two clades is likely connected to historical human demographic processes in Japan, with one hypothesis proposing the introduction of a continental Asian *Anaerolineaceae* lineage to Japan by migrants arriving from mainland Asia (Eisenhofer *et al.*, 2020).

Although some evidence of genetic population structure in the human microbiome has been found, studying the population structure of the ancient human microbiome would contribute to a better understanding of this topic. This is because; contrary to ancient populations, modern globalized societies are more connected to each other, with a more similar diet and lifestyle despite living in different geographical regions. Globalization processes have directly or indirectly affected even populations with traditional lifestyles. In contrast, ancient human populations were isolated, separated into different environments and with a diet and lifestyle adapted to the environment where they settled. This probably promoted genetic structural differentiation of some species of the human microbiome across different geographic regions. All of this considering that diet, genetics of the host, the lifestyle, and the geography play a determinant role in the structure and composition of the human microbiome (Conlon and Bird, 2015). Despite the above, this approach has not been explored in the analysis of the ancient microbiome. This is probably due to the lack of a large number of ancient samples.

Recovery of ancient microbiome from sediments and other sources

Analyzing DNA in sediments is rapidly becoming an important strategy in aDNA studies. With DNA sequencing of sediments from caves and other environments, it has been possible to identify different species of extinct animals (Zavala *et al.*, 2021). These works include the successful reconstruction of a Neanderthal mitochondrial genome (Slon *et al.*, 2017). Under this approach, investigations have attempted to sequence and identify some members of the gut microbiome of Neanderthals and humans from sediments of archaeological sites (Sabin *et al.*, 2020; Rampelli *et al.*, 2021). Although these works were able to successfully identify species of the gut microbiome, it is still necessary to corroborate that the information generated is not the result of different sources of contamination, since unlike coprolites, the sediments are more exposed and in direct contact with the environment. The use of bioinformatic tools that integrate the analysis of bacterial communities and the DNA sequences of the potential host should be essential in this new approach (Borry *et al.*, 2020). However, in the future, this line of research promises to generate valuable information about the ancient microbiome, especially in places where environmental conditions do not allow the preservation of coprolites or paleofeces.

Finally, a novel approach involving the analysis of chewed birch pitch from a 5700-year-old human has been proposed for the study of ancient oral microbiome (Jensen *et al.*, 2019). By applying metagenomics to the chewed birch pitch, the successful recovery of the ancient microbiome and the human ancient genome was achieved. This analysis also revealed various species associated with pneumococcal disease, such as *Streptococcus viridans* and multiple *Streptococcus pneumoniae* strains (Jensen *et al.*, 2019). The confirmation of the oral microbiome in chewed birch pitch expands the possibility of studying the ancient human microbiome using sources beyond coprolites, paleofeces, teeth, and calculus.

Conclusion

Despite the long journey studying the ancient human microbiome, it is now that we can exploit the great informative potential of ancient samples (coprolites, paleofeces, dental calculus), thanks to the knowledge generated both in microbial ecology and in the characterization and recovery of ancient molecules. In this review, we explored a series of approaches that have been applied in current human microbiome research but less explored in the ancient microbiome. Although they have methodological limitations, some of them have been successfully applied to ancient samples, promising to generate knowledge that supports this line of research. All the techniques discussed above generate relevant information without one being more important than the other, answering different questions from different perspectives. In fact, comprehensive use contributes to a better understanding of the topic, delving into the microbial groups and strains that were potentially in the microbiome of ancient human populations, as well as their possible metabolic functions. In addition to the above, it is important to note that most of the information on the ancient gut microbiome has been restricted to a limited number of coprolites. However, it has to be considered that the human microbiome is highly variable between individuals and between populations, so a greater effort is needed in the identification and characterization of a broader range of ancient human microbiome sources that cover different time scales and different geographical regions. Analyzing a broad range of samples from different populations and time scales let us understand general and specific characteristics of the different ancient populations, without assuming that all ancient populations present similar microbiome. Furthermore, through these new techniques we can even learn about the socio-cultural and health processes of the different human groups: their diet; migration processes, and diseases caused by infectious agents. It is important to highlight that the study of the ancient microbiome should not be restricted to the analysis of bacterial communities, but rather to other microorganisms that comprise the human microbiome, such as viruses, protozoa, fungi, and nematodes. All this together opens the possibility of being able to study how the ecological and evolutionary processes led to the association with the different microorganisms that are part of our body from the perspective of the holobiont.

Acknowledgements

Thanks the Posgrado en Ciencias Biologicas, UNAM and acknowledges the doctoral scholarship supported by the Consejo Nacional de Ciencia y Tecnología (CONACyT) (CVU: 776199).

Conflict of Interest

The authors of this article declare that the research was conducted in the absence of any commercial or financial relationships that could be construed as a potential conflict of interest.

Author Contributions

All three authors have made substantial and equal contributions to the development and enhancement of this research article. Santiago Rosas-Plaza led the conceptualization and development of the research article, taking charge of the initial draft and laying out the main ideas. Ximena Rosas-Plaza collaborated extensively in the refinement of the manuscript, providing critical intellectual input, revising content, and contributing to the overall improvement of the article. Rene Cerritos actively participated in the review and revision process, offering valuable insights, conducting additional analyses, and complementing the work with diverse perspectives.

Open Research Statement

No data were collected for this study. Empirical data were not used for this research.

References

Abu-Ali, G.S., Mehta, R.S., Lloyd-Price, J., Mallick, H., Branck, T. *et al.* (2018) Metatranscriptome of human faecal microbial communities in a cohort of adult men. *Nature Microbiology* 3(3), 356–366. DOI: 10.1038/s41564-017-0084-4.

Adler, C.J., Dobney, K., Weyrich, L.S., Kaidonis, J., Walker, A.W. *et al.* (2013) Sequencing ancient calcified dental plaque shows changes in oral microbiota with dietary shifts of the neolithic and industrial revolutions. *Nature Genetics* 45(4), 450–455. DOI: 10.1038/ng.2536.

Afouda, P., Dubourg, G., Levasseur, A., Fournier, P.E., Delerce, J. *et al.* (2020) Culturing ancient bacteria carrying resistance genes from permafrost and comparative genomics with modern isolates. *Microorganisms* 8(10), 1–13. DOI: 10.3390/microorganisms8101522.

Andam, C.P., Challagundla, L., Azarian, T., Hanage, W.P. and Robinson, D.A. (2017) *Population Structure of Pathogenic Bacteria. Genetics and Evolution of Infectious Diseases: Second Edition*. Elsevier Inc, Amsterdam, Netherlands. DOI: 10.1016/B978-0-12-799942-5.00003-2.

Angelakis, E., Bachar, D., Yasir, M., Musso, D., Djossou, F. *et al.* (2019) *Treponema* species enrich the gut microbiota of traditional rural populations but are absent from urban individuals. *New Microbes and New Infections* 27, 14–21. DOI: 10.1016/j.nmni.2018.10.009.

Appelt, S., Armougom, F., Le Bailly, M., Robert, C. and Drancourt, M. (2014) Polyphasic analysis of a middle ages coprolite microbiota, Belgium. *PloS ONE* 9(2), 1–8. DOI: 10.1371/journal.pone.0088376.

Ayeni, F.A., Biagi, E., Rampelli, S., Fiori, J., Soverini, M. *et al.* (2018) Infant and adult gut microbiome and metabolome in rural bassa and urban settlers from Nigeria. *Cell Reports* 23(10), 3056–3067. DOI: 10.1016/j.celrep.2018.05.018.

Borry, M., Cordova, B., Perri, A., Wibowo, M., Honap, T.P. *et al.* (2020) CoprolD predicts the source of coprolites and paleofeces using microbiome composition and host DNA content. *PeerJ* 2020(4), 1–23. DOI: 10.7717/peerj.9001.

Briggs, A.W., Stenzel, U., Meyer, M., Krause, J., Kircher, M. *et al.* (2009) Removal of deaminated cytosines and detection of *in vivo* methylation in ancient DNA. *Nucleic Acids Research* 38(6), e87–e87. DOI: 10.1093/nar/gkp1163.

Browne, H.P., Forster, S.C., Anonye, B.O., Kumar, N., Neville, B.A. *et al.* (2016) Culturing of 'unculturable' human microbiota reveals novel taxa and extensive sporulation. *Nature* 533(7604), 543–546. DOI: 10.1038/nature17645.

Brownstein, K.J., Tushingham, S., Damitio, W.J., Nguyen, T. and Gang, D.R. (2020) An ancient residue metabolomics-based method to distinguish use of closely related plant species in ancient pipes. *Frontiers in Molecular Biosciences* 7(Jun), 1–14. DOI: 10.3389/fmolb.2020.00133.

Cano, R.J., Tiefenbrunner, F., Ubaldi, M., Del Cueto, C., Luciani, S. *et al.* (2000) Sequence analysis of bacterial DNA in the colon and stomach of the Tyrolean iceman. *American Journal of Physical Anthropology* 112(3), 297–309. DOI: 10.1002/1096-8644(200007)112:3<297::AID-AJPA2>3.0.CO;2-0.

Cano, R.J., Rivera-Perez, J., Toranzos, G.A., Santiago-Rodriguez, T.M., Narganes-Storde, Y.M. *et al.* (2014) Paleomicrobiology: Revealing fecal microbiomes of ancient indigenous cultures. *PloS ONE* 9(9), 1–15. DOI: 10.1371/journal.pone.0106833.

Caporaso, J.G., Kuczynski, J., Stombaugh, J., Bittinger, K., Bushman, F.D. *et al.* (2010) QIIME allows analysis of high-throughput community sequencing data. *Nature Publishing Group* 7(5), 335–336. DOI: 10.1038/nmeth0510-335.

Carøe, C., Gopalakrishnan, S., Vinner, L., Mak, S.S.T., Sinding, M.H.S. *et al.* (2018) Single-tube library preparation for degraded DNA. *Methods in Ecology and Evolution* 9(2), 410–419. DOI: 10.1111/2041-210X.12871.

Chaumeil, P., Mussig, A.J., Parks, D.H. and Hugenholtz, P. (2020) GTDB- tk: A toolkit to classify genomes with the genome taxonomy database. *Bioinformatics* 36(6), 1925–1727. DOI: 10.1093/bioinformatics/btz848.

Chen, Y., Ye, W., Zhang, Y. and Xu, Y. (2015) High speed BLASTN: An accelerated megablast search tool. *Nucleic Acids Research* 43(16), 7762–7768. DOI: 10.1093/nar/gkv784.

Cole, J.R., Wang, Q., Fish, J.A., Chai, B., McGarrell, D.M. *et al.* (2014) Ribosomal database project: Data and tools for high throughput RRNA analysis. *Nucleic Acids Research* 42(D1), 633–642. DOI: 10.1093/nar/gkt1244.

Conlon, M.A. and Bird, A.R. (2015) The impact of diet and lifestyle on gut microbiota and human health. *Nutrients* 7(1), 17–44. DOI: 10.3390/un7010017.

Dabney, J., Meyer, M. and Pääbo, S. (2013) Ancient DNA damage. *Cold Spring Harbor Perspectives in Biology* 5(7), 1–7. DOI: 10.1101/cshperspect.a012567.

Daliri, E.B.M., Wei, S., Oh, D.H. and Lee, B.H. (2017) The human microbiome and metabolomics: Current concepts and applications. *Critical Reviews in Food Science and Nutrition* 57(16), 3565–3576. DOI: 10.1080/10408398.2016.1220913.

Daliri, E.B.M., Ofosu, F.K., Chelliah, R., Lee, B.H. and Oh, D.H. (2021) Challenges and perspective in integrated multi-omics in gut microbiota studies. *Biomolecules* 11(2), 1–10. DOI: 10.3390/biom11020300.

De Filippo, C., Cavalieri, D., Paola, M.D., Ramazzotti, M., Poullet, J.B. *et al.* (2010) Impact of diet in shaping gut microbiota revealed by a comparative study in children from Europe and rural Africa. *Proceedings of the National Academy of Sciences of the United States of America* 107(33), 14691–14696. DOI: 10.1073/pnas.1005963107.

Der Sarkissian, C., Ermini, L., Jónsson, H., Alekseev, A.N., Crubezy, E. *et al.* (2014) Shotgun microbial profiling of fossil remains. *Molecular Ecology* 23(7), 1780–1798. DOI: 10.1111/mec.12690.

Eisenhofer, R., Kanzawa-Kiriyama, H., Shinoda, K.I. and Weyrich, L.S. (2020) Investigating the demographic history of Japan using ancient oral microbiota: Ancient Japanese dental calculus. *Philosophical Transactions of the Royal Society B: Biological Sciences* 375(1812), 1–11. DOI: 10.1098/rstb.2019.0578.

Ellegaard, K.M. and Engel, P. (2016) Beyond 16S RRNA community profiling: Intra-species diversity in the gut microbiota. *Frontiers in Microbiology* 7(Sep), 1–16. DOI: 10.3389/fmicb.2016.01475.

Fordyce, S.L., Ávila-Arcos, M.C., Rasmussen, M., Cappellini, E., Romero-Navarro, J.A. *et al.* (2013a) Deep sequencing of RNA from ancient maize kernels. *PLoS ONE* 8(1), 1–9. DOI: 10.1371/journal.pone.0050961.

Fordyce, S.L., Kampmann, M.L., Doorn, N.L. and Gilbert, M.T.P. (2013b) Long-term RNA persistence in postmortem contexts. *Investigative Genetics* 4(1), 1–7. DOI: 10.1186/2041-2223-4-7.

Franzosa, E.A., Mciver, L.J., Rahnavard, G., Thompson, L.R., Schirmer, M. *et al.* (2018) Species-level functional profiling of metagenomes and metatranscriptomes. *Nature Methods* 15(Nov), 962–968. DOI: 10.1038/s41592-018-0176-y.

Ginolhac, A., Rasmussen, M., Gilbert, M.T.P., Willerslev, E. and Orlando, L. (2011) MapDamage: Testing for damage patterns in ancient DNA sequences. *Bioinformatics* 27(15), 2153–2155. DOI: 10.1093/bioinformatics/btr347.

Glassing, A., Dowd, S.E., Galandiuk, S., Davis, B. and Chiodini, R.J. (2016) Inherent bacterial DNA contamination of extraction and sequencing reagents may affect interpretation of microbiota in low bacterial biomass samples. *Gut Pathogens* 8(1), 1–12. DOI: 10.1186/s13099-016-0103-7.

Gordo, I. (2019) Evolutionary change in the human gut microbiome: From a static to a dynamic view. *PLoS Biology* 17(2), 1–5. DOI: 10.1371/journal.pbio.3000126.

Granehäll, L., Huang, K.D., Tett, A., Manghi, P., Paladin, A. *et al.* (2021) Metagenomic analysis of ancient dental calculus reveals unexplored diversity of oral archaeal methanobrevibacter. *Microbiome* 9(1), 1–18. DOI: 10.1186/s40168-021-01132-8.

Grigorenko, A.P., Borinskaya, S.A., Yankovsky, N.K. and Rogaev, E.I. (2009) Achievements and peculiarities in studies of ancient DNA and DNA from complicated forensic specimens. *Acta Naturae* 1(3), 58–69. DOI: 10.32607/actanaturae.10766.

Hagan, R.W., Hofman, C.A., Hübner, A., Reinhard, K., Schnorr, S. *et al.* (2020) Comparison of extraction methods for recovering ancient microbial DNA from paleofeces. *American Journal of Physical Anthropology* 171(2), 275–284. DOI: 10.1002/ajpa.23978.

Hansen, M.E.B., Rubel, M.A., Bailey, A.G., Ranciaro, A., Thompson, S.R. *et al.* (2019) Population structure of human gut bacteria in a diverse cohort from rural Tanzania and Botswana. *Genome Biology* 20(16), 1–21. DOI: 10.1186/s13059-018-1616-9.

Hendy, J. (2021) Ancient protein analysis in archaeology. *Science Advances* 7(3), 1–11. DOI: 10.1126/sciadv.abb9314.

Henneberger, K., Barlow, A. and Paijmans, J.L.A. (2019) Double-stranded library preparation for ancient and other degraded samples. In: Shapiro, B., Barlow, A., Heintzman, P.D., Hofreiter, M., Paijmans, J.L.A. et al. (eds) *Authentication and Assessment of Contamination in Ancient DNA*. Springer, Hatfield, Hertfordshire, pp. 65–73.

Herbig, A., Maixner, F., Bos, K.I., Zink, A., Krause, J. *et al.* (2016) MALT: Fast alignment and analysis of metagenomic DNA sequence data applied to the Tyrolean iceman. *BioRxiv*.

Hübler, R., Key, F.M., Warinner, C., Bos, K.I., Krause, J. *et al.* (2019) HOPS: Automated detection and authentication of pathogen DNA in archaeological remains. *Genome Biology* 20(280), 1–13.

Huynh, H.T.T., Nkamga, V.D., Signoli, M., Tzortzis, S., Pinguet, R. *et al.* (2016) Restricted diversity of dental calculus methanogens over five centuries, France. *Nature Publishing Group* 6(1), 4–9. DOI: 10.1038/srep25775.

Jacobson, D.K., Honap, T.P., Monroe, C., Lund, J., Houk, B.A. *et al.* (2020) Functional diversity of microbial ecologies estimated from ancient human coprolites and dental calculus: Ecology and ancient human microbiota. *Philosophical Transactions of the Royal Society B: Biological Sciences* 375(1812), 1–11. DOI: 10.1098/rstb.2019.0586.

Jensen, T.Z.T., Niemann, J., Iversen, K.H., Fotakis, A.K., Gopalakrishnan, S. *et al.* (2019) A 5700 year-old human genome and oral microbiome from chewed birch pitch. *Nature Communications* 10(1), 1–10. DOI: 10.1038/s41467-019-13549-9.

Jernberg, C., Lofmark, S., Edlund, C. and Jansson, J.K. (2010) Long- term impacts of antibiotic exposure on the human intestinal microbiota. *Microbiology* 156(11), 3216–3223. DOI: 10.1099/mic.0.040618-0.

Jersie-Christensen, R.R., Lanigan, L.T., Lyon, D., Mackie, M., Belstrøm, D. *et al.* (2018) Quantitative metaproteomics of medieval dental calculus reveals individual oral health status. *Nature Communications* 9(1), 1–12. DOI: 10.1038/s41467-018-07148-3.

Jha, A.R., Davenport, E.R., Gautam, Y., Bhandari, D., Tandukar, S. *et al.* (2018) Gut microbiome transition across a lifestyle gradient in Himalaya. *PLoS Biology* 16(11), 1–30. DOI: 10.1371/journal.pbio.2005396.

Johnson, C.H. and Gonzalez, F.J. (2012) Challenges and opportunities of metabolomics. *Journal of Cellular Physiology* 227(8), 2975–2981. DOI: 10.1002/jcp.24002.

Kang, D.D., Li, F., Kirton, E., Thomas, A., Egan, R. *et al.* (2019) MetaBAT 2: An adaptive binning algorithm for robust and efficient genome reconstruction from metagenome assemblies. *PeerJ* 2019(7), 1–13. DOI: 10.7717/peerj.7359.

Kazarina, A., Petersone-Gordina, E., Kimsis, J., Kuzmicka, J., Zayakin, P. *et al.* (2021) The postmedieval latvian oral microbiome in the context of modern dental calculus and modern dental plaque microbial profiles. *Genes* 12(2), 1–16. DOI: 10.3390/genes12020309.

Kim, M., Wilpiszeski, R.L., Wells, M., Wymore, A.M., Gionfriddo, C.M. *et al.* (2021) Metagenome-assembled genome sequences of novel prokaryotic species from the mercury-contaminated east fork poplar creek. *Microbiology Resource Announcements* 10(17), 1–5. DOI: 10.1128/mra.00153-21.

Knights, D., Kuczynski, J., Charlson, E.S., Zaneveld, J., Mozer, M.C. *et al.* (2011) Bayesian community-wide culture-independent microbial source tracking. *Nature Methods* 8(9), 761–765. DOI: 10.1038/nmeth.1650.

Kuhlwilm, M., Gronau, I., Hubisz, M.J., Filippo, C., Prado-Martinez, J. *et al.* (2016) Ancient gene flow from early modern humans into eastern neanderthals. *Nature* 530(7591), 429–433. DOI: 10.1038/nature16544.

Lagier, J.C., Khelaifia, S., Alou, M.T., Ndongo, S., Dione, N. *et al.* (2016) Culture of previously uncultured members of the human gut microbiota by culturomics. *Nature Microbiology* 1(Dec), 1–8. DOI: 10.1038/nmicrobiol.2016.203.

Li, D., Liu, C.M., Luo, R., Sadakane, K. and Lam, T.W. (2015) MEGAHIT: An ultra-fast single-node solution for large and complex metagenomics assembly via succinct de Bruijn graph. *Bioinformatics* 31(10), 1674–1676. DOI: 10.1093/bioinformatics/btv033.

Lin, H., He, Q.Y., Shi, L., Sleeman, M., Baker, M.S. *et al.* (2019) Proteomics and the microbiome: Pitfalls and potential. *Expert Review of Proteomics* 16(6), 501–511. DOI: 10.1080/14789450.2018.1523724.

Lindqvist, C. and Rajora, O.P. (eds) (2019) *Paleogenomics: Genome- Scale Analysis of Ancient DNA*. Springer, Switzerland.

Lloyd-Price, J., Abu-Ali, G. and Huttenhower, C. (2016) The healthy human microbiome. *Genome Medicine* 8(1), 1–11. DOI: 10.1186/s13073-016-0307-y.

Luciani, S., Fornaciari, G., Rickards, O., Labarga, C.M. and Rollo, F. (2006) Molecular characterization of a pre-columbian mummy and *in situ* coprolite. *American Journal of Physical Anthropology* 129(4), 620–629. DOI: 10.1002/ajpa.

Mackie, M., Hendy, J., Lowe, A.D., Sperduti, A., Holst, M. *et al.* (2017) Preservation of the metaproteome: Variability of protein preservation in ancient dental calculus. *Science and Technology of Archaeological Research* 3(1), 58–70. DOI: 10.1080/20548923.2017.1361629.

Maurice, C.F., Haiser, H.J. and Turnbaugh, P.J. (2013) Xenobiotics shape the physiology and gene expression of the active human gut microbiome. *Cell* 152(1–2), 39–50. DOI: 10.1016/j.cell.2012.10.052.

McDonald, D., Price, M.N., Goodrich, J., Nawrocki, E.P., DeSantis, T.Z. *et al.* (2012) An improved greengenes taxonomy with explicit ranks for ecological and evolutionary analyses of bacteria and archaea. *The ISME Journal* 6(3), 610–618. DOI: 10.1038/ismej.2011.139.

Meyer, M. and Kircher, M. (2010) Illumina sequencing library preparation for highly multiplexed target capture and sequencing. *Cold Spring Harbor Protocols* 2010(6), 1–11. DOI: 10.1101/pdb.prot5448.

Mohanty, R., Asopa, S.J., Joseph, M.D., Singh, B., Rajguru, J.P. *et al.* (2019) Red complex: Polymicrobial conglomerate in oral flora: A review. *Journal of Family Medicine and Primary Care* 8(11), 3480–3486. DOI: 10.4103/jfmpc.jfmpc.

Muth, T., Behne, A., Heyer, R., Kohrs, F., Benndorf, D. *et al.* (2015) The metaproteomeanalyzer: A powerful open-source software suite for metaproteomics data analysis and interpretation. *Journal of Proteome Research* 14(3), 1557–1565. DOI: 10.1021/pr501246w.

Neukamm, J., Pfrengle, S., Molak, M., Seitz, A., Francken, M. *et al.* (2020) 2000-year-old pathogen genomes reconstructed from metagenomic analysis of Egyptian mummified individuals. *BMC Biology* 18(1), 1–18. DOI: 10.1186/s12915-020-00839-8.

Neukamm, J., Peltzer, A. and Nieselt, K. (2021) DamageProfiler: Fast damage pattern calculation for ancient DNA. *Bioinformatics* 37(20), 3652–3653. DOI: 10.1093/bioinformatics/btab190.

Nicholson, W.L., Munakata, N., Horneck, G., Melosh, H.J. and Setlow, P. (2000) Resistance of bacillus endospores to extreme terrestrial and extraterrestrial environments. *Microbiology and Molecular Biology Reviews* 64(3), 548–572. DOI: 10.1128/mmbr.64.3.548-572.2000.

Nurk, S., Meleshko, D., Korobeynikov, A. and Pevzner, P.A. (2017) MetaSPAdes: A new versatile metagenomic assembler. *Genome Research* 27(5), 824–834. DOI: 10.1101/gr.213959.116.

Parks, D.H., Imelfort, M., Skennerton, C.T., Hugenholtz, P. and Tyson, G.W. (2015) CheckM: Assessing the quality of microbial genomes recovered from isolates, single cells, and metagenomes. *Genome Research* 25, 1043–1055. DOI: 10.1101/gr.186072.114.Freely.

Pasolli, E., Asnicar, F., Manara, S., Zolfo, M., Karcher, N. *et al.* (2019) Extensive unexplored human microbiome diversity revealed by over 150,000 genomes from metagenomes spanning age, geography, and lifestyle. *Cell* 176(3), 649–662. DOI: 10.1016/j.cell.2019.01.001.

Pati, A., Heath, L.S., Kyrpides, N.C. and Ivanova, N. (2011) ClaMS: A classifier for metagenomic sequences Amrita. *Standards in Genomic Sciences* 5, 248–253. DOI: 10.4056/sigs.2075298.

Pérez-Cobas, A.E., Gomez-Valero, L. and Buchrieser, C. (2020) Metagenomic approaches in microbial ecology: An update on whole- genome and marker gene sequencing analyses. *Microbial Genomics* 6(8), 1–22. DOI: 10.1099/mgen.0.000409.

Peyrégne, S. and Peter, B.M. (2020) AuthentiCT: A model of ancient DNA damage to estimate the proportion of present-day DNA contamination. *Genome Biology* 21(1), 1–16. DOI: 10.1186/s13059-020-02123-y.

Peyrégne, S. and Prüfer, K. (2020) Present-day DNA contamination in ancient DNA datasets. *BioEssays* 42(9), 1–11. DOI: 10.1002/bies.202000081.

Philips, A., Stolarek, I., Handschuh, L., Nowis, K., Juras, A. *et al.* (2020) Analysis of oral microbiome from fossil human remains revealed the significant differences in virulence factors of modern and ancient *Tannerella forsythia*. *BMC Genomics* 21(1), 1–14. DOI: 10.1186/s12864-020-06810-9.

Pochon, Z., Bergfeldt, N., Kırdök, E., Vicente, M., Naidoo, T. *et al.* (2023) AMeta: An accurate and memory-efficient ancient metagenomic profiling workflow. *Genome Biology* 24(242), 1–30. DOI: 10.1186/s13059-023-03083-9.

Porru, E., Giorgi, E., Turroni, S., Helg, R., Silani, M. *et al.* (2021) Bile acids and oxo-metabolites as markers of human faecal input in the ancient Pompeii ruins. *Scientific Reports* 11(1), 1–7. DOI: 10.1038/s41598-021-82831-y.

Quagliariello, A., Modi, A., Innocenti, G., Zaro, V., Barbaro, C.C. *et al.* (2022) Ancient oral microbiomes support gradual neolithic dietary shifts towards agriculture. *Nature Communications* 13(1), 1–14. DOI: 10.1038/s41467-022-34416-0au.

Rampelli, S., Turroni, S., Mallol, C., Hernandez, C., Galván, B. *et al.* (2021) Components of a neanderthal gut microbiome recovered from fecal sediments from el salt. *Communications Biology* 4(1), 1–10. DOI: 10.1038/s42003-021-01689-y.

Reiman, D., Layden, B.T. and Dai, Y. (2021) MiMeNet: Exploring microbiome-metabolome relationships using neural networks. *PLoS Computational Biology* 17(5), 1–25. DOI: 10.1371/journal.pcbi.1009021.

Reinhard, K.J. and Vaughn, B. (1992) Coprolite analysis: A biological perspective on archaeology. *Archaeological Method and Theory* 4, 245–288.

Renaud, G., Schubert, M., Sawyer, S. and Orlando, L. (2019) Authentication and assessment of contamination in ancient DNA. In: Shapiro, B., Barlow, A., Heintzman, P.D., Hofreiter, M., Paijmans, J.L.A. et al. (eds) *Authentication and Assessment of Contamination in Ancient DNA*, 2nd edn. Springer, pp. 163–194. DOI: 10.1007/978-1-4939-9176-1_17.

Rifkin, R.F., Vikram, S., Ramond, J.-B., Rey-Iglesia, A., Brand, T.B. *et al.* (2020) Multi-proxy analyses of a mid-15th century middle iron age bantu-speaker palaeo-faecal specimen elucidates the configuration of the 'ancestral' sub-Saharan African intestinal microbiome. *Microbiome* 8(1), 1–23. DOI: 10.1186/s40168-020-00832-x.

Rohland, N., Harney, E., Mallick, S., Nordenfelt, S. and Reich, D. (2015) Partial uracil – DNA – glycosylase treatment for screening of ancient DNA. *Philosophical Transactions of the Royal Society B: Biological Sciences* 370(1660), 1–11. DOI: 10.1098/rstb.2013.0624.

Rollo, F., Luciani, S., Marota, I., Olivieri, C. and Ermini, L. (2007) Persistence and decay of the intestinal microbiota's DNA in glacier mummies from the alps. *Journal of Archaeological Science* 34(8), 1294–1305. DOI: 10.1016/j.jas.2006.10.019.

Rosas-Plaza, S., Hernández-Terán, A., Navarro-Díaz, M., Escalante, A.E., Morales-Espinosa, R. *et al.* (2022) Human gut microbiome across different lifestyles: From hunter-gatherers to urban populations. *Frontiers in Microbiology* 13(Apr), 1–10. DOI: 10.3389/fmicb.2022.843170.

Sabin, S., Yeh, H.Y., Pluskowski, A., Clamer, C., Mitchell, P.D. *et al.* (2020) Estimating molecular preservation of the intestinal microbiome via metagenomic analyses of latrine sediments from two medieval cities: Metagenomic analyses of ancient latrines. *Philosophical Transactions of the Royal Society B: Biological Sciences* 375(1812), 1–15. DOI: 10.1098/rstb.2019.0576rstb20190576.

Santiago-Rodriguez, T.M., Narganes-Storde, Y.M., Chanlatte, L., Crespo-Torres, E., Toranzos, G.A. *et al.* (2013) Microbial communities in pre-columbian coprolites. *PLoS ONE* 8(6), 1–12. DOI: 10.1371/journal.pone.0065191.

Santiago-Rodriguez, T.M., Fornaciari, G., Luciani, S., Dowd, S.E., Toranzos, G.A. *et al.* (2015) Gut microbiome of an 11th century a.d. *Pre-Columbian Andean Mummy. PLoS ONE* 10(9), 1–23. DOI: 10.1371/journal.pone.0138135.

Santiago-Rodriguez, T.M., Fornaciari, G., Luciani, S., Dowd, S.E., Toranzos, G.A. *et al.* (2016) Taxonomic and predicted metabolic profiles of the human gut microbiome in pre-columbian mummies. *FEMS Microbiology Ecology* 92(11), fiw182. DOI: 10.1093/femsec/fiw182.

Santiago-Rodriguez, T.M., Narganes-Storde, Y., Toranzos, G.A. and Cano, R.J. (2017) Insights of the dental calculi microbiome of pre-columbian inhabitants from Puerto Rico. *PeerJ* 1–24. DOI: 10.7717/peerj.3277.

Santiago-Rodriguez, T.M., Fornaciari, A., Fornaciari, G., Luciani, S., Marota, I. *et al.* (2019) Commensal and pathogenic members of the dental calculus microbiome of Badia Pozzeveri individuals from the 11th to 19th centuries. *Genes* 10(299), 1–15.

Sarhan, M.S., Lehmkuhl, A., Straub, R., Tett, A. and Wieland, G. (2021) Ancient DNA diffuses from human bones to cave stones. *IScience* 24(12), 103397. DOI: 10.1016/j.isci.2021.103397.

Scanlan, P.D. (2019) Microbial evolution and ecological opportunity in the gut environment. *Proceedings of the Royal Society B: Biological Sciences* 286(1915), 1–9. DOI: 10.1098/rspb.2019.1964.

Schloissnig, S., Arumugam, M., Sunagawa, S., Mitreva, M., Tap, J. *et al.* (2013) Genomic variation landscape of the human gut microbiome. *Nature* 493(7430), 45–50. DOI: 10.1038/nature11711.

Schloss, P.D., Westcott, S.L., Ryabin, T., Hall, J.R., Hartmann, M. *et al.* (2009) Introducing mothur: Open-source, platform-independent, community-supported software for describing and comparing microbial communities. *Applied and Environmental Microbiology* 75(23), 7537–7541. DOI: 10.1128/AEM.01541-09.

Schnorr, S.L., Candela, M., Rampelli, S., Centanni, M., Consolandi, C. *et al.* (2014) Gut microbiome of the Hadza hunter-gatherers. *Nature Communications* 5(3654), 1–12. DOI: 10.1038/ncomms4654.

Schubert, M., Ermini, L., Sarkissian, C., Jónsson, H., Ginolhac, A. *et al.* (2014) Characterization of ancient and modern genomes by SNP detection and phylogenomic and metagenomic analysis using PALEOMIX. *Nature Protocols* 9(5), 1056–1082. DOI: 10.1038/nprot.2014.063.

Schubert, O.T., Röst, H.L., Collins, B.C., Rosenberger, G. and Aebersold, R. (2017) Quantitative proteomics: Challenges and opportunities in basic and applied research. *Nature Protocols* 12(7), 1289–1294. DOI: 10.1038/nprot.2017.040.

Selber-Hnativ, S., Rukundo, B., Ahmadi, M., Akoubi, H., Al-Bizri, H. *et al.* (2017) Human gut microbiota: Toward an ecology of disease. *Frontiers in Microbiology* 8(1265), 1–19. DOI: 10.3389/fmicb.2017.01265.

Shaffer, M., Thurimella, K., Quinn, K., Doenges, K., Zhang, X. *et al.* (2019) AMON: Annotation of metabolite origins via networks to integrate microbiome and metabolome data. *BMC Bioinformatics* 20(1), 1–11. DOI: 10.1186/s12859-019-3176-8.

Shenhav, L., Thompson, M., Joseph, T.A., Briscoe, L., Furman, O. *et al.* (2019) FEAST: Fast expectation-maximization for microbial source tracking. *Nature Methods* 16(7), 627–632. DOI: 10.1038/s41592-019-0431-x.

Slon, V., Hopfe, C., Weiß, C.L., Mafessoni, F., Rasilla, M. *et al.* (2017) Neandertal and denisovan DNA from Pleistocene sediments Viviane. *Science* 356(6338), 605–608.

Smith, O., Clapham, A., Rose, P., Liu, Y., Wang, J. *et al.* (2014) A complete ancient RNA genome: Identification, reconstruction and evolutionary history of archaeological barley stripe mosaic virus. *Scientific Reports* 4, 1–6. DOI: 10.1038/srep04003.

Smith, O., Dunshea, G., Sinding, M.H.S., Fedorov, S., Germonpre, M. *et al.* (2019) Ancient RNA from late pleistocene permafrost and historical canids shows tissue-specific transcriptome survival. *PLoS Biology* 17(7), 1–28. DOI: 10.1371/journal.pbio.3000166.

Sorbara, M.T., Littmann, E.R., Fontana, E., Moody, T.U., Kohout, C.E. *et al.* (2020) Functional and genomic variation between human-derived isolates of lachnospiraceae reveals inter- and intra-species diversity. *Cell Host and Microbe* 28(1), 134–146. DOI: 10.1016/j.chom.2020.05.005.

Spyrou, M.A., Bos, K.I., Herbig, A. and Krause, J. (2019) Ancient pathogen genomics as an emerging tool for infectious disease research. *Nature Reviews Genetics* 20(6), 323–340. DOI: 10.1038/s41576-019-0119-1.

Tett, A., Huang, K.D., Asnicar, F., Fehlner-Peach, H., Pasolli, E. *et al.* (2019) The prevotella copri complex comprises four distinct clades underrepresented in westernized populations. *Cell Host and Microbe* 26(5), 666–679. DOI: 10.1016/j.chom.2019.08.018.

Tito, R.Y., Knights, D., Metcalf, J., Obregon-Tito, A.J., Cleeland, L. *et al.* (2012) Insights from characterizing extinct human gut microbiomes. *PLoS ONE* 7(12), 1–8. DOI: 10.1371/journal.pone.0051146.

Truong, D.T., Franzosa, E.A., Tickle, T.L., Scholz, M., Weingart, G. *et al.* (2015) MetaPhlAn2 for enhanced metagenomic taxonomic profiling. *Nature Methods* 12(10), 902–903. DOI: 10.1038/nmeth.3589.

Truong, D.T., Tett, A., Pasolli, E. and Huttenhower, C. (2017) Microbial strain-level population structure and genetic diversity from metagenomes. *Genome Research* 27(4), 626–638. DOI: 10.1101/gr.216242.116.Freely.

Ubaldi, M., Luciani, S., Marota, I., Fornaciari, G., Cano, R.J. *et al.* (1998) Sequence analysis of bacterial DNA in the colon of an andean mummy. *American Journal of Physical Anthropology* 107(3), 285–295. DOI: 10.1002/(SICI)1096-8644(199811)107:3<285::AID-AJPA5>3.0.CO;2-U.

van de Guchte, M., Blottière, H.M. and Doré, J. (2018) Humans as holobionts: Implications for prevention and therapy. *Microbiome* 6(1), 81. DOI: 10.1186/s40168-018-0466-8.

Velsko, I.M., Overmyer, K.A., Speller, C., Klaus, L., Collins, M.J. *et al.* (2017) The dental calculus metabolome in modern and historic samples. *Metabolomics* 13(11), 1–17. DOI: 10.1007/s11306-017-1270-3.

Velsko, I.M., Frantz, L.A.F., Herbig, A., Larson, G. and Warinner, C. (2018) Selection of appropriate metagenome taxonomic classifiers for ancient microbiome research. *MSystems* 3(4), 1–23. DOI: 10.1128/msystems.00080-18.

Velsko, I.M., Fellows Yates, J.A., Aron, F., Hagan, R.W., Frantz, L.A.F. *et al.* (2019) Microbial differences between dental plaque and historic dental calculus are related to oral biofilm maturation stage. *Microbiome* 7(1), 1–20. DOI: 10.1186/s40168-019-0717-3.

Wadsworth, C., Procopio, N., Anderung, C., Carretero, J.M., Iriarte, E. *et al.* (2017) Comparing ancient DNA survival and proteome content in 69 archaeological cattle tooth and bone samples from multiple European sites. *Journal of Proteomics* 158, 1–8. DOI: 10.1016/j.jprot.2017.01.004.

Wakefield, E.G. and Dellinger, S.C. (1936) Diet of the bluff dwellers of the ozark mountains, and its skeletal effects. *Annals of Internal Medicine* 9(10), 1412–1418.

Wang, Y., Hu, Y., Liu, F., Cao, J., Lv, N. *et al.* (2020) Integrated metagenomic and metatranscriptomic profiling reveals differentially expressed resistomes in human, chicken, and pig gut microbiomes. *Environment International* 138(Dec 2019), 1–12. DOI: 10.1016/j.envint.2020.105649.

Warinner, C., Matias Rodrigues, J.F., Vyas, R., Trachsel, C., Shved, N. *et al.* (2014) Pathogens and host immunity in the ancient human oral cavity. *Nature Genetics* 46(4), 336–344. DOI: 10.1038/ng.2906.

Warinner, C., Speller, C., Collins, M.J. and Lewis, C.M. (2015) Ancient human microbiomes. *Journal of Human Evolution* 79, 125–136. DOI: 10.1016/j.jhevol.2014.10.016.

Weyrich, L.S., Farrer, A.G., Eisenhofer, R., Arriola, L.A., Young, J. *et al.* (2019) Laboratory contamination over time during low-biomass sample analysis. *Molecular Ecology Resources* 19(4), 982–996. DOI: 10.1111/1755-0998.13011.

White, A.E., De-Dios, T., Carrión, P., Bonora, G.L., Llovera, L. *et al.* (2021) Genomic analysis of 18th-century Kazakh individuals and their oral microbiome. *Biology* 10(1324), 1–21.

Wibowo, M.C., Yang, Z., Borry, M., Hübner, A., Huang, K.D. *et al.* (2021) Reconstruction of ancient microbial genomes from the human gut. *Nature* 594, 234–239. DOI: 10.1038/s41586-021-03532-0.

Wilkins, L.G.E., Ettinger, C.L., Jospin, G. and Eisen, J.A. (2019) Metagenome-assembled genomes provide new insight into the microbial diversity of two thermal pools in Kamchatka, Russia. *Scientific Reports* 9(1), 1–15. DOI: 10.1038/s41598-019-39576-6.

Wood, D.E. and Salzberg, S.L. (2014) Kraken: Ultrafast metagenomic sequence classification using exact alignments. *Genome Biology* 15(46), 1–12.

Wu, G.D., Compher, C., Chen, E.Z., Smith, S.A., Shah, R.D. *et al.* (2016a) Comparative metabolomics in vegans and omnivores reveal constraints on diet-dependent gut microbiota metabolite production. *Gut* 65(1), 63–72. DOI: 10.1136/gutjnl-2014-308209.

Wu, Y.-W., Simmons, B.A. and Singer, S.W. (2016b) MaxBin 2.0: An automated binning algorithm to recover genomes from multiple metagenomic datasets. *Bioinformatics* 32(4), 605–607. DOI: 10.1093/bioinformatics/btv638.

Xu, J. and Yang, Y. (2021) Gut microbiome and its meta-omics perspectives: Profound implications for cardiovascular diseases. *Gut Microbes* 13(1), 1–25. DOI: 10.1080/19490976.2021.1936379.

Yatsunenko, T., Rey, F.E., Manary, M.J., Trehan, I., Dominguez-Bello, M.G. *et al.* (2012) Human gut microbiome viewed across age and geography. *Nature* 486, 222–227. DOI: 10.1038/nature11053.

Yilmaz, P., Parfrey, L.W., Yarza, P., Gerken, J., Pruesse, E. *et al.* (2014) The SILVA and 'All-species living tree project (LTP)' taxonomic frameworks. *Nucleic Acids Research* 42(D1), 643–648. DOI: 10.1093/nar/gkt1209.

Youngblut, N.D., Cuesta-Zuluaga, J., Reischer, G.H., Dauser, S., Schuster, N. *et al.* (2020) Large-scale metagenome assembly reveals novel animal-associated microbial genomes, biosynthetic gene clusters, and other genetic diversity. *MSystems* 5(6), 1–15. DOI: 10.1128/msystems.01045-20.

Zavala, E.I., Jacobs, Z., Vernot, B., Shunkov, M.V., Kozlikin, M.B. *et al.* (2021) Pleistocene sediment DNA reveals hominin and faunal turnovers at Denisova cave. *Nature* 595(7867), 399–403. DOI: 10.1038/s41586-021-03675-0.

Zhao, C., Dimitrov, B., Goldman, M., Nayfach, S. and Pollard, K.S. (2023) MIDAS2: Metagenomic intra-species diversity analysis system. *Bioinformatics (Oxford, England)* 39(1), 3–4. DOI: 10.1093/bioinformatics/btac713.

Zhou, Z., Luhmann, N., Alikhan, N.F., Quince, C. and Achtman, M. (2017) Accurate reconstruction of microbial strains from metagenomic sequencing using representative reference genomes. *BioRxiv* 1–12.

Ziesemer, K.A., Mann, A.E., Sankaranarayanan, K., Schroeder, H., Ozga, A.T. *et al.* (2015) Intrinsic challenges in ancient microbiome reconstruction using 16S rRNA gene amplification. *Scientific Reports* 5(1), 16498. DOI: 10.1038/srep16498.

5 More Than Food: Why Restoring the Cycle of Organic Matter in Sustainable Plant Production is Essential for the One Health Nexus

Cindy E. Morris[1*], Andrea Radici[2], Christine N. Meynard[3], Nicolas Sauvion[4], Claire Nedellec[5], Ghislain Geniaux[6] and Samuel Soubeyrand[2]
[1]INRAE, Pathologie Végétale, F-84140, Montfavet, France; [2]INRAE, BioSP, F-84914 Avignon, France; [3]CBGP,INRAE, CIRAD, IRD, Montpellier SupAgro, Univ Montpellier, Montpellier, France; [4]PHIM, Univ Montpellier, INRAE, CIRAD, IRD, Institut Agro, Montpellier, France; [5]Université Paris-Sacl, INRAE, MaIAGE, F-78352 Jouy-en-Josas, France; [6]INRAE, Ecodéveloppement UR 767, F-84914, Avignon, France

Abstract
One Health professes that the health of organisms is interconnected through the exploitation of planetary resources, trade, and transportation, in particular. The impetus for the emergence of this concept in the early 2000s was knowledge of the epidemiology of zoonotic diseases that put humans at risk of diseases carried by animals. In spite of the intended comprehensiveness of One Health, the place of plant health in this concept is vague, and few issues about plant health are debated in the scientific literature related to One Health. Here, we explore the history of concepts related to One Health in an attempt to understand why there is this schism between the plant sciences and the medical and veterinary sciences beyond the prism of zoonotic diseases. We illustrate the rich history of concepts in the plant sciences concerning the oneness of plants, animals and humans, and the debates about the definition and scope of sustainability that are precursors to One Health. These concepts continue to be foundations for research and development, particularly for food security and food safety. The emergence of these concepts from plant sciences was based on fundamental understanding of the food web – where plants are food for humans and animals whose digestive processes create important resources for plant growth and health. Yet, this latter part of the food web – recycling of manures in particular – was ruptured during modernization of agriculture. We explain how attaining sustainable One Health depends on restoring this part of the food web via soil stewardship, whose principal guarantors are the ensemble of actors in plant production.

Keywords: plant health, sustainability, soil health, agriculture, food security, global change, agricultural history

*Corresponding author: cindy.morris@inrae.fr

Introduction

One Health is a concept that professes that the health of humans, animals, and the environment are interconnected as part of one world (Gruetzmacher *et al.*, 2021). Although One Health might be construed as a philosophical outlook on nature, it is saliently pragmatic. In practical terms for science, this concept provides a framework to understand the epidemiology of diseases and, in particular, the systemic causes of disease emergence beyond simple etiology and identification of pre-disposing factors. It is applicable not only to diseases caused by microorganisms but also to ailments caused by chemical agents, allergens, microplastics, etc. Insight from One Health can be deployed to establish surveillance and management practices to avoid disease and to establish governance for these practices to be implemented at large geographic scales in the case of major pandemics (Li *et al.*, 2023). The particularity of One Health is its goal to be very comprehensive by identifying the processes and phenomena in systems whose interconnections have impacts on the health of the system components. It defends the need for collaboration of multiple disciplines and a wide range of stakeholders working locally, nationally, and globally to attain optimal health for people, animals, and the environment and thus to be conducive to sustainable societies.

The foundation for today's predominant One Health perspective initially arose from the concern that there could be links between human health and animal health. While numerous historical texts suggest that this link was understood for the first time in the late 1700s or mid-1800s (Bresalier *et al.*, 2020), the earliest traces of this perception date back to the beginning of animal domestication at the time of the transition toward agriculture about 8000–10,000 years ago, thereby highlighting the relative intuitive and conspicuous nature of this link. The increased opportunities for the observation of animals that resulted from domestication likely led to intuitive perceptions of this connection (Currier and Steele, 2011). As early as the 18th century BC, this perception was formalized in the Babylonian Laws of Eshnunna (Hubálek and Rudolf, 2010) that required owners of rabid dogs to pay fines for sickness caused to victims of bites (Wu, 2001). Nevertheless, Pasteur's germ theory of disease, announced in 1861, was essential for understanding the mechanistic link between diseases of humans and animals. This new paradigm of microbiology and many of the other important discoveries of the mid-19th century (theories of evolution and natural selection, the cell theory, laws of inheritance of traits, etc.) occurred as the system of knowledge about the natural world was being compartmentalized into distinct scientific disciplines reigned by specialists in search of novelty (Stichweh, 2001). However, by the mid-20th century, unusual health crises including HIV, Legionnaire's disease, SARS, cryptococcal meningoencephalitis, and others up to the COVID-19 pandemic sparked calls for interdisciplinary solutions. These crises made it more and more apparent that the consequences of the stresses being put on our planet – including globalized trade, increasing human travel, and deforestation due to the need for agricultural and urban spaces – were exacerbating the processes of spill-over of zoonotic diseases from animals and from environmental reservoirs to humans (Morris *et al.*, 2022). This led to specific calls for comprehensive, interdisciplinary approaches that account for the various and interwoven processes of zoonotic spill-over, culminating in fledgling One Health initiatives. From the first official One Health conference held in 2004, a set of principles arose that were updated in 2019 as the ten Berlin principles intended to orient policies and other actions of economic, social, research, and academic organizations to reconnect the health of humans, animals, and ecosystems in a sustainable economic and socio-political context (Gruetzmacher *et al.*, 2021). The intense interest in One Health since these initiatives is illustrated by the increase in the numbers of scientific publications that specifically mention One Health in the title or the abstract (according to the Web of Science) from 22 in 2005 to 265 in 2015, and to 1195 in 2022, for example.

A few decades before the calls for One Health actions, international development organizations and agencies were founding concepts and frameworks that were precursors of One Health in the effort to confront concerns about the future of planetary ecosystems and resources. There was considerable debate around the definition and scope of one important concept – 'sustainability' (Becker, 1997). The debate opposed proponents of a biocentric view, who called for a holistic accounting of the impacts of development on all ecosystem components, to those who defended a more focused anthropocentric view. The anthropocentric perspective dominated the 1992 declaration by the United Nations Conference on Environment and Development where 'human beings are at the center of concern for sustainable development.' With a slightly different nuance, the Consultative Group on International Agricultural Research used 'sustainability' in their 1989 mission statement to mean 'successful management of resources for agriculture to satisfy changing human needs while maintaining or enhancing the quality of the environment and conserving natural resources' (Becker, 1997). When the anthropocentric One Health movement took form in 2004, it is possible that the idea was not perceived as particularly novel in some circles depending on their understanding of sustainable development principles. This is likely to be the case for scientists involved in managing plant health where sustainability has been an important issue for decades (He *et al.*, 2021). In addition to sustainability, plant production sciences have been inspired by questions analogous to those addressed by One Health such as the ecological relationships within agro-food systems and their link to socio-economic contexts. This interest is manifested by research in diverse approaches to agroecology including organic agriculture, biodynamic production, Integrated Pest Management, permaculture, and eco-agriculture (Merrill, 1983; Baker *et al.*, 2020; Knorr, 2023). In face of this rich context for holistic approaches for plant sciences, One Health might have seemed pale. Whatever the real cause, the status of plant health in One Health is perceived as vague (Vittecoq, 2022), and the scientific literature shows little debate on plant health as an issue for One Health. Specifically, for publications that mention One Health in the title or abstract, we found only 10 in 2022 and 6 in 2023, indexed in the Web of Science, that specifically address plant disease epidemiology and/or management of plant health, thereby constituting less than 1% of the publications on One Health in this period (Table 5.1). This rate is similar to that reported for the time period before 2022 (Andrivon *et al.*, 2022).

This article is based on our opinion that plant health management should be an integral part of One Health concepts, policies, actions, and governance. One of our objectives is to convey historical details and perspectives from scientific culture to understand why there is a schism between the plant sciences and the medical and veterinary sciences concerning One Health. As described above, the parallel evolution of the concepts of sustainable development and of One Health – and the respective alignment of the plant sciences vs the medical and veterinary sciences – might offer some explanation about this schism. However, here, we will focus on another factor that underlies this schism, *viz.* the lack of appreciation of the multiple facets of the relationship between plants, animals, and humans that are inherent to their ecology in Earth's biosphere. One obvious facet of this relationship is that plants provide direct services for humans and animals as food and feed. From a One Health perspective, this food and feed should be nutritious and produced with minimal contamination of the environment from chemicals that are detrimental to human and animal health (Hoffmann *et al.*, 2022). In light of concern about food security as the world population grows and as the ravages of climate change put considerable stress on plant production (Savary *et al.*, 2019), it is easy to understand that this is the dominant perspective on how plant, animal, and human health are related. The second facet of the plant-animal-human relationship, which is rarely evoked explicitly, is that as primary and secondary consumers in the food web, humans and animals digest organic matter, thereby transforming it into essential resources for plants. Whereas this relationship had been fundamental for plant production for millennia, its importance was ultimately forsaken during industrialization and urbanization. Our objective is to describe how this basic principle of ecology was abandoned and why its comeback is critical for achieving *bona fide* One Health.

Table 5.1. Publications in 2022 and 2023 that specifically address plant health from a One Health perspective from the total 2298 publications about One Health indexed in the Web of Science in these 2 years (published before December 4, 2023).

Year	Journal	Title	Reference
2022	Plant Pathology	Plant Health in a One Health world: missing links and hidden treasures	(Andrivon *et al.*, 2022)
2022	Nature Reviews Microbiology	Soil microbiomes and one health	(Banerjee and van der Heijden, 2023)
2022	Frontiers in Public Health	Operationalizing One Health as One Digital Health through a global framework that emphasizes fair and equitable sharing of benefits from the use of artificial intelligence and related digital technologies	(Ho, 2022)
2022	CABI Agriculture and Bioscience	A one health approach to plant health	(Hoffmann *et al.*, 2022)
2022	JMIR Public Health and Surveillance	The landscape of participatory surveillance systems across the One Health spectrum: Systematic review	(McNeil *et al.*, 2022)
2022	Environmental Health	Risk and asset-based strategies in health: priorities in biomedical, life and environmental science literature since the early twentieth century. A rapid review	(Migeot *et al.*, 2022)
2022	Agriculture	Antimicrobial use and resistance in plant agriculture: A One Health perspective	(Miller *et al.*, 2022)
2022	Frontiers in Sustainable Food Systems	Integrated Soil Health Management for Plant Health and One Health: Lessons From Histories of Soil-borne Disease Management in California Strawberries and Arthropod Pest Management	(Muramoto *et al.*, 2022)
2022	Environnement Risques et Sante	Mettre en pratique l'approche ≪ Une seule sante ≫	(Vittecoq, 2022)
2022	Plant Pathology	One Health concepts and challenges for surveillance, forecasting, and mitigation of plant disease beyond the traditional scope of crop production	(Morris *et al.*, 2022)
2023	Symbiosis	Missing symbionts – emerging pathogens? Microbiome management for sustainable agriculture	(Berg *et al.*, 2023)
2023	Kafkas Universitesi Veteriner Fakultesi Dergisi	Thiamethoxam Toxicity: A Review in One-Health Perspective	(Qamar *et al.*, 2023)
2023	Nature Microbiology	Soil microbiomes must be explicitly included in One Health policy	(Singh *et al.*, 2023)
2023	Environmental Research	Glyphosate and environmental toxicity with One Health approach, a review	(Ferrante *et al.*, 2023)
2023	Cahiers Agriculture	Crop protection practices and risks associated with human fungal infectious diseases: a One Health perspective	(Ratnadass and Sester, 2023)
2023	Food and Chemical Toxicology	Aflatoxins posing threat to food safety and security in Pakistan: Call for a one health approach	(Ashraf *et al.*, 2023)

Review Methodology

To assess trends in the frequency of publications concerning One Health, we searched the Web of Science using the query 'One Health' for titles and abstracts of papers published in 2005, 2015, 2022, and 2023. To determine the frequency of publications that specifically concerned plant health, we manually screened the results of this query for the years 2022 and 2023. Papers were noted as pertinent to plant health if they specifically addressed plant health concerns in the body of the paper. Literature to support the other parts of the text of this article was found via queries of the Web of Science and Google Scholar for subjects related to soil health, agroecology, sewage management, the history of science, sustainable agriculture, etc. via discussions with colleagues and thanks to recommendations of the reviewers.

Breaking the Food Web

For about 4000–6000 years, crop production was generally self-sufficient, in terms of the cycle of nutrients, and consequently sustainable (Knorr, 2023). Various compilations of historical crop production practices point out that the sustainability was founded on efficient use of resources and their recycling back into the production system as exemplified by agricultural practices in ancient China or by various indigenous peoples elsewhere (King and Percy, 1911; FAO, 2021). The input of manure, particularly from livestock, has been a key component of plant cultivation as early as the Neolithic period and onward (Jones, 2012; Bogaard *et al.*, 2013), thereby contributing to the reciprocity of the food web between plants, animals, and humans. With the transition of societies toward industrialization and urbanization that distanced populations from farms, the recycling of resources back to agricultural fields decreased markedly. This led to a major environmental crisis for agriculture in the early 19th century – the severe decline of soil fertility in North America and Europe between about 1830 and 1870 (Foster and Magdoff, 1998) – that set off an international scramble to secure fertilizers for crop production.

Two major quests to secure fertilizers for crop production were launched at the onset of the soil exhaustion crisis. One quest focused on the synthetic production of mineral fertilizers starting with superphosphate of lime from bones, of sulfur from diverse types of rocks, of potassium from wood ashes and culminating in the energy-intensive Haber-Bosch process that succeeded in producing ammonia from atmospheric nitrogen at industrial scales by 1913 (Russel and Williams, 1977). The other quest was the rush to harvest organic materials in the form of bird guano, especially from South American atolls. This guano rush started in 1840, leading to the creation of an elite business class dubbed the 'guanopreneurs' (Snyders, 2019) and the Guano Island Act of 1856, whereby the USA annexed, occupied, and exploited over 100 islands for this precious resource (Burnett, 2005). The companies and labor contracts established by the guanopreneurs assured the transportation of millions of metric tons of nitrogen fertilizer and more than 100,000 workers across the globe, producing significant changes in environmental habitats[1] and in labor conditions throughout the world. This was a major paradigm shift for agriculture in that farming was no longer a closed system in which nitrogen was cycled among soil, plants, animals, and people at the local scale. Farming became an open, energy-intensive system for which nitrogen and other mineral resources could come from distant places (Melillo, 2012). This scurry for new resources and the change of paradigm were set in the backdrop of accumulating sewage in urban centers – the cause of numerous outbreaks of cholera epidemics in London from 1817 to 1854 and the Great Stink of 1858 (De Feo *et al.*, 2014), for example. As a so-called solution to the urban sewage problem, sewage was dumped into major rivers such as the Thames and Seine and put on a path out to sea.

The paradox of massive amounts of nitrogen-rich feces being dumped into rivers and oceans in the face of a major fertility crisis for crop production did not escape the attention of intellectuals of the early 19th century. For example, in volume 5 of *Les Misérables*, the influential writer and French parliamentarian Victor Hugo decried the wastefulness displayed in Paris by the dumping of sewage – a resource more valuable than guano in his opinion – into the Seine river (Hugo, 1862). Various intellectuals in Victorian England engaged in a decades' long debate on sewage as a valuable commodity (Goddard, 1996). In *Das Kapital*, the German philosopher, historian, and economist Karl Marx noted the contradiction to sustainable societies of dumping sewage into the Thames River. He exclaimed that the 'conscious and rational treatment of the land as permanent communal property is the inalienable condition for the existence and reproduction of the chain of human generations' (Foster, 1999). Likewise, German chemist Justus von Liebig argued in his *Letters on Modern Agriculture* and on *Utilization of Municipal Sewage* that soil nutrients were carried away by modern agricultural practices as a form of robbery of environmental wealth. He noted that the pollution of cities with human and animal excrement and the depletion of the natural fertility of the soil were connected and that organic recycling of nutrients back to the soil was an indispensable part of a rational society with urban and agricultural components (Foster, 1999).

The early efforts to valorize human waste from urban centers were mostly unsuccessful, plagued by the high volume of sewage due to the use of water as the carrier for wastes by the sewage systems that were adopted in Europe and the USA (Hamlin, 1980; Goddard, 1996). Furthermore, the promise of economic gains from the value of the wastes as fertilizers could not overcome the costs and fear of health hazards linked to sanitation issues (i.e. fears of dissemination of diseases such as cholera) and the stigma of these wastes as dirty (Hamlin, 1980; Goddard, 1996). Whatever the advantages of the practices that emerged in the 19th century for capturing and dumping human wastes, they reinforced the societal processes that deprived crop production of an abundant source of organic matter that evidently is beneficial to crop health and productivity (Feller *et al.*, 2012; Goldan *et al.*, 2023). The rupture of the plant-animal-human food web also contributed to the conception of linear – rather than circular – economies (Rodríguez-Espinosa *et al.*, 2023) where resources for sustaining an agricultural system could come from far away.

The Farm as an Organism and the Living Bridge of Soil: The First One Health Concepts

The push to recycle nutrients back to the soil continued in the 20th century with publications by Rudolf Steiner in 1924 defending the idea that the soil had properties of an organism (Paull, 2010) and the 1926 publication of Franklin H. King who defended principles of recycling organic materials back to the soil. King's ideas had a remarkable influence. As a soil physicist at the University of Wisconsin, he published '*Farmers of Forty Centuries, or Permanent Agriculture in China, Korea, and Japan*' in 1926 (Paull, 2011; Heckman, 2013). This book was a reaction to his dissatisfaction with the agricultural practices promoted by the US Department of Agriculture at the time where he pointed out the importance of returning composted wastes, especially composted fecal wastes, to agricultural soils. Inspired by King's work and by his own decades of farming experience, the British agricultural scientist Albert Howard formulated the notion of The Law of Return in '*An Agricultural Testament*' published in 1943 (Heckman, 2006). He advocated for the recycling of all organic waste materials including sewage sludge back to agricultural soils, and he described precise conditions for composting as a means to foster 'humus farming.' The objective of the Law of Return was to build humus and the 'living bridge' of soil life that supported the health of plants, livestock, and humans (Heckman, 2006). Paradoxically, and in spite of his proclamation that modern agriculture was robbing soil of its nutrients, Liebig contested the notion that plants could obtain nutrients from the organic constituents of soil. He perceived the Law of Return as an opposition – rather than a complement – to his theory on the Law of the Minimum that focused on soil chemistry and inorganic nutrition, especially for the elements N, P, and K (Heckman, 2013). This 'mineralist' doctrine has continued to the present times to dominate agricultural practices, with the role of organic matter and soil structure receiving renewed acceptance only since the early 2000s (Feller *et al.*, 2012). Mineral nutrients can indeed be limiting factors for plant productivity. However and paradoxically, their natural abundance in soils can far surpass the amounts provided by synthetic fertilizers and even the total synthetic production capacity as in the case of phosphorus (Gerke, 2022). Organic matter is essential for the chemical and biological reactions that mobilize the soil-bound and recalcitrant forms into bio-available forms that can be assimilated by plants (Gerke, 2022).

This debate on soil quality led to a movement to promote 'organic farming,' a name coined by polymath and Oxford University lecturer Walter J. Northbourne in his 1940 manifesto '*Look to the Land*' (Paull, 2014). Northbourne intended for the term 'organic' to reflect a philosophical perspective where the farm was an organism 'having a complex and necessary interrelationship of parts, similar to that in living things' (Heckman, 2006; Paull, 2014). Reflecting Howard's living bridge of soil, Northbourne stressed that 'the soil and the micro-organisms in it together with the plants growing on it form an organic whole' (Paull, 2014). The organic farming movement was further propelled in the UK by the foundation of the Soil Association in 1946 (Conford and Holden, 2007), and in the USA by farming practices popularized in the *Organic Farming and Gardening* magazine published by Jerome Rodale starting in 1942 (Heckman, 2006). Notably, one of the objectives of the Soil Association was 'to bring together all those working for a fuller understanding of the vital relationships between soil, plant, animal and man' (Conford and Holden, 2007). Overall, this fervor to restore soil and promote a holistic vision of agriculture was not just a farming priority. In the backdrop of the great Dust Bowl catastrophe in North America in the 1930s and 1940s (McLeman *et al.*, 2014), it was a cry in the defense of civilization (Reed, 2001).

This surge of defense for organic farming spurred the rise of advocacy groups in the USA, in Australia, and across Europe in particular to promote organic farming practices. In 1974, a meeting of several advocacy groups convened in Versailles, France, under the leadership of the French advocacy group *Nature et Progrès*, thereby fostering the creation of the International Federation of Organic Agriculture Movements (IFOAM) (now called Organics International[2]). Since the beginning of the organic farming movement, its history has been marked by recurrent conflict with what has become conventional agriculture. Its major critics insist that organic farming cannot produce sufficient food for the growing world population (Heckman, 2006). The advocacy groups were created to disseminate knowledge about organic farming practices and to bolster its credibility as a means of sustainable food production. But notably, the origins of organic farming were founded on explicit notions of One Health. This was epitomized by the famous quotation from Eve Balfour, the chair of the inaugural meeting of the Soil Association, that 'the health of soil, plant, animal and man is one and indivisible' (Vieweger and Döring, 2015). It has evolved more fully as expressed in the FAO's definition of organic agriculture,[3] adopted in 1999, as a 'holistic production management system which promotes and enhances agro-ecosystem health, including biodiversity, biological cycles, and soil biological activity. FAO's definition of organic agriculture emphasizes the use of management practices in preference to the use of off-farm inputs, taking into account that regional conditions require locally adapted systems. This is accomplished by using, where possible, agronomic, biological, and mechanical methods, as opposed to using synthetic materials, to fulfil any specific function within the system.' The principles of organic agriculture promoted by IFOAM go a step farther in their comprehensiveness by proclaiming that 'organic agriculture should sustain and enhance the health of soil, plant, animal, human and planet as one and indivisible' (Paull, 2010). This holistic approach has not been confined to organic farming. It is also espoused in tenants of various strategies of agroecology including permaculture, syntropic agriculture, and regenerative agriculture, for example. Permaculture principles were formulated in the late 1970s and advocate for a more comprehensive understanding of yield where self-regulation and feedback of ecosystem services come into play (Ferguson and Lovell, 2014; Krebs and Bach, 2018). Syntropic agriculture, proposed in 1992 (Cossel *et al.*, 2020), professed that soil-physical cultivation parameters including humus cover, fertility, water infiltration, and erosion control are enhanced through management of plant diversity and reliance on within-system material input. Regenerative agricultural principles were developed as an offshoot of organic farming practices that targeted productivity but were founded on both biological and socio-economic stability (Giller *et al.*, 2021). These ideas are part of the efforts to deploy agroecological principles to achieve sustainability by leveraging the diverse dimensions of food production. These dimensions include soil quality management, water and energy conservation, reduction of pesticides, forecasting technological innovations, fostering cooperation and value-creation in the food chain, and deploying climate-smart farming – all to promote ecological resilience and social responsibility (Marchetti *et al.*, 2020). The ensemble of these perspectives are precursors to and are fully coherent with the current principles of One Health (Gruetzmacher *et al.*, 2021).

One Health in the Face of Unsustainability

Whatever the capacity of conventional farming to produce sufficient food and feed for the world population of humans and livestock that has exploded since the end of World War II, it is being achieved at the cost of the quasi-total alienation of the One Health principles promoted by the sustainable agroecological approaches described in the previous sections. This alienation is expressed not only in terms of technical practices but also in terms of the loss of domains of competence among farmers, agronomists, and other practitioners. The resulting imbalances in the ecological processes that could assure plant nutrition and that could mitigate the explosion of populations of pathogens or weeds, for example, have been compensated for with synthetic chemicals (fertilizers, pesticides, herbicides). Synthetic nitrogen fertilizers epitomize this imbalance through the intensive capture of gaseous nitrogen from the atmosphere to create reactive nitrogen for conventional farming, thereby seriously disrupting the nitrogen balance of the planet. Via the Haber-Bosch process, the USA, for example, captures 13,100 kt of atmospheric nitrogen per year that is turned into reactive nitrogen. This is equivalent to the total annual 13,200 kt of reactive nitrogen already available in wastes from livestock, food wastes, and sewage wastewater in the USA (Lavallais and Dunn, 2023). On a worldwide scale, the fabrication of synthetic fertilizer for crop production and the modern practice of intensified legume cultivation convert around 120 million tons of nitrogen from the atmosphere annually into reactive forms of nitrogen. This quantity is greater than the combined forms of reactive nitrogen generated from all of Earth's terrestrial processes leading to an excessive – and unnecessary – overload of reactive nitrogen in the environment with devastating consequences on Earth system processes and resource quality (Liu *et al.*, 2020). This led Rockström and colleagues to declare more than a decade ago that this disequilibrium is outside the 'safe operating space for humans' on planet Earth (Rockström *et al.*, 2009). The safe operating space defined by these authors identifies the thresholds of nine Earth system processes that are likely to have irreversible consequences if they are crossed – i.e. planetary boundaries. These include processes that lead to climate change, biodiversity loss, ocean acidification, global freshwater availability, nitrogen and phosphorus distribution in the environment. Since the initial definition of these planetary boundaries, six of the nine boundaries have been crossed as of 2023 (Richardson *et al.*, 2023).

Since the soil exhaustion crisis of the 19th century, changes in soil fertilization practices reinforced by the invention of the Haber-Bosch process have markedly altered soil physics and biology as well as soil chemistry (Toor *et al.*, 2021). The physical and biological properties of soil are now recognized as critically important to plant health (Feller *et al.*, 2012; Nwokolo *et al.*, 2021; Kopittke *et al.*, 2022; Allen *et al.*, 2023). These soil qualities have degraded during the abandonment of traditional farming practices that had focused on maintaining and cycling soil nutrients (Toor *et al.*, 2021). For example, the complexity of microbial communities in soil can keep plant pathogens in check. The addition of manure to soil has been repeatedly shown to contribute to the establishment of these microbial communities and to the concomitant disease-suppressive capacity of soil (Janvier *et al.*, 2007; Nwokolo *et al.*, 2021). Changes in the functions of soil microbial communities due to the impoverishing organic matter are being exacerbated by the use of antimicrobials (pesticides, antibiotics) and herbicides (Kang *et al.*, 2021; Liao *et al.*, 2021; van Bruggen *et al.*, 2021), leading to dramatic and worrisome proliferation of resistance to antimicrobials among bacterial and fungal pathogens of humans and animals (Hernando-Amado *et al.*, 2020). These imbalances in microbial communities are contributing to the crossing of yet another of the Earth system thresholds, *viz.* the functional component of biosphere integrity (Richardson *et al.*, 2023). If humans are indeed part of the functional component of biosphere integrity, it is critical to note that pesticide exposure also deteriorates farmer health and thus reduces farm productivity (Athukorala *et al.*, 2023; Kitole *et al.*, 2023). By diminishing farmer health, pesticides further exacerbate the negative effects of poverty and poor education on the capacity of farmers to implement good agronomic practices that assure crop yields (Guest *et al.*, 2023). The deleterious effects of synthetic pesticides on human health permeate beyond farmers to the neighboring residents and into the food chain (Dereumeaux *et al.*, 2020; Lombardi *et al.*, 2021). The social costs are enormous. In France, for example, the social costs attributable to the use of synthetic pesticides (372 million euros) amount to more than 10% of the 2017 annual budget of the Ministry of Agriculture due primarily to the significant effects on the environment and human health (Alliot *et al.*, 2022), thereby diminishing resources that could otherwise contribute to farm productivity.

The structure of soil is assured in large part by the maintenance of organic content, allowing the soil to confer its major services to plants and the environment (including water holding and filtration, nutrient cycling, decomposition and recycling of organic materials, and production of biomass) (Hu *et al.*, 2023). Yet, in 2015, about one-third of the world's soils had been classified as 'degraded' (Toor *et al.*, 2021). Unfortunately, efforts to rectify soil health are increasingly in conflict with other uses of biomass in the multitude of initiatives to recycle biomass. The use of biomass as an energy source alternative to fossil fuels is a leading competitor (Chojnacka *et al.*, 2022). Although fertilizers can be extracted from the combusted biomass, this mode of recycling continues to reinforce the outmoded mineralist doctrine of plant nutrition that hampers the full scope of ecosystem services, thereby limiting the potential of those natural services that contribute to the health of plants, animals, and humans.

Following the wake of the catastrophic dust storms of North America, US President F.D. Roosevelt declared in 1937 that the 'nation that destroys its soil destroys itself' (Toor *et al.*, 2021). Since then, multiple initiatives have been launched to alert to the importance of renewing and protecting soils. This culminated in the declaration by the United Nations that 2015–2024 would be the International Decade of Soils (Singh *et al.*, 2017). Soils are considered as the 'single most important common variable in sustaining life on our planet' (Kopittke *et al.*, 2022). This re-awakening about the centrality of soils to sustainability has also brought attention to their centrality to One Health because of their roles as habitats and havens of passage of microorganisms with direct impacts on the health of plants, humans, and animals. A recent report brilliantly points to examples of microorganisms in soil that (i) are pathogens of plants, humans, or animals, (ii) promote plant growth, (iii) produce antibiotics, (iv) assure basic soil functions such nutrient cycling, (v) mitigate consequences of climate change including adaptation to drought and so on, and that can even (vi) influence levels of anxiety via their role in gut health (Banerjee and van der Heijden, 2023). Many of the microorganisms found in soil are in passage between other habitats making soil a hub for exchange and interconnectedness among habitats (van Bruggen *et al.*, 2019; Sessitsch *et al.*, 2023). The state of the microbial biodiversity in soils is directly impacted by land use and agricultural practices, with conventional agricultural practices leading to diminished biodiversity in contrast with organic or conservation practices that are linked to enriched biodiversity (Tahat *et al.*, 2020; Barros-Rodríguez *et al.*, 2021).

Managing Soil Quality for Crop Production to Facilitate the Future of One Health

One of the major contributions of modern One Health initiatives has been to elucidate the new connections among disparate ecosystems and habitats that have arisen via population growth, urbanization, industrialization, transportation, and the concomitant exploitation of Earth's resources that have become root causes of disease emergence. Pointing out and surveying these new connections are important goals of One Health. Nevertheless, importantly, the ensemble of insight gained from One Health-based analyses of the root causes of disease emergence can be deployed to reconstruct a more sustainable world where some of these root causes are diminished. Multiple authors before us have clearly defended the position that attending to soil quality is essential for sustainability and for assuring human health in the context of One Health (Keith *et al.*, 2016; Singh *et al.*, 2017; van Bruggen *et al.*, 2019; Yan *et al.*, 2022; Banerjee and van der Heijden 2023; Kopittke *et al.* 2023; Singh *et al.*, 2023). According to a 2022 study by the FAO, the soil microbiome in particular – a key component of soil quality – is a 'game changer' for food security, and human and planetary health (Kendzior *et al.*, 2022). Among the key findings of this study was the role of manures and compost in nurturing the soil microbiome and in maintaining long-term soil fertility and functions. However, in stark contrast to this perspective, a 260-page report on '*The State of Food Security in the World*' issued by the WHO in the same year mentioned soils only four times, mostly to indicate policies that did not take soils into account (Flaxman, 2023). These examples reveal the striking disparity in perspectives of a major organization focused on human health vs that of its counterpart organization focused on food production. These organizations (UN, FAO, WHO) and the World Organization for Animal Health united their efforts, again in 2022, produce a 70-page plan of action for One Health (FAO *et al.*, 2022). In a rather telling outcome, soils were mentioned only six times in this report. These mentions concerned precautions about soil pollution and sources of contaminants but not about fertility or soil health, reflecting an important ambiguity by the main international forces behind One Health policies in their consensus opinion on organic practices to manage soil quality.

Independently from motivations inspired by One Health, actions to close the gap on the life cycle of fecal wastes – from the farm to the consumer and back to the farm – are increasing. In the European Union (EU), for example, actions are emerging from the EU's commitment to the United Nations' Sustainable Development Goals, for which seven concern soil either directly or indirectly. From 2014 to 2022, the EU's Common Agricultural Policy encouraged improvements in soil and manure management through various incentives. Legislative initiatives are currently being prepared for monitoring and to assure their high standards, with the recommendation by auditors to avoid derogations and conflicts with other policies that could hinder the goal of restoring soil quality (ECA, 2023). Soil quality can be improved by amending with various sources of fecal matter including manures and bio-solids derived from sewage sludge. There are various advantages (fertility, circular economy, etc.) and disadvantages (chemical pollutants, pathogenic microorganisms, etc.) of applying waste-based amendments to soil (Houot *et al.*, 2016) that need to be addressed. The EU has a growing body of legislation for the use of bio-solids from sewage in agricultural fields as dumping into landfills is becoming widely prohibited (Collivignarelli *et al.*, 2019). However, the management of fecal wastes from centralized waste management systems such as sewers concerns less than half of the world's population. Currently, 3.6 billion people live outside of centralized waste management systems (Allen *et al.*, 2023). Although most of these people are in the developing world, rural and mountainous settings in Europe and elsewhere also require decentralized waste management systems (Risch *et al.*, 2021). There is need for innovation in waste treatment to respond to these different socio-economic contexts, and, fortunately, there are more and more technological solutions (Shukla *et al.*, 2023). Furthermore, the EU has established and is continuously updating its regulations about effluent quality from decentralized wastewater management systems because of the abundance of European rural habitations that are not connected to centralized systems (Falipou *et al.*, 2022). In light of the fact that human excreta could meet between 9% and 22% of agricultural demand for the three essential plant macronutrients – nitrogen, phosphorus, and potassium – it is becoming untenable to ignore the value of the almost 1 billion tons of feces generated each year (Allen *et al.*, 2023). An extensive review of the literature concerning tests of the effect of fecal amendments on crops found that amendments derived from on-site sanitation systems had a positive impact on crop yields when compared to unamended control treatments and also produced yields equivalent to those for treatments with synthetic nitrogen-based fertilizers (Allen *et al.*, 2023). These experimental results weaken the argument that organic farming cannot be as productive as conventional farming. However, they need to add considerations about the necessary caveats for adoption in different ecosystems (e.g. dry vs tropical contexts) and landscapes (e.g. polyculture vs monoculture) to bolster their applicability. Cost-benefit analyses could be performed in these different situations at the level of individual farms and from a more holistic perspective encompassing indirect or non-intentional positive and negative effects to assess cost-benefits for society. Furthermore, these analyses should be conducted in the context of prospection on future agricultural landscapes and agronomic practices that facilitate circular economies.

If soils are indeed central to One Health, then the stewards of soil quality should be central actors of One Health initiatives. Who are these actors? Farmers who produce crops and those involved in the scientific disciplines that support them are the central players for managing soil quality. Based on the rich history of practices and scientific literature concerning organic agricultural and of agro-ecological methods for crop production, this corps of actors can foster practices that are founded on century-old concepts of the oneness of the health of humans, animals, and plants. This insight needs to be leveraged to address questions of how to restore the food web in plant production and on how to reinforce methods of assuring plant health without synthetic pesticides (Fig. 5.1). This will need to be accomplished all while fostering the ecosystem services of soil that, for example, mitigate the impacts of drought, detoxify pollutants in soils, liberate soil-bound mineral reserves for plant nutrition, limit the proliferation of antibiotic resistance (Banerjee and van der Heijden, 2023), foster the storage of carbon (Gerke, 2022), etc. Part of the transformation of soil management will indeed need to promote an 'underground revolution' via ecological engineering to assure specific soil activities and functions (Bender *et al.*, 2016).

Overall, our relationship with soil and our understanding of its role in the health of humans, animals, plants, and the biosphere in general, can be markedly modernized. Such a dramatic change in understanding has a well-known precedent, embodied in the functions of the human gut. The human gut has been transmogrified from something dirty to foundational for good health. For the upcoming transition in our relationship with soil, we call on scientists and practitioners to find indicators of soil health, to conceive advice for feeding and caring for soil, to reveal soil's protective role for plant and animal health, and to elucidate the range of environmental functions soil assures directly or indirectly – in the same manner as we have come to understand these for the human gut. For soil, the scope of the actions and innovations needed for this transformation will also need to encompass the full extent of the food web, calling into play engineers and economists, in particular, to establish production and value chains for organic matter (Fig. 5.1). Therefore, farmers who cultivate crops, alongside professionals in scientific disciplines supporting agriculture, possess essential knowledge to contribute to building a world aligned with modern One Health principles. Recognizing and encouraging their pivotal role in One Health initiatives, practices, and policies is crucial.

Conclusion

The adaptation of agriculture to industrialization and urbanization ruptured a fundamental part of the food web related to the production of plants. This robbed plant production of an important resource and led to serious disruption of planetary mineral cycles, overexploitation and waste of resources, habitat destruction, and other major global changes. This major alteration of planetary ecology occurred despite knowledge about the importance of food web

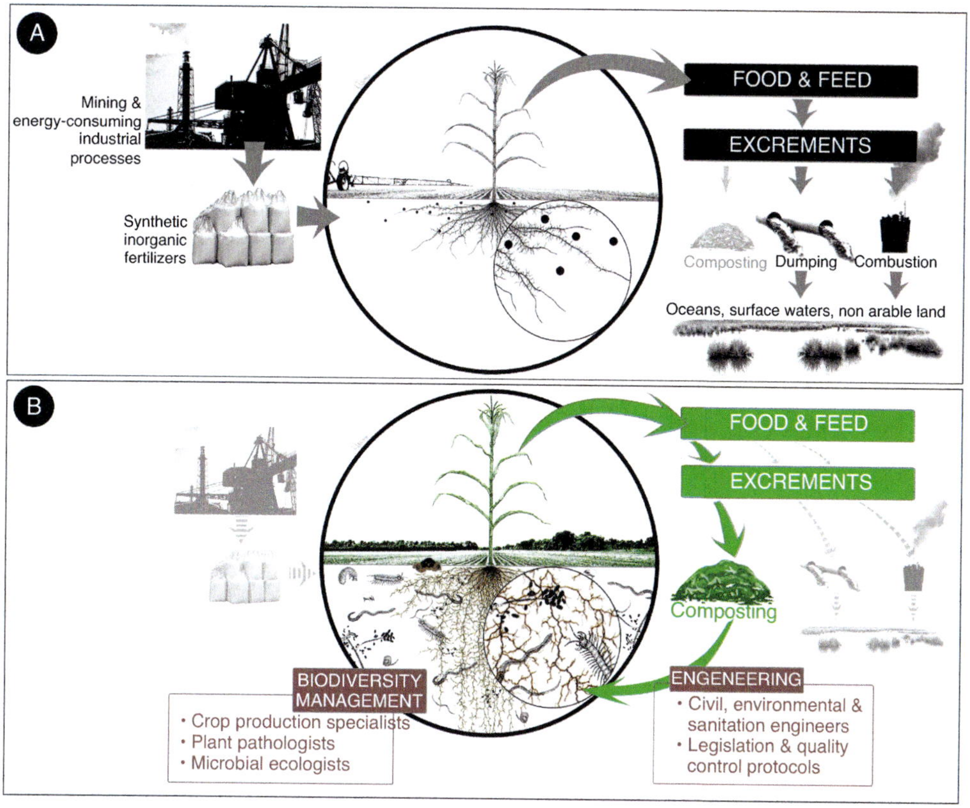

Fig. 5.1. Component processes and actors for diverting the disuse of organic wastes (A) toward the restoration of the cycle of organic matter (B) for sustainable plant production that strengthens the One Health nexus of plants, animals, humans, and the environment. In general, conventional plant production practices (A) resort to mining and energy-consuming industrial processes to produce synthetic fertilizer all while wasting a large part of excrements from food and feed digestion that hold resources for plant production. The One Health nexus of plants, animals, humans, and the environment can be strengthened by reducing the need for synthetic fertilizers via the valorization of excrements from digestion of food and feed and hence averting their loss or their negative impacts on the environment (B). This will bring into play a range of actors to assure the hygienic qualities of composts and their suitability as fertilizers and to deploy them for optimizing the ecosystem functions of the soil microbiome that contribute to the health of plants, animals, and humans.

processes and the rational use of resources for sustainability and, importantly, despite the existence of well-formulated concepts of the interconnectedness of the health of organisms that were precursors to the modern One Health concept. These concepts centered on the role of soil – with its physical and chemical properties as well as its microbiology – as a hub that links the health of plants, animals, and humans. As the modern One Health concept emerged in the 2000s, the precursor concepts from agriculture were mostly ignored. Today, the position of plant health in the One Health concept is unclear, and few scientific publications in the field of One Health directly treat issues related to plant production apart from the role of plants as food and feeds. Here, we have addressed the history of how plant health became disconnected from the One Health nexus. We propose a central role for the major stewards of soil quality – farmers who produce crops and those involved in the scientific disciplines that support them – in strengthening and rendering sustainable One Health initiatives, practices, and policies.

Notes

[1] An example of extreme destruction of an entire island and a way of life of its indigenous people occurred on the Micronesian island Nauru that was mined for its rich deposits of phosphate that had accumulated from millions of years of bird migrations. See Gowdy and McDaniel (1999).
[2] Extensive details on the history of organic agriculture are available on the IFOAM website https://www.ifoam.bio/ (accessed 29 November 2023).
[3] Available at: https://www.fao.org/3/X0075e/X0075e.htm (accessed 29 November 2023).

Acknowledgments

The authors acknowledge the support of funding from the French National Research Agency (ANR) for the BEYOND project (contract # 20-PCPA-0002) that has facilitated the regular interactions of all authors and that led to the conception and realization of this publication.

Conflict of Interest

The authors have no conflicts of interest to declare.

Author Contributions

CEM conceived the initial idea for this work; CNM, GG, and SS contributed to defining its scope; CN, AR, and NS contributed to the elaboration of precise technical information and coherence of the manuscript content. CEM wrote the initial version and all authors contributed to revising subsequent versions. CEM and NS conceived the figure and NS made the figure. All authors approve the content of the manuscript.

References

Allen, K., Rodríguez López, E.L., Banwart, S.A. and Evans, B. (2023) A systematic review of the effects of fecal sludge derived amendments on crop growth and soil health. *ACS ES&T Engineering* 3, 746–761. DOI: 10.1021/acsestengg.2c00438.

Alliot, C., Mc Adams-Marin, D., Borniotto, D. and Baret, P.V. (2022) The social costs of pesticide use in France. *Frontiers in Sustainable Food Systems* 6, 1027583. DOI: 10.3389/fsufs.2022.1027583.

Andrivon, D., Montarry, J. and Fournet, S. (2022) Plant health in a one health world: Missing links and hidden treasures. *Plant Pathology* 71, 23–29. DOI: 10.1111/ppa.13463.

Ashraf, W., Rehman, A., Rabbani, M., Shaukat, W. and Wang, J.-S. (2023) Aflatoxins posing threat to food safety and security in Pakistan: Call for a one health approach. *Food and Chemical Toxicology* 180, 114006. DOI: 10.1016/j.fct.2023.114006.

Athukorala, W., Lee, B.L., Wilson, C., Fujii, H. and Managi, S. (2023) Measuring the impact of pesticide exposure on farmers' health and farm productivity. *Economic Analysis and Policy* 77, 851–862. DOI: 10.1016/j.eap.2022.12.007.

Baker, B.P., Green, T.A. and Loker, A.J. (2020) Biological control and integrated pest management in organic and conventional systems. *Biological Control* 140, 104095. DOI: 10.1016/j.biocontrol.2019.104095.

Banerjee, S. and van der Heijden, M.G.A. (2023) Soil microbiomes and one health. *Nature Reviews Microbiology* 21, 6–20. DOI: 10.1038/s41579-022-00779-w.

Barros-Rodríguez, A., Rangseekaew, P., Lasudee, K., Pathom-Aree, W. and Manzanera, M. (2021) Impacts of agriculture on the environment and soil microbial biodiversity. *Plants* 10, 2325. DOI: 10.3390/plants10112325.

Becker, B. (1997) *Sustainability Assessment: A review of Values, Concepts, and Methodological Approaches*. CGIAR 1–63.

Bender, S.F., Wagg, C. and van der Heijden, M.G.A. (2016) An underground revolution: Biodiversity and soil ecological engineering for agricultural sustainability. *Trends in Ecology & Evolution* 31, 440–452. DOI: 10.1016/j.tree.2016.02.016.

Berg, G., Schweitzer, M., Abdelfattah, A., Cernava, T. and Wassermann, B. (2023) Missing symbionts – Emerging pathogens? Microbiome management for sustainable agriculture. *Symbiosis* 89, 163–171. DOI: 10.1007/s13199-023-00903-1.

Bogaard, A., Fraser, R., Heaton, T.H., Wallace, M., Vaiglova, P. *et al.* (2013) Crop manuring and intensive land management by Europe's first farmers. *Proceedings of the National Academy of Sciences of the United States of America* 110, 12589–12594. DOI: 10.1073/pnas.1305918110.

Bresalier, M., Cassidy, A., Woods, A. *et al.* (2020) One health dans l'histoire. In: Zinsstag, J. (ed.) *One Health, Une Seule Santé*. Quae, Versailles, pp. 21–40.

Burnett, C.D. (2005) The edges of empire and the limits of sovereignty: American Guano Islands. *American Quarterly* 57, 779–803. DOI: 10.2307/40068316.

Chojnacka, K., Moustakas, K. and Mikulewicz, M. (2022) Valorisation of agri-food waste to fertilisers is a challenge in implementing the circular economy concept in practice. *Environmental Pollution* 312, 119906. DOI: 10.1016/j.envpol.2022.119906.

Collivignarelli, M.C., Abbà, A., Frattarola, A., Carnevale Miino, M., Padovani, S. *et al.* (2019) Legislation for the reuse of biosolids on agricultural land in Europe: Overview. *Sustainability* 11, 6015. DOI: 10.3390/su11216015.

Conford, P. and Holden, P. (2007) The soil association. In: Lockeretz, W. (ed.) *Organic Farming: An International History*. CAB International, Wallingford, UK, pp. 187–200.

Cossel, M.V., Ludwig, H., Cichocki, J., Fesani, S., Guenther, R. *et al.* (2020) Adapting syntropic permaculture for renaturation of a former quarry area in the temperate zone. *Agriculture* 10, 603. DOI: 10.3390/agriculture10120603.

Currier, R.W. and Steele, J.H. (2011) One health—one medicine: Unifying human and animal medicine within an evolutionary paradigm. *Annals of the New York Academy of Sciences* 1230, 4–11. DOI: 10.1111/j.1749-6632.2011.06138.x.

De Feo, G., Antoniou, G., Fardin, H.F., El-Gohary, F., Zheng, X.Y. *et al.* (2014) The historical development of sewers worldwide. *Sustainability* 6, 3936–3974. DOI: 10.3390/su6063936.

Dereumeaux, C., Fillol, C., Quenel, P. and Denys, S. (2020) Pesticide exposures for residents living close to agricultural lands: A review. *Environment International* 134, 105210. DOI: 10.1016/j.envint.2019.105210.

ECA (2023) EU efforts for sustainable soil management: Unambitious standards and limited targeting. In: ECA, dd (ed.) Brussels.

Falipou, E., Favre, C., Lacasse, R. and Boutin, C. (2022) Prediction of household wastewater treatment systems' *in situ* performance based on standardized tests. *Water Science and Technology* 85, 1090–1106. DOI: 10.2166/wst.2022.025.

FAO (2021) *The White/Wiphala Paper on Indigenous Peoples' Food Systems*. FAO, Rome, p. 143.

FAO, UNEP, WHO, and WOAH (2022) *One Health Joint Plan of Action (2022–2026). Working Together for the Health of Humans, Animals, Plants and the Environment*. FAO, Rome.

Feller, C., Blanchart, E., Bernoux, M., Lal, R. and Manlay, R. (2012) Soil fertility concepts over the past two centuries: The importance attributed to soil organic matter in developed and developing countries. *Archives of Agronomy and Soil Science* 58, S3–S21. DOI: 10.1080/03650340.2012.693598.

Ferguson, R.S. and Lovell, S.T. (2014) Permaculture for agroecology: Design, movement, practice, and worldview. A review. *Agronomy for Sustainable Development* 34, 251–274. DOI: 10.1007/s13593-013-0181-6.

Ferrante, M., Rapisarda, P., Grasso, A., Favara, C. and Oliveri Conti, G. (2023) Glyphosate and environmental toxicity with "One Health" approach, a review. *Environmental Research* 235, 116678. DOI: 10.1016/j.envres.2023.116678.

Flaxman, M. (2023) Food security and the soil microbiome. One Health Newsletter. Available at: https://www.vet.k-state.edu/about/news-eventspublications/OneHealth/Vol15-Iss1/food-security.html (accessed 29 November 2023).

Foster, J.B. (1999) Marx's theory of metabolic rift: Classical foundations for environmental sociology. *American Journal of Sociology* 105, 366–405.

Foster, J.B. and Magdoff, F. (1998) Liebig, Marx, and the depletion of soil fertility: Relevance for today's agriculture. *Monthly Review* p. 32.

Gerke, J. (2022) *The central role of soil organic matter in soil fertility and carbon storage*. Soil Systems.

Giller, K.E., Hijbeek, R., Andersson, J.A. and Sumberg, J. (2021) Regenerative agriculture: An agronomic perspective. *Outlook on Agriculture* 50, 13–25. DOI: 10.1177/0030727021998063.

Goddard, N. (1996) "A mine of wealth"? The victorians and the agricultural value of sewage. *Journal of Historical Geography* 22, 274–290. DOI: 10.1006/jhge.1996.0017.

Goldan, E., Nedeff, V., Barsan, N., Culea, M., Panainte-Lehadus, M. *et al.* (2023) Assessment of manure compost used as soil amendment – A review. *Processes* 11, 1167. DOI: 10.3390/pr11041167.

Gowdy, J.A. and McDaniel, C.N. (1999) The physical destruction of Nauru: An example of weak sustainability. *Land Economics* 75, 333–338.

Gruetzmacher, K., Karesh, W.B., Amuasi, J.H., Arshad, A., Farlow, A. *et al.* (2021) The berlin principles on one health – Bridging global health and conservation. *Science of The Total Environment* 764, 142919. DOI: 10.1016/j.scitotenv.2020.142919.

Guest, D., Butubu, J., Ogtrop, F., Hall, J., Vinning, G. *et al.* (2023) Poverty, education and family health limit disease management and yields on smallholder cocoa farms in Bougainville. *CABI One Health*. DOI: 10.1079/cabionehealth.2023.0009.

Hamlin, C. (1980) Sewage: Waste or resource? *Environment: Science and Policy for Sustainable Development* 22, 16–42. DOI: 10.1080/00139157.1980.9932440.

He, D.-C., Burdon, J.J., Xie, L.-H. and Zhan, J. (2021) Triple bottom-line consideration of sustainable plant disease management: From economic, sociological and ecological perspectives. *Journal of Integrative Agriculture* 20, 2581–2591. DOI: 10.1016/S2095-3119(21)63627-4.

Heckman, J.R. (2006) A history of organic farming: Transitions from sir Albert Howard's war in the soil to USDA national organic program. *Renewable Agriculture and Food Systems* 21, 143–150. DOI: 10.1079/RAF2005126.

Heckman, J.R. (2013) Soil fertility management a century ago in farmers of forty centuries. *Sustainability* 5, 2796–2801. DOI: 10.3390/su5062796.

Hernando-Amado, S., Coque, T.M., Baquero, F. and Martínez, J.L. (2020) Antibiotic resistance: Moving from individual health norms to social norms in one health and global health. *Frontiers in Microbiology* 11, 547252. DOI: 10.3389/fmicb.2020.01914.

Ho, C.W.-L. (2022) Operationalizing "One Health" as "One Digital Health" through a global framework that emphasizes fair and equitable sharing of benefits from the use of artificial intelligence and related digital technologies. *Frontiers in Public Health* 10, 768977. DOI: 10.3389/fpubh.2022.768977.

Hoffmann, V., Paul, B., Falade, T., Moodley, A., Ramankutty, N. *et al.* (2022) A one health approach to plant health. *CABI Agriculture and Bioscience* 3, 62. DOI: 10.1186/s43170-022-00118-2.

Houot, S., Pons, M.-N., Pradel, M. and Tibi, A. (2016) Recyclage de déchets organiques en agriculture – Effets agronomiques et environnementaux de leur épandage editions quae. Paris.

Hu, W., Cichota, R., Beare, M., Müller, K., Drewry, J. *et al.* (2023) Soil structural vulnerability: Critical review and conceptual development. *Geoderma* 430, 116346. DOI: 10.1016/j.geoderma.2023.116346.

Hubálek, Z. and Rudolf, I. (2010) A history of Zoonoses and Sapronoses and research into them. In: *Microbial Zoonoses and Sapronoses*. Springer, Dordrecht, pp. 9–24.

Hugo, V. (1862) *Les Misérables A.* Lacroix, Verboeckhoven & Cie, Belgium.

Janvier, C., Villeneuve, F., Alabouvette, C., Edel-Hermann, V., Mateille, T. *et al.* (2007) Soil health through soil disease suppression: Which strategy from descriptors to indicators? *Soil Biology and Biochemistry* 39, 1–23. DOI: 10.1016/j.soilbio.2006.07.001.

Jones, R. (ed.) (2012) *Manure Matters: Historial, Archaeological and Ethnographic Perspectives*. Routledge, New York, p. 249.

Kang, S.E., Sumabat, L.G., Melie, T., Mangum, B., Momany, M. *et al.* (2021) Evidence for the agricultural origin of resistance to multiple antimicrobials in *Aspergillus fumigatus*, a fungal pathogen of humans. *G3 Genes|Genomes|Genetics* jkab427. DOI: 10.1093/g3journal/jkab427.

Keith, A.M., Schmidt, O. and McMahon, B.J. (2016) Soil stewardship as a nexus between ecosystem services and one health. *Ecosystem Services* 17, 40–42. DOI: 10.1016/j.ecoser.2015.11.008.

Kendzior, J., Warren Raffa, D. and Bogdanski, A. (2022) *The Soil Microbiome: A Game Changer for Food and Agriculture – Executive Summary for Policymakers and Researchers*. FAO, Rome. Available at: 10.4060/cc0717en

King, F.H. and Percy, B. (1911) *Farmers of Forty Centuries; or, Permanent Agriculture in China, Korea and Japan*. Organic Gardening Press, Emmaus, PA.

Kitole, F.A., Lihawa, R.M. and Nsindagi, T.E. (2023) Agriculture productivity and farmers' health in Tanzania: Analysis on maize subsector. *Global Social Welfare* 10, 197–206. DOI: 10.1007/s40609-022-00243-w.

Knorr, D. (2023) Organic agriculture and foods: Advancing process-product integrations. *Critical Reviews in Food Science and Nutrition* 1–13. DOI: 10.1080/10408398.2023.2200829.

Kopittke, P.M., Berhe, A.A., Carrillo, Y., Cavagnaro, T.R., Chen, D. *et al*. (2022) Ensuring planetary survival: The centrality of organic carbon in balancing the multifunctional nature of soils. *Critical Reviews in Environmental Science and Technology* 52, 4308–4324. DOI: 10.1080/10643389.2021.2024484.

Kopittke, P.M., Minasny, B., Pendall, E., Rumpel, C. and McKenna, B.A. (2023) Healthy soil for healthy humans and a healthy planet. *Critical Reviews in Environmental Science and Technology* 1–12. DOI: 10.1080/10643389.2023.2228651.

Krebs, J. and Bach, S. (2018) Permaculture—Scientific evidence of principles for the agroecological design of farming systems. *Sustainability* 10, 3218. DOI: 10.3390/su10093218.

Lavallais, C.M. and Dunn, J.B. (2023) Developing product level indicators to advance the nitrogen circular economy. *Resources, Conservation and Recycling* 198, 107167. DOI: 10.1016/j.resconrec.2023.107167.

Li, O.Y., Wang, X., Yang, K., Liu, D. and Shi, H. (2023) The approaching pilot for one health governance index. *Infectious Diseases of Poverty* 12, 16. DOI: 10.1186/s40249-023-01067-2.

Liao, H., Li, X., Yang, Q., Bai, Y., Cui, P. *et al*. (2021) Herbicide selection promotes antibiotic resistance in soil microbiomes. *Molecular Biology and Evolution* 38, 2337–2350. DOI: 10.1093/molbev/msab029.

Liu, X.J., Xu, W., Du, E.Z., Tang, A.H., Zhang, Y. *et al*. (2020) Environmental impacts of nitrogen emissions in China and the role of policies in emission reduction. *Philosophical Transactions of the Royal Society A: Mathematical, Physical and Engineering Sciences* 378, 20190324. DOI: 10.1098/rsta.2019.0324.

Lombardi, C., Thompson, S., Ritz, B., Cockburn, M. and Heck, J.E. (2021) Residential proximity to pesticide application as a risk factor for childhood central nervous system tumors. *Environmental Research* 197, 111078. DOI: 10.1016/j.envres.2021.111078.

Marchetti, L., Cattivelli, V., Cocozza, C., Salbitano, F. and Marchetti, M. (2020) Beyond sustainability in food systems: Perspectives from agroecology and social innovation. *Sustainability* 12, 7524. DOI: 10.3390/su12187524.

McLeman, R.A., Dupre, J., Berrang Ford, L., Ford, J., Gajewski, K. *et al*. (2014) What we learned from the dust bowl: Lessons in science, policy, and adaptation. *Population and Environment* 35, 417–440. DOI: 10.1007/s11111-013-0190-z.

McNeil, C., Verlander, S., Divi, N. and Smolinski, M. (2022) The landscape of participatory surveillance systems across the one health spectrum: Systematic review. *JMIR Public Health Surveill* 8, e38551. DOI: 10.2196/38551.

Melillo, E.D. (ed.) (2012) The first green revolution: Debt peonage and the making of the nitrogen fertilizer trade, 1840–1930. *The American Historical Review* 117, 1028–1060. DOI: 10.1093/ahr/117.4.1028.

Merrill, M.C. (1983) Eco-agriculture: A review of its history and philosophy. *Biological Agriculture & Horticulture* 1, 181–210. DOI: 10.1080/01448765.1983.9754395.

Migeot, V., Guihenneuc, J., Ouazzani, H.E., Albouy, M., Dupuis, A. *et al*. (2022) Risk and asset-based strategies in health: Priorities in biomedical, life and environmental science literature since the early twentieth century. A rapid review. *Environmental Health* 21, 22. DOI: 10.1186/s12940-022-00833-3.

Miller, S.A., Ferreira, J.P. and LeJeune, J.T. (2022) Antimicrobial use and resistance in plant agriculture: A one health perspective. *Agriculture*.

Morris, C.E., Géniaux, G., Nédellec, C., Sauvion, N. and Soubeyrand, S. (2022) One health concepts and challenges for surveillance, forecasting, and mitigation of plant disease beyond the traditional scope of crop production. *Plant Pathology* 71, 86–97. DOI: 10.1111/ppa.13446.

Muramoto, J., Parr, D.M., Perez, J. and Wong, D.G. (2022) Integrated soil health management for plant health and one health: Lessons from histories of soil-borne disease management in California strawberries and arthropod pest management. *Frontiers in Sustainable Food Systems* 6, 839648. DOI: 10.3389/fsufs.2022.839648.

Nwokolo, N.L., Enebe, M.C., Chigor, C.B., Chigor, V.N. and Dada, O.A. (2021) The contributions of biotic lines of defence to improving plant disease suppression in soils: A review. *Rhizosphere* 19, 100372. DOI: 10.1016/j.rhisph.2021.100372.

Paull, J. (2010) From france to the world: The international organization of organic agriculture movements (IFOAM). *Journal of Social Research and Policy* 1, 93–102.

Paull, J. (2011) The making of an agricultural classic: Farmers of forty centuries or permanent agriculture in China, Korea and Japan, 1911–2011. *Agricultural Sciences* 2, 175–180. DOI: 10.4236/as.2011.23024.

Paull, J. (2014) Lord northbourne, the man who invented organic farming, a biography. *Journal of Organic Systems* 9, 31–53.

Qamar, W., Shahid, M.U., Irfan, M., Abbas, R.Z., Faraz, A. *et al.* (2023) Thiamethoxam toxicity: A review in one-health perspective. *Kafkas Univ Vet Fak Derg* 29, 557–570. DOI: 10.9775/kvfd.2023.30161.

Ratnadass, A. and Sester, M. (2023) Crop protection practices and risks associated with human fungal infectious diseases: A one health perspective. *Cahiers Agricultures* 32, 7.

Reed, M. (2001) Fight the future! How the contemporary campaigns of the UK organic movement have arisen from their composting of the past. *Sociologia Ruralis* 41, 131–145. DOI: 10.1111/1467-9523.00173.

Richardson, K., Steffen, W., Lucht, W., Bendtsen, J., Cornell, S.E. *et al.* (2023) Earth beyond six of nine planetary boundaries. *Science Advances* 9, eadh2458. DOI: 10.1126/sciadv.adh2458.

Risch, E., Boutin, C. and Roux, P. (2021) Applying life cycle assessment to assess the environmental performance of decentralised versus centralised wastewater systems. *Water Research* 196, 116991. DOI: 10.1016/j.watres.2021.116991.

Rockström, J., Steffen, W., Noone, K., Persson, Å., Chapin, F.S. *et al.* (2009) A safe operating space for humanity. *Nature* 461, 472–475. DOI: 10.1038/461472a.

Rodríguez-Espinosa, T., Papamichael, I., Voukkali, I., Gimeno, A.P., Candel, M.B.A. *et al.* (2023) Nitrogen management in farming systems under the use of agricultural wastes and circular economy. *Science of The Total Environment* 876, 162666. DOI: 10.1016/j.scitotenv.2023.162666.

Russel, D.A. and Williams, G.G. (1977) History of chemical fertilizer development. *Soil Science Society of America* 41, 260–265.

Savary, S., Willocquet, L., Pethybridge, S.J., Esker, P., McRoberts, N. *et al.* (2019) The global burden of pathogens and pests on major food crops. *Nature Ecology & Evolution* 3, 430–439. DOI: 10.1038/s41559-018-0793-y.

Sessitsch, A., Wakelin, S., Schloter, M., Maguin, E., Cernava, T. *et al.* (2023) Microbiome interconnectedness throughout environments with major consequences for healthy people and a healthy planet. *Microbiology and Molecular Biology Reviews* 87, e00212-22. DOI: 10.1128/mmbr.00212-22.

Shukla, A., Patwa, A., Parde, D. and Vijay, R. (2023) A review on generation, characterization, containment, transport and treatment of fecal sludge and septage with resource recovery-oriented sanitation. *Environmental Research* 216, 114389. DOI: 10.1016/j.envres.2022.114389.

Singh, B.K., Yan, Z.-Z., Whittaker, M., Vargas, R. and Abdelfattah, A. (2023) Soil microbiomes must be explicitly included in one health policy. *Nature Microbiology* 8, 1367–1372. DOI: 10.1038/s41564-023.

Singh, B.R., McLaughlin, M.J. and Brevik, E. (eds) (2017) *The Nexus of Soils, Plants, Animals and Human Health*. Shweitzerbartz Science Publishers, Stuttgart, Germany, p. 163.

Snyders, H. (2019) Guanopreneurs and the dynamics of policymaking in the cape colony, 1843–1845. *New Contree: A Journal of Historical and Human Sciences for Southern Africa* 83, 1–23.

Stichweh, R. (2001) Scientific disciplines, history of. In: Smelser, N.J. and Baltes, P.B. (eds) *International Encyclopedia of the Social & Behavioral Sciences*. Pergamon, Oxford, UK, pp. 13727–13731.

Tahat, M.M., Alananbeh, K.M., Othman, Y.A. and Leskovar, D.I. (2020) Soil health and sustainable agriculture. *Sustainability* 12, 4859. DOI: 10.3390/su12124859.

Toor, G.S., Yang, Y.-Y., Das, S., Dorsey, S. and Felton, G. (2021) Chapter four – soil health in agricultural ecosystems: Current status and future perspectives. In: Sparks, D.L. (ed.) *Advances in Agronomy*. Academic Press, Amsterdam, pp. 157–201.

van Bruggen, A.H.C., Goss, E.M., Havelaar, A., Diepeningen, A.D., Finckh, M.R. *et al.* (2019) One health – Cycling of diverse microbial communities as a connecting force for soil, plant, animal, human and ecosystem health. *Science of The Total Environment* 664, 927–937. DOI: 10.1016/j.scitotenv.2019.02.091.

van Bruggen, A.H.C., Finckh, M.R., He, M., Ritsema, C.J., Harkes, P. *et al.* (2021) Indirect effects of the herbicide glyphosate on plant, animal and human health through its effects on microbial communities. *Frontiers in Environmental Science* 9. DOI: 10.3389/fenvs.2021.763917.

Vieweger, A. and Döring, T.F. (2015) Assessing health in agriculture – Towards a common research framework for soils, plants, animals, humans and ecosystems. *Journal of the Science of Food and Agriculture* 95, 438–446. DOI: 10.1002/jsfa.6708.

Vittecoq, M. (2022) Mettre en pratique l'approche « une seule santé ». Audelà du « comment » se poser la question du « pourquoi». *Environnement, Risques & Santé* 21, 201–204. DOI: 10.1684/ers.2022.1646.

Wu, Y. (2001) Rabies and rabid dogs in Sumerian and Akkadian literature. *Journal of the American Oriental Society* 121, 32–43.

Yan, Z., Xiong, C., Liu, H. and Singh, B.K. (2022) Sustainable agricultural practices contribute significantly to One Health. *Journal of Sustainable Agriculture and Environment* 1, 165–176. DOI: 10.1002/sae2.12019.

6 Foodborne Pathogens and their Association with Well-Known Enteric Infections and Emerging Non-Communicable Disorders

Asma Afshari[1], Ramin Rezaee[2,3] and Golshan Shakeri[1,4*]

[1]Department of Nutrition, Faculty of Medicine, Mashhad University of Medical Sciences, Mashhad, Iran; [2]Clinical Research Development Unit, Imam Reza Hospital, Faculty of Medicine, Mashhad University of Medical Sciences, Mashhad, Iran; [3]Applied Biomedical Research Center, Mashhad University of Medical Sciences, Mashhad, Iran; [4]The German Federal Institute for Risk Assessment, Diedersdorfer Weg 1, D-12277 Berlin, Germany

Abstract

Annually, numerous new cases of communicable and non-communicable diseases are diagnosed, and consumption of food/ water contaminated with different levels of microbial and chemical agents is responsible for a considerable portion of this burden. Generally, acute foodborne diseases are readily identified, while chronic deleterious effects are often neglected and rarely blamed for health consequences. The present work narrates a journey from consuming foods containing bacteria/bacterial toxins to developing chronic diseases, making humans more susceptible to emerging diseases. We aim to shed light on the chronic effects of foodborne diseases, particularly gastrointestinal disorders (GIDs) and inflammatory bowel diseases (IBDs), which are common chronic symptoms of most foodborne diseases.

Keywords: food, foodborne pathogens, bacterial contamination, chronic disease, IBD, GID

Introduction

According to the most recent estimation of the burden of foodborne diseases published by the WHO, consumption of unsafe food can globally lead to 600 million cases of foodborne illness and 420,000 deaths per year, which result in losing 33 million years of life (WHO, 2021). In 2018, in the United states, FoodNet (The Foodborne Diseases Active Surveillance Network) identified 25,606 foodborne cases with 5893 hospitalizations and 120 deaths, which overpassed those of the previous years (Tack *et al.*, 2019; Kingsbury *et al.*, 2020). The burden of foodborne diseases is heavier in low- and middle-income countries (WHO, 2021). However, generally, the burden of foodborne illnesses to public health, welfare, and economy is often underestimated due to under-reporting and the difficulty to establish causal relationships between food contamination and

*Corresponding author: golshan.shakeri@gmail.com

health outcomes/death (Kuchenmüller *et al.*, 2009). Of note, while there are over 250 foodborne diseases, caused by bacteria, viruses, and parasites and also chemicals, it is still challenging to attribute a chronic disease to exposure to such agents (WHO, 2021). Microbial contaminants can cause various health problems ranging from self-limiting gastroenteritis to fatal complications including hepatic, renal, and neurological syndromes. Chronic effects of exposure to food contaminants might be far more dangerous than the acute ones, and for many of these long-term effects, contributing factors and underlying mechanisms have been described (Batz *et al.*, 2013).

Depending on the number and duration of foodborne infections that an individual has experienced during his/her life, exposure to infectious agents can alter the gut flora, increase intestinal permeability, and trigger inappropriate immune responses (Thabane and Marshall, 2009). Even low levels of bacterial contamination in food may cause foodborne infections and initiate a cascade of reactions that may result in chronic inflammations like inflammatory bowel diseases (IBDs) and colitis which recently demonstrated an increasing trend of incidence and prevalence (Yang *et al.*, 2017). Indeed, repeated exposure and recurrent infections debilitate normal host protection over time (Yang *et al.*, 2017). Furthermore, repeated exposure to low levels of toxins should be taken into serious account as bio-accumulation and damage due to chronic exposure may occur, especially in the case of lipophilic and stable toxins (Rajkovic, 2014). Although long-term exposure to low-to-moderate levels of bacterial toxins has not been widely studied, they may substantially influence our health.

Cancers might be another life-threatening sequela of foodborne diseases. Based on the literature, there are relationships between certain bacterial infections and cancer etiology (Mager, 2006). In this regard, WHO considers bacteria a CLASS I carcinogen (Eyvazi *et al.*, 2020). Globally, over 15% of malignancies could be attributed to infections induced by viruses, bacteria, and parasites (Pisani *et al.*, 1997). Bacteria are supposed to have several indirect carcinogenic actions in the gut. The mechanism of action may be related to the deconjugation of bile acids that produces cytotoxic deoxycholate and lithocholic acid, activating exogenous mutagen precursors, fermentation of polysaccharides and glycoproteins to volatile fatty acids, and attaching and effacing lesions of the large intestine. (Parsonnet, 1995). Therefore, intramucosal bacteria, particularly enteropathogenic *Escherichia coli* (*E. coli*), which induce inflammatory conditions, may pose a potential risk of cancer to humans. For instance, IBD can significantly increase the risk of colorectal cancer, and bacteria may be involved in the pathogenesis of gastric lymphomas and immunoproliferative small intestinal disease (Parsonnet, 1995). Table 6.1 presents foodborne bacteria that were shown to be associated with cancer induction.

Foodborne diseases constitute a significant public health concern worldwide, affecting populations across different socioeconomic strata. Despite progress in addressing acute foodborne

Table 6.1. Foodborne bacterial species and their roles in particular cancers.

Bacterial species	Induced cancers	Reference
Clostridium spp.	Mainly colon cancer	Fukugaiti *et al.* (2015)
Salmonella typhi	Melanoma, colon and bladder cancers, gallbladder and hepatobiliary carcinoma	Caygill *et al.* (1995); Shukla *et al.* (2000); Mager (2006)
Escherichia coli	Colon cancer	Martin *et al.* (2004)
Streptococci	Colon cancer	Boleij *et al.* (2011)
Helicobacter pylori	Stomach cancer	Zamani *et al.* (2017)
Staphylococcus aureus	Bladder cancer	Sheweita and Alsamghan (2020)
Mycobacterium tuberculosis	Lung cancer	Steinitz (1965)

illnesses, the chronic effects resulting from consuming contaminated food have received limited attention. This article aims to bridge this knowledge gap by elucidating the chronic consequences of foodborne diseases, focusing on GID, IBD, and their potential role in the development of other chronic conditions.

Review Methodology

The following databases were searched by two separate authors (AA and GS): *Web of Science, PubMed,* and *Google Scholar*. Keyword search terms used were as follows: bacterial food borne; disease; chronic; Salmonella spp; Listeria spp; enteropathogenic Ecoli; *Clostridium perfringens; Bacillus cereus; Shigella spp; Yersinia spp; Vibrio spp*. In addition, to check for additional relevant articles, we used the references of the included articles. Any inconsistency was solved by the third author (RR).

Microbial Foodborne Pathogens: Bacteria as Leading Agent

Bacteria (66%) followed by viruses (4%) and parasites (4%) are the leading causes of microbial foodborne illnesses (Addis and Sisay, 2015). For decades, foodborne bacterial diseases have demonstrated high impact on public health (Adley and Ryan, 2016; Abebe *et al.*, 2020). Following the growth of bacteria under favorable conditions, they may produce toxins in the food and produce mild-to-moderate disorders. Toxins could be absorbed through the gastrointestinal tract's epithelial membrane and cause local tissue damage or may reach distant organs such as the kidney, liver, and central nervous system (Schuchat *et al.*, 1991; Addis and Sisay, 2015).

According to the European Food Safety Authority (EFSA) and Centers for Disease Control and Prevention (CDC), major foodborne pathogens in Europe and the United States are *Campylobacter*, *Salmonella*, Shiga toxin-producing *E. coli* (*STEC*), *Shigella*, *Yersinia*, *Listeria*, and *Vibrio* (Marder *et al.*, 2018; WHO, 2021). Other bacteria including *Staphylococcus aureus* and *Clostridium* were also reported as causative agents of food- or water-borne diseases (Adley and Ryan, 2016; Abebe *et al.*, 2020).

Late health sequelae of foodborne infections can predispose for emerging health threats. Importantly, several investigations showed that presence of comorbidities such as hypertension, diabetes, chronic lung and renal diseases, cardio-cerebrovascular diseases, and cancer led to poor clinical outcomes, highlighting the importance of controlling such predisposing factors in population (Guan *et al.*, 2020; Hussain *et al.*, 2020).

In this review, we highlight the significance of specific bacteria known to cause foodborne illnesses, including *Campylobacter*, *Salmonella*, enteropathogenic *E. coli*, *Shigella*, *Yersinia*, *Listeria*, *Vibrio*, *Staphylococcus aureus*, and *Clostridium*, by emphasizing their sequelae as potential predisposing factors for emerging health threats.

Long-Term Effects of Exposure to Food Contaminated by Bacterial Pathogens

Campylobacter

Campylobacter infections constitute most of foodborne infections in humans in Europe and the United States (Marder *et al.*, 2018; European Food Safety Authority, and European Centre for Disease Prevention and Control, 2021). Clinical outcome of *C. jejuni* infection ranges from mild to severe diarrheal disease and some post-infection sequelae including Guillain–Barré syndrome (GBS), and reactive arthritis (Backert *et al.*, 2017). *C. jejuni* induces GBS through the production of autoantibodies that target both the bacterial ganglioside-like lipooligosaccharide (LOS) structures and human peripheral nerve gangliosides. Consequently, axonal degeneration and demyelination of the peripheral nerves may occur and eventually result in muscular weakness (Nyati and Nyati, 2013) (Fig. 6.1).

C. jejuni can also cause pancreatitis (Kobayashi *et al.*, 2014) due to direct spread of inflammation from the small intestine to the pancreas and pancreatic duct via the blood and lymphatic vessels (Kobayashi *et al.*, 2014). Postinfectious irritable bowel syndrome

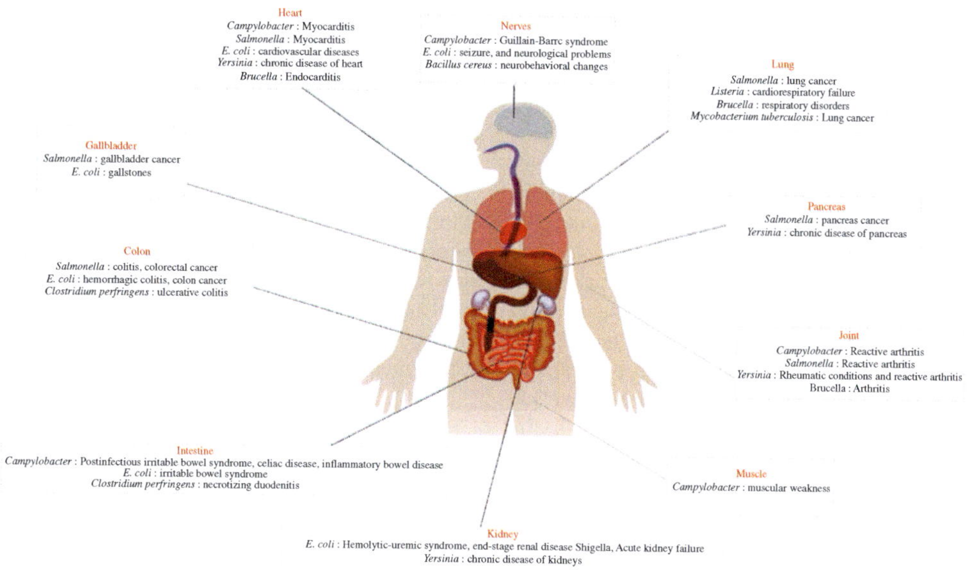

Fig. 6.1. Chronic effects of bacterial infections on different organs.

(PI-IBS) and myocarditis are other important sequelae of *Campylobacter* infection (Jess *et al.*, 2011; Ayyildiz *et al.*, 2018; Walter *et al.*, 2019). Myocarditis can be a rare but severe complication of campylobacteriosis, as well as other infectious diseases such as salmonellosis and shigellosis (Olsen, 2001). In addition, *C. jejuni* as an infectious agent can contribute to the pathogenesis of celiac disease (Verdu *et al.*, 2007; Riddle *et al.*, 2013). *Campylobacter* may also contribute to the development of IBD. For example, a study by Bernstein *et al.* found that exposure to *Campylobacter* was associated with an increased risk of developing Crohn's disease (Bernstein *et al.*, 1999). Furthermore, evidence suggests that *C. jejuni* infection may be associated with an increased risk of colorectal cancer (Fox and Wang, 2007; Duijster *et al.*, 2021).

Salmonella

Salmonella is the second leading cause of foodborne infections in Europe and the United States (Marder *et al.*, 2018; European Food Safety Authority, and European Centre for Disease Prevention and Control, 2021). The symptoms of infection include fever, diarrhea, gastroenteritis, and sepsis (Chiller, 2019). Bacteremia, endovascular, and localized infections may also occur in individuals with low gastric pH. Furthermore, *Salmonella* can develop tolerance against gastric acid, making it more invasive, as a number of bacteria become able to survive in gastric environments, multiply, and translocate to other organs (Zha *et al.*, 2019).

It was reported that each year in the United States, approximately 1.4 million people are infected with *Salmonella* (Rohekar *et al.*, 2008), and infected people were reported to be at a higher risk of immune-related diseases such as arthritis (Rohekar *et al.*, 2008) and IBD (Axelrad *et al.*, 2019). It was shown that repeated episodes of food poisoning by low and non-lethal *Salmonella enterica* Typhimurium levels may lead to chronic inflammation of the intestine and colitis (Yang *et al.*, 2017). *Salmonella* may induce inflammation through intestinal alkaline phosphatase (IAP) degradation by neuraminidase 3 (Neu3) production in the duodenum (Yang *et al.*, 2017). In addition, results of a study suggest that non-typhoidal *Salmonella* infection may contribute to the generation of autoantibodies and may play a role in autoimmune diseases (Ktsoyan *et al.*, 2019). Furthermore, non-typhoidal *Salmonella* infection has been linked to an increased risk of colorectal cancer, particularly in individuals with underlying IBD (Duijster *et al.*, 2021). Research showed that *Salmonella* infection might induce carcinogenesis through various pathways as it can cause persistent intestinal infection, imbalance in the gut flora, and chronic inflammation, which further induces DNA damage through the production of cytolethal distending toxins (CDT) (Zha *et al.*, 2019). Cluster genes of *Salmonella* pathogenicity islands (SPI) regulate the invasion to host cells and type 3 secretion system (T3SS) variation coded by SPI-1 and SPI-2, which plays an essential role in host cell pathways (Zha *et al.*, 2019; Lerminiaux *et al.*, 2020). In fact, the effectors of the T3SS activate essential host cell pathways causing immune regulation disorders and dysbiosis, which can contribute to colitis-associated cancer (Zha *et al.*, 2019). Repetitive exposure to non-typhoidal *Salmonella* may lead to chronic inflammation in the colon, which can promote the development and growth of tumors. Furthermore, gut microbiota may play a role in modulating the host response to non-typhoidal *Salmonella* infection and the subsequent risk of colon cancer (van Elsland *et al.*, 2022). Additionally, probability of intestinal fibrosis in mice through the Cox-2 and MyD88 signaling pathway was shown (Månsson *et al.*, 2012). Moreover, although the evidence was limited to suggest association between *Salmonella* and gallbladder cancer (Parry *et al.*, 2002), some recent results strengthened this hypothesis (Koshiol *et al.*, 2016; Mughini-Gras *et al.*, 2018; Zha *et al.*, 2019). A review suggested a possible connection between chronic *Salmonella* Typhi infection and the development of gallbladder cancer due to the high incidence of gallbladder cancer in certain parts of the world, particularly in areas where *Salmonella* Typhi is endemic. The bacteria could possibly cause chronic inflammation, DNA damage, and alterations in cellular signaling pathways that could lead to the development of cancer (Upadhayay *et al.*, 2022). Sequelae of *Salmonella* infection can also result in a high risk of pancreas and lung cancer (Zha *et al.*, 2019). Non-typhoidal infection may lead to chronic inflammation and immune system dysfunction, which can promote the development and progression of hematological malignancies. In a nationwide population-based cohort study in Taiwan, it has been found that individuals with a history of non-typhoidal infection had an increased risk of developing hematological malignancies, such as leukemia and lymphoma. Moreover, the risk was higher among those who had multiple episodes of non-typhoidal infection and those who were infected with certain serotypes of non-typhoidal infection (Yun *et al.*, 2022) . In searching the literature, we encountered a recently reported case of invasive *Salmonella* which developed extraintestinal focal infections (EFIs) with mycotic aneurysm and spinal osteomyelitis in a 39-year-old male (Castlemain and Castlemain, 2022).

Enteropathogenic *E. coli*

Shiga toxin (verotoxin)-producing *E. coli* (STEC) is the third most-reported foodborne pathogen in Europe and the fourth in the United States (Marder *et al.*, 2018; WHO, 2021). STEC produces two types of Shiga toxins (Stx) including Stx1 and Stx2. Previous investigations showed a higher toxicity for Stx1 compared to Stx2 (Tesh *et al.*, 1993; Louise and Obrig, 1995; Terajima *et al.*, 2017).

Contamination of meat during slaughter plays the principal role in transferring STEC to human via food (Terajima *et al.*, 2017). In many outbreaks throughout the world, infections with one of the most threatening STEC, *E. coli* O157, were associated with a range of human illnesses ranging from mild diarrhea to complications such as hemorrhagic colitis, hemolytic-uremic syndrome (HUS), and thrombotic thrombocytopenic purpura (Fernandez, 2008; Farah *et al.*, 2014). Although *E. coli* is mostly associated with HUS which often occurs in children, it can cause chronic organ dysfunction and external dysfunction (Ameer *et al.*, 2021). Results of a case study demonstrated the importance of considering STEC as a causative agent of microangiopathic hemolytic anemia in older people (Ko *et al.*, 2016).

Adults recovered from *E. coli* O157:H7 infections had increased risks of high blood pressure, kidney problems, and cardiovascular diseases (Clark *et al.*, 2010). Result of a study showed the host-bacterial interactions of *E. coli* O157:H7 strain with initiation and progression of cardiovascular diseases in the host (Miryala *et al.*, 2021). It should be noted that

E. coli O157:H7 is resistant to acidic conditions and most antibiotics, and it carries a 60-MDa plasmid and an attaching (*eae*) gene, all contributing to STEC pathogenicity (Fernandez, 2008). In addition, Shiga-like toxin (SLT) is toxic to human colon and ileum cells (Buchanan and Doyle, 1997). A study on the carcinogenic properties of colon cancer-associated *E. coli* strain in multiple intestinal neoplasia in mice showed that pathogenic strains of *E. coli* can produce toxins and induce chronic inflammation which has a role in carcinogenesis (Bonnet *et al.*, 2014). Enterotoxigenic *E. coli* strains have been also associated with colorectal cancer, and some studies have suggested a possible role for diffusely adherent *E. coli* strains as well (Arthur *et al.*, 2012; Duijster *et al.*, 2021). A study that analyzed data from two large prospective cohort studies, proposed possible mechanisms by which PKs island-carrying *E. coli* could contribute to the development of cancer, including activation of cellular signaling pathways, chronic inflammation, and DNA damage (Arima *et al.*, 2022).

Shigella

According to the CDC, *Shigella* was the third most-reported foodborne pathogen in the United States during 2017 (Marder *et al.*, 2018). Shigellosis is caused through the bacterial invasion to the epithelium lining of the terminal ileum, colon, and rectum. Clinical manifestations of shigellosis vary from acute watery diarrhea to fulminant dysentery characterized by frequent scant bloody stools with fever, prostration, and abdominal cramps (Kotloff *et al.*, 2018). Many of the lethal toxins produced by *Shigella* are cytotoxic when injected parenterally, and if produced in the intestine, they will presumably cause necrosis and ulceration in the mucosa and, consequently, diarrhea or dysentery. This may explain the mechanism by which the cytotoxic enterotoxin of *Shigella dysenteriae* exerts its effect. *Shigella*'s neurotoxin is substantially inactivated in the stomach. Adhesion and invasion plasmid antigens are virulence factors of *Shigella*, allowing its entrance into target cells (Addis and Sisay, 2015).

Acute kidney failure may be a sequela of *Shigella* spp. infection which occurs subsequent to binding to the tubular epithelium and glomerular endothelial cells and under the effect of Shiga toxins which induce apoptosis, necrosis, and thrombotic microangiopathy (Mayer *et al.*, 2012). Results of a study reported a pediatric case of MERS (mild encephalitis with reversible splenial lesion of the corpus callosum) associated with *Shigella flexneri* infection in a 5-year-old boy with no history of disease (Le Soudéer *et al.*, 2022).

Yersinia

Yersinia has been identified as the fourth foodborne pathogen in Europe and the fifth in the United States (European Food Safety Authority, and European Centre for Disease Prevention and Control, 2021). Infection due to *Yersinia enterocolitica* is characterized by symptoms like abdominal pain, ileitis, diarrhea, fever, and rash, and rarely, it has been associated with sepsis. Generally, it causes a self-limiting mesenteric lymphadenitis that mimics appendicitis. Yersiniosis complications include reactive arthritis, autoimmune thyroid disease (Graves' disease), and erythema nodosum (Effraimidis *et al.*, 2011; Shoaib *et al.*, 2019; Brady *et al.*, 2023). In a study, 458 patients with yersiniosis were followed for 4–14 years (1974–1987). Rheumatic conditions and chronic diseases of the liver, kidneys, heart, pancreas, thyroid, or nervous system were observed in some patients, indicating that sequelae of yersiniosis could lead to malignant diseases or even death (Sæbos and Lassen, 1991). Results of a case report in a patient with previously undiagnosed liver cirrhosis with splenic abscesses, a case of myopericarditis infection in a 50-year-old man, showed *Yersinia pseudotuberculosis* and *Yersinia enterocolitica* as causative agents, respectively (Nehoff *et al.*, 2022; Zewude *et al.*, 2022). The role of *Y. enterocolitica* in Crohn's disease (CD) pathogenesis is also of interest but remains unclear, although evidence indicated a correlation between *Y. enterocolitica* infection and CD in clinical symptoms and pathological manifestations (Fang *et al.*, 2023).

Listeria

Listeria is the fifth most-reported foodborne pathogen in Europe. However, it was demonstrated to have the highest fatality rate among other foodborne zoonosis (European Food Safety Authority, and European Centre for Disease Prevention and Control, 2021). It is a facultative intracellular bacterium that enters non-phagocytic cells and spreads cell to cell via an actin-based motility process (Zewude *et al.*, 2022). *L. monocytogenes* can be found in soil or water (Schlech, 2019) and cause listeriosis (Ramaswamy *et al.*, 2007) and rarely sepsis, meningitis, rhombencephalitis, and cardiorespiratory failure particularly in immunocompromised patients such as those suffering from cancer, leukemia, or transplant patients (Schlech, 2019). The fatality rate in immunocompromised individuals can reach 30% (Schlech, 2019). Moreover, in some case reports, abdominal aortic aneurysm (Murphy *et al.*, 2013) as well as peritonitis (Sin *et al.*, 2021) were attributed to listeriosis.

Results of a Danish nationwide cohort study in 2012 showed an increased risk of death due to cancer in patients (at ages of >50 years) diagnosed with *L. monocytogenes* meningitis in the first 5 years of their follow-up (Roed *et al.*, 2012). In pregnant women, the symptoms range from mild chills to severe illness like premature delivery (20–25% of perinatal cases) or mental retardation, hearing loss, or brain damage in the newborn (Ramaswamy *et al.*, 2007). In a severe case of listeriosis, a 62-year-old male with an unremarkable medical history exhibited acute hepatitis and experienced multiple organ dysfunction syndromes (Teodor *et al.*, 2012). Furthermore, another notable case of listeriosis, specifically neurolisteriosis, was diagnosed in a 50-year-old male presenting with facial neuritis (Cao *et al.*, 2021).

Clostridium perfringens

Clostridium perfringens types A, B, C, D, and E generate at least 12 different toxins (McDonel, 1980). Enterotoxin, necrotic enteritis B-like toxin (NetB), and beta-2 toxin play significant role in the pathogenesis of *C. perfringens*-associated diseases (Miyamoto *et al.*, 2009). Symptoms include abdominal cramps and watery diarrhea that usually heal within 24 hour. Sometimes less severe symptoms may last for 1 or 2 weeks (Hailegebreal, 2017). Sulfate-reducing bacteria (SRB) including *C. perfringens* are known to initiate inflammatory processes leading to organ dysfunction like ulcerative colitis (Kushkevych *et al.*, 2016). A study showed that levels of H_2S due to high SRB counts were in correlation with ulcerative colitis formation (Ulcerative Colitis–Pathophysiology, 2003).

C. perfringens type C, which is mostly observed during outbreaks or in underdeveloped countries, causes a fatal disease characterized by hemorrhagic or ischemic necrosis in the jejunum (Acheson, 2009). Fatal cases of *C. perfringens* infection were reported in adults with type 2 diabetes in both developed and developing countries (Gui *et al.*, 2002; Smith *et al.*, 2011). A report from Japan stated a death due to necrotizing duodenitis caused by *C. perfringens* type C (Hagiya *et al.*, 2012). Some studies have suggested a possible association between *Clostridium* spp. and colorectal cancer, but the evidence is limited and inconsistent (Rolhion and Chassaing, 2016).

Bacillus cereus

The emetic toxin of *Bacillus cereus*, cereulide (a heat-stable cyclic depsipeptide) produced in food before ingestion, was linked to clinical symptoms including acute liver failure and acute encephalopathy (Stenfors Arnesen *et al.*, 2008; Tschiedel *et al.*, 2015). Cereulide-producing *B. cereus* can produce spores resistant to temperatures around 90°C (Carlin *et al.*, 2006). Such spores are likely to survive and accumulate in food processed by repeated heating. Cereulide negatively affects mitochondrial function and cell respiration by inhibiting the oxidation of fatty acids, which causes liver failure. Indeed, the toxin influences aerobic ATP production pathways and, consequently, causes an increase in plasma lactate levels, and thus a reduction in blood pH (Stenfors Arnesen *et al.*, 2008; Naranjo *et al.*, 2011). Therefore, long-term exposure to this toxin can potentially contribute to the development of diabetes

(Vangoitsenhoven *et al.*, 2014). Moreover, exposure to low-dose cereulide was reported to be associated with a detrimental effect on pancreatic beta cells. It was shown that insulin-producing pancreatic islet beta cells (MIN-6) are susceptible to cereulide-induced cytolysis (Hoornstra *et al.*, 2013). In addition, an investigation based on the porcine model demonstrated cereulide accumulation in some organs, such as the liver and kidney. Cereulide is also capable of passing through the blood-brain barrier and causing cerebral intoxication with neurobehavioral changes (Bauer *et al.*, 2018). Besides, toxic effects of cereulide have been documented in other cells such as sperms, hepatocytes, and human epithelial type 2 cells (Vangoitsenhoven *et al.*, 2015). There is a very recent report of bloodstream infection (BSI) caused by *Bacillus cereus*. Although *B. cereus* is not typically associated with bloodstream infections, it should be considered as a possible cause of BSI in patients with a recent history of consuming contaminated food (Maslar *et al.*, 2023). A severe case of *Bacillus cereus* food poisoning due to pre-formed exotoxin in fried rice was associated with sepsis, multi-organ failure, rhabdomyolysis, and coagulopathy (Colaco *et al.*, 2021), and also infective endocarditis (i.e.) was reported in a 58-year-old Sri Lankan male (Nallarajah and Mujahieth, 2020).

Vibrio

Vibrio spp. are Gram-negative, motile rods with a facultative anaerobic metabolism and ecologically significant aquatic bacteria. Vibriosis can be either cholera or non-cholera infection. Cholera is caused by the consumption of water or food containing toxigenic

V. cholerae (serogroups O1 and O139) and has been reported in developed countries. Non-cholera *Vibrio* infections typically result from the consumption of contaminated shellfish, and symptoms are characteristically gastroenteritis, wound or ear infection, and/ or septicemia (Brumfield *et al.*, 2021). The pathogenesis of *Vibrio cholerae* involves its capability to induce extra-intestinal infections, including otitis media, wound infections, skin and soft tissue infections, cholangitis, peritonitis, meningitis, and septicemia (Van Bonn *et al.*, 2020). *Vibrio parahaemolyticus*, another vibrio species, causing Guillain-Barré Syndrome (GBS) by the consumption of contaminated oysters was reported in a case study. This infection is a type of inflammatory and immune reaction that links gastrointestinal illness with GBS (Freeman, 2019).

Foodborne Diseases and Susceptibility to Emerging Diseases

Foodborne diseases expose people to infections, augment malnutrition, and make a circle of debilitation and mortality. Sometimes people who survive may suffer from delayed physical and mental development (Newell *et al.*, 2010; WHO, 2015). Many of these long-term manifestations are challenging to characterize, and therefore, they are too often missed by clinicians and public health authorities.

Gastrointestinal disorders (GIDs) and IBDs are common chronic symptoms of most foodborne diseases (Batz *et al.*, 2013). On the other hand, recent studies suggest that there might be a link between sequelae of foodborne diseases and an increased susceptibility to emerging diseases such as COVID-19. For instance, the inflamed intestinal lining in IBD patients demonstrates higher number of ACE II receptors (Verstockt *et al.*, 2021). Therefore, there is a concern that there may be an increased risk of developing COVID-19 in IBD patients as SARS-CoV-2 binds to target cells through ACE II receptors. Moreover, autoimmune diseases are another concern to increase the susceptibility to COVID-19, and as mentioned earlier, many foodborne diseases such as nontyphoidal salmonellosis are involved in the development of autoimmune diseases. In general, Gram-negative enteric pathogens such as some species of *Salmonella*, *Shigella*, *Yersinia*, and *Campylobacter* are reported to be associated with reactive arthritis as an autoimmune disease (Soloski and Metcalf, 2007; Huţanaşu *et al.*, 2009). On the other hand, infection with foodborne pathogens is also introduced as a cofactor in the pathogenesis of colorectal cancer and can provoke start of autoimmune responses, weeks after emergence of acute illness, and may lead to reactive arthritis, GBS, autoimmune thyroid disease, and possibly IBS.

Additionally, microbial exposure is considered a potential environmental factor in celiac disease. However, further research is required for a deep understanding of how infectious agents might stimulate celiac disease in susceptible individuals (Riddle *et al.*, 2013; Petersen *et al.*, 2020). However, it was shown that celiac patients are not at a greater risk for COVID-19 compared to others (Gokden *et al.*, 2020; Lebwohl *et al.*, 2021), but it was hypothesized that genetically predisposed COVID-19-infected individuals may be at a higher risk of developing celiac (Trovato *et al.*, 2021).

The extent of threat of foodborne diseases and their implications in human morbidity and mortality are not clearly understood, especially because of the underdiagnosed and underreported cases as well as the emergence of new pathogens. It should be also noted that many species have become resistant to antimicrobial therapies, which make foodborne diseases a perennial issue in the era when antimicrobial resistance is another emerging health threat.

Conclusion

According to our review, repeated exposure to low levels of bacterial contaminants, particularly *Campylobacter* and *Salmonella*, can lead to chronic inflammations and various health risks including Guillain-Barré syndrome, reactive arthritis, pancreatitis, irritable bowel syndrome, myocarditis, celiac disease, and IBD. Additionally, long-term exposure to bacterial toxins should be considered due to their potential implications for human health. The potential link between foodborne diseases and cancer, specifically colorectal cancer and gastric lymphomas, has been also discussed, with bacteria such as *E. coli* being implicated in increasing the risk of these malignancies.

In conclusion, the review highlights the significant burden of foodborne diseases on global health and the often-neglected chronic consequences of consuming contaminated food. Our study could raise awareness, promote further investigation, and facilitate the implementation of effective control strategies to protect public health.

Acknowledgements

We would like to thank Mashhad University of Medical sciences.

Funding

Mashhad University of Medical Sciences, Department of Nutrition.

Conflict of interest

The authors declare no conflict of interest.

Author Contributions

AA suggested the topic, performed the literature review and wrote the first draft. RR and GS revised the manuscript. All authors read and approved the final manuscript.

References

Abebe, E., Gugsa, G. and Ahmed, M. (2020) Review on major food-borne zoonotic bacterial pathogens. *Journal of Tropical Medicine* 4674235.

Acheson, D.W.K. (2009) Food and waterborne illnesses. *Encyclopedia of Microbiology* 365–381.

Addis, M. and Sisay, D. (2015) A review on major food borne bacterial illnesses. *International Journal of Tropical Diseases* 3(4), 176–183.

Adley, C. and Ryan, M. (2016) The nature and extent of foodborne disease. In: *Antimicrobial Food Packaging*. Academic Press, Cambridge, MA, pp. 1–10.

Ameer, M.A., Wasey, A. and Salen, P. (2021) *Escherichia Coli (E Coli 0157 H7)*. StatPearls Publishing, Treasure Island, FL.

Arima, K., Zhong, R., Ugai, T., Zhao, M., Haruki, K. *et al.* (2022) Western-Style diet, PKs island-carrying *Escherichia coli*, and colorectal cancer: Analyses from two large prospective cohort studies. *Gastroenterology* 163(4), 862–874.

Arthur, J.C., Perez-Chanona, E., Mühlbauer, M., Tomkovich, S. *et al.* (2012) Intestinal inflammation targets cancer-inducing activity of the microbiota. *Science* 338(6103), 120–123.

Axelrad, J.E., Olén, O., Askling, J., Lebwohl, B., Khalili, H. *et al.* (2019) Gastrointestinal infection increases odds of inflammatory bowel disease in a nationwide case–control study. *Clinical Gastroenterology and Hepatology* 17(7), 1311–1322.

Ayyildiz, H., Kalayci, M., Bozkurt, M. and Karadag, M.K. (2018) Myocarditis case associated with *Campylobacter jejuni*. *Turkish Journal of Biochemistry* 43(5), 568–570.

Backert, S., Tegtmeyer, N., Cróinín, T.Ó., Boehm, M. and Heimesaat, M.M. (2017) Human campylobacteriosis. In: *Campylobacter*. Academic Press, Cambridge, MA, pp. 1–25.

Batz, M.B., Henke, E. and Kowalcyk, B. (2013) Long-term consequences of foodborne infections. *Infectious Disease Clinics* 27(3), 599–616.

Bauer, T., Sipos, W., Stark, T.D., Käser, T., Knecht, C. *et al.* (2018) First insights into within host translocation of the *Bacillus cereus* toxin cereulide using a porcine model. *Frontiers in Microbiology* 9, 2652.

Bernstein, C.N., Blanchard, J.F., Rawsthorne, P. and Wajda, A. (1999) Epidemiology of crohn's disease and ulcerative colitis in a central Canadian province: A population-based study. *American Journal of Epidemiology* 149(10), 916–924.

Boleij, A., Gelder, M.M., Swinkels, D.W. and Tjalsma, H. (2011) Clinical importance of *Streptococcus gallolyticus* infection among colorectal cancer patients: Systematic review and meta-analysis. *Clinical Infectious Diseases* 53(9), 870–878.

Bonnet, M., Buc, E., Sauvanet, P., Darcha, C., Dubois, D. *et al.* (2014) Colonization of the human gut by *E. Coli* and colorectal cancer risk. *Clinical Cancer Research* 20(4), 859–867.

Brady, M.F., Yarrarapu, S.N.S. and Anjum, F. (2023) *Yersinia Pseudotuberculosis*. StatPearls Publishing, Tampa, FL.

Brumfield, K.D., Usmani, M., Chen, K.M., Gangwar, M., Jutla, A.S. *et al.* (2021) Environmental parameters associated with incidence and transmission of *Pathogenic vibrio* spp. *Environmental Microbiology* 23(12), 7314–7340.

Buchanan, R.L. and Doyle, M.P. (1997) Foodborne disease significance of *Escherichia coli* O157: H7 and other enterohemorrhagic *E. Coli*. *Food Technology (Chicago)* 51(10), 69–76.

Cao, L., Lin, Y., Jiang, H. and Wei, J. (2021) Severe invasive *Listeria monocytogenes* rhombencephalitis mimicking facial neuritis in a healthy middle-aged man: A case report and literature review. *Journal of International Medical Research* 49(1), 0300060520982653.

Carlin, F., Fricker, M., Pielaat, A., Heisterkamp, S., Shaheen, R. *et al.* (2006) Emetic toxin-producing strains of *Bacillus cereus* show distinct characteristics within the *Bacillus cereus* group. *International Journal of Food Microbiology* 109(1–2), 132–138.

Castlemain, B.M. and Castlemain, B.D. (2022) Case report: Post-salmonellosis abscess positive for *Salmonella oranienburg*. *BMC Infectious Diseases* 22(1), 1–4.

Caygill, C., Braddick, M., Hill, M., Knowles, R. and Sharp, J. (1995) The association between typhoid carriage, typhoid infection and subsequent cancer at a number of sites. *European Journal of Cancer Prevention: The Official Journal of the European Cancer Prevention Organisation (ECP)* 4(2), 187–193.

Chiller, T.M. (2019) Salmonella/foodborne outbreaks in USA. *Pathology* 51, S59–S60.

Clark, W.F., Sontrop, J.M., Macnab, J.J., Salvadori, M., Moist, L. *et al.* (2010) Long term risk for hypertension, renal impairment, and cardiovascular disease after gastroenteritis from drinking water contaminated with *Escherichia coli* O157: H7: A prospective cohort study. *Bmj* 341, c6020.

Colaco, C.M., Basile, K., Draper, J. and Ferguson, P.E. (2021) Fulminant *Bacillus cereus* food poisoning with fatal multi-organ failure. *BMJ Case Reports CP* 14(1), e238716.

Duijster, J.W., Franz, E., Neefjes, J. and Mughini-Gras, L. (2021) Bacterial and parasitic pathogens as risk factors for cancers in the gastrointestinal tract: A review of current epidemiological knowledge. *Frontiers in Microbiology* 12, 790256.

Effraimidis, G., Tijssen, J., Strieder, T. and Wiersinga, W. (2011) No causal relationship between *Yersinia enterocolitica* infection and autoimmune thyroid disease: Evidence from a prospective study. *Clinical & Experimental Immunology* 165(1), 38–43.

European Food Safety Authority, and European Centre for Disease Prevention and Control (2021) The European Union one health 2019 Zoonoses report. *EFSA Journal* 19(2), 6406.

Eyvazi, S., Vostakolaei, M.A., Dilmaghani, A., Borumandi, O., Hejazi, M.S. *et al.* (2020) The oncogenic roles of bacterial infections in development of cancer. *Microbial Pathogenesis* 141, 104019.

Fang, X., Kang, L., Qiu, Y.-F., Li, Z.-S. and Bai, Y. (2023) *Yersinia enterocolitica* in Crohn's disease. *Frontiers in Cellular and Infection Microbiology* 13, 1129996.

Farah, M., Hildebrand, A.M., Huang, S., Dammas, H. and Clark, W.F. (2014) Thrombotic *Thrombocytopenic purpura* and *Hemolytic uremic* syndrome in 2014—Current knowledge and outcomes with plasma exchange. *Oncology & Hematology Review (US)* 10(2), 82.

Fernandez, T.F. (2008) *E. coli* O157: H7. *Veterinary World* 1(3), 83.

Fox, J.G. and Wang, T.C. (2007) Inflammation, atrophy, and gastric cancer. *The Journal of Clinical Investigation* 117(1), 60–69.

Freeman, M.D. (2019) Medicolegal investigation of *Vibrio parahaemolyticus*-related foodborne illness as the most probable cause of Guillain-Barré syndrome. *Forensic Science International: Reports* 1, 100004.

Fukugaiti, M.H., Ignacio, A., Fernandes, M.R., Ribeiro Júnior, U., Nakano, V. *et al.* (2015) High occurrence of *Fusobacterium nucleatum* and *Clostridium difficile* in the intestinal microbiota of colorectal carcinoma patients. *Brazilian Journal of Microbiology* 46(4), 1135–1140.

Gokden, Y., Hot, S., Adas, M., Koc, D.O., Atak, S. *et al.* (2020) Celiac disease and COVID-19 pandemic: Should we worry. *Acta Gastro-Enterologica Belgica* 83, 517–525.

Guan, W.-J., Liang, W.-H., Zhao, Y., Liang, H.-R., Chen, Z.-S. *et al.* (2020) Comorbidity and its impact on 1590 patients with covid-19 in China: A nationwide analysis. *European Respiratory Journal* 55(5), 2000547.

Gui, L., Subramony, C., Fratkin, J. and Hughson, M.D. (2002) Fatal enteritis necroticans (pigbel) in a diabetic adult. *Modern Pathology* 15(1), 66–70.

Hagiya, H., Naito, H., Sugiyama, J., Nojima, H., Hagioka, S. *et al.* (2012) Necrotizing duodenitis caused by *Clostridium perfringens* type a in a Japanese young man. *Internal Medicine* 51(20), 2973–2976.

Hailegebreal, G. (2017) A review on *Clostridium perfringens* food poisoning. *Global Research Journal of Public Health and Epidemiology* 4(3), 104–109.

Hoornstra, D., Andersson, M.A., Teplova, V.V., Mikkola, R., Uotila, L.M. *et al.* (2013) Potato crop as a source of emetic *Bacillus cereus* and cereulide-induced mammalian cell toxicity. *Applied and Environmental Microbiology* 79(12), 3534–3543.

Hussain, A., Bhowmik, B. and Vale Moreira, N.C. (2020) COVID-19 and diabetes: Knowledge in progress. *Diabetes Research and Clinical Practice* 108142.

Huţanaşu, C., Sfarti, C., Trifan, A., Huţanaşu, M. and Stanciu, C. (2009) Aflatoxin contamination of food: Additional risk factor for chronic liver diseases. *Revista Medico-Chirurgicala a Societatii de Medici Si Naturalisti Din Iasi* 113(4), 1061–1065.

Jess, T., Simonsen, J., Nielsen, N.M., Jørgensen, K.T., Bager, P. *et al.* (2011) Enteric *Salmonella* or *Campylobacter* infections and the risk of inflammatory bowel disease. *Gut* 60(3), 318–324.

Kingsbury, J., Lake, R., Hewitt, J., Smit, E. and King, N. (2020) Potential for foodborne transmission of Covid-19: Literature review update. Update.

Ko, H., Maymani, H. and Rojas-Hernandez, C. (2016) Hemolytic uremic syndrome associated with *Escherichia coli* O157: H7 infection in older adults: A case report and review of the literature. *Journal of Medical Case Reports* 10(1), 1–4.

Kobayashi, R., Matsumoto, S. and Yoshida, Y. (2014) Case of acute pancreatitis associated with *Campylobacter enteritis*. *World Journal of Gastroenterology: WJG* 20(23), 7514.

Koshiol, J., Wozniak, A., Cook, P., Adaniel, C., Acevedo, J. *et al.* (2016) *Salmonella enterica* serovar Typhi and gallbladder cancer: A case–control study and meta-analysis. *Cancer Medicine* 5(11), 3310–3235.

Kotloff, K.L., Riddle, M.S., Platts-Mills, J.A., Pavlinac, P. and Zaidi, A.K.M. (2018) Shigellosis. *Lancet* 391(10122), 801–812.

Ktsoyan, Z., Budaghyan, L., Agababova, M., Mnatsakanyan, A., Arakelova, K. *et al.* (2019) Potential involvement of *Salmonella* infection in autoimmunity. *Pathogens* 8(3), 96.

Kuchenmüller, T., Hird, S., Stein, C., Kramarz, P., Nanda, A. *et al.* (2009) Estimating the global burden of foodborne diseases-a collaborative effort. *Eurosurveillance* 14(18), 19195.

Kushkevych, I., Kollar, P., Ferreira, A.L., Palma, D., Duarte, A. *et al.* (2016) Antimicrobial effect of salicylamide derivatives against intestinal sulfate-reducing bacteria. *Journal of Applied Biomedicine* 14(2), 125–130.

Lebwohl, B., Larsson, E., Söderling, J., Roelstraete, B., Murray, J.A. *et al.* (2021) Risk of severe covid-19 in patients with celiac disease: A population-based cohort study. *Clinical Epidemiology* 13, 121.

Lerminiaux, N.A., MacKenzie, K.D. and Cameron, A.D. (2020) Salmonella pathogenicity island 1 (SPI-1): The evolution and stabilization of a core genomic type three secretion system. *Microorganisms* 8(4), 576.

Le Soudéer, L., Truong, J., Le Gal, J. and Escoda, S. (2022) *Shigella*-associated mild encephalitis with reversible splenial lesion in hospital center Delafontaine, Saint-Dentis, France. *BMC Pediatrics* 22(1), 421.

Louise, C.B. and Obrig, T.G. (1995) Specific interaction of *Escherichia* coli O157:H7-derived Shiga-like toxin II with human renal endothelial cells. *The Journal of Infectious Diseases* 172(5), 1397–1401.

Mager, D. (2006) Bacteria and cancer: Cause, coincidence or cure? A review. *Journal of Translational Medicine* 4(1), 14.

Månsson, L.E., Montero, M., Zarepour, M., Bergstrom, K.S., Ma, C. *et al.* (2012) MyD88 signaling promotes both mucosal homeostatic and fibrotic responses during salmonella-induced colitis. *American Journal of Physiology-Gastrointestinal and Liver Physiology* 303(3), G311–23.

Marder, E.P., Griffin, P.M., Cieslak, P.R., Dunn, J., Hurd, S. *et al.* (2018) Preliminary incidence and trends of infections with pathogens transmitted commonly through food—foodborne diseases active surveillance network, 10 US sites, 2006–2017. *Morbidity and Mortality Weekly Report* 67(11), 324.

Martin, H.M., Campbell, B.J., Hart, C.A., Mpofu, C., Nayar, M. *et al.* (2004) Enhanced *Escherichia coli* adherence and invasion in Crohn's disease and colon cancer. *Gastroenterology* 127(1), 80–93.

Maslar, A., Kullar, R. and Usiak, S. (2023) An uncommon culprit, *Bacillus cereus*, as a foodborne bloodstream infection (BSI). *American Journal of Infection Control* 51(7), S12.

Mayer, C.L., Leibowitz, C.S., Kurosawa, S. and Stearns-Kurosawa, D.J. (2012) Shiga toxins and the pathophysiology of hemolytic uremic syndrome in humans and animals. *Toxins* 4(11), 1261–1287.

McDonel, J.L. (1980) Clostridium perfringens toxins (type a, b, c, d, e). *Pharmacology & Therapeutics* 10(3), 617–655.

Miryala, S.K., Anbarasu, A. and Ramaiah, S. (2021) Gene interaction network to unravel the role of gut bacterial species in cardiovascular diseases: *E. coli* O157: H7 host-bacterial interaction study. *Computers in Biology and Medicine* 133, 104417.

Miyamoto, K., Li, J. and McClane, B.A. (2009) Enterotoxigenic *Clostridium perfringens*: Detection and identification. *Microbes and Environments* 1204110375.

Mughini-Gras, L., Schaapveld, M., Kramers, J., Mooij, S., Neefjes-Borst, E.A. *et al.* (2018) Increased colon cancer risk after severe *Salmonella* infection. *PloS One* 13(1), e0189721.

Murphy, K., Al-Jundi, W. and Nawaz, S. (2013) Mycotic aneurysms of the abdominal aorta due to Listeria monocytogenes. *International Journal of Surgery Case Reports* 4(7), 626–628.

Nallarajah, J. and Mujahieth, M. (2020) *Bacillus cereus* subacute native valve infective endocarditis and its multiple complications. *Case Reports in Cardiology* 8826956.

Naranjo, M., Denayer, S., Botteldoorn, N., Delbrassinne, L., Veys, J. *et al.* (2011) Sudden death of a young adult associated with *Bacillus cereus* food poisoning. *Journal of Clinical Microbiology* 49(12), 4379–4381.

Nehoff, H., Henley, E., Hamblin, R., Isenman, H. and Crozier, I. (2022) *Yersinia enterocolitica* associated myopericarditis: Case report and review of the literature. *The New Zealand Medical Journal* 135(1549), 113–116.

Newell, D.G., Koopmans, M., Verhoef, L., Duizer, E., Aidara-Kane, A. *et al.* (2010) Food-borne diseases—The challenges of 20 years ago still persist while new ones continue to emerge. *International Journal of Food Microbiology* 139, S3–S15.

Nyati, K.K. and Nyati, R. (2013) Role of *Campylobacter jejuni* infection in the pathogenesis of Guillain-Barré syndrome: An update. *BioMed Research International* 852195.

Olsen, P.W.B. (2001) Myocarditis in a patient with *Salmonella* and *Campylobacter enteritis*. *Scandinavian Journal of Infectious Diseases* 33(11), 860–862.

Parry, C.M., Hein, T.T., Dougan, G., White, N.J. and Farrar, J.J. (2002) Typhoid fever. *The New England Journal of Medicine* 347, 1770–1782.

Parsonnet, J. (1995) Bacterial infection as a cause of cancer. *Environmental Health Perspectives* 103(suppl 8), 263–268.

Petersen, J., Ciacchi, L., Tran, M.T., Loh, K.L., Kooy-Winkelaar, Y. *et al.* (2020) T cell receptor cross-reactivity between gliadin and bacterial peptides in celiac disease. *Nature Structural & Molecular Biology* 27(1), 49–61.

Pisani, P., Parkin, D.M., Muñoz, N. and Ferlay, J. (1997) Cancer and infection: Estimates of the attributable fraction in 1990. *Cancer Epidemiology and Prevention Biomarkers* 6(6), 387–400.

Rajkovic, A. (2014) Microbial toxins and low level of foodborne exposure. *Trends in Food Science & Technology* 38(2), 149–157.

Ramaswamy, V., Cresence, V.M., Rejitha, J.S., Lekshmi, M.U., Dharsana, K. *et al.* (2007) Listeria-review of epidemiology and pathogenesis. *Journal of Microbiology Immunology and Infection* 40(1), 4.

Riddle, M.S., Murray, J.A., Cash, B.D., Pimentel, M. and Porter, C.K. (2013) Pathogen-specific risk of celiac disease following bacterial causes of foodborne illness: A retrospective cohort study. *Digestive Diseases and Sciences* 58(11), 3242–3245.

Roed, C., Engsig, F.N., Omland, L.H., Skinhoj, P. and Obel, N. (2012) Long-term mortality in patients diagnosed with *Listeria* monocytogenes meningitis: A danish nationwide cohort study. *Journal of Infection* 64(1), 34–40.

Rohekar, S., Tsui, F.W., Tsui, H.W., Xi, N., Riarh, R. *et al.* (2008) Symptomatic acute reactive arthritis after an outbreak of *Salmonella*. *The Journal of Rheumatology* 35(8), 1599–1602.

Rolhion, N. and Chassaing, B. (2016) When pathogenic bacteria meet the intestinal microbiota. *Philosophical Transactions of the Royal Society B: Biological Sciences* 371(1707), 20150504.

Schlech, W.F. (2019) Epidemiology and clinical manifestations of *Listeria* monocytogenes infection. *Microbiology Spectrum* 7(3). DOI: 10.1128/microbiolspec.GPP3-0014-2018.

Schuchat, A., Swaminathan, B. and Broome, C.V. (1991) Epidemiology of human listeriosis. *Clinical Microbiology Reviews* 4(2), 169–183.

Sheweita, S.A. and Alsamghan, A.S. (2020) Molecular mechanisms contributing bacterial infections to the incidence of various types of cancer. *Mediators of Inflammation* 4070419.

Shoaib, M., Shehzad, A., Raza, H., Niazi, S., Khan, I.M. *et al.* (2019) A comprehensive review on the prevalence, pathogenesis and detection of *Yersinia enterocolitica*. *RSC Advances* 9(70), 41010–41021.

Shukla, V.K., Singh, H., Pandey, M., Upadhyay, S. and Nath, G. (2000) Carcinoma of the gallbladder—Is it a sequel of typhoid? *Digestive Diseases and Sciences* 45(5), 900–903.

Sin, H.K., Cheuk, A., Lee, W., Yim, K.F., Poon, C. *et al.* (2021) *Listeria monocytogenes* peritonitis in a patient receiving continuous ambulatory peritoneal dialysis: A case report and review of the literature. *Case Reports in Nephrology* 6681629.

Smith, A.M., Thomas, J. and Mostert, P.J. (2011) Fatal case of *Clostridium perfringens* enteritis and bacteraemia in South Africa. *The Journal of Infection in Developing Countries* 5(5), 400–402.

Soloski, M.J. and Metcalf, E.S. (2007) Salmonella as an inducer of autoimmunity. *EcoSal Plus* 2(2). DOI: 10.1128/ecosalplus.8.8.13.

Steinitz, R. (1965) Pulmonary tuberculosis and carcinoma of the lung: A survey from two population-based disease registers. *American Review of Respiratory Disease* 92(5), 758–766.

Stenfors Arnesen, L.P., Fagerlund, A. and Granum, P.E. (2008) From soil to gut: *Bacillus cereus* and its food poisoning toxins. *FEMS Microbiology Reviews* 32(4), 579–606.

Sæbos, A. and Lassen, J. (1991) A survey of acute and chronic disease associated with *Yersinia enterocolitica* infection: A Norwegian 10-year follow-up study on 458 hospitalized patients. *Scandinavian Journal of Infectious Diseases* 23(5), 517–527.

Tack, D.M., Marder, E.P., Griffin, P.M., Cieslak, P.R. *et al.* (2019) Preliminary incidence and trends of infections with pathogens transmitted commonly through food—foodborne diseases active surveillance network, 10 US sites, 2015–2018. *Morbidity and Mortality Weekly Report* 68(16), 369.

Teodor, A., Teodor, D., Miftode, E., Prisăcaru, D., Leca, D. *et al.* (2012) Severe invasive listeriosis—Case report. *Rev Med Chir Soc Med Nat Iasi* 116(3), 808–811.

Terajima, J., Izumiya, H., Hara-Kudo, Y. and Ohnishi, M. (2017) Shiga toxin (Verotoxin)-producing *Escherichia coli* and foodborne disease: A review. *Food Saf (Tokyo)* 5(2), 35–53.

Tesh, V.L., Burris, J.A., Owens, J.W., Gordon, V.M., Wadolkowski, E.A. *et al.* (1993) Comparison of the relative toxicities of Shiga-like toxins type i and type II for mice. *Infection and Immunity* 61(8), 3392–3402.

Thabane, M. and Marshall, J.K. (2009) Post-infectious irritable bowel syndrome. *World Journal of Gastroenterology: WJG* 15(29), 3591.

Trovato, C.M., Montuori, M., Pietropaoli, N. and Oliva, S. (2021) COVID-19 and celiac disease: A pathogenetic hypothesis for a celiac outbreak. *International Journal of Clinical Practice* e14452.

Tschiedel, E., Rath, P.M., Steinmann, J., Becker, H., Dietrich, R. *et al.* (2015) Lifesaving liver transplantation for multi-organ failure caused by *Bacillus cereus* food poisoning. *Pediatric Transplantation* 19(1), E11–E14.

Ulcerative Colitis–Pathophysiology, U. (2003) Inflammatory bowel disease part I: Ulcerative colitis–pathophysiology and conventional and alternative treatment options. *Alternative Medicine Review* 8(3), 247–283.

Upadhayay, A., Pal, D. and Kumar, A. (2022) *Salmonella typhi* induced oncogenesis in gallbladder cancer: Co-relation and progression. *Advances in Cancer Biology-Metastasis* 4, 100032.

Van Bonn, S.M., Schraven, S.P., Schuldt, T., Heimesaat, M.M., Mlynski, R. *et al.* (2020) Chronic otitis media following infection by non-O1/ non-O139 *Vibrio cholerae*: A case report and review of the literature. *European Journal of Microbiology and Immunology* 10(3), 186–191.

van Elsland, D.M., Duijster, J.W., Zhang, J., Stévenin, V. *et al.* (2022) Repetitive non-typhoidal *Salmonella* exposure is an environmental risk factor for colon cancer and tumor growth. *Cell Reports Medicine* 3, 12.

Vangoitsenhoven, R., Rondas, D., Crèvecoeur, I., D'Hertog, W., Baatsen, P. *et al.* (2014) Foodborne cereulide causes beta-cell dysfunction and apoptosis. *PLoS One* 9(8), e104866.

Vangoitsenhoven, R., Maris, M., Overbergh, L., Loco, J., Mathieu, C. *et al.* (2015) Cereulide food toxin, beta cell function and diabetes: Facts and hypotheses. *Diabetes Research and Clinical Practice* 109(1), 1–5.

Verdu, E., Mauro, M., Bourgeois, J. and Armstrong, D. (2007) Clinical onset of celiac disease after an episode of *Campylobacter jejuni* enteritis. *Canadian Journal of Gastroenterology and Hepatology* 21(7), 453–455.

Verstockt, B., Verstockt, S., Abdu Rahiman, S., Ke, B.-J., Arnauts, K. *et al.* (2021) Intestinal receptor of SARS-cov-2 in inflamed IBD tissue seems downregulated by HNF4A in ileum and upregulated by interferon regulating factors in colon. *Journal of Crohn's and Colitis* 15(3), 485–498.

Walter, E.J.S., Crim, S.M., Bruce, B.B. and Griffin, P.M. (2019) Postinfectious irritable bowel syndrome after *Campylobacter* infection. *American Journal of Gastroenterology* 114(10), 1649–1656.

World Health Organization (WHO) (2015) WHO estimates of the global burden of foodborne diseases: Foodborne disease burden epidemiology reference group 2007–2015: World Health Organization.

World Health Organization (WHO) (2021) Estimating the burden of foodborne diseases: A practical handbook for countries: Slide set 1 of 3 belonging to the handbook. Module 1. World Health Organisation.

Yang, W.H., Heithoff, D.M., Aziz, P.V., Sperandio, M., Nizet, V. *et al.* (2017) Recurrent infection progressively disables host protection against intestinal inflammation. *Science* 358(6370), eaao5610.

Yun, C.-H., Kao, W.-C., Hsu, C.Y., Chang, R., Cheng, M.-F. *et al.* (2022) Nontyphoidal salmonella infection associated with subsequent risk of hematological malignancies: A nationwide population-based cohort study. *International Journal of Environmental Research and Public Health* 19(19), 12943.

Zamani, M., Vahedi, A., Maghdouri, Z. and Shokri-Shirvani, J. (2017) Role of food in environmental transmission of *Helicobacter pylori*. *Caspian Journal of Internal Medicine* 8(3), 146–152.

Zewude, R.T., Alem, Z. and Stefanovic, A. (2022) *Yersinia pseudotuberculosis* bacteremia with splenic abscesses: A case report. *Access Microbiology* 1, 000525.

Zha, L., Garrett, S. and Sun, J. (2019) Salmonella infection in chronic inflammation and gastrointestinal cancer. *Diseases* 7(1), 28.

7 Current Perspectives for the Use of Medical Ozone in Veterinary Medicine

Haytham Aamer[1], Eman Nour[1], Ayman Refaie[2], Mohamed Youssef[3] and Maged El-Ashker[3]*

[1]Faculty of Medicine, Urology & Nephrology Centre, Animal Research Facility, Mansoura University, Mansoura, Egypt; [2]Nephrology and Transplantation Unit, Urology and Nephrology Center, Mansoura University, Mansoura, Egypt; [3]Faculty of Veterinary Medicine, Department of Internal Medicine and Infectious Diseases, Mansoura University, Mansoura, 35516, Egypt

Abstract

Although ozone has been used in veterinary medicine for more than 30 years, it is still inadequate and limited to certain areas and breeds. Medical ozone has gained popularity worldwide as current medical treatments have become more expensive, and there are growing concerns about antibiotic-resistant infections. In this review, we present current perspectives on the application of ozone in veterinary diseases, highlighting its mechanisms of action, how it is generated, and how it acts in living tissues. Furthermore, we address the impact of medical ozone on various diseases in animals, including renal ischemia-reperfusion injury. We also report the inherent biases and limitations of clinical studies and case series related to ozone therapy in veterinary medicine, without control groups. Although the information provided in this review is promising and confirms the potential of medical ozone therapy in the treatment of animal diseases, the accuracy of the results of this therapeutic modality is of vital importance in view of the objections identified in the authorization of ozone therapy and the existence of some limitations associated with relevant studies, which offer the possibility of potential biases.

Keywords: animal diseases, ozone therapy, uses, routes, pathophysiology, renal ischemia-reperfusion injury

Introduction

Two decades ago, it seemed paradoxical to suggest the use of some gasses for therapeutic purposes, but there is now extensive literature pointing to the importance of several other gasses besides oxygen, such as nitric oxide (NO), carbon monoxide (CO), hydrogen (H_2), hydrogen sulfide (H_2S), xenon (Xe), and ozone (O_3) (Nakao *et al.*, 2009; Bocci *et al.*, 2011; Inal *et al.*, 2011).

Ozone is a naturally occurring compound consisting of three oxygen atoms. In nature, it occurs as a colorless gas in the stratosphere at concentrations of 1–10 ppm, where it is constantly formed from and destroyed by molecular O_2 (Grootveld *et al.*, 2004). Stratospheric ozone is also essential to both thermal structure of the stratosphere and the ecological framework of life on Earth. Its ability to filter UV radiation makes it one of the most important gasses in the stratosphere, but in the troposphere, it is toxic

*Corresponding author: magid_rez@mans.edu.eg

if chronically inhaled. This protective layer is visible as blue sky (Bocci *et al.*, 2011). However, it is a critical issue to differentiate ozone as pollutant or disinfectant on the surfaces and in environments (Orlandin *et al.*, 2021).

So far, there has been little attention paid to the clinical use of ozone in animal diseases (Ogata and Nagahata, 2000). Although ozone has been used in veterinary medicine for over 30 years, it is still inadequate and limited to certain areas and breeds. The use of ozone appears to be empirical, with few studies providing histological and biochemical evidence of its effects (Iliakis *et al.*, 2008).

Ozone was first used to disinfect operating rooms in a hospital in 1856, and the first ozone water treatment plant was built in Monaco in 1860 to disinfect water (Iliakis *et al.*, 2008). In the late 1980s, it was reported that HIV patients in Germany were successfully treated with ozone autohemotherapy (O_3-AHT). Since there was no pharmacological treatment for HIV at that time, the Canadian government approved the testing of O_3-AHT for safety and efficacy in the treatment of AIDS patients (Elvis and Ekta, 2011).

In this review, we present the current perspectives on the application of ozone in veterinary diseases, highlighting its mechanisms of action, how it is generated, and how it acts in living tissues. Furthermore, we address the impact of medical ozone on various diseases in animals, including renal ischemia-reperfusion injury. We also report the inherent biases and limitations of clinical studies and case series related to ozone therapy in veterinary medicine without control groups.

Review Methodology

We searched databases including CAB Abstracts, Google Scholar, Science Direct, PubMed, and ISI Web of Knowledge (Keyword search terms used: animal diseases, ozone therapy, uses, routes, pathophysiology, renal ischemia-reperfusion injury, etc.). We used the references from the articles obtained by this method to check for additional relevant material. The database results were combined with EndNote (version X7; Thomson Reuters).

Medical Ozone Production

Highly specific devices known as ozone generators (silent electrical discharge generators) have been used to produce ozone for medical purposes (Manjunath *et al.*, 2015). Werner von Siemens put into practice the idea that ozone is created from pure oxygen when a voltaic arc produces an electrical discharge. The super induction tube (Siemens tube) invented by Siemens consists of two interconnected electrode plates set to high voltages of 4000–14,000 V that can produce ozone in the presence of oxygen (Bocci, 2005).

Ozone concentration can range from 1 to 100 μg/ml depending on the application. Only 5% of the gas produced by the generator is O_3, the rest is oxygen. It consists of a mixture of 0.05% ozone, 99.95% O_2, or 5% O_3 to 95% O_2 from 100% pure oxygen (Kozat and Okman, 2019).

The energy in the generators causes the individual O_2 molecules to break down into oxygen atoms, which combine with a free O_2 molecule to form an O_3 molecule. Since normal air contains a high concentration of nitrogen and releases toxic nitrogen dioxide (N_2O_2), ozone generators are recommended for applications that slow down this transformation. Medical ozone is always generated on-site with a special generator and applied immediately, because after 1 hour only half of the original ozone remains; the rest decays to oxygen (Kozat and Okman, 2019). Non-reactive materials (such as steel, especially anodized aluminum, ceramics, glass, or Teflon) should also be used for ozone devices.

Indications for Ozone Therapy

Ozone therapy has recently gained popularity as current medical treatments become more expensive and antibiotic-resistant infections attract more attention worldwide. This therapy is extremely cost-effective and does not lead to antibiotic resistance (Kozat and Okman, 2019). Ozone therapy has been used in medical practice to treat a variety of diseases, including infected wounds, chronic skin ulcers, early and advanced-stage ischemic gangrene, abscesses, anal fissures, bedsores, gingivitis, peritonitis, vulvo-vaginitis, sinusitis, stomatitis, and periodontitis (Zobel *et al.*, 2012; Szponder *et al.*, 2017). Subsequently, physicians learned about medical ozone and discovered that it had therapeutic, hemodynamic, and anti-inflammatory properties and could be used to treat hypoxic and ischemic conditions (Bocci, 2006). Several diseases were treated with ozone in German soldiers during World War I, including facial paralysis, lumbar disk herniation, periodontitis, infections, and hepatitis (Gupta, 2012).

Ozone Therapy in Veterinary Medicine

The clinical application of ozone to animal diseases has received little attention (Ogata and Nagahata, 2000). Although ozone has been used in veterinary medicine for over 30 years, it is still inadequate and limited to specific areas and breeds, such as the treatment of mastitis, endometritis, fetal membrane retention, vaginitis, urovagina, enteritis, and laminitis, as well as the local treatment of various lesions and neuromuscular disorders (Teixeira *et al.*, 2013). To enhance reader understanding, we provide a quick and clear reference for the different application techniques of medical ozone in different animal species (Table 7.1).

Medical ozone has recently been studied as a preventive and therapeutic agent in the treatment of puerperal diseases in ruminants and to improve reproductive performance (Zobel *et al.*, 2012; Zobel *et al.*, 2014; Đuričić *et al.*, 2015; Szponder *et al.*, 2017). When applied rectally in bitches after ovariohysterectomy, ozone had a strong analgesic effect (Teixeira *et al.*, 2013; Đuričić *et al.*, 2015; Szponder *et al.*, 2017).

Ozone therapy had no side effects and was quite reliable due to its natural origin and may be a promising, effective, and residue-free treatment option. Ozone therapy has been shown to reduce inflammation in rabbits with experimentally induced endophthalmitis (Lake *et al.*, 2004), and induce bactericidal effects in rats with pneumoperitoneum (Silva *et al.*, 2009). In another study, ozone therapy was found to modulate the anti-inflammatory response in rats with intra-abdominal infections (Souza *et al.*, 2010). On the other hand, ozone cannot be stored for a long period of time. It can be combined with an aqueous vehicle to accelerate the decomposition of ozone into oxygen or with a viscous vehicle to slow it down (Nogales *et al.*, 2008).

Methods of Ozone Application

Medical ozone can be administered in several ways, although there are some limitations to intravenous administration as a gas due to the risk of oxygen embolism, as the gas mixture always contains at least 95% O_2 (Zanardi *et al.*, 2016). Systemic administration of ozone is done via various injection methods such as autologous blood therapy or direct injection into a vein, artery, muscle, joint, or directly into a tumor. Insufflation – into the rectum, ear, vagina, and urethra. Inhalation – bubbled through olive oil. Ingestion – ozonated water. Transdermal – sub-atmospheric body suit of ozonated olive oil, cupping with a funnel and steam sauna (Bocci *et al.*, 2011).

Major autohemotherapy (major O_3-AHT)

This is an extracorporeal ozone gas blood treatment followed by intravenous re-infusion of the patient's treated blood (Nogales *et al.*, 2008). As in humans, a volume of blood equal to 1/20–1/25 of the total mass is drawn from a superficial vein in Na citrate 3.8% (1.5 ml every 9 ml), which is then mixed without bubbling with an equal volume of ozone gas, the concentration of which varies according to the species (i.e. in cats and dogs, 10–40 μg/ml; in sheep and pigs, 20–50 μg/ml; in horses and cows, 20–50 μg/ml (Bocci, 2002).

Ozone therapy is indicated for the treatment of arterial circulatory disorders, infections, and rheumatoid arthritis; it is also useful for promoting immune activation and as adjunctive therapy for patients with geriatric carcinoma (Nogales *et al.*, 2008; Viebahn-Hänsler *et al.*, 2012).

Table 7.1. Application of ozone therapy in different animal species.

Species	Disease	Form of application	Formulation	Concentration	Volume	Treatment frequency	References
Bovine	Mastitis	Intramammary	Gas	6 to 30 mg equivalent to 6 mg/ml	1–5 L	Single dose	Ogata and Nagahata (2000)
Bovine	Urovagina	Intrauterine and IVG	Foam spray	Not informed	10 ml	Single dose	Zobel *et al.* (2012)
Bovine	Retained fetal membranes	Intrauterine	Foam spray	Not informed	Not informed	Single dose	Djuricic *et al.* (2015)
Bovine		Intrauterine	Ozone pearls	Not informed	six pearls	Single dose	Djuricic *et al.* (2012)
Bovine	Metritis	Intrauterine	Foam spray	Not informed	Not informed	Single dose	Đuričić *et al.* (2014)
Bovine		Intrauterine	Foam spray	Not informed	Not informed	1 × per week for 1 month	Constantin *et al.* (2016)
Bovine	Uterine infection	Intrauterine	Foam spray	Not informed	Not informed	Single dose	Durrani *et al.* (2017)
Bovine		Intramammary	Oil	600 units/kg	10 ml	3 days straight	Quintana *et al.* (2019)
Bovine		Intrauterine	Gas	55 μg/ml	60 ml	2 days straight	Mali *et al.* (2020)
Bovine	Endometritis	Intrauterine	Ozonized water	50 μg/ml	50 ml	Single dose	Escandón *et al.* (2020)
Equine	Antioxidant capacity	Autohemotherapy	Gas	20 μg/Kg in 400 mL			Tsuzuki *et al.* (2015)
Ovine	Retained fetal membranes	Intrauterine	Foam spray	Not informed	Not informed	Single dose	Đuričić *et al.* (2016); Szponder *et al.* (2017)
Canine	POA	O_2-O_3 mixture gas	Intrarectally and acupoints	30 μg/mL			Teixeira *et al.* (2013)

Note: IVG: Intravaginal; and POA: Postoperative analgesia.

Minor autohemotherapy (minor O_3-AHT)

This is an extracorporeal blood treatment and intramuscular injection method commonly used in pets. It involves exposing 3–5 ml of blood to 3–5 ml of gas (ozone concentration 40–80 µg/ml) and immediately re-injecting it IM. It is indicated for allergies, acne, furunculosis, and adjuvant cancer therapy (Nogales *et al.*, 2008). The mechanism of action involves non-specific activation and general stimulation of the immune system (Bocci, 2010).

Intra- or peri-articular injections

In this method, 1–3 ml of gas (ozone concentration µg/ml) was delivered followed by ozonized water flushing. Following the gas, 1 ml of sterile ozonized oil can be injected. These administrations are used in dogs with infectious arthritis and coxo-femoral arthrosis (Bocci, 2002).

Intra-lesion gas injection

High concentrations of ozone (60–80 µg/ml) were initially delivered to the lesion (e.g. abscesses, superficial tumors, osteomyelitis, and cysts), then gradually decreasing concentrations (40–10 µg/ml). The lesion is washed with ozonated water if necessary. For skin infections (i.e. decubitus, chronic wounds, ulcers, mycoses, etc.), the animal is placed in a strong polyethylene bag with some water, with the head well insulated on the outside (Bocci, 2002).

The ozone concentration can range from 60 to 20 µg/ml for 15–20 min, depending on the severity of the disease. Bag treatment must be performed for several days until the infection has cleared. This method is suitable for the treatment of gangrene, diabetic foot ulcers, bad wounds, tick bites, and all wounds that are infected or slow to heal. It is also used for the treatment of extremities and local skin lesions (Fathi *et al.*, 2012).

Intravaginal and endometrial

Ozonated water is applied to the infected vagina or uterus and followed by gas (ozone concentration 20 µg/ml) infusion and sterile ozonated oil (Bocci, 2002).

Intraurethral and bladder infections

In dogs and cats, the infected urethra and urinary bladder were treated by gentle washing with ozonized water, insufflation of gas with ozone concentration of 15 µg/ml (volume 20–50 ml) (Bocci, 2002).

Intramammary injection

Gas can be slowly injected into the infected bovine udder at a low concentration (10–20 µg/ml) followed by sterile ozonized oil, the total infusion volume was 1–5 l/quarter depending on the capacity of the quarter (Ogata and Nagahata, 2000).

Rectal insufflation

Rectal ozone insufflation (RI-Ozone) is considered one of the oldest systemic and local methods of applying ozone therapy. It is noninvasive, simple, inexpensive, and virtually free of side effects (Beck *et al.*, 1998). RI-ozone has shown therapeutic success in preclinical and clinical studies with standardized clinical protocols (Martínez-Sánchez and Re, 2012). Based on animal studies and a comprehensive experimental study, RI-ozone has been shown to protect against hepatic ischemia-reperfusion injury and reduce reactive oxygen species by stimulating and/or preserving endogenous antioxidant systems in an experimental liver and kidney ischemia-reperfusion model (Peralta *et al.*, 1999; Peralta *et al.*, 2000).

It has been suggested that ozone products pass through the intestinal walls into the bloodstream. Thus, the blood removes the byproducts of ozone depletion and its reactions with various biomolecules from all systems. This procedure is painless and generally results in an increased sense of vitality and well-being (Beck *et al.*, 1998). It is used to treat arterial circulatory disorders, heart disease, general immune activation, adjuvant cancer therapy, and hepatitis A, B, and C (Viebahn-Hänsler and León Fernández, 2021). It is commonly performed in companion animals for intestinal and systemic infections using a 20–30 cm polyethylene catheter. Depending on the size of the animal, the gas volume can range from 25 to 600 ml, and the ozone concentration from 20 to 35 μg/ml (Bocci, 2002).

A previous study in dogs undergoing elective ovariohysterectomy found that RI-ozone and ozone injections into acupoints were as effective as meloxicam in providing postoperative analgesia (Teixeira *et al.*, 2013). In this study, the generator was set to produce an oxygen-ozone mixture with a concentration of 30 μg/ml, and the mixture was prepared immediately before application. A 10-ml syringe was connected to a three-way stopcock and a urethral catheter was inserted into the rectum, then ozone was applied for approximately 30 s. After the urethral catheter was removed from the rectum, the anus was gently squeezed for approximately 60 s.

Ozone Inside the Body

Like any other gas, ozone physically dissolves in water and body fluids, whether in blood plasma, extracellular fluids, or the thin layer of water covering the skin and especially the mucous membranes of the respiratory tract, intestines, and vagina (Bocci, 2005). When ozone enters the body and decays to oxygen, it releases some of the energy to the body, while another part is absorbed and stimulates cells. It prepares the host to experience pathophysiological events mediated by reactive oxygen species (ROS) (Inal *et al.*, 2011). Ozone, a powerful oxidant, reacts instantly with a variety of molecules found in biological fluids, proteins, carbohydrates, and preferably polyunsaturated fatty acids (PUFAs), namely antioxidants, producing atomic oxygen, a highly reactive atom (Bocci, 2010).

Ozone can be endogenously produced in the inflammation and antibacterial response of the immune system. Similar to medical ozone, endogenous ozone has not been fully embraced because of the limited understanding of its formation mechanisms (Onyango, 2023). In fact, medical ozone has several beneficial biological effects, including (a) enhancement of oxygen, glucose, and ATP supply in ischemic tissues through NO, CO, and increased levels of intra-erythrocytic 2,3-diphosphoglycerate (DPG); (b) promotion of neoangiogenesis and possibly facilitation of implantation of bone marrow-derived stem cells that can provide neovascularization and tissue regeneration; (c) elicitation of the phenomenon of preconditioning by upregulating the expression of antioxidant enzymes and heme oxygenase I; (d) elicitation of mild activation of the immune system and increase in the release of growth factors; and (e) induction of a surprising sense of well-being in most patients, most likely by stimulating the neuroendocrine system (Bocci, 2006; Tufekci *et al.*, 2011).

In order of priority, ozone reacts with PUFA, antioxidants such as ascorbic acid and uric acid, thiol compounds with – SH groups such as cysteine, reduced glutathione (GSH), and albumin (Bocci, 2006). Ozone also has virucidal and bactericidal properties and can be used for disinfection, sterilization, and destruction of malignant cells (Eliakim *et al.*, 2001).

Hydrogen peroxide (H_2O_2) is a non-radical oxidant produced during ozone therapy as a result of oxidative stress and lipid oxidation and mediates the biological effects of ozone therapy by acting as a second messenger responsible for triggering various biological and therapeutic effects (Inal *et al.*, 2011). Repeated exposure to ozone therapy can lead to resistance to oxidative stress by inducing the antioxidant system. During ozone therapy, transmembrane oxygen flux is stimulated and superoxide dismutase (SOD) is activated, which is responsible for protecting the body from processes related to superoxide overproduction, and peroxidases and catalases are also improved, as well as oxygen utilization in the mitochondrial respiratory chain (Madej *et al.*, 2007).

Ozone therapy increases the rate of glycolysis in red blood cells. This stimulates 2,3-DPG, which leads to an increase in the amount of oxygen delivered to tissues (Mandhare *et al.*, 2012). Ozone stimulates ATP production by increasing oxidative carboxylation of pyruvate in the Krebs cycle. It also significantly reduces NADH and supports the oxidation of cytochrome C (Farias *et al.*, 2020). It increases the production of enzymes that act as free radical scavengers and cell wall protectors, such as glutathione peroxidase (GSH-Px), catalase (CAT), and SOD (Di Mauro *et al.*, 2019; Travagli and Iorio, 2023).

Ozone reduces or eliminates the clumping of red blood cells in small capillaries, restores red blood cell flexibility, and improves blood flow and oxygen-carrying capacity; tissue oxygenation improves as arterial partial pressure increases and blood viscosity decreases. Ozone also oxidizes plaque in the arteries, removing the degradation products and decongesting the blood vessels (Helal, 2014).

Mechanism of ozone action

Ozone is identified as a ROS with a high oxidizing capacity. ROS are categorized into free radicals and non-radicals (with one or more uncoupled electrons), while ozone is among the non-radical ones (Halliwell and Gutteridge, 2015; Travagli and Iorio, 2023). Animal and clinical studies of ozone therapy have shown that the basic mechanism of ozone action depends on oxidative stress and nuclear transcription factors, as oxidative stress acts as a second messenger in various intracellular signaling pathways (Sagai and Bocci, 2011).

Ozone dissociates rapidly in water and releases a reactive form of oxygen that can oxidize cells. It can react directly with biological structures such as amino acids, enzymes, DNA, membrane glycoproteins, and lipids (Delgadillo-Valero *et al.*, 2023). However, due to its instability, ozone can dissolve in a chain reaction to form a variety of free radicals, such as hydroxyl radicals (•OH) and superoxide radicals (O2•−), which acquire missing electrons by oxidizing biological components. Cells can also rapidly initiate biological responses against oxidative stress to maintain biological homeostasis and adapt to such stresses (Sagai and Bocci, 2011). Some nuclear factors can also trigger various biological responses against oxidative stress.

Previous studies suggested that the mechanisms of action of ozone therapy involve the activation of antioxidant defense systems, with moderate oxidative stress inducing the activation of nuclear transcription factors such as Nrf2, hypoxia-inducible factor-1a (HIF-1a), nuclear factor of activated T-cells (NFAT), and activated protein-1 (AT-1) (Sagai and Bocci, 2011).

The ROS created from the interactions of ozone and ozone itself oxidizes the cysteinyl thiols of Kelch-like ECH-associated protein1 (KEAP1), a protein that keeps nuclear erythroid factor2 (Nrf2) ubiquitinated and, therefore, destroyed by the proteasome. Such an event leads Nrf2, a transcription factor, to translocate to the nucleus, where it regulates oxidative damage by inducing antioxidant response elements (ARE) (Ma, 2013), including antioxidant enzymes that serve as protective responses that delay, prevent, or remove oxidative damage, via catalytic or scavenger activity of free radicals. Examples of upregulated antioxidant proteins include CAT, SOD, GSH-Px, glutathione S-transferase (GSTr), hemeoxygenase-1(HO-1), NADPH quinone oxido-reductase1 (NQO1), and heat shock protein-70 (HSP70) (Hidalgo-Tallón *et al.*, 2022).

Ozone therapy also works by inducing a controlled oxidation of PUFAs found in cell membranes. This creates ozonated lipid products (LOPs), which are important signal transducers and regulators of inflammation (Smith *et al.*, 2017). The LOPs (specifically hydroxy-hydroperoxides) exacerbate Nrf2 nuclear translocation by oxidizing cysteine residues, promoting KEAP1-Nrf2 dissociation and activation of Nrf2-ARE pathways (Viebahn-Hänsler *et al.*, 2012). Furthermore, they increase the phosphorylation of Nrf2 by casein kinase 2 (CK2) (Delgado-Roche *et al.*, 2017). In addition, LOPs have a hormetic response since, at low concentrations, they downregulate activation of nuclear factor kappa B (NF-XB) and inflammatory cytokines and increase antioxidant and anti-inflammatory compounds (Viebahn-Hänsler *et al.*, 2012).

High concentrations stimulate potential antimicrobial and chemotactic responses by activating phospholipase A2 and phospholipase C, which via intracellular cascades, including that of the arachidonic acid, stimulate the synthesis of NF-XB and, therefore, pro inflammatory cytokines e.g., interleukins (IL) 1 and 6 and tumor necrosis factor alpha (TNF-α), transforming growth factor beta (TGF-β), as well as the cyclooxygenase (COX) (Cenci *et al.*, 2022). This could explain how controlled and non-toxic oxidation by ozone mediates the upregulation of antioxidant and anti-inflammatory defenses.

Ozone may influence the immune system by stimulating the proliferation of B and T lymphocytes, monocytes, and neutrophils, causing them to release cytokines such as interferons α, β, γ, tumor necrosis factor α, interleukins 1, 2, 4, 6, 8 and 10, granulo-poietine and transforming growth factor β (Ohtsuka *et al.*, 2006). These cytokines reestablish cellular immunity during inflammatory processes (Travagli *et al.*, 2009).

There have been no negative effects associated with the use of ozone in veterinary medicine (Đuričić *et al.*, 2015). The advantages of using ozone over antibiotics in the treatment of various pathological conditions include the following: no prescription required, no side effects, no residues in milk, meat, or other tissues, and thus no microbial resistance (Zobel *et al.*, 2014). Ozone has no discernible effect on milk production or GIT contents, whereas the effectiveness of certain antibiotics decreases or is completely absent, also it has no negative interactions with other drugs or the gastrointestinal microbiota. There are no allergic reactions observed after using therapeutic concentrations of ozone preparations, whereas all antibiotics can cause adverse reactions to some extent. There is no withdrawal period with ozone therapy (Đuričić *et al.*, 2015).

Acute Kidney Injury in Pet Animals

Acute kidney injury (AKI) is a serious and progressive disease that affects dogs and cats and is considered to be one of the most common clinical scenarios seen in small animal practices (McGrotty, 2008). It can occur at any age, with a 0.5 and 4.5% incidence in dogs and cats, respectively (Bartges and Polzin, 2011). The disease is characterized by an abrupt onset of renal parenchymal damage, followed by a decline in renal tissue function, and is frequently associated with uremia, and the clinical course is often unfavorable (Ross, 2011; Osman *et al.*, 2020). As a result, tracking the progression of the disease is essential under field conditions.

The etiology of AKI is found to be multifactorial, and animal models of AKI do not always mimic those of humans (Vanmassenhove *et al.*, 2015), but in general, AKI can be divided into three major categories based on the cause: (1) pre-renal; where the kidneys do not receive an adequate blood supply, for example, as a result of a drop in systemic blood pressure after a hemorrhage; (2) intrinsic; where the failure is renal in origin, possibly due to nephrotoxic drugs; and (3) post-renal; where impaired urine outflow occurs, such as ureteral or bladder obstruction and prostate cancer (Makris and Spanou, 2016).

The cause of kidney disorders in pets and other species is frequently unknown. Dogs with severe glomerular damage (i.e. glomerulonephritis or amyloidosis) frequently exhibit marked proteinuria, and some of its causes are thought to be due to an immune mechanism (Vaden, 2011). However, the etiology of the more common forms of chronic kidney disease in dogs is purely speculative, in which tubule-interstitial lesions predominate and only mild to moderate proteinuria exists.

AKI in dogs and cats can be caused by toxins, ischemia, inflammation, obstruction, or infection (McGrotty, 2008). The mortality rate following AKI in cats is also high, and the most common cause of the disease is nephrotoxicity (i.e. ingestion of lily, ethylene glycol, or non-steroidal anti-inflammatory drugs), though the cause of AKI in affected cats is generally unknown in clinical practice (Segev *et al.*, 2013).

The Impact of Ozone Therapy on Renal Ischemia-Reperfusion Injury Using Canine Model

Renal ischemia is still one of the leading causes of AKI in dogs and cats and is a major issue in human renal transplantation (McGrotty, 2008). It is caused by a generalized or local impairment in the supply of oxygen and nutrients to the kidney cells, as well as waste elimination (Le Dorze *et al.*, 2009).

Renal ischemia with subsequent renal ischemia-reperfusion injury (IRI) is purposely created in normal urologic practice during kidney transplantation, partial nephrectomy, and anatrophic nephrolithotomy with subsequent early kidney injury. In canine model, it has shown that an ischemic preconditioning schedule of 5-min ischemia and 10-min reperfusion improves IRI from subsequent prolonged ischemia (Salehipour *et al.*, 2007).

The term 'IRI' refers to two stages of damage in a transplanted kidney. The first phase, which occurs immediately after transplantation, is associated with ischemic injury, whereas the second phase, which occurs later, is associated with activation of the innate and adaptive immune response, which may result in either antibody-mediated rejection (ABMR) or cell-mediated rejection (CMR) (Fuquay *et al.*, 2013). Ischemic reperfusion injury is a complicated process that manifests clinically as delayed graft function (DGF) or primary non-function (PNF) following transplantation (Chun-Cheng *et al.*, 2015). Organ damage in kidney transplantation begins with severe hemodynamic instability caused by physiological changes associated with brain death or circulatory death and continues throughout the transplantation process (Chun-Cheng *et al.*, 2015).

Renal artery clamping causes a brief but severe renal ischemia during the harvesting operation. In addition to the cold ischemia during the allograft, kidney storage may also cause a further ischemic damage (Dong and Tilney, 2001). Warm ischemia can result from arterial clamping in allograft kidney transplantation from heart-beating donors, but brain death-related disorders are absent, and cold ischemia is also shorter. The final and most severe stage of injury occurs during reperfusion following revascularization (Gulec, 2011).

Following the removal of a cadaveric donor's kidney, it is briefly kept under non-physiological conditions before being re-perfused at the time of transplantation, resulting in a complex pathophysiological process that begins with disturbed perfusion and ischemia associated with organ retrieval and preservation and continues with post-reperfusion injury from the pro-inflammatory milieu (Chun-Cheng *et al.*, 2015).

The pathophysiology of IRI is a very complex condition involving depletion of ATP, accumulation of intracellular Ca^{+2} and ROS, production of pro-inflammatory cytokines, and activation of the apoptotic pathway. At present, a protagonist role has been appointed to free radicals, in that increasing prooxidant substances produces an imbalance with antioxidant substances, creating oxidative stress (Annuk *et al.*, 2001). The main oxidative products in biological systems are the ROS which include superoxide anion, hydrogen peroxide, hydroxyl radical, singlet oxygen, and hypochlorous acid (Bocci, 2010). Ultimately this leads to mitochondrial damage, tubular and endothelial cell injury, obstructive cast formation, and widespread vascular damage (Shokeir *et al.*, 2015).

In spite of improvements in prevention strategies and support measures, AKI is associated with high morbidity and mortality and follows progress of chronic kidney disease. Presently, there is no specific medication for acute kidney injury arising from IRI in clinical use. However, because both inflammation and apoptosis occur together in renal IRI, the optimal therapeutic or preventive approach should target both pathways (Lempiäinen *et al.*, 2014).

In the last decades, urologic literature is replete with data supporting the use of medical ozone in cases of IRI insult in humans using lower and higher animal models. Several studies have demonstrated that ozone has therapeutic properties as an antimicrobial, anti-inflammatory, modulator of antioxidant defense system, and apoptosis (Wu *et al.*, 2013). Clinical studies have demonstrated that ozone increases antioxidant enzyme activities such as GSH-Px, SOD, and CAT, preparing the host to face physio-pathological conditions mediated by ROS/RNS (Bocci, 2006).

Ozone oxidative therapies applied in I/R treatment include preconditioning and post-conditioning treatments, which have shown beneficial effects of ozone on I/R injury in different organs and tissues (León Fernández *et al.*, 2008; Stadlbauer *et al.*, 2008; Fernández Iglesias *et al.*, 2011). Several studies have focused on the protective effects of ozone oxidative preconditioning against inflammation, apoptosis, and oxidative stress during I/R, both *in vivo* and *in vitro* (Wang *et al.*, 2018). It has been associated with elevated nitrous oxide production, decreased tissue oxidative stress parameters (such as lipid peroxidation, protein oxidation, and nitrite plus nitrate), and increased antioxidant enzyme activities (Ajamieh *et al.*, 2005).

Ozone preconditioning can promote oxidative stress by increasing the activity of antioxidant endogenous systems, which helps to keep the cell's redox state stable, it promotes cellular antioxidant systems and prevents septic shock by mediating ROS/RNS expression (Zamora *et al.*, 2005). In IRI, mononuclear cellular infiltration, glomerulotubular changes, and total damage scores can be reduced by using ozone alone or in combination (Kal *et al.*, 2016). In renal IRI, ozone prevents apoptosis and has an anti-inflammatory effect (Zamora *et al.*, 2005). It reduces long-term renal fibrosis after IR injury (Wang *et al.*, 2014).

It has been clearly demonstrated that ozone oxidative preconditioning has a cytoprotective effect in the liver and kidneys subjected to ischemia-reperfusion stress, as well as activating the endogenous antioxidant defense system (Borrego *et al.*, 2004; Ajamieh *et al.*, 2005). Although the beneficial effects of ozone oxidative post-conditioning have been reported in various animal models such as diabetes or the use of nephrotoxic drugs such as Adriamycin or cisplatin (Al-Dalain *et al.*, 2001; Calunga Fernández *et al.*, 2004). Rectal ozone treatment after cisplatin challenge (ozone oxidative post-conditioning) effectively prevented the drug's detrimental effect on the renal antioxidant defense system (González *et al.*, 2004).

Ozone post-conditioning is more clinically applicable and attracts greater attention than preconditioning because the occurrence of ischemia is often not predictable (Wang *et al.*, 2019). Ozone oxidative treatment showed a protective effect in preserving renal function and reducing overall histological damage induced by I/R in the proximal tubules (Fernández Iglesias *et al.*, 2011). Furthermore, treatment of I/R in rats with ozone post-conditioning showed significantly reduced serum Cr and BUN levels and improved renal pathology at early phase (Jiang *et al.*, 2020).

Clinical Studies and Evidence of Inherent Biases and Limitations

The therapeutic use of ozone and its derivatives in veterinary medicine is still in its infancy. Several factors hinder the use of ozone under field conditions, such as the instability of ozone, variability of ozone application in different animal species, limited case reports, a lack of consistent evaluation of their results, and a lack of standardization of treatment modalities (Orlandin *et al.*, 2021). All these factors pose an open question for the dissemination and official accreditation of ozone.

Ozone cannot be equated with any other drug, although the biochemical basis for its use in veterinary medicine has been verified (Tsuzuki *et al.*, 2015; Sciorsci *et al.*, 2020). Several studies using different application methods have been conducted to investigate the effect of ozone on mammalian species and in veterinary practice. Although the statistics obtained are promising and confirm the potential of medical ozone therapy in the treatment of animal diseases, the accuracy of the results of this therapeutic modality is of vital importance in view of the objections identified in the authorization of ozone therapy and the existence of some limitations associated with these studies, which offer the possibility of potential bias.

In this context, Ogata and Nagahata (2000) compared the use of ozone and antibiotics in the treatment of acute clinical mastitis in cattle, while Quintana *et al.* (2019) evaluated the use of ozone in the treatment of cows with subclinical mastitis. The studies provided an opportunity for potential bias in ozone therapy, as there was no randomization or control group. Similarly, Shinozuka *et al.* (2008) argued in favor of ozone therapy over antibiotics. Researchers hypothesized that ozone could increase white blood cell function and respiratory bursts. Nevertheless, this study did not provide robust evidence that ozone could aid in the reversal of the local and systemic signs of acute clinical mastitis.

In a study conducted on cows that underwent urovaginal surgery (Xiao *et al.*, 2017), the authors recommended the use of ozone because it improves wound healing. However, this is a case study, the results are provided from the author's perspective, and the data are not yet published. Some other authors recommend that the use of ozone in the form of foam is effective during the first puerperium and improves reproductive performance in dairy cows, but they do not provide convincing evidence and abandon confounding factors (Djuricic *et al.*, 2012).

The effectiveness of intrauterine ozone therapy has been compared with that of conventional antibiotics in sheep and goat species with retained fetal membranes (Djuricic *et al.*, 2015; Đuričić *et al.*, 2016). Based on their results, the authors advocated the use of ozone therapy for the treatment of retained fetal membranes in these animal species; however, the studies were limited to randomized and controlled groups. Another study showed that the therapeutic association of ozone with platelet-rich plasma has been advocated for the treatment of acute foot root disease. The study lacked quality of evidence despite the finding of good recovery without experiencing adverse effects (Szponder *et al.*, 2017).

Another study evaluated the potential impact of ozonated autohemotherapy on the redox status of horses before exercise (Tsuzuki *et al.*, 2015). The authors found that ozone could improve the antioxidant capacity of the horses studied; however, the lack of randomization in this study may limit the quality of the evidence.

In a recent study, the effects of intra-articular ozone therapy on inflammation and cartilage catabolism biomarkers were evaluated in horses with orthopedic diseases (Vendruscolo *et al.*, 2018). Because there were no discernible changes in the concentrations of the selected biomarkers, the authors advocated the use of ozone in horses with osteoarthritis. However, this study overlooked contributing factors that could cause bias.

Ozone therapy has been evaluated for the management of chronic grade IV laminitis in horses (Coelho *et al.*, 2015). The therapeutic regimen included hoof trimming, followed by intramuscular, peritendinous, and intrarectal administration of medical ozone for 10 weeks. After 6 months, the horses partially recovered from laminitis and reached Obel grade II. However, the absence of gold standards for establishing treatment efficacy can lead to bias.

In a study conducted on 30 horses with back pain, they were treated with a mixture of oxygen and ozone via local infiltration into the affected muscle in the intervertebral and paravertebral regions (Ballardini, 2005). According to their findings, ozone had an analgesic effect because the animals did not experience pain during palpation at a later stage. Therefore, the authors recommend the use of medical ozone for pain control. However, this study lacked an appropriate research design and may be subject to bias.

In canine models, the analgesic effects of rectal or acupoint ozone therapy have been evaluated in ovariectomized female dogs and compared with meloxicam (Teixeira *et al.*, 2013). The authors reported no statistically significant differences in pain severity among the three analgesic regimens. This clinical study demonstrated promising results of ozone in reducing ovariohysterectomy pain.

Avilés *et al.* (2016) reported four cases of dogs with different neoplastic processes (lymphoma, chondrosarcoma, adenocarcinoma, and osteosarcoma). Three dogs received chemotherapy and one underwent surgery. All dogs were treated with ozone therapy. Although there was a significant improvement in dogs treated with ozone and chemotherapy, it was not possible to deduce a clear understanding of the positive effects of ozone application.

Conclusion

Although the information provided in this review is promising and confirms the potential of medical ozone therapy in the treatment of animal diseases, the accuracy of the results of this therapeutic modality is of vital importance in view of the objections identified in the authorization of ozone therapy and the existence of some limitations associated with relevant studies, which offer the possibility of potential biases. Several factors might hinder the use of ozone under field conditions, such as the instability of ozone, variability of ozone application in different animal species, limited case reports, lack of consistent evaluation of their results, and lack of standardization of treatment modalities. All these factors pose an open question for the dissemination and official accreditation of ozone.

Funding

This research did not receive any specific funding.

Conflicts of Interest

The authors declare that they have no conflict of interest.

Consent for Publication

All contributing authors approved the manuscript for publication

Availability of Data and Material

All data presented in this study are available in the text.

References

Ajamieh, H.H., Berlanga, J., Merino, N., Sanchez, G.M., Carmona, A.M. *et al.* (2005) Role of protein synthesis in the protection conferred by ozone-oxidative-preconditioning in hepatic ischaemia/reperfusion. *Transplant International* 18(5), 604–612.

Al-Dalain, S.M., Martínez, G., Candelario-Jalil, E., Menéndez, S., Re, L. *et al.* (2001) Ozone treatment reduces markers of oxidative and endothelial damage in an experimental diabetes model in rats. *Pharmacological Research* 44(5), 391–396.

Annuk, M., Fellström, B., Akerblom, O., Zilmer, K., Vihalemm, T. *et al.* (2001) Oxidative stress markers in pre-uremic patients. *Clinical Nephrology* 56(4), 308–314.

Avilés, M., Rojo, A. and González, R. (2016) Ozone therapy as a coadjuvant treatment in veterinary oncology. Case Reports, *Ozone Therapy Global Journal* 6(1), 231–236.

Ballardini, E. (2005) Oxygen-ozone therapy for spinal muscle. *Rivista Italiana Di Ossigeno-Ozonoterapia* 4, 70–73.

Bartges, J. and Polzin, D. (2011) Nephrology and Urology of Small Animals. John Wiley & Sons. Blackwell Publishing Limited, UK.

Beck, E., Wasser, G. and Viebahn-Hänsler, R. (1998) The current status of ozone therapy. Empirical developments. Basic research. Medicinal society for the use of ozone in prevention therapy. *Forsch Komplementärmed* 5, 61–75.

Bocci, V. (2002) Ozone therapy in veterinary medicine. In: *Oxygen-Ozone Therapy*. Springer, Dordrecht, pp. 337–339. DOI: 10.1007/978-94-015-9952-8_28.

Bocci, V. (2005) *Ozone: A new Medical Drug*, 2nd edn. Springer Dordrecht Heidelberg, London New York. DOI: 10.1007/978-90-481-9234-2.

Bocci, V. (2006) Scientific and medical aspects of ozone therapy. State of the art. *Archives of Medical Research* 37(4), 425–435.

Bocci, V. (2010) *How does ozone act? How and why can we avoid ozone toxicity? Ozone: A New Medical Drug*. Springer, Dordrecht, pp. 17–26. DOI: 10.1007/978-90-481-9234-2_4.

Bocci, V., Zanardi, I. and Travagli, V. (2011) Oxygen/ozone as a medical gas mixture. A critical evaluation of the various methods clarifies positive and negative aspects. *Medical Gas Research* 1(1), 6.

Borrego, A., Zamora, Z.B., González, R., Romay, C., Menéndez, S. *et al.* (2004) Protection by ozone preconditioning is mediated by the antioxidant system in cisplatin-induced nephrotoxicity in rats. *Mediators of Inflammation* 13(1), 13–19.

Calunga Fernández, J.L., Bello Ferro, M., Chaple La Hoz, M., Barber Gutiérrez, E., Menéndez Cepero, S. *et al.* (2004) Ozonoterapia en la glomerulonefritis tóxica experimental por adriamicina. *Revista Cubana de Investigaciones Biomédicas* 23(3), 139–143.

Cenci, A., Macchia, I., La Sorsa, V., Sbarigia, C., Di Donna, V. *et al.* (2022) Mechanisms of action of ozone therapy in emerging viral diseases: Immunomodulatory effects and therapeutic advantages with reference to SARS-CoV. *Frontiers in Microbiology* 13, 871645. DOI: 10.3389/fmicb.2022.871645.

Chun-Cheng, C., William, C.C. and Hanto, D.W. (2015) Ischemia-reperfusion injury in kidney transplantation. *Frontiers in Bioscience, Elite* 7, 134–154.

Coelho, C., Abreu-Bernadi, W., Ginelli, A., Spagnol, T., Gardel, L. *et al.* (2015) Use of ozone therapy in chronic laminitis in a horse. *Journal of Ozone Therapy* 1(1).

Constantin, T., Bîrţoiu, I. and Procedia, A. (2016) Prelliminary study on ozone therapy in postpartum endometritis of dairy cows. *Agriculture and Agricultural Science Procedia* 10, 384–389.

Delgadillo-Valero, L., Hernández-Cruz, E. and Pedraza-Chaverri, J. (2023) The protective role of ozone therapy in kidney disease: A review. *Life (Basel)* 13(3), 752. DOI: 10.3390/life13030752.

Delgado-Roche, L., Riera-Romo, M., Mesta, F., Hernández-Matos, Y., Barrios, J. *et al.* (2017) Medical ozone promotes NrF2 phosphorylation reducing oxidative stress and pro-inflammatory cytokines in multiple sclerosis patients. *European Journal of Pharmacology* 811, 148–154.

Di Mauro, R., Cantarella, G., Bernardini, R., Di Rosa, M., Barbagallo, I. *et al.* (2019) The biochemical and pharmacological properties of ozone: The smell of protection in acute and chronic diseases. *International Journal of Molecular Sciences* 20(3), 634.

Djuricic, D., Vince, S., Ablondi, M., Dobranic, T. and Samardzija, M. (2012) Effect of preventive intrauterine ozone application on reproductive efficiency in Holstein cows. *Reproduction in Domestic Animals* 47(1), 87–91.

Djuricic, D., Valpotic, H. and Samardzija, M. (2015) The intrauterine treatment of the retained foetal membrane in dairy goats by ozone: Novel alternative to antibiotic therapy. *Reproduction in Domestic Animals* 50(2), 236–239.

Dong, V. and Tilney, N. (2001) Reduction of ischemia/reperfusion injury in organ transplants by cytoprotective strategies. *Current Opinion in Organ Transplantation* 6, 69–74. DOI: 10.1097/00075200-200103000-00013.

Đuričić, D., Lipar, M. and Samardžija, M. (2014) Ozone treatment of metritis and endometritis in Holstein cows. *Veterinarski Arhiv* 84(2), 103–110.

Đuričić, D., Valpotić, H. and Samardžija, M. (2015) Prophylaxis and therapeutic potential of ozone in buiatrics: Current knowledge. *Animal Reproduction Science* 159, 1–7.

Đuričić, D., Valpotić, H., Žura Žaja, I. and Samardžija, M. (2016) Comparison of intrauterine antibiotics versus ozone medical use in sheep with retained placenta and following obstetric assistance. *Reproduction in Domestic Animals* 51(4), 538–540.

Durrani, A., Raza, M. and Channa, A. (2017) An alternative therapy with ozone to avoid antimicrobial resistence (AMR) in uterine infections in dairy cattle. *Journal of Scientific and Technical Research* 1(1), 774–778.

Eliakim, R., Karmeli, F., Rachmilewitz, D., Cohen, P. and Zimran, A. (2001) Ozone enema: A model of microscopic colitis in rats. *Digestive Diseases and Sciences* 46(11), 2515–2520.

Elvis, A. and Ekta, J. (2011) Ozone therapy: A clinical review. *Journal of Natural Science, Biology, and Medicine* 2(1), 66.

Escandón, B., Espinoza, J., Perea, F., Quito, F., Ochoa, R. *et al.* (2020) Intrauterine therapy with ozone reduces subclinical endometritis and improves reproductive performance in postpartum dairy cows managed in pasture-based systems. *Tropical Animal Health and Production* 52, 2523–2528.

Farias, J., Farias, A. and Souza, A. (2020) Ozone therapy as an adjunct in the treatment to COVID-19. *Revista Brasileira de Fisiologia Do Exercício* 19(2suppl), S5–S8.

Fathi, A., Mawsouf, M. and Viebahn-Hänsler, R. (2012) Ozone therapy in diabetic foot and chronic, non-healing wounds. *Ozone: Science Engineering* 34(6), 438–450. DOI: 10.1080/01919512.2012.718700.

Fernández Iglesias, A., González Núñez, L., Calunga Fernández, J.L., Rodríguez Salgueiro, S. and Santos Febles, E. (2011) Ozone postconditioning in renal ischaemia-reperfusion model functional and morphological evidences. *Nefrologia* 31(4), 464–470. DOI: 10.3265/Nefrologia.pre2011.

Fuquay, R., Renner, B., Kulik, L., McCullough, J.W., Amura, C. *et al.* (2013) Renal ischemia-reperfusion injury amplifies the humoral immune response. *Journal of the American Society of Nephrology* 24(7), 1063–1072.

González, R., Borrego, A., Zamora, Z., Romay, C., Hernández, F. *et al.* (2004) Reversion by ozone treatment of acute nephrotoxicity induced by cisplatin in rats. *Mediators of Inflammation* 13(5–6), 307–312.

Grootveld, M., Baysan, A., Sidiiqui, N., Sim, J., Silwood, C. *et al.* (2004) History of the clinical applications of ozone. Ozone: The Revolution in Dentistry. Quintessence Publishing Co, London, pp. 23–30.

Gulec, B. (2011) Ischemia reperfusion injury in kidney transplantation. In: *Kidney Transplantation-New Perspectives*. IntechOpen, London. DOI: 10.5772/18289.

Gupta, M. (2012) Ozone: An emerging prospect in dentistry. *Indian Journal of Dental Sciences* 4(1), 47–50.

Halliwell, B. and Gutteridge, J.M. (2015) *Free radicals in biology and medicine*, 5th edn. Oxford Academic, USA. DOI: 10.1093/acprof:oso/9780198717478.001.0001.

Helal, S. (2014) Oxygen therapy. *Egyptian Journal of Occupational Medicine* 38(1), 111–123.

Hidalgo-Tallón, F., Torres-Morera, L., Baeza-Noci, J., Carrillo-Izquierdo, M. and Pinto-Bonilla, R. (2022) Updated review on ozone therapy in pain medicine. *Frontiers in Physiology* 13, 840623.

Iliakis, E., Petropoulos, I., Iliaki, A., Agapitos, E. and Agrogiannis, G. (2008) Is medical ozone safe when injected intra articularly. A comparative histological study in rat. *International Journal of Ozone Therapy* 7, 7–15.

Inal, M., Dokumacioglu, A., Özcelik, E. and Ucar, O. (2011) The effects of ozone therapy and coenzyme Q 10 combination on oxidative stress markers in healthy subjects. *Irish Journal of Medical Science* 180(3), 703–707.

Jiang, B., Su, Y., Chen, Q., Dong, L., Zhou, W. *et al.* (2020) Protective effects of ozone oxidative postconditioning on long-term injury after renal ischemia/reperfusion in rat. *Transplant Proceedings* 52(1), 365–372. DOI: 10.1016/j.transproceed.2019.10.004.

Kal, O., Akillioglu, I., Kal, A., Celik, E., Yilmaz, M. *et al.* (2016) Prophylactic ozone administration reduces renal ischemia-reperfusion injury in the rat. *International Journal of Clinical and Experimental Medicine* 9(7), 13677–13688.

Kozat, S. and Okman, E.N. (2019) Has ozone therapy a future in veterinary medicine. *Journal of Animal Husbandry and Dairy Science* 3(3), 25–34.

Lake, J., Felberg, S., Malavazzi, G., Goulart, D., Nishiwaki-Dantas, M. *et al.* (2004) Efeito terapêutico da aplicação intra-ocular de ozônio em modelo experimental de endoftalmite por Staphylococcus epidermidis em coelhos. *Arquivos Brasileiros de Oftalmologia* 67(4), 575–579.

Le Dorze, M., Legrand, M., Payen, D. and Ince, C. (2009) The role of the microcirculation in acute kidney injury. *Journal of Current Opinion in Critical Care* 15(6), 503–508.

Lempiäinen, J., Finckenberg, P., Mervaala, E.E., Storvik, M., Kaivola, J. *et al.* (2014) Dexmedetomidine preconditioning ameliorates kidney ischemia-reperfusion injury. *Pharmacology Research & Perspectives* 2(3), e00045. DOI: 10.1002/prp2.45.

León Fernández, O., Ajamieh, H., Berlanga, J., Menéndez, S., Viebahn-Hánsler, R. *et al.* (2008) Ozone oxidative preconditioning is mediated by A1 adenosine receptors in a rat model of liver ischemia/reperfusion. *Transplant International* 21(1), 39–48. DOI: 10.1111/j.1432-2277.2007.00568.x.

Ma, Q. (2013) Role of nrf2 in oxidative stress and toxicity. *Annual Review of Pharmacology* 53, 401–426.

Madej, P., Plewka, A., Madej, J.A., Nowak, M., Plewka, D. *et al.* (2007) Ozonotherapy in an induced septic shock. I. effect of ozonotherapy on rat organs in evaluation of free radical reactions and selected enzymatic systems. *Inflammation* 30(1–2), 52.

Makris, K. and Spanou, L. (2016) Acute kidney injury: Definition, pathophysiology and clinical phenotypes. *The Clinical Biochemist Reviews* 37(2), 85.

Mali, S., Rangnekar, M., Amle, M., Khillare, K., Mali, A. *et al.* (2020) Efficacy of intrauterine ozone therapy in repeat breeder cows with subclinical uterine infection. *Haryana Veterinarian* 59(Special Issue), 83–86.

Mandhare, M., Jagdale, D., Gaikwad, P., Gandhi, P. and Kadam, V. (2012) Miracle of ozone therapy as an alternative medicine. *International Journal of Pharmaceutical, Chemical, and Biological Sciences* 2(1), 63–71.

Manjunath, S., Singla, D. and Singh, A. (2015) Ozone revisited. *Journal of Advanced Oral Research* 6(2), 5–9.

Martínez-Sánchez, G. and Re, L. (2012) Rectal administration and its application in ozone therapy. *International Journal of Ozone Therapy* 11, 41–49.

McGrotty, Y. (2008) Diagnosis and management of chronic kidney disease in dogs and cats. *In Practice* 30(9), 502–507.

Nakao, A., Sugimoto, R., Billiar, T. and McCurry, K. (2009) Therapeutic antioxidant medical gas. *Journal of Clinical Biochemistry and Nutrition* 44(1), 1–13.

Nogales, C.G., Ferrari, P.H., Kantorovich, E.O. and Lage-Marques, J. (2008) Ozone therapy in medicine and dentistry. *The Journal of Contemporary Dental Practice* 9(4), 75–84.

Ogata, A. and Nagahata, H. (2000) Intramammary application of ozone therapy to acute clinical mastitis in dairy cows. *Journal of Veterinary Medical Science* 62(7), 681–686.

Ohtsuka, H., Ogata, A., Terasaki, N., Koiwa, M. and Kawamura, S. (2006) Changes in leukocyte population after ozonated autohemoadministration in cows with inflammatory diseases. *Journal of Veterinary Medical Science* 68(2), 175–178.

Onyango, A.N. (2023) Endogenous ozone as a regular reactive oxygen species in (patho) physiology. *Advances in Redox Research* 9, 100075.

Orlandin, J., Machado, L., Ambrosio, C. and Travagli, V. (2021) Ozone and its derivatives in veterinary medicine: A careful appraisal. *Veterinary and Animal Science* 13, 100191. DOI: 10.1016/j.vas.2021.100191.

Osman, Y., Hamed, S.M., Barakat, N.M., Khater, S., Gabr, M. *et al.* (2020) Prophylaxis against renal ischemia-reperfusion injury in canine model: Stem cell approach. *Indian Journal of Urology* 36(1), 44.

Peralta, C., Leon, O., Xaus, C., Prats, N., Jalil, E. *et al.* (1999) Protective effect of ozone treatment on the injury associated with hepatic ischemia-reperfusion: Antioxidant-prooxidant balance. *Free Radical Research* 31(3), 191–196.

Peralta, C., Xaus, C., Bartrons, R., Leon, O.S., Gelpí, E. *et al.* (2000) Effect of ozone treatment on reactive oxygen species and adenosine production during hepatic ischemia-reperfusion. *Free Radical Research* 33(5), 595–605.

Quintana, M., Domingues, I. and Ribeiro, A. (2019) Use of ozonized oil in the treatment of subclinical mastitis in Jersey cow: Case report. *Pubvet* 13(5).

Ross, L. (2011) Acute kidney injury in dogs and cats. *Veterinary Clinics: Small Animal Practice* 41(1), 1–14.

Sagai, M. and Bocci, V. (2011) Mechanisms of action involved in ozone therapy: Is healing induced via a mild oxidative stress? *Medical Gas Research* 1(1), 29.

Salehipour, M., Khezri, A., Monabbati, A., Jalaeian, H., Kroup, M. *et al.* (2007) Ischemic preconditioning protects the dog kidney from ischemia-reperfusion injury. *Urologia Internationalis* 79(4), 328–331.

Sciorsci, R., Lillo, E., Occhiogrosso, L. and Rizzo, A. (2020) Ozone therapy in veterinary medicine: A review. *Research in Veterinary Science* 130, 240–246.

Segev, G., Nivy, R., Kass, P.H. and Cowgill, L. (2013) A retrospective study of acute kidney injury in cats and development of a novel clinical scoring system for predicting outcome for cats managed by hemodialysis. *Journal of Veterinary Internal Medicine* 4, 830–839.

Shinozuka, Y., Uematsu, K., Takagi, M. and Taura, Y. (2008) Comparison of the amounts of endotoxin released from *Escherichia coli* after exposure to antibiotics and ozone: An *in vitro* evaluation. *Journal of Veterinary Medical Science* 70(4), 419–422.

Shokeir, A., Barakat, N., Hussein, A., Awadalla, A., Harraz, A. *et al.* (2015) Activation of Nrf2 by ischemic preconditioning and sulforaphane in renal ischemia/reperfusion injury: A comparative experimental study. *Physiological Research* 64(3), 313–323.

Silva, R., Garotti, J., Silva, R., Navarini, A. and Pacheco, M. (2009) Analysis of the bactericidal effect of ozone pneumoperitoneum. *Acta Cirurgica Brasileira* 24(2), 124–127.

Smith, N., Wilson, A., Gandhi, J., Vatsia, S. and Khan, S. (2017) Ozone therapy: An overview of pharmacodynamics, current research, and clinical utility. *Medical Gas Research* 7(3), 212–219. DOI: 10.4103/2045-9912.215752.

Souza, Y., Fontes, B., Martins, J., Sannomiya, P., Brito, G. *et al.* (2010) Evaluation of the effects of ozone therapy in the treatment of intra-abdominal infection in rats. *Clinics (Sao Paulo)* 65(2), 195–202. DOI: 10.1590/S1807-59322010000200012.

Stadlbauer, T., Eisele, A., Heidt, M., Tillmanns, H. and Schulz, S. (2008) Preconditioning with ozone abrogates acute rejection and prolongs cardiac allograft survival in rats. *Transplantation Proceedings* 40(4), 974–977.

Szponder, T., Wessely-Szponder, J., Świeca, M., Smolira, A. and Gruszecki, T. (2017) The combined use of ozone therapy and autologous platelet-rich plasma as an alternative approach to foot rot treatment for sheep. A preliminary study. *Small Ruminant Research* 156, 50–56.

Teixeira, L., Luna, S., Taffarel, M., Lima, A., Sousa, N. *et al.* (2013) Comparison of intrarectal ozone, ozone administered in acupoints and meloxicam for postoperative analgesia in bitches undergoing ovariohysterectomy. *The Veterinary Journal* 197(3), 794–799.

Travagli, V. and Iorio, E.L. (2023) The biological and molecular action of ozone and its derivatives: State-of-the-art, enhanced scenarios, and quality insights. *International Journal of Molecular Sciences* 24(10), 8465.

Travagli, V., Zanardi, I. and Bocci, V. (2009) Topical applications of ozone and ozonated oils as anti-infective agents: An insight into the patent claims. *Recent Patents on Anti-Infective Drug Discovery* 4(2), 130–142.

Tsuzuki, N., Endo, Y., Kikkawa, L., Korosue, K., Kaneko, Y. *et al.* (2015) Effects of ozonated autohemotherapy on the antioxidant capacity of Thoroughbred horses. *Journal of Veterinary Medical Science* 77(12), 1647–1650. DOI: 10.1292/jvms.15-0225.

Tufekci, K., Civi Bayin, E., Genc, S. and Genc, K. (2011) The Nrf2/ARE pathway: A promising target to counteract mitochondrial dysfunction in Parkinson's disease. *Parkinson's Disease* 314082. DOI: 10.4061/2011/314082.

Vaden, S. (2011) Glomerular disease. *Topics in Companion Animal Medicine* 26(3), 128–134.

Vanmassenhove, J., Veys, N. and Biesen, W. (2015) Prevention and conservative management of acute kidney injury. *The Italian Journal of Urology and Nephrology* 68(1), 58–71.

Vendruscolo, C., Moreira, J., Seidel, S., Fülber, J., Neuenschwander, H. *et al.* (2018) Effects of medical ozone upon healthy equine joints: Clinical and laboratorial aspects. *PLoS One* 13(5), e0197736. DOI: 10.1371/journal.pone.0197736.

Viebahn-Hänsler, R. and León Fernández, O. (2021) Ozone in medicine. The low-dose ozone concept and its basic biochemical mechanisms of action in chronic inflammatory diseases. *International Journal of Molecular Sciences* 22(15), 7890.

Viebahn-Hänsler, R., León Fernández, O.S. and Fahmy, Z. (2012) Ozone in medicine: The low-dose ozone concept—guidelines and treatment strategies. *Ozone: Science & Engineering* 34(6), 408–424. DOI: 10.1080/01919512.2012.717847.

Wang, L., Chen, H., Liu, X.-H., Chen, Z.-Y., Weng, X.-D. *et al.* (2014) Ozone oxidative preconditioning inhibits renal fibrosis induced by ischemia and reperfusion injury in rats. *Experimental Therapeutic Medicine* 8(6), 1764–1768. DOI: 10.3892/etm.2014.2004.

Wang, L., Chen, Z., Liu, Y., Du, Y. and Liu, X. (2018) Ozone oxidative postconditioning inhibits oxidative stress and apoptosis in renal ischemia and reperfusion injury through inhibition of MAPK signaling pathway. *Drug Design, Development and Therapy* 12, 1293.

Wang, L., Chen, Z., Weng, X., Wang, M., Du, Y. *et al.* (2019) Combined ischemic postconditioning and ozone postconditioning provides synergistic protection against renal ischemia and reperfusion injury through inhibiting pyroptosis. *Urology* 123(296), e291–296.

Wu, X., Li, Z., Liu, X., Peng, H., Huang, Y. *et al.* (2013) Major ozonated autohemotherapy promotes the recovery of upper limb motor function in patients with acute cerebral infarction. *Neural Regeneration Research* 8(5), 461.

Xiao, W., Tang, H., Wu, M., Liao, Y., Li, K. *et al.* (2017) Ozone oil promotes wound healing by increasing the migration of fibroblasts via PI3K/Akt/ mTOR signaling pathway. *Bioscience Reports* 37(6), BSR20170658. DOI: 10.1042/BSR20170658.

Zamora, Z.B., Borrego, A., López, O.Y., Delgado, R., González, R. *et al.* (2005) Effects of ozone oxidative preconditioning on TNF-α release and antioxidant-prooxidant intracellular balance in mice during endotoxic shock. *Mediators of Inflammation* 2005(1), 16–22.

Zanardi, I., Borrelli, E., Valacchi, G., Travagli, V. and Bocci, V. (2016) Ozone: A multifaceted molecule with unexpected therapeutic activity. *Current Medicinal Chemistry* 23(4), 304–314. DOI: 10.2174/0929867323666151221150420.

Zobel, R., Tkalčić, S., Štoković, I., Pipal, I. and Buić, V. (2012) Efficacy of ozone as a novel treatment option for urovagina in dairy cows. *Reproduction in Domestic Animals* 47(2), 293–298.

Zobel, R., Jurčić, G. and Perak, M. (2014) Ozone in veterinary medicine: A review. *Hrvatski Veterinarski Vjesnik* 22(3/4).

8 Dengue a Global Threat: An Insight Into Management and Control

Muhammad Jamil[1]*, Ashiq Saleem[1], Rida Naz[2], Sajad Ahmad[2], Faiqah Ramzan[3], Mubarik Ali[4] and Norina Jabeen[5]

[1]PARC Arid Zone Research Centre, Dera Ismail Khan, 29050, Pakistan; [2]Regional Blood Centre, Dera Ismail Khan, 29050, Pakistan; [3]Faculty of Veterinary and Animal Sciences, Gomal University Dera Ismail Khan, 29050, Pakistan; [4]Animal science Institute, National Agricultural Research Center, Islamabad, 54000, Pakistan; [5]Department of Rural Sociology, University of Agriculture Faisalabad, 37000, Pakistan

Abstract

Background: Dengue, whose severe forms have the potential to be fatal, is the most prevalent and rapidly proliferating vector-borne viral disease worldwide. It is evolving as a significant public health and economic dilemma for both rural and urban communities. *Objectives*: Given the urgent need for control measures, the purpose of this study is to evaluate both traditional and contemporary preventive strategies. *Results*: Traditional dengue control measures, while somewhat effective, tend to provide only temporary relief. In contrast, biotechnological innovations such as paratransgenesis, sterile insect technology, and genetically modified vectors have increased the effectiveness of conventional methods. In addition, the novel discovery of vaccines and immunotherapies offers a promising avenue for the management of dengue. *Discussion & Conclusion:* Integration of time-tested techniques with the most recent biotechnological interventions emerges as a crucial dengue-prevention strategy. While these developments offer cause for optimism, additional research is required to determine the long-term implications and viability of these techniques. *Implications*: The findings have significant implications for theory, policymaking, and medical practice, highlighting the need for a combined approach to dengue management.

Keywords: dengue, global threat, disease, management, control

Introduction

Dengue

Arthropod-borne disease dengue is a serious health concern, particularly in the tropics and subtropics. Since the 1960s, incidences have increased globally by more than 30-fold, affecting more than 100 nations on all continents. Every year, it is thought that 390 million dengue illnesses take place. A total of 70% of this global burden is carried by Asia. Over the past 20 years, the incidence of dengue has drastically increased, rising 505,430 cases in 2000 to over 2.4 and 4.2 million in 2009 and 2010, respectively. Mosquitoes transmit dengue virus (DENV-1 through DENV-4), the

*Corresponding author: jamilmatrah@gmail.com

most common virus transmitted by mosquitoes. DENV infection can cause a variety of clinical symptoms such as flu-like symptoms and even cause death. There is a high mortality rate associated with dengue shock syndrome (DSS) due to serious hemorrhage, shock, and rash, as well as nausea, fever, vomiting, and aches.

Classification of dengue

Dengue hemorrhagic fever (DHF) was divided into several categories, with grades III–IV being categorized as DSS. In 2009, the WHO revised its case classification system for dengue to reduce the number of different classifications (Kalayanarooj, 2011; Hadinegoro, 2012).

Causes of dengue

Aedes albopictus and *Aedes aegypti* mosquitoes transmit dengue, a fever sickness brought on by one of the serotypes of Flavivirus (DENV1-4), after a blood meal. Mosquitoes feed during the day and have an urban habitat. Due to global trade, *A. albopictus* is currently spreading to many developing and developed countries such as North America, Europe, India, Iran, China, and Pakistan. A dengue outbreak has been reported in five other European countries as well as the Portuguese island of Madeira.

The *A. aegypti* mosquito is a holometabolous insect, meaning it undergoes a full metamorphosis that includes an egg, larvae, pupae, and ultimately an adult stage. When an infected mosquito bites, the virus is spread. Following a mosquito bite, the virus spreads to the keratinocytes, which are adjacent skin cells. When infected, people act as a reservoir and source for additional viruses produced during viral replication in hosts.

Pakistan dengue species distribution

Pakistan has reported the presence of both dengue-causing mosquito species, *A. aegypti* and *A. albopictus*, but little is known about their diversity or how their populations disperse. Pakistan and Bangladesh have reported 104 species of mosquitoes.

Distribution of dengue

The vector-borne viral disease dengue, which is currently a concern to public health, has a significant socio-economic impact on many tropical, subtropical, and temperate regions of the world. According to estimates, 50% of the world's population currently resides in dengue-prone countries and locations where individuals are at risk of contracting the dengue arboviral disease. Over 390 million individuals globally have a possibility of contracting dengue each year, and there are roughly 100 million reported cases of the disease.

Dengue has been documented throughout recorded history for many millennia. A dengue-like illness was originally mentioned in the China Medical Encyclopedia over 992 AD. Although there is disagreement on DENV's geographic spread also known as 'water poison' as it is related to insects. West India and Central America experienced dengue-related illness outbreaks in 1635 and 1699, respectively. Consequently, there was some evidence that showed mosquito-borne viruses were present in Asian and African forests, with severe epidemics affecting residents of Asia, Africa, Philadelphia, and North America in 1780. An epidemic also occurred in New Orleans in 1945. Prior to 1970, dengue epidemics were only observed in nine countries. The global distribution of dengue is given in Table 8.1.

Etiology and pathogenesis

Dengue fever is a serious flu-like condition that affects people of all ages (infants, children, adolescents, and adults). The mosquito *A. aegypti* transmits the disease to people, and in the rainy season it is most prevalent. Four different single-stranded RNA viruses of the genus Flavivirus can cause dengue fever. Direct epidermal infection by the virus, viral replication that occurs largely in macrophages, and immunological and chemical mechanisms triggered by host-viral

Table 8.1. Distribution of dengue around the globe.

Serial number	Countries	References
1	Pakistan, India	Bhatt *et al.* (2013); Khan *et al.* (2020); Gupta *et al.* (2021)
2	America	Messina *et al.* (2019)
3	China	Wu *et al.* (2021)
4	Bangkok	Pongsiri *et al.* (2012); Khormi and Kumar (2014); Chen (2018)
5	Philippines	Pongsiri *et al.* (2012); Khormi and Kumar (2014); Chen (2018)
6	Thailand, Taiwan	Pongsiri *et al.* (2012); Khormi and Kumar (2014); Chen (2018)
7	Europe	Pongsiri *et al.* (2012); Khormi and Kumar (2014); Chen (2018)
8	Malaysia	Ong (2016)

interaction are the hypothesized causes of dengue virus infection.

Review Methodology

This investigation adhered to the PRISMA guidelines, with predetermined eligibility criteria steering our exhaustive database search. Our focus included both rural and urban communities affected by dengue. The search strategy was created to incorporate both traditional and contemporary dengue control methods.

Objectives

- To understand the historical, epidemiological, and transmission dynamics of dengue.
- To delve into its clinical presentations and current preventive measures.
- To analyze the socio-economic implications of dengue in affected regions and globally.
- To highlight research gaps and advocate for improved disease management.

Methodology

Data sources

The search was carried out using the PRISMA (Preferred Reporting Items for Systematic Reviews and Meta-Analyses) guidelines to ensure a rigorous and transparent review process. The databases utilized for this review were:

- PubMed
- Scopus
- Web of Science
- Google Scholar
- Cochrane Library

Search strategy

The following search terms were used in combination to ensure a comprehensive retrieval of relevant articles:

- 'Dengue'
- 'Management'
- 'Control'
- 'Epidemiology'
- 'Global Impact'
- 'Prevention'
- 'Treatment'

Boolean operators ('AND', 'OR') were employed to combine various search terms. An example search query would be: 'Dengue' AND 'Management' OR 'Control'.

Eligibility Criteria

Inclusion criteria

- Peer-reviewed original research articles and reviews published in the English language.

- Studies focusing on the management, control, and global impact of dengue.
- Publications dated from 2000 to 2023 to ensure relevance and updated information.

Exclusion criteria

- Non-peer-reviewed articles, opinion pieces, letters to the editor, and commentaries.
- Studies not published in the English language.
- Research articles that do not provide a clear methodology or results section.

Study selection

Initial search results were first screened by title and abstract to remove any irrelevant studies. Subsequently, full-text articles were examined to determine their suitability based on the inclusion and exclusion criteria. Any discrepancies in the selection process were resolved through discussion or by involving a third reviewer.

Quality assessment

The quality of the included studies was assessed using the Newcastle-Ottawa Scale for observational studies and the Cochrane Risk of Bias tool for randomized controlled trials. Studies were rated as low, moderate, or high quality based on their scores.

Data synthesis

The extracted data were synthesized to highlight the main findings related to the management, control, and global implications of dengue. Both qualitative and quantitative analyses were conducted to present a comprehensive review.

Transmission

Transmission through mosquito bite

Viruses spread to humans when infected female mosquitoes, particularly the Aegypti mosquito, bite them. *A. aegypti* is the primary vector, but other members of the *Aedes* genus can also transmit the disease. Infected mosquitoes reproduce virus in their midgut after feeding on an infected host with DENV, which then spreads to secondary tissues like their salivary glands. A virus is infectious for a period of time before it can spread to a new host (extrinsic incubation period [EIP]). It typically takes 8–12 days for the EIP to complete when the outside temperature is between 25 and 28°C.

Different variables such as the magnitude of daily temperature fluctuations, the virus genotype, and initial viral concentration affect the EIP. The mosquito can continue to spread viruses for the remainder of its life after becoming infected.

Human-to-mosquito transmission

Infected individuals can transmit the DENV to mosquitoes. Symptomatic individuals, presymptomatic individuals who have not yet developed symptoms, and those who are completely healthy (asymptomatic individuals) can be included here. Human- to-mosquito transmission can occur up to 2 days before or after someone stops having a fever. In contrast, fever as well as viremia in the patient are positively correlated with mosquito infection, while DENV-specific antibodies are connected with a reduced threat of mosquito poison. Most of the patients remain viremic for about 4–5 days, although the virus can persist for up to 12 days in some cases.

Maternal transmission

Mosquito vectors are the main means of DENV transmission between people. However, there is proof that maternal transfer could occur. Although the risk of vertical transmission seems to be correlated with the period of the dengue infection during pregnancy, vertical transmission rates do appear to be minimal. Babies who have mothers who have DENV infections during pregnancy run the risk of preterm birth, low birth weight, and fetal discomfort.

Other mode of transmission

Rare instances of transmission by transfusions, organ donation, and blood products have been documented. Similar to that, records of the virus being transmitted transovarially within mosquitoes also exist.

Signs and symptoms

A patient often reaches the crucial period 3–7 days after the onset of their illness. In a small number of individuals, the first 24–48 hour of the critical phase may see a severe worsening of symptoms. When the patient's fever is dropping (below 38°C/100°F) at this stage, the warning signs of severe dengue can start to manifest. Severe dengue is a potentially fatal outcome due to plasma leakage, fluid accumulation, breathing problems, severe bleeding, or organ malfunction.

Doctors should keep an eye out for the following warning signs:

1. Acute stomach discomfort
2. Continuous vomiting
3. Fast breathing
4. Bleeding
5. Exhaustion
6. Restlessness
7. Liver enlargement
8. Fatigue

Epidemiology and prevalence

It is the viral disease with the fastest global spread transmitted by mosquitoes with an annual impact of more than 100 million people. Dengue is another disease that affects more than 100 nations and kills 20–25,000 people annually, mostly children. Epidemiological outbreaks occur annually in the Americas, Asia, Africa, and Australia. There are two cycles of transmission that keep the dengue virus alive: (1) transfer from non-human primate to non-human primate by mosquito and (2) transmission from human to human by mosquito. The human-mosquito cycle is especially prominent in urban areas. The virus may or may not pass from person to mosquito, depending on the viral load of the mosquito's blood meal. The primary disease-carrying mosquito species are female *A. aegypti* and *A. albopictus* insects. Although *A. aegypti* is linked to the majority of diseases, *A. albopictus* range is growing, it can withstand cold environments better, it feeds aggressively but less frequently, and it may be linked to an increase in population. These mosquito species typically reside indoors and are active throughout the day. There have been reports of transmission by prenatal contact, blood transfusions, breast milk, and organ transplantation.

Akhtar *et al.* (2016) reported DENV-2 serotype from Khyber Pakhtunkhwa, Pakistan, while many other scientists had reported incidences of dengue from different areas of the country like Balochistan, Karachi, and Multan (Akram *et al.*, 1998; Jamil *et al.*, 2007; Ahmad *et al.*, 2017) as given in Table 8.2.

Results and Discussion

Relationship of dengue with age and sex of dengue affected patients

According to reports from Faisalabad in 2011, 38% of all cases were reported to be between the ages of 21 and 30. According to a brief publication on the epidemiology of dengue fever in Pakistan, patients' median ages are 32 years and 23 months; however, our study found that the median age was 37.95 years and 16.32 months. According to Gupta *et al.* (2021), the majority of cases from India occurred in people between the ages of 21 and 30. The young adults were the main group affected by DHF. The relationship is shown in Fig. 8.1 (Ahuja *et al.*, 2013).

Table 8.2. Prevalence of serotype-reported dengue cases during different years in Pakistan.

Year	Prevalent serotype	References	Year	Prevalent serotype	References
1994	DENV-1–2	Suleman *et al.* (2017)	2013	DENV-1–4	Ali *et al.* (2016)
1995	DENV-1–2	Khanani *et al.* (2011)	2014	DENV-1–3	Ali *et al.* (2013)
2003	DENV-2	Khanani *et al.* (2011)	2015	DENV-1–4	Mahmood *et al.* (2012)
2005	DENV-2–3	Khanani *et al.* (2011)	2016	DENV-1–4	Ahmad *et al.* (2017)
2006	DENV-2–3	Khan *et al.* (2018)	2017	DENV-1–4	Ahmad *et al.* (2017)
2007	DENV-2–3	Khan *et al.* (2018)	2018	DENV-1–4	Khan *et al.* (2018)
2008	DENV-2–4	Fatima *et al.* (2011); Khan *et al.* (2018)	2019	DENV-1–4	Shahid *et al.* (2017); Khan *et al.* (2018)
2009	DENV-2–3	Mahmood *et al.* (2012); Khan *et al.* (2018)	2020	DENV-1–4	Khan *et al.* (2018)
2010	DENV-1–2	Mahmood *et al.* (2012)	2021	DENV-1–4	Khan *et al.* (2018)
2011	DENV-2–4	Humayoun *et al.* (2010); Khanani *et al.* (2011)			

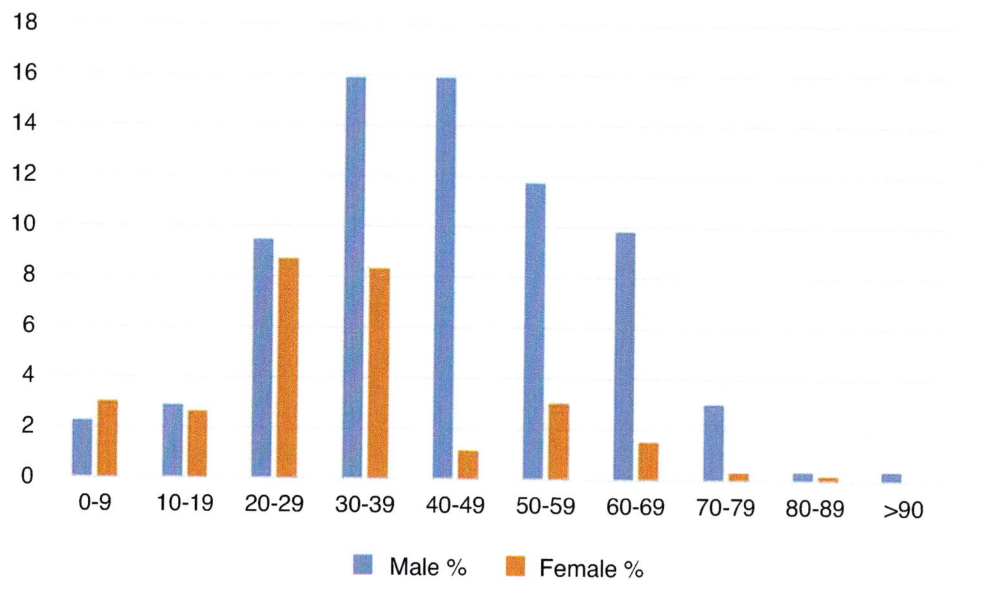

Fig. 8.1. Relationship of dengue with age and sex.

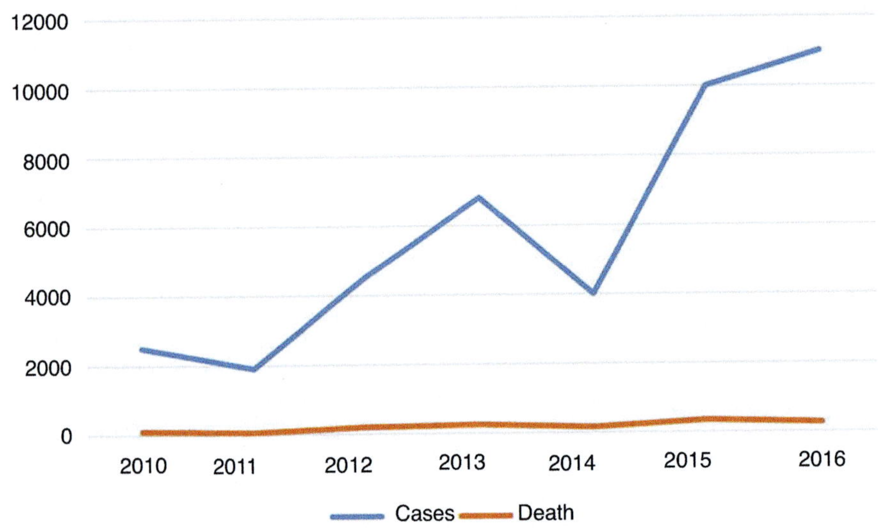

Fig. 8.2. The dengue cases and deaths reported in India.

Table 8.3. Factors influencing the incidence of or epidemics of dengue.

Factors	References
High occupancy rate per room, unscreened homes, insufficient showers, inadequate water storage for the home, a lack of waste collection system, a lack of air conditioning, and the direct discharge of sewage into ponds or street drainage are all problems.	Villabona-Arenas and Zanotto (2013)
Increased container and Breteau indices.	Braga *et al*. (2010)
Housing in close proximity to marketplaces, slums, or locations with exposed sewers.	Stewart-Ibarra *et al*. (2014)
Lack of knowledge.	Selck *et al*. (2014)
Mosquito breeding areas in the courtyard, presence of plastic containers and cans, tyre casings, pools of temporary water in plants, gutters for collecting rainwater, open water storage containers, and pans for food or water for animals.	Hayes *et al*. (2006)

Factors associated with dengue

There are different factors which link with dengue and cause mortality (Fig. 8.2). Some are given in Table 8.3.

Prognosis and complications

A total of 10%–20% of people who have severe dengue fever who go untreated may pass away. Proper supportive treatment brings the death rate down to about 1%. Liver injury, seizures, pneumonia, encephalopathy, cardiomyopathy, orchitis, oophoritis, and encephalitis (Grange *et al.*, 2014; Hasan *et al.*, 2016; Rathore *et al.*, 2020; Thach *et al.*, 2021; Lefebvre *et al.*, 2022).

Global implications

Grasping the multifaceted challenges posed by dengue is essential not just for the healthcare sector but also for global economies and communities at large. This review seeks to empower its readers with a comprehensive understanding of dengue's threats and the measures needed for its control.

Vector Control and Prevention Strategies

Prevention

Prevent mosquito bites

Different preventive techniques have been used to control the dispersal or spread of dengue disease such as avoiding mosquito bites to minimize the vector population which ultimately reduces the disease threat. Put on protective gear and reduce mosquito habitat by using insect repellent are the best dengue protection tools (Onen *et al.*, 2023).

Cultural control/physical control

Modification or changes in man-made breeding sites of vector

The threat of disease can be reduced by changes in man-made breeding sites. The reduction in the pest population can occur by improving house designs which stop the entry of mosquitoes; draining and cleaning roof gutters, installing outdoor sinks and condensate collection units under refrigerators and air conditioners, and chlorinating ornamental pools or fountain management can minimize the vector threat.

Environmental management

This is the most efficient method of controlling vectors, and it involves preventing and reducing vector reproduction and human-vector contact by destroying, changing, discarding, or recycling containers that are responsible for the greatest amount of adult mosquito production (Wilson *et al.*, 2020).

Reducing vector breeding sites and solid waste management

Drums, overhead tanks, and jars should not be used to store water. If they must be used, they should be covered with screens or tight-fitting lids. By keeping mosquitoes from laying their eggs on the surface of water tanks, the use of polystyrene beads helps decrease mosquito breeding. Solid waste is the term for non-biodegradable components of municipal, industrial, and domestic garbage. Regular recycling of solid waste, including used tires, bottles, and cans, is recommended (Curtis *et al.*, 2002).

Health education

It is the most crucial tool in the war against dengue. For the dengue control programs to be implemented effectively, detailed public education about dengue is required. Mass awareness campaigns or audiovisual media can be used to sensitize the public.

Community participation

It is crucial to educate the public so that they can actively participate in dengue control initiatives.

Effective surveillance

Fundamental data on risk assessment, epidemic response, program evaluation, and guidance, as well as prompt interventions to prevent and control dengue, are provided via surveillance. The understanding of the spatiotemporal distribution of dengue cases is made possible through surveillance, which also gives entomological and epidemiological correlations for improved planning. However, these initiatives do not prioritize eradicating the dengue vector (Abbas *et al.*, 2014). After decades of observation, the dengue outbreak revealed unsustainable vector control tactics and poor surveillance in 2005. Controlling vector species will benefit from an efficient surveillance system, giving the necessary data regarding vector concentration, breeding habitats, and identification (Scarpino *et al.*, 2017).

Biological control

Predator

Dragonflies and damselflies – commonly referred to as 'mosquito hawks' in India – feed on mosquitoes, as well as frogs, toads, and their tadpoles, birds – particularly swallows, martins, and swifts, ducks, and other waterfowl – fish, and tadpoles of frogs and toads (including goldfish, guppies, bass, bluegill, and catfish) are the most effective predators of mosquito larvae.

Fish

Gambusia affinis and *Poecilia reticulata*, a viviparous species, have been used in limited freshwater wells and huge water tanks. Use should only be made of natural larvicidal fishes.

Endosymbiotic and predatory copepod control

An internal parasite, Wolbachia feeds on mosquitoes, thus DENV infection reduces with parasite infection. Only certain container habitats have shown potential for mosquito control by tiny predatory freshwater crustaceans.

Entomopathogenic fungi

A potential biological control agent could be entomopathogenic ascomycetes. Once germinated, the conidia of these fungi directly enter the adult mosquito's cuticle and then release a mixture of organic substances that kill the insect by depleting its nutrients and inflicting internal mechanical injury. These fungi have been used successfully in the field to kill malaria vectors and alter the behavior of wild mosquitoes that feed on blood (Howard *et al.*, 2011).

Fungi such as *Metarhizium anisopliae* and *Beauveria bassiana* are the two main species that are now being employed by many laboratories worldwide, despite the fact that a wide variety of these fungi have been used in research with dengue vectors (Scholte *et al.*, 2007). *M. anisopliae* caused *A. albopictus* to die significantly, according to Scholte *et al.* (2007), who also discovered high levels of infection. Studies have shown that exposure to *M. anisopliae* and *B. bassiana* considerably enhanced the mortality of *A. aegypti* (Garcia-Munguia *et al.*, 2011; Reyes-Villanueva *et al.*, 2011). Unfortunately, after a blood meal, sensitivity to fungal infection is greatly reduced, but after digestion, susceptibility reverted to pre-feeding levels (De Paula *et al.*, 2011a). Additionally, wild strains might be less prone to fungal infection than other commonly utilized colony strains (De Paula *et al.*, 2011b). Nevertheless, co-exposure to an insecticide can boost fungal virulence (De Paula *et al.*, 2011a).

Parasitoids

Parasitoids are organisms that go through a larva-like juvenile stage before destroying their host mosquito host. The protozoan *Ascogregarina culicis*, a parasitoid of *A. aegypti* larvae that negatively impacts the mosquito population, is a good example. Under laboratory circumstances, *Wolbachia pipientis*, a different bacterial parasite, has been shown to shorten *A. aegypti's* life span.

Chemical control

Larvicidal agents can be used in large breeding vessels or insecticides sprayed as aerosols and thermal fogs. Formulations made of oil are recommended because they prevent evaporation. Organophosphorus compounds (fenitrothion and malathion) and pyrethroids are a couple of the regularly used insecticides (Table 8.4).

Residual treatment

With hand-operated compression sprayers, suitable pesticides with larvicidal and adulticidal properties can be used. Insecticides are sprayed on the human houses and animals in a given region using an indoor residual spraying (IRS) technique. The adult vector mosquitoes are killed when they land on the treated place (Wahid *et al.*, 2019).

Table 8.4. List of chemicals used against dengue vector.

No.	Chemical name	References
1	Fenitrothion	Ong (2016)
	Cyphenothrin	Ong (2016)
2	Temephos	Ong (2016)
3	Fenthion	Ong (2016)
4	d-tetramethrin +cyphenothrin	Ong (2016)
5	s-bioallethrin +permethrin + piperonyl butoxide	Ong (2016)
	Cypermethrin	Ong (2016)
	Bioresmethrin	Ong (2016)
	Spinosad	Darriet *et al*. (2010)
	Pyriproxyfen	Phuanukoonnon *et al*. (2005)
	Temephos	Phuanukoonnon *et al*. (2005)

Table 8.5. Candidates for a dengue vaccine are presently undergoing various stages of clinical studies.

Type of vaccine	Developer	Phase
DNA vaccine expressing prM and E protein	WRAIR, Naval Medical Research Centre	I
Chimeric yellow virus dengue vaccine (CYD)	Sanofi Pasteur	Licensed
Cell culture based LAV	WRAIR-GSK	II
Intertypic chimera-DENVax	CDC-Inviragen/Takeda	III
Recombinant subunit vaccine-V180	Hawaii Biotech, Merck and Co.	I
Targeted mutagenesis based LAV-TetraVax-DV	NIH	III

Use of pheromones as 'Attract-And-Kill' approach

Pheromones have a long history of use in a variety of sectors, including integrated pest control (IPM) (Nagpal *et al*., 2015).

Use of insect growth regulators (IGRs)

Insect growth regulators (IGRs), among other well-known chemical substances, are employed to thwart insect growth and development. IGRs cause early developmental alterations that cause the insect to die before reaching an adult. Many IGRs, including methoprene, endotoxins, and diflubenzuron, have been utilized to combat viral infections caused by *A. aegypti* (Abbas *et al*., 2014). In their investigation, Lau *et al*. discovered that cyromazine was effective at reducing the larval population indices of *A. aegypti*. They claim that field populations of vector species develop resistance to several IGRs (Lau *et al*., 2015).

Vaccine

Dengvaxia is the main dengue fever vaccine that has been used all over the globe to control dengue fever. Candidates for a dengue vaccine are presently undergoing various stages of clinical studies (Table 8.5). The major strategy for preventing dengue illnesses is vector control. Environmental changes, chemical control employing insecticides and larvicides, and biological control can all be used to achieve this. Environmental interventions involve reducing or eliminating vector breeding grounds that are both natural and created by humans, such as trash cans and improperly run waste facilities. The effect of environmental interventions on reducing larval populations was shown to be modest, despite the fact that they are thought of as safe measures, according to a recent systematic review and meta-analysis.

Efficiency of Latest Vector Control Strategies: A Spotlight on Wolbachia

Vector control remains a cornerstone in the fight against mosquito-borne diseases, including dengue, Zika, and chikungunya. Recent strategies have shifted from conventional measures like insecticides to innovative biological interventions. One such promising strategy is the introduction of the Wolbachia bacterium into *A. aegypti* mosquitoes, the primary vector for many arboviruses (Wilson *et al.*, 2020).

Wolbachia is a naturally occurring bacterium found in up to 60% of insect species but notably absent in the *A. aegypti* mosquito. When introduced into these mosquitoes, Wolbachia interferes with the mosquito's ability to transmit viruses to humans. The mechanisms include reducing the mosquito's lifespan (thus limiting their potential to transmit diseases), and directly inhibiting the replication of the virus inside the mosquito (Iturbe-Ormaetxe *et al.*, 2011).

Several pilot projects have released Wolbachia-infected mosquitoes into the environment with promising results. For instance, trials in parts of Australia have shown a significant reduction in dengue transmissions following the release of Wolbachia-infected mosquitoes. Furthermore, these mosquitoes have the ability to pass Wolbachia to their offspring, ensuring the sustainability of the approach (Wilson *et al.*, 2020).

Beyond its direct impact on disease transmission, the Wolbachia method offers several advantages:

1. Environmentally friendly: Unlike insecticides, which can harm ecosystems and beneficial insects, Wolbachia is a natural method that targets only specific mosquito populations.
2. Resistance management: The overuse of insecticides can lead to resistance in mosquito populations. Wolbachia provides an alternative approach that can be integrated with other methods to delay or manage resistance.
3. Cost-effective: Once established in a mosquito population, Wolbachia can sustain itself without constant reintroductions, potentially reducing long-term control costs.
4. Safety: Wolbachia is not known to cause harm to humans, animals, or the wider environment (Iturbe-Ormaetxe *et al.*, 2011).

However, challenges remain. The establishment of Wolbachia in mosquito populations requires strategic releases and consistent monitoring. Moreover, its efficiency may vary based on local ecological and climatic conditions. There is also a need to gauge community acceptance and address any concerns related to releasing modified mosquitoes.

Conclusion

The enduring challenge posed by the dengue virus (DENV) underscores the urgency and significance of continued research and innovation. Although strides have been made in raising awareness about dengue prevention, we are still confronted with multiple impediments. One major challenge is the absence of a cohesive strategy that addresses the growing incidence of dengue outbreaks in ever-expanding regions. Additionally, the constraint of inadequate funding and resources further exacerbates the situation. However, with collaborative efforts, the integration of new methodologies, and a commitment to research, it is plausible to envision a future where dengue's threat is considerably diminished and where communities are better equipped to manage and prevent outbreaks.

Recommendations

To tackle the pressing issue of dengue, it is imperative to invest in research that delves into innovative methods and tools for its control and prevention. Enhanced understanding of the disease, its vectors, and the nuances of its transmission is vital. Moreover, the design and implementation of a comprehensive, multifaceted strategy is paramount. This approach should not only address the core challenges of dengue control but should also be adaptable to the changing dynamics of disease transmission in various regions. Given the multifaceted nature of the dengue threat, collaborations across sectors, ministries, and agencies are essential. By ensuring a cohesive and well-organized response, it becomes feasible to pool resources, expertise, and knowledge. Such coordinated efforts can pave the way for effective dengue management, facilitating the efficient utilization of available resources, and fostering an environment where preventive measures are prioritized and executed seamlessly.

Conflict of Interest

The authors have no conflicts of interest to declare.

References

Abbas, A., Abbas, R.Z., Khan, J.A., Iqbal, Z., Bhatti, M.M.H. *et al.* (2014) Integrated strategies for the control and prevention of dengue vectors with particular reference to *Aedes aegypti*. *Pakistan Veterinary Journal* 34, 1–10.

Ahmad, S., Aziz, M.A., Aftab, A., Ullah, Z., Ahmad, M.I. *et al.* (2017) Epidemiology of dengue in Pakistan, present prevalence and guidelines for future control. *International Journal of Mosquito Research* 4(6), 25–32.

Ahuja, G., Sheikh, S., Zubairi, A., Mansoor, K., Khawaja, S. *et al.* (2013) Prevalence of dengue in patients presenting to a tertiary care hospital of Karachi. *Editorial Board* 2(1), 27.

Akhtar, N., Saeed, K., Rafiq, N. and Khan, N. (2016) Prevalence of dengue serotype (DENV-2) in Pakistan. *Journal of Genes and Cells* 2(1), 8.

Akram, D.S., Igarashi, A. and Takasu, T. (1998) Dengue virus infection among children with undifferentiated fever in Karachi. *The Indian Journal of Pediatrics* 65(5), 735–740.

Ali, A., Ahmad, H., Idrees, M., Zahir, F. and Ali, I. (2013) Dengue virus serotype 2 and 3 causing high morbidity and mortality in Swat, Pakistan. *Biohelikon: Immunity and Diseases* 1, 11–13.

Ali, A., Ahmad, H., Idrees, M., Zahir, F. and Ali, I. (2016) Circulating serotypes of dengue virus and their incursion into non-endemic areas of Pakistan; A serious threat. *Virology Journal* 13, 144.

Bhatt, S., Gething, P.W., Brady, O.J., Messina, J.P., Farlow, A.W. *et al.* (2013) The global distribution and burden of dengue. *Nature* 496(7446), 504–507.

Braga, C., Luna, C.F., Martelli, C.M., Souza, W.V., Cordeiro, M.T. *et al.* (2010) Seroprevalence and risk factors for dengue infection in socio-economically distinct areas of Recife, Brazil. *Acta Tropica* 113, 234–240.

Chen, W.J. (2018) Dengue outbreaks and the geographic distribution of dengue vectors in Taiwan: A 20-year epidemiological analysis. *Biomedical Journal* 41(5), 283–289.

Curtis, C.F., Malecela-Lazaro, M., Reuben, R. and Maxwell, C.A. (2002) Use of floating layers of polystyrene beads to control populations of the filaria vector Culex quinquefasciatus. *Annals of Tropical Medicine and Parasitology* 96(Suppl 2), S97–S104.

Darriet, F., Marcombe, S., Etienne, M., Yebakima, A., Agnew, P. *et al.* (2010) Field evaluation of pyriproxyfen and spinosad mixture for the control of insecticide resistant *Aedes aegypti* in Martinique (French West Indies). *Parasites & Vectors* 3, 88.

De Paula, A.R., Carolino, A.T., Paula, C.O. and Samuels, R.I. (2011a) The combination of the entomopathogenic fungus *Metarhizium anisopliae* with the insecticide imidacloprid increases virulence against the dengue vector *Aedes aegypti* (Diptera: Culicidae). *Parasites & Vectors* 4, 8.

De Paula, A.R., Carolino, A.T., Silva, C.P. and Samuels, R.I. (2011b) Susceptibility of adult female *Aedes aegypti* (Diptera: Culicidae) to the entomopathogenic fungus *Metarhizium anisopliae* is modified following blood feeding. *Parasites & Vectors* 4, 91.

Fatima, Z., Idrees, M., Bajwa, M.A., Tahir, Z., Ullah, O. *et al.* (2011) Serotype and genotype analysis of dengue virus by sequencing followed by phylogenetic analysis using samples from three mini outbreaks-2007-2009 in Pakistan. *BMC Microbiology* 11(1), 1–8.

Garcia-Munguia, A.M., Garza-Hernandez, J.A., Rebollar-Tellez, E.A., Rodriguez Perez, M.A. and Reyes-Villanueva, F. (2011) Transmission of *Beauveria bassiana* from male to female *Aedes aegypti* mosquitoes. *Parasites & Vectors* 4, 24.

Grange, L., Simon-Loriere, E., Sakuntabhai, A., Gresh, L., Paul, R. *et al.* (2014) Epidemiological risk factors associated with high global frequency of inapparent dengue virus infections. *Frontiers in Immunology* 5, 280.

Gupta, A., Rijhwani, P., Pahadia, M.R., Kalia, A., Choudhary, S. *et al.* (2021) Prevalence of dengue serotypes and its correlation with the laboratory profile at a tertiary care hospital in Northwestern India. *Cureus* 13(5), e15030.

Hadinegoro, S.R.S. (2012) The revised WHO dengue case classification: Does the system need to be modified? *Paediatrics and International Child Health* 32(Sup1), 33–38.

Hasan, S., Jamdar, S.F., Alalowi, M. and Al Beaiji, S.M.A.A. (2016) Dengue virus: A global human threat: Review of literature. *Journal of International Society of Preventive & Community Dentistry* 6(1), 1.

Hayes, J.M., Rigau-Perez, J.G., Reiter, P., Paul, V.E., Lorrin, P. *et al.* (2006) Risk factors for infection during a dengue-1 outbreak in Maui, Hawaii, 2001. *Transactions of the Royal Society of Tropical Medicine and Hygiene* 100, 559–566.

Howard, A.F.V., Adongo, E.A., Vulule, V. and Githure, J. (2011) Effects of a botanical larvicide derived from *Azadirachta indica* (the neem tree) on oviposition behaviour in *Anopheles gambiae* s.s. mosquitoes. *Journal of Medicinal Plants Research* 5, 1948–1954.

Humayoun, M.A., Waseem, T., Jawa, A.A., Hashmi, M.S. and Akram, J. (2010) Multiple dengue serotypes and high frequency of dengue hemorrhagic fever at two tertiary care hospitals in Lahore during the 2008 dengue virus outbreak in Punjab, Pakistan. *International Journal of Infectious Diseases* 14, e54–e59.

Iturbe-Ormaetxe, I., Walker, T. and O'Neill, S.L. (2011) Wolbachia and the biological control of mosquito-borne disease. *EMBO Reports* 12(6), 508–518.

Jamil, B., Hasan, R., Zafar, A., Bewley, K., Chamberlain, J. *et al.* (2007) Dengue virus serotype 3, Karachi, Pakistan. *Emerging Infectious Diseases* 13(1), 182. DOI: 10.3201/eid1301.060376.

Kalayanarooj, S. (2011) Dengue classification: Current WHO vs. the newly suggested classification for better clinical application. *Journal of the Medical Association of Thailand* 94(Suppl 3), S74–S84.

Khan, J., Khan, I., Ghaffar, A. and Khalid, B. (2018) Epidemiological trends and risk factors associated with dengue disease in Pakistan (1980–2014): A systematic literature search and analysis. *BMC Public Health* 18, 1–13.

Khan, N.U., Danish, L., Khan, H.U., Shah, M., Ismail, M. *et al.* (2020) Prevalence of dengue virus serotypes in the 2017 outbreak in Peshawar, KP, Pakistan. *Journal of Clinical Laboratory Analysis* 34(9), e23371.

Khormi, H.M. and Kumar, L. (2014) Climate change and the potential global distribution of *Aedes aegypti*: Spatial modelling using geographical information system and CLIMEX. *Geospatial Health* 8(2), 405–415.

Lau, K.W., Chen, C.D., Lee, H.L., Norma-Rashid, Y. and Sofian-Azirun, M. (2015) Evaluation of insect growth regulators against field-collected *Aedes aegypti* and *Aedes albopictus* (Diptera: Culicidae) from Malaysia. *Journal of Medical Entomology* 52, 199–206. DOI: 10.1093/jme/tju019.

Khanani, R.M., Arif, A. and Shaikh, R. (2011) Dengue in Pakistan: Journey from a disease free to a hyper endemic nation. *Journal of the Dow University of Health Sciences (JDUHS)* 5(3), 81–84.

Lefebvre, B., Karki, R., Misslin, R., Nakhapakorn, K., Daudé, E. *et al.* (2022) Importance of public transport networks for reconciling the spatial distribution of dengue and the association of socio-economic factors with dengue risk in Bangkok, Thailand. *International Journal of Environmental Research and Public Health* 19(16), 10123.

Mahmood, N., Rana, M.Y., Qureshi, Z., Mujtaba, G. and Shaukat, U. (2012) Prevalence and molecular characterization of dengue viruses serotypes in 2010 epidemic. *The American Journal of the Medical Sciences* 343, 61–64.

Messina, J.P., Brady, O.J., Golding, N., Kraemer, M.U., Wint, G.R. *et al.* (2019) The current and future global distribution and population at risk of dengue. *Nature Microbiology* 4(9), 1508–1515.

Nagpal, B.N., Ghosh, S.K., Eapen, A., Srivastava, A., Sharma, M.C. *et al.* (2015) Control of *Aedes aegypti* and *Ae. albopictus*, the vectors of dengue and chikungunya, by using pheromone C21 with an insect growth regulator: Results of multicentric trials from 2007–12 in India. *Journal of Vector Borne Diseases* 52, 224–231.

Onen, H., Luzala, M.M., Kigozi, S., Sikumbili, R.M., Muanga, C.-J.K. *et al.* (2023) Mosquito-borne diseases and their control strategies: An overview focused on green synthesized plant-based metallic nanoparticles. *Insects* 14, 221.

Ong, S.Q. (2016) Dengue vector control in Malaysia: A review for current and alternative strategies. *Sains Malays* 45(5), 777–785.

Phuanukoonnon, S., Mueller, I. and Bryan, J.H. (2005) Effectiveness of dengue control practices in household water containers in Northeast Thailand. *Tropical Medicine and International Health* 10, 755–763.

Pongsiri, P., Themboonlers, A. and Poovorawan, Y. (2012) Changing pattern of dengue virus serotypes in Thailand between 2004 and 2010. *Journal of Health, Population, and Nutrition* 30(3), 366.

Rathore, A.P., Farouk, F.S. and John, A.L.S. (2020) Risk factors and biomarkers of severe dengue. *Current Opinion in Virology* 43, 1–8.

Reyes-Villanueva, F., Garza-Hernandez, J.A., Garcia-Munguia, A.M., Tamez-Guerra, P., Howard, A.F.V. *et al.* (2011) Dissemination of *Metarhizium anisopliae* of low and high virulence by mating behavior in *Aedes aegypti*. *Parasites & Vectors* 4, 171.

Scarpino, S.V., Meyers, L.A. and Johansson, M.A. (2017) Design strategies for efficient arbovirus surveillance. *Emerging Infectious Diseases* 23, 642–644. DOI: 10.3201/eid2304.160944.

Scholte, E.-J., Takken, W. and Knols, B.G.J. (2007) Infection of adult *Aedes aegypti* and *Ae. albopictus* mosquitoes with the entomopathogenic fungus *Metarhizium anisopliae*. *Acta Tropica* 102, 151–158.

Selck, F.W., Adalja, A.A. and Boddie, C.R. (2014) An estimate of the global health care and lost productivity costs of dengue. *Vector-Borne and Zoonotic Diseases* 14, 824–826.

Shahid, M., Amin, I., Afzal, S., Fatima, Z., Zahid, S. *et al.* (2017) Prevalence and molecular detection of dengue virus in 2013 outbreak in KPK and Punjab, Pakistan. *Pakistan Journal of Zoology* 49(3), 1–7.

Stewart-Ibarra, A.M., Munoz, A.G., Ryan, S.J., Ayala, E.B. *et al.* (2014) Spatiotemporal clustering, climate periodicity, and social-ecological risk factors for dengue during an outbreak in Machala, Ecuador, in 2010. *BMC Infectious Diseases* 14, 610–618.

Suleman, M., Faryal, R., Alam, M.M., Sharif, S., Shaukat, S. *et al.* (2017) Dengue virus serotypes circulating in Khyber Pakhtunkhwa province, Pakistan, 2013–2015. *Annals of Laboratory Medicine* 37(2), 151.

Thach, T.Q., Eisa, H.G., Hmeda, A.B., Faraj, H., Thuan, T.M. *et al.* (2021) Predictive markers for the early prognosis of dengue severity: A systematic review and meta-analysis. *PLoS Neglected Tropical Diseases* 15(10), e0009808.

Tsheten, T., Clements, A.C., Gray, D.J., Adhikary, R.K., Furuya-Kanamori, L. *et al.* (2021) Clinical predictors of severe dengue: A systematic review and meta-analysis. *Infectious Diseases of Poverty* 10(1), 1–10.

Villabona-Arenas, C.J. and Zanotto, P.M. (2013) Worldwide spread of dengue virus type 1. *PLoS ONE* 8, e62649.

Wahid, I., Ishak, H., Hafid, A., Fajri, M., Sidjal, S. *et al.* (2019) Integrated vector management with additional pre-transmission season thermal fogging is associated with a reduction in dengue incidence in Makassar, Indonesia: Results of an 8-year observational study. *PLOS Neglected Tropical Diseases* 13(8), e0007606.

Wilson, A.L., Courtenay, O., Kelly-Hope, L.A., Scott, T.W., Takken, W. *et al.* (2020) The importance of vector control for the control and elimination of vector-borne diseases. *PLOS Neglected Tropical Diseases* 14(1), e0007831.

Wu, W., Ren, H. and Lu, L. (2021) Increasingly expanded future risk of dengue fever in the Pearl River Delta, China. *PLoS Neglected Tropical Diseases* 15(9), e0009745.

9 Impacts of Climate Change on Animal Welfare

Joe Joseph[1], Renae Charalambous[1], Harsh Pahuja[1], Dylan Fox[1], Jiwoo Jeon[1], Ning-Yuan Ko[1], Nishit Rao[1], Zhiheng Wang[1], Sneh Kashinath Nerurkar[1], Sharvari Avinash Sherekar[1], Yifei Yang[2], Kate Dutton-Regester[1] and Edward Narayan[3]*

[1]School of Agriculture and Food Sustainability, The University of Queensland, Gatton Campus, QLD 4343, Australia; [2]School of Veterinary Sciences, The University of Queensland, Gatton Campus, QLD 4343, Australia; [3]Queensland Alliance for Agriculture and Food Innovation, The University of Queensland, St Lucia, QLD 4072, Australia

Abstract

Climate change has a significant impact on domesticated and wildlife animals globally. Projections for a 2°C rise in atmospheric temperature will result in catastrophic impacts globally. Animal welfare is an integral component of human-animal interaction and it is of paramount importance for wildlife rehabilitation and domestic animals. Animal welfare can be assessed using the five domains model, which includes nutrition, environment, physical health, behaviour, and mental attributes of an animal's response to environmental change. Researchers use some of these domain attributes to evaluate the effects of stress on their animals and to improve the management and welfare of animals. Although there are variations in how animals respond biologically to stress, in general, the five domains model provides a robust tool for research use, and to evaluate the proximate effects of climatic variability on animals. In this review, our research group (The Stress Lab; www.edwardstresslab.org) presents a series of wildlife and domesticated animal examples to showcase how climate change impacts animal welfare. We provide examples of animals from various countries, across both aquatic and terrestrial systems, and provide an overview of the impacts of climate change on each of the five domains of animal welfare. We hope that future researchers will apply the animal welfare domains to evaluate how climate change impacts animals, and further research will pave the way to the protection of animals from the catastrophic impacts of climate change.

Keywords: extinction crisis, global warming, human-animal-interaction, stress, welfare domains

Introduction

Climate change poses an unprecedented global crisis for humans and biodiversity. In recent years, extreme climatic events such as droughts and floods have profoundly impacted human populations. To address this, scientists have been enhancing weather prediction technology and preparing communities for the impending climate crisis (Hennessy *et al.*, 2005). While humans have support mechanisms to cope with climate change, animals require human

*Corresponding author: e.narayan@uq.edu.au

intervention to mitigate climate risks. Many wildlife species exhibit remarkable abilities to naturally forecast and adapt to the imminent dangers of climate change through behavioural and physiological changes. For instance, migrating sea turtles demonstrate these adaptive strategies (Pike *et al.*, 2006). According to the World Wildlife Fund (WWF), climate change drives nature loss through elevated temperatures, rising sea levels, and the exacerbation of extreme events (WWF, 2022). Global warming, primarily caused by human-induced factors such as increased levels of greenhouse gases (e.g. carbon dioxide, methane, and nitrous oxide) in the atmosphere, results from activities like agriculture, forestry, and other land use practices (Yoro and Daramola, 2020). The challenges posed by climate change are not limited to environmental concerns alone. Animals play a crucial role in meeting human needs, such as food security (e.g. animal-based protein, manufacturing, clothing) and fulfilling aesthetic desires like zoos and nature recreational parks (Argent, 2022). Consequently, climate change has detrimental effects on animal welfare, impacting their biology, ecology, and survival directly and indirectly, which will be discussed in this review.

In layman's terms, animal welfare can be defined as the genuine state of well-being and condition of the animal, independent of human expectations or desires for their prosperity. If climate stress is prolonged, it can have severe consequences on the health, well-being, and/or productivity of animals. There are various reviews on the topic of animal welfare, which can be referred here (Hamann *et al.*, 2007; Marsh *et al.*, 2007; Adams and Hayes, 2008; Adams, 2010; Narayan *et al.*, 2012; Huey and Kingsolver, 2019). While researchers have extensively examined the effects of climate change on animals, the direct correlation between climate change and animal welfare, particularly in the context of wild animals, remains relatively scarce in existing studies.

Therefore, the aim of this review is to utilize the five welfare domains (see Fig. 9.1) (Broom, 2014; Hemsworth *et al.*, 2015; Mellor *et al.*, 2020) to discuss the potential impacts of climate change on animal welfare. Our review provides a broad overview of the impacts of climate change on animal welfare, drawing on examples from various animal groups across terrestrial and aquatic habitats, encompassing both wildlife and domesticated species.

Methods

The data presented in this work were obtained through comprehensive searches conducted on various web and scientific search engines including Google Scholar, PubMed, and Science Direct. Primary search terms comprised the animal welfare domains (nutrition, environment, physical health, behaviour, and mental), environmental temperature as the surrogate for climate change, and the model animal species, which included invertebrates, fishes, amphibians, reptiles, birds, and small and large mammals. It is a non-systematic review. Table 9.1 provides an overview of the animal welfare domains and dimensions covered by the research.

Invertebrates

Diversity and importance

'Invertebrate' is a term of convenience and refers to a group of animals that do not develop a spine (vertebral column) and are not members of the Vertebrata (Agassiz, 2013). They are a diverse group, having a greater number and variety of species than all known vertebrates (Richards and Davies, 2013); it is estimated that they compose 90% of the existing animal species. They have a wide range of uses, such as research, aquaculture, farming, and displays in aquariums for conservation and educational purposes (Carere *et al.*, 2011). Many familiar invertebrates serve as major food sources and are economically viable, such as shrimps, clams, squids, locusts, termites, grasshoppers, and beetle grubs, as well as honey from bees. Other invertebrates are valued for their ability to make luxuries, such as silk, pearls, and shells (Kellert, 1993). Due to their diversity, abundance, accessibility, quick generation times, and large number of offspring compared to vertebrates, they are also of scientific significance. Despite this, invertebrates are frequently overlooked by

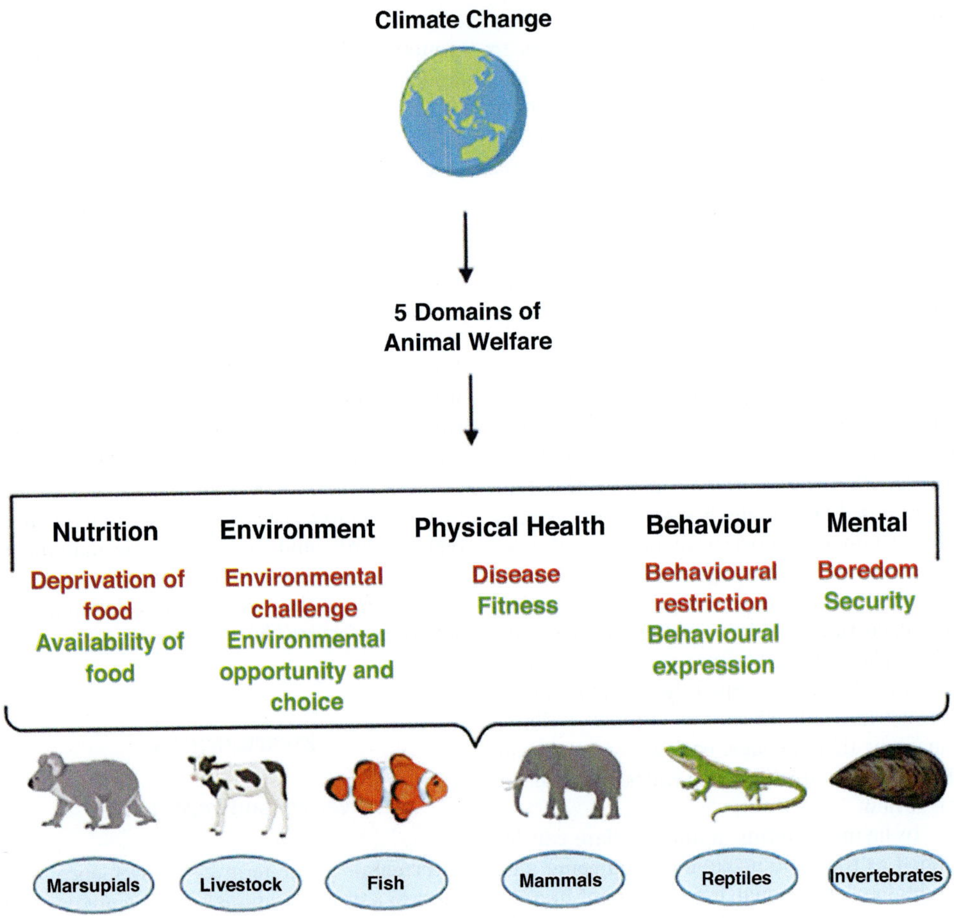

Fig. 9.1. The framework of the study which uses the five domains model (Mellor *et al.*, 2020) to explore the impacts of climate change on various animal groups.

the public and scientific community and often kept with limited animal care and supervision. Unfortunately, the majority of invertebrates are disliked or feared due to concerns of disease (Kellert, 1993). Consequently, the focus tends to be on charismatic species that capture the public attention, while the welfare of vital invertebrate species often goes unnoticed.

Invertebrates are ectotherms, and their growth rates are strongly affected by environmental factors such as temperature, humidity (Forrest, 2017), and water properties (Culler-Juarez and Onthank, 2021). Hence, there are substantial concerns surrounding the effects of global warming and the acidification of oceans on invertebrates (Raven *et al.*, 2005). Changes in temperature and rainfall patterns brought on by climate change are predicted to have a significant direct impact on the distribution of invertebrates and indirect effects on food plant ranges and phenologies. For instance, compared to data from a few decades ago, the first flight of butterflies has advanced by as much as a month (Roy and Sparks, 2000).

Many invertebrate species, particularly insects, are adapted to specific ecosystems all over the world. Many of these species are restricted to relatively small climatic ranges, and their response to climate change is dependent on whether individuals are able to adapt to the new conditions and the genetic diversity among populations (Butterfield and Coulson, 1997).

Table 9.1. An overview of the animal welfare domains and dimensions covered by the research.

Animal group and management system	Welfare dimension and dimension attribute	Methods used	Key results	Conclusion	References
Invertebrate; unspecified	Nutrition; food quantity	Review paper	Elevated temperatures weaken the symbiotic relationship between cnidarians and algae, resulting in the loss of their primary food source.	The loss of symbiotic algae decreases energy available to cnidarians resulting in death and the phenomenon known as coral bleaching.	Cziesielski *et al.* (2019)
Fish; intensive	Environment; temperature	Measured steroidogenesis markers, immunity status, and ovarian tissue of female Nile tilapia (*Oreochromis niloticus*) experiencing heat stress	Reproductive hormones and cortisol significantly declined due to heat stress; further, gene expression was downregulated, and ovary tissues were injured.	Heat stress has harmful effects on female tilapia physiology through modulation of steroidogenesis-related gene expression and immunity	Mahmoud *et al.* (2020)
Fish; intensive	Nutrition; food quantity	Measured the effects of dietary nano-selenium on organizational structure, lipid changes, and biochemical parameters as well as heat-shock protein- and selenoprotein-related gene expression in rainbow trout (*Oncorhynchus mykiss*).	Stress began to increase significantly when trout experienced heat stress.	Supplementation with 5 mg/kg nano-Se effectively alleviates stress damage in rainbow trout.	Mahmoud *et al.* (2020)
Fish; unspecified	Environment; temperature	Measured transcriptomic profile, histopathology, and oxidative stress in the liver samples of pikeperch (*Sander lucioperca*) experiencing heat stress.	The most significant heat-stress-related pathway was the protein processing in the endoplasmic reticulum; liver histology was changed due to heat stress.	Heat stress at 29°C caused oxidative damage and dysfunction in the pikeperch liver between 3 hour and 48 hour.	Wang *et al.* (2019)

Continued

Table 9.1. Continued

Animal group and management system	Welfare dimension and dimension attribute	Methods used	Key results	Conclusion	References
Fish; unspecified	Behaviour; temperature	Measured the performance of zebrafish (*Danio rerio*) exposed to different environmental temperatures and subject to four behavioural tests.	Heat treatment reduced anxiety and increases the boldness of zebrafish.	The increase in ambient temperature may compromise zebrafish survival rate in the natural environment.	Angiulli *et al.* (2020)
Amphibian; intensive	Health; disease	Measured urinary corticosterone levels of Chytridiomycosis positive and negative Stony Creek Frogs (*Litoria wilcoxii*) *via* enzyme-immunoassay.	Elevated corticosterone concentrations result in the reduction of eosinophils and lymphocytes.	Corticosterone elevation induced by heat stress increases susceptibility to diseases such as chytridiomycosis.	Kindermann *et al.* (2012)
Amphibian; intensive	Environment; temperature	Measured urinary corticosterone levels of Cane Toads (*Rhinella marina*) *via* enzyme-immunoassay.	Elevated environmental temperatures induce excessive corticosterone production in amphibians.	Excess production of corticosterone results in alterations to metabolic rate and other physiological traits in amphibians.	Narayan *et al.* (2012)
Reptile; unspecified	Nutrition; food quality	Review chapter	Variability in environmental temperature could influence the distribution and quality of seagrasses, which green sea turtles are reliant on as a food source.	Variability in the quality and distribution of seagrasses because of climate change can influence the ability of green sea turtles to satisfy their nutritional requirements.	Hamann *et al.* (2007)
Wildlife mammal; captive	Nutrition; food intake	Investigated whether koalas adjust the number and/or the size of their meals when offered eucalypt foliage with varying concentrations of formylated phloroglucinol compounds (FPC).	High FPC reduced the total intake of foliage.	Climate change results in increased toxic content and reduced nitrogen levels in eucalypts.	Marsh *et al.* (2007)

Continued

Table 9.1. Continued

Animal group and management system	Welfare dimension and dimension attribute	Methods used	Key results	Conclusion	References
Wildlife mammal; free-ranging	Health; limitations	Trapping of wild bats and monitoring against climatic data, analysis utilized principal component analysis.	Elevated temperature and dry weather lead to decreased reproductive performance in female bats.	Environmental conditions have a significant effect on bat reproduction.	Adams (2010)
Wildlife mammal; free-ranging	Nutrition; water intake	Capturing and tagging female bats to monitor activity and behaviour around an artificial water source.	Lactating females have a higher water requirement as compared to their non-lactating counterparts.	Increased temperatures will reduce water availability, increasing the chance of bat population reduction	Adams and Hayes (2008)
Wildlife mammal; free-ranging	Environment; choices	Measuring bat activity against environmental variables. Data analysed using generalized linear mixed model (GLMM).	Moonlight and temperature have the highest effect on insectivorous bat activity.	The ways in which bat species respond to environmental variables are predictable.	Appel *et al.* (2019)
Wildlife mammal; free-ranging	Environment; limitations	Trapping of bats, and comparing data with similar studies done on bats.	The number of reproducing female bats was lower in years with higher precipitation.	Higher precipitation delays or prevents reproduction in female bats.	Grindal *et al.* (1992)
Wildlife mammal; free-ranging	Behaviour; thermal comfort	Conducted behavioural observations of female bats in elevated temperatures.	Nursing female bats exposed to extreme temperatures demonstrated an increase in fanning and grooming behaviour concurrent with reduced resting behaviour. Further, nursing females were at increased risk of death.	Nursing female bats are more susceptible to heat-stress compared to their non-lactating counterparts.	Snoyman *et al.* (2013)
Wildlife mammal; free-ranging	Nutrition: water and food intake	Analysed elephant carcasses in Kenya to determine the cause of death.	Most elephant deaths could be classified under natural causes (i.e. nutritional deficiency), poaching or human conflict.	Drought and resource scarcity, as a result of climate change, are key contributors to elephant mortality rates.	Mukeka *et al.* (2022)

Continued

Table 9.1. Continued

Animal group and management system	Welfare dimension and dimension attribute	Methods used	Key results	Conclusion	References
Wildlife mammal; unspecified	Mental; thermal comfort	Observation and analysis of the impacts of climate change on elephants.	Elephants perform evaporative water loss through their skin for thermoregulation, even at low temperatures. Consequently, they require large amounts of drinking water to support thermoregulatory processes within the body.	Reduced water availability and intake result in reduced effectiveness of elephants to thermoregulate, thereby increasing heat stress.	Fuller *et al.* (2016)
Domesticated species, captive	Health; disease	Autopsies were conducted on broiler chickens kept under hot conditions for 4 days.	Elevated temperatures result in greater concentrations of reactive oxygen, which can react with the cells of the animals and cause necrosis.	Higher cases of necrosis among broiler chickens will reduce the animals' quality of life and reduce the quality of their meat.	Santos *et al.* (2015)
Domesticated species; intensive	Environment; temperature	Measured feed intake and milk production of dairy cows.	Heat stress resulted in a 35% reduction in milk production.	The extent of milk yield decline observed in heat-stressed cows depends on various factors that interact with high air temperature.	Bernabucci *et al.* (2010)

Additionally, the atmospheric carbon dioxide levels in the ocean, which have been increasing at a rate of around 0.5% per year primarily due to human activity, have recently experienced the most rapid change in CO_2 concentrations (Raven *et al.*, 2005; Fabry *et al.*, 2008). The ocean's acidity has increased by 26% after absorbing nearly one-third of the human CO_2 produced (Sabine *et al.*, 2004); a further 250% increase in acidity is expected by the end of this century (Pachauri and Meyer, 2014). The ocean absorbs surplus heat from a warming world and serves as a 'sink' for atmospheric carbon dioxide, with land and ocean surface temperatures already increasing by 0.85°C (Pachauri and Meyer, 2014). The coastal sea surface temperature is likely to rise 1–3°C more than what has already been recorded if more CO_2 emission mitigation measures are not taken (Parry *et al.*, 2007; Pachauri and Meyer, 2014).

Stress response in invertebrates

As invertebrates are important to many ecosystems and play a vital role in maintaining the balance of nature, understanding their stress physiology can help us to better protect these animals and their habitats. Invertebrates have a variety of mechanisms for responding to stress; the mechanism utilized depends on their specific physiology and the type of stress they are experiencing (Butterfield and Coulson, 1997).

For example, some invertebrates may respond to physical stress, such as extreme temperatures or changes in salinity, by regulating their body fluids or by moving to a more favourable environment (Jin *et al.*, 2022). Others may respond to biological stress, such as the presence of predators or changes in their food supply, by changing their behaviour or by using chemical defences (Horwitz *et al.*, 2020). Overall, the stress response in invertebrates is like that of vertebrates, involving the activation of hormones and neurotransmitters that help the animal to cope with the stressor. However, the specific mechanisms involved may differ among different types of invertebrates. For example, insects and other arthropods may use hormones called ecdysteroids to help them cope with stress (Moen *et al.*, 2022), while molluscs may use molecules called opisthobranch peptides (Roggatz *et al.*, 2016).

Biogenic amines and heat stress in insects

The biosynthesis of biogenic amines and other compounds is a crucial process in insects. Biogenic amines, such as dopamine and serotonin, are neurotransmitters that play important roles in the nervous system (Neven, 2000). They are released in response to various stimuli, including heat stress. Other neuroendocrine factors, such as adipokinetic hormone, are also released in response to heat and serve to mobilize the insect's energetic reserves (González-Tokman *et al.*, 2020). However, the exact role of these hormones in the response to heat stress is not yet well understood. Heat stress can have synergistic effects when combined with other stressors, such as insecticides. For example, in the moth *Plodia interpunctella*, heat and insecticide exposure have a synergistic effect that greatly increases the stress response and mortality (González-Tokman *et al.*, 2020). These synergistic effects are common in nature, but the mechanisms underlying them are not yet fully understood.

Heat can have significant effects on insect physiology, including changes in metabolism, respiration, nervous and endocrine systems, and the elicitation of heat shock proteins (HSPs). In order to be effective, heat treatments used to disinfect fresh and stored products must take into account the sensitivity of insects to high temperatures (Neven, 2000). Insects can be transferred from one temperature to another in a step-wise or ramp-wise manner. The former demonstrates how quickly an insect can respond to a thermal challenge while the latter reveals mechanisms involved in thermal tolerance and indicates whether tolerance limits are wider in response to a ramp-wise or step-wise function (Neven, 2000). Heat treatments can also cause damage to insect cells and tissues, leading to death.

HSPs are a highly conserved class of proteins that display elevated transcription during periods of stress, playing important roles in protecting the cell and its components from damage. Different insects have different sets of HSPs, and the specific HSPs that are upregulated in response to heat vary among species (González-Tokman *et al.*, 2020). Heat stress can have a range of negative effects on insects, including reducing their ability to fly, reproduce, and feed (González-Tokman *et al.*, 2020). It can also affect their immune function, making them more susceptible to diseases. However, some insects have evolved mechanisms to tolerate or even benefit from heat stress. For example, desert locusts can increase their body temperature by sunbathing, which enhances their metabolism and immune function.

Conversely, heat shock has negative effects on male reproductive success in the springtail *Orchesella cincta* (Zizzari and Ellers, 2011). Researchers exposed male springtails to four temperature treatments: heat hardening (35.2°C for 1 hour), heat shock (37.2°C for 1 hour), heat hardening plus heat shock (35.2°C for 1 hour followed by 37.2°C for 1 hour), and control (20°C). Significant mortality was only found in the treatment with heat shock, with and without heat hardening. A direct effect of heat treatment was found for time to first reproduction, which was significantly longer after heat shock (with or without heat hardening) than in the control treatment. There was no difference among treatments in the number of spermatophores produced in the first reproductive instar. The mechanism of stress physiology in this study is the induction of HSPs in response to heat stress. Exposure to heat shock causes the expression of the heat shock gene Hsp70 to increase, indicating that the treatments induced thermal stress. This increase in HSPs may help protect the organism against the detrimental effects of heat stress, but it does not protect against all negative effects (Zizzari and Ellers, 2011).

Stress in crustaceans

Chang (2005) has developed methods for the quantification of stress in crustaceans. They have observed increases in crustacean hyperglycemic hormone (CHH) under conditions of acute hypoxia, elevated temperature, and altered salinity. In addition, elevated CHH concentrations were observed in Norway lobsters that were parasitized with the dinoflagellate *Hematodinium* sp. Further, they examined the influence of heat-shock, osmotic stress, and the moult cycle on HSP expression at the protein and mRNA levels. When comparing claw and abdominal muscles during moulting, a tissue-specific HSP response was observed (Chang, 2005). Quantification of these different stress responses may serve as early indicators of the degradation of environmental health. The CHH ELISA may also be useful for the quantification of circulating CHH levels following exposure to endocrine-disrupting compounds (Chang, 2005).

Chronic heat stress can negatively impact the growth, survival, and feeding of the sea urchin *Strongylocentrotus intermedius* (Zhan *et al.*, 2019). Researchers cultured the sea urchins in the northern Yellow Sea in China under two conditions: 20°C and 25°C. After 28 days, they found that the specific growth and ingestion rates of the sea urchins reared under high-temperature conditions decreased compared to those reared under optimal temperature conditions. In addition, the study identified 2125 differentially expressed genes in the sea urchins reared under high-temperature conditions compared to those subjected to optimal temperature conditions, which included 1015 upregulated and 1100 downregulated genes (Zhan *et al.*, 2019). The findings provide new insight into the molecular mechanism of echinoid species in response to heat stress (Zhan *et al.*, 2019).

Coral bleaching

Coral bleaching is a process that occurs when corals experience extreme and prolonged heat stress. This can cause the symbiotic relationship between corals and the algae of the family Symbiodiniaceae to break down (Cziesielski *et al.*, 2019). The algae provide most of the energetic requirements of the coral host, enabling them to effectively calcify and become the foundation of modern reefs. When the symbiotic relationship is disrupted, the coral experiences an energetic deficit that can lead to its death. The loss and degradation of coral reefs because of bleaching events is a major concern. Initial research into bleaching began in the early 1900s, but it was not until the 1990s that mass bleaching events were recorded (Cziesielski *et al.*, 2019). Since then, research into the mechanisms underlying coral bleaching has advanced rapidly, with the use of omics tools providing new insights. Despite these advances, the underlying molecular mechanisms of host and symbiont heat stress response are still not fully understood.

In conclusion, heat stress is a significant environmental factor that can have negative effects on insects. It can affect their behaviour, physiology, and immune function. However, the specific mechanisms underlying these effects are not yet fully understood, and further research is needed to better understand how insects respond to heat stress and other climatic stressors more broadly.

Fish

The welfare of fish is relatively novel in the field of animals. Indeed, the term 'fish welfare' was rarely used by fish researchers until 2000 (Kristiansen and Bracke, 2020), but the Medway report is believed to be the first report that specifically related to fish welfare (Medway, 1980). Today, fish have become an important food source for humans (Martos-Sitcha *et al.*, 2020). According to the Food and Agriculture

Organisation of the United Nations (FAO), finfish (including freshwater, diadromous, and marine fish) had the greatest share of the total fisheries and aquaculture production, reaching 135 million tonnes in 2019 (FAO, 2021). The main change in aquatic source production was that aquaculture has gradually replaced wild catch with 48% of contribution in global fisheries and aquaculture production in 2019 (FAO, 2021). Therefore, this section will focus on the impact of climate change on farmed fish because of the substantial number of them kept for food purposes; both marine and freshwater species are discussed.

In recent years, climate change has become one of the major threats to fish production. Climatic variables include cyclones, drought, flood, global warming, ocean acidification, salinity, rainfall variation, and rising sea level (Ahmed *et al.*, 2019). Temperature rise due to global warming can have a profound impact on fish farming as water temperature is a primary factor in fish welfare (Cochrane *et al.*, 2009). Increased water temperature (refer to heat stress in land animals) is a core stressor to ectothermic animals. Researchers have found that elevated water temperatures (> 30°C) have harmful effects on female Nile tilapia (*Oreochromis niloticus*) physiology through modulation of steroidogenesis markers, immunity function and ovarian tissue (Mahmoud *et al.*, 2020). More specifically, when the temperature exceeds 32°C, significant increases were found in serum stress indicators and enzyme activities, in addition to mRNA expression of HSP (Mahmoud *et al.*, 2020). Further, many cold-water fish species such as rainbow trout (*Oncorhynchus mykiss*) are even more vulnerable to heat stress (Wang *et al.*, 2019). The addition of appropriate dietary selenium (Se) provides one solution to enhance heat resistance in rainbow trout (Li, 2022). In addition to physiological effects, temperature can either directly or indirectly alter the swimming performance of fish (Domenici *et al.*, 2019). For example, zebrafish (*Danio rerio*) were more mobile in warm water (34°C) compared to cold water (26°C), showing much higher swimming speed and total distance travelled (Angiulli *et al.*, 2020). Temperature also affects the selection of depths and habitats of marine fish. For example, Atlantic cod (*Gadus morhua*) swim to colder and deeper water areas during the summer when sea surface temperatures are high (Freitas *et al.*, 2021).

Cyclones, floods, ocean acidification, salinity changes, and sea level rise pose additional risks to coastal and marine aquaculture (Ahmed *et al.*, 2019). Climatic events affect not only infrastructure but also fish productivity, particularly outdoor operations. Recently, a land-based, indoor, and controlled farming system known as the 'Recirculating Aquaculture System' (RAS), has been developed to adapt to environmental challenges (Bueno and Soto, 2017; Ahmed *et al.*, 2019). The RAS, initially conceived in Japan in the 1950s, was first commercially used in Denmark, and then further developed in North America, Asia, Europe, and other countries (Ying *et al.*, 2015). This fish-rearing facility is purpose-built for eco-friendly and intensive farming, which eliminates the effects of climate change on fish welfare (Ying *et al.*, 2015; Ahmed and Turchini, 2021). However, costly operations, greenhouse gas emissions, energy consumption, and engineering approaches are still the main challenges of the RAS (Ying *et al.*, 2015).

Global warming, water temperature rise, and any other alteration of water parameters can pose many risks to fish. As an ectotherm, fish are more vulnerable to climate change. Increased water temperatures not only have an impact on fish physiology but also their behaviour and habitat selection.

Amphibians

Amphibians are an ancient class of animals, vestigial of the first terrestrial vertebrates, and can be identified by their use of their skin as their primary organ for respiration (Wake and Koo, 2018). Currently, there are an estimated 8000 extant species, separated into three orders: (i) the Anurans, which includes frogs and toads. This is the most successful order, found on all continents excluding Antarctica and comprising approximately 7000 of the surviving amphibian species (Wake and Koo, 2018); (ii) Caudates, including salamanders and newts which are found throughout the northern hemisphere and South America; finally, (iii) Gymniophones which include caecilians. This is the least studied order which is constrained to the tropics (Wake and Koo, 2018; Stebbins and Cohen, 2021). This section will specifically focus on the impacts of climate change on the physical health, nutritional, and environmental domain of amphibian welfare.

Amphibians are far more sensitive to the quality of their environment than other terrestrial vertebrates due to their reliance on water for maintaining their skin moisture for respiration, reproduction, ion exchange, and a variety of other physiological processes. This makes them susceptible to rapid changes in the environment (Wake and Koo, 2018; Stebbins and Cohen, 2021). Environmental temperature has been shown to be integral in modulating metabolism, and performance and fitness traits such as locomotion and reproduction (Moore and Zoeller, 1985; Seebacher *et al.*, 2005; Narayan *et al.*, 2012; Narayan and Hero, 2014a). As such, increasing mean temperatures approaching and exceeding the thermal stress tolerances of many amphibian taxa, and erratic weather patterns resulting in extended periods of drought, flood, and fire instigated by climate change have resulted in the exposure of amphibians to the greatest risk of extinction of any vertebrate class (Bernardo and Spotila, 2006; Wake and Koo, 2018; CSIRO, 2020).

Amphibians are ectotherms; animals that are reliant on external sources of heat for the regulation of their body temperature which in turn controls their metabolic rate, behaviour, immunity, and other physiological qualities (Narayan *et al.*, 2012; Beltrán *et al.*, 2021). One pathway through which environmental temperature can influence the physiology of amphibians is through the synthesis of the stress hormone corticosterone. Corticosterone typically induces a short-term stress response; for example, corticosterone can increase lipid, amino acid, and glucose mobilization and availability, to provide additional energy and increase the organism's metabolic activity (Narayan *et al.*, 2012). In general, stress hormones are known to influence immune cell distribution and corticosterone is no exception as it decreases concentrations of lymphocytes and eosinophils (Kindermann *et al.*, 2012). Elevated environmental temperatures have been shown to elevate corticosterone concentrations in amphibians and these concentrations do not decrease unless the temperature declines (Narayan *et al.*, 2012). The positive relationship between mean temperature and corticosterone concentrations and the ongoing impacts of climate change on temperature may result in permanent impairment of amphibian health, nutrition requirements, and behaviour (Narayan *et al.*, 2012).

The resultant increase in metabolic activity from elevated corticosterone is detrimental to the nutritional and behavioural welfare of amphibians, as the mobilization of fats, glucose, and amino acids results in the reduction of the animals' energy reserves while simultaneously increasing the nutritional requirement of the animal, thereby increasing their susceptibility to periods of food scarcity (Narayan *et al.*, 2012; Huey and Kingsolver, 2019). Furthermore, the impacts of mean temperature elevation are likely to increase amphibian susceptibility to disease (Narayan *et al.*, 2012). Absence of lymphocytes and eosinophils will weaken the adaptive immune system and increase the predisposition to infection from fungi and parasites (Narayan *et al.*, 2012; Figueiredo and Neves, 2018; Flajnik, 2018). Chytridiomycosis is an amphibian-targeting fungal disease caused by *Batrachochytrium dendrobatidis* (Bd) and has been responsible for declines in amphibian populations throughout the world (Kindermann *et al.*, 2012). As a disease of fungal origin, the reduction in eosinophil concentration further increases the vulnerability of amphibians to chytridiomycosis (Kindermann *et al.*, 2012; Figueiredo and Neves, 2018). Furthermore, extended exposure to heat stress can decrease the sensitivity of the endocrine system to acute stressors such as pathogens, resulting in greater loss of amphibians to chytridiomycosis and other diseases (Narayan and Hero, 2014b).

The prevalence of heat stress among amphibians due to climate change and increasing mean temperatures has resulted in a decrease in amphibian welfare, with the health of amphibians being heavily impacted due to the suppression of their immune systems (Narayan *et al.*, 2012).

Reptiles

There are over 9000 species that form the class Reptilia. This includes more than 8000 species of snakes and lizards (order Squamata). Threats to these species include invasive species, habitat destruction, disease, pollution, and overexploitation, all of which have resulted in around 22% of reptiles becoming threatened or extinct (Cabrelli, 2013). One of the most important challenges for reptiles, however, is climate change. Cabrelli (2013) reported that, over the past five decades there has been a global rise in temperature of around 0.46°C, along with variations in water temperature, sea level, rainfall patterns, and frequency and intensity of extreme climatic conditions. This section will specifically focus on the broad-headed snake (*Hoplocephalus bungaroides*) and the impact climate change has on its welfare regarding the environmental and behavioural domains.

Global temperature rise leads to an environment, which is extremely stressful for reptiles (Hall, 2020). Reptiles are commonly found in dry environments and can do so as their integuments are thick and scaly which reduces water loss. However, excessive heating of habitats could restrict lizards to cooler microhabitats and alter behavioural patterns such as periods of activity (Gunn, 1942; Cooper, 2000). Reptiles are ectotherms and are the most vulnerable species to climate warming. The fluctuation in temperature can generate 'realized' thermal reactions i.e. fitness norms that are different from the fundamental norms in standard temperature conditions (Paaijmans *et al.*, 2013).

Reptiles, like all animals, have a thermal threshold within which they are comfortable. Physiological markers such as HSPs can determine the physiological responses of reptiles to thermal stress. In some reptiles, such as sea turtles, which rely on temperature for sex determination, the thermal environment becomes more important for gender-balanced population dynamics (Hamann *et al.*, 2007). By the year 2050, the global temperature range will increase by 1.1–1.2°C. The changes that take place in ultraviolet light and radiation will also have drawbacks on food availability and quality for species such as the green sea turtle, which is an herbivore. This consequence is a direct example of the impact of climate change on the nutritional domain of reptiles (see Fig. 9.1) (Hamann *et al.*, 2007).

The broad-headed snake is the most endangered snake species in Australia (Penman, 2010; Cogger, 2014). This species has specific habitat requirements for thermoregulation. For example, when temperatures are decreasing they are observed to reside in crevices and under rocks in locations which are exposed; conversely, in summer they move into hollow trees (Pringle *et al.*, 2003). The broad-headed snake is distributed throughout climatically suitable areas, otherwise known as the bioclimatic envelope. These locations are restricted for species that are threatened by habitat degradation and collection from the wild (Schlesinger and Shine, 1994; Shine et al., 1998; Webb *et al.* 2002a, b; Penman, 2010). The distribution of the broad-headed snake has resulted in a loss of genetic variation (Cabrelli, 2013). These changes may alter various biological traits of the reptiles such as their reproductive cycle, sex ratio, breeding pattern, site selection, habitat use, and rates of survival (Forchhammer *et al.*, 1998; Crick and Sparks, 1999; Winkler *et al.*, 2002; Visser and Both, 2005; Pike *et al.*, 2006; Telemeco *et al.*, 2009; Penman, 2010). The effects of these changes might benefit some animals by extending their ranges to unexplored areas, while others may suffer due to lack of connectivity to the area to provide suitable conditions for survival (Penman, 2010). However, it was reported that climate change, wildfire, extinction of fauna, and modifications in anthropogenic landscapes drive changes in vegetation.

It can be concluded that rising temperatures adversely impact the broad-headed snake. It alters biological traits such as site selection, habitat use, survival rates, reproductive cyclicity, and genetic variations. Climate change has impacted the ecology of reptiles in the wild and researchers have assessed the eco-physiological responses of species *in situ* using physiology, behavioural, and other methods. However, there has been limited work done to link the impacts directly to welfare domains. As climate change drives more wild populations to their ecological limits, there will be potential welfare consequences and considerations that need to be accounted for.

Birds

The impact of climate change on birds has been well documented. It is expected that one-eighth of species of birds will become extinct in the coming decades due to climate change. It is projected that increases in temperature by 3.5°C will lead to the extinction of approximately 900 bird species, with over 80% in the tropic region (Şekercioğlu *et al.*, 2012). Climate change impacts wild bird species in many ways such as habitat distribution, breeding season and migration, and the gross morphology of some bird species. Tropical birds such as northern snowbirds will be highly vulnerable to climate change due to limited access to high-elevation habitats. Birds are homeotherms; however, heat stress due to climate change can impact birds both physiologically and behaviourally. Excess heat dissipation due to exposure to acute heat stress can be costly for birds and trade-off with crucial life-history stages such as growth, development, and reproduction. Effects of heat stress can have significant consequences on breeding success and parental behaviour. Recent research has shown that seabirds are impacted by significant heat stress during breeding. For example, seabird breeding habitats and nests can be impacted by high coastal temperatures resulting in nest abandonment (Olin *et al.*, 2023). Researchers have highlighted the direct and indirect effects of climate change on food resources and disease transmission (e.g. avian influenza and malaria) will increase extinction risks for wild birds (Crick, 2004; Auer and Martin, 2013).

Marsupials

Marsupials are a subclass of mammals that are characterized by premature birth and continued development of the newborn while attached to the nipples on the mother's lower belly within a pouch (Kennedy, 1992; Britannica, 1999). Of the over 250 species of marsupials, most can be found in Australia and New Guinea, with the rest being found in America (Kennedy, 1992; Tyndale-Biscoe, 2005). Tooth dentition provides information relating to the type of food an animal eats and, therefore, can indicate their role within the ecosystem (Tyndale-Biscoe, 2005). Marsupial tooth dentition varies, indicating that some marsupials are herbivorous (i.e. the koala *Phascolarctos cinereus*), some are omnivorous (i.e. the common brushtail possum *Trichosurus vulpecula*), and others are carnivorous (i.e. the Tasmanian devil *Sarcophilus harrisii*) (Tyndale-Biscoe, 2005). Here, we will explore how climate change affects the welfare of marsupials, with a focus on the koala and their environmental and nutritional domain.

Climate change has been recognized as a major factor driving population decline across many species of marsupial, including the koala (Adams-Hosking *et al.*, 2011; Lunney *et al.*, 2014). Although Australian marsupials have been traditionally well adapted to the country's erratic climatic patterns, in modern times their survival is threatened by extreme weather events (Tyndale-Biscoe, 2005; CSIRO, 2020), including increasing mean temperatures, rainfall extremes such as prolonged rain and drought, and more frequent and longer fire seasons (Woinarski and Burbidge, 2016; CSIRO, 2020).

Koalas maintain their body temperature at a fairly consistent level (35.5°C) (Tyndale-Biscoe, 2005). They do this by expending the least amount of energy when the surrounding temperature is nearly the same as their body temperature (Tyndale-Biscoe, 2005). Essentially, when their surrounding temperature is lower, more energy is required to generate heat, and when their surrounding temperature is higher, more energy is expended to cool down (Tyndale-Biscoe, 2005). Koalas are a highly specialized species with a specific diet of around 40 eucalyptus species out of the almost 600 species that grow in Australia (Phillips and Callaghan, 2000; Phillips *et al.*, 2000). Eucalyptus is a highly tolerant tree species (Booth, 2013), and contains low levels of nitrogen and high toxic metabolites such as formylated phloroglucinol compounds (Moore *et al.*, 2005; Hovenden and Williams, 2010). However, current climate change projections indicate poor outcomes for eucalyptus leaf quality (Hovenden and Williams, 2010). Increasing mean temperatures influenced by climate change mean marsupial species such as the koala will be required to expend more energy to maintain their body temperature, using a food source that is reduced in quality.

Koalas use dietary water derived from foliage to meet their water requirements (Ellis,

1995). Leaf water is normally sufficient to meet the moisture requirements of koalas; however, minimum thresholds are much higher when their surrounding temperature is higher (Hume and Esson, 1993; Clifton *et al.*, 2007). This means that as temperatures become more extreme, the leaf water content may not be sufficient to meet the needs of koalas (Mella *et al.*, 2019), and large-scale mortality events may occur due to dehydration (Gordon *et al.*, 1988; Seabrook *et al.*, 2011; Lunney *et al.*, 2012). Furthermore, eucalyptus is considered the most proficient and successful epicormic resprouter in the incidence of bushfires (Burrows, 2013), which potentially means only short-term loss of food for koalas (Matthews *et al.*, 2007). However, the recovery of eucalyptus post-fire is dependent on a number of factors such as forest composition, seasonal conditions before and after the fire, and the patchiness and intensity of the fire (Heath *et al.*, 2016). This means that the incidence of more frequent and longer fire seasons influenced by climate change could result in long-term loss of food for koalas (Beale *et al.*, 2022).

With the loss of quality food, and potentially food altogether, climate change has already begun to, and will continue to affect the welfare of marsupials, including the iconic koala.

Bats

Bats (Chiropterans) are considered to be the second most diverse mammalian order, with more than 1400 documented species, having a one-fifth contribution to the worldwide mammalian diversity (Simmons and Cirranello, 2020). Bats have a major role to play in the ecosystem, primarily as pollen transporters and seed disposers across many plant species in different parts of the world (Fujita and Tuttle, 1991); for example, bats act as a major pollinator of ferns in New Zealand (Brock and Collier, 2020).

Climate change is having a significant effect on the survival, population density, and reproductive performance of many different animal species (Mawdsley *et al.*, 2009). A study conducted by Appel *et al.* (2019) investigated the major environmental factors affecting insectivorous bat activity. They reported that moonlight and temperature had the highest impact on bat activity followed by rainfall, which affected the activity patterns of a very limited proportion of species. This section will explore the impacts of climate change on the environmental, nutritional, and behavioural domains of bat welfare.

Due to the absence of sweat glands and a high surface-volume ratio, bats are unable to dissipate heat efficiently making them extremely vulnerable to the ill effects of high temperatures (Downs *et al.*, 2012; Korine *et al.*, 2016). One such instance was observed in New South Wales when temperatures reached up to 42°C (Welbergen *et al.*, 2008). This led to the death of around 3500 bats across nine different species from separate colonies (Welbergen *et al.*, 2008). The temperature increase was linked to a set of behaviours observed in bats, including fanning, increased saliva-spreading, and panting, which were presumably employed as mechanisms to dissipate heat (Welbergen *et al.*, 2008). However, these behaviours were followed by individuals falling from trees and subsequently dying (Welbergen *et al.*, 2008).

Insectivorous bats can be severely affected by climate change as the insects that they consume require very specific climatic conditions for their growth and development (Burles *et al.*, 2009). Temperatures below 10°C can reduce insect activity, which eventually leads to delayed development (Cryan *et al.*, 2000). Consequently, this disruption in the insect life cycle leaves insectivorous bats with less food, which can ultimately compromise their reproductive performance (Cryan *et al.*, 2000). Frick *et al.* (2012) observed that the time of emergence of bats from their caves for foraging was partially dependent on climatic conditions. Bats emerged earlier in years with extremely dry conditions as compared to the years with high moisture, which may increase their chances of predation. Conversely, when the surface temperature was higher the bats emerged later in search of food.

Highly variable habitat temperature because of climate change has an adverse effect on many different bat behavioural patterns. Downs *et al.* (2012) studied the effects of different seasons on the sleep patterns of the bats, observing that bats slept less in summer than in winter. They reported that high temperatures reduce sleep duration considerably as the bats spent most of their time trying to cool themselves. An increase in fanning behaviour was observed by Snoyman *et al.* (2013) in response to high temperatures. Additionally, females with young pups showed an increase in grooming behaviour compared to other individuals in the same group, indicating their vulnerability to high temperatures. Moreover, female bats consumed more water with increased ambient temperature (Adams and Hayes, 2008).

Finally, the effects of climate change are also seen in the reproductive success of female bats. Elevated temperatures and dry weather have an adverse effect on the reproductive patterns of bats (Adams, 2010). Increased rainfall has also been shown to reduce reproductive success in female bats due to reduced foraging activities and prey detection capacity (Grindal *et al.*, 1992; Lučan *et al.*, 2013). In summary, climate change proposes to be a significant threat to the survival of bats and will continue to have adverse effects if mitigation strategies are not established.

Production Animal Examples

Broiler chickens

Chicken meat has become a dietary staple for Australians due to its affordability and versatility (ACMF, 2022). The price per kilogram has remained stable since the mid-1990s, around AUS $5.50, making it the cheapest meat available for consumers (Phibbs *et al.*, 2021). While many Australians are reflecting on their meat consumption behaviours, ABARES have forecast a per capita consumption of 48.8 kg for FY 2021/22, with consumption expected to continue to increase year after year (ACMF, 2022). Decades of genetic selection of broilers has created highly efficient feed converters, which have a rapid growth rate (Phibbs *et al.*, 2021). Selective breeding has led to many morphological changes, especially in highly marketable carcase traits, namely more breast muscle. However, these breeding efforts have negatively impacted leg health, resulting in altered gait and an increase in leg-related issues (Danbury *et al.*, 2000). This raises significant animal welfare concerns for broiler chickens.

A survey by Taylor and Signal (2009) revealed that Australian consumers are aware of broiler welfare concerns; however, the public's overall knowledge of production methods is poorly understood. Additionally, they also show that while consumers advocate for more ethical production methods, consumers are typically unwilling to pay more. This situation gives rise to a complex dilemma, wherein producers lack sufficient incentives to embrace more ethical production methods. To address this issue, a deeper understanding of consumer motivations is needed to encourage the adoption of ethical production methods.

Commercial broiler systems typically opt for caged or floor-based methods (Shields and Greger, 2013). While uncommon in Australia, caged broilers are known to have higher instances of flesh wounds due to abrasion against the cage floor, which reduces meat quality (Slepukhin *et al.*, 2000; Shane, 2001). Caged systems often incur greater labour costs compared to floor systems (Reece *et al.*, 1971). Such systems significantly limit free space per bird and thus reduce the range of natural behaviours, such as dustbathing, that animals can partake in (Olsson and Keeling, 2005). As such, cage broilers are known to have weaker bones as a consequence of their inability to exercise (Wabeck and Littlefield, 1972; Travis *et al.*, 1983). Floor systems enable broilers to access deep litter, where they are free to express natural behaviours, which are otherwise limited in caged production systems (Shields and Greger, 2013). In floor systems, the birds are provided with ample space and therefore sufficient opportunity to exercise as they grow, and thus strengthen their bones, ultimately reducing bone health concerns. Free-range systems, where birds are raised in houses with voluntary access to the outdoors (Martínez-Pérez *et al.*, 2017), are becoming popular in Australia, and are seen as a more proactive approach to animal welfare and meat chicken production. Similar to floor systems, free-range enterprises enable birds to explore natural behaviours, which reduces stress, and improves health and animal performance (Abouelezz *et al.*, 2012).

In Australia, state and territory governments have implemented legislation that provides a broad scope of the minimum animal welfare standards required in broiler production systems (Phibbs *et al.*, 2021), while additional, best practise protocols exist at the federal level (Pisc, 2002). Animal welfare organizations such as the RSPCA offer accreditation programmes that producers can opt into, including their Approved Farming Scheme, and the Free Range Egg and Poultry Australia (FREPA) scheme (Phibbs *et al.*, 2021). Both accreditors provide elevated animal welfare standards to ensure producers outperform current minimum requirements, with the RSPCA encouraging the use of perches for enrichment and bone health (RSPCA, 2016). In return, successful producers are able to advertise their meat as 'RSPCA Approved' (RSPCA, 2020). About 70% of Australian chicken meat is produced according to the RSPCA Scheme, including chicken products sold by two major Australian supermarket chains (RSPCA, 2018). The FREPA standards offer fewer specific requirements for producers and account for ~20% of Australian meat production. The adoption of improved animal welfare practices into commercial farms has not significantly affected the producer's bottom line nor the cost to the consumer, with chicken meat prices remaining stable during the transition (Phibbs *et al.*, 2021).

Strong domestic and international demand for Australian chicken meat will inevitably result in a significant increase in resource requirements throughout the supply chain, including additional water and land for feed production, increased energy requirements for climate regulation within growing sheds, and labour costs (Izar-Tenorio *et al.*, 2020). Climatic changes, which are expected to result in elevated temperatures, translate to greater energy expenditure per unit of production. The welfare of birds, especially mature broilers, under warmer conditions, is of great concern. Birds have a limited capacity for heat regulation as they lack sweat glands, and regulate temperature by panting, limiting their activity, and drinking more (Fairchild, 2009; Izar-Tenorio *et al.*, 2020). Depending on the season, young chicks are provided with additional heating between 32 and 35°C for the first ~20 days, until they are of sufficient size to regulate their own body temperature (Xin *et al.*, 2001). Energy-expensive heating systems may be required during winter and cooler nights to ensure growing sheds are kept at ~21°C (Fairchild, 2009). During summer, mechanical ventilation and fans are commonly used to encourage air circulation and decrease environmental temperature (Izar-Tenorio *et al.*, 2020). As stated by Fairchild (2009), in warm climates, air conditioning units may be required to maintain an optimal production temperature.

In summary, chicken meat is a popular and affordable choice in Australia, but broiler welfare concerns persist. Consumers desire ethical production methods but are unwilling to pay higher prices, creating a dilemma for producers. Different production systems have varying impacts on animal welfare, with cage-free systems offering better conditions. Accreditation programmes and legislation aim to improve standards without significantly affecting costs. However, the industry faces resource challenges and climate change risks. Balancing ethics, affordability, and sustainability is crucial for the future of Australian chicken meat.

Ruminants

Climate change has a negative impact on livestock, affecting their productivity and physical health. Ruminants suffer from heat stress, which can alter their dry matter intake and impact forage crops and grazing practices. Climate change leads to variations in greenhouse gas concentrations and temperature, causing changes in forage growth, shifts in forage composition, and fluctuations in nitrogen content (Slepukhin *et al.*, 2000).

In Australia, the world's largest apparel wool growing country, climate change poses risks to livestock welfare, including reproductive potential and hormonal function. Rising temperatures and thermal stress can result in embryo loss and chronic stress in Merino sheep. Heat stress reduces feed intake and reproductive output, posing animal welfare concerns and affecting nutrition and health (Olsson and Keeling, 2005). Previous research from our lab revealed that heat stress (THI >75) and elevated glucocorticoid levels (indexed using faecal glucocorticoid metabolites) are linked to embryo loss in Merino ewes (Narayan *et al.*, 2018). Chronic stress can also be assessed in livestock such as Merino sheep using wool profiles of glucocorticoids (Wabeck and Littlefield, 1972).

Heat stress has been shown to reduce feed intake and reproductive output in livestock, raising animal welfare concerns and impacting nutrition and health domains (Martínez-Pérez *et al.*, 2017).

Livestock's thermal comfort zone is challenged when temperatures surpass their optimal range, leading to changes in endocrine status, ruminant activity frequency, nutrient uptake, and feed intake behaviour. Energy use efficiency declines in animals experiencing heat stress, necessitating dietary modifications to minimize heat production. Maintaining consistent acid detergent fibre (ADF) and total plant fibre levels is crucial for optimal rumen function (Abouelezz *et al.*, 2012). According to RSPCA (2018), the efficiency of conversion to milk in diets containing 100%, 75%, or 50% hay is 54%, 61%, and 65%, respectively. Researchers have also found that the addition of alfalfa and dietary fibre both increase the heat load and exacerbate heat stress (Izar-Tenorio *et al.*, 2020). To ensure optimal rumen function, it is advisable to maintain ADF and total plant fibre at a consistent level of 18% and 28%, respectively (RSPCA, 2020).

Ruminants respond to climate change through behaviour adjustments such as seeking shade and increasing standing time for cooling. Heat stress significantly impacts lactation performance, immune function, and calf health. Monitoring cows' activity and rumination time helps detect heat stress, and appropriate heat dissipation strategies such as sunshades and sprinklers can mitigate its effects. Techniques like embryo transfer can increase conception rates during the hot season (Fairchild, 2009). In animal husbandry, the monitoring of cows' activity time and rumination time serves as an early warning system for detecting heat stress (3BL, 2022). During lactation, there is evidence of a correlation between the temperature-humidity index (THI) and conception rate (CR) in dairy cows (WHO, 2020). According to the relationship between mean THI and CR, the threshold at which heat stress can have the most significant effect on CR is when the THI value is 73 (WHO, 2020). Studies have also shown that cows living in milder climates are more susceptible to heat stress than those in tropical and subtropical climates (Castrica *et al.*, 2018). Further, cows are most susceptible to heat stress during the first 1–21 days before breeding. It is, therefore, important to develop appropriate heat dissipation strategies to avoid the effects of heat stress (German *et al.*, 2018). Heat stress can affect production levels and physical fitness of livestock, but breeders can provide equipment and techniques to help them recover (Miller *et al.*, 2018). It has also been shown that embryo transfer can be used during the hot season to increase the chances of conception and counteract the negative effects of heat stress (Packer *et al.*, 2019).

In conclusion, heat stress can affect production levels and physical fitness of livestock. But breeders can provide equipment and techniques to help them recover.

Companion Animals

Companion animals, including cats and dogs, play a significant and influential role in societies across the world, with an estimated population of hundreds of millions serving as companions to people worldwide (AVMA, 2022).

In contemporary society, the realm of pet food has grown increasingly sophisticated, with a significant rise in expenditure, underscoring the paramount significance and elevated status bestowed upon pets in today's world. Several studies have highlighted the connection between companion animals and their environmental impact, revealing that the allocation of additional resources to these animals can potentially contribute to the escalation of climate change (Protopopova *et al.*, 2021). This connection stems from the often overlooked factor of food production for companion animals, which contributes to environmental damage (Su *et al.*, 2018). In the USA, the environmental impact of the pet dog and cat diets can reach 30% (Okin, 2017), and while these impacts may be lower on a global scale, the trend is continuing for pet food to be of increasingly high standards, almost comparable to that of human food (3BL, 2022). These high standards of pet food could also further exacerbate the global food crisis (WHO, 2020). Overfeeding companion animals can also have detrimental environmental consequences and jeopardize their own health (Su *et al.*, 2018). To alleviate environmental stress, companion animal food can be sourced from human food remnants or waste (Castrica *et al.*, 2018). By embracing these measures, companion animal owners can play an active role in reducing the ecological impact of their pets while simultaneously improving their welfare.

For dogs, exercise forms an important part of their health and welfare. About 50% of dogs in the UK are overweight. There are dietary reasons for this, but insufficient exercise is also an important cause of obesity and overweight status (German *et al.*, 2018). Factors such as weather conditions can be a potential hindrance to dog walking. For example, about 87% of owners report that they exercise their dogs less during hot weather (Hall *et al.*, 2021); therefore, extreme heat may contribute to increased rates of canine obesity. Further, heat stress can affect the performance and physical health of working dogs. For example, studies have shown that heat-related diseases are a leading cause of death in military working dogs (Miller *et al.*, 2018). Physical exercise is a major contributor to heat-related illness in the UK and Israel (Packer *et al.*, 2019). Therefore, the gradual increase in global temperature has the potential to decline the level of welfare for dogs, which may also lead to changes in the role of dogs in human society. In the case of cats and other animals in shelters, environmental changes can induce stress (Stella and Croney, 2016).

To safeguard the well-being of companion animals amidst the challenges posed by global warming, it is crucial to consider the behaviour and breeding practices of pet owners. For instance, one important measure is to refrain from leaving pets unattended in vehicles without proper air conditioning, as this can pose a significant risk. Additionally, certain breeds, particularly those with short-headed characteristics, are more susceptible to heat stroke despite their popularity (Hall *et al.*, 2020). Hence, responsible pet ownership entails being mindful of these factors to protect the health of companion animals in a warming world (Hall *et al.*, 2020).

The stark reality that the climate is moving in a direction that is detrimental to both humans and companion animals is already in front of human eyes, and it is necessary for humans to see companion animals as an important link in influencing climate change. This is because companion animals can, to some extent, contribute to climate warming, while climate warming can also affect the survival of companion animals, especially canines.

Large Wildlife Mammals

While most of this review has focused on endemic Australian species, it is important to acknowledge that climate change has a variety of differing influences in different regions, and ecosystems, and on organisms that cannot be represented with a restricted focus on Australian animals. An example of this is the African bush elephant (*Loxodonta africana*), a large herbivore endemic to many dryland environments in the African continent (Fuller *et al.*, 2021). This section will focus on the impacts of climate change on African elephant welfare, and compare these impacts to the red kangaroo (*Macropus rufus*), another herbivore endemic to dryland habitats (Fuller *et al.*, 2021).

As the largest, extant terrestrial land mammal, the African elephant has significant daily food and water requirements (Fuller *et al.*, 2021). However, with the effects of climate change compounding with every passing day, the ability of elephants to meet their nutritional needs decreases (Mukeka *et al.*, 2022). As droughts become more frequent and unpredictable, the availability of water and vegetation cover declines, increasing elephant heat and nutrition stress, contributing to the elevated elephant mortality we are currently witnessing (Mukeka *et al.*, 2022).

A mature African elephant requires up to 200 l of water and 90 kg of dry matter per day to reach their nutritional and metabolic requirements (Ullrey *et al.*, 1997; Greene *et al.*, 2019). Elephants require large quantities of daily drinking water as a physiological adaptation to endure the heat of their environment, while maintaining their large body size. Due to their size, elephants are far more inefficient at maintaining homeostatic thermoregulation when compared to smaller animals. As a result, elephants have evolved adaptations such as highly vascularized ears and a high surface-to-volume ratio, to expedite their ability to cool themselves (Tattersall *et al.*, 2012). One of these adaptations utilizes their excess skin to increase evaporative water loss, a process similar to sweating (Fuller *et al.*, 2016). Even under climatic temperatures of 10°C, elephants have been reported to have a greater rate of cutaneous evaporative cooling than other animals (Mitchell *et al.*, 2018). With the current patterns of increased drought and elevated temperatures, elephants will have to find other methods to regulate their body temperatures, while also meeting their water and nutritional needs with reduced access to water and foliage.

The implications of increased drought frequency directly reduce the nutritional welfare of elephants through decreased water availability and thereby decreased foliage density (Mukeka *et al.*, 2022). The severity of nutritional and water stress is further exacerbated by the tendency of mammals to catabolize endogenous proteins to extract water, during periods of low water availability, resulting in greater degradation of body condition (McCue *et al.*, 2017). These nutritional issues develop into mental and environmental welfare issues as a result of reduced vegetation for utilization as shelter from the sun, as well as an increase in heat stress from the animals' inability to achieve their water requirements and thereby being unable to effectively thermoregulate (Dunkin, 2013; Fuller *et al.*, 2016).

In comparison with elephants, kangaroos are far more adapted to erratic weather patterns and periodic drought (Tyndale-Biscoe, 2005; Mukeka *et al.*, 2022). Kangaroos undergo periods of population growth and decline, dictated by environmental factors, particularly the absence or abundance of food and water (Caughley *et al.*, 1985; McLeod, 2021). However, despite this, ultimately both species are prone to elevated mortality rates as a result of drought (Caughley *et al.*, 1985; Douglas-Hamilton, 1987). From an ecological perspective, this process of drought-induced die-offs and rain-induced population booms is natural. However, complexity arises when the issue is examined through a welfare-centric lens (Wilson and Edwards, 2019; Zanker, 2021). The process of die-offs is induced by the starvation of animals as a result of insufficient vegetation to support the population, greatly impacting the nutritional welfare of the animals (Wilson and Edwards, 2019).

As a result of climatic variability, elephants are no longer able to acquire their nutritional requirements, and as a result their environmental and mental welfare suffers (Mukeka *et al.*, 2022). In comparison, the kangaroo while also suffering from nutritional disparity is involved in a complex balancing act between ecological balance and animal welfare maintenance, highlighting the complexities that are associated with the effects of climate change on animal welfare (Caughley *et al.*, 1985; Wilson and Edwards, 2019; Zanker, 2021).

Conclusion

As demonstrated in our review, climate change has impacted the welfare of animals in both the wild and domestic settings. Researchers have assessed the eco-physiological responses of species using physiology, behavioural, and other methods. Although common themes regarding the methods and measurements are emerging, we believe that thus far, there has been limited work done to link the impacts of climate change directly to welfare domains, especially in wildlife. As climate change drives more wild populations to ecological limitations, there will be potential welfare consequences and considerations to explore; for example, when vulnerable species would need to be transferred to new environments (e.g. captive breeding), should food and habitat become limiting resources. Likewise, production animals and other domesticated species will be impacted by the extreme environmental changes with consequences on each of the dimensions within the five domains of animal welfare (Fig. 9.1). We believe that the impacts of climate change will be multi-faceted, whereby there could be cascading effects across all domains. Researchers need to carefully consider which domains are immediate and future priorities to safeguard animal longevity and welfare.

Acknowledgements

We would like to thank all the team members of The Stress Lab who contributed to the initial discussion regarding the formation of the article.

Funding

This review article did not receive any form of funding from funding agencies in the public, commercial, or not-for-profit sectors.

Conflict of Interest

There are no conflicts of interest to disclose.

Author Contributions

All authors contributed to the conceptualization of the presented article, curation of data, analysis of data, conduction of the research process, formation of the methodology, presentation of the final work, construction of the final draft and review, and editing of the final work. EN was responsible for project administration and supervision.

References

3BL (2022) Humanization of pet food' driving new capacity for manufacturers, CRB report finds. In: *3BL Blogs – 3BL Media*. Proquest.

Abouelezz, F. *et al*. (2012) Outdoor egg production using local forages in the tropics. *World's Poultry Science Journal* 68(4), 679–692.

Adams, R.A. (2010) Bat reproduction declines when conditions mimic climate change projections for western North America. *Ecology* 91(8), 2437–2445.

Adams, R.A. and Hayes, M.A. (2008) Water availability and successful lactation by bats as related to climate change in arid regions of western North America. *Journal of Animal Ecology* 77(6), 1115–1121.

ACMF (2022) Facts and figures. Available at: https://www.chicken.org.au/ (accessed 8 December 2022).

Adams-Hosking, C. *et al*. (2011) Modelling climate-change-induced shifts in the distribution of the koala. *Wildlife Research* 38(2), 122–130.

Agassiz, L. (2013) *Essay on Classification*. Dover Publications, Mineola, NY.

Ahmed, N. and Turchini, G.M. (2021) Recirculating aquaculture systems (RAS): Environmental solution and climate change adaptation. *Journal of Cleaner Production* 297, 126604.

Ahmed, N., Thompson, S. and Glaser, M. (2019) Global aquaculture productivity, environmental sustainability, and climate change adaptability. *Environmental Management* 63(2), 159–172.

Angiulli, E. *et al*. (2020) Increase in environmental temperature affects exploratory behaviour, anxiety and social preference in Danio rerio. *Scientific Reports* 10(1), 1–12.

Appel, G. *et al*. (2019) Temperature, rainfall, and moonlight intensity effects on activity of tropical insectivorous bats. *Journal of Mammalogy* 100(6), 1889–1900.

Argent, G. (2022) Human-animal relationships and welfare in the Anthropocene: Pandemics, climate change, and other disasters. *Journal of Applied Animal Welfare Science* 25(2), 115–118.

Auer, S.K. and Martin, T.E. (2013) Climate change has indirect effects on resource use and overlap among coexisting bird species with negative consequences for their reproductive success. *Global Change Biology* 19(2), 411–419.

AVMA (2022) U.S. Pet Ownership Statistics. Available at: https://www.avma.org/resources-tools/reports-statistics/us-pet-ownership-statistics (accessed 14 December 2022).

Beale, P., Youngentob, K. and Marsh, K. (2022) *Effects of Fire on Koalas and Their Habitat*. The Australian National University, Canberra.

Beltrán, I. *et al.* (2021) Are ectotherm brains vulnerable to global warming? *Trends in Ecology & Evolution* 36(8), 691–699.

Bernabucci, U. *et al.* (2010) Metabolic and hormonal acclimation to heat stress in domesticated ruminants. *Animal* 4(7), 1167–1183.

Bernardo, J. and Spotila, J.R. (2006) Physiological constraints on organismal response to global warming: Mechanistic insights from clinally varying populations and implications for assessing endangerment. *Biology Letters* 2(1), 135–139.

Booth, T.H. (2013) Eucalypt plantations and climate change. *Forest Ecology and Management* 301, 28–34.

Brock, J.M.R. and Collier, K. (2020) Bat dispersal of fern spores in New Zealand. *New Zealand Journal of Ecology* 44(2), 1–3.

Broom, D.M. (2014) *Sentience and Animal Welfare*. CAB International, Wallingford, UK.

Bueno, P.B. and Soto, D. (2017) Adaptation strategies of the aquaculture sector to the impacts of climate change 12. *Fisheries & Aquaculture Circular* 99, 1–28.

Burles, D.W. *et al.* (2009) Influence of weather on two insectivorous bats in a temperate pacific northwest rainforest. *Revue Canadienne De Zoologie* 87(2), 132–138.

Burrows, G. (2013) Buds, bushfires and resprouting in the Eucalypts. *Australian Journal of Botany* 61(5), 331–349.

Butterfield, J.E. and Coulson, J.C. (1997) Terrestrial invertebrates and climate change: Physiological and life-cycle adaptations. In: *Past and Future Rapid Environmental Changes*. Springer, UK, pp. 401–412.

Cabrelli, A. (2013) *The Impacts of Climate Change on Australian Reptiles*. Faculty of Science, Department of Biological Sciences, Macquarie University.

Carere, C., Wood, J.B. and Mather, J. (2011) Species differences in captivity: Where are the invertebrates? *Trends in Ecology & Evolution* 26(5), 211.

Castrica, M. *et al.* (2018) Pet food as the most concrete strategy for using food waste as feedstuff within the European context: A feasibility study. *Sustainability* 10(6), 2035.

Caughley, G., Grigg, G.C. and Smith, L. (1985) The effect of drought on kangaroo populations. *The Journal of Wildlife Management* 679–685.

Chang, E.S. (2005) Stressed-out lobsters: Crustacean hyperglycemic hormone and stress proteins. *Integrative and Comparative Biology* 45(1), 43–50.

Clifton, I.D. *et al.* (2007) Water turnover and the northern range of the koala (*Phascolarctos cinereus*). *Australian Mammalogy* 29(1), 85–88.

Cochrane, K. *et al.* (2009) Climate change implications for fisheries and aquaculture. *FAO Fisheries and Aquaculture Technical Paper* 530, 212.

Cogger, H. (2014) *Reptiles and Amphibians of Australia*. CSIRO Publishing, Clayton, Victoria.

Cooper, W. (2000) Effect of temperature on escape behaviour by an ectothermic vertebrate, the keeled earless lizard (*Holbrookia propinqua*). *Behaviour* 137(10), 1299–1315.

Crick, H.Q.P. (2004) The impact of climate change on birds. *Ibis* 146(s1), 48–56.

Cryan, P.M., Bogan, M.A. and Altenbach, J.S. (2000) Effect of elevation on distribution of female bats in the Black hills, South Dakota. *Journal of Mammalogy* 81(3), 719–725.

Crick, H.Q. and Sparks, T.H. (1999) Climate change related to egg-laying trends. *Nature* 399(6735), 423–423.

CSIRO (2020) State of the Climate Report 2020. Available at: https://www.csiro.au/en/research/environmental-impacts/climate-change/State-of-the-Climate/Previous/State-of-the-Climate-2020

Culler-Juarez, M.E. and Onthank, K.L. (2021) Elevated immune response in *Octopus rubescens* under ocean acidification and warming conditions. *Marine Biology* 168(9), 1–10.

Cziesielski, M.J., Schmidt-Roach, S. and Aranda, M. (2019) The past, present, and future of coral heat stress studies. *Ecology and Evolution* 9(17), 10055–10066.

Danbury, T. *et al.* (2000) Self-selection of the analgesic drug carprofen by lame broiler chickens. *Veterinary Record* 146(11), 307–311.

Domenici, P. *et al.* (2019) The effect of climate change on the escape kinematics and performance of fishes: Implications for future predator– prey interactions. *Conservation Physiology* 7(1), coz078.
Douglas-Hamilton, I. (1987) African elephants: Population trends and their causes. *Oryx* 21(1), 11–24.
Downs, C.T., Zungu, M.M. and Brown, M. (2012) Seasonal effects on thermoregulatory abilities of the Wahlberg's epauletted fruit bat (*Epomophorus wahlbergi*) in Kwazulu-Natal, South Africa. *Journal of Thermal Biology* 37(2), 144–150.
Dunkin, R.C. *et al.* (2013) Climate influences thermal balance and water use in African and Asian elephants: Physiology can predict drivers of elephant distribution. *Journal of Experimental Biology* 216(15), 2939–2952.
Ellis, W. *et al.* (1995) Seasonal-variation in water flux, field metabolic-rate and food-consumption of free-ranging koalas (*Phascolarctos cinereus*). *Australian Journal of Zoology* 43(1), 59–68.
Encyclopaedia Britannica (1999) *Marsupial*. Encyclopaedia Britannica, Chicago, IL.
Fabry, V.J. *et al.* (2008) Impacts of ocean acidification on marine fauna and ecosystem processes. *ICES Journal of Marine Science* 65(3), 414–432.
Fairchild, B.D. (2009) *Environmental Factors to Control When Brooding Chicks*.
FAO (2021) *World Food and Agriculture – Statistical Yearbook 2021*. FAO, Rome.
Figueiredo, R.T. and Neves, J.S. (2018) Eosinophils in fungal diseases: An overview. *Journal of Leukocyte Biology* 104(1), 49–60.
Flajnik, M.F. (2018) A cold-blooded view of adaptive immunity. *Nature Reviews Immunology* 18(7), 438–453.
Forchhammer, M.C., Post, E. and Stenseth, N.C. (1998) Breeding phenology and climate. *Nature* 391(6662), 29–30.
Forrest, J.R. (2017) Insect pollinators and climate change. In: *Global Climate Change and Terrestrial Invertebrates*. John Wiley, Hoboken, NJ, pp. 69–91.
Freitas, C. *et al.* (2021) Sea temperature effects on depth use and habitat selection in a marine fish community. *Journal of Animal Ecology* 90(7), 1787–1800.
Frick, W.F. *et al.* (2012) Climate and weather impact timing of emergence of bats. *PLoS One* 7(8), e42737.
Fujita, M.S. and Tuttle, M.D. (1991) Flying foxes (*Chiroptera: pteropodidae*): Threatened animals of key ecological and economic importance. *Conservation Biology* 5(4), 455–463.
Fuller, A. *et al.* (2016) Towards a mechanistic understanding of the responses of large terrestrial mammals to heat and aridity associated with climate change. *Climate Change Responses* 3(1), 1–19.
Fuller, A. *et al.* (2021) How dryland mammals will respond to climate change: The effects of body size, heat load and a lack of food and water. *Journal of Experimental Biology* 224(Suppl_1), jeb238113.
German, A.J. *et al.* (2018) Dangerous trends in pet obesity. *The Veterinary Record* 182(1), 25.
González-Tokman, D. *et al.* (2020) Insect responses to heat: Physiological mechanisms, evolution and ecological implications in a warming world. *Biological Reviews* 95(3), 802–821.
Gordon, G., Brown, A. and Pulsford, T. (1988) A koala (*Phascolarctos cinereus Goldfuss*) population crash during drought and heatwave conditions in south-western Queensland. *Australian Journal of Ecology* 13(4), 451–461.
Greene, W., Dierenfeld, E.S. and Mikota, S. (2019) A review of Asian and African elephant gastrointestinal anatomy, physiology, and pharmacology: Elephant gastrointestinal anatomy, physiology, and pharmacology. *Journal of Zoo and Aquarium Research* 7(1), 1–14.
Grindal, S.D. *et al.* (1992) The influence of precipitation on reproduction by myotis bats in British Columbia. *The American Midland Naturalist* 128(2), 339–344.
Gunn, D. (1942) Body temperature in poikilothermal animals. *Biological Reviews* 17(4), 293–314.
Hall, J.M. (2020) *Heat Tolerance of Reptile Embryos in A Changing World: Physiological Mechanisms and Ecological Effects*. Nature Portfolio, UK.
Hall, E.J., Carter, A.J. and O'Neill, D.G. (2020) Incidence and risk factors for heat-related illness (heat-stroke) in UK dogs under primary veterinary care in 2016. *Scientific Reports* 10(1), 1–12.
Hall, E.J., Carter, A.J. and Farnworth, M.J. (2021) Exploring owner perceptions of the impacts of seasonal weather variations on canine activity and potential consequences for human–canine relationships. *Animals* 11(11), 3302.
Hamann, M., Limpus, C.J. and Read, M.A. (2007) *Vulnerability of Marine Reptiles in the Great Barrier Reef to Climate Change*. The Great Barrier Reef Marine Park Authority, Townsville, Australia.
Heath, J.T. *et al.* (2016) Post-fire recovery of eucalypt-dominated vegetation communities in the Sydney Basin, Australia. *Fire Ecology* 12(3), 53–79.

Hemsworth, P. *et al*. (2015) Scientific assessment of animal welfare. *New Zealand Veterinary Journal* 63(1), 24–30.

Hennessy, K. *et al*. (2005) *Climate Change Impacts on Fire-Weather in South-East Australia*. Climate Impacts Group, CSIRO Atmospheric Research and the Australian Government Bureau of Meteorology, Aspendale.

Horwitz, R. *et al*. (2020) Near-future ocean warming and acidification alter foraging behaviour, locomotion, and metabolic rate in a keystone marine mollusc. *Scientific Reports* 10(1), 5461.

Hovenden, M.J. and Williams, A.L. (2010) The impacts of rising CO_2 concentrations on Australian terrestrial species and ecosystems. *Austral Ecology* 35(6), 665–684.

Huey, R.B. and Kingsolver, J.G. (2019) Climate warming, resource availability, and the metabolic meltdown of ectotherms. *The American Naturalist* 194(6), E140–E150.

Hume, I. and Esson, C. (1993) Nutrients, antinutrients and leaf selection by captive koalas (*Phascolarctos cinereus*). *Australian Journal of Zoology* 41(4), 379–392.

Izar-Tenorio, J. *et al*. (2020) Impacts of projected climate change scenarios on heating and cooling demand for industrial broiler chicken farming in the Eastern US. *Journal of Cleaner Production* 255, 120306.

Jin, X. *et al*. (2022) Editorial: Homeostasis and physiological regulation in the aquatic animal during osmotic stress. *Frontiers in Physiology* 13, 977185.

Kellert, S.R. (1993) Values and perceptions of invertebrates. *Conservation Biology* 7(4), 845–855.

Kennedy, M. (1992) *Australasian Marsupials and Monotremes: An Action Plan for Their Conservation*. IUCN, Switzerland.

Kindermann, C., Narayan, E.J. and Hero, J.-M. (2012) Urinary corticosterone metabolites and chytridiomycosis disease prevalence in a free-living population of male stony creek frogs (*Litoria wilcoxii*). *Comparative Biochemistry and Physiology Part A: Molecular & Integrative Physiology* 162(3), 171–176.

Korine, C. *et al*. (2016) Bats and water: Anthropogenic alterations threaten global bat populations. In: *Bats in the Anthropocene: Conservation of Bats in a Changing World*. Springer, Cham, pp. 215–241.

Kristiansen, T.S. and Bracke, M. (2020) A brief look into the origins of fish welfare science. In: *The Welfare of Fish*. Springer, pp. 1–17.

Li, L. *et al*. (2022) Dietary nanoselenium supplementation for heat-stressed rainbow trout: Effects on organizational structure, lipid changes, and biochemical parameters as well as heat-shock-protein- and selenoprotein-related gene expression. *Fish Physiology and Biochemistry* 48(3), 707–722.

Lučan, R.K., Weiser, M. and Hanák, V. (2013) Contrasting effects of climate change on the timing of reproduction and reproductive success of a temperate insectivorous bat. *Journal of Zoology* 290(2), 151–159.

Lunney, D. *et al*. (2014) Extinction in eden: Identifying the role of climate change in the decline of the koala in south-eastern NSW. *Wildlife Research* 41(1), 22–34.

Lunney, D. *et al*. (2012) Koalas and climate change: A case study on the Liverpool Plains, north-west new South Wales. In: Lunney, D. and Hutchings, P. (eds) *Wildlife and Climate Change: Towards Robust Conservation Strategies for Australian Fauna, Royal Zoological Society of New South Wales*. Mosman, Australia, pp. 150–168.

Mahmoud, S. *et al*. (2020) Deleterious impacts of heat stress on steroidogenesis markers, immunity status and ovarian tissue of Nile tilapia (*Oreochromis niloticus*). *Journal of Thermal Biology* 91, 102578.

Marsh, K.J., Wallis, I.R. and Foley, W.J. (2007) Behavioural contributions to the regulated intake of plant secondary metabolites in koalas. *Oecologia* 154(2), 283–290.

Martos-Sitcha, J.A. *et al*. (2020) Welfare and stressors in fish: Challenges facing aquaculture. *Frontiers Media SA* 11, 162.

Martínez-Pérez, M. *et al*. (2017) Poultry meat production in free-range systems: Perspectives for tropical areas. *World's Poultry Science Journal* 73(2), 309–320.

Matthews, A. *et al*. (2007) Tree use by koalas (*Phascolarctos cinereus*) after fire in remnant coastal forest. *Wildlife Research* 34(2), 84–93.

Mawdsley, J.R., O'Malley, R. and Ojima, D.S. (2009) Review of climate-change adaptation strategies for wildlife management and biodiversity conservation. *Conservation Biology* 23(5), 1080–1089.

McCue, M.D. *et al*. (2017) Dehydration causes increased reliance on protein oxidation in mice: A test of the protein-for-water hypothesis in a mammal. *Physiological and Biochemical Zoology* 90(3), 359–369.

McLeod, S.R. *et al*. (2021) Assessing the spatial and temporal organization of Red Kangaroo, Western Grey Kangaroo and Eastern Grey Kangaroo populations in eastern Australia using multivariate autoregressive state-space models. *Ecological Management & Restoration* 22, 106–123.

Medway, L. (1980) *Report of the Panel of Enquiry into Shooting and Angling (1976–79)*. Horsham, UK.

Mella, V.S. *et al*. (2019) Needing a drink: Rainfall and temperature drive the use of free water by a threatened arboreal folivore. *PLoS One* 14(5), e0216964.

Mellor, D.J. *et al*. (2020) The 2020 five domains model: Including human– animal interactions in assessments of animal welfare. *Animals* 10(10), 1870.

Miller, L. *et al*. (2018) Causes of death in military working dogs during operation iraqi freedom and operation enduring freedom, 2001–2013. *Military Medicine* 183(9–10), e467–e474.

Mitchell, D. *et al*. (2018) Revisiting concepts of thermal physiology: Predicting responses of mammals to climate change. *Journal of Animal Ecology* 87(4), 956–973.

Moen, C., Johnson, J.C. and Hackney Price, J. (2022) Ecdysteroid responses to urban heat island conditions during development of the western black widow spider (*Latrodectus hesperus*). *PLoS One* 17(4), e0267398.

Moore, B.D. *et al*. (2005) Eucalyptus foliar chemistry explains selective feeding by koalas. *Biology Letters* 1(1), 64–67.

Moore, F.L. and Zoeller, R.T. (1985) Stress-induced inhibition of reproduction: Evidence of suppressed secretion of LH-RH in an amphibian. *General and Comparative Endocrinology* 60(2), 252–258.

Mukeka, J. *et al*. (2022) Long-term trends in elephant mortality and their causes in Kenya. *Frontiers in Conservation Science* 3, 82.

Narayan, E.J. and Hero, J.-M. (2014a) Acute thermal stressor increases glucocorticoid response but minimizes testosterone and locomotor performance in the cane toad (*Rhinella marina*). *PLoS One* 9(3), e92090.

Narayan, E.J. and Hero, J.-M. (2014b) Repeated thermal stressor causes chronic elevation of baseline corticosterone and suppresses the physiological endocrine sensitivity to acute stressor in the cane toad (*Rhinella marina*). *Journal of Thermal Biology* 41, 72–76.

Narayan, E., Sawyer, G. and Parisella, S. (2018) Faecal glucocorticoid metabolites and body temperature in Australian merino ewes (*Ovis aries*) during summer artificial insemination (AI) program. *PloS One* 13(1), e0191961.

Narayan, E.J., Cockrem, J.F. and Hero, J.-M. (2012) Effects of temperature on urinary corticosterone metabolite responses to short-term capture and handling stress in the cane toad (*Rhinella marina*). *General and Comparative Endocrinology* 178(2), 301–305.

Neven, L.G. (2000) Physiological responses of insects to heat. *Postharvest Biology and Technology* 21(1), 103–111.

Okin, G.S. (2017) Environmental impacts of food consumption by dogs and cats. *PLoS One* 12(8), e0181301.

Olin, A.B. *et al*. (2023) Breeding failures and reduced nest attendance in response to heat stress in a high-latitude seabird. *Marine Ecology Progress Series* heat, HEATav3.

Olsson, I.A.S. and Keeling, L.J. (2005) Why in earth? Dustbathing behaviour in jungle and domestic fowl reviewed from a Tinbergian and animal welfare perspective. *Applied Animal Behaviour Science* 93(3–4), 259–282.

Paaijmans, K.P. *et al*. (2013) Temperature variation makes ectotherms more sensitive to climate change. *Global Change Biology* 19(8), 2373–2380.

Pachauri, R. and Meyer, L. (2014) *Climate Change 2014: Synthesis Report. Contribution of Working Groups I, II and III to the Fifth Assessment Report of the Intergovernmental Panel on Climate Change*. Intergovernmental Panel on Climate Change (IPCC), Geneva.

Packer, R.M. *et al*. (2019) Great expectations, inconvenient truths, and the paradoxes of the dog-owner relationship for owners of brachycephalic dogs. *PLoS One* 14(7), e0219918.

Parry, M.L. *et al*. (2007) *Climate Change 2007-Impacts, Adaptation and Vulnerability: Working Group II Contribution to the Fourth Assessment Report of the IPCC*, Vol. 4. Cambridge University Press, Cambridge, UK.

Penman, T.D. *et al*. (2010) Predicting the impact of climate change on Australia's most endangered snake, *Hoplocephalus bungaroides*. *Diversity and Distributions* 16(1), 109–118.

Phibbs, D., Groves, P. and Muir, W. (2021) Leg health of meat chickens: Impact on welfare, consumer behaviour, and the role of environmental enrichment. *Animal Production Science* 61(12), 1203–1212.

Phillips, S. and Callaghan, J. (2000) Tree species preferences of koalas (*Phascolarctos cinereus*) in the Campbelltown area south-west of Sydney, New South Wales. *Wildlife Research* 27(5), 509–516.

Phillips, S., Callaghan, J. and Thompson, V. (2000) The tree species preferences of koalas (*Phascolarctos cinereus*) inhabiting forest and woodland communities on Quaternary deposits in the Port Stephens area, New South Wales. *Wildlife Research* 27, 1–10.

Pike, D.A., Antworth, R.L. and Stiner, J.C. (2006) Earlier nesting contributes to shorter nesting seasons for the loggerhead seaturtle, *Caretta caretta*. *Journal of Herpetology* 40(1), 91–94.

Pisc (2002) *Model Code of Practice for the Welfare of Animals: Domestic Poultry. Vol. 83*, Vol. 83. CSIRO Publishing, Clayton, Victoria.

Pringle, R.M., Webb, J.K. and Shine, R. (2003) Canopy structure, microclimate, and habitat selection by a nocturnal snake, *Hoplocephalus bungaroides*. *Ecology* 84(10), 2668–2679.

Protopopova, A. *et al*. (2021) Climate change and companion animals: Identifying links and opportunities for mitigation and adaptation strategies. *Integrative and Comparative Biology* 61(1), 166–181.

Raven, J. *et al*. (2005) *Ocean Acidification Due to Increasing Atmospheric Carbon Dioxide*. The Royal Society, London.

Reece, F. *et al*. (1971) Cage versus floor rearing of broiler chickens. *Poultry Science* 50(6), 1786–1790.

Richards, O.W. and Davies, R.G. (2013) *Imms General Textbook of Entomology: Volume 2: Classification and Biology. Springer Science*. Business Media, Zurich, Switzerland.

Roggatz, C.C. *et al*. (2016) Ocean acidification affects marine chemical communication by changing structure and function of peptide signalling molecules. *Global Change Biology* 22(12), 3914–3926.

Roy, D. and Sparks, T. (2000) Phenology of british butterflies and climate change. *Global Change Biology* 6(4), 407–416.

RSPCA (2016) *RSPCA Approved Farming Scheme Impact Report 2016*. RSPCA, Canberra.

RSPCA (2018) *RSPCA Approved Farming Scheme*. RSPCA, Canberra.

RSPCA (2020) *RSPCA Impact Report 2020*. RSPCA, Canberra.

Sabine, C.L. *et al*. (2004) The oceanic sink for anthropogenic CO2. *Science* 305(5682), 367–371.

Santos, R.R. *et al*. (2015) Quantitative histo-morphometric analysis of heat-stress-related damage in the small intestines of broiler chickens. *Avian Pathology* 44(1), 19–22.

Schlesinger, C.A. and Shine, R. (1994) Choosing a rock: Perspectives of a bush-rock collector and a saxicolous lizard. *Biological Conservation* 67(1), 49–56.

Seabrook, L. *et al*. (2011) Drought-driven change in wildlife distribution and numbers: A case study of koalas in south west Queensland. *Wildlife Research* 38(6), 509–524.

Seebacher, F. *et al*. (2005) A falsification of the thermal specialization paradigm: Compensation for elevated temperatures in Antarctic fishes. *Biology Letters* 1(2), 151–154.

Shane, S. (2001) Versatility of broiler growing cages. *Zootecnica International* 8, 18–19.

Shields, S. and Greger, M. (2013) Animal welfare and food safety aspects of confining broiler chickens to cages. *Animals* 3(2), 386–400.

Shine, R. *et al*. (1998) The impact of bush-rock removal on an endangered snake species, *Hoplocephalus bungaroides (Serpentes: Elapidae)*. *Wildlife Research* 25(3), 285–295.

Simmons, N. and Cirranello, A. (2020) Bat species of the world: A taxonomic and geographic database. *Accessed On* 7(10), 2020.

Slepukhin, V., Galpern, I. and Cherepanov, S. (2000) Breeding Russian broilers to adapt them to the cage environment. *World Poultry* 16(10), 25–27.

Snoyman, S., Muhic, J. and Brown, C. (2013) Corrigendum to "Nursing females are more prone to heat stress: Demography matters when managing flying-foxes for climate change". [Appl. Anim. Behav. Sci. 142 (December (1–2)) (2012) 90–97], *Applied Animal Behaviour Science* 145(3–4), 138–138.

Stebbins, R.C. and Cohen, N.W. (2021) *A Natural History of Amphibians*. Princeton University Press, Princeton, NJ.

Stella, J.L. and Croney, C.C. (2016) Environmental aspects of domestic cat care and management: Implications for cat welfare. *Scientific World Journal* 6296315.

Su, B., Martens, P. and Enders-Slegers, M.-J. (2018) A neglected predictor of environmental damage: The ecological paw print and carbon emissions of food consumption by companion dogs and cats in china. *Journal of Cleaner Production* 194, 1–11.

Tattersall, G.J. *et al*. (2012) Coping with thermal challenges: Physiological adaptations to environmental temperatures. *Comprehensive Physiology* 2(3), 2151–2202.

Taylor, N. and Signal, T.D. (2009) Willingness to pay: Australian consumers and "on the farm" welfare. *Journal of Applied Animal Welfare Science* 12(4), 345–359.

Telemeco, R.S., Elphick, M.J. and Shine, R. (2009) Nesting lizards (*Bassiana duperreyi*) compensate partly, but not completely, for climate change. *Ecology* 90(1), 17–22.

Travis, D., Sloan, D. and Hughes, B. (1983) Bone fragility in broilers as affected by pen height, sex, and a comparison of left and right humeri. *Poultry Science* 62(10), 2117–2119.

Tyndale-Biscoe, C.H. (2005) *Life of Marsupials*. CSIRO Publishing, Clayton, Victoria.

Ullrey, D.E., Crissey, S.D. and Hintz, H.F. (1997) *Elephants: Nutrition and Dietary Husbandry*. Nutrition Advisory Group East Lansing, Brookfield, IL.

Visser, M.E. and Both, C. (2005) Shifts in phenology due to global climate change: The need for a yard-stick. *Proceedings of the Royal Society B: Biological Sciences* 272(1581), 2561–2569.

Wabeck, C. and Littlefield, L. (1972) Bone strength of broilers reared in floor pens and in cages having different bottoms. *Poultry Science* 51(3), 897–899.

Wake, D.B. and Koo, M.S. (2018) Amphibians. *Current Biology* 28(21), R1237–R1241.

Wang, Y. *et al*. (2019) Alterations to transcriptomic profile, histopathology, and oxidative stress in liver of pikeperch (*Sander lucioperca*) under heat stress. *Fish & Shellfish Immunology* 95, 659–669.

Webb, J.K., Brook, B.W. and Shine, R. (2002a) Collectors endanger Australia's most threatened snake, the broad-headed snake *Hoplocephalus bungaroides*. *Oryx* 36(2), 170–181.

Webb, J.K., Brook, B.W. and Shine, R. (2002b) What makes a species vulnerable to extinction? Comparative life-history traits of two sympatric snakes. *Ecological Research* 17(1), 59–67.

Welbergen, J.A. *et al*. (2008) Climate change and the effects of temperature extremes on australian flying-foxes. *Proceedings of the Royal Society B* 275(1633), 419–425.

WHO (2020) *The State of Food Security and Nutrition in the World 2020: Transforming Food Systems for Affordable Healthy Diets*, Vol. 2020. FAO.

Wilson, G.R. and Edwards, M. (2019) Professional kangaroo population control leads to better animal welfare, conservation outcomes and avoids waste. *Australian Zoologist* 40(1), 181–202.

Winkler, D.W., Dunn, P.O. and McCulloch, C.E. (2002) Predicting the effects of climate change on avian life-history traits. *Proceedings of the National Academy of Sciences* 99(21), 13595–13599.

Woinarski, J. and Burbidge, A. (2016) *Phascolarctos cinereus. The IUCN Red List of Threatened Species 2016* e. T16892A21960344.

WWF (2022) *Effects of Climate Change*. WWF, Gland, Switzerland.

Xin, H. *et al*. (2001) Heat and moisture production of poultry and their housing systems: Broilers. *Transactions of the ASAE* 44(6), 1851.

Ying, L. *et al*. (2015) Recirculating aquaculture systems in China-current application and prospects. *Fisheries and Aquaculture Journal* 6(3), 1.

Yoro, K.O. and Daramola, M.O. (2020) CO_2 emission sources, greenhouse gases, and the global warming effect. In: *Advances in Carbon Capture*. Elsevier, pp. 3–28.

Zanker, L. (2021) Kangaroos, drought and a frustrated landowner. *Ecological Management & Restoration* 22, 66.

Zhan, Y. *et al*. (2019) The impact of chronic heat stress on the growth, survival, feeding, and differential gene expression in the sea urchin *Strongylocentrotus intermedius*. *Frontiers in Genetics* 10, 301.

Zizzari, Z.V. and Ellers, J. (2011) Effects of exposure to short-term heat stress on male reproductive fitness in a soil arthropod. *Journal of Insect Physiology* 57(3), 421–426.

Şekercioğlu, Ç.H., Primack, R.B. and Wormworth, J. (2012) The effects of climate change on tropical birds. *Biological Conservation* 148(1), 1–18.

10 Tuberculosis Vaccines for Cattle

Federico Blanco, Julia Sabio y García and Fabiana Bigi*
Instituto de Biotecnología, CICVA, Instituto Nacional de Tecnología Agropecuaria, Argentina (INTA) and Instituto de Agrobiotecnología y Biología Molecular, (IABIMO) INTA-CONICET, Hurlingham CP1686, Buenos Aires, Argentina

Abstract

Bovine tuberculosis (bTB) is a zoonotic disease caused by *Mycobacterium bovis* that mainly affects cattle. The traditional bTB control strategy is to slaughter animals positive for the official diagnostic test. This method, however, may not be economically feasible in developing countries and is less effective when cattle are in contact with wildlife reservoirs of infection. In these scenarios, cattle vaccination could be an important strategy to control bTB.

In this review, we describe the diversified vaccine development against bTB and identify gaps in current knowledge. We discuss progress made in live attenuated (including BCG), inactivated and subunit vaccines tested in preclinical models and field trials. We also provide an overview of existing knowledge in the correlates and biomarkers of protection after vaccination against bTB, as well as the most recent advances in the understanding of the protective immune response against tuberculosis.

The similarities between the mechanisms of the immune protection elicited by humans and cattle against TB and bTB, respectively, make any advance in human TB and bTB vaccines mutually beneficial. In accordance with the One Health concept, this mutual benefit is expected to progress in the future.

Keywords: bovine tuberculosis, vaccine, field trials, *Mycobacterium bovis*, BCG

Introduction

Mycobacterium bovis, a member of the *Mycobacterium tuberculosis* complex (MTBC), is the causative agent of bovine tuberculosis (bTB). bTB is a chronic respiratory disease that may affect a wide range of mammals, including humans, and its chronic nature makes this disease highly complex (Viale *et al*., 2016). This disease also affects other production animals such as sheep, goats and pigs, apart from cattle, and this may aggravate the epidemiological status of productive livestock. Furthermore, the absence of clinical signs during the early stages of infection makes quick identification of bTB-infected animals difficult.

Regarding its zoonotic nature, bTB mainly affects rural workers who are in close contact with animals. Contaminated food, mainly unpasteurized dairy products or their derivatives, represents also a risk of bTB transmission (Sabio y García *et al*., 2020).

Therefore, bTB has three main impacts: (a) direct economic losses because of a reduction in livestock productivity, (b) indirect economic losses caused by restrictions on livestock trade, and negative impact on public health.

*Corresponding author: bigi.fabiana@inta.gob.ar

This disease is endemic in many low-middle-income countries owing to the failure or absence of control programs. The test-and-slaughter strategies are the most efficient bTB control policies but their high monetary cost makes them unfeasible in low-income countries.

Although vaccination is undoubtedly the best strategy for the control of infectious diseases, there is still no accepted vaccine for the control of bTB. Most bTB vaccine trials have been conducted with the human tuberculosis vaccine, the Bacillus Calmette-Guérin (BCG) vaccine. This vaccination strategy, however, interferes with the tuberculin test, which is the most widely used diagnostic test for bTB and whose basic screening component is the purified protein derivative (PPD) (Vordermeier *et al.*, 2016b).

In recent years, researchers have developed and evaluated numerous bTB vaccination strategies in animal models and in the natural hosts of *M. bovis* (Vordermeier *et al.*, 2006; Waters *et al.*, 2012; Buddle *et al.*, 2018). Likewise, several studies have focused on the improvement of diagnostic strategies that allow differentiating between vaccinated and infected animals (Bayissa *et al.*, 2022). In this review, we attempt to collect all available data regarding the protective efficacy of the BCG vaccine as well as of new experimental vaccines against bTB in both preclinical and field trials. We also describe the state-of-the-art immune correlates of bTB protection that may assist in the selection of the most promising vaccine candidates.

Review Methodology

We searched for articles published between 1995 and 2022 in PubMed to identify publications on the development of bovine tuberculosis vaccines. The key words or terms used in the search were 'bovine tuberculosis', 'vaccines', 'attenuated strain', 'subunit vaccine' or 'cattle'. We reviewed articles resulting from these searches and their references.

Vaccination with BCG

BCG is a live-attenuated vaccine derived from *M. bovis*. This strain was obtained in 1908 by Albert Calmette and Camille Guérin by culturing a virulent bovine strain on potato slices impregnated with ox bile and glycerine and performing successive passages of this culture. The result was an *M. bovis* strain that failed to cause disease in guinea pigs, rabbits, cattle, and horses. Finally, in 1921, this strain, named BCG, was first administered to an infant via the oral route (Setiabudiawan *et al.*, 2022).

In 1996, Mahairas *et al.* determined the genomic differences between the different BCG substrains and *M. bovis* or *M. tuberculosis* (Mahairas *et al.*, 1996). They identified three DNA segments absent from BCG. These regions are named RD1 (9.5 kb), RD2 (10.7 kb) and RD3 (9.3 kb). RD1 was absent from all BCG substrains but conserved in all virulent laboratory and clinical strains of *M. bovis* and *M. tuberculosis* tested. In the case of RD2, it was absent from BCG Pasteur substrains obtained after 1925. Finally, RD3 was also deleted in a minority of *M. tuberculosis* clinical isolates.

In humans, BCG vaccine is administered soon after birth. The vaccine is extensively applied in countries with a high burden of TB and in high-risk groups from low-burden TB countries. Since its first use in 1921 over 4 billion doses have been administered, thus making BCG one of the most widespread vaccines. It is well documented that BCG vaccination protects against severe forms of the disease, such as disseminated or meningeal TB in infants, but this protection is partial or incomplete against pulmonary TB in adolescents and adults. A meta-analysis of the performance of BCG has reported impaired immunity after ten years of vaccination in seven of ten trials and an average efficacy of 14% (Sterne *et al.*, 1998). This variable efficacy is explained by different factors, including chronic helminth infections, viral co-infections and exposure to environmental mycobacteria (Ottenhoff and Kaufmann, 2012).

Calmette and Guérin have also performed the first vaccination trials with BCG in cattle. Over the past decades, several countries have made investments to study BCG vaccination in cattle within their territory. BCG vaccination has been tested via subcutaneous or oral administration and in different doses. In this regard, parenteral administration of BCG in doses ranging from 10e4 to 10e6 colony forming units (CFU) has shown similar results of protection, while its oral administration has required higher doses (10e8 CFU). Detailed information about the latest results in BCG cattle vaccination has been reviewed previously by Buddle *et al.* (2018).

Another aspect usually discussed in BCG trials in cattle is the type of *M. bovis* challenge. Historically, the administration route for a challenge with high doses of virulent *M. bovis* has been the intravenous, subcutaneous or oral administration but these routes have led to atypical pathology. In efforts to mimic the natural *M. bovis* infection, researchers from New Zealand and UK have performed intranasal, intratonsillar or intratracheal/endobronchial inoculation using relatively low doses of the pathogen (10e3–10e4 CFU) (Vordermeier *et al.*, 2014). The evaluation of the resulting protection was performed according to gross lesions in the lungs and associated lymph nodes to establish a pathology score. These trials often included bacterial loads in tissue samples.

During the last decade, researchers have focused their research on field trials. These trials consist of exposing vaccinated animals to naturally infected herds with different prevalences of bTB. Knowledge about how BCG vaccination of cattle performs against natural exposure to *M. bovis* infection is crucial in assessing the utility of the vaccine in field situations. One disadvantage of these procedures is that natural exposure is time-consuming in comparison with experimental challenges. A summarised description of the different vaccine trials reviewed in this article, including the last experiment described by Buddle *et al.* in the 2018 review (Buddle *et al.*, 2018), is depicted in Table 10.1.

In 2017, Nugent *et al.* published part of their results from a four-year trial involving more than 1000 animals located in a low-density area. In this first publication, they focused on the protective capacity of BCG administered orally. According to the authors, this route of administration has the advantage of having a relatively lower interference with the diagnostic test but requires higher doses than the subcutaneous route to confer protection. Another particular characteristic of this trial was the presence of wildlife reservoirs in the study area, particularly brushtail possums and introduced sentinel feral pigs, whose prevalence of bTB infection was followed by the researchers across several years (Nugent *et al.*, 2017). Of the 1286 animals studied, 675 were vaccinated with BCG orally. The proportion of animals with positive culture and/or TB lesions was 4.8% among the vaccinated animals and 11.9% among the unvaccinated animals (Nugent *et al.*, 2017). This gives a vaccination efficacy for oral BCG of 67.4%. Overall, the vaccination efficacy achieved by oral BCG was similar to that recorded using subcutaneous BCG. This experiment was the first vaccine trial conducted in a field with monitoring of wildlife intervention.

In parallel, the same group of researchers conducted a low-dose subcutaneous BCG vaccination trial between 2014 and 2018 (Nugent *et al.*, 2018). Based on previous results, a dose of BCG 10-fold lower than that administered regularly induced similar levels of protection, thus reducing production costs. The lower dose of BCG, however, failed to reduce cross reaction with the intradermal test (Buddle *et al.*, 2013). This particular trial consisted of inoculating a dose of BCG equivalent to that used in human BCG vaccination. Regarding the efficacy of BCG in this trial, only few animals displayed macroscopic lesions. In comparison with the previous trial, the authors observed a lower rate of transmission between cattle, which made it difficult to infer the effect of BCG in preventing infection. Instead, they observed protection against macroscopic lesions.

Two other relevant vaccination trials were conducted in Chile. In those cases, the administration of BCG was subcutaneous and the doses applied were similar to those previously used in the New Zealand study. The first vaccination trial involved 122 heifers (Retamal *et al.*, 2022), whereas the second involved seven dairy herds with different prevalences of bTB and included a large cohort of vaccinated and control animals (Ábalos *et al.*, 2022). Unfortunately, the researchers of both studies were unable to perform postmortem examination and tissue cultures owing to logistical and legal reasons and had to perform DIVA-IGRA test instead, in order to identify the infected animals and calculate the

Table 10.1. Summary of BCG vaccination trials in cattle conducted after 2018.

Country	BCG strain	Route	Dose (CFU)	% prevalence of bTB in the infected herd (source of infection)	Number of animals (control; vaccinated)	Cattle breed/age (months)	% of infected animals (BCG/control)	Vaccine trial time (years)	References
New Zealand	Danish	oral-sb	1 × 10e8–2 × 10e7 oral, 3 × 10e5 sb	5–10%	77; 675 (oral), 34 (sb)	Hereford/7–28	65/85	4.0	(Nugent *et al.*, 2017)
New Zealand	Danish	sb	3 × 10e5	5–10%	297; 520	Hereford/12–24	0.38/2.69 (culture confirmed TB lesions)	3.7	(Nugent *et al.*, 2018)
Chile	Russia	sb	2–8 × 10e5	24% of TB infection	60; 62	Holstein-Friesian/11	11.3/28.3(DIVA IGRA)	1.5	(Retamal *et al.*, 2022)
Ethiopia	Russia	sb	1 × 10e6	60 SICCT +animals, 100% prevalence	18; 22	Crossbreed (HF x Zebu)/ 1 week	68.2/88.9 (Visible lesions)	1.0	(Bayissa *et al.*, 2021)
Chile	Russia	sb	2–8 × 10e5	7 herds 76–15%	514; 575	Holstein/1	vaccine efficacy 22.4% (DIVA IGRA)	1.5	(Ábalos *et al.*, 2022)

Note: sb: subcutaneous; and CFU: colony forming units.

vaccine efficacy. The several protein cocktails used to assess whole blood samples included synthetic peptides of ESAT-6, CFP-10 and Rv3615c. The overall calculated vaccine efficacy was 66.5% for the first trial and 22.4% for the last one. These results may be controversial as determining the infection status only by IGRA, instead of using the accepted postmortem visual examination and *M. bovis* detection in tissue samples, is a limitation.

The last study took place in Ethiopia (Bayissa *et al.*, 2021). In this region, crossbred cattle are commonly employed in dairy herds. This trial consisted of monitoring groups of vaccinated and control Holstein-Friesian zebu (HF x zebu) crossbred cattle throughout one year of exposure to tuberculin-positive reactors in a ratio of 1:1. Direct protective efficacy of BCG determined by gross TB lesions observed at necropsy was 23%. The authors argued that the low level of protection was due to the high pressure of infection since the study was conducted in a herd with 100% of prevalence. The efficacy analysis comprised premortem determinations, including the DIVA skin test. None of the vaccinated calves were positive at the 6th week of vaccination; which demonstrates the usefulness of this test to differentiate vaccinated from infected animals. However, the diagnostic sensitivity of the DIVA skin test was lower than the single intradermal comparative cervical tuberculin (SICCT) test.

Finally, it is worth mentioning the efforts made by some of the countries that conducted BCG trials in wildlife reservoirs. As discussed before, New Zealand and the UK are two major examples of the intense and comprehensive evaluation of *M. bovis*-infected wild animals and their impact on livestock. During the past decades, researchers from New Zealand and UK have experimented with oral baits to vaccinate badgers and possums. In the study of the last published article after the 2018 review, which was performed in Great Britain (Lesellier *et al.*, 2020), the researchers employed bioreactor-grown BCG to vaccinate badgers by direct administration into the mouth and in baits. According to the results of that study, unlike manual vaccination, voluntarily-consumed baits apparently failed to protect. As confirmed by IFN-gamma determinations, the manual delivery of the vaccine seems to reach tonsils and underlying lymphoid-associated tissue of the oropharynx, thus inducing a protective immune response.

Altogether, different groups of researchers have documented a large range of protection efficacies obtained in cattle trials. The most discussed variables are variation in experiment settings, BCG strain, disease severity, number of experimental calves, transmission pressure (bTB prevalence in the herd), calf age at vaccination, calf breed, parameters used to determine infection and time of exposure of experimental animals, to mention a few of the most relevant. The advantage and good results of the DIVA skin test, as documented in the Ethiopian trial, are remarkable. The main future goal regarding these tests should be the improvement of their sensitivity. Other remarkable output shared by the mentioned experiments is that the immune protection conferred by BCG declines after an average period of two years and that vaccination with BCG appeared to slow the progression of bTB, as evidenced by the lower lesions scores in infected animals that had been previously vaccinated.

Vaccines Based on Live Attenuated Mutant Strains

In calves, the *M. bovis* Ravenel strain deleted in RD1 region (ΔRD1) induced protection against *M. bovis* infection three months after vaccination and the level of this protection was similar to that of BCG, at least for all the parameters evaluated (Waters *et al.*, 2009). By contrast, an *M. bovis* mutant deleted in two *mce-2* genes (Blanco *et al.*, 2012; Klepp and Sabio y Garcia, 2022) protected calves better than BCG against an experimental challenge with virulent *M. bovis* (Blanco *et al.*, 2013), as evidenced by pulmonary and lymph node histopathological score levels. However, the use of Mb Δmce2 led to positive reactions to tuberculin intradermal tests after vaccination, thus indicating that this vaccine candidate may interfere with the official bTB diagnostic test. In this respect, ancillary tests may overcome the interference of some vaccine strategies with the diagnostic tests, to differentiate vaccinated from infected animals (DIVA) properly.

ESAT-6 and CFP-10 are the most promising DIVA antigens (Vordermeier *et al.*, 2016a) and, therefore, the rationale of bTB vaccine development seems to favour the omission of these antigens. In this line, however, the evaluation of an *M. bovis* with a deletion of *esat-6* and *cfp-10* (Mb Δmce2) has shown that the new genomic deletion significantly reduces the protective capacity of the resulting double mutant strain in mice (García *et al.*, 2020). This finding highlights the importance of ESAT-6 and CFP-10 in the mechanisms of protection induced by rationally attenuated *M. bovis* mutant strains when used as vaccine candidates to control *M. bovis* infections and reveals the need of evaluating different strategies to compensate for the lack of these DIVA antigens in new vaccine formulations.

The elimination of the virulence gene *phoP* (García *et al.*, 2018) from MbΔmce2 yielded a more attenuated strain. In this case, vaccination with the double mutant or BCG showed similar protection levels against a challenge with a virulent *M. bovis* strain in mice (García *et al.*, 2015; García *et al.*, 2021).

Two attenuated transposon mutants of *M. bovis*, WAg553 and WAg563, have been tested as vaccine candidates against bTB in the guinea pig that was sensitised or not with *Mycobacterium avium*. As a result, WAg553 showed an efficacy similar to that of BCG, whereas WAg563 displayed a higher efficacy (Collins *et al.*, 2011). However, an evaluation in the possum (*Trichosurus vulpecula*), which is the main wildlife reservoir for *M. bovis* infection in New Zealand, showed opposite results: WAg553 induced higher protection than BCG and the protection induced by WAg563 was similar to that of BCG. These results highlight the importance of testing the vaccine candidates in the target species.

MTBVAC is an attenuated *Mycobacterium tuberculosis* vaccine that contains two independent unmarked stable deletion mutations in the virulence genes *phoP* and *fadD26*, without antibiotic resistance markers (Tameris *et al.*, 2019). This vaccine candidate has shown similar protection to BCG against natural exposure to *Mycobacterium caprae* in goats (Roy *et al.*, 2019).

Variants of BCG strains deleted in genes encoding for *fdr8*, *leuCD pks16*, *mmaA4*, and *metA* have shown lower virulence than wild-type BCG in immunocompromised mice and similar to BCG in protected calves after an *M. bovis* experimental challenge (Waters *et al.*, 2016). Although these mutant BCG strains do not provide advantages for the vaccination of cattle, they may be considered as TB vaccines for immunocompromised humans.

To date, few vaccine candidates based on live attenuated *M. bovis* strains have been evaluated in cattle (Table 10.2) or laboratory models and, therefore, there is insufficient evidence to define whether or not they are a promising alternative to bTB control.

According to the mentioned studies, only one vaccine candidate surpassed BCG (in only one protection parameter), while the rest induced the same protection levels as BCG in cattle (Table 10.2). Thus, despite not having a very good performance, BCG vaccination seems to be still the most appropriate option because of its advantages in terms of biosafety and its possible adaptation to a DIVA diagnosis. Regarding live attenuated vaccines against human TB, MTBVAC is the only vaccine that has been tested in neonates as a preventive vaccine. The results of a clinical trial in adults and neonates from South Africa have shown that MTBVAC induced higher CD4T cell responses than BCG, when both vaccines were used at the same dose, and also suggested that this vaccine candidate was as safe as BCG (Tameris *et al.*, 2019). Although these results are encouraging, the efficacy of MTBVAC has not yet been demonstrated. Therefore, so far, no live attenuated vaccine has shown a superlative improvement to the protection conferred by BCG in humans or in cattle.

A better understanding of the mycobacterial components that should be present in a vaccine candidate and the molecular, cellular and immune mechanisms that must be triggered to induce protective innate and adaptive responses will undoubtedly assist in the development of superior vaccines based on live attenuated strains of *M. bovis*.

Inactivated Vaccines

Killed mycobacterial vaccines are often considered safer than live attenuated *M. bovis* vaccines,

Table 10.2. Summary of anti-bTB vaccination assays in cattle.

Vaccine strategy	Route	Dose	Challenge	Number of animals (control/ vaccinated)	Cattle breed/age (months)	Challenge time[a]/ post-challenge time (months)	Superior protection than BCGb	References
M. bovis Ravenel strain deleted in RD1 region (ΔRD1)	sc	1 × 10e6 CFU	Aerosol	11/11	Holstein bull/0.5	3.0/4.5	NO	(Waters *et al.*, 2009)
M. bovis strain deleted in two *mce-2* genes (Δmce2)	sc	1 × 10e6 CFU	Intratracheal	5/5	Holstein-Fresian/3–4	2.0/3.2	YES	(Blanco *et al.*, 2013)
BCG strains deleted in *fdr8*, *leuCD pks16*, *mmaA4*, and *metA*	sc	1 × 10e6 CFU	-	10/10	Holstein steers/0.5–0.75	~3.0/4.0	NO	(Waters *et al.*, 2016)
Killed *Mycobacterium vaccae*	id	2 × 10e9 killed *M. vaccae*	Intratrachea	12/12	Friesian or Friesian-cross/5–6	1.5/~5.0–5.5	NO	(Buddle *et al.*, 1995)
BGC/ protein-CPF-Emulsigen™ /CpG-ODN	sb	0.4 mg CFP/0.25 mg ODN 2007/Emulsigen 50% and 1 × 10e6 CFU BCG	Intratracheal	10/10	Friesian cross/6	5.25/3.75–4	YES	(Wedlock *et al.*, 2005a)
BCG/DNA encoding Ag85B, MPT64 and MPT83	im	0.5 mg of each plasmid and 1 × 10e6 BCG CFU	Intratracheal	5/5	-/6	5.5/5.5	YES	(Cai *et al.*, 2006)
BCG/DNA encoding Hsp65, Hsp70, and Apa	im/id	0.5 mg of each plasmid and 1 × 10e6 BCG CFU	Intratracheal	10–11/11	Friesiancross/0.03–0.07	4.25–4.5/4	YES	(Skinner *et al.*, 2005)
DNA encoding MPB70 or DNA encoding MPB83 or DNA encoding MPB70/ MPB70protein	im/sc	1 mg (DNA or protein) per dose	Intratracheal	10/10	Friesian-cross/6–9	3.25/4.25	NOa	(Wedlock *et al.*, 2003)
DNA encoding ESAT-6, CD80 and CD86	im	2 mg of total plasmid and 1 mg ODN 2006/IFA	Aerosol	4–5/5	Mixed breed/-	-/~3.5	NO	(Maue *et al.*, 2004)

BCG/MVA85A or BCG/Ad85A	sc/id	1 × 10e6 BCG CFU and 10^9–2×10^9 PFU	Intratracheal	10/10	Friesian/6	3.5/3.5	YES	(Vordermeier *et al.*, 2009)
BCG/multi-valent viral vaccine expressing Ag85A, Rv0287, Rv0288 and Rv0251 (Ad5-TBF)	sc/id	1 × 10e6 BCG CFU and 2 × 10e9 PFU	Endobronchial	10/10	Friesian/4–6	3/3.5	NO	(Dean *et al.*, 2014)
BCG/multi-valent Ag85A, Rv0287, Rv0288 and Rv0251 protein vaccine (Adj-TBF)	sc/id	1 × 10e6 BCG CFU and 100 mg of each protein in Montanide ISA 7	Endobronchial	10/10	Friesian/4–6	3/3.5	NO	(Dean *et al.*, 2014)
BCG/ viral vaccine expressing Ag85A	sc/id	1 × 10e6 BCG CFU and 2 × 10e9 PFU	Endobronchial	10/10	Friesian/4–6	3/3.5	YES	(Dean *et al.*, 2014)
BCG/ Ag85A	sc/eb	1 × 10e6 BCG CFU and 2 × 10e9 PFU	Endobronchial	10/9	Holstein-Friesian/5–7	3/6	YES	(Dean *et al.*, 2015)

Note: sc: subcutaneous; id: intradermal; im: intramuscular; and eb: endobronchial.
[a]Challenge time after first inoculation in multiple doses vaccine scheme.
[b]Data statistically different at least in one protection parameter.
[c]p-value < 0.05.

because they do not contain any infectious microorganisms. In this line, heat-inactivated *M. bovis* administered by the parenteral route have been shown to reduce the prevalence of *M. bovis* in wild boar piglets (Díez-Delgado *et al.*, 2017). Similarly, in an experimental challenge model, pigs vaccinated with heat-inactivated *M. bovis* by the oral route showed a reduction in some parameters of pathology, in comparison to the unvaccinated animals (Nol *et al.*, 2020). In a deer model of bTB, however, killed BCG in a mineral-oil adjuvant failed to protect animals against *M. bovis* challenge (Griffin *et al.*, 1999).

Killed *Mycobacterium vaccae* has been shown to be safe when administered orally to humans in a phase II trial (Butov *et al.*, 2013) and some evidence of efficacy as a therapeutic TB vaccine has been reported (Bourinbaiar *et al.*, 2020). In the possum, killed *M. vaccae* vaccine has improved the protection conferred by live BCG (Skinner *et al.*, 2002). However, this vaccine has failed to protect cattle against *M. bovis* challenge (Buddle *et al.*, 1995) (Table 10.2).

The results obtained so far highlight the use of inactivated mycobacteria in therapies for TB and probably for bTB, but do not support their use as a prophylactic vaccine for cattle. In bTB reservoir animals such as the possum, the use of inactivated mycobacteria vaccines seems to be very beneficial for bTB eradication and control programs. Also, this vaccine strategy could be an attractive option to control bTB in pigs.

Subunit Vaccines

Live vaccines raise great concern regarding biosafety and are still rejected because of the interference with the bTB diagnosis. Conversely, vaccines based on simple subunits or defined antigenic complexes are an attractive alternative for the control of bTB, since they may overcome these issues. The main advantage of subunit vaccines is that it is relatively simple to identify antigens for use in a DIVA diagnostic test to differentiate vaccinated from infected animals. For example, the diagnostic antigen ‘PPD’ used in the intradermal test may be produced from a strain of *M. bovis* AN5 deleted in the genes that encode for the vaccine proteins.

Researchers have developed and evaluated numerous protein subunit vaccines for the control of TB in animal models and observed different degrees of protection depending on the antigen, the delivery system and the route of inoculation (Khademi *et al.*, 2018). Several protein-based TB vaccines formulated in different adjuvants are currently in clinical trials (Whitlow *et al.*, 2020; Franco and Peri, 2021). Among these subunit vaccine candidates, the adjuvanted protein vaccine M72/AS01E has shown 49.7% efficacy as a vaccine in a final analysis of a phase IIb clinical trial (Tait *et al.*, 2019). Despite the substantial advance in the generation of knowledge and vaccine tools for TB, as evidenced by the numerous clinical trials coordinated and supported by Tuberculosis Vaccine Initiative (TBVI, 2015), the transfer to the field of vaccinology against bTB remains limited and only very few new candidate vaccines have been developed and evaluated so far.

Subunit vaccines may be classified as adjuvanted protein subunit vaccines, recombinant viral vector vaccines and DNA vaccines. Regarding adjuvanted proteins as bTB vaccine candidates, researchers have evaluated only four vaccine strategies in animal models so far. The immunogenic protein MPB70 emulsified with incomplete Freund's adjuvant failed to confer protection to calves challenged with *M. bovis* when used to boost an MPB70-DNA vaccine (Wedlock *et al.*, 2003). By contrast, Ag85A and ESAT-6 formulated with a synthetic mycobacterial phosphatidylinositol di-mannoside induced moderate protection in *M. bovis* challenged mice (Parlane *et al.*, 2012). In addition, H65, a fusion protein of three pairs of ESX-secreted antigens, adjuvanted with the liposome CAF01, conferred protection against *M. bovis* infection in a mouse model of bTB (Blanco *et al.*, 2021b). Finally, total proteins from *M. bovis* culture supernatant (called culture filtrate protein-CPF) formulated with Emulsigen™ in combination with CpG oligodeoxynucleotide (ODN) and injected simultaneously with BCG protected calves better than BCG alone, in terms of macroscopic lesions and *M. bovis* culture-positive animals (Wedlock *et al.*, 2005a). However, although vaccination with CPF/Emulsigen/CpG (ODN) alone showed a moderate level of protection in one trial (Wedlock *et al.*, 2005b), it failed to protect in another similar trial (Wedlock *et al.*, 2005a).

The authors argued that these differences were due to the different proportions of the adjuvant used in each formulation.

As mentioned above, one promising vaccine candidate for the control of TB is the fusion protein M72 formulated in AS01E adjuvant. This adjuvant includes bacterially derived monophosphoryl lipid A (MPL) from *Salmonella minnesota* and saponin QS-21. This vaccine, which has finished phase IIb trials in humans, has conferred 49.7% of protection against the progression of TB disease (Tait *et al.*, 2019), as mentioned above. Given the similarities between bTB and human TB, it would be valuable to test this vaccine in cattle. However, the high cost of the AS01E adjuvant could constrain the use of this vaccine formulation in cattle, particularly in developing countries.

Although the vaccination schemes that include boosting live attenuated *M. bovis* strains with subunit vaccines, have been developed and tested at a low degree in bTB, the data availability in the field of TB vaccination is enormous. For instance, in the rhesus macaque model, boosting BCG with proteins/adjuvants has not enhanced protection against primary infection with *M. tuberculosis* compared with BCG alone (Darrah *et al.*, 2019). Conversely, vaccination of cynomolgus macaques with BCG and boosted with H56/IC31 has resulted in the efficient control of *M. tuberculosis* infection, with reduced rates of clinical disease and improved survival of the animals, in comparison with BCG alone (Lin *et al.*, 2012). In mouse models of TB, the results of BCG prime and adjuvanted protein/s boost schemes have been variable (Khademi *et al.*, 2018).

Similarly, in mouse models of bTB, heterologous prime-boost vaccination schemes have shown different degrees of success. The protein ArgF formulated in poly lactic-co-glycolic acid copolymers improved the protection conferred by BCG in *M. bovis* challenged mice (Ni *et al.*, 2021). In addition, mice vaccinated with BCG/H65 +CAF01 and boosted with H65 +CAF01 developed better protection against *M. bovis* than mice vaccinated with any of the vaccines given alone (Blanco *et al.*, 2021b). However, when mice were vaccinated with a live *M. bovis* mutant strain, instead of BCG, the co-administration and subsequent boosts of H65 +CAF01 failed to improve the protection elicited by the mutant strain (García *et al.* 2021) Thus, although the results are scarce, they would indicate that the success of the prime-boost strategies in bTB vaccines depends on the live strain used for the priming (where BCG showed better results), the antigen, and the formulation of the boost vaccines.

Probably, the lack of consistency in the outcome of the bTB vaccine assays highlights the existing gaps in the knowledge of the complex immune response against bTB. In this respect, most studies have only focused on the *M. bovis* -antigen-specific CD4 +Th-1 arm of the immune system. Although that approach is important, little is known about innate immune responses involving neutrophils, monocytes (macrophages and dendritic cells) or NK cells (Larsen *et al.*, 2022), or about the *M. bovis* -antigen-specific B cell responses (Tanner *et al.*, 2019).

DNA naked and viral vector-based vaccines have been widely evaluated for the control of various infectious diseases, including TB and COVID-19, but very little progress has been made in this field regarding bTB vaccinology.

DNA vaccines based on different gene fusions of *ag85B*, *mpb64*, and *esat-6* showed equivalent protection to BCG in mice that were infected with *M. bovis* five weeks after the first vaccination (Liu *et al.*, 2008). Moreover, mouse vaccination with DNA expressing MPB83 exceeded the protection conferred by BCG against infection with *M. bovis* about 10 weeks after the first vaccination (Chambers *et al.*, 2000). Another study showed that DNA vaccines expressing ESAT-6 and Ag85A required 24 weeks to induce protection in mice when challenged with *M. bovis*. However, these ESAT-6 and Ag85A DNA vaccines did not enhance the protection conferred by BCG vaccination (Skinner *et al.*, 2003). Altogether, these findings indicate that the outcome of DNA vaccination against bTB in mouse models seems to be highly dependent on the experimental condition established in each assay.

In cattle (Table 10.2), the BCG prime-boost schemes of multivalent DNA vaccines with plasmids encoding Ag85B, MPT64 and MPT83 (Cai *et al.*, 2006) and plasmids encoding for Hsp65, Hsp70, and Apa (Skinner *et al.*, 2003; Skinner *et al.*, 2005) have improved the protection efficacy of BCG. However, when used alone, immunisation with DNA vaccines encoding MPB70 or MPB83 failed to protect cattle against bovine tuberculosis (Wedlock *et al.*, 2003). Co-administration of plasmids expressing the costimulatory molecules CD80 (B7-1) and CD86 (B7-2) seems to have enhanced the protection, in cattle (Table 10.2), conferred by an ESAT-6 DNA vaccine at the level of lung and lymph node pathology; however, the results were not completely reproducible between two similar trials (Maue *et al.*, 2004).

Therefore, despite the initial enthusiasm that prevailed in the first decade of 2000 and some encouraging results, the development and use of vaccines based on plasmid DNA have waned and their value has not been properly established.

An adenovirus vaccine expressing the mycobacterial antigen TB10.4 as a boost of BCG vaccination conferred better protection than BCG alone to mice challenged with *M. bovis* but this increased protection was not sustained in a year-long survival study. These findings suggest that the viral vaccine failed to boost T memory cells (Kaveh *et al.*, 2016).

Boosting BCG with MVA85A or Ad85A viral vector vaccines led to lower gross pathology scores than BCG alone in calves infected with *M. bovis* (Vordermeier *et al.*, 2009). In a second trial, Ad85A failed to enhance the protection conferred by BCG vaccination in terms of gross pathology scores. However, this study showed that vaccination in calves either with Ad85A or multi-valent viral vaccines expressing Ag85A, Rv0287, Rv0288 and Rv0251 reduced the degree of pathology at the histological level in BCG prime-boost schemes compared to BGC alone (Dean *et al.*, 2014). In addition, BCG-vaccinated calves that were simultaneously administered with Ag85A by the endobronchial route showed better protection against *M. bovis* than animals vaccinated with BCG alone (Dean *et al.*, 2015).

Overall, virus-vectored vaccines are a promising strategy for bTB control when used in BCG prime-boost immunisation schemes. However, there are doubts about the efficacy of these vaccines over time and long-term evaluations are mandatory to clarify this.

New Vaccine Antigens

In recent studies, researchers have developed novel rational strategies to search for new vaccine antigens. Benedictus *et al.* have found that *M. bovis* BCG lipopeptides induced specific memory T cells with immune phenotypes associated with protection against bTB in *M. bovis* BCG-vaccinated and *M. bovis*-challenged calves (Benedictus *et al.*, 2020). However, studies with individual lipoproteins have shown that the impact on the immune response can be antagonistic, depending on the mycobacterial lipoprotein. For example, in mice, the lipoprotein LprG induces immunosuppression, whereas LppZ induces proinflammatory cytokines (Hovav *et al.*, 2006; Chen *et al.*, 2019).

In another study, by selecting a BCG transposon mutant library in naïve and BCG-vaccinated cattle, Smith *et al.* identified ten BCG proteins as a vaccine candidates and determined that YrbE1B, PPE20 and Mb0086 induced the production of cytokines associated with protection against bTB in samples from BCG-vaccinated cattle (Smith *et al.*, 2020).

As mentioned before, an important aspect to take into account for the design of new bTB vaccines is that ESAT-6 and CFP-10 should not be included in vaccine formulations because of their importance as diagnostic antigens (Vordermeier *et al.*, 2016b).

Biomarkers and Correlates of Protection

The cellular responses characterised by interferon gamma-producing T helper cells (CD4+) are essential to contain the tubercle bacillus. Cytotoxic T cells (CD8+) also play a role in the control of tuberculosis mycobacterial infection, especially in the late stages of the disease (Larsen *et al.*, 2022). However, other components of the adaptive immune response, as well as the innate and trained innate responses, are also critical in anti-TB immunity, since humans and cattle, for example, can mount potent IFN-γ responses against *M. tuberculosis* or *M. bovis* infection and develop active disease.

The field trials of anti-bTB vaccines are very expensive and time-consuming. Furthermore, if the challenge is experimental, these trials require housing infected cattle in containments with high levels of biosecurity. The identification of protective correlates of immunity against bTB would facilitate the selection of the best candidate vaccines to be analysed in clinical trials.

Undoubtedly, IFN-γ is a key cytokine to respond efficiently to *M. bovis* infection and therefore it would be a useful biomarker of vaccine protection against bTB. However, according to early studies, the amount of IFN-γ produced after specific stimulation of cattle blood from vaccinated cattle did not correlate with protection (Buddle *et al.*, 2005). Conversely, the frequency of IFN-γ-producing T lymphocytes determined with the IFN-γ ELISPOT assays, a method that quantifies the frequency of IFN-γ secretion for a single cell, has shown to correlate very well with the protection conferred by vaccination, according to lesion score analyses of one vaccine assay in cattle (Hope *et al.*, 2011). The study of Blunt *et al.* has revealed that the central-memory-like T cells (Tcm) (CD45RO(+) CD62L(hi)) secreting IFN-γ is the dominant cell population that increases in frequency in vaccinated and protected cattle, in relation to unprotected animals. However, according to Biffar *et al.*, the percentage of CD4 +Tcm cells expressing both IFN-γ and IL-2 was not statistically different between protected and unprotected cattle in a bovine BCG challenge model (Biffar *et al.*, 2020). The model used by Biffar *et al.* consisted of a challenge performed with BCG into the prescapular lymph node and an assessment of the bacterial loads within the lymph nodes to evaluate the protection level.

On the other hand, Maggioli *et al.* have demonstrated that, early after *M. bovis* infection of vaccinated cattle, polyfunctional Tcm cells expressing IFN-γ/TNF-α/IL-2 are indicative of a protective response (Maggioli *et al.*, 2016). Although these findings highlight the role of Tcm in the protective immune responses against bTB, more studies are needed to consolidate this first evidence and to determine which subsets of polyfunctional Tcm should be stimulated for a vaccine to be effective.

The expression of the gene encoding granulysin and perforin in blood from vaccinated cattle increases after vaccination; which suggests these proteins as biomarkers of protection. However, whether this vaccine-induced gene expression negatively correlates with the progression of the disease after *M. bovis* infection remains unclear (Capinos Scherer *et al.*, 2009).

According to a transcriptomic analysis using *Bos taurus* DNA microarrays, the expression of *ERAP1* and *PDE8A* was significantly downregulated before the experimental *M. bovis* challenge in PPD-stimulated PBMC from vaccinated and protected cattle (Blanco *et al.*, 2017). Both genes encode proteins that are negatively associated with immune protection against bTB.

Bhuju *et al.* have defined the transcriptome of PPD-stimulated PBMC of vaccinated and protected cattle. According to their study, IL-22 expression is the dominant surrogate of bTB protection. The genes encoding for IFN-γ, CCL3, IL13 and MT-3, to mention a few, are also upregulated in protected animals. The upregulation of *MT-3* and *CCL3* could be due to the strong IFN-γ responses induced in protected animals. The gene encoding for VCAM1, CXCL12 and CCL14 were the most downregulated genes associated with protection (Bhuju *et al.*, 2012).

Researchers have also proposed IL-17 as a biomarker of protection against bTB in cattle. In two cattle vaccine assays, the expression of IL-17 in stimulated PBMC (before experimental challenge) correlated with protection against bTB (Rizzi *et al.*, 2012; Blanco *et al.*, 2013).

Altogether, the reports analysed in this section indicate that the expression of IL-22 and IL-17 is a good correlate of protection after vaccination. Regarding the protective importance of the IFN-γ expression after vaccination, the results are not conclusive. However, robust data indicate that the frequency of central-memory-like T cells secreting IFN-γ, rather than total peripheral IFN-γ production, is critical to protect against bTB. Although other biomarker candidates of protection such as ERAP, PDE8A, MT-3, CCL3, VCAM 1, CXCL12 and CCL14 are promising, more experiments are essential to confirm their potential.

Timing and location of the immune responses against tuberculosis

Timing and location seem to be crucial variables in the effectiveness of the immune response against tuberculosis. As mentioned above, strong immunological responses (Thacker *et al.*, 2007) with higher expression of IFN-γ and IL-17 (Blanco *et al.*, 2011; Waters *et al.*, 2016) seem to be associated with increased pathology.

Paradoxically, the expression level of IL-17 and IFN-γ after cattle vaccination has also been positively associated with protection against *M. bovis* infection (Bhuju *et al.*, 2012; Blanco *et al.*, 2013). These facts lead us to believe that early induction of a proinflammatory immune response with an effective production of IL-17 and IFN-γ, could rapidly suppress bacterial replication and, thus, the progression of the disease. By contrast, a high inflammatory response associated with pathology could be due to a less controlled bacterial replication at the beginning of the infection. This lower control leads to exacerbation of the inflammatory response, which eventually increases tissue damage.

Thus, protection against bTB seems to be highly dependent on the timing of the initial immune response after infection by *M. bovis* or *M. tuberculosis* and the innate and trained innate immune responses may play key roles in these scenarios (Blanco *et al.*, 2021a). It is possible that an appropriate innate, and likely trained, immune response capable of rapidly counteracting the evasion mechanisms deployed by mycobacteria will allow the necessary time to mount an effective and controlled adaptive immune response to finally diminish the tissue damage.

The location of the T cells within the infected site is also critical to the outcome of tuberculosis infections (Robinson *et al.*, 2015). This is in part due to the fact that T-lymphocytes (TL) need to interact directly with macrophages to efficiently control mycobacterial replication (Robinson *et al.*, 2015). Only a subset of *M. tuberculosis* specific CD4T cells may be able to enter the lungs. The ability of CD4T cells to migrate to the lungs and confer protection against *M. tuberculosis* infection is determined by the expression of chemokine receptors (Robinson *et al.*, 2015). TLs express two mutually exclusive markers associated with terminal differentiation: killer cell lectin-like receptor subfamily G member 1 (KLRG1) and programmed cell death 1 (PD1). In the context of TB infection, while KLRG1 seems to be a marker of terminal differentiation (Lindenstrøm *et al.*, 2013; Hu *et al.*, 2018), a body of evidence suggests that PD1 is not strictly a marker of exhaustion; however, the data can be contradictory and the mechanistic details are still unclear (Sallin *et al.*, 2017).

Several studies in humans and mouse models of TB have shown that only less-differentiated CD4T cells expressing PD1 migrate into the lung parenchyma and confer protection against *M. tuberculosis*, whereas terminally-differentiated effector CD4T cells expressing high levels of KLRG1 reside in the vasculature without conferring protection against *M. tuberculosis* infection (Robinson *et al.*, 2015). Therefore, many publications highlight the role of the local response in the protection against TB and the importance of avoiding terminal differentiation of CD4T cells (Hu *et al.*, 2018).

Particularly, the level of CD4 +KLRG1T cells in the lung parenchyma seems to be an indicator of protection status against TB in mouse models (Sallin *et al.*, 2017; Clemmensen *et al.*, 2021). Therefore, an important feature of protective immunity against TB seems to be the induction of a less differentiated CD4T cell response, at least in mouse models.

In this sense, heterologous prime-boost vaccine strategies should have the advantage of avoiding continuous antigenic stimulation of T cells and therefore induce less-differentiated CD4 +T cells, in comparison to homologous prime-booster vaccines. However, more research is necessary to precise the role of CD4T cell differentiation in local lung protection against TB and bTB, since poor penetration of CD4T cells, rather than terminally-differentiated CD4 cells, into the granulomas has been associated with a lack of protection against TB in rhesus macaques (Kauffman *et al.*, 2018).

Conclusions

Researchers have made significant progress in developing bTB vaccines as well as in identifying biomarkers and immune correlates of protection against bTB. However, most of the studies have focused on BCG, which is the only currently approved vaccine for human TB. In a similar way to human BCG vaccination, cattle BCG vaccination has been shown to confer variable protection levels when tested in field trials settled in regions with different prevalences of bTB. This may be explained in part because of pre-exposure to *Mycobacterium* species in regions with high bTB prevalence, which may mask the protective effects of vaccination. In any case, the protection conferred by BCG on cattle would not be sufficient for the effective control of bTB in these high-prevalence regions. Thus, live attenuated vaccines with higher protective efficacy than BCG would be desirable.

The main limitation to the use of bTB vaccines is their interference with the official diagnosis. Fortunately, researchers have made significant advances in the design of DIVA diagnostics, particularly in ancillary tests, in order to differentiate infected animals from those vaccinated with BCG.

Although promising subunit vaccines for TB, such as M72/AS01E vaccine, are now in clinical assays in humans, few protein-or DNA-based bTB vaccine candidates have been developed and pre-clinically evaluated, and even fewer have been tested in clinical field trials. The advantage of subunit vaccines compared to live attenuated strains is their compatibility with DIVA diagnostic methods based on multiple antigens. The disadvantage is that they may be less protective than live vaccines such as BCG.

Different aspects of the immune response against bTB that remain neglected and overshadowed by the centrality of the adaptive Th1 response in TB and bTB should be explored to achieve a better vaccine than BCG.

Studies in humans, non-human primates and other animal models have indicated that less-studied arms of the immune response such as the innate, trained innate immune responses and humoral responses are key elements for the induction of protection after vaccination against TB. The location of the initial immune response appears to be also relevant and therefore different routes of administration should be evaluated.

In addition, heterologous prime-boost schemes are attractive vaccine strategies to improve the efficacy of vaccination against bTB.

Individual Contributions for Authors

FCB wrote part of the manuscript and contributed with ideas; JSG wrote part of the manuscript, review and editing activities; FB designed and wrote part of the manuscript.

Funding

Ministerio de Ciencia, Tecnología e Innovación Productiva, (Grant/Award Number: 'PITES 43') Instituto Nacional de Técnica Aeroespacial, (Grant/Award Number: 'i102') Fondo para la Investigación Científica y Tecnológica, (Grant/Award Numbers: 'PICT2017-1721' and 'PICT2018-01113/04692').

Conflict of Interest

The authors have declared no conflict of interest.

References

Ábalos, P., Valdivieso, N., Pérez de Val, B., Vordermeier, M., Benavides, M.B. *et al.* (2022) Vaccination of calves with the *Mycobacterium bovis* BCG strain induces protection against bovine tuberculosis in dairy herds under a natural transmission setting. *Animals (Basel)* 12, 1083. DOI: 10.3390/ani12091083.

Bayissa, B., Sirak, A., Worku, A., Zewude, A., Zeleke, Y. *et al.* (2021) Evaluation of the efficacy of BCG in protecting against contact challenge with bovine tuberculosis in Holstein-Friesian and zebu crossbred calves in Ethiopia. *Frontiers in Veterinary Science* 8, 702402. DOI: 10.3389/fvets.2021.702402.

Bayissa, B., Sirak, A., Zewude, A., Worku, A., Gumi, B. *et al.* (2022) Field evaluation of specific mycobacterial protein-based skin test for the differentiation of *Mycobacterium bovis*-infected and Bacillus Calmette Guerin-vaccinated crossbred cattle in Ethiopia. *Transboundary and Emerging Diseases* 69, e1–e9. DOI: 10.1111/tbed.14252.

Benedictus, L., Steinbach, S., Holder, T., Bakker, D., Vrettou, C. *et al.* (2020) Hydrophobic mycobacterial antigens elicit polyfunctional T cells in *Mycobacterium bovis* immunized cattle: Association with protection against challenge? *Frontiers in Immunology* 11, 588180. DOI: 10.3389/fimmu.2020.588180.

Bhuju, S., Aranday-Cortes, E., Villarreal-Ramos, B., Xing, Z., Singh, M. *et al.* (2012) Global gene transcriptome analysis in vaccinated cattle revealed a dominant role of IL-22 for protection against bovine tuberculosis. *PLoS Pathogens* 8, e1003077. DOI: 10.1371/journal.ppat.1003077.

Biffar, L., Blunt, L., Atkins, W., Anderson, P., Holder, T. *et al.* (2020) Evaluating the sensitivity of the bovine BCG challenge model using a prime boost Ad85A vaccine regimen. *Vaccine* 38, 1241–1248. DOI: 10.1016/j.vaccine.2019.11.005.

Blanco, F.C., Bianco, M.V., Meikle, V., Garbaccio, S., Vagnoni, L. *et al.* (2011) Increased IL-17 expression is associated with pathology in a bovine model of tuberculosis. *Tuberculosis* 91, 57–63. DOI: 10.1016/j.tube.2010.11.007.

Blanco, F.C., Soria, M., Gravisaco, M.J., Bianco, M.V., Meikle, V. *et al.* (2012) Assessment of the immune responses induced in cattle after inoculation of a *Mycobacterium bovis* strain deleted in two mce2 genes. *Journal of Biomedicine and Biotechnology* 258353. DOI: 10.1155/2012/258353.

Blanco, F.C., Bianco, M.V., Garbaccio, S., Meikle, V., Gravisaco, M.J. *et al.* (2013) *Mycobacterium bovis* δmce2 double deletion mutant protects cattle against challenge with virulent *M. bovis*. *Tuberculosis* 93, 363–372. DOI: 10.1016/j.tube.2013.02.004.

Blanco, F.C., Soria, M.A., Klepp, L.I. and Bigi, F. (2017) ERAP1 and PDE8A are downregulated in cattle protected against bovine tuberculosis. *Journal of Molecular Microbiology and Biotechnology* 27, 237–245. DOI: 10.1159/000479183.

Blanco, F.C., Sabio y Garcia, J. and Bigi, F. (2021a) Recent advances in non-specific immune memory against bovine tuberculosis. *Comparative Immunology, Microbiology and Infectious Diseases* 75, 101615. DOI: 10.1016/j.cimid.2021.101615.

Blanco, F.C., García, E.A., Aagaard, C. and Bigi, F. (2021b) The subunit vaccine H65 + CAF01 increased the BCG-protection against *Mycobacterium bovis* infection in a mouse model of bovine tuberculosis. *Research in Veterinary Science* 136, 595–597. DOI: 10.1016/j.rvsc.2021.04.014.

Bourinbaiar, A.S., Batbold, U., Efremenko, Y., Sanjagdorj, M., Butov, D. *et al.* (2020) Phase III, placebo-controlled, randomized, double-blind trial of tableted, therapeutic TB vaccine (V7) containing heat-killed *M. vaccae* administered daily for one month. *Journal of Clinical Tuberculosis and Other Mycobacterial Diseases* 18, 100141. DOI: 10.1016/j.jctube.2019.100141.

Buddle, B.M., Keen, D., Thomson, A., Jowett, G., McCarthy, A.R. *et al.* (1995) Protection of cattle from bovine tuberculosis by vaccination with BCG by the respiratory or subcutaneous route, but not by vaccination with killed *Mycobacterium vaccae*. *Research in Veterinary Science* 59, 10–16. DOI: 10.1016/0034-5288(95)90023-3.

Buddle, B.M., Wedlock, D.N., Denis, M. and Skinner, M.A. (2005) Identification of immune response correlates for protection against bovine tuberculosis. *Veterinary Immunology and Immunopathology* 108, 45–51. DOI: 10.1016/j.vetimm.2005.08.002.

Buddle, B.M., Hewinson, R.G., Vordermeier, H.M. and Wedlock, D.N. (2013) Subcutaneous administration of a 10-fold-lower dose of a commercial human tuberculosis vaccine, *Mycobacterium bovis* bacillus Calmette-Guerin Danish, induced levels of protection against bovine tuberculosis and responses in the tuberculin intradermal test similar to those induced by a standard cattle dose. *Clinical and Vaccine Immunology* 20, 1559–1562. DOI: 10.1128/CVI.00435-13.

Buddle, B.M., Vordermeier, H.M., Chambers, M.A. and de Klerk-Lorist, L.M. (2018) Efficacy and safety of BCG vaccine for control of tuberculosis in domestic livestock and wildlife. *Frontiers in Veterinary Science* 5, 259. DOI: 10.3389/fvets.2018.00259.

Butov, D.A., Efremenko, Y., Prihoda, N.D., Zaitzeva, S.I. and Yurchenko, L. (2013) Randomized, placebo-controlled Phase II trial of heat-killed *Mycobacterium vaccae* (Immodulon batch) formulated as an oral pill (V7). *Immunotherapy* 5, 1047–1054. DOI: 10.2217/imt.13.110.

Cai, H., Yu, D.H., Hu, X.D., Li, S.X. and Zhu, Y.X. (2006) A combined DNA vaccine-prime, BCG-boost strategy results in better protection against *Mycobacterium bovis* challenge. *DNA Cell Biology* 25, 438–447. DOI: 10.1089/dna.2006.25.438.

Capinos Scherer, C.F., Endsley, J.J., Aguiar, J.B., Jacobs, W.R., Larsen, M.H. *et al.* (2009) Evaluation of granulysin and perforin as candidate biomarkers for protection following vaccination with *Mycobacterium bovis* BCG or M. bovisδRD1. *Transboundary Emerging Diseases* 56, 228–239. DOI: 10.1111/j.1865-1682.2008.01058.x.

Chambers, M.A., Vordermeier, H.M., Whelan, A., Commander, N., Tascon, R. *et al.* (2000) Vaccination of mice and cattle with plasmid DNA encoding the *Mycobacterium bovis* antigen MPB83. *Clinical Infectious Diseases* 30(3), S283–287. DOI: 10.1086/313875.

Chen, Y., Xiao, J.N., Li, Y., Xiao, Y.J., Xiong, Y.Q. *et al.* (2019) Mycobacterial lipoprotein Z triggers efficient innate and adaptive immunity for protection against *Mycobacterium tuberculosis* infection. *Frontiers in Immunology* 9, 3190. DOI: 10.3389/fimmu.2018.03190.

Clemmensen, H.S., Dube, J.Y., McIntosh, F., Rosenkrands, I., Jungersen, G. *et al.* (2021) *In vivo* antigen expression regulates cd4 t cell differentiation and vaccine efficacy against *Mycobacterium tuberculosis* infection. *mBio* 12, e00226-21. DOI: 10.1128/mBio.00226-21.

Collins, D.M., Buddle, B.M., Kawakami, R.P., Hotter, G., Mildenhall, N. *et al.* (2011) Newly attenuated *Mycobacterium bovis* mutants as vaccines against bovine tuberculosis, particularly for possums. *Veterinary Microbiology* 151, 99–103. DOI: 10.1016/j.vetmic.2011.02.031.

Darrah, P.A., DiFazio, R.M., Maiello, P., Gideon, H.P., Myers, A.J. *et al.* (2019) Boosting BCG with proteins or rAd5 does not enhance protection against tuberculosis in *Rhesus macaques*. *NPJ Vaccines* 4, 21. DOI: 10.1038/s41541-019-0113-9.

Dean, G., Whelan, A., Clifford, D., Salguero, F.J., Xing, Z. *et al.* (2014) Comparison of the immunogenicity and protection against bovine tuberculosis following immunization by BCG-riming and boosting with adenovirus or protein based vaccines. *Vaccine* 32, 1304–1310. DOI: 10.1016/j.vaccine.2013.11.045.

Dean, G.S., Clifford, D., Whelan, A.O., Tchilian, E.Z., Beverley, P.C.L. *et al.* (2015) Protection induced by simultaneous subcutaneous and endobronchial vaccination with BCG/BCG and BCG/adenovirus expressing antigen 85A against *Mycobacterium bovis* in cattle. *PLoS One* 10, e0142270. DOI: 10.1371/journal.pone.0142270.

Díez-Delgado, I., Rodríguez, O., Boadella, M., Garrido, J.M., Sevilla, I.A. *et al.* (2017) Parenteral vaccination with heat-inactivated *Mycobacterium bovis* reduces the prevalence of tuberculosis-compatible lesions in farmed wild boar. *Transboundary Emerging Diseases* 64, e18–e21. DOI: 10.1111/tbed.12526.

Franco, A.R. and Peri, F. (2021) Developing new anti-tuberculosis vaccines: Focus on adjuvants. *Cells* 10, 78. DOI: 10.3390/cells10010078.

García, E., Bianco, M.V., Gravisaco, M.J., Rocha, R.V., Blanco, F.C. *et al.* (2015) Evaluation of *Mycobacterium bovis* double knockout mce2-phoP as candidate vaccine against bovine tuberculosis. *Tuberculosis* 95, 186–189. DOI: 10.1016/j.tube.2015.01.001.

García, E., Blanco, F., Muñiz, X., Eirin, M., Klepp, L. *et al.* (2020) Elimination of ESAT-6 and CFP-10 from a candidate vaccine against bovine tuberculosis impaired its protection efficacy in the BALBc mouse model. *International Journal of Mycobacteriology* 9, 417–421. DOI: 10.4103/ijmy.ijmy-180-20.

García, E., Blanco, F. and Bigi, F. (2021) H65 fusion protein fails to improve the protection of a rationally attenuated live vaccine candidate against bovine tuberculosis in a mouse model of tuberculosis. *International Journal of Mycobacteriology* 10, 411–413. DOI: 10.4103/ijmy.ijmy_201_21.

García, E.A., Blanco, F.C., Bigi, M.M., Vazquez, C.L., Forrellad, M.A. *et al.* (2018) Characterization of the two component regulatory system PhoPR in *Mycobacterium bovis*. *Veterinary Microbiology* 222, 30–38. DOI: 10.1016/j.vetmic.2018.06.016.

Griffin, J.F.T., Mackintosh, C.G., Slobbe, L., Thomson, A.J. and Buchan, G.S. (1999) Vaccine protocols to optimise the protective efficacy of BCG. *Tubercle and Lung Disease* 79, 135–143. DOI: 10.1054/tuld.1998.0202.

Hope, J.C., Thom, M.L., McAulay, M., Mead, E., Vordermeier, H.M. *et al.* (2011) Identification of surrogates and correlates of protection in protective immunity against *Mycobacterium bovis* infection induced in neonatal calves by vaccination with *M. bovis* BCG pasteur and *M. bovis* BCG Danish. *Bovis BCG Pasteur and M. Bovis BCG Danish. Clinical and Vaccine Immunology* 18, 373–379. DOI: 10.1128/CVI.00543-10.

Hovav, A.H., Mullerad, J., Maly, A., Davidovitch, L., Fishman, Y. *et al.* (2006) Aggravated infection in mice co-administered with *Mycobacterium tuberculosis* and the 27-kDa lipoprotein. *Microbes and Infection* 8, 1750–1757. DOI: 10.1016/j.micinf.2006.02.011.

Hu, Z., Zhao, H.M., Li, C.L., Liu, X.H., Barkan, D. *et al.* (2018) The role of KLRG1 in human CD4+ t-cell immunity against tuberculosis. *Journal of Infectious Diseases* 217, 1491–1503. DOI: 10.1093/infdis/jiy046.

Kauffman, K.D., Sallin, M.A., Sakai, S., Kamenyeva, O., Kabat, J. *et al.* (2018) Defective positioning in granulomas but not lung-homing limits CD4 t-cell interactions with *Mycobacterium tuberculosis*-infected macrophages in *Rhesus macaques*. *Mucosal Immunology* 11, 462–473. DOI: 10.1038/mi.2017.60.

Kaveh, D.A., Garcia-Pelayo, M.C., Webb, P.R., Wooff, E.E., Bachy, V.S. *et al.* (2016) Parenteral adenoviral boost enhances BCG induced protection, but not long term survival in a murine model of bovine TB. *Vaccine* 34, 4003–4011. DOI: 10.1016/j.vaccine.2016.06.032.

Khademi, F., Derakhshan, M., Yousefi-Avarvand, A., Tafaghodi, M. and Soleimanpour, S. (2018) Multi-stage subunit vaccines against *Mycobacterium tuberculosis*: An alternative to the BCG vaccine or a BCG-prime boost? *Expert Review of Vaccines* 17, 31–44. DOI: 10.1080/14760584.2018.1406309.

Klepp, L.I. and Sabio y Garcia, J. (2022) Mycobacterial MCE proteins as transporters that control lipid homeostasis of the cell wall. *Tuberculosis* 132, 102162. DOI: 10.1016/j.tube.2021.102162.

Larsen, S.E., Williams, B.D., Rais, M., Coler, R.N. and Baldwin, S.L. (2022) It takes a village: The multi-faceted immune response to *Mycobacterium tuberculosis* infection and vaccine-induced immunity. *Frontiers in Immunology* 13, 840225. DOI: 10.3389/fimmu.2022.840225.

Lesellier, S., Birch, C.P.D., Davé, D., Dalley, D., Gowtage, S. *et al.* (2020) Bioreactor-grown bacillus of calmette and guérin (BCG) vaccine protects badgers against virulent *Mycobacterium bovis* when administered orally: Identifying limitations in baited vaccine delivery. *Pharmaceutics* 12, 782. DOI: 10.3390/pharmaceutics12080782.

Lin, P.L., Dietrich, J., Tan, E., Abalos, R.M., Burgos, J. *et al.* (2012) The multistage vaccine H56 boosts the effects of BCG to protect cynomolgus macaques against active tuberculosis and reactivation of latent *Mycobacterium tuberculosis* infection. *Journal of Clinical Investigation* 122, 303–314. DOI: 10.1172/JCI46252.

Lindenstrøm, T., Knudsen, N.P.H., Agger, E.M. and Andersen, P. (2013) Control of chronic *Mycobacterium tuberculosis* infection by CD4 KLRG1 – IL-2–Secreting central memory cells. *The Journal of Immunology* 190, 6311–6319. DOI: 10.4049/jimmunol.1300248.

Liu, S., Gong, Q., Wang, C., Liu, H., Wang, Y. *et al.* (2008) A novel DNA vaccine for protective immunity against virulent *Mycobacterium bovis* in mice. *Immunology Letters* 117, 136–145. DOI: 10.1016/j.imlet.2008.01.008.

Maggioli, M.F., Palmer, M., Thacker, T.C., Vordermeier, H.M., McGill, J.L. *et al.* (2016) Increased TNF-α/IFN-γ/IL-2 and decreased TNF-α/ IFN-γ production by central memory t cells are associated with protective responses against bovine tuberculosis following BCG vaccination. *Frontiers in Immunology* 7, 421. DOI: 10.3389/fimmu.2016.00421.

Mahairas, G.G., Sabo, P.J., Hickey, M.J., Singh, D.C. and Stover, C.K. (1996) Molecular analysis of genetic differences between *Mycobacterium bovis* BCG and virulent *M. bovis*. *Journal of Bacteriology* 178, 1274–1282. DOI: 10.1128/jb.178.5.1274-1282.1996.

Maue, A.C., Waters, W.R., Palmer, M., Whipple, D.L., Minion, F.C. *et al.* (2004) CD80 and CD86, but not CD154, augment DNA vaccine-induced protection in experimental bovine tuberculosis. *Vaccine* 23, 769–779. DOI: 10.1016/j.vaccine.2004.07.019.

Ni, J., Liu, Y., Hussain, T., Li, M., Liang, Z. *et al.* (2021) Recombinant ArgF PLGA nanoparticles enhances BCG induced immune responses against *Mycobacterium bovis* infection. *Biomedicine and Pharmacotherapy* 137, 111341. DOI: 10.1016/j.biopha.2021.111341.

Nol, P., Wehtje, M.E., Bowen, R.A., Robbe-Austerman, S., Thacker, T.C. *et al.* (2020) Effects of inactivated *Mycobacterium bovis* vaccination on molokai-origin wild pigs experimentally infected with virulent *M. bovis*. *Bovis. Pathogens* 9, 199. DOI: 10.3390/pathogens9030199.

Nugent, G., Yockney, I.J., Whitford, J., Aldwell, F.E. and Buddle, B.M. (2017) Efficacy of oral BCG vaccination in protecting free-ranging cattle from natural infection by *Mycobacterium bovis*. *Veternary Microbiology* 208, 181–189. DOI: 10.1016/j.vetmic.2017.07.029.

Nugent, G., Yockney, I.J., Cross, M.L. and Buddle, B.M. (2018) Low-dose BCG vaccination protects free-ranging cattle against naturally-acquired bovine tuberculosis. *Vaccine* 36, 7338–7344. DOI: 10.1016/j.vaccine.2018.10.025.

Ottenhoff, T.H.M. and Kaufmann, S.H.E. (2012) Vaccines against tuberculosis: Where are we and where do we need to go? *PLoS Pathogens* 8, e1002607. DOI: 10.1371/journal.ppat.1002607.

Parlane, N.A., Compton, B.J., Hayman, C.M., Painter, G.F., Basaraba, R.J. *et al.* (2012) Phosphatidylinositol di-mannoside and derivates modulate the immune response to and efficacy of a tuberculosis protein vaccine against *Mycobacterium bovis* infection. *Vaccine* 30, 580–588. DOI: 10.1016/j.vaccine.2011.11.055.

Retamal, P., Ábalos, P., Alegría-Morán, R., Valdivieso, N., Vordermeier, M. *et al.* (2022) Vaccination of Holstein heifers with *Mycobacterium bovis* BCG strain induces protection against bovine tuberculosis and higher milk production yields in a natural transmission setting. *Transboundary Emerging Diseases* 69, 1419–1425. DOI: 10.1111/tbed.14108.

Rizzi, C., Bianco, M.V., Blanco, F.C., Soria, M., Gravisaco, M.J. *et al.* (2012) Vaccination with a BCG strain overexpressing Ag85B protects cattle against *Mycobacterium bovis* challenge. *PLoS One* 7, e51396. DOI: 10.1371/journal.pone.0051396.

Robinson, R.T., Orme, I.M. and Cooper, A.M. (2015) The onset of adaptive immunity in the mouse model of tuberculosis and the factors that compromise its expression. *Immunological Reviews* 264, 46–59. DOI: 10.1111/imr.12259.

Roy, A., Tomé, I., Romero, B., Lorente-Leal, V., Infantes-Lorenzo, J.A. *et al.* (2019) Evaluation of the immunogenicity and efficacy of BCG and MTBVAC vaccines using a natural transmission model of tuberculosis. *Veterinary Research* 50, 82. DOI: 10.1186/s13567-019-0702-7.

Sabio y García, J., Bigi, M.M., Klepp, L.I., García, E.A., Blanco, F.C. *et al.* (2020) Does *Mycobacterium bovis* persist in cattle in a non-replicative latent state as *Mycobacterium tuberculosis* in human beings. *Veterinary Microbiology* 247, 108758. DOI: 10.1016/j.vetmic.2020.108758.

Sallin, M.A., Sakai, S., Kauffman, K.D., Young, H.A., Zhu, J. *et al.* (2017) Th1 differentiation drives the accumulation of intravascular, non-protective CD4 t cells during tuberculosis. *Cell Reports* 18, 3091–3104. DOI: 10.1016/j.celrep.2017.03.007.

Setiabudiawan, T.P., Reurink, R.K., Hill, P.C., Netea, M.G., Crevel, R. *et al.* (2022) Protection against tuberculosis by Bacillus Calmette-Guérin (BCG) vaccination: A historical perspective. *Med* 3, 6–24. DOI: 10.1016/j.medj.2021.11.006.

Skinner, M.A., Keen, D.L., Parlane, N.A., Yates, G.F. and Buddle, B.M. (2002) Increased protection against bovine tuberculosis in the Brushtail possum (*Trichosurus vulpecula*) when BCG is administered with killed *Mycobacterium vaccae*. *Tuberculosis* 82, 15–22. DOI: 10.1054/tube.2001.0318.

Skinner, M.A., Ramsay, A.J., Buchan, G.S., Keen, D.L., Ranasinghe, C. *et al.* (2003) A DNA prime-live vaccine boost strategy in mice can augment IFN-γ responses to mycobacterial antigens but does not increase the protective efficacy of two attenuated strains of *Mycobacterium bovis* against bovine tuberculosis. *Immunology* 108, 548–555. DOI: 10.1046/j.1365-2567.2003.01589.x.

Skinner, M.A., Wedlock, D.N., de Lisle, G.W., Cooke, M.M., Tascon, R.E. *et al.* (2005) The order of prime-boost vaccination of neonatal calves with *Mycobacterium bovis* BCG and a DNA vaccine encoding mycobacterial proteins Hsp65, Hsp70, and Apa is not critical for enhancing protection against bovine tuberculosis. *Infection and Immunity* 73, 4441–4444. DOI: 10.1128/IAI.73.7.4441-4444.2005.

Smith, A.A., Villarreal-Ramos, B., Mendum, T.A., Williams, K.J., Jones, G.J. *et al.* (2020) Genetic screening for the protective antigenic targets of BCG vaccination. *Tuberculosis* 124, 101979. DOI: 10.1016/j.tube.2020.101979.

Sterne, J.A.C., Rodrigues, L.C. and Guedes, I.N. (1998) Does the efficacy of BCG decline with time since vaccination? *The International Journal of Tuberculosis and Lung Disease* 2, 200–207. Available at: https://www.ingentaconnect.com/content/iuatld/ijtld/1998/00000002/00000003;jsessionid=8p05m39kaq4ja.x-ic-live-03)

Tait, D.R., Hatherill, M., van der Meeren, O., Ginsberg, A.M., Van Brakel, E. *et al.* (2019) Final analysis of a trial of M72/AS01 e vaccine to prevent tuberculosis. *New England Journal of Medicine* 381, 2429–2439. DOI: 10.1056/nejmoa1909953.

Tameris, M., Mearns, H., Penn-Nicholson, A., Gregg, Y., Bilek, N. *et al.* (2019) Live-attenuated mycobacterium tuberculosis vaccine MTBVAC versus BCG in adults and neonates: A randomised controlled, double-blind dose-escalation trial. *Lancet Respiratory Medicine* 7, 757–770. DOI: 10.1016/S2213-2600(19)30251-6.

Tanner, R., Villarreal-Ramos, B., Vordermeier, H.M. and McShane, H. (2019) The humoral immune response to BCG vaccination. *Frontiers in Immunology* 10, 1317. DOI: 10.3389/fimmu.2019.01317.

Thacker, T.C., Palmer, M.V. and Waters, W.R. (2007) Associations between cytokine gene expression and pathology in *Mycobacterium bovis* infected cattle. *Veterinary Immunology and Immunopathology* 119, 204–213. DOI: 10.1016/j.vetimm.2007.05.009.

TuBerculosis Vaccine Initiative (TBVI) (2015). Available at: https://www.tbvi.eu/ (accessed 14 March 2023).

Viale, M.N., Zumárraga, M.J., Araújo, F.R., Zarraga, A.M., Cataldi, A.A. *et al.* (2016) The genomics of mycobacteria. *Scientific and Technical Review. International Office of Epizootics* 35, 215–240. DOI: 10.20506/rst.35.1.2429.

Vordermeier, H.M., Chambers, M.A., Buddle, B.M., Pollock, J.M. and Hewinson, R.G. (2006) Progress in the development of vaccines and diagnostic reagents to control tuberculosis in cattle. *Veterinary Journal* 171, 229–244. DOI: 10.1016/j.tvjl.2004.11.001.

Vordermeier, H.M., Villarreal-Ramos, B., Cockle, P.J., McAulay, M., Rhodes, S.G. *et al.* (2009) Viral booster vaccines improve *Mycobacterium bovis* BCG-induced protection against bovine tuberculosis. *Infection and Immunity* 77, 3364–3373. DOI: 10.1128/IAI.00287-09.

Vordermeier, H.M., Pérez de Val, B., Buddle, B.M., Villarreal-Ramos, B., Jones, G.J. *et al.* (2014) Vaccination of domestic animals against tuberculosis: Review of progress and contributions to the field of the TBSTEP project. *Research in Veterinary Science* 97, S53–60. DOI: 10.1016/j.rvsc.2014.04.015.

Vordermeier, H.M., Jones, G.J., Buddle, B.M. and Hewinson, R.G. (2016a) Development of immune-diagnostic reagents to diagnose bovine tuberculosis in cattle. *Veterinary Immunology and Immunopathology* 181, 10–14. DOI: 10.1016/j.vetimm.2016.02.003.

Vordermeier, H.M., Jones, G.J., Buddle, B.M., Hewinson, R.G. and Villarreal-Ramos, B. (2016b) Bovine tuberculosis in cattle: Vaccines, DIVA tests, and host biomarker discovery. *Annual Review of Animal Biosciences* 4, 87–109. DOI: 10.1146/annurev-animal-021815-111311.

Waters, W.R., Palmer, M., Nonnecke, B.J., Thacker, T.C., Scherer, C.F.C. *et al.* (2009) Efficacy and immunogenicity of *Mycobacterium bovis* δRD1 against aerosol *M. bovis* infection in neonatal calves. *Vaccine* 27, 1201–1209. DOI: 10.1016/j.vaccine.2008.12.018.

Waters, W.R., Palmer, M.V., Buddle, B.M. and Vordermeier, H.M. (2012) *Bovine tuberculosis* vaccine research: Historical perspectives and recent advances. *Vaccine* 30, 2611–2622. DOI: 10.1016/j.vaccine.2012.02.018.

Waters, W.R., Maggioli, M.F., Palmer, M.V., Thacker, T.C., McGill, J.L. *et al.* (2016) Interleukin-17A as a biomarker for bovine tuberculosis. *Clinical and Vaccine Immunology* 23, 168–180. DOI: 10.1128/CVI.00637-15.

Wedlock, D.N., Skinner, M.A., Parlane, N.A., Vordermeier, H.M., Hewinson, R.G. *et al.* (2003) Vaccination with DNA vaccines encoding MPB70 or MPB83 or a MPB70 DNA prime-protein boost does not protect cattle against bovine tuberculosis. *Tuberculosis* 83, 339–349. DOI: 10.1016/S1472-9792(03)00055-6.

Wedlock, D.N., Denis, M., Skinner, M.A., Koach, J., Lisle, G.W. *et al.* (2005a) Vaccination of cattle with a CpG oligodeoxynucleotide-formulated mycobacterial protein vaccine and *Mycobacterium bovis* BCG induces levels of protection against bovine tuberculosis superior to those induced by vaccination with BCG alone. *Infection and Immunity* 73, 3540–3546. DOI: 10.1128/IAI.73.6.3540-3546.2005.

Wedlock, D.N., Skinner, M.A., Lisle, G.W., Vordermeier, H.M., Hewinson, R.G. *et al.* (2005b) Vaccination of cattle with *Mycobacterium bovis* culture filtrate proteins and CpG oligodeoxynucleotides induces protection against bovine tuberculosis. *Veterinary Immunology and Immunopathology* 106, 53–63. DOI: 10.1016/j.vetimm.2005.01.002.

Whitlow, E., Mustafa, A.S. and Hanif, S.N.M. (2020) An overview of the development of new vaccines for tuberculosis. *Vaccines* 8, 586. DOI: 10.3390/vaccines8040586.

11 How Agricultural Practices Affect the Risk of Human Contamination by Infectious Pathogens: The Need for a 'One Health' Perspective

Alain Ratnadass[1,2]* and Samira Sarter[3,4]

[1]CIRAD, UPR Aïda, F-97410 Saint-Pierre, Réunion, France; [2]Aïda, Univ Montpellier, CIRAD, Montpellier, France; [3]CIRAD, UMR ISEM, F-34398 Montpellier, France; [4]ISEM, Univ Montpellier, CNRS, EPHE, IRD, Montpellier, France

Abstract

We conducted a comprehensive literature review with a global geographic scope, of interactions between agricultural crop production practices (excluding crop protection practices) and biological human health hazards. The majority of relevant references dealt with bacterial contaminations and infections, largely due to the important public health issue of antibiotic resistance. Indicator coliforms were particularly significant (only a minority mentioned harmful *Escherichia coli* strains), followed by species belonging to *Salmonella*, *Campylobacter*, *Clostridia*, *Pseudomonas*, and *Listeria* genera. Protozoan *Cryptosporidium* spp. and *Giardia* spp., and helminthic *Ascaris* spp. and *Trichuris* spp. dominated the references to parasites. Enteric viruses largely dominated the references to viruses (particularly noroviruses and rotaviruses). Very few references mentioned human fungal pathogens. Fresh vegetables were the most commonly mentioned crops, particularly leafy greens and those eaten raw, due to the use of wastewater for irrigation, and fertilization with livestock manure and human excreta/sewage sludge, potentially unsafe practices. While earlier literature reviews have shown that crop protection practices are central to the One Health concept, this review shows that other agricultural practices can also contribute to human and environmental health *via* different pathways, including better soil health, water quality, better food safety, and human nutrition. Our review underlines that besides tradeoffs, synergies should be sought, between, on the one hand, saving/preserving freshwater and organic waste recycling (affecting environmental health and some aspects of human health), and health hazards associated with the use of potentially contaminated waste on the other (affecting other aspects of human health), from both agroecological and One Health perspectives.

Keywords: bacteria, parasites, antibiotic resistance, wastewater, livestock manure, human excreta, sewage sludge

Introduction

The agricultural sector contributes greatly to human health and well-being, notably *via* the provision of safe food of high nutritional quality in sufficient quantities. However, some agricultural practices may have adverse effects on human health, either *via* intoxication or

*Corresponding author: alain.ratnadass@cirad.fr

poisoning (e.g. pesticides, mycotoxins) or by favoring infectious diseases (e.g. zoonoses) (Han *et al.*, 2016). Indeed, the growth of agriculture and the intensification of livestock farming have been shown to increase pathogen emergence and transmission at the wildlife–livestock–human interface (Jones *et al.*, 2013). For instance, recent viral zoonotic epidemics have been ascribed to human activities, including agricultural practices (Jones *et al.*, 2013; Morand *et al.*, 2019; Plowright *et al.*, 2021). As for animal farming, it was estimated that of the 202 EIZDs (emerging infectious zoonotic diseases) identified between 1940 and 2004, 74 (36.6%) were associated with animals kept for food production, with 70.3% caused by bacteria, 13.5% by viruses and the remaining 16.2% by protozoa, fungi or helminths (Otte and Pica-Ciamarra, 2021). Contamination of water resources by these infectious pathogens of humans constitutes a high public health burden throughout the world (Jones *et al.*, 2008; Pandey *et al.*, 2014). The importance of a global 'One Health' (OH) approach to control waterborne pathogens and microbial hazards associated with agriculture has been underlined; this will address these challenges from multiple perspectives (FAO *et al.*, 2020; Otte and Pica-Ciamarra, 2021).

It should be noted that plant health was never fully part of the OH concept, which mainly encompasses human, animal, and environmental health. The inclusion of ecosystem health has so far pertained mainly to that of wild fauna as potential or confirmed reservoirs of zoonotic diseases (Destoumieux-Garzón *et al.*, 2018). While wild plants are considered part of natural ecosystems, cultivated plants (or crops) within agroecosystems are largely ignored (van Bruggen *et al.*, 2019). Some organizational efforts have been made to bring plant and animal health together under the OH framework, e.g. Plant Clinics promoted by CABI (Boa *et al.*, 2015; Rushton *et al.*, 2018; Danielsen *et al.*, 2019), or shared methodological approaches, e.g. the impact of biodiversity on human and animal health, and plant health (Van Bruggen and Finckh, 2016; Ratnadass *et al.*, 2021).

With a view to better integration of crop (plant) health into the OH concept, we conducted a series of literature reviews on the interactions between crop protection (CP) practices and human infectious diseases, which, to the best of our knowledge, had never been done before. These reviews pertained to viral zoonotic diseases (Ratnadass and Deguine, 2021), bacterial diseases (Ratnadass and Deberdt, 2021), parasitic diseases (Ratnadass and Martin, 2022), and fungal diseases (Ratnadass and Sester, 2023) of humans.

Not all agricultural practices were considered in these reviews, and only those that explicitly aim for better plant health *via* alleviation of crop pest and pathogen aggressions were considered. However, agricultural practices not aimed at CP *per se* have been reported to have impacts on infectious disease risk to humans. Indeed, many such agricultural practices may affect plant health by indirectly affecting pests or pathogens (or their natural enemies), while others may affect plant health as they have a beneficial effect on plant physiology, directly or indirectly *via* what is referred to as 'soil health' (Lehmann *et al.*, 2020). A comprehensive review was conducted to analyze the interactions between agricultural practices aimed at crop production other than CP practices, and risks of human exposure to viral, bacterial, parasitic, or fungal pathogenic agents. After describing the review methodology, we summarize the general bibliometrics: type of pathogens, geographical scope of reviewed papers and crops, with a focus on general levers driving human exposure to pathogens. We then review each of these levers in depth, by type of pathogen, associated risks of human exposure, and levers for mitigating the specific type of hazard exposure. Finally, we discuss the outcomes of our review against those of our earlier reviews on CP practices and against other references relevant to the topic that did not emerge from our systematic review.

Review Methodology

The data source for this study was Clarivate Analytics' Web of Science Core collection (WoSCC) (Clarivate Analytics, 2021). A systematic review was performed in July 2022. The search equation used was ('agricultur*' OR 'crop*' OR 'farm*') AND ('practic*' OR 'manag*' OR 'irrig*' OR 'fertil*' OR 'manur*' OR 'deforest*') AND ('infectio*' OR 'diseas*'

OR 'pathoge*') AND ('huma*' OR 'medic*' OR 'public') AND ('health') AND ('vir*' OR 'parasit*' OR 'bacteri*' OR 'fung*').

The terms of the equation were chosen based on references that emerged during our previous reviews on crop protection (Ratnadass and Deguine, 2021; Ratnadass and Deberdt, 2021; Ratnadass and Martin, 2022; Ratnadass and Sester, 2023). No restrictions were placed on publication date or language.

The second step was to review the relevance of all references (both research and review articles) based on their title and abstract, then on the full text. References dealing specifically with CP were discarded as those aspects had been covered by our previous reviews (e.g. Léchenault-Bergerot *et al.*, 2019; Fraaije *et al.*, 2020).

Results

General bibliometrics

The query resulted in a total of 2178 references. Of these, we identified a total of 242 (174 research articles and 68 review articles) as relevant. A publication was considered as relevant if it actually addressed, at least partly, the effects of agricultural practices other than those specifically aiming at crop pest or pathogen control, on exposure to human infectious diseases.

Types of pathogens

Both types of articles focused primarily on bacteria, followed by parasites and viruses (at par), with barely any references to fungi (Fig. 11.1). Some references dealt with multiple pathogens. Evidently, quite a few references dealt with two types of pathogens. Only two research articles dealt with bacteria, parasites, and viruses however, while nine review articles dealt with these three types of pathogens.

BACTERIUM GENERA/SPECIES. One hundred and thirteen research articles and 45 review articles dealt with bacteria. The main genera (namely the 20 first most cited, in at least four articles) addressed in both research and review articles are shown in Fig. 11.2. Nine research articles did not refer to any particular genus of bacterium (Duan *et al.*, 2017; Cui *et al.*, 2018; Gou *et al.*, 2018; Bougnom *et al.*, 2020; Cui *et al.*, 2020; Sun *et al.*, 2020; Xu *et al.*, 2021; Bech *et al.*, 2022; Zhang *et al.*, 2022) as well as 11 review articles (Williams-Nguyen *et al.*, 2016; Youngquist *et al.*, 2016; Such *et al.*, 2019; Urra *et al.*, 2019; Checcucci *et al.*, 2020; He *et al.*, 2020; Iwu *et al.*, 2020; Inyinbor *et al.*, 2021; Sorinolu *et al.*, 2021; Miller *et al.*, 2022; Wang *et al.*, 2022). These 20 articles pertained to antimicrobial resistance (AMR), with references to genes rather than specific bacterial organisms.

A majority of articles pertained to coliforms [particularly fecal coliforms (FC) such as *E. coli*], not necessarily pathogenic but rather commensal, used as microbial indicators of fecal contamination (hence, the potential presence of other pathogens). Some papers focused specifically on the relevance of such microbial indicators (e.g. Blumenthal *et al.*, 2000; Campos, 2008; Jokinen *et al.*, 2020). Those pertaining exclusively to pathogenic, virulent or antibiotic-resistant (ABR) *E. coli* (e.g. EHEC O157:H7, including the Shiga toxin-producing pathotypes (STEC), or commensal *E. coli* with virulence genes, or with ABR), were much less numerous: Only 26 research articles (Duffy *et al.*, 2004; Westrell *et al.*, 2004; Williams *et al.*, 2006; Trang *et al.* (2007); Duriez *et al.*, 2008; Hutchison *et al.*, 2008; Forslund *et al.*, 2011; Fahrenfeld *et al.*, 2013; Olivieri *et al.*, 2014; Du Plessis *et al.*, 2015; Scheinemann *et al.*, 2015; Givens *et al.*, 2016; Jongman and Korsten, 2016b; Mikhail *et al.*, 2018; Ye *et al.*, 2018; Chen *et al.*, 2019; Miller *et al.*, 2019; O'Flaherty *et al.*, 2019; Deepnarain *et al.*, 2020; Eissenberger *et al.*, 2020; Touati *et al.*, 2020; Amato *et al.*, 2021; Nag *et al.*, 2021; Bonetta *et al.*, 2022; Fatoba *et al.*, 2022; Iwu *et al.*, 2022) and 16 review articles (Geldreich, 1996; Jones, 1999; Bicudo and Goyal, 2003; Heinonen-Tanski *et al.*, 2006; Avery *et al.*, 2012; Uyttendaele *et al.*, 2015; Fijalkowski *et al.*, 2017; Adegoke *et al.*, 2018; Alegbeleye *et al.*, 2018; Al-Gheethi *et al.*, 2018; Iwu and Okoh, 2019; Kintz *et al.*, 2019; Nag *et al.*, 2019; Alegbeleye and Sant'Ana, 2020; Zalewska *et al.*, 2021; Lin *et al.*, 2022) were linked to these phenomena.

As regards *Salmonella*, 21 research articles and 13 review articles referred only to *Salmonella* spp., which is also used as a microbial indicator, but considered as pathogenic. They were thus

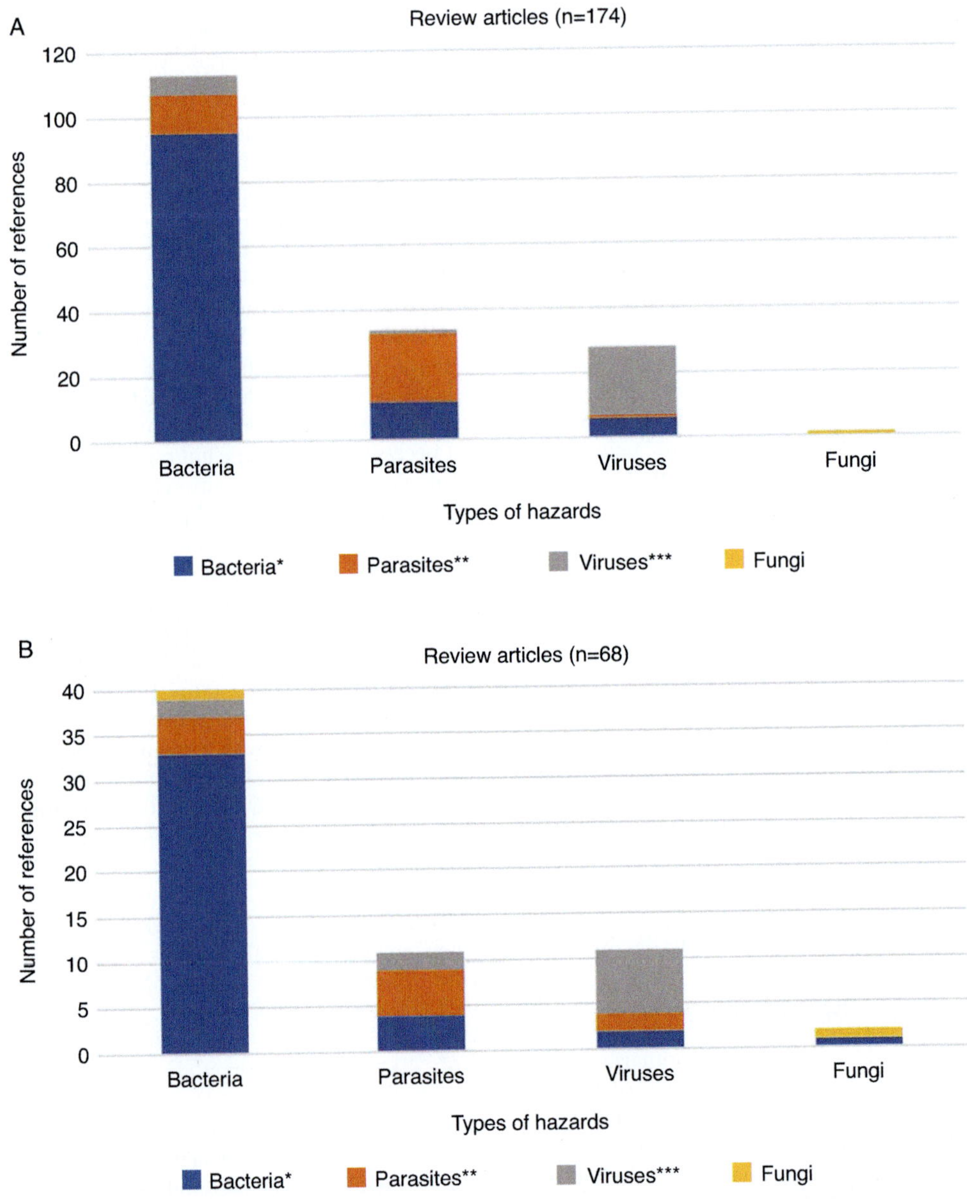

Fig. 11.1. Distribution of references [both research (a) and review (b) articles] across types of human biological hazards. * Bacteria (alone when in the bacteria bar, along with other pathogen types when in other bars). ** Parasites (alone when in the parasites bar, along with other pathogen types when in other bars). *** Viruses (alone when in the viruses bar, along with other pathogen types when in other bars)

at par with pathogenic, or potentially human infectious *E. coli*. However, the highly pathogenic *S. enterica* was also addressed in two research articles (Hutchison *et al.*, 2008; Obayomi *et al.*, 2019) and one review article (Uyttendaele *et al.*, 2015), as well as serovar *S.* Typhimurium, in one review article (Bicudo and Goyal, 2003).

As regards *Campylobacter* spp., highly pathogenic *C. jejuni* was specifically mentioned in three research articles (Hutchison *et al.*, 2008;

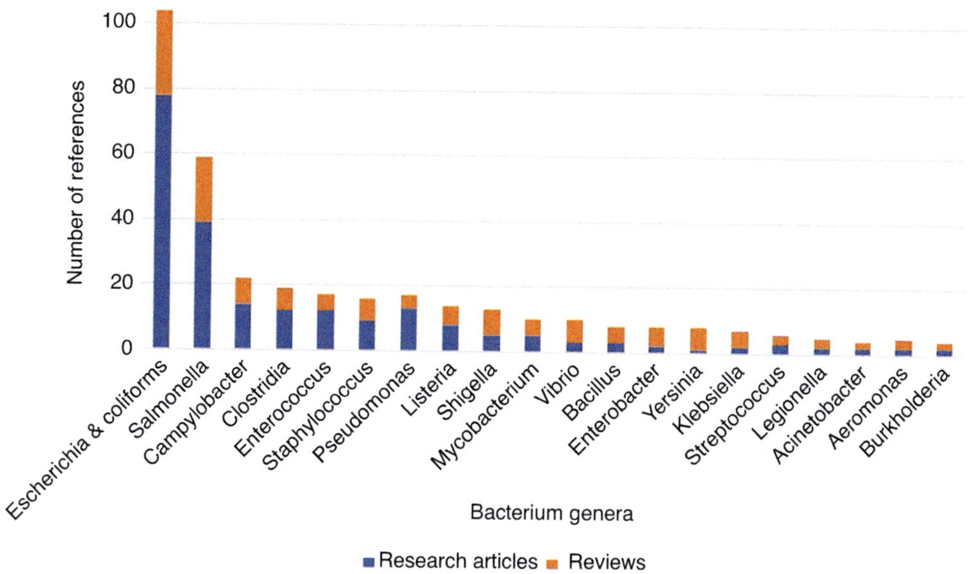

Fig. 11.2. Main bacterium genera addressed in selected references (*n*=158).

Forslund *et al.*, 2011; Givens *et al.*, 2016) and two review articles (Bicudo and Goyal, 2003; Zhao and Liu, 2019). Regarding *Clostridia*, three research articles (Barbour *et al.*, 2002; Scheinemann *et al.*, 2015; Le Maréchal *et al.*, 2019) and three review articles (Al-Gheethi *et al.*, 2018; Zhao and Liu, 2019; Alegbeleye and Sant'Ana, 2020) referred to *C. perfringens*, while three research articles referred to *Clostridioides difficile* (Le Maréchal *et al.*, 2019; Kabelitz *et al.*, 2020; Kabelitz *et al.*, 2021).

Regarding enterococci, three research articles referred to pathogenic strains (Givens *et al.*, 2016; Kabelitz *et al.*, 2020; Kabelitz *et al.*, 2021), the latter two articles focused specifically on antibiotic-resistant strains, the first on *Enterococcus faecalis*. The *Staphylococcus* genus was mainly represented by *S. aureus* (five research articles: (Barbour *et al.*, 2002; Scheinemann *et al.*, 2015; Givens *et al.*, 2016; Kabelitz *et al.*, 2020; Kabelitz *et al.*, 2021), the latter two focusing on antibiotic-resistant strains.

The *Pseudomonas* genus was mainly represented by *P. aeruginosa*, with one review article (Ramakrishna *et al.*, 2019), and five research articles (Fahrenfeld *et al.*, 2013; Ye *et al.*, 2018; Obayomi *et al.*, 2019; Kabelitz *et al.*, 2020; Cruz *et al.*, 2021), the latter two focusing on antibiotic-resistant strains. *Listeria* spp. were mentioned in eight research articles and six review articles; pathogenic *L. monocytogenes* were specifically addressed in six research articles (Du Plessis *et al.*, 2015; Scheinemann *et al.*, 2015; Jongman and Korsten, 2016a; Allard *et al.*, 2019; Kabelitz *et al.*, 2020; Nag *et al.*, 2021) and three review articles (Alegbeleye *et al.*, 2018; Iwu and Okoh, 2019; Alegbeleye and Sant'Ana, 2020). It should also be noted that *Clostridia* were sometimes used as surrogate microbial indicators for sporulating protozoa.

PARASITE (PROTOZOA AND HELMINTHS) GENERA. Parasite genera (protozoa and helminths) addressed in both research and review articles are shown in Fig. 11.3. Four references mentioned only 'helminth eggs', as indicators of contamination, without reference to specific genera (*viz* Mirhosseini *et al.*, 2008; Forslund *et al.*, 2012; Fuhrimann *et al.*, 2016a; de França *et al.*, 2021).

VIRUS GENERA. Virus genera addressed in both research and review articles are shown in Fig. 11.4.

Enteric viruses, encompassing the first five genera (namely *Norovirus*, *Rotavirus*, *Mastadenovirus*, *Hepatovirus*, and *Enterovirus*),

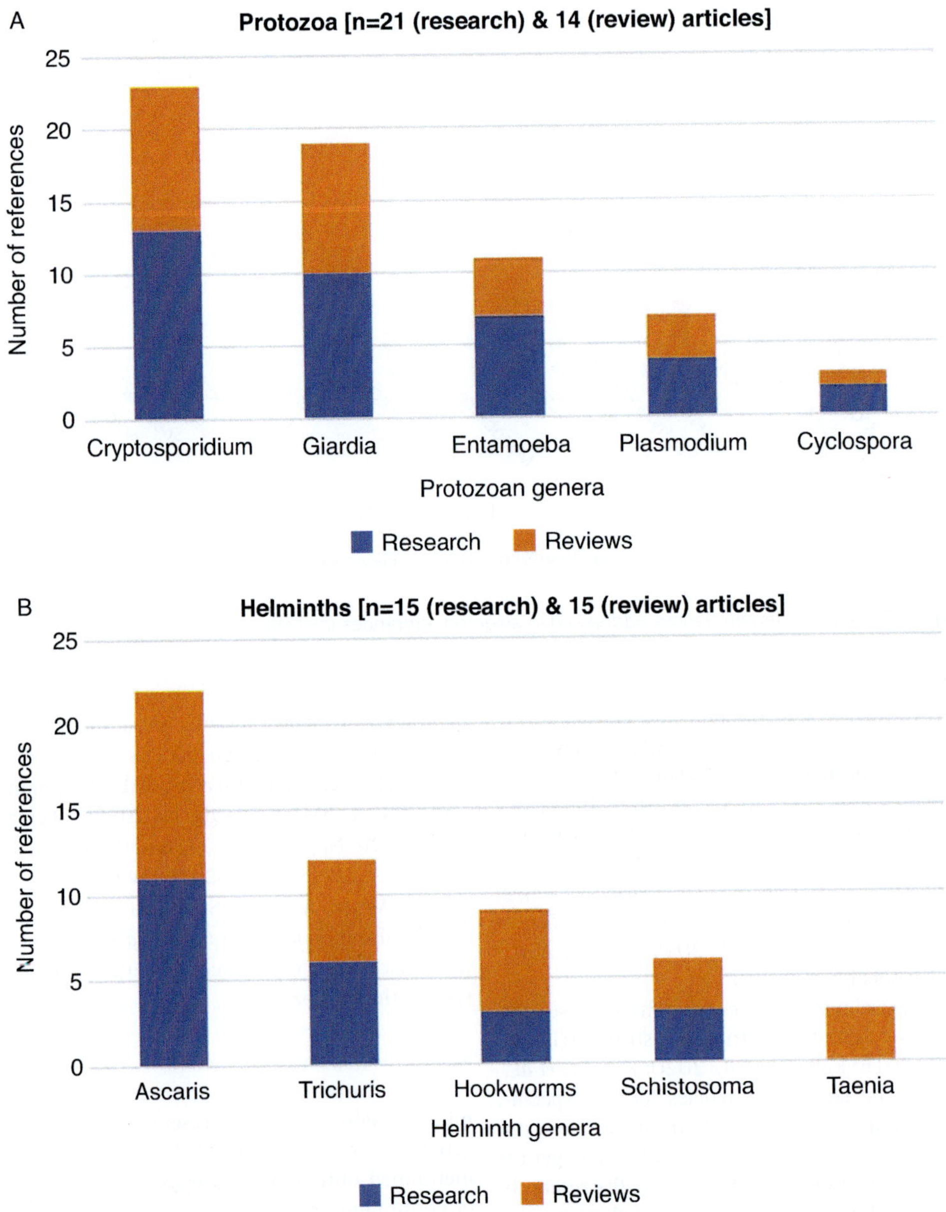

Fig. 11.3. Distribution of references (both research and review articles) across human parasitic pathogen genera (*n*=33), both protozoan (a) and helminthic (b). Note: 'Hookworms' may signify either *Ancylostoma duodenale* or *Necator americanus*.

were largely dominant, particularly *Norovirus* (Campos, 2008; Wei and Kniel, 2010; Mok *et al.*, 2014; Lim *et al.*, 2015; Uyttendaele *et al.*, 2015; Beaudequin *et al.*, 2016; Courault *et al.*, 2017; Jaramillo and Restrepo, 2017; Kobayashi *et al.*, 2017; Adegoke *et al.*, 2018; Alegbeleye *et al.*, 2018; Chandrasekaran and Jiang, 2018; Prez *et al.*, 2018; Gonzales-Gustavson *et al.*, 2019; Nag *et al.*, 2019; Chacón *et al.*, 2020; Alam and Ali, 2021; Nag *et al.*, 2021; Ofori

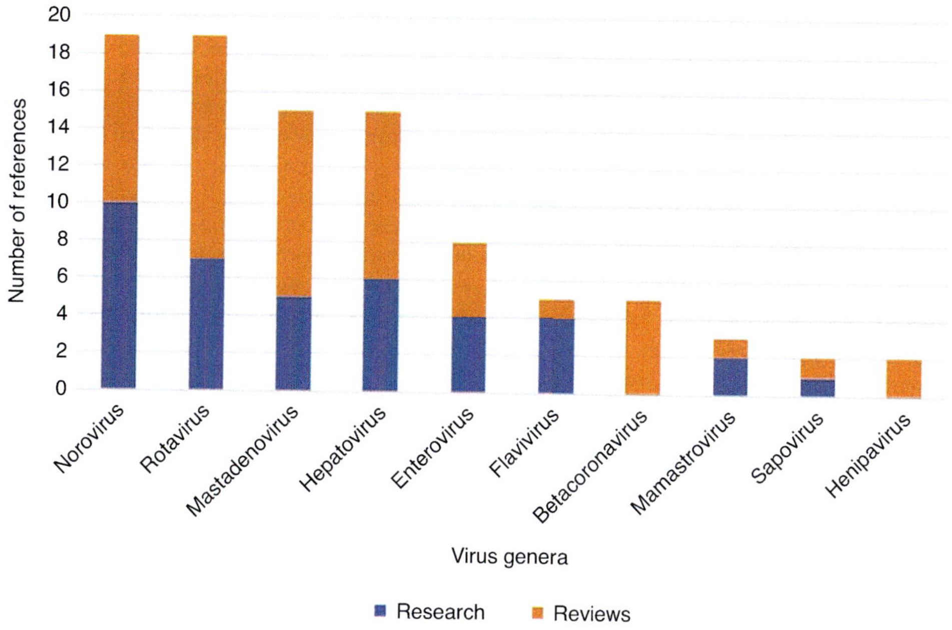

Fig. 11.4. Distribution of main references across human viral pathogen genera: research (*n*=27) and review (*n*=18) articles

et al., 2021) and *Rotavirus* (Höglund *et al.*, 2002; Hamilton *et al.*, 2007; Campos, 2008; Wei and Kniel, 2010; García *et al.*, 2013; Pavione *et al.*, 2013; Anchang *et al.*, 2014; Bischel *et al.*, 2015; Uyttendaele *et al.*, 2015; Jaramillo and Restrepo, 2017; Kobayashi *et al.*, 2017; Adegoke *et al.*, 2018; Alegbeleye *et al.*, 2018; Prez *et al.*, 2018; Alegbeleye and Sant'Ana, 2020; Chacón *et al.*, 2020; Alam and Ali, 2021; Ofori *et al.*, 2021), at par. The *Mastadenovirus* genus that encompasses human adenoviruses followed (Hamilton *et al.*, 2007; Campos, 2008; Wei and Kniel, 2010; Bischel *et al.*, 2015; Uyttendaele *et al.*, 2015; Jaramillo and Restrepo, 2017; Adegoke *et al.*, 2018; Fongaro *et al.*, 2018; Gonzales-Gustavson *et al.*, 2019; Nag *et al.*, 2019; Zhao and Liu, 2019; Alegbeleye and Sant'Ana, 2020; Alam and Ali, 2021; Ofori *et al.*, 2021; Gholipour *et al.*, 2022), at par with the *Hepatovirus* genus.

The *Hepatovirus* genus was mainly represented by Hepatitis A (Hamilton *et al.*, 2007; Campos, 2008; Wei and Kniel, 2010; Uyttendaele *et al.*, 2015; Jaramillo and Restrepo, 2017; Kobayashi *et al.*, 2017; Alegbeleye *et al.*, 2018; Nag *et al.*, 2019; Alegbeleye and Sant'Ana, 2020; Chacón *et al.*, 2020; Alam and Ali, 2021; Ofori *et al.*, 2021) and Hepatitis E viruses (Wei and Kniel, 2010; García *et al.*, 2013; Givens *et al.*, 2016; Jaramillo and Restrepo, 2017; Kobayashi *et al.*, 2017; Moazeni *et al.*, 2017; Alegbeleye and Sant'Ana, 2020; Ofori *et al.*, 2021). The *Enterovirus* genus encompassed *Enterovirus* (Campos, 2008; Kobayashi *et al.*, 2017; Prez *et al.*, 2018; Zhao and Liu, 2019; Chacón *et al.*, 2020), *Poliovirus* (Hamilton *et al.*, 2007), and *Coxsackievirus* (Alegbeleye *et al.*, 2018; Alegbeleye and Sant'Ana, 2020) viruses. The *Flavivirus* genus encompassed mainly the West Nile virus (responsible for Japanese encephalitis) (Ghimire and Dhakal, 2015; Marcantonio *et al.*, 2015; Tian *et al.*, 2015) and Dengue viruses (Catenacci *et al.*, 2021; Gregory *et al.*, 2022). The *Betacoronavirus* genus was mainly represented by SARS-Cov-2 (Zhao and Liu, 2019; Alam and Ali, 2021; Mancuso *et al.*, 2021; Ofori *et al.*, 2021; Usman *et al.*, 2021).

One should note that bacterial phages (particularly coliphages) were also sometimes used as surrogate microbial indicators for enteric viruses (Höglund *et al.*, 2002; Campos, 2008; Decrey *et al.*, 2011; Forslund *et al.*, 2011; Young *et al.*, 2016; Fongaro *et al.*, 2018; Chacón *et al.*,

2020). There were also six references (not shown in Fig. 11.4) with unspecified virus genera (Petterson *et al.*, 2001; Munoz *et al.*, 2010Van Ginneken and Oron, 2000; Okubo *et al.*, 2019; Summerlin III *et al.*, 2021; Singh, 2021).

FUNGUS GENERA. There were only three mentions of human pathogenic fungi in research articles, namely *Candida* (de Oliveira *et al.*, 2016; Lüneberg *et al.*, 2019) and *Cryptococcus* (Jongman and Korsten, 2016a), and two in review articles, specifically *Histoplasma* (Jayasvati and Jayasvati, 2018) and *Aspergillus* (Avery *et al.*, 2012). Many articles referring to *Aspergillus fumigatus* were discarded since they pertained to AMR induced by the use of azole fungicides (as crop protection), e.g. (Léchenault-Bergerot *et al.*, 2019; Fraaije *et al.*, 2020; Garcia-Rubio *et al.*, 2021), which had already been included in one of our earlier reviews (Ratnadass and Sester, 2023).

Geographical scope

Research was mainly conducted in the USA, China, and South Africa (≥10 references each), but also in Spain, Israel, Iran, Brazil, Australia, Germany, the UK and Vietnam (≥5 references from each of these countries) (Fig. 11.5). A few articles covered several countries, in which case each country concerned was allotted a fraction. Only one article referred to 'Europe' as a whole (Fongaro *et al.*, 2018).

These figures pertain only to research articles since reviews had a wider scope, with a small number having a more limited scope, *viz.* one targeting 'arid and semi-arid regions' (Bernstein, 2011), another 'low-income nations', with a focus on sub-Saharan Africa (Inyinbor *et al.*, 2021), the 'Middle East' (Al-Gheethi *et al.*, 2018), 'Latin America' (Domínguez *et al.*, 2021), and 'the European Union' (Such *et al.*, 2019), and only seven were country-specific, with scopes limited to, respectively, Bolivia (Verbyla *et al.*, 2015), Canada (Topp *et al.*, 2009), Chile (Geldreich, 1996), Ireland (Nag *et al.*, 2019), Spain (Herrero-Cófreces *et al.*, 2021), the UK (Jones, 1999), and the USA (Oliver *et al.*, 2020).

It should be noted that research on bacteria was predominant in most countries, particularly in the Global North (e.g. USA), while parasites

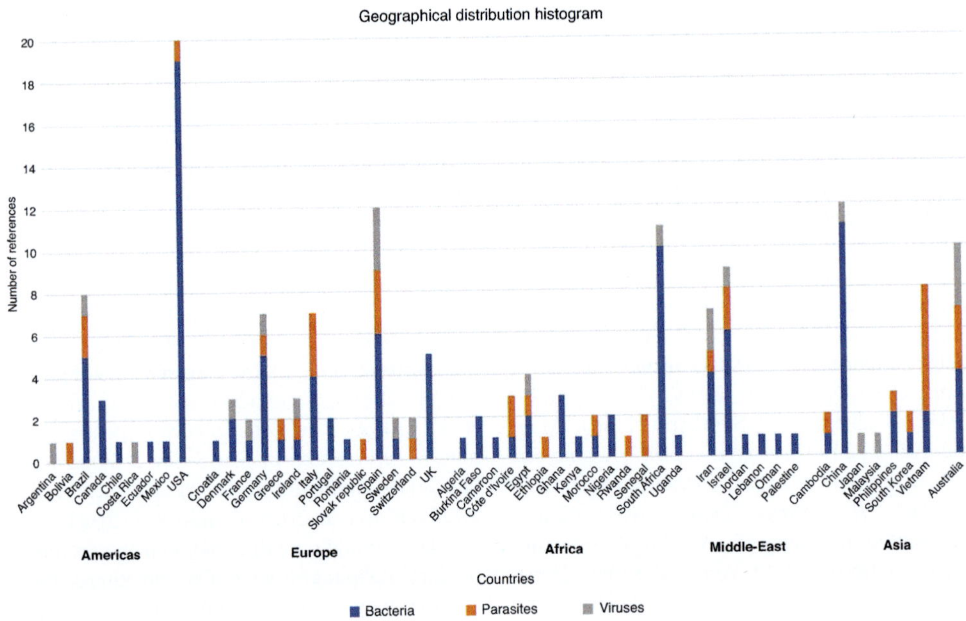

Fig. 11.5. Geographical distribution of research articles dealing with bacteria, parasites, and viruses, identified for this review (*n*=173).

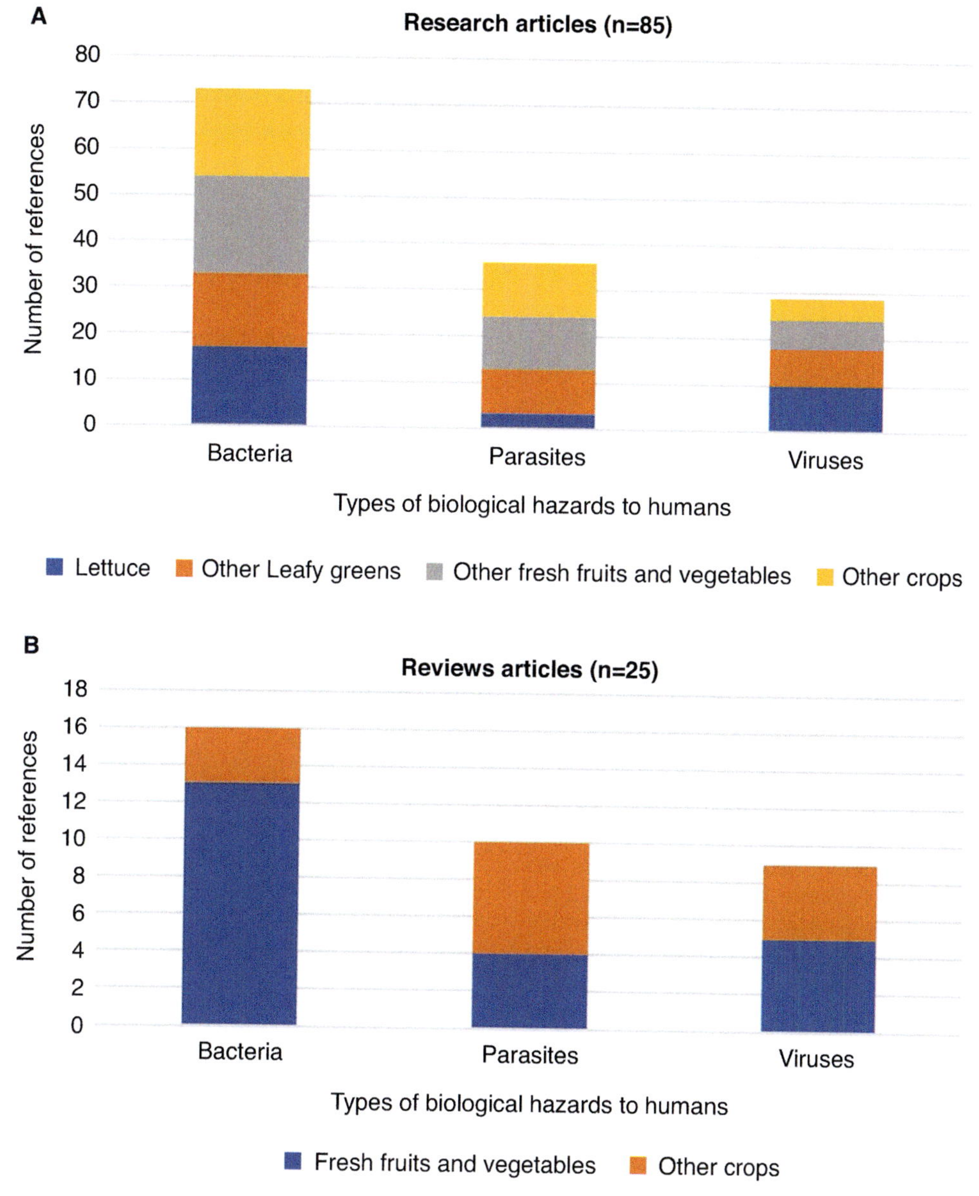

Fig. 11.6. Main crops addressed in both research (a) and review (b) articles.

were more present in the Global South, particularly in Vietnam.

Crops

Crops (either groups of crops or specific crops) addressed in both research and review articles are shown in Fig. 11.6.

For bacterial pathogens, of the 73 mentions of crops in research articles, 54 pertained to vegetable crops, of which 33 pertained to leafy greens (including 17, which focused specifically on lettuce (and to a lesser extent other salad crops, cabbage and pakchoi)). Thirteen mentions were made to grass food or forage crops (mainly maize), one to a flower crop (roses) and two to fruit tree crops (apple and nectarine). Many articles did not refer to crops, mainly those dealing with antibiotic resistance, or treatment of wastewater, animal manure, human waste, and sewage sludge. Similarly, many review articles did not refer to crops (for the same reason as research articles), while 13 mentions were made of fresh vegetables and fruits, and three to grass food or forage crops.

Thus, vegetable crops, namely leafy greens and eaten raw (and to a lesser extent soft fruits), are the most at risk in terms of food safety, since the major hazard is linked to by-products such as the use of wastewater (or surface water contaminated by wastewater) for irrigation, and animal or human waste as a fertilizer.

Similarly, for parasites, 36 research articles mentioned crops. Twenty-four pertained to vegetable crops, of which 13 focused mainly on leafy greens (three of which lettuce). Of the review articles, three out of the 10 mentioned vegetable crops, one fresh fruits, and one, a spice (cardamom).

For viruses, 28 research articles mentioned crops. Vegetables were largely dominant, with 24 mentions, of which 18 mentioned leafy greens, and 10 lettuce specifically. As for other crops, there was only one mention each for lucerne, maize, potato, and rice. Viruses were mentioned in nine review articles, of which fresh fruits and vegetables accounted for five, with no further details, except for mango. Other crops were mentioned once each, namely palm, maize, soybean, and rice. With regard to fungi, only one research article mentioned crops, namely forage crops (Lüneberg *et al.*, 2019).

Overall, fresh vegetables were the most prevalent crops, particularly leafy greens and those eaten raw (particularly lettuce), due to the dominance of wastewater/sewage sludge/livestock manure concerns. The presence of water bodies for irrigation and deforestation pertained respectively to rice and maize/soybean, and to some perennial crops.

Levers

The main lever addressed in both research and review articles was the use of wastewater for irrigation, followed by the use of livestock manure as a fertilizer. The use of human excreta or sewage sludge for fertilization came in third, followed by the use of other organic amendments for fertilization (Fig. 11.7). Conversely, the presence of water bodies for irrigation as a source of human contamination by pathogens with invertebrate vectors or reservoirs was in a minority. This was the same for some of those related to deforestation.

Major outcomes

Use of wastewater for crop irrigation

PATHOGENIC BACTERIA

Associated risk of human exposure to pathogenic bacteria Research articles providing data on pathogenic bacteria-related human health hazards associated with the use of wastewater for crop irrigation are listed in Table 11.1. Most studies stated that fresh vegetables irrigated with wastewater contained bacterial loads above acceptable levels, translated into a human health hazard.

In the case of *E. coli* and coliforms, there were 13 cases of increased risk and four cases of no evidence. One should note that these results were based on total coliforms (TCs), fecal coliforms (FCs), or *E. coli* used as hygiene indicators only, with four articles referring to pathogenic or antibiotic resistant *E. coli* from South Africa (Du Plessis *et al.*, 2015), Spain (Amato *et al.*, 2021), the USA (Olivieri *et al.*, 2014), and Vietnam (Tran *et al.*, 2020). For the other six bacterial genera, there were nine cases of increased risk and four cases of no evidence. There was no geographical trend.

In Accra, Ghana, *E. coli* concentrations in all stream, drain, and waste stabilization pond waters used for irrigation exceeded WHO limits (10^3 and 10^4 fecal indicator *E. coli* CFU/100 mL for root and leaf crops, respectively (Silverman *et al.*, 2013)). Similarly, wastewater-irrigated fresh vegetables suffered from bacterial contamination by both *E. coli* and *Salmonella*, above acceptable standards of $<1{,}0^3{,}100\,g^{-1}$ fresh weight of food in Kumasi, Ghana (Abass *et al.*, 2016). Moreover, it was found to be more efficient to manage bacterial risk factors (based on contamination levels by fecal indicator *E. coli*) on lettuce and cabbage

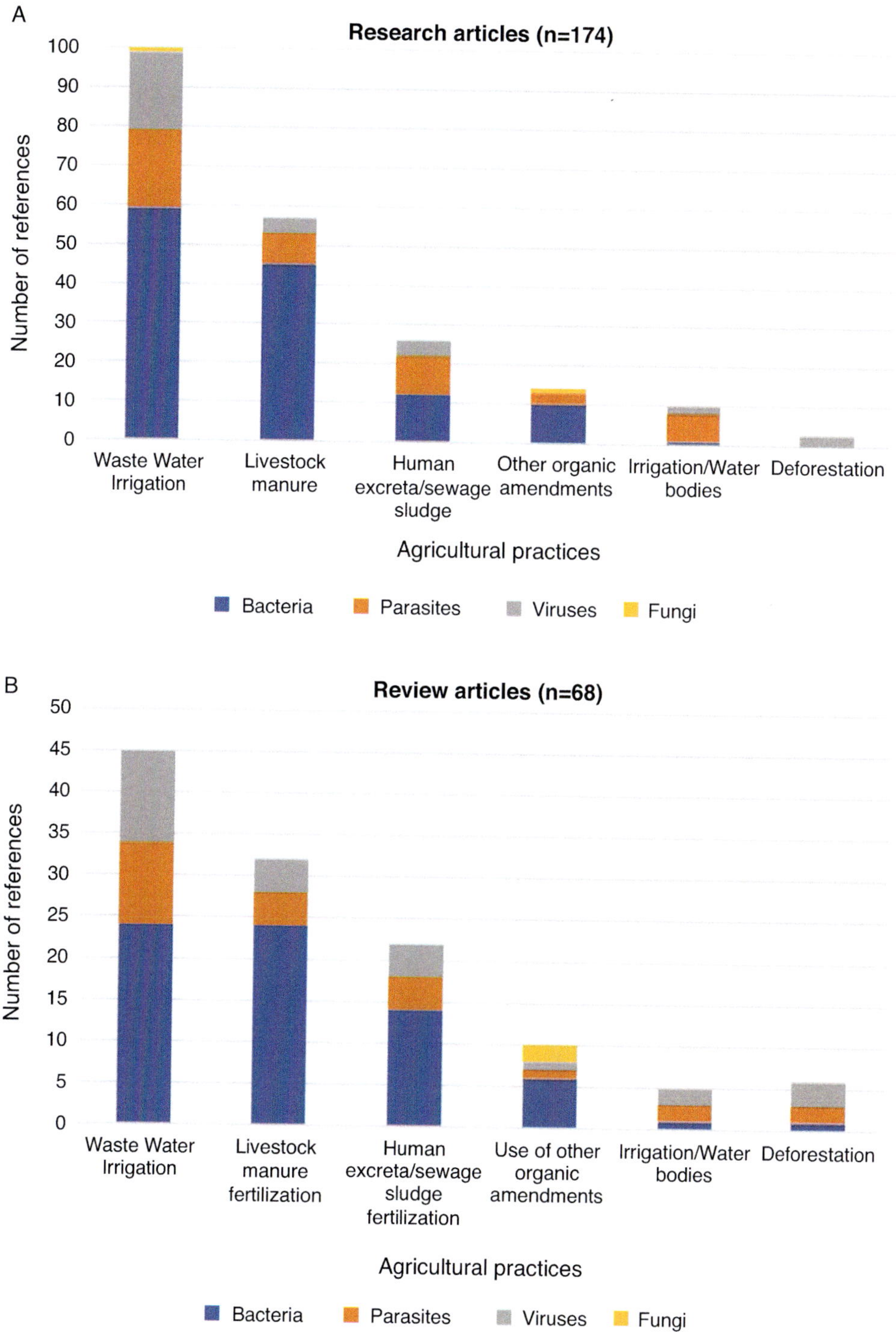

Fig. 11.7. Distribution of research (a) and review (b) articles across agricultural practices (excluding those dealing solely with crop protection).

Table 11.1. Risk of human contamination by human pathogens linked to the use of wastewater for crop irrigation as reflected by selected references (figures in brackets).

Countries													
Pathogens	Argentina	Australia	Bolivia	Brazil	Costa Rica	Egypt	France	Ghana	Greece	Iran	Israel	Italy	Japan
Bacteria													
E. coli and coliforms						+(Abdelhafiz *et al.*, 2021)		+(Abass *et al.*, 2016); (−155)	+(Forslund *et al.*, 2012)		+(Armon *et al.*, 1994)	−(Forslund *et al.*, 2012)	
Salmonella spp								+(Abass *et al.*, 2016)			+(Armon *et al.*, 1994)		
Listeria spp													
Streptococcus spp						+(Abdelhafiz *et al.*, 2021)							
Bacillus spp.													
Campylobacter spp	±(Ayuso-Gabella *et al.*, 2011)									−(Farhadkhani *et al.*, 2020)	±(Ayuso-Gabella *et al.*, 2011)	±(Ayuso-Gabella *et al.*, 2011)	
Mycobacterium spp													
Parasites													
Cryptosporidium spp.											+(Armon *et al.*, 2002)		
Giardia spp.		+(Verbyla *et al.*, 2015)									+(Armon *et al.*, 2002)		
Entamoeba spp.			+(Cutolo *et al.*, 2012)										
Cyclospora spp.												+(Giangaspero *et al.*, 2015)	
Ascaris spp.			+(Cutolo *et al.*, 2012)										
Trichuris spp.													
Hookworms[b]													
Viruses													
Norovirus	+(Prez *et al.*, 2018)	−(Mok *et al.*, 2014)			−(Chacón *et al.*, 2020)		−(Courault *et al.*, 2017)						+(Kobayashi *et al.*, 2017)
Hepatovirus	+(Lim *et al.*, 2015)				−(Mirhosseini *et al.*, 2008)					+(García *et al.*, 2013)			
Rotavirus	+(Prez *et al.*, 2018)				−(Chacón *et al.*, 2020)								
Mastadenovirus										±(Gholipour *et al.*, 2022)			
Mamastrovirus	+(Prez *et al.*, 2018)												
Enterovirus	−(Prez *et al.*, 2018)												

Continued

Table 11.1. Continued

Countries											
Pathogens	Kenya	Mexico	Morocco	Nigeria	Oman	Philippines	South Africa	South Korea	Spain	USA	Vietnam
Bacteria											
E. coli and coliforms			+(Ouarrak *et al.*, 2019)	+(Chigor *et al.*, 2022)	−(Mothershaw *et al.*, 2013)	+(Garcia *et al.*, 2015)	+(Iwu and Okoh, 2020); −(Du Plessis *et al.*, 2015)	+(An *et al.*, 2007)	+(Amato *et al.*, 2021)	−(Olivieri *et al.*, 2014; Allard *et al.*, 2019)	+(Fuhrimann *et al.*, 2016a; Tran *et al.*, 2020)
Salmonella spp			+(Ouarrak *et al.*, 2019)				+(Iwu and Okoh, 2020)			−(Allard *et al.*, 2019)	+(Fuhrimann *et al.*, 2016a; Tran *et al.*, 2020)
Listeria spp										−(Allard *et al.*, 2019)	
Streptococcus spp			+(Ouarrak *et al.*, 2019)								
Bacillus spp.					−(Mothershaw *et al.*, 2013)						
Campylobacter spp									±(Ayuso-Gabella *et al.*, 2011)		+(Tran *et al.*, 2020)
Mycobacterium spp	+(Gregson *et al.*, 2022)										
Parasites											
Cryptosporidium spp.		+(Di Giovanni *et al.*, 2006)						+(Hong *et al.*, 2014)		−(Olivieri *et al.*, 2014)	
Giardia spp.		−(Di Giovanni *et al.*, 2006)	+(Amahmid *et al.*, 2022)							−(Olivieri *et al.*, 2014)	−(Fuhrimann *et al.*, 2016b)
Entamoeba spp.			+(Amahmid *et al.*, 2022)						+(Reyes-Batlle *et al.*, 2021)[a]		+(Trang *et al.*, 2007); −(Fuhrimann *et al.*, 2016b)
Cyclospora spp.											
Ascaris spp.			+(Amahmid *et al.*, 2022)								+(Pham-Duc *et al.*, 2013); (Fuhrimann *et al.*, 2016b, 176)
Trichuris spp.											+(Pham-Duc *et al.*, 2013); −(Fuhrimann *et al.*, 2016b; Trang *et al.*, 2007)
Hookworms[b]											+(Pham-Duc *et al.*, 2013); −(Fuhrimann *et al.*, 2016b)
Viruses											
Norovirus									+(Gondim-Porto *et al.*, 2016)	+(Lim *et al.*, 2015; Chandrasekaran and Jiang, 2018)	
Hepatovirus											
Rotavirus											
Mastadenovirus									+(Gondim-Porto *et al.*, 2016)		
Mamastrovirus											
Enterovirus											

+: increased risk; −: no documented evidence of risk; ±: conflicting results.
[a]Other amoeba species.
[b]'Hookworms' stand for either *Ancylostoma duodenale* or *Necator americanus*.

at markets and in kitchens than during the production process in Accra (Antwi-Agyei *et al.*, 2015). In Southeast Nigeria, a high prevalence of multidrug-resistant *E. coli* was found on vegetable samples (Chigor *et al.*, 2022).

Potential pathogens, notably *Mycobacterium fortuitum*, were identified in one of the water-harvesting irrigation ponds used by rural smallholder farmers in the County of Laikipia, Kenya (Gregson *et al.*, 2022). In Eastern Cape Province, South Africa, irrigation with contaminated water was found to be a potential transmission route of multidrug-resistant *Listeria monocytogenes* and consequently a threat to public health (Iwu and Okoh, 2020). In Eastern Cape, high levels of multi-drug resistant *E. coli* pathovars were found in irrigation water (Iwu *et al.*, 2022). However, despite river water being contaminated, *E. coli* O157:H7 was not detected in onions using overhead (Du Plessis *et al.*, 2015).

In Spain, all water samples taken from agricultural irrigation ditches around Valencia contained very high levels of resistant fecal coliforms, presenting an increased risk of transfer of antibiotic-resistant bacteria (ARBs) and antibiotic-resistant genes (ARGs) to food crops in the event that these contaminated waters were used for irrigation (Amato *et al.*, 2021). The Quantitative Microbial Risk Assessment (QMRA) model adopted by WHO found that the consumption of tomatoes in the Po valley (northern Italy) and Crete (Greece) was considered safe, while tap water and treated wastewater used for irrigation were shown to exceed permissible limits of farmers exposure to contaminated soil (1.0×10^{-3} disease risk per person per year) (Forslund *et al.*, 2012). The study highlighted then the need to upgrade the QMRA model with accurate ratios between fecal indicator *E. coli* and pathogen species.

In Israel, a clear link was found between the quality of the effluents used for irrigation and the degree of residual microbial contamination found on irrigated vegetables (Armon *et al.*, 1994). Wastewater irrigation was not found to result in a significant *Campylobacter* spp. risk for vegetable consumers in Iran (Farhadkhani *et al.*, 2020). It was also found that median risks for *Campylobacter* were acceptable ($<10^{-6}$ disability adjusted life years, (DALYs)) at all sites studied in Israel, Apulia (Italy), Catalonia (Spain), and South Australia, with the exception of hazards from accidental aerosol ingestion (Ayuso-Gabella *et al.*, 2011).

In Oman, although microbial load (*E. coli* and *Bacillus* spp.) was higher in treated wastewater (as opposed to tap water), it had no effect on cucumber quality (Mothershaw *et al.*, 2013). In Meknes (Central-South Morocco), the use of wastewater for irrigating vegetables resulted in bacterial loads (*E. coli*, *Salmonella* sp., *Streptococcus* sp.), which exceeded local standards (Ouarrak *et al.*, 2019).

In Metro Manila, Philippines, highly contaminated irrigation water and vegetables (with *E. coli* in particular) were noted (Garcia *et al.*, 2015). Similarly, bacterial contamination of water used in agricultural fields in Hanoi (Vietnam) was found to exceed safe limits (Fuhrimann *et al.*, 2016a). The concentrations of total coliforms (TC), *Escherichia coli* and *Salmonella* spp. were 110 times the Vietnamese discharge limits for agricultural reuse (5000 CFU TC/100 mL) and 260 times the World Health Organization's safe limits (10^3–10^4 CFU *E. coli*/100 mL) for unrestricted irrigation.

In addition, it should be mentioned that soils irrigated with wastewater in three African cities (Ouagadougou, Burkina Faso, and Ngaoundere and Yaounde, Cameroon) were found to represent a potential vector for the spread of antibiotic resistance, threatening human and animal health (Bougnom *et al.*, 2020).

Levers for mitigating risks of exposure to pathogenic bacteria The levers and associated practices/technologies are listed in Table 11.2.

The first lever is the quality of irrigation water. This can be improved by mixing reclaimed water and tap water (Cui *et al.*, 2020), improving the wastewater conveyance system (Fuhrimann *et al.*, 2016a), or through various treatments, namely managed aquifer recharge (MAR) (Ayuso-Gabella *et al.*, 2011), natural wastewater treatment systems (Verbyla *et al.*, 2015), high-rate algal ponds (HRAP) treatment (Young *et al.*, 2016), ultraviolet (UV) disinfection (An *et al.*, 2007; Deepnarain *et al.*, 2020; Monteiro and Santos, 2020), chlorination (Bernstein *et al.*, 2008; Fahrenfeld *et al.*, 2013; Deepnarain *et al.*, 2020), ozonation disinfection (Deepnarain *et al.*, 2020), electro-oxidation (Ungureanu *et al.*, 2019), use of a membrane

Table 11.2. Levers and associated practices/technologies to mitigate risk of human exposure to pathogenic bacteria, parasites and viruses, linked with the use of wastewater for crop irrigation as reflected by selected references.

Levers	Associated practices	References/bacteria	References/parasites	References/viruses
Quality of irrigation water	Mixing reclaimed water and tap water	(Cui *et al.*, 2020)		
	Wastewater conveyance system	(Fuhrimann *et al.*, 2016a)		
	Managed aquifer recharge (MAR)	(Ayuso-Gabella *et al.*, 2011)	(Ayuso-Gabella *et al.*, 2011)	
	Natural wastewater treatment systems (Stabilization ponds)	(Verbyla *et al.*, 2015)	(Cutolo *et al.*, 2012)	(Pavione *et al.*, 2013; Gondim-Porto *et al.*, 2016; Alam and Ali, 2021)
	High rate algal ponds (HRAP) treatment	(Young *et al.*, 2016)		(Murayama *et al.*, 2010)
	UV disinfection	(An *et al.*, 2007; Deepnarain *et al.*, 2020; Monteiro and Santos, 2020)	(Forslund *et al.*, 2012)	(Mok *et al.*, 2014; Gondim-Porto *et al.*, 2016)
	Chlorination	(Bernstein *et al.*, 2008; Fahrenfeld *et al.*, 2013; Deepnarain *et al.*, 2020)		(Mok *et al.*, 2014; Gondim-Porto *et al.*, 2016)
	Ozonation disinfection	(Deepnarain *et al.*, 2020)		(Mok *et al.*, 2014)
	Electro-oxidation	(Ungureanu *et al.*, 2019)		
	Membrane bioreactor system	(Bonetta *et al.*, 2022)	(Forslund *et al.*, 2012)	
	Multiple-barrier treatment	(Cutolo *et al.*, 2012)	(Cutolo *et al.*, 2012)	
	Flocculation			(Gondim-Porto *et al.*, 2016)
	DHS (down-flow hanging sponge) reactor			(Kobayashi *et al.*, 2017)
	Gravel infiltration		(Forslund *et al.*, 2012)	
	Sludge removal		(Walsh *et al.*, 1993)	

Table 11.2. Continued

Levers	Associated practices	References/bacteria	References/parasites	References/viruses
Type of irrigation system	Subsurface *vs* surface *vs* sprinkler irrigation	(Forslund *et al.*, 2011; Sacks and Bernstein, 2011; Forslund *et al.*, 2012; Uyttendaele *et al.*, 2015; Allard *et al.*, 2019; Obayomi *et al.*, 2019; Esteves *et al.*, 2020; Ofori *et al.*, 2021; Perulli *et al.*, 2021)		(Forslund *et al.*, 2011)
	Irrigation regime (leaching)	(Bernstein *et al.*, 2007)		
Bioremediation in soil	Biochar	(Cui *et al.*, 2018)		
Selection of use	According to soil type	(Uyttendaele *et al.*, 2015; Eissenberger *et al.*, 2020)		(Forslund *et al.*, 2011)
	According to crop type	(Scheinemann *et al.*, 2015; Perulli *et al.*, 2021)		

bioreactor system (Bonetta *et al.*, 2022), and multiple-barrier treatment (Cutolo *et al.*, 2012). For instance, it was found that HRAPs were able to remove viral and bacterial indicators to levels acceptable for subsurface irrigation of nonfood crops (Young *et al.*, 2016).

MAR could reduce the human health hazards of irrigation using reclaimed water (Ayuso-Gabella *et al.*, 2011). In South Korea, it was found that in rice fields, risk was lowered when UV disinfection was used (An *et al.*, 2007). Chlorination was found to be effective in suppressing *E. coli* and coliform populations in a soilless greenhouse production system (Bernstein *et al.*, 2008). However, an membrane bioreactor system was found to be more efficient than chlorination for suppressing *E. coli*, *Salmonella* spp., *Campylobacter* spp., and *Legionella* spp. in wastewater (Bonetta *et al.*, 2022).

Another approach is to target the irrigation system (i.e. subsurface, surface or sprinkler) (Petterson *et al.*, 2001; Forslund *et al.*, 2011; Forslund *et al.*, 2012; Uyttendaele *et al.*, 2015; Allard *et al.*, 2019; Obayomi *et al.*, 2019; Esteves *et al.*, 2020; Ofori *et al.*, 2021; Perulli *et al.*, 2021), or irrigation regime (e.g. leaching (Bernstein *et al.*, 2007)). This would benefit both consumer and farmer/farm worker health. For instance, in kale and radish, no bacterial pathogen transfer to crops *via* drip irrigation was detected in the Mid-Atlantic region, USA (Allard *et al.*, 2019). In Israel, it was found that leaching could reduce *Salmonella* spp. concentration in the rhizosphere (Bernstein *et al.*, 2007).

In addition to irrigation system and regime, a form of bioremediation may be exerted by biochar (Cui *et al.*, 2018). Also, wastewater, depending on its quality, may be used only on certain types of crops or soils (Obayomi *et al.*, 2019; Eissenberger *et al.*, 2020; Perulli *et al.*, 2021). A different approach is 'farm to fork MRA', resulting in targeting the postharvest phase (Antwi-Agyei *et al.*, 2015), but that does not take into consideration the safety of farmers or farm workers.

PATHOGENIC PARASITES

Associated risk for human exposure to pathogenic parasites The outcome was mixed regarding the effect of wastewater irrigation on the presence of protozoan or helminthic parasites (Table 11.1).

In Israel, a high prevalence of *Cryptosporidium* oocysts (80–10,000/0.5 kg), and to a lesser extent, *Giardia* cysts, was found on zucchini, due to its sticky and hairy outer surface (Armon *et al.*, 2002). In South Korea, it was deemed necessary to reduce *Cryptosporidium* infection in farm soil and vegetables due to the risk to public health (Hong *et al.*, 2014). In the Juarez Valley, Mexico, high levels of pathogens were found in reclaimed wastewater, with 183 to >7000 *Giardia* cysts and 9–762 *Cryptosporidium* oocysts detected per liter, but these pathogens were rarely found on forage plants, and there was no evidence of zooanthroponotic transmission from sheep (Di Giovanni *et al.*, 2006). Similarly, current agricultural and public health water recycling regulations in California (USA) were not found to measurably increase risk of infection by *Cryptosporidium parvum* and *Giardia lamblia* (Olivieri *et al.*, 2014).

In Morocco, the presence of pathogenic *Giardia* spp. and *Entamoeba* spp. cysts, and *Ascaris* spp. and *Trichuris* spp. eggs entailed health risks for farmers, produce handlers, and consumers (Amahmid *et al.*, 2022). Exposure to wastewater was not directly associated with helminth infection (e.g. *Ascaris* spp., hookworms, and *Trichuris* spp.) or intestinal protozoa infection (e.g. *Giardia* spp., *Entamoeba* spp.) in different population groups in Hanoi (Vietnam) (Fuhrimann *et al.*, 2016a). In São Paulo State, Brazil, the presence of *Ascaris* spp. and *Entamoeba coli* was detected in treated wastewater with an average density of 6.4 eggs L^{-1} and 1.7 cysts L^{-1}, respectively, which is above the tolerable level recommended by WHO (≤1 egg L^{-1}) (Cutolo *et al.*, 2012).

In Spain, the coexistence observed in water and soil of pathogenic bacteria and free-living amoebas (FLAs) could indicate an increased risk of human infection in agroecosystems (Reyes-Batlle *et al.*, 2021). FLAs are considered an emerging group of opportunistic pathogens with the potential of causing numerous diseases in humans (e.g. cutaneous and ocular infections, lung, bone, or adrenal gland conditions, or fatal encephalitis). In Hanoi (North Vietnam), contact with wastewater was found to be the principal risk factor for diarrhea, mainly due to the enteric pathogen *Entamoeba histolytica* (Trang *et al.*, 2007).

In the Apulia region of southern Italy, *Cyclospora cayetanensis* was detected in treated irrigation water, well water, soil, vegetables (particularly fennel), and human stools (Giangaspero *et al.*, 2015). These results suggest that irrigation water, soil, and vegetables may represent a source of *C. cayetanensis* infection to humans, requiring monitoring by health authorities.

The high infection rate (47%) of the population of the Hanam province, northern Vietnam, with intestinal helminths (*Ascaris*, *Trichuris*, and hookworms) was ascribed to exposure to wastewater, used for crop irrigation (Pham-Duc *et al.*, 2013). In contrast, household tap water use was a protective factor against helminth infection. In contrast, in a peri-urban area in Hanoi, wastewater exposure did not pose a major risk for helminth infection (*Ascaris*, *Trichuris*, and hookworms) (Trang *et al.*, 2007).

Moreover, no helminth eggs (indicators for pathogenic helminthic parasite contamination) were found in irrigation water or on tomatoes from Crete (Greece), whereas two tomato samples out of 36 from the Po Valley (Italy) were contaminated by helminth eggs (mean: 0.18 eggs L^{-1}), which had been irrigated with treated wastewater and tap water, respectively (Forslund *et al.*, 2012). It was found that in Hanoi, Vietnam, mean helminth egg concentrations in agricultural irrigation water were below WHO tolerable levels in all study systems (<1 egg L^{-1}) (World Health Organization, 2006; Fuhrimann *et al.*, 2016a). In two Bolivian wastewater stabilization ponds, the helminth egg concentrations calculated for treated wastewater samples were between 31 and 130 eggs L^{-1}, and between 69 and 352 eggs L^{-1}, respectively (Verbyla *et al.*, 2015). These values exceeded the maximum concentration of 1 egg L^{-1} recommended by WHO and greatly exceeded the limit of 0.1 eggs L^{-1} recommended for children.

Levers for mitigating risks of exposure to pathogenic parasites All levers pertained to the improvement of irrigation water quality with associated practices or technologies: wastewater conveyance systems; gravel filtration; managed aquifer recharge (MAR); UV disinfection; membrane bioreactor systems; waste stabilization ponds; high-rate algal ponds (cf. Table 11.2).

In Hanoi, mean helminth egg concentrations in wastewater used in agriculture were below WHO tolerable levels in all study systems (<1 egg L^{-1}) (Fuhrimann *et al.*, 2016a). Wastewater treatment by either membrane bio reactor (MBR) technology, gravel filtration, or UV treatment before irrigation resulted in tomatoes safe for human consumption (Forslund *et al.*, 2012).

MAR resulted in a reduction of risk to human health when reclaimed water was used for irrigation and could potentially be an important tool in water recycling *via* aquifers and for irrigation management, particularly for pathogenic protozoa (e.g. *Cryptosporidium*) (Ayuso-Gabella *et al.*, 2011). Sludge accumulation in ponds was found to potentially limit removal of helminths (and to a lesser extent protozoan parasites) more than *E. coli*, stressing the importance of maintenance such as sludge removal (Verbyla *et al.*, 2015). Similarly, the low removal efficiency of the stabilization ponds of helminth (e.g. *Ascaris* sp.) eggs and protozoa (e.g. *Entamoeba coli*) cysts was stressed, calling for technologies such as multiple barriers to reduce and, if possible, eliminate parasites from treated wastewater (Cutolo *et al.*, 2012).

Additional environmental sources and the potential for regrowth made aerobic spore-forming bacteria (ASFB) unsuitable indicators for pathogenic protozoa in natural pond systems (Young *et al.*, 2016).

PATHOGENIC VIRUSES

Associated risk for human exposure to pathogenic viruses The outcome was mixed regarding the effect of wastewater irrigation on pathogenic viruses (Table 11.1).

It should be noted that the *Hepatovirus* genus encompasses the Hepatitis A and Hepatitis E viruses, and the *Enterovirus* genus encompasses *Poliovirus* and *Coxsackievirus*, and the genus *Flavivirus* encompasses the West Nile and Dengue viruses.

In Costa Rica, human enteric viruses (*viz. Enterovirus* (EV), Hepatitis A virus (HAV), *Norovirus* (NoV) GI and GII, and *Rotavirus* (RV)) were frequently detected in WWTP influent and effluent (Chacón *et al.*, 2020). RV was the most frequently detected virus in both influent and effluent samples (47 and 39%, respectively), followed by NoVGI (39 and 36%, respectively). Globally, NoVGI was detected twice as frequently as NoVGII. Less than 25% of the samples tested positive for EV, and less than 10% of the samples tested positive for HAV.

In the USA, noroviruses internalized in lettuce were found to pose a risk to consumers. Hydroponically-grown lettuce posed a much higher risk than soil-grown lettuce (Chandrasekaran and Jiang, 2018). Near Clermont-Ferrand, France, enteric viruses were measured in water and air in the vicinity of a wastewater treatment plant and in fields irrigated with wastewater (Courault *et al.*, 2017). The health risk of inhaled noroviruses (which were most abundant in raw sewage water (with >10e^4 GC/L)) was assessed. Low quantities of airborne viruses were detected (<10e^3 GC/m^3).

In Catalonia, Spain, the disease burden of NoV GII and Human adenovirus (HAdV) for the consumption of lettuce irrigated with tertiary effluent from two wastewater treatment plants was higher than the WHO recommendation of 10^{-6} DALYs for both viruses (Gondim-Porto *et al.*, 2016). In Japan, LRs ($\log_{10}$ reduction values) of 2.6 and 3.7 for Norovirus GII are required in treated municipal wastewater in order to remain within the tolerable disease burden of 10^{-4} and 10^{-6} DALYs per person per year (pppy), respectively, for 95% of the population exposed to wastewater *via* irrigation (Kobayashi *et al.*, 2017). In Iran, the mean probability of illness from consumption of wastewater-irrigated vegetables was 4×10^{-1} pppy, which was about two orders of magnitude higher than the WHO safe level (10^{-3} pppy) for reuse of wastewater (Gholipour *et al.*, 2022). HAdV-F was detected in 74% of wastewater samples with a mean concentration of 38 Genomic Copy (GC)/mL. HAdV was also detected in wastewater-irrigated soil (2×102 GC/g) and crop (<10 GC/g) samples.

In the USA, food crop irrigation using captured urban stormwater was found to have a high annual viral infection risk (median range: 6.8×10^{-4}–9.7×10^{-1} pppy), exceeding the WHO recommended disease burdens of $\leq 10^{-6}$ DALYs pppy (Lim *et al.*, 2015). In north-central Victoria, Australia, the use of wastewater stabilization pond (WSP) effluent resulted in a range of 10^{-5} to 10^{-3} DALYs pppy (Mok *et al.*, 2014), with all median values exceeding the WHO (World Health Organization, 2006) and Australian (NRMMC *et al.*, 2006) guideline threshold of $< 10^{-6}$ DALYs pppy for acceptable level of risk from wastewater reuse. In central Argentina, Nov, RV and Human astroviruses (HAstV) were detected in almost all irrigation waters, while iEV (infective enterovirus) was only sporadically detected, more often on leafy vegetables (Prez *et al.*, 2018).

Levers for mitigating risks of exposure to pathogenic viruses Levers and associated practices/technologies are listed in Table 11.2.

Using an F-RNA bacteriophage as a viral indicator in a study conducted in South Australia, HRAPs were found to be able to reduce viral indicators to levels acceptable for subsurface irrigation of nonfood crops (Young *et al.*, 2016). Conversely, it was found in Japan that the DHS (down-flow hanging sponge) effluent should not be used directly for agricultural irrigation because ~49% and 69% of 10,000 DALY values exceeded the tolerable disease burden of 10^{-4} and 10^{-6} DALY loss pppy, respectively (Kobayashi *et al.*, 2017).

Using the virus indicator *Salmonella* Typhimurium bacteriophage 28 on potato samples in a soil lysimeter study conducted in Denmark, it was suggested that the main risk associated with subsurface drip irrigation using low-quality water was fecal contamination of root crops, in particular those consumed raw (Forslund *et al.*, 2011). Also, after 27 days, phage 28B continued to be present in similar concentrations in leachate from lysimeters containing coarse sand, while no phage was found in lysimeters with sandy loam soil. In Brazil, it was found that irrigation with effluents containing 10^3–10^4 *E. coli* per 100 ml resulted in a median rotavirus infection risk of approximately 10^{-3} and 10^{-4} pppy for low- and high-growing salad crops, respectively (Fongaro *et al.*, 2018).

PATHOGENIC FUNGI. The composition of soil fungal community and diversity of natural shrubland was analyzed and compared with agricultural systems irrigated with water of differing quality, namely rainwater, freshwater, and dam-stored and untreated wastewater in the Mezquital Valley, Mexico (Lüneberg *et al.*, 2019). Potentially harmful human pathogens (particularly of the *Candida* genus), a human

Table 11.3. Risk of human exposure to pathogenic bacteria associated with the use of livestock manure in crop fertilization as reflected by selected references.

Bacterium genera	Country	Risk[a]	References
E. coli	USA	+	(Givens *et al.*, 2016; Chen *et al.*, 2019)
	South Africa	+	(Fatoba *et al.*, 2022)
	UK	–	(Murayama *et al.*, 2010)
	Algeria	+	(Touati *et al.*, 2020)
Salmonella	USA	+	(Givens *et al.*, 2016; Pornsukarom and Thakur, 2016; Chen *et al.*, 2019)
	UK	–	(Murayama *et al.*, 2010)
	Cambodia	+	(Ström *et al.*, 2018)
Staphylococcus	USA	+	(Casey *et al.*, 2013; Fatoba *et al.*, 2022)
Enterococcus	USA	+	(Givens *et al.*, 2016)
Campylobacter	USA	+	(Givens *et al.*, 2016)
	UK	–	(Murayama *et al.*, 2010)
Yersinia	UK	–	(Murayama *et al.*, 2010)
Pseudomonas	USA	+	(Udikovic-Kolic *et al.*, 2014)
Brevundimonas and *Brachybacterium*	China	+	(Yang *et al.*, 2016)

[a]+: increased risk; -: no documented evidence of risk.

health risk, were identified. In crops irrigated with roof-harvested rainwater in South Africa, fungal sequences were identified belonging to *Cryptococcus* spp., a species known to cause fever, coughing, and shortness of breath in humans (Jongman and Korsten, 2016a).

Use of livestock manure for crop fertilization

PATHOGENIC BACTERIA

Associated risk for human exposure to pathogenic bacteria References (research articles only), providing data on risks of human contamination by pathogenic bacteria associated with use of livestock manure for crop fertilization, are listed in Table 11.3.

In California, it was found that solid bovine manure was a source of *E. coli* O157 and *Salmonella* spp. and that the application of untreated manure as biological soil amendments might pose potential risks to public health (Chen *et al.*, 2019). Similarly, in Iowa, several zoonotic pathogens, including Shiga-toxin producing *E. coli*, *Campylobacter jejuni*, pathogenic enterococci, and *Staphylococcus aureus*, were detected in both manure samples and in corresponding surface water following swine manure applications (Givens *et al.*, 2016). All of these pathogens can pose mild to serious health risks to swine, humans, and other wildlife.

In South Africa, soil amendment with chicken litter significantly increased the number of antibiotic-resistant *E. coli* in the soil. The application of chicken litter thus appeared to transfer antibiotic-resistant *E. coli* to the soil, enhancing the soil resistome and highlighting the risks of such agricultural practices to public health (Fatoba *et al.*, 2022). Similarly, in Algeria, farms were found to be an important reservoir of colistin-resistant *E. coli* as well as other antimicrobial resistance genes such as extended-spectrum beta-lactamase (ESBL) genes. Transfer of manure from animals to soil and use of irrigation water may disseminate multiple resistances, posing a worrying threat to human health (Touati *et al.*, 2020).

In the UK, no gastrointestinal pathogens were detected in air sampled immediately adjacent to the agricultural spreading of bovine slurry (air was examined for the presence of culturable *Salmonella* spp., *Campylobacter* spp., *Yersinia enterocolitica*, and *E. coli* O157:H7) (Murayama *et al.*, 2010). Among the diverse bacteria detected, only a few have been shown to be opportunistically pathogenic to humans and none of these organisms have been described as having an inhalational infection route and therefore were not deemed to pose a significant health threat for immunocompetent individuals.

In Cambodia, *Salmonella enterica* was detected in 9.7% of manure samples collected in a study conducted in urban and peri-urban areas of Phnom Penh (Ström *et al.*, 2018). The survey revealed a difference in management between cattle and pig manure. Cattle manure was most commonly used as fertilizer for crop production (66%), whereas pig manure was most commonly dumped in the environment (46%). In Pennsylvania (USA), proximity to swine manure application to crops was found to be associated with MRSA and skin and soft-tissue infection by *Staphylococcus aureus* (Casey *et al.*, 2013). In Connecticut (USA), manure amendment was found to induce a bloom of certain antibiotic-resistant bacteria in soil independent of antibiotic exposure of the cows from which the manure was derived, e.g. antibiotic-resistant *Pseudomonas* spp. (Udikovic-Kolic *et al.*, 2014).

In the suburbs of Xinxiang City (China), chicken manure or organic fertilizer application increased the populations of multiple antibiotic-resistant bacteria (MARB) in soil and multiple antibiotic-resistant endophytic bacteria (MAREB) in pakchoi (Yang *et al.*, 2016). The cointroduction of antibiotics into the soils *via* irrigation and manure application and/or the sustained selection pressure of antibiotics from these sources was also found to facilitate the proliferation of ARGs in agricultural soils from the Yangtze River Delta (Sun *et al.*, 2020). Similarly, in the suburb of Tianjin, the application of composted pig manure significantly increased the pollution load of ARGs in farmland soil and plant, and promoted their proliferation (Xu *et al.*, 2021).

Levers for mitigating risks of exposure to pathogenic bacteria The levers and associated practices/technologies are listed in Table 11.4.

Evidently, an ideal manure would be antibiotic-free. But this is not the purpose of this review as it does not cover livestock farming. A novel approach would be to establish exclusion periods between manure fertilization and crop grazing/harvesting, through risk-based approaches incorporating differences in climate, soil management, and initial levels of bacteria during application (Tariq *et al.*, 2022).

The choice of manure source is important. In Portugal, higher frequencies of AB resistance phenotypes in isolates were found from manured soil than in the manure itself, and higher resistance in poultry manure than in dairy cattle manure (Amador *et al.*, 2018). It was also found in North Dakota, South Dakota, and Nebraska that beef cattle manure amendment minimally affected antimicrobial resistance gene levels (Miller *et al.*, 2019), while in Connecticut, cow manure amendment induced a bloom of some antibiotic-resistant bacteria in the soil (Udikovic-Kolic *et al.*, 2014). Swine farm management schemes in south-east USA positively and negatively affected microbial and antibiotic-resistant populations in confined animal feeding operation (CAFO) wastewater (Brooks *et al.*, 2014). In the suburb of Xinxiang City (China), it was found that the application of chicken manure increased populations of multiple antibiotic-resistant bacteria (MARB) in soils and multiple antibiotic-resistant endophytic bacteria (MAREB) in pakchoi (Yang *et al.*, 2016).

The use of copper and zinc in pig fodder was found to be closely associated with the presence of MDR *Salmonella* spp (Zalewska *et al.*, 2021). This required a range of prevention strategies such as vaccination, the addition to fodder of probiotics, prebiotics, or bioactive compounds such as antimicrobial peptides to protect herds from infection. It was also argued that the prevalence of *Salmonella* spp. in pig feces might depend on the production system, namely all-in/all-out management vs farrow-to-finish systems, or raising on slotted floors vs with raising on dirt lots (Bicudo and Goyal, 2003). The composition of manure was considered to be influenced to a large extent by the animal

Table 11.4. Levers and associated practices/technologies to mitigate risk of human exposure to pathogenic bacteria, parasites and viruses linked to the use of livestock manure in crop fertilization as reflected by selected references.

Levers	Practices/technologies	References/bacteria	References/parasites	References/viruses
Quality of manure	Source of manure	(Bicudo and Goyal, 2003; Brooks *et al.*, 2014; Amador *et al.*, 2018; Iwu and Okoh, 2019; Miller *et al.*, 2019; Zalewska *et al.*, 2021)		
Manure storage	Commercial storage	(Duriez *et al.*, 2008; Topp *et al.*, 2009)		
	Anaerobic storage	(Bicudo and Goyal, 2003; Fongaro *et al.*, 2018)		
	Cold temperature	(Johnston *et al.*, 2003)		
	High dry matter	(Kabelitz *et al.*, 2020; Münch *et al.*, 2020; Kabelitz *et al.*, 2021)		
Treatment of livestock manure	Chemical treatments	(Bicudo and Goyal, 2003; Heinonen-Tanski *et al.*, 2006; Avilez *et al.*, 2019)		
	Solarization	(Barbour *et al.*, 2002)		
	Addition of organic matter/biochar	(Duffy *et al.*, 2004; Iwu *et al.*, 2020)		
	Aerobic composting	(Heinonen-Tanski *et al.*, 2006; Youngquist *et al.*, 2016; Karimi *et al.*, 2017; Gou *et al.*, 2018; Iwu and Okoh, 2019; Urra *et al.*, 2019; Alegbeleye and Sant'Ana, 2020; Checcucci *et al.*, 2020; Iwu *et al.*, 2020; Oliver *et al.*, 2020; Liu *et al.*, 2021; Wang *et al.*, 2022)	(Karimi *et al.*, 2017)	(García *et al.*, 2013)
	Anaerobic digestion	(Bicudo and Goyal, 2003; Heinonen-Tanski *et al.*, 2006; Saunders *et al.*, 2012; Manyi-Loh *et al.*, 2014; Youngquist *et al.*, 2016; Le Maréchal *et al.*, 2019; Nag *et al.*, 2019; Urra *et al.*, 2019; Checcucci *et al.*, 2020; Oliver *et al.*, 2020; Nag *et al.*, 2021; Zhang *et al.*, 2021; Lin *et al.*, 2022; Wang *et al.*, 2022)	(Nag *et al.*, 2021)	(Nag *et al.*, 2021)
	Pasteurization	(Heinonen-Tanski *et al.*, 2006; Nag *et al.*, 2021)	(Nag *et al.*, 2021)	

	Lactic acid fermentation	(Scheinemann *et al*., 2015)	(Scheinemann *et al*., 2015)	(Scheinemann *et al*., 2015)
	Aeration	(Bicudo and Goyal, 2003; Iwu and Okoh, 2019)		
	Electrolytic treatment	(Bicudo and Goyal, 2003)		
	Ozonation	(Bicudo and Goyal, 2003; Checcucci *et al*., 2020)		
	Thermophilic aerobic stabilization	(Bicudo and Goyal, 2003)		
	Aerobic sequencing batch reactor	(Bicudo and Goyal, 2003)		
Method of application	Rain gun sprayer	(Gou *et al*., 2018)		
	Surface application vs soil incorporation	(Truhlar *et al*., 2015)		
Soil and field management	No-till	(Jenkins *et al*., 2014)		
	Earthworms	(Murry Jr and Hinckley, 1992)		
	Vegetative filter strips	(Bicudo and Goyal, 2003)		
	Biochar	(He *et al*., 2020)		

feed, which also determines the type of pathogens in the manure as well as their capacity to survive treatment (Iwu and Okoh, 2019). It has been suggested that the incidence of pathogens such as *Salmonella* spp. and *E. coli* O157:H7 in cattle is influenced by the nature of the animals' diet; a diet high in energy and poor in fiber aids these pathogens to survive in the manure.

Besides the importance of the type of animal being reared and the concentration of pathogenic microorganisms in animal manure, an additional concern is the ability of pathogens to survive treatments and for long periods, thus remaining infective in the environment until ingested by human or animal hosts. For instance, a significant reduction in the carriage of virulence genes by *E. coli* during commercial manure storage in a Canadian swine farm was found (Duriez *et al.*, 2008). Similarly, the importance of the length and method of storage of manure on microbial composition and pathogen survival was stressed (Topp *et al.*, 2009).

While storage of digestate (sludge and effluent) in tropical areas was considered an effective post-sanitation treatment based on a study conducted in Santa Catarina state, Brazil (Fongaro *et al.*, 2018), it was found in Minnesota (USA) that *S. anatum* could survive in liquid swine manure containing ground piglet carcass for up to 109 days when stored in cold environmental temperatures (<10°C) (Johnston *et al.*, 2003). A study conducted on poultry and pig farms in Germany found that a high manure dry matter (DM) effectively reduced pathogen numbers, but resulted in an elevated amount of particulate matter (PM) emissions and vice versa (Kabelitz *et al.*, 2020). Therefore, optimal DM is a tradeoff between the amount of viable microorganisms and low levels of PM release. The optimal DM of poultry manure for PM emissions and microbial dispersion was found to be 50–70%, which corresponds to the natural DM level of fresh poultry manure (Kabelitz *et al.*, 2021). In another study conducted on German farms, particles of manure origin in the PM10 fraction were found to be small and light enough to be carried over long distances and therefore presents a potential risk of antibiotic-resistant bacteria dispersal in human settlements, when they can be deposited (Münch *et al.*, 2020).

Lime products are the main chemical compounds used to reduce pathogenic microorganisms in manure. This increases pH, inactivating microbial cells (Heinonen-Tanski *et al.*, 2006). Ammonia release at high pH (over 10) also inhibits many enteric bacteria. Lime products have been used to destroy *Salmonella* strains and other pathogens present in manure. For chemical treatment of slurry, it was found that 3% CaO treatment (but not NaOH, H_2SO_4, or $KMnO_4$) had a statistically significant negative effect on *Mycobacterium avium* subsp. *paratuberculosis* viability in cattle slurry, based on a study conducted in southern Chile. *Clostridia* were among the most common bacteria remaining following the application of most chemical treatments (Avilez *et al.*, 2019).

Solarization of chicken manure-treated soil in Lebanon resulted in reductions of potentially pathogenic bacteria, e.g. 26.3% for *S. aureus*, 81.8% for *Clostridium perfringens*, and 92.6% for fecal coliforms (Barbour *et al.*, 2002). Moreover, a Californian study showed that the use of molasses as an amendment to compost teas to stimulate beneficial microbial populations also increased numbers of fast-growing, pathogenic *Salmonella* spp. and *E. coli* (Duffy *et al.*, 2004). Conversely, it was highlighted that the incorporation of bulking agents (e.g. biochar) during manure composting could enhance the degradation of antibiotics and prevent the spread of ARGs within the manure (Iwu *et al.*, 2020).

A study in Victoria, Australia, demonstrated that composting was an effective approach to mitigate ARG dispersal associated with the application of organic waste to fields (Gou *et al.*, 2018). The results of a study conducted in Iran showed a significant reduction in number of FCs in cow manure–organic waste; 350,000 MPN/g in the raw sample decreased to 800 MPN/g within an 8-week period, while in cow manure–sewage sludge, it decreased from 6,500,000 MPN/g to 2400 MPN/g (Karimi *et al.*, 2017). A study of large-scale open-air composting (OC) in the UK showed that pathogenic bacteria (PB) levels in livestock manure were significantly greater than that in the surrounding topsoil, while the distribution of bacteria resistant to amoxicillin (AMX), tetracycline (TC), and amoxicillin-tetracycline (AMX-TC) was lower due to long-term resistance selection pressure (Liu *et al.*, 2021). *E. coli* and *Enterococcus* spp. were the dominant pathogens in faeces and surrounding soil, respectively, and AMX-resistant bacteria dominated in soil, compost, and vegetable samples.

Many efficient and recommended manure treatments like composting have been demonstrated to satisfactorily inactivate enteric pathogens in manure (Alegbeleye and Sant'Ana, 2020). Composting can substantially reduce the antibiotic load, especially during the thermophilic phase, but recalcitrant antibiotics accumulate in compost products and in amended soil (Checcucci *et al.*, 2020). Heap composting of 2–3 months done in an area protected against rain can result in useful reductions in the numbers of enteric microorganisms in cattle manure (Heinonen-Tanski *et al.*, 2006). Composting is ordinarily considered as sufficient to terminate bacteria at 55°C for 3 days (Iwu and Okoh, 2019). With aerobic composting and anaerobic digestion, residues of antibiotics and ARGs are effectively reduced in manure before it is applied to soil (Iwu *et al.*, 2020). However, antibiotic and ARG elimination rates in manure vary between different treatment procedures, manure types, and sites.

It was stressed that manure treatment systems had not been specifically designed to mitigate AMR (Oliver *et al.*, 2020). Well-managed aerobic compost treatments reaching higher peak temperatures (>60°C) are more effective at lowering antibiotic residues than static stockpiles. Both composting and anaerobic digestion repeatedly showed good potential for the removal of ARGs (Urra *et al.*, 2019). Nevertheless, some authors revealed inconsistent results on the beneficial effects of composting on ARG reduction.

Aerobic composting and anaerobic and aerobic digestion of manure are considered to be effective in reducing the introduction of antibiotic resistance into agricultural soils (Wang *et al.*, 2022). Composting was found to significantly reduce levels of extractable antibiotics in livestock manure in nearly all cases (Youngquist *et al.*, 2016). There was, however, more limited evidence that levels of ARB are reduced by composting. Studies of ARGs revealed mixed evidence for their removal during thermophilic composting.

In a survey conducted in France, levels of pathogenic bacteria in both manure and digestate suggested that some (spore-forming) bacteria could remain after anaerobic digestion (Le Maréchal *et al.*, 2019). A study conducted in Eastern Cape (South Africa) showed that bacterial pathogens in manure could be considerably reduced through anaerobic digestion after 133 days (Manyi-Loh *et al.*, 2014). In a study conducted in Washington State (USA), anaerobic digestion of dairy waste was found to have the potential to reduce pathogenic bacteria loading on crops (Saunders *et al.*, 2012). In Guangdong Province, southern China, high-density polyethylene covered biogas digesters (HDPE-BD) were found to be the most eco-friendly and effective anaerobic digester in reducing antibiotic resistance risks in swine wastewater (Zhang *et al.*, 2021).

Heat treatment such as pasteurization has been claimed to be an effective way of reducing enteric microorganisms to an acceptable level of risk (Heinonen-Tanski *et al.*, 2006). In Ireland, the Irish pasteurization process (60°C for 4 days), though energy-intensive, was found to be more effective than EU pasteurization (70°C for 1 hour), with post-AD pasteurization most likely to assure the safety of the digestate (Nag *et al.*, 2021).

A study conducted in Germany showed that bacterial pathogens were inactivated within 3 days of lactic acid fermentation (Scheinemann *et al.*, 2015). Other physical methods have been discussed, namely aeration, ozonation, electrolytic treatment, thermophilic aerobic stabilization, or aerobic sequencing batch reactors (Bicudo and Goyal, 2003).

In terms of the methods of application of treated or untreated manure, the risk to public health from the aerosolized spread of bacteria during slurry spreading by rain gun sprayer was found to be low in a UK study (Hutchison *et al.*, 2008). In Ithaca, New York (USA), surface application of manure resulted in significantly higher numbers of curli-producing *E. coli* than incorporation of manure into soil (Truhlar *et al.*, 2015).

In terms of soil and field management methods, prior or post-manure application did not result in significant differences in total load of *E. coli* and *Salmonella* spp. or the percent of total loads of *E. coli* and *Salmonella* spp. recovered in runoff between tillage systems in Georgia, USA (Jenkins *et al.*, 2014). Results of a study conducted in Connecticut showed that earthworm biotechnology may be beneficial in the management of animal manure by decreasing pathogen persistence (Murry Jr and Hinckley, 1992).

It was also concluded that vegetative filter strips could be used as a best management practice to control microorganism transport in overland flow, based on studies on fecal coliforms and streptococci (Bicudo and Goyal, 2003). It was also stressed that manures were not only a major source of ARGs but could also promote the growth of potential ARG-carrying bacteria by providing nutrients (He *et al.*, 2020). It was also underlined that processes such as using biochar for soil remediation and manure composting could greatly reduce the level and potential spread of ARGs.

PATHOGENIC PARASITES. Few research articles dealt with the risk of human contamination by pathogenic parasites linked to the use of livestock manure in crop fertilization. Although there has yet been no report of foodborne outbreaks of cryptosporidiosis in South Korea, the potential risk exists (Hong *et al.*, 2014). In Phnom Penh, Cambodia, *Ascaris suum* and *Trichuris suis* were detected, respectively, in 1.6 and 2.4% of the 287 samples collected from 176 households during a socio-economic survey of manure handling practices (Ström *et al.*, 2018). It was concluded that manure management in urban and peri-urban households may pose a threat to public health and the environment.

Likewise, few references addressed levers and associated practices/technologies to reduce risk of human contamination by pathogenic parasites linked to crop fertilization using livestock manure (cf. Table 11.4). Relevant studies mentioned treatment of livestock manure by anaerobic digestion and/or pasteurization (Nag *et al.*, 2021), lactic acid fermentation (Scheinemann *et al.*, 2015) or the addition of OM and vermicomposting (Karimi *et al.*, 2017).

PATHOGENIC VIRUSES. Studies dealing with the risk of human contamination by pathogenic viruses from the use of livestock manure in crop fertilization only mentioned the Hepatitis E virus (HEV, an *Hepatovirus*). In Spain, HEV was not detected in any final compost destined to be sold as fertilizer, suggesting that composting is an effective method of eliminating HEV and thus, reducing transmission of HEV from pigs to humans (García *et al.*, 2013). Conversely, in the USA, the occurrence of HEV in both manure samples and in surface water following manure application suggested swine manure as a potential route in the spreading of zoonotic pathogens to the surrounding environment (Givens *et al.*, 2016).

Studies on levers and associated practices/technologies to reduce risk of human contamination by pathogenic viruses from the use of livestock manure in crop fertilization only mentioned treatment of livestock manure by lactic acid fermentation (Scheinemann *et al.*, 2015), composting (García *et al.*, 2013), or anaerobic digestion (Nag *et al.*, 2021) (cf. Table 11.4).

Use of human excreta or sewage sludge for crop fertilization

PATHOGENIC BACTERIA

Associated risk of human exposure to pathogenic bacteria All studies on human contamination by pathogenic bacteria linked to human excreta or sewage sludge used for crop fertilization showed an increased risk. In South Africa, discharge of sewage onto agricultural soil was found to be a potential transmission route to the food web of pathogenic *E. coli* and multidrug-resistant *Listeria monocytogenes* and consequently a threat to public health (Iwu and Okoh, 2020). In Iran, it was concluded that the treatment processes of WWTPs needed to improve in order to produce a higher quality agricultural sludge, since TC and FC coliform counts placed the sludge of the two WWTPs examined into Class B of USEPA 40 CFR Part 503 regulations (Mirhosseini *et al.*, 2008). In Sweden, it was found that the largest number of bacterial infections linked to sludge handling and application, particularly from EHEC (since the risk from *Salmonella* spp. was found to be negligible), was through vegetables fertilized with sludge and eaten raw (Westrell *et al.*, 2004). However, this practice is banned in Sweden.

Levers for mitigating risks of exposure to pathogenic bacteria Levers and associated practices/technologies are listed in Table 11.5.

Table 11.5. Levers and associated practices/technologies to mitigate risk of human exposure to pathogenic bacteria, parasites, and viruses, linked to the use of human excreta or sewage in crop fertilization as reflected by selected references.

Levers	Practices	References/bacteria	References/parasites	References/ viruses
Separation of excreta	Collection of urine	(Bischel *et al.*, 2015)		(Höglund *et al.*, 2002)
Selection of use	Use on selected crops	(Al-Gheethi *et al.*, 2018; de França *et al.*, 2021)	(de França *et al.*, 2021)	
Storage	Storage time		(Jensen *et al.*, 2009)	(Höglund *et al.*, 2002)
Treatment of sludge/ excreta	Aerobic vs anaerobic digestion	(World Health Organization, 2006)		
	Aerobic composting	(Youngquist *et al.*, 2016; Karimi *et al.*, 2017; Urra *et al.*, 2019; Wang *et al.*, 2022)	(Szabová *et al.*, 2010; Amorós *et al.*, 2016)	
	Anaerobic digestion	(Owamah *et al.*, 2014; Youngquist *et al.*, 2016; Fijalkowski *et al.*, 2017; Urra *et al.*, 2019; Zhao and Liu, 2019; McCord *et al.*, 2020; Wang *et al.*, 2022)		
	Addition of organic matter/ livestock manure/ food waste	(Owamah *et al.*, 2014; Karimi *et al.*, 2017)	(Karimi *et al.*, 2017)	
	'Green' composting of human waste	(Liu *et al.*, 2021)		
	Dried sludge	(Mirhosseini *et al.*, 2008)		
	Lactic acid fermentation	(Scheinemann *et al.*, 2015)	(Scheinemann *et al.*, 2015)	
	High temperature	(Fijalkowski *et al.*, 2017)	(Decrey *et al.*, 2011)	
	Trickling filters (TF)	(Fijalkowski *et al.*, 2017)		
	Autothermal thermophilic aerobic digestion (ATAD)	(Fijalkowski *et al.*, 2017)		

Source separation of human excreta is a lever for reducing human infectious disease risk. Collection of urine in South Africa had the benefit of sequestering contaminants prior to environmental release and allowed for targeted treatment of potential health hazards prior to agricultural application (Bischel *et al.*, 2015). This was notably the case for bacteria *Aeromonas* spp., *Shigella* spp. and *Clostridium perfringens*, antibiotics sulfamethoxazole and trimethoprim, and sulfonamide antibiotic resistance gene *sul1*.

In Santa Catarina, Brazil, the use of sewage sludge was found to be acceptable for application on coffee plants, forestry, culture to fibre, and oil production, based on FC counts placing the sludge into class B, although *Salmonella* counts (as well as viruses and viable helminth eggs), would have led to classification as class A (Du Plessis *et al.*, 2015). Selecting the plant species grown in soils fertilized with biosolids issued from sewage treatment (*viz.* processed food crops and non-food crops, vs food crops eaten raw) was also suggested as a means to reduce health risks in Middle Eastern countries, notably from pathogenic and AR *E. coli*, and from *Salmonella*, *Shigella*, and *Clostridium* (Al-Gheethi *et al.*, 2018).

In terms of treatment of sewage sludge and human excreta, in Spain, fecal bacterial markers (fecal coliforms and enterococci, *Clostridium* spores) and ampicillin-resistant bacteria increased in soils amended with high amounts of biosolids. Their decay was different depending on dose and type of biosolid (more rapid decay with anaerobic compared to aerobic sludge) (Gondim-Porto *et al.*, 2016). As for aerobic vermicomposting, in Iran, a significant reduction in number of FCs was observed in cow manure–organic waste: the initial figure of 350,000 MPN/g in the raw sample decreased to 800 MPN/g within 8-weeks, and FC in cow manure–sewage sludge was reduced from 6,500,000 MPN/g to 2400 MPN/g (Karimi *et al.*, 2017).

As indicated in Section 'Levers for mitigating risks of exposure to pathogenic bacteria' for livestock manure, although composting and anaerobic digestion show good potential for ARG removal, there is no overall consensus among scientists (Urra *et al.*, 2019). Aerobic composting and anaerobic and aerobic digestion of sludge were found to be effective in reducing the introduction of antibiotic resistance into agricultural soils (Wang *et al.*, 2022). The literature on the fate of antibiotics, ARB, and ARGs during anaerobic digestion and composting of biosolids, i.e. the solid or semi-solid by-products of municipal wastewater treatment, was reviewed (Williams-Nguyen *et al.*, 2016); while biosolid processing and management are based in part on pathogen removal and removal of antibiotics, ARBs and ARGs are not part of the current decision matrix.

As regards anaerobic digestion specifically, micro-scale biogas systems using proper post-digestion treatment, with potential to improve waste handling and meet fertilizer standards were presented in Uganda (McCord *et al.*, 2020). However, fecal coliform and *E. coli* concentrations of digester effluent exceeded WHO guidelines for unrestricted agricultural field application of excreta-based biosolids ($<1 \times 10^3$ CFU *E. coli* g^{-1}), indicating that digestate poses a risk to human health and should not be field applied.

The residual total coliforms of 2.10x 10^8 CFU/100 ml in the digestate of food waste and human excreta was found to exceed tolerable limits for direct application to fields in Nigeria (Owamah *et al.*, 2014). Microbial analysis of the digestate biofertilizer revealed the presence of bacterial strains from different genera: *Klebsiella*, *Bacillus*, *Bacteroides*, *Pseudomonas*, *Clostridium* and *Salmonella*. *Klebsiella* spp., *Bacillus* spp., and *Pseudomonas* spp. can boost the efficiency of the biofertilizer through nitrogen fixation and soil nutrient solubility but *Klebsiella* spp. and *Salmonella* spp. are potential health hazards.

The presence of antibiotics in the environment may result in antibiotic-resistant strains, such as multi-resistant *E. coli*, occurring in sewage sludge (Fijalkowski *et al.*, 2017). Very little is also known about the ability of pathogenic strains, such as EHEC pathogen O104:H4, to survive in sewage sludge and then in soil. All of these threats should lead to strict limits on the direct use of sewage sludge as a fertilizer on soils. Sewage sludge processing, mainly hygienization with the use of high-temperature, anaerobic digestion, trickling filters (TF), or autothermal thermophilic aerobic digestion (ATAD), may reduce the presence of pathogens such as *E. coli* or *Salmonella* spp.

According to Zhao and Liu, *Escherichia coli*, *Salmonella* spp., *Yersinia enterocolitica*, and

Enterococcus spp. were vulnerable to AD, while *Campylobacter jejuni*, *Streptomyces* spp., *Collinsella aerofaciens*, *Streptococcus salivarius*, and *Gordonia bronchialis* were reported to be much more resistant to and barely removed by AD (Zhao and Liu, 2019). Furthermore, some spore-forming pathogens, e.g. *Clostridium* spp. and *Bacillus* spp. with high resistance to acute stresses, can survive mesophilic or even thermophilic anaerobic digestion, therefore creating a biohazard when biosolids are spread. There was also evidence showing that most ARGs were barely reduced by AD.

In the UK, composting toilet systems (CT) offered faster throughput with improved removal of antibiotic-resistant bacteria (ARB) but a higher number of pathogenic bacteria as compared to large-scale open-air composting (OC) of livestock manure (Liu *et al.*, 2021). In Iran, based on TC and FC counts, wastewater treatment plants needed improvement to produce dried sewage sludge suitable for agricultural spreading (Mirhosseini *et al.*, 2008). Finally, in a study conducted in Germany, bacterial pathogens (*E. coli* EHEC O:157, *Salmonella*, *Listeria*, *Staphylococcus*, *Clostridium*) were inactivated within 3 days of lactic acid fermentation (Scheinemann *et al.*, 2015).

PATHOGENIC PARASITES

Associated risk of human exposure to pathogenic parasites All studies on the risk of human contamination by pathogenic parasites with the use of human excreta/sewage sludge as crop fertilizer drew attention to the increased risk. In Spain, *Cryptosporidium* and *Giardia* (oo) cysts were present in sewage sludge-end products from wastewater treatment, a public health hazard (Jensen *et al.*, 2009). In Switzerland, the risk of contamination by *Ascaris* eggs when using source-separated human urine as fertilizer was highlighted (Decrey *et al.*, 2011). On farms in Vietnam, the use of human excreta as fertilizer was found to be a major risk factor for helminth infection (*Ascaris*, *Trichuris*, and hookworms) (Pham-Duc *et al.*, 2013; Trang *et al.*, 2007).

Levers for mitigating risks of exposure to pathogenic parasites The levers and associated practices/technologies are listed in Table 11.5.

Based on helminth eggs counts in Brazil, the use of sewage sludge was deemed acceptable for application on coffee plants, forestry, culture for fiber, and oil production (see Section 'Levers for mitigating risks of exposure to pathogenic bacteria') (de França *et al.*, 2021). It was also found that by inactivating > 99% of all *A. suum* eggs in human excreta over a three-month storage period, the commonly used Double Vault Composting (DVC) latrine, in which urine is not separated, could potentially provide a safe and hygienic fertilizer in Vietnam (Jensen *et al.*, 2009).

In aerobic sanitation composting, it was only in samples from composting plants that no *Cryptosporidium* and *Giardia* (oo) cysts were detected in Spain (Amorós *et al.*, 2016). In the Slovak Republic, total devitalization of *A. suum* eggs between day 4–5 of a composting experiment in the winter and on day 6 in the summer was observed, and it was concluded that the final product was suitable for agricultural spreading with no risk of transmitting pathogens to the environment (Szabová *et al.*, 2010).

As for aerobic vermicomposting, in Iran, a mixture of cow manure–sludge and cow manure–organic waste had the highest number of parasite eggs (22/g) in the raw samples (Karimi *et al.*, 2017); this was completely removed in the second week of the vermicomposting process. In Germany, *Ascaris suum* eggs were inactivated within 56 days of lactic acid fermentation (Scheinemann *et al.*, 2015).

As regards the microbiological risks struvite fertilizer presents to producers and consumers, *Ascaris* eggs require high temperatures, preferably combined with low relative humidity, for short-term inactivation in Switzerland (Decrey *et al.*, 2011). For temperatures below 35°C, inactivation may occur if the fertilizer cake is stored for several weeks. However, this assumption remains to be tested.

PATHOGENIC VIRUSES. Only two references, both from South Africa, dealt with the risk of human contamination by pathogenic viruses linked to the use of human excreta as a crop fertilizer. The most frequently detected viral pathogens in urine storage tanks in three regions of eThekwini were JC polyomavirus, rotavirus, and human adenovirus in 100%, 34%, and 31% of samples, respectively (Bischel *et al.*, 2015).

In the case of enteroviruses, urine collection had the benefit of sequestering contaminants prior to environmental release and allowed targeted treatment of potential health hazards prior to agricultural application. Finally, by following viral persistence of the Rhesus rotavirus in Sweden over time, it was found that if stored at 20°C for at least 6 months, urine was safe to use as a fertilizer for any crop (Höglund *et al.*, 2002).

Use of other organic amendments for crop fertilization

In Brazil, a wide range of opportunistic fungal pathogens (particularly *Cryptococcus* spp.) were identified in fresh pressmud (a residue derived from sugarcane juice filtrate, used as fertilizer). It was found that the pressmud composting process significantly reduced the pathogenic fungal load (de Oliveira *et al.*, 2016). Pathogenic fungi such as *A. fumigatus* were found to have greater resistance to the composting process for manures and other routinely applied organic waste (Avery *et al.*, 2012). It was also shown that amendment of agricultural soils in Burkina Faso with untreated urban waste led to an increase of some opportunistic human pathogens (*P. aeruginosa* and *Stenotrophomonas maltophilia*) including multi-drug antibiotic resistant isolates (Youenou *et al.*, 2016). A literature review also warned about microbial hazards associated with the application of food waste to soil, while taking stock of processes that can inactivate pathogens, such as thermal destruction, natural die-off, depletion of nutrients, and by-product toxicity (Avery *et al.*, 2012; O'Connor *et al.*, 2022).

As regards bat guano, a literature review called for a compromise between its use as a fertilizer which compensates for the lack of sources of phosphorus, and the risk of fungal infection of workers harvesting the guano in the caves or those mixing, drying, and bagging it, as well as those buying the guano at the cave sites (Jayasvati and Jayasvati, 2018). They suggested mitigation levers such as cave zone management, guano collection training, establishment of veterinary services as well as exposure reduction (Jayasvati and Jayasvati, 2018).

Although microbial inoculants can be differentiated from organic waste-derived organic amendments or organic fertilizers, these are undeniably organic in nature and may potentially exert beneficial effects on plant growth and health (Urra *et al.*, 2019). This is notably the case for Plant Growth Promoting Bacteria (PGPB), which may have negative sanitary effects (Ramakrishna *et al.*, 2019). The application of biofertilizers containing living or dormant PGPB could bring humans into contact with pathogenic bacteria inhabiting the soil rhizosphere, e.g. *Pseudomonas aeruginosa* and *Burkholderia cepacia* and soil bacteria, e.g. *Stenotrophomonas* and *Enterobacter* genera (Tariq *et al.*, 2022).

Irrigation infrastructures (proximity to water bodies)

PATHOGENIC BACTERIA. A national study on the link between epidemiological data for Buruli ulcer disease (BU) cases (caused by the bacterium *Mycobacterium ulcerans*) and environmental and socio-economic data was conducted in Côte d'Ivoire (Brou *et al.*, 2008). It showed that irrigated rice field cultures areas, and, to a lesser extent, banana fields as well as areas in the vicinity of dams used for irrigation and aquaculture purposes, represented high-risk zones for the human population to contract BU.

A literature review on the relationship between common voles (*Microtus arvalis*) population fluctuations and tularemia (a disease caused by the bacterium *Francisella tularensis*) was conducted in North-West Spain (Herrero-Cófreces *et al.*, 2021). It suggested that the colonization of farming environments by common voles was triggered by the transformation and irrigation of agricultural habitats creating a novel terrestrial-aquatic interface. This irruptive rodent host was found to be a major amplifier of the *F. tularensis* bacterium during vole population explosions, with human tularemia episodes being closely linked in time and space to periodic (cyclic) variations in vole abundance.

PATHOGENIC PARASITES. A higher prevalence of malaria (caused by the protozoan parasite *Plasmodium falciparum* and transmitted mainly by the *Anopheles gambiae* complex and by *A. funestus*) was highlighted in villages of northern Côte d'Ivoire involved in double annually cropping of rice (De Plaen *et al.*, 2004). In addition, socio-economic, entomological/ parasitological, and epidemiological surveys were conducted in central Côte d'Ivoire to assess and quantify the effect of malaria, on the performance of farms, with an emphasis on drip-irrigated vegetable farming (Girardin *et al.*, 2004). The results of these surveys showed that well-maintained drip irrigation of vegetable crops (*viz* okra and cabbage) was less associated with transmission of water-related parasitic diseases when compared to traditional surface irrigation, due to the absence of open water bodies.

A descriptive ecological study was conducted in a district of western Ethiopia. The study reviewed health service records to extract data on malaria morbidity, mortality, and prevention and control methods (Haileselassie *et al.*, 2022). It highlighted an abrupt rise in cases immediately following the intensification of rice production and the implementation of an irrigation system by a private agricultural development company. Increased transmission of malaria was thus ascribed to the creation of favorable conditions for mosquito breeding. This ecological transformation is due to agricultural development, particularly irrigation-based rice cultivation. Similarly, a large-scale survey of rural households conducted in eastern Rwanda showed that rice-cultivating households faced a significantly higher malaria risk, as evidenced by a higher incidence of fever. This confirmed the negative externality of agricultural intensification on public health by creating a habitat for malaria-transmitting mosquito species (Rulisa *et al.*, 2022).

It was also highlighted that malaria was 54% more prevalent in the Hola cotton and vegetable irrigation scheme in Kenya than in non-irrigated surrounding areas (Anchang *et al.*, 2014). The authors suggested that farmers may be exposed to mosquito bites when using stagnant water for irrigation or simply as a result of having pools of stagnant water around the farmstead.

An anthropological study was conducted on the prevalence of schistosomiasis (caused by *Schistosoma mansoni*) comprising immunologic examinations of desiccated tissue samples from two ancient Nubian populations (southern Egypt) (Hibbs *et al.*, 2011). These parasitic flatworms are prevalent in aquatic environments such as lakes, stagnant ponds, and paddy fields. One population used canal irrigation. This compounds the risk of exposure to schistosomes by increasing the available habitat for the aquatic snails (intermediate hosts required by the parasitic worm that requires the snails to release its larvae into water), while the other used only annual flood irrigation. The study clearly showed the impact of human environmental alteration on parasite transmission, i.e. that irrigated agriculture contributed in a significant and negative way to schistosomiasis transmission.

In the Diama Dam region (northern Senegal), a team-based theme analysis was conducted to investigate perception of schistosomiasis risk and reported preventive behaviors (Lund *et al.*, 2019). It has been shown that rural villagers understood the risk of schistosomiasis. Accordingly, they adopted some preventive behaviors, but ultimately, exposure persisted because of the unavoidability of contact with water and therefore exposure to schistosome parasites in rural areas. A cross-sectional epidemiological study of the relationship between irrigated area and the prevalence and intensity of schistosome infection was conducted in the same region (Lund *et al.*, 2021). It showed that engagement in irrigated agriculture increased individual risk of *Schistosoma haematobium* but not *S. mansoni* infection. Increased contact with irrigated landscapes was likely the source of exposure, with greater impacts on farming households. Another review also highlighted the fact that rice farmers in sub-Saharan Africa are more exposed to schistosomiasis-causing trematodes than non-farmers (Anchang *et al.*, 2014).

An opinion paper underlined China's remarkable achievements in integrated schistosomiasis control programs, associated experiences and lessons, and the resulting service to those combating the disease, particularly in sub-Saharan Africa (Liang *et al.*, 2018). It highlighted that the key to the success of control programs in China was intervention from the public health sector with environmental management programs sponsored by agricultural and hydrological departments, for instance contamination source management (e.g. human waste and livestock) and agricultural development (e.g. crop structure shifting and irrigation system development that controls disease transmission).

PATHOGENIC VIRUSES. Remote sensing and GIS were used to collate multiple types of environmental data over a continental spatial scale in order to model annual West Nile Fever (WNF) incidence across Europe and neighbouring countries in Asia and North Africa (Marcantonio *et al.*, 2015). Among land use variables, the most significant predictors of WNF incidence were the percentage of area of irrigated croplands, or populated forests, both of which were positively correlated with WNF incidence. An increase of 5% of cultivated irrigated croplands predicted an increase of 113 cases per 100,000 people.

Generalized threshold models were constructed to project vector mosquito (*Culex* spp.) and Japanese encephalitis (JE, caused by a *Flavivirus* species) dynamics in China (Tian *et al.*, 2015). Although (perhaps surprisingly) wetness of rice paddies (assessed by temperature vegetation dryness index) did not significantly impact mosquito density, the normalized difference vegetation index, which measured rice field conditions and could reflect the lushness of the vegetation and biomass level, was both closely associated with mosquito density and number of cases of JE. Rice paddies were thus suspected to provide favorable habitats for mosquito development.

Similarly, irrigated rice farming systems favorable to mosquito development in higher altitudes are a probable risk factor for emergence and re-emergence of JE in Nepal (Ghimire and Dhakal, 2015). *Culex tritaeniorhynchus*, the primary vector of JEV, was mainly found in irrigated rice fields.

Deforestation/habitat fragmentation

PATHOGENIC BACTERIA. Only one reference relating to this practice and pathogen emerged from our review. It was a literature review highlighting that clearing primary forest to develop subsistence farming or more intensive agriculture, e.g. rice farming in Côte d'Ivoire, resulted in increased human exposure to the bacterial pathogen *M. ulcerans*, which causes Buruli ulcer disease (Guégan *et al.*, 2019).

PATHOGENIC PARASITES. In one literature review, the 1940s Trinidad malaria epidemic that struck following forest clearance to create plantations of cocoa, grown in agroforestry systems under *Erythrina* trees, was spotlighted (Walsh *et al.*, 1993). Unfortunately, these nurse trees were ideal sites for epiphytic bromeliads, of which 20 species provided favorable breeding sites for the principal vector of malaria, *Anopheles bellator*. The same review highlighted that destruction of the primary forest in Thailand, followed by planting of coffee and rubber crops, favored the resurgence of *Anopheles minimus*, an important local malaria vector.

Conversely, the review underlined the link in Tanzania between deforestation and a decline of human onchocerciasis (caused by the filarial worm *Onchocerca volvulus*, vector: blackflies of the *Simulium damnosum* complex and the *S. neavei* group, e.g. *S. woodi*). The timber industry and increased agricultural activity are the major causes of deforestation, exposing small, sheltered forest streams and rendering them less suitable breeding sites for *S. woodi*. However, the rapid expansion of cardamom cultivation in small forest clearings translated into increased human exposure to vector bites as a result of their entering the forest more frequently to farm the small patches (Walsh *et al.*, 1993).

PATHOGENIC VIRUSES. An eco-epidemiological survey of arboviruses (particularly the genus *Flavivirus*, e.g. Dengue or WNV) was conducted in Bahia State, Brazil, using multivariate logistic regression models (Catenacci *et al.*, 2021). It highlighted that the presence of forest and free-living monkeys in the areas close to communities had a 'protective' effect on the human population (i.e. lower seroprevalence). The dilution effect was considered as one explanation. A study combined the analysis of fine-scale field temperature data, published temperature responses of *Aedes albopictus* mosquitoes (vectors of the *Flavivirus* species causing Dengue fever), and field data on adult mosquito populations in Malaysia (Gregory *et al.*, 2022). They found that land-use change from forest to oil palm plantation could increase vectorial capacity by 50%. On the same note, an increase of 5% in the area of forests with scattered, low-density human populations predicted an increase of 36 cases of WNF per 100,000 people across Europe and neighbouring Asian and North African countries (Marcantonio *et al.*, 2015).

Rapid deforestation, shrinking buffer zone areas between humans and animals, and hence increased human–animal contact, all create favorable conditions for the emergence of zoonotic diseases and epidemics, notably in Asia, e.g. *Henipavirus* in Malaysia (Debnath *et al.*, 2021). For instance, loss of tropical forests caused fruit bats to change their feeding habits and they shifted to new fruit resources, increasing their contact with humans and the opportunities for disease transmission (Guégan *et al.*, 2019). In Argentina, the emergence in the 1950s of Argentine haemorrhagic fever (AHF) caused by the Junin virus (JV, a *Mammarenavirus*) was hypothesized to have resulted from human alterations to habitats as a result of agricultural intensification (Enria *et al.*, 1998). Such changes in the environment reportedly resulted in the population growth of the main JV reservoir, the rodent *Calomys musculinus*.

Discussion

Crop protection practices are central to the One Health concept insofar as they aim for better crop health through regulation of plant pests and pathogens. They may have either positive or negative impacts on human and environmental health. In particular, protection practices may positively or negatively affect human health *via* their impact on human viral, bacterial, parasitic, or fungal pathogens (Ratnadass and Deberdt, 2021; Ratnadass and Deguine, 2021; Ratnadass and Martin, 2022; Ratnadass and Sester, 2023). However, many other agricultural practices are also relevant to the One Health concept as they contribute equally to human and environmental health *via* different pathways, including soil health, water quality, and better food safety and human nutrition. Hence, the timeliness of the present comprehensive review on interactions between agricultural crop production practices (excluding crop protection practices) and biological risks to human health.

In terms of levers for mitigating human infectious hazards, there were few references in this review on irrigation systems and regimes (i.e. presence of water bodies for irrigation as sources of human infection with pathogens with invertebrate vectors or reservoirs). Many were discarded because they dealt directly with crop protection practices and were thus considered 'out of scope', while some others dealing with malaria and bilharzia, and relevant to the topic of this review (e.g. De Clercq *et al.*, 2000; Haileselassie *et al.*, 2021) surprisingly did not emerge.

On the other hand, some references relate to deforestation and land-use change (but with no reference to crop protection), and as such, which were discarded from our earlier reviews, did not emerge either in this review, despite being relevant to the topic. For instance, in Argentina, deforestation for agricultural purposes other than crop protection resulted in the infestation of maize fields by drylands vesper mouse *Calomys musculinus* and small vesper mouse *C. laucha*, and infestation of soybean and alfalfa plots by Azara's grass mouse *Akodon azarae* and dark bolo mouse *Necromys obscurus*, all rodent pests, and reservoirs of the Junin virus (*Mammarenavirus*, Arenaviridae), responsible for transmission to rural workers, causing Argentine viral hemorrhagic fever outbreaks (Tapia-Ramírez *et al.*, 2022). This was exacerbated by agricultural intensification and mechanization, part of the 'Efficiency-based' approach of the Efficiency-Substitution-Redesign (E-S-R) conceptual framework (Hill and MacRae, 1996) used in our earlier reviews. Combine harvesters currently used in corn monoculture (Enria *et al.*, 1998) not only produce clouds of infectious dust, but also create an aerosol of infectious blood when animals are accidentally crushed.

Conversely, references to the re-use of wastewater for crop irrigation, and on the use of livestock manure and human wastes for crop fertilization were prevalent in this review. Although it may serve crop protection objectives (e.g. animal manure against nematodes: Renčo and Kováčik, 2012; Amulu and Adekunle, 2018), and was therefore considered as such in our earlier reviews, manure application generally serves other purposes, e.g. crop fertilization/nutrition. This was especially the case with wastewater irrigation, or the use of human excreta for fertilization (or as waste disposal practices).

Our study showed that fresh vegetables and those eaten raw were most at risk of contamination from wastewater, sewage sludge, or livestock manure. In this regard, wastewater reuse and surface water contaminated by animal or human feces used in crop irrigation contribute to the dissemination of hazardous waterborne pathogens (e.g. enteric bacteria, viruses, protozoa). Wastewater treatments give mixed results in terms of microbial/parasitic load reduction; protozoa for instance are more resistant to treatment than bacteria or viruses (Partyka and Bond, 2022).

Bacteria were very numerous in the references retrieved, unlike other types of pathogenic organisms. This is mainly because of the burden of foodborne diseases and antibiotic resistance as a public health concern, particularly as a 'One Health' issue (Newell *et al.*, 2010; Otte and Pica-Ciamarra, 2021). The fact that research on bacteria was predominant in most countries was partly due to the bias of microbial indicators, partly due to the burden of opportunistic bacterial pathogens, particularly in the Global North. Discrepancy between research in the Global North and the Global South may also be due to unavailability of research material, funding disparity, lack of critical mass of available researchers.

Despite the value of using indicator bacteria (*E. coli*/coliforms) for monitoring water quality, it is worth noting that these indicators do not necessarily correlate with the presence or concentration of specific pathogenic bacterial, viral, or parasitic strains. In addition, many studies have stressed the need for improving guidelines and risk-based standards to achieve a more effective risk assessment and monitoring (e.g. Forslund *et al.*, 2012; Partyka and Bond, 2022).

Conversely, there were very few references addressing human fungal diseases (mycoses) in this review, other than those (out of scope) dealing with antimicrobial resistance from the use of azole fungicides for crop protection. The outcome of our literature review regarding wastewater irrigation, livestock manure fertilization, and human sewage sludge fertilization is highlighted in Figs. 11.8–11.10. They underline the need for tradeoffs between freshwater saving/ preservation measures and organic waste recycling on the one hand (environmental health), and health hazards on the other (human health).

This issue does not, however, necessarily entail a conflict between the WHO, working towards human infectious disease control, and the FAO, as a defender of food security. This has similarities with the issue of misuse of insecticide-treated mosquito bednets in agriculture (and, worse, in fishing) (Ratnadass and Martin, 2022). But it undeniably sheds light on the multifaceted/ polysemous aspects of health issues.

Further to the need to widely re-use grey water for crop irrigation under certain (if not most) situations, instead of rare and precious drinking water, the use of source-separated and sanitized human urine could, for instance, partly compensate for the lack of nitrogen-based fertilizers, including in the Global South (cf. Moussa *et al.*, 2021). Figs. 11.8–11.10 also

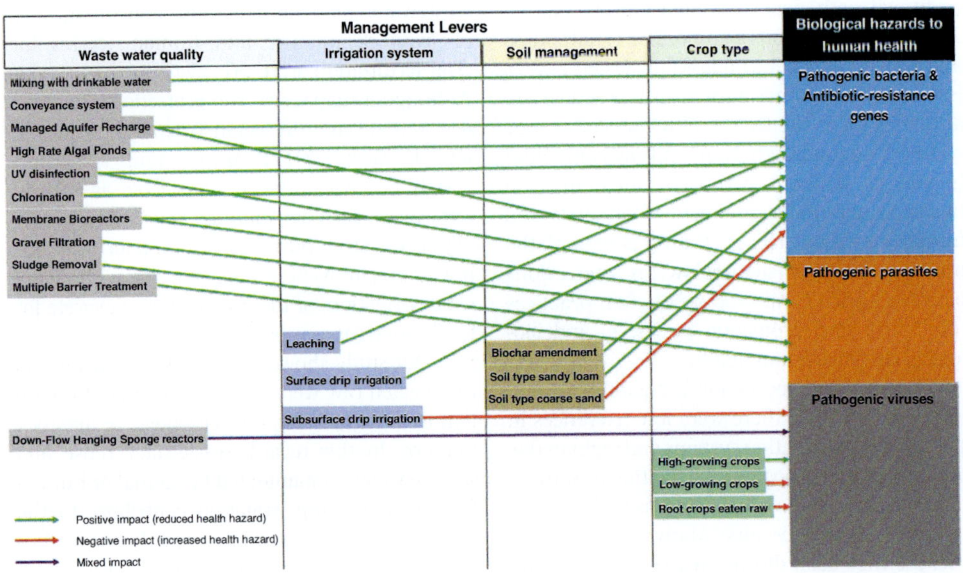

Fig. 11.8. Impacts of irrigation with wastewater on biological hazards to human health.

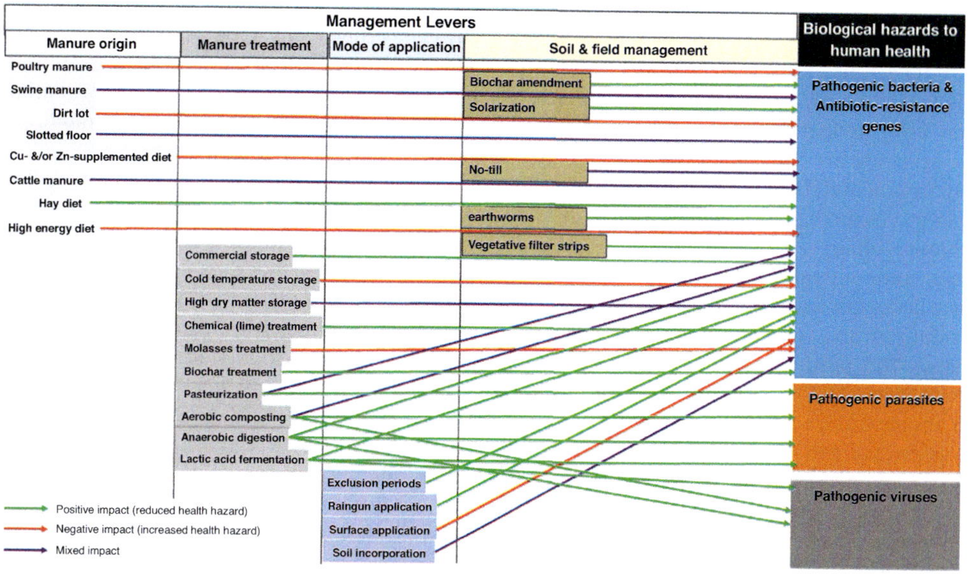

Fig. 11.9. Impacts of fertilization with livestock manure on biological hazards to human health.

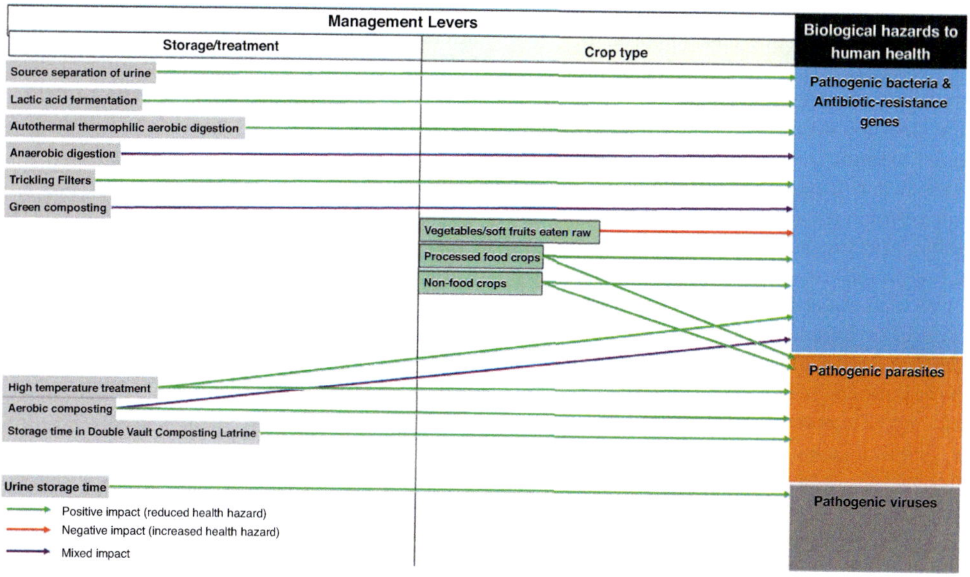

Fig. 11.10. Impacts of fertilization with human excreta or sewage sludge on biological hazards to human health.

underline the many ways available to optimize these uses.

The reuse/recycling of wastewater and that of human and domestic animal waste for crop irrigation and crop fertilization, respectively, are considered critical ecological/ environmental issues, in a context of fresh water resource shortage (notably due to climate change, in terms of both adaptation and mitigation), and over-reliance on synthetic fertilizers (which causes increased pollution and greenhouse gas emissions), hence the need to efficiently and economically dispose of this waste within a circular economy framework. In this respect, recycling wastewater and human and animal organic waste should be viewed as agroecological at the production or food system level, *via* a redesign-based approach, or at least a substitution-based approach. Conversely, drinking water can no longer be considered a truly renewable resource (groundwater certainly is not (Bierkens and Wada, 2019)), so its use pertains to a conventional approach, or at most (e.g. with water-saving drip-irrigation systems), an efficiency-based approach.

Nevertheless, some decontamination processes require energy, many using fuels that are not necessarily renewable, operating under extreme hot and dry climatic conditions. Wastewater treatment in stabilization ponds may result in undesirable losses by water evaporation and nitrogen volatilization. Conversely, although the risk of biological contamination is lower with mineral fertilizers than with animal manure or human waste, their use is not sustainable since it may result in eutrophication in the aquatic environment (e.g. Slavik *et al.*, 2004) and may indirectly promote the emergence of disease, including bilharzias, *via* increased numbers of host snails (Johnson *et al.*, 2007; Halstead *et al.*, 2014).

Further to tradeoffs, synergies can be found from a 'One Health' standpoint. For instance, treatment of irrigation water could target plant-parasitic nematodes as well as human pathogenic helminths (Santos *et al.*, 2014; Benito *et al.*, 2020; Inga López *et al.*, 2020). Soil nematodes along with other soil biota should suppress human pathogens introduced by fertilization and irrigation practices, rather than disseminating them (Roth *et al.*, 2015). Crops, soil types, wastewater, and animal/human waste application techniques should be chosen depending on the contamination level of grey water and whether it has been treated or not.

It should be noted that neither our earlier reviews nor the present review focused on cropping practices resulting in better physiological plant health, directly or *via* what is referred to as 'soil health' (Lehmann *et al.*, 2020), which is central to agroecology. Although this has a beneficial effect on human health, *via* improved access to high quality food in sufficient quantities, this aspect was deemed as beyond the scope of this review since it does not involve organisms pathogenic to humans. Similarly, for non-infectious diseases such as mycotoxin intoxications/ poisoning by plant pathogenic or entomopathogenic fungi, which can be caused by inadequate harvest or postharvest practices, and result in acute or chronic food and fodder safety issues (e.g. Bankole and Adebanjo, 2003; Neme and Mohammed, 2017). It is therefore necessary to broaden the scope of analysis of interactions between agricultural practices and human health, to include non-communicable diseases, in a truly extended 'One Health' perspective.

Conclusion

Our comprehensive literature review of interactions between agricultural practices (excluding crop protection practices) and biological human health hazards, highlighted the following:

- Bacteria (particularly *Escherichia coli* and *Salmonella* spp.), parasitic protozoa (particularly *Cryptosporidium* spp. and *Giardia* spp.), and helminths (particularly *Ascaris* spp. and *Trichuris* spp.), as well as enteric viruses as major biological threats;
- Fresh vegetables, particularly leafy greens, and those eaten raw, as particularly unsafe;
- Irrigation with wastewater and fertilization with livestock manure and human excreta/ sewage sludge as potentially hazardous practices.

However, the recycling of wastewater and human and animal organic waste is essential from an environmental health perspective, and even for some aspects of human health. Further to tradeoffs, synergies and optimal pathways must be sought to reconcile all dimensions of crop production with human, animal, and environmental health, both from agroecological and 'One Health' perspectives.

Acknowledgments

The authors thank Andrew Hobson for the English editing of the manuscript. This study and English editing were supported by the CIRAD DPP SantéBiodiv agronomical research program (period: 2022–2024) from the European Union (ERDF) and the Conseil Régional de La Réunion.

Conflict of Interest

The authors have no conflicts of interest to declare.

References

Abass, K., Ganle, J.K. and Adaborna, E. (2016) Coliform contamination of peri-urban grown vegetables and potential public health risks: Evidence from Kumasi, Ghana. *Journal of Community Health* 41(2), 392–397. DOI: 10.1007/s10900-015-0109-y.

Abdelhafiz, M.A., Elnazer, A.A., Seleem, E.M.M., Mostafa, A., Al-Gamal, A.G. *et al.* (2021) Chemical and bacterial quality monitoring of the Nile River water and associated health risks in Qena–Sohag sector, Egypt. *Environmental Geochemistry and Health* 43(10), 4089–4104. DOI: 10.1007/s10653-021-00893-3.

Adegoke, A.A., Amoah, I.D., Stenström, T.A., Verbyla, M.E. and Mihelcic, J.R. (2018) Epidemiological evidence and health risks associated with agricultural reuse of partially treated and untreated wastewater: A review. *Frontiers in Public Health* 6, 337. DOI: 10.3389/fpubh.2018.00337.

Alam, A. and Ali, L. (2021) Prospects and risks related to potential transmission of COVID-19 and other viruses and disinfection in sewage effluent. *Pakistan Journal of Zoology* 53(2). DOI: 10.17582/journal.pjz/20200821130834.

Alegbeleye, O.O. and Sant'Ana, A.S. (2020) Manure-borne pathogens as an important source of water contamination: An update on the dynamics of pathogen survival/transport as well as practical risk mitigation strategies. *International Journal of Hygiene and Environmental Health* 227, 113524. DOI: 10.1016/j.ijheh.2020.113524.

Alegbeleye, O.O., Singleton, I. and Sant'Ana, A.S. (2018) Sources and contamination routes of microbial pathogens to fresh produce during field cultivation: A review. *Food Microbiology* 73, 177–208. DOI: 10.1016/j.fm.2018.01.003.

Al-Gheethi, A.A., Efaq, A.N., Bala, J.D., Norli, I. and Abdel-Monem, M.O. (2018) Removal of pathogenic bacteria from sewage-treated effluent and biosolids for agricultural purposes. *Applied Water Science* 8(2), 1–25. DOI: 10.1007/s13201-018-0698-6.

Allard, S.M., Callahan, M.T., Bui, A., Ferelli, A.M.C., Chopyk, J. *et al.* (2019) Creek to table: Tracking fecal indicator bacteria, bacterial pathogens, and total bacterial communities from irrigation water to kale and radish crops. *Science of the Total Environment* 666, 461–471. DOI: 10.1016/j.scitotenv.2019.02.179.

Amador, P., Duarte, I.M., Costa, R.R., Fernandes, R. and Prudêncio, C. (2018) Characterization of antibiotic resistance in *Enterobacteriaceae* from agricultural manure and soil in Portugal. *Soil Science* 182(8), 292–301. DOI: 10.1097/SS.0000000000000222.

Amahmid, O., Asmama, S. and Bouhoum, K. (2022) Pathogenic parasites in sewage irrigated crops and soil: Pattern of occurrence and health implications. *International Journal of Environmental Health Research* 32(7), 1594–1608. DOI: 10.1080/09603123.2021.1898551.

Amato, M., Dasí, D., González, A., Ferrús, M.A. and Castillo, M.Á. (2021) Occurrence of antibiotic resistant bacteria and resistance genes in agricultural irrigation waters from Valencia city (Spain). *Agricultural Water Management* 256, 107097. DOI: 10.1016/j.agwat.2021.107097.

Amorós, I., Moreno, Y., Reyes, M., Moreno-Mesonero, L. and Alonso, J.L. (2016) Prevalence of *Cryptosporidium oocysts* and *Giardia cysts* in raw and treated sewage sludges. *Environmental Technology* 37(22), 2898–2904. DOI: 10.1080/09593330.2016.1168486.

Amulu, L.U. and Adekunle, O.K. (2018) Comparative effects of poultry manure, cow dung, and carbofuran on yield of *Meloidogyne incognita*-infested okra. *Journal of Agricultural Science and Technology* 17, 495–504.

Anchang, K.Y., Avery, L. and Pertiwiningrum, A. (2014) A commentary on occupational infectious diseases due to agricultural practices in Sub-Saharan Africa. *Biomass and Bioenergy* 70, 99–111. DOI: 10.1016/j.biombioe.2014.02.037.

Antwi-Agyei, P., Cairncross, S., Peasey, A., Price, V., Bruce, J. *et al.* (2015) A farm to fork risk assessment for the use of wastewater in agriculture in Accra, Ghana. *PloS One* 10(11), e0142346. DOI: 10.1371/journal.pone.0142346.

An, Y.J., Yoon, C.G., Jung, K.W. and Ham, J.H. (2007) Estimating the microbial risk of *E. coli* in reclaimed wastewater irrigation on paddy field. *Environmental Monitoring and Assessment* 129(1), 53–60. DOI: 10.1007/s10661-006-9425-0.

Armon, R., Dosoretz, C.G., Azov, Y. and Shelef, G. (1994) Residual contamination of crops irrigated with effluent of different qualities: A field study. *Water Science and Technology* 30(9), 239.

Armon, R., Gold, D., Brodsky, M. and Oron, G. (2002) Surface and subsurface irrigation with effluents of different qualities and presence of *Cryptosporidium oocysts* in soil and on crops. *Water Science and Technology* 46(3), 115–122.

Avery, L.M., Booth, P., Campbell, C., Tompkins, D. and Hough, R.L. (2012) Prevalence and survival of potential pathogens in source-segregated green waste compost. *Science of the Total Environment* 431, 128–138. DOI: 10.1016/j.scitotenv.2012.05.020.

Avilez, C., Alfaro, M.A., Salazar, F., Encina, C., Verdugo, C. *et al.* (2019) Fate of *Mycobacterium avium* subsp. *paratuberculosis* and changes in bacterial diversity populations in dairy slurry after chemical treatments. *Journal of Applied Microbiology* 127(2), 370–378. DOI: 10.1111/jam.14288.

Ayuso-Gabella, N., Page, D., Masciopinto, C., Aharoni, A., Salgot, M. *et al.* (2011) Quantifying the effect of Managed Aquifer Recharge on the microbiological human health risks of irrigating crops with recycled water. *Agricultural Water Management* 99(1), 93–102. DOI: 10.1016/j.agwat.2011.07.014.

Bankole, S.A. and Adebanjo, A. (2003) Mycotoxins in food in West Africa: Current situation and possibilities of controlling it. *African Journal of Biotechnology* 2(9), 254–263. DOI: 10.5897/AJB2003.000-1053.

Barbour, E.K., Husseini, S.A., Farran, M.T., Itani, D.A., Houalla, R.H. *et al.* (2002) Soil solarization: A sustainable agriculture approach to reduce microorganisms in chicken manure-treated soil. *Journal of Sustainable Agriculture* 19(4), 95–104. DOI: 10.1300/J064v19n04_09.

Beaudequin, D., Harden, F., Roiko, A. and Mengersen, K. (2016) Utility of Bayesian networks in QMRA-based evaluation of risk reduction options for recycled water. *Science of the Total Environment* 541, 1393–1409. DOI: 10.1016/j.scitotenv.2015.10.030.

Bech, T.B., Badawi, N. and Rosenbom, A.E. (2022) Impact of surface-applied liquid manure on the drainage resistance profile of an agricultural tile-drained clay till field. *Journal of Environmental Quality* 51(4), 656–669. DOI: 10.1002/jeq2.20354.

Benito, M., Menacho, C., Chueca, P., Ormad, M.P. and Goñi, P. (2020) Seeking the reuse of effluents and sludge from conventional wastewater treatment plants: Analysis of the presence of intestinal protozoa and nematode eggs. *Journal of Environmental Management* 261, 110268. DOI: 10.1016/j.jenvman.2020.110268.

Bernstein, N. (2011) Potential for contamination of crops by microbial human pathogens introduced into the soil by irrigation with treated effluent. *Israel Journal of Plant Sciences* 59(2–4), 115–123. DOI: 10.1560/IJPS.59.2-4.115.

Bernstein, N., Sela, S. and Neder-Lavon, S. (2007) Effect of irrigation regimes on persistence of *Salmonella enterica* serovar Newport in small experimental pots designed for plant cultivation. *Irrigation Science* 26(1), 1–8. DOI: 10.1007/s00271-006-0059-3.

Bernstein, N., Guetsky, R., Friedman, H., Bar-Tal, A. and Rot, I. (2008) Monitoring bacterial populations in an agricultural greenhouse production system irrigated with reclaimed wastewater. *The Journal of Horticultural Science and Biotechnology* 83(6), 821–827. DOI: 10.1080/14620316.2008.11512467.

Bicudo, J.R. and Goyal, S.M. (2003) Pathogens and manure management systems: A review. *Environmental Technology* 24(1), 115–130. DOI: 10.1080/09593330309385542.

Bierkens, M.F. and Wada, Y. (2019) Non-renewable groundwater use and groundwater depletion: A review. *Environmental Research Letters* 14(6), 063002. DOI: 10.1088/1748-9326/ab1a5f.

Bischel, H.N., Duygan, B.D.Ö., Strande, L., McArdell, C.S., Udert, K.M. *et al.* (2015) Pathogens and pharmaceuticals in source-separated urine in Ethekwini, South Africa. *Water Research* 85, 57–65. DOI: 10.1016/j.watres.2015.08.022.

Blumenthal, U.J., Mara, D.D., Peasey, A., Ruiz-Palacios, G. and Stott, R. (2000) Guidelines for the microbiological quality of treated wastewater used in agriculture: Recommendations for revising WHO guidelines. *Bulletin of the World Health Organization* 78, 1104–1116.

Boa, E., Danielsen, S. and Haesen, S. (2015) Better together: Identifying the benefits of a closer integration between plant health, agriculture and One Health. In: Zinsstag, J., Schelling, E., Waltner-Toews, D., Whittaker, M. and Tanner, M. (eds) *One Health: The Theory and Practice of Integrated Health Approaches*. CABI, Wallingford, UK, pp. 258–271. DOI: 10.1079/9781780643410.0258.

Bonetta, S., Pignata, C., Gasparro, E., Richiardi, L., Bonetta, S. *et al.* (2022) Impact of wastewater treatment plants on microbiological contamination for evaluating the risks of wastewater reuse. *Environmental Sciences Europe* 34(1), 1–13. DOI: 10.1186/s12302-022-00597-0.

Bougnom, B.P., Thiele-Bruhn, S., Ricci, V., Zongo, C. and Piddock, L.J.V. (2020) Raw wastewater irrigation for urban agriculture in three African cities increases the abundance of transferable antibiotic resistance genes in soil, including those encoding extended spectrum β-lactamases (ESBLs). *Science of the Total Environment* 698, 134201. DOI: 10.1016/j.scitotenv.2019.134201.

Brooks, J.P., Adeli, A. and McLaughlin, M.R. (2014) Microbial ecology, bacterial pathogens, and antibiotic resistant genes in swine manure wastewater as influenced by three swine management systems. *Water Research* 57, 96–103. DOI: 10.1016/j.watres.2014.03.017.

Brou, T., Broutin, H., Elguero, E., Asse, H. and Guegan, J.F. (2008) Landscape diversity related to Buruli ulcer disease in Cote d'Ivoire. *PLoS Neglected Tropical Diseases* 2(7), e271. DOI: 10.1371/journal.pntd.0000271.

Campos, C. (2008) New perspectives on microbiological water control for wastewater reuse. *Desalination* 218(1–3), 34–42. DOI: 10.1016/j.desal.2007.08.002.

Casey, J.A., Curriero, F.C., Cosgrove, S.E., Nachman, K.E. and Schwartz, B.S. (2013) High-density livestock operations, crop field application of manure, and risk of community-associated methicillin-resistant *Staphylococcus aureus* infection in Pennsylvania. *JAMA Internal Medicine* 173(21), 1980–1990. DOI: 10.1001/jamainternmed.2013.10408.

Catenacci, L.S., Ferreira, M.S., Fernandes, D., Padda, H., Travassos-da-Rosa, E.S. *et al.* (2021) Individual, household and environmental factors associated with arboviruses in rural human populations, Brazil. *Zoonoses and Public Health* 68(3), 203–212. DOI: 10.1111/zph.12811.

Chacón, L., Barrantes, K., Santamaría-Ulloa, C., Solano, M., Reyes, L. *et al.* (2020) A somatic coliphage threshold approach to improve the management of activated sludge wastewater treatment plant effluents in resource-limited regions. *Applied and Environmental Microbiology* 86(17), e00616–20. DOI: 10.1128/AEM.00616-20.

Chandrasekaran, S. and Jiang, S.C. (2018) A dynamic transport model for quantification of norovirus internalization in lettuce from irrigation water and associated health risk. *Science of the Total Environment* 643, 751–761. DOI: 10.1016/j.scitotenv.2018.06.158.

Checcucci, A., Trevisi, P., Luise, D., Modesto, M., Blasioli, S. *et al.* (2020) Exploring the animal waste resistome: The spread of antimicrobial resistance genes through the use of livestock manure. *Frontiers in Microbiology* 11, 1416. DOI: 10.3389/fmicb.2020.01416.

Chen, Z., Biswas, S., Aminabadi, P., Stackhouse, J.W., Jay-Russell, M.T. *et al.* (2019) Prevalence of *Escherichia coli* O157 and *Salmonella* spp. in solid bovine manure in California using real-time quantitative PCR. *Letters in Applied Microbiology* 69(1), 23–29. DOI: 10.1111/lam.13156.

Chigor, C.B., Ibangha, I.A.I., Nweze, N.O., Onuora, V.C., Ozochi, C.A. *et al.* (2022) Prevalence of integrons in multidrug-resistant *Escherichia coli* isolates from waters and vegetables in Nsukka and Enugu, Southeast Nigeria. *Environmental Science and Pollution Research* 29(40), 60952. DOI: 10.1007/s11356-022-20254-6.

Clarivate Analytics (2021) *Web of Science Databases*. Available at: https://clarivate.com/products/web-of-science/databases/ (accessed 15 July 2022).

Courault, D., Albert, I., Perelle, S., Fraisse, A., Renault, P. *et al.* (2017) Assessment and risk modeling of airborne enteric viruses emitted from wastewater reused for irrigation. *Science of the Total Environment* 592, 512–526. DOI: 10.1016/j.scitotenv.2017.03.105.

Cruz, D., Cisneros, R., Benítez, Á., Zúñiga-Sarango, W., Peña, J. *et al.* (2021) Gram-negative bacteria from organic and conventional agriculture in the hydrographic basin of Loja: Quality or pathogen reservoir? *Agronomy* 11(11), 2362. DOI: 10.3390/agronomy11112362.

Cui, E.P., Gao, F., Liu, Y., Fan, X.Y., Li, Z.Y. *et al.* (2018) Amendment soil with biochar to control antibiotic resistance genes under unconventional water resources irrigation: Proceed with caution. *Environmental Pollution* 240, 475–484. DOI: 10.1016/j.envpol.2018.04.143.

Cui, B., Hu, C., Fan, X., Cui, E., Li, Z. *et al.* (2020) Changes of endophytic bacterial community and pathogens in pepper (*Capsicum annuum* L.) as affected by reclaimed water irrigation. *Applied Soil Ecology* 156, 103627. DOI: 10.1016/j.apsoil.2020.103627.

Cutolo, S.A., Piveli, R.P., Santos, J.G., Montes, C.R., Sundefeld, G. *et al.* (2012) Parasitological risk assessment from wastewater reuse for disposal in soil in developing countries. *Water Science and Technology* 65(8), 1357–1367. DOI: 10.2166/wst.2012.012.

Danielsen, S., Kajura, C., Mulema, J., Taylor, R., Kansiime, M. *et al.* (2019) Reaching for the low hanging fruits: One health benefits of joint crop-livestock services for small-scale farmers. *One Health* 7, 100082. DOI: 10.1016/j.onehlt.2019.100082.

Debnath, F., Chakraborty, D., Deb, A.K., Saha, M.K. and Dutta, S. (2021) Increased human-animal interface and emerging zoonotic diseases: An enigma requiring multi-sectoral efforts to address. *The Indian Journal of Medical Research* 153(5–6), 577. DOI: 10.4103/ijmr.IJMR_2971_20.

Decrey, L., Udert, K.M., Tilley, E., Pecson, B.M. and Kohn, T. (2011) Fate of the pathogen indicators phage φX174 and *Ascaris suum* eggs during the production of struvite fertilizer from source-separated urine. *Water Research* 45(16), 4960–4972. DOI: 10.1016/j.watres.2011.06.042.

Deepnarain, N., Nasr, M., Amoah, I.D., Enitan-Folami, A.M., Reddy, P. *et al.* (2020) Impact of sludge bulking on receiving environment using quantitative microbial risk assessment (QMRA)-based management for full-scale wastewater treatment plants. *Journal of Environmental Management* 267, 110660. DOI: 10.1016/j.jenvman.2020.110660.

Destoumieux-Garzón, D., Mavingui, P., Boetsch, G., Boissier, J., Darriet, F. *et al.* (2018) The one health concept: 10 years old and a long road ahead. *Frontiers in Veterinary Science* 5, 14. DOI: 10.3389/fvets.2018.00014.

De Clercq, D., Vercruysse, J., Sène, M., Seck, I., Sall, C.S.M. *et al.* (2000) The effects of irrigated agriculture on the transmission of urinary schistosomiasis in the Middle and Upper Valleys of the Senegal River basin. *Annals of Tropical Medicine and Parasitology* 94(6), 581–590.

de França, M., Emmerich, M., Oliveira, T.M.N., Franczack, P. and Oliveira Maia, B.G. (2021) Toxicity study of the sanitary wastewater treatment plant sludge aiming its reuse in agriculture. *Water, Air and Soil Pollution* 232(6), 1–12. DOI: 10.1007/s11270-021-05192-2.

de Oliveira, T.B., Lopes, V.C.P., Barbosa, F.N., Ferro, M., Meirelles, L.A. *et al.* (2016) Fungal communities in pressmud composting harbour beneficial and detrimental fungi for human welfare. *Microbiology* 162(7), 1147–1156. DOI: 10.1099/mic.0.000306.

De Plaen, R., Seka, M.L. and Koutoua, A. (2004) The paddy, the vector and the caregiver: Lessons from an ecosystem approach to irrigation and malaria in Northern Côte d'Ivoire. *Acta Tropica* 89(2), 135–146. DOI: 10.1016/j.actatropica.2003.09.018.

Di Giovanni, G.D., Betancourt, W.Q., Hernandez, J., Assadian, N.W., Flores Margez, J.P. *et al.* (2006) Investigation of potential zooanthroponotic transmission of cryptosporidiosis and giardiasis through agricultural use of reclaimed wastewater. *International Journal of Environmental Health Research* 16(6), 405–418. DOI: 10.1080/09603120601095100.

Domínguez, D.C., Chacón, L.M. and Wallace, D.J. (2021) Anthropogenic activities and the problem of antibiotic resistance in Latin America: A water issue. *Water* 13(19), 2693. DOI: 10.3390/w13192693.

Du Plessis, E.M., Duvenage, F. and Korsten, L. (2015) Determining the potential link between irrigation water quality and the microbiological quality of onions by phenotypic and genotypic characterization of *Escherichia coli* isolates. *Journal of Food Protection* 78(4), 643–651. DOI: 10.4315/0362-028X.JFP-14-486.

Duan, M., Li, H., Gu, J., Tuo, X., Sun, W. *et al.* (2017) Effects of biochar on reducing the abundance of oxytetracycline, antibiotic resistance genes, and human pathogenic bacteria in soil and lettuce. *Environmental Pollution* 224, 787–795. DOI: 10.1016/j.envpol.2017.01.021.

Duffy, B., Sarreal, C., Ravva, S. and Stanker, L. (2004) Effect of molasses on regrowth of *E. coli* O157: H7 and Salmonella in compost teas. *Compost Science and Utilization* 12(1), 93–96.
Duriez, P., Zhang, Y., Lu, Z., Scott, A. and Topp, E. (2008) Loss of virulence genes in *Escherichia coli* populations during manure storage on a commercial swine farm. *Applied and Environmental Microbiology* 74(13), 3935–3942. DOI: 10.1128/AEM.02710-07.
Eissenberger, K., Drissner, D., Walsh, F., Weiss, A. and Schmidt, H. (2020) Plant variety and soil type influence *Escherichia coli* O104: H4 strain C227/11ϕcu adherence to and internalization into the roots of lettuce plants. *Food Microbiology* 86, 103316. DOI: 10.1016/j.fm.2019.103316.
Enria, D.A., Briggiler, A.M. and Feuillade, M.R. (1998) An overview of the epidemiological, ecological and preventive hallmarks of Argentine haemorrhagic fever (Junin virus). *Bulletin de l'Institut Pasteur* 96(2), 103–114.
Esteves, R.G.R., Gerba, C.P. and Slack, D.C. (2020) Evaluation of subsurface irrigation on microorganism contamination of romaine lettuce. *E3S Web of Conferences* 187, 04009. DOI: 10.1051/e3sconf/202018704009.
Fahrenfeld, N., Ma, Y., O'Brien, M. and Pruden, A. (2013) Reclaimed water as a reservoir of antibiotic resistance genes: Distribution system and irrigation implications. *Frontiers in Microbiology* 4, 130. DOI: 10.3389/fmicb.2013.00130.
FAO, CIRAD, CIFOR and WCS (2020) *White paper: Build back better in a post-COVID-19 world – Reducing future wildlife-borne spillover of disease to humans: Sustainable Wildlife Management (SWM) Programme*. FAO, Rome. DOI: 10.4060/cb1503en.
Farhadkhani, M., Nikaeen, M., Hadi, M., Gholipour, S. and Yadegarfar, G. (2020) Campylobacter risk for the consumers of wastewater-irrigated vegetables based on field experiments. *Chemosphere* 251, 126408. DOI: 10.1016/j.chemosphere.2020.126408.
Fatoba, D.O., Amoako, D.G., Abia, A.L.K. and Essack, S.Y. (2022) Transmission of antibiotic-resistant *Escherichia coli* from chicken litter to agricultural soil. *Frontiers in Environmental Science* 9, 751732. DOI: 10.3389/fenvs.2021.751732.
Fijalkowski, K., Rorat, A., Grobelak, A. and Kacprzak, M.J. (2017) The presence of contaminations in sewage sludge–the current situation. *Journal of Environmental Management* 203, 1126–1136. DOI: 10.1016/j.jenvman.2017.05.068.
Fongaro, G., Kunz, A., Magri, M.E., Viancelli, A., Schissi, C.D. *et al.* (2018) Evaluation of the effective inactivation of enteric bacteria and viruses from swine effluent and sludge at tropical temperatures. *Water, Air and Soil Pollution* 229(7), 1–8. DOI: 10.1007/s11270-018-3878-y.
Forslund, A., Andersen, M.N., Markussen, B. and Dalsgaard, A. (2011) Leaching of human pathogens in repacked soil lysimeters and contamination of potato tubers under subsurface drip irrigation in Denmark. *Water Research* 45(15), 4367–4380. DOI: 10.1016/j.watres.2011.05.009.
Forslund, A., Ensink, J.H.J., Markussen, B., Battilani, A., Psarras, G. *et al.* (2012) *Escherichia coli* contamination and health aspects of soil and tomatoes (*Solanum lycopersicum* L.) subsurface drip irrigated with on-site treated domestic wastewater. *Water Research* 46(18), 5917–5934. DOI: 10.1016/j.watres.2012.08.011.
Fraaije, B., Atkins, S., Hanley, S., Macdonald, A. and Lucas, J. (2020) The multi-fungicide resistance status of aspergillus fumigatus populations in arable soils and the wider European environment. *Frontiers in Microbiology* 11, 599233. DOI: 10.3389/fmicb.2020.599233.
Fuhrimann, S., Pham-Duc, P., Cissé, G., Tram, N.T., Ha, H.T. *et al.* (2016a) Microbial contamination along the main open wastewater and storm water channel of Hanoi, Vietnam, and potential health risks for urban farmers. *Science of the Total Environment* 566, 1014–1022. DOI: 10.1016/j.scitotenv.2016.05.080.
Fuhrimann, S., Winkler, M.S., Pham-Duc, P., Do-Trung, D., Schindler, C. *et al.* (2016b) Intestinal parasite infections and associated risk factors in communities exposed to wastewater in urban and peri-urban transition zones in Hanoi, Vietnam. *Parasites and Vectors* 9(1), 1–14. DOI: 10.1186/s13071-016-1809-6.
García, M., Fernandez-Barredo, S. and Pérez-Gracia, M.T. (2013) Detection of hepatitis E virus (HEV) through the different stages of pig manure composting plants. *Microbial Biotechnology* 7(1), 26–31. DOI: 10.1111/1751-7915.12064.
Garcia, B.C.B., Dimasupil, M.A.Z., Vital, P.G., Widmer, K.W. and Rivera, W.L. (2015) Fecal contamination in irrigation water and microbial quality of vegetable primary production in urban farms of Metro Manila, Philippines. *Journal of Environmental Science and Health, Part B* 50(10), 734–743. DOI: 10.1080/03601234.2015.1048107.

Garcia-Rubio, R., Gonzalez-Jimenez, I., Lucio, J. and Mellado, E. (2021) *Aspergillus fumigatus* cross-resistance between clinical and demethylase inhibitor azole drugs. *Applied Environmental Microbiology* 87, e02539–20. DOI: 10.1128/AEM.02539-20.

Geldreich, E.E. (1996) Pathogenic agents in freshwater resources. *Hydrological Processes* 10(2), 315–333.

Ghimire, S. and Dhakal, S. (2015) Japanese encephalitis: Challenges and intervention opportunities in Nepal. *Veterinary World* 8(1), 61–65. DOI: 10.14202/vetworld.2015.61-65.

Gholipour, S., Hosseini, M., Nikaeen, M., Hadi, M., Sarmadi, M. *et al.* (2022) Quantification of human adenovirus in irrigation water-soil-crop continuum: Are consumers of wastewater-irrigated vegetables at risk? *Environmental Science and Pollution Research* 29(36), 54561–54570. DOI: 10.1007/s11356-022-19588-y.

Giangaspero, A., Marangi, M., Koehler, A.V., Papini, R., Normanno, G. *et al.* (2015) Molecular detection of cyclospora in water, soil, vegetables and humans in southern Italy signals a need for improved monitoring by health authorities. *International Journal of Food Microbiology* 211, 95–100. DOI: 10.1016/j.ijfoodmicro.2015.07.002.

Girardin, O., Dao, D., Koudou, B.G., Essé, C., Cissé, G. *et al.* (2004) Opportunities and limiting factors of intensive vegetable farming in malaria endemic Côte d'Ivoire. *Acta Tropica* 89(2), 109–123. DOI: 10.1016/j.actatropica.2003.08.004.

Givens, C.E., Kolpin, D.W., Borchardt, M.A., Duris, J.W., Moorman, T.B. *et al.* (2016) Detection of hepatitis e virus and other livestock-related pathogens in Iowa streams. *Science of the Total Environment* 566, 1042–1051. DOI: 10.1016/j.scitotenv.2016.05.123.

Gondim-Porto, C., Platero, L., Nadal, I. and Navarro-García, F. (2016) Fate of classical faecal bacterial markers and ampicillin-resistant bacteria in agricultural soils under mediterranean climate after urban sludge amendment. *Science of the Total Environment* 565, 200–210. DOI: 10.1016/j.scitotenv.2016.04.160.

Gonzales-Gustavson, E., Rusiñol, M., Medema, G., Calvo, M. and Girones, R. (2019) Quantitative risk assessment of norovirus and adenovirus for the use of reclaimed water to irrigate lettuce in Catalonia. *Water Research* 153, 91–99. DOI: 10.1016/j.watres.2018.12.070.

Gou, M., Hu, H.W., Zhang, Y.J., Wang, J.T., Hayden, H. *et al.* (2018) Aerobic composting reduces antibiotic resistance genes in cattle manure and the resistome dissemination in agricultural soils. *Science of the Total Environment* 612, 1300–1310. DOI: 10.1016/j.scitotenv.2017.09.028.

Gregory, N., Ewers, R.M., Chung, A.Y.C. and Cator, L.J. (2022) Oil palm expansion increases the vectorial capacity of dengue vectors in Malaysian Borneo. *PLOS Neglected Tropical Diseases* 16(3), e0009525. DOI: 10.1371/journal.pntd.0009525.

Gregson, B.H., Bani, A., Steinfield, L., Holt, D. and Whitby, C. (2022) Anaerobes and methanogens dominate the microbial communities in water harvesting ponds used by Kenyan rural smallholder farmers. *Science of the Total Environment* 819, 153040. DOI: 10.1016/j.scitotenv.2022.153040.

Guégan, J.F., Thoisy, B., Ayouba, A. and Cappelle, J. (2019) Forêts tropicales, changements d'usage des sols et risques infectieux émergents. *Santé Publique* 1(HS), 91–106. DOI: 10.3917/spub.190.0091.

Haileselassie, W., Zemene, E., Lee, M.C., Zhong, D., Zhou, G. *et al.* (2021) The effect of irrigation on malaria vector bionomics and transmission intensity in Western Ethiopia. *Parasites and Vectors* 14, 1–11. DOI: 10.1186/s13071-021-04993-y.

Haileselassie, W., Parker, D.M., Taye, B., David, R.E., Zemene, E. *et al.* (2022) Burden of malaria, impact of interventions and climate variability in Western Ethiopia: An area with large irrigation based farming. *BMC Public Health* 22(1), 1–11. DOI: 10.1186/s12889-022-12571-9.

Halstead, N.T., McMahon, T.A., Johnson, S.A., Raffel, T.R., Romansic, J.M. *et al.* (2014) Community ecology theory predicts the effects of agrochemical mixtures on aquatic biodiversity and ecosystem properties. *Ecology Letters* 17(8), 932–941. DOI: 10.1111/ele.12295.

Hamilton, A.J., Stagnitti, F., Kumarage, S.C. and Premier, R.R. (2007) RIRA: A tool for conducting health risk assessments for irrigation of edible crops with recycled water. *Computers and Electronics in Agriculture* 57(1), 80–87. DOI: 10.1016/j.compag.2007.02.004.

Han, B.A., Kramer, A.M. and Drake, J.M. (2016) Global patterns of zoonotic disease in mammals. *Trends in Parasitology* 32(7), 565–577. DOI: 10.1016/j.pt.2016.04.007.

Heinonen-Tanski, H., Mohaibes, M., Karinen, P. and Koivunen, J. (2006) Methods to reduce pathogen microorganisms in manure. *Livestock Science* 102(3), 248–255. DOI: 10.1016/j.livsci.2006.03.024.

Herrero-Cófreces, S., Mougeot, F., Lambin, X. and Luque-Larena, J.J. (2021) Linking zoonosis emergence to farmland invasion by fluctuating herbivores: Common vole populations and tularemia outbreaks in NW Spain. *Frontiers in Veterinary Science* 8, 698454. DOI: 10.3389/fvets.2021.698454.

He, J., Yan, Z. and Chen, Q. (2020) Transmission of antibiotic resistance genes in agroecosystems: An overview. *Frontiers of Agricultural Science and Engineering* 7(3), 329–332. DOI: 10.15302/J-FASE-2020333.

Hibbs, A.C., Secor, W.E., Gerven, D. and Armelagos, G. (2011) Irrigation and infection: The immunoepidemiology of schistosomiasis in ancient Nubia. *American Journal of Physical Anthropology* 145(2), 290–298. DOI: 10.1002/ajpa.21493.

Hill, S.B. and MacRae, R.J. (1996) Conceptual framework for the transition from conventional to sustainable agriculture. *Journal of Sustainable Agriculture* 7, 81–87. DOI: 10.1300/J064v07n01_07.

Höglund, C., Ashbolt, N., Stenström, T.A. and Svensson, L. (2002) Viral persistence in source-separated human urine. *Advances in Environmental Research* 6(3), 265–275. DOI: 10.1016/S1093-0191(01)00057-0.

Hong, S., Kim, K., Yoon, S., Park, W.Y., Sim, S. *et al.* (2014) Detection of *Cryptosporidium parvum* in environmental soil and vegetables. *Journal of Korean Medical Science* 29(10), 1367–1371. DOI: 10.3346/jkms.2014.29.10.1367.

Hutchison, M.L., Avery, S.M. and Monaghan, J.M. (2008) The air-borne distribution of zoonotic agents from livestock waste spreading and microbiological risk to fresh produce from contaminated irrigation sources. *Journal of Applied Microbiology* 105(3), 848–857. DOI: 10.1111/j.1365-2672.2008.03811.x.

Inga López, J., Meza Contreras, V., Rodríguez Delfín, A., Ponce Álvarez, S., Paredes Larroca, F.H. *et al.* (2020) Treatment of irrigation water infested with nematodes using a solar photoreactor. *Desalination and Water Treatment* 174, 161–170. DOI: 10.5004/dwt.2020.24842.

Inyinbor, A.A., Tsopmo, A. and Udenigwe, C.C. (2021) Antibiotics threats on vegetables and the perils of low income nations practices. *Sustainable Chemistry and Pharmacy* 21, 100448. DOI: 10.1016/j.scp.2021.100448.

Iwu, C.D. and Okoh, A.I. (2019) Preharvest transmission routes of fresh produce associated bacterial pathogens with outbreak potentials: A review. *International Journal of Environmental Research and Public Health* 16(22), 4407. DOI: 10.3390/ijerph16224407.

Iwu, C.D. and Okoh, A.I. (2020) Characterization of antibiogram fingerprints in listeria monocytogenes recovered from irrigation water and agricultural soil samples. *PLoS One* 15(2), e0228956. DOI: 10.1371/journal.pone.0228956.

Iwu, C.D., Korsten, L. and Okoh, A.I. (2020) The incidence of antibiotic resistance within and beyond the agricultural ecosystem: A concern for public health. *MicrobiologyOpen* 9(9), e1035. DOI: 10.1002/mbo3.1035.

Iwu, C.D., Kayode, A.J., Igere, B.E. and Okoh, A.I. (2022) High levels of multi drug resistant *Escherichia coli* pathovars in preharvest environmental samples: A ticking time bomb for fresh produce related disease outbreak. *Frontiers in Environmental Science* 10, 858964. DOI: 10.3389/fenvs.2022.858964.

Jaramillo, M.F. and Restrepo, I. (2017) Wastewater reuse in agriculture: A review about its limitations and benefits. *Sustainability* 9(10), 1734. DOI: 10.3390/su9101734.

Jayasvati, I. and Jayasvati, M. (2018) Bat guano as the component of fertilizer or the health hazard? *Southeast Asian Journal of Tropical Medicine* 49, 331–339.

Jenkins, M.B., Truman, C.C., Franklin, D.H., Potter, T.L., Bosch, D.D. *et al.* (2014) Fecal bacterial losses in runoff from conventional and no-till pearl millet fertilized with broiler litter. *Agricultural Water Management* 134, 38–41. DOI: 10.1016/j.agwat.2013.11.013.

Jensen, P.K., Phuc, P.D., Konradsen, F., Klank, L.T. and Dalsgaard, A. (2009) Survival of ascaris eggs and hygienic quality of human excreta in Vietnamese composting latrines. *Environmental Health* 8(1), 1–9. DOI: 10.1186/1476-069X-8-57.

Johnston, L.J., Clanton, C.J., Ajariyakhajorn, C. and Goyal, S.M. (2003) Survival of pathogenic indicator organisms in stored swine manure containing ground piglet carcasses during cold temperatures. *Applied Engineering in Agriculture* 19(4), 491. DOI: 10.13031/2013.14921.

Johnson, P.T., Chase, J.M., Dosch, K.L., Hartson, R.B., Gross, J.A. *et al.* (2007) Aquatic eutrophication promotes pathogenic infection in amphibians. *Proceedings of the National Academy of Sciences* 104(40), 15781–15786. DOI: 10.1073/pnas.0707763104.

Jokinen, C.C., Cook, S.R., Reuter, T. and Tymensen, L. (2020) Assessing enterococci as an alternative fecal indicator for irrigation water quality. *Agricultural Water Management* 233, 106098. DOI: 10.1016/j.agwat.2020.106098.

Jones, D.L. (1999) Potential health risks associated with the persistence of *Escherichia coli* O157 in agricultural environments. *Soil Use and Management* 15(2), 76–83.

Jones, K.E., Patel, N.G., Levy, M.A., Storeygard, A., Balk, D. *et al.* (2008) Global trends in emerging infectious diseases. *Nature* 451(7181), 990–993. DOI: 10.1038/nature06536.

Jones, B.A., Grace, D., Kock, R., Alonso, S., Rushton, J. *et al.* (2013) Zoonosis emergence linked to agricultural intensification and environmental change. *Proceedings of the National Academy of Sciences* 110(21), 8399–8404. DOI: 10.1073/pnas.1208059110.

Jongman, M. and Korsten, L. (2016a) Microbial quality and suitability of roof-harvested rainwater in rural villages for crop irrigation and domestic use. *Journal of Water and Health* 14(6), 961–971. DOI: 10.2166/wh.2016.058.

Jongman, M. and Korsten, L. (2016b) Genetic diversity and antibiotic resistance of *Escherichia coli* isolates from different leafy green production systems. *Journal of Food Protection* 79(11), 1846–1853. DOI: 10.4315/0362-028X.JFP-16-117.

Kabelitz, T., Ammon, C., Funk, R., Münch, S., Biniasch, O. *et al.* (2020) Functional relationship of particulate matter (PM) emissions, animal species, and moisture content during manure application. *Environment International* 143, 105577. DOI: 10.1016/j.envint.2020.105577.

Kabelitz, T., Biniasch, O., Ammon, C., Nübel, U., Thiel, N. *et al.* (2021) Particulate matter emissions during field application of poultry manure - The influence of moisture content and treatment. *Science of the Total Environment* 780, 146652.

Karimi, H., Mokhtari, M., Salehi, F., Sojoudi, S. and Ebrahimi, A. (2017) Changes in microbial pathogen dynamics during vermicomposting mixture of cow manure–organic solid waste and cow manure–sewage sludge. *International Journal of Recycling of Organic Waste in Agriculture* 6(1), 57–61. DOI: 10.1007/s40093-016-0152-4.

Keesing, F., Holt, R.D. and Ostfeld, R.S. (2006) Effects of species diversity on disease risk. *Ecology Letters* 9(4), 485–498. DOI: 10.1111/j.1461-0248.2006.00885.x.

Kintz, E., Byrne, L., Jenkins, C., McCarthy, N., Vivancos, R. *et al.* (2019) Outbreaks of Shiga toxin–producing *Escherichia coli* linked to sprouted seeds, salad, and leafy greens: A systematic review. *Journal of Food Protection* 82(11), 1950–1958. DOI: 10.4315/0362-028X.JFP-19-014.

Kobayashi, N., Oshiki, M., Ito, T., Segawa, T., Hatamoto, M. *et al.* (2017) Removal of human pathogenic viruses in a down-flow hanging sponge (DHS) reactor treating municipal wastewater and health risks associated with utilization of the effluent for agricultural irrigation. *Water Research* 110, 389–398. DOI: 10.1016/j.watres.2016.10.054.

Léchenault-Bergerot, C., Morin-Crini, N., Rocchi, S., Lichtfouse, E., Chanet, G. *et al.* (2019) Hemp to limit diffusion of difenoconazole in vegetable garden soils. *Heliyon* 5(9), e02392. DOI: 10.1016/j.heliyon.2019.

Lehmann, J., Bossio, D.A., Kögel-Knabner, I. and Rillig, M.C. (2020) The concept and future prospects of soil health. *Nature Reviews Earth and Environment* 1(10), 544–553. DOI: 10.1038/s43017-020-0080-8.

Le Maréchal, C., Druilhe, C., Repérant, E., Boscher, E., Rouxel, S. *et al.* (2019) Evaluation of the occurrence of sporulating and nonsporulating pathogenic bacteria in manure and in digestate of five agricultural biogas plants. *MicrobiologyOpen* 8(10), e872. DOI: 10.1002/mbo3.872.

Liang, S., Abe, E.M. and Zhou, X.N. (2018) Integrating ecological approaches to interrupt schistosomiasis transmission: Opportunities and challenges. *Infectious Diseases of Poverty* 7(1), 1–6. DOI: 10.1186/s40249-018-0506-4.

Lim, K.Y., Hamilton, A.J. and Jiang, S.C. (2015) Assessment of public health risk associated with viral contamination in harvested urban stormwater for domestic applications. *Science of the Total Environment* 523, 95–108. DOI: 10.1016/j.scitotenv.2015.03.077.

Lin, M., Wang, A., Ren, L., Qiao, W., Wandera, S.M. *et al.* (2022) Challenges of pathogen inactivation in animal manure through anaerobic digestion: A short review. *Bioengineered* 13(1), 1149–1161. DOI: 10.1080/21655979.2021.2017717.

Liu, N., Xu, L., Han, L., Huang, G. and Ciric, L. (2021) Microbiological safety and antibiotic resistance risks at a sustainable farm under large-scale open-air composting and composting toilet systems. *Journal of Hazardous Materials* 401, 123391. DOI: 10.1016/j.jhazmat.2020.123391.

Lund, A.J., Sam, M.M., Sy, A.B., Sow, O.W., Ali, S. *et al.* (2019) Unavoidable risks: Local perspectives on water contact behavior and implications for schistosomiasis control in an agricultural region of northern Senegal. *The American Journal of Tropical Medicine and Hygiene* 101(4), 837. DOI: 10.4269%2Fajtmh.19-0099.

Lund, A.J., Rehkopf, D.H., Sokolow, S.H., Sam, M.M., Jouanard, N. *et al.* (2021) Land use impacts on parasitic infection: A cross-sectional epidemiological study on the role of irrigated agriculture in schistosome infection in a dammed landscape. *Infectious Diseases of Poverty* 10(1), 1–10. DOI: 10.1186/s40249-021-00816-5.

Lüneberg, K., Schneider, D., Brinkmann, N., Siebe, C. and Daniel, R. (2019) Land use change and water quality use for irrigation alters drylands soil fungal community in the Mezquital Valley, Mexico. *Frontiers in Microbiology* 10, 1220. DOI: 10.3389/fmicb.2019.01220.

Mancuso, G., Perulli, G.D., Lavrni´c, S., Morandi, B. and Toscano, A. (2021) SARS-CoV-2 from urban to rural water environment: Occurrence, persistence, fate, and influence on agriculture irrigation. *A Review. Water* 13, 764. DOI: 10.3390/w13060764.

Manyi-Loh, C.E., Mamphweli, S.N., Meyer, E.L., Okoh, A.I., Makaka, G. *et al.* (2014) Inactivation of selected bacterial pathogens in dairy cattle manure by mesophilic anaerobic digestion (balloon type digester). *International Journal of Environmental Research and Public Health* 11(7), 7184–7194. DOI: 10.3390/ijerph110707184.

Marcantonio, M., Rizzoli, A., Metz, M., Rosà, R., Marini, G. *et al.* (2015) Identifying the environmental conditions favouring West Nile Virus outbreaks in Europe. *PLoS ONE* 10(3), e0121158. DOI: 10.1371/journal.pone.0121158.

McCord, A.I., Stefanos, S.A., Tumwesige, V., Lsoto, D., Kawala, M. *et al.* (2020) Anaerobic digestion in Uganda: Risks and opportunities for integration of waste management and agricultural systems. *Renewable Agriculture and Food Systems* 35(6), 678–687. DOI: 10.1017/S1742170519000346.

Mikhail, A.F.W., Jenkins, C., Dallman, T.J., Inns, T., Douglas, A. *et al.* (2018) An outbreak of Shiga toxin-producing *Escherichia coli* O157: H7 associated with contaminated salad leaves: Epidemiological, genomic and food trace back investigations. *Epidemiology and Infection* 146(2), 187–196. DOI: 10.1017/S0950268817002874.

Miller, E., Spiehs, M., Arthur, T.M., Woodbury, B., Cortus, E. *et al.* (2019) Cropland amendment with beef cattle manure minimally affects antimicrobial resistance. *Journal of Environmental Quality* 48(6), 1683–1693. DOI: 10.2134/jeq2019.02.0042.

Miller, S.A., Ferreira, J.P. and LeJeune, J.T. (2022) Antimicrobial use and resistance in plant agriculture: A one health perspective. *Agriculture* 12(2), 289. DOI: 10.3390/agriculture12020289.

Mirhosseini, G., Moghaddam, M.R.A. and Maknoon, R. (2008) Assessment of sewage sludge characteristics in Tehran municipal wastewater treatment plants. *Journal of Residuals Science and Technology* 5(3), 145–150.

Moazeni, M., Nikaeen, M., Hadi, M., Moghim, S., Mouhebat, L. *et al.* (2017) Estimation of health risks caused by exposure to enteroviruses from agricultural application of wastewater effluents. *Water Research* 125, 104–113. DOI: 10.1016/j.watres.2017.08.028.

Mok, H.F., Barker, S.F. and Hamilton, A.J. (2014) A probabilistic quantitative microbial risk assessment model of norovirus disease burden from wastewater irrigation of vegetables in Shepparton, Australia. *Water Research* 54, 347–362. DOI: 10.1016/j.watres.2014.01.060.

Monteiro, S. and Santos, R. (2020) Incidence of enterococci resistant to clinically relevant antibiotics in environmental waters and in reclaimed waters used for irrigation. *Journal of Water and Health* 18(6), 911–924. DOI: 10.2166/wh.2020.020.

Morand, S., Blasdell, K., Bordes, F., Buchy, P., Carcy, B. *et al.* (2019) Changing landscapes of Southeast Asia and rodent-borne diseases: Decreased diversity but increased transmission risks. *Ecological Applications* 29(4), e01886. DOI: 10.1002/eap.1886.

Mothershaw, A.S., Kharousi, Z.A., Mumtaz Khan, M., Al-Mahruki, Y.A. and Said, F.A. (2013) Microbial analysis of cucumbers (*Cucumis sativus*) produced with tap or treated waste water. *Annals of Applied Biology* 163(2), 281–287. DOI: 10.1111/aab.12054.

Moussa, H.O., Nwankwo, C.I., Aminou, A.M., Stern, D.A., Haussmann, B.I. *et al.* (2021) Sanitized human urine (Oga) as a fertilizer auto-innovation from women farmers in Niger. *Agronomy for Sustainable Development* 41(4), 1–13. DOI: 10.1007/s13593-021-00675-2.

Münch, S., Papke, N., Thiel, N., Nübel, U., Siller, P. *et al.* (2020) Effects of farmyard manure application on dust emissions from arable soils. *Atmospheric Pollution Research* 11(9), 1610–1624. DOI: 10.1016/j.apr.2020.06.007.

Munoz, I., Tomas, N., Mas, J., Garcia-Reyes, J.F., Molina-Diaz, A. *et al.* (2010) Potential chemical and microbiological risks on human health from urban wastewater reuse in agriculture. Case study of wastewater effluents in Spain. *Journal of Environmental Science and Health Part B* 45(4), 300–309. DOI: 10.1007/s13593-021-00675-2.

Murayama, M., Kakinuma, Y., Maeda, Y., Rao, J.R., Matsuda, M. *et al.* (2010) Molecular identification of airborne bacteria associated with aerial spraying of bovine slurry waste employing 16S rRNA gene PCR and gene sequencing techniques. *Ecotoxicology and Environmental Safety* 73(3), 443–447. DOI: 10.1016/j.ecoenv.2009.10.003.

Murry Jr, A.C. and Hinckley, L.S. (1992) Effect of the earthworm (*Eisenia foetida*) on *Salmonella enteritidis* in horse manure. *Bioresource Technology* 41(2), 97–100.

Nag, R., Auer, A., Markey, B.K., Whyte, P., Nolan, S. *et al.* (2019) Anaerobic digestion of agricultural manure and biomass–critical indicators of risk and knowledge gaps. *Science of the Total Environment* 690, 460–479. DOI: 10.1016/j.scitotenv.2019.06.512.

Nag, R., Auer, A., Nolan, S., Russell, L., Markey, B.K. *et al.* (2021) Evaluation of pathogen concentration in anaerobic digestate using a predictive modelling approach (ADRISK). *Science of the Total Environment* 800, 149574. DOI: 10.1016/j.scitotenv.2021.149574.

Neme, K. and Mohammed, A. (2017) Mycotoxin occurrence in grains and the role of postharvest management as a mitigation strategies. *A Review. Food Control* 78, 412–425. DOI: 10.1016/j.foodcont.2017.03.012.

Newell, D.G., Koopmans, M., Verhoef, L., Duizer, E., Aidara-Kane, A. *et al.* (2010) Food-borne diseases—the challenges of 20 years ago still persist while new ones continue to emerge. *International Journal of Food Microbiology* 139, S3–S15. DOI: 10.1016/j.ijfoodmicro.2010.01.021.

NRMMC, EPHC and AHMC (2006) Australian guidelines for water recycling: Managing health and environmental risks. Phase 1. *National Water Quality Management Strategy 21*. In: *Natural Resource Management Ministerial Council, Environment Protection and Heritage Council, and the Australian Health Ministers' Conference*, Canberra, Australia.

Obayomi, O., Bernstein, N., Edelstein, M., Vonshak, A., Ghazayarn, L. *et al.* (2019) Importance of soil texture to the fate of pathogens introduced by irrigation with treated wastewater. *Science of the Total Environment* 653, 886–896. DOI: 10.1016/j.scitotenv.2018.10.378.

O'Connor, J., Mickan, B., Siddique, K.H., Rinklebe, J., Kirkham, M.B. *et al.* (2022) Physical, chemical, and microbial contaminants in food waste management for soil application: A review. *Environmental Pollution* 300, 118860. DOI: 10.1016/j.envpol.2022.118860.

O'Flaherty, E., Solimini, A.G., Pantanella, F., Giusti, M. and Cummins, E. (2019) Human exposure to antibiotic resistant-*Escherichia coli* through irrigated lettuce. *Environment International* 122, 270–280. DOI: 10.1016/j.envint.2018.11.022.

Ofori, S., Puškáčová, A., Růžičková, I. and Wanner, J. (2021) Treated wastewater reuse for irrigation: Pros and cons. *Science of the Total Environment* 760, 144026. DOI: 10.1016/j.scitotenv.2020.144026.

Okubo, T., Iguchi, A., Tanaka, S., Uchida, S., Tagawa, T. *et al.* (2019) Health impact of agricultural drainage water for farmers in the West Nile Delta. *International Journal of Environmental Research* 13(2), 319–325. DOI: 10.1007/s41742-019-00176-x.

Oliver, J.P., Gooch, C.A., Lansing, S., Schueler, J., Hurst, J.J. *et al.* (2020) Invited review: Fate of antibiotic residues, antibiotic-resistant bacteria, and antibiotic resistance genes in US dairy manure management systems. *Journal of Dairy Science* 103(2), 1051–1071. DOI: 10.3168.jds.2019-16778.

Olivieri, A.W., Seto, E., Cooper, R.C., Cahn, M.D., Colford, J. *et al.* (2014) Risk-based review of California's water-recycling criteria for agricultural irrigation. *Journal of Environmental Engineering* 140(6), 04014015. DOI: 10.1061/(ASCE)EE.1943-7870.0000833.

Otte, J. and Pica-Ciamarra, U. (2021) Emerging infectious zoonotic diseases: The neglected role of food animals. *One Health* 13, 100323. DOI: 10.1016/j.onehlt.2021.100323.

Ouarrak, K., Chahlaoui, A., Taouraout, A. and Taha, I. (2019) Impacts of the reuse of wastewater from the Bouishak wadi in the city of Meknes (central-south Morocco) in urban agriculture. In: Mohamed, B.A., Karaşo, I.R., Saadane, R., Mtalaa, W. and Abdelhakim, B.A. (eds) *Proceedings of the 4th International Conference on Smart City Applications. October 2–4, 2019*, Association for Computing Machinery, pp. 1–4. DOI: 10.1145/3368756.3368999.

Owamah, H.I., Dahunsi, S.O., Oranusi, U.S. and Alfa, M.I. (2014) Fertilizer and sanitary quality of digestate biofertilizer from the co-digestion of food waste and human excreta. *Waste Management* 34(4), 747–752. DOI: 10.1016/j.wasman.2014.01.017.

Pandey, P.K., Soupir, M.L. and Ikenberry, C. (2014) Modelling animal waste pathogen transport from agricultural land to streams 19(1), 012014. DOI: 10.1088/1755-1315/19/1/012014/meta.

Partyka, M.L. and Bond, R.F. (2022) Wastewater reuse for irrigation of produce: A review of research, regulations, and risks. *Science of the Total Environment* 154385. DOI: 10.1016/j.scitotenv.2022.154385.

Pavione, D.M.S., Bastos, R.K.X. and Bevilacqua, P.D. (2013) Quantitative microbial risk assessment applied to irrigation of salad crops with waste stabilization pond effluents. *Water Science and Technology* 67(6), 1208–1215. DOI: 10.2166/wst.2013.674.

Perulli, G.D., Gaggia, F., Sorrenti, G., Donati, I., Boini, A. *et al.* (2021) Treated wastewater as irrigation source: A microbiological and chemical evaluation in apple and nectarine trees. *Agricultural Water Management* 244, 106403. DOI: 10.1016/j.agwat.2020.106403.

Petterson, S.R., Ashbolt, N.J. and Sharma, A. (2001) Microbial risks from wastewater irrigation of salad crops: A screening-level risk assessment. *Water Environment Research* 73(6), 667–672. DOI: 10.2175/106143001X143402.

Pham-Duc, P., Nguyen-Viet, H., Hattendorf, J., Zinsstag, J., Phung-Dac, C. *et al.* (2013) *Ascaris lumbricoides* and *Trichuris trichiura* infections associated with wastewater and human excreta use in agriculture in Vietnam. *Parasitology International* 62(2), 172–180. DOI: 10.1016/j.parint.2012.12.007.

Plowright, R.K., Reaser, J.K., Locke, H., Woodley, S.J., Patz, J.A. *et al.* (2021) Land use-induced spillover: A call to action to safeguard environmental, animal, and human health. *The Lancet Planetary Health* 5(4), e237–e245. DOI: 10.1016/S2542-5196(21)00031-0.

Pornsukarom, S. and Thakur, S. (2016) Assessing the impact of manure application in commercial swine farms on the transmission of antimicrobial resistant *Salmonella* in the environment. *PloS One* 11(10), e0164621. DOI: 10.1371/journal.pone.0164621.

Prez, V.E., Martinez, L.C., Victoria, M., Giordano, M.O., Masachessi, G. *et al.* (2018) Tracking enteric viruses in green vegetables from central Argentina: Potential association with viral contamination of irrigation waters. *Science of the Total Environment* 637, 665–671. DOI: 10.1016/j.scitotenv.2018.05.044.

Ratnadass, A. and Deberdt, P. (2021) Pratiques de protection des cultures en agroécosystèmes tropicaux et risques de maladies humaines et animales d'origine bactérienne. *Cahiers Agricultures* 30, 42. DOI: 10.1051/cagri/2021028.

Ratnadass, A. and Deguine, J.P. (2021) Crop protection practices and viral zoonotic risks within a one health framework. *Science of the Total Environment* 774, 145172. DOI: 10.1016/j.scitotenv.2021.145172.

Ratnadass, A. and Martin, T. (2022) Crop protection practices and risks associated with infectious tropical parasitic diseases. *Science of the Total Environment* 823, 153633. DOI: 10.1016/j.scitotenv.2022.153633.

Ratnadass, A. and Sester, M. (2023) Crop protection practices and risks associated with human fungal infectious diseases: A one health perspective. DOI: 10.1051/cagri/2022036.

Ratnadass, A., Fernandes, P., Avelino, J. and Habib, R. (2012) Plant species diversity for sustainable management of crop pests and diseases in agroecosystems: A review. *Agronomy for Sustainable Development* 32, 273–303. DOI: 10.1007/s13593-011-0022-4.

Ramakrishna, W., Yadav, R. and Li, K. (2019) Plant growth promoting bacteria in agriculture: Two sides of a coin. *Applied Soil Ecology* 138, 10–18. DOI: 10.1016/j.apsoil.2019.02.019.

Ratnadass, A., Avelino, J., Fernandes, P., Letourmy, P., Babin, R. *et al.* (2021) Synergies and tradeoffs in natural regulation of crop pests and diseases under plant species diversification. *Crop Protection* 146, 105658. DOI: 10.1016/j.cropro.2021.105658.

Renčo, M. and Kováčik, P. (2012) Response of plant parasitic and free living soil nematodes to composted animal manure soil amendments. *Journal of Nematology* 44(4), 329.

Reyes-Batlle, M., Díaz, F.J., Sifaoui, I., Rodríguez-Expósito, R., Rizo-Liendo, A. *et al.* (2021) Free living amoebae isolation in irrigation waters and soils of an insular arid agroecosystem. *Science of the Total Environment* 753, 141833. DOI: 10.1016/j.scitotenv.2020.141833.

Roth, E., Samara, N., Ackermann, M., Seiml-Buchinger, R., Saleh, A. *et al.* (2015) Fertilization and irrigation practice as source of microorganisms and the impact on nematodes as their potential vectors. *Applied Soil Ecology* 90, 68–77. DOI: 10.1016/j.apsoil.2015.02.002.

Rulisa, A., Kempen, L. and Koch, D.-J. (2022) When local trade-offs between SDGs turn out to be wealth-dependent: Interaction between expanding rice cultivation and eradicating malaria in Rwanda. *Sustainability* 14, 2100. DOI: 10.3390/su14042100.

Rushton, J., Nielsen, L.R., Cornelsen, L., Queenan, K., Rüegg, S.R. *et al.* (2018) Evaluation of integrated approaches to health with a focus on one health. In: Rüegg, S., Häsler, B. and Zinsstag, J. (eds) *Integrated Approaches to Health: A Handbook for the Evaluation of One Health*. Wageningen Academic Publishers, pp. 14–21. DOI: 10.3920/978-90-8686-875-9.

Sacks, M. and Bernstein, N. (2011) Utilization of reclaimed wastewater for irrigation of field-grown melons by surface and subsurface drip irrigation. *Israel Journal of Plant Sciences* 59(2–4), 159–169. DOI: 10.1560/IJPS.59.2-4.159.

Santos, M.C., Martín, I. and Trujillo, E.M. (2014) Nematodes as a factor for consideration in the wastewater treatment and water reuse process. *Desalination and Water Treatment* 52(25–27), 4715–4720. DOI: 10.1080/19443994.2013.815734.

Saunders, O., Harrison, J., Fortuna, A.M., Whitefield, E. and Bary, A. (2012) Effect of anaerobic digestion and application method on the presence and survivability of *E. coli* and fecal coliforms in dairy waste applied to soil. *Water, Air and Soil Pollution* 223(3), 1055–1063. DOI: 10.1007/s11270-011-0923-5.

Scheinemann, H.A., Dittmar, K., Stöckel, F.S., Müller, H. and Krüger, M.E. (2015) Hygienisation and nutrient conservation of sewage sludge or cattle manure by lactic acid fermentation. *PLoS One* 10(3), e0118230. DOI: 10.1371/journal.pone.0118230.

Silverman, A.I., Akrong, M.O., Amoah, P., Drechsel, P. and Nelson, K.L. (2013) Quantification of human norovirus GII, human adenovirus, and fecal indicator organisms in wastewater used for irrigation in Accra, Ghana. *Journal of Water and Health* 11(3), 473–488. DOI: 10.2166/wh.2013.025.

Singh, A. (2021) A review of wastewater irrigation: Environmental implications. *Resources, Conservation and Recycling* 168, 105454. DOI: 10.1016/j.resconrec.2021.105454.

Slavik, K., Peterson, B.J., Deegan, L.A., Bowden, W.B., Hershey, A.E. *et al.* (2004) Long-term responses of the Kuparuk River ecosystem to phosphorus fertilization. *Ecology* 85(4), 939–954. DOI: 10.1890/02-4039.

Sorinolu, A.J., Tyagi, N., Kumar, A. and Munir, M. (2021) Antibiotic resistance development and human health risks during wastewater reuse and biosolids application in agriculture. *Chemosphere* 265, 129032. DOI: 10.1016/j.chemosphere.2020.129032.

Ström, G., Albihn, A., Jinnerot, T., Boqvist, S., Andersson-Djurfeldt, A. *et al.* (2018) Manure management and public health: Sanitary and socio-economic aspects among urban livestock-keepers in Cambodia. *Science of the Total Environment* 621, 193–200. DOI: 10.1016/j.scitotenv.2017.11.254.

Such, N., Husveth, F., Marton, A., Koltay, I., Szoko, Z. *et al.* (2019) The effect and accumulation of antibiotics and their residues in horticultural plants: A review. *Journal of Central European Agriculture* 20(1), 431–446. DOI: 10.5513/JCEA01/20.1.2045.

Summerlin III, H.N., Pola, C.C., Chamakura, K.R., Young, R., Gentry, T. *et al.* (2021) Fate of enteric viruses during leafy greens (romaine lettuce) production using treated municipal wastewater and AP205 bacteriophage as a surrogate. *Journal of Environmental Science and Health, Part A* 56(10), 1138–1144. DOI: 10.1080/10934529.2021.1968231.

Sun, J., Jin, L., He, T., Wei, Z., Liu, X. *et al.* (2020) Antibiotic resistance genes (ARGs) in agricultural soils from the Yangtze River Delta, China. *Science of the Total Environment* 740, 140001. DOI: 10.1016/j.scitotenv.2020.140001.

Szabová, E., Juriš, P. and Papajová, I. (2010) Sanitation composting process in different seasons. *Ascaris Suum as Model. Waste Management* 30(3), 426–432. DOI: 10.1016/j.wasman.2009.09.035.

Tapia-Ramírez, G., Lorenzo, C., Navarrete, D., Carrillo-Reyes, A., Retana, Ó. *et al.* (2022) A review of mammarenaviruses and rodent reservoirs in the Americas. *Ecohealth* 1–18. DOI: 10.1007/s10393-022-01580-0.

Tariq, M., Jameel, F., Ijaz, U., Abdullah, M. and Rashid, K. (2022) Biofertilizer microorganisms accompanying pathogenic attributes: A potential threat. *Physiology and Molecular Biology of Plants* 1–14. DOI: 10.1007/s12298-022-01138-y.

Tian, H.Y., Bi, P., Cazelles, B., Zhou, S. and Huang, S.Q. (2015) How environmental conditions impact mosquito ecology and *Japanese encephalitis*: An eco-epidemiological approach. *Environment International* 79, 17–24. DOI: 10.1016/j.envint.2015.03.002.

Topp, E., Scott, A., Lapen, D.R., Lyautey, E. and Duriez, P. (2009) Livestock waste treatment systems for reducing environmental exposure to hazardous enteric pathogens: Some considerations. *Bioresource Technology* 100(22), 5395–5398. DOI: 10.1016/j.biortech.2008.11.001.

Touati, M., Hadjadj, L., Berrazeg, M., Baron, S.A. and Rolain, J.M. (2020) Emergence of *Escherichia coli* harbouring mcr-1 and mcr-3 genes in North West Algerian farmlands. *Journal of Global Antimicrobial Resistance* 21, 132–137. DOI: 10.1016/j.jgar.2019.10.001.

Tran, D.T., Bradbury, M.I., Ogtrop, F.F.V., Bozkurt, H., Jones, B.J. *et al.* (2020) Environmental drivers for persistence of *Escherichia coli* and *Salmonella* in manure-amended soils: A meta-analysis. *Journal of Food Protection* 83(7), 1268–1277. DOI: 10.4315/0362-028X.JFP-19-460.

Trang, D.T., Mølbak, K., Cam, P.D. and Dalsgaard, A. (2007) Helminth infections among people using wastewater and human excreta in peri-urban agriculture and aquaculture in Hanoi, Vietnam. *Tropical Medicine and International Health* 12, 82–90. DOI: 10.1111/j.1365-3156.2007.01945.x.

Trang, D.T., Hien, B.T.T., Mølbak, K., Cam, P.D. and Dalsgaard, A. (2007) Epidemiology and aetiology of diarrhoeal diseases in adults engaged in wastewater-fed agriculture and aquaculture in Hanoi, Vietnam. *Tropical Medicine and International Health* 12, 23–33. DOI: 10.1111/j.1365-3156.2007.01938.x.

Truhlar, A.M., Salvucci, A.E., Walter, M.T., Warnick, L.D., Hay, A.G. *et al.* (2015) Effects of manure-application practices on curli production by *Escherichia coli* transported through soil. *Environmental Science and Technology* 49(4), 2099–2104. DOI: 10.1021/es5053039.

Udikovic-Kolic, N., Wichmann, F., Broderick, N.A. and Handelsman, J. (2014) Bloom of resident antibiotic-resistant bacteria in soil following manure fertilization. *Proceedings of the National Academy of Sciences* 111(42), 15202–15207. DOI: 10.1073/pnas.1409836111.

Ungureanu, N., Vlăduţ, V., Istrate, I.A., Zăbavă, B. Ş., Tociu, C. *et al.* (2019) Advanced electrochemical treatment of the wastewater from cattle farm. In: Kovačěv, I. and Bilandžija, N. (eds) *Proceedings of the 47th International Symposium Actual Tasks on Agricultural Engineering*, Opatija, Croatia. University of Zagreb, Zagreb, March 5–7, 2019, pp. 147–157.

Urra, J., Alkorta, I. and Garbisu, C. (2019) Potential benefits and risks for soil health derived from the use of organic amendments in agriculture. *Agronomy* 9(9), 542. DOI: 10.3390/agronomy9090542.

Usman, M., Farooq, M., Farooq, M. and Anastopoulos, I. (2021) Exposure to SARS-CoV-2 in aerosolized wastewater: Toilet flushing, wastewater treatment, and sprinkler irrigation. *Water* 13(4), 436. DOI: 10.3390/w13040436.

Uyttendaele, M., Jaykus, L.A., Amoah, P., Chiodini, A., Cunliffe, D. *et al.* (2015) Microbial hazards in irrigation water: Standards, norms, and testing to manage use of water in fresh produce primary production. *Comprehensive Reviews in Food Science and Food Safety* 14(4), 336–356. DOI: 10.1111/1541-4337.12133.

Van Bruggen, A.H.C. and Finckh, M.R. (2016) Plant diseases and management approaches in organic farming systems. *Annual Review of Phytopathology* 54(1), 25–54. DOI: 10.1146/annurev-phyto-080615-100123.

Van Ginneken, M. and Oron, G. (2000) Risk assessment of consuming agricultural products irrigated with reclaimed wastewater: An exposure model. *Water Resources Research* 36(9), 2691–2699. DOI: 10.1029/2000WR900106.

van Bruggen, A.H., Goss, E.M., Havelaar, A., Diepeningen, A.D., Finckh, M.R. *et al.* (2019) One health-cycling of diverse microbial communities as a connecting force for soil, plant, animal, human and ecosystem health. *Science of the Total Environment* 664, 927–937. DOI: 10.3389/fenvs.2021.763917.

Verbyla, M.E., Caims, M.R., Gonzalez, P.A., Whiteford, L.M. and Mihelcic, J.R. (2015) Emerging challenges for pathogen control and resource recovery in natural wastewater treatment systems. *Wiley Interdisciplinary Reviews: Water* 2(6), 701–714. DOI: 10.1002/wat2.1101.

Walsh, J.F., Molyneux, D.H. and Birley, M.H. (1993) Deforestation: Effects on vector-borne disease. *Parasitology* 106(S1), S55–S75.

Wang, J., Wang, L., Zhu, L., Wang, J. and Xing, B. (2022) Antibiotic resistance in agricultural soils: Source, fate, mechanism and attenuation strategy. *Critical Reviews in Environmental Science and Technology* 52(6), 847–889. DOI: 10.1080/10643389.2020.1835438.

Wei, J. and Kniel, K.E. (2010) Pre-harvest viral contamination of crops originating from fecal matter. *Food and Environmental Virology* 2(4), 195–206. DOI: 10.1007/s12560-010-9050-5.

Westrell, T., Schönning, C., Stenström, T.A. and Ashbolt, N.J. (2004) QMRA (quantitative microbial risk assessment) and HACCP (hazard analysis and critical control points) for management of pathogens in wastewater and sewage sludge treatment and reuse. *Water Science and Technology* 50(2), 23–30.

Williams, A.P., Roberts, P., Avery, L.M., Killham, K. and Jones, D.L. (2006) Earthworms as vectors of *Escherichia coli* O157: H7 in soil and vermicomposts. *FEMS Microbiology Ecology* 58(1), 54–64. DOI: 10.1111/j.1574-6941.2006.00142.x.

Williams-Nguyen, J., Sallach, J.B., Bartelt-Hunt, S., Boxall, A.B., Durso, L.M. *et al.* (2016) Antibiotics and antibiotic resistance in agroecosystems: State of the science. *Journal of Environmental Quality* 45(2), 394–406. DOI: 10.2134/jeq2015.07.0336.

World Health Organization (2006) *WHO Guidelines for the Safe Use of Wasterwater Excreta and Greywater*, Vol. 1. World Health Organization, Geneva.

Xu, Y., Li, H., Shao, Z., Li, X., Zheng, X. *et al.* (2021) Fate of antibiotic resistance genes in farmland soil applied with three different fertilizers during the growth cycle of pakchoi and after harvesting. *Journal of Environmental Management* 289, 112576. DOI: 10.1016/j.jenvman.2021.112576.

Yang, Q., Zhang, H., Guo, Y. and Tian, T. (2016) Influence of chicken manure fertilization on antibiotic-resistant bacteria in soil and the endophytic bacteria of pakchoi. *International Journal of Environmental Research and Public Health* 13(7), 662. DOI: 10.3390/ijerph13070662.

Ye, M., Sun, M., Zhao, Y., Jiao, W., Xia, B. *et al.* (2018) Targeted inactivation of antibiotic-resistant *Escherichia coli* and *Pseudomonas aeruginosa* in a soil-lettuce system by combined polyvalent bacteriophage and biochar treatment. *Environmental Pollution* 241, 978–987. DOI: 10.1016/j.envpol.2018.04.070.

Youenou, B., Hien, E., Deredjian, A., Brothier, E., Favre-Bonté, S. *et al.* (2016) Impact of untreated urban waste on the prevalence and antibiotic resistance profiles of human opportunistic pathogens in agricultural soils from Burkina Faso. *Environmental Science and Pollution Research* 23(24), 25299–25311. DOI: 10.1007/s11356-016-7699-5.

Young, P., Buchanan, N. and Fallowfield, H.J. (2016) Inactivation of indicator organisms in wastewater treated by a high rate algal pond system. *Journal of Applied Microbiology* 121(2), 577–586. DOI: 10.1111/jam.13180.

Youngquist, C.P., Mitchell, S.M. and Cogger, C.G. (2016) Fate of antibiotics and antibiotic resistance during digestion and composting: A review. *Journal of Environmental Quality* 45(2), 537–545. DOI: 10.2134/jeq2015.05.0256.

Zalewska, M., Błażejewska, A., Czapko, A. and Popowska, M. (2021) Antibiotics and antibiotic resistance genes in animal manure–consequences of its application in agriculture. *Frontiers in Microbiology* 12, 610656. DOI: 10.3389/fmicb.2021.610656.

Zhang, M., Liu, Y.S., Zhao, J.L., Liu, W.R., Chen, J. *et al.* (2021) Variations of antibiotic resistome in swine wastewater during full-scale anaerobic digestion treatment. *Environment International* 155, 106694. DOI: 10.1016/j.envint.2021.106694.

Zhang, Y., Zhou, J., Wu, J., Hua, Q. and Bao, C. (2022) Distribution and transfer of antibiotic resistance genes in different soil–plant systems. *Environmental Science and Pollution Research* 29(39), 59159–59172. DOI: 10.1007/s11356-021-17465-8.

Zhao, Q. and Liu, Y. (2019) Is anaerobic digestion a reliable barrier for deactivation of pathogens in biosludge. *Science of the Total Environment* 668, 893–902. DOI: 10.1016/j.scitotenv.2019.03.063.

12 The Role of Agriculture in Human Infectious Disease Outbreaks

Serge Morand[1,2,3*]

[1]MIVEGEC, CNRS-IRD, Montpellier University, Montpellier, France; [2]Faculty of Veterinary Technology, Kasetsart University, Bangkok, Thailand; [3]Faculty of Tropical Medicine, Mahidol University, Bangkok, Thailand

Abstract

This study uses the available data to explore the temporal and geographical patterns of infectious diseases and their links between human demography, human-induced land-use change, livestock and poultry expansion, and biodiversity loss. Over the last decades, the number of outbreaks of zoonotic and vector-borne diseases increased mostly in the intertropical zone. The increase in cropland, grassland, tree plantation, livestock, poultry, biodiversity at threat (using the Red List index) mostly occurred in the intertropical zone. Using structural equation modeling, significant relationships were observed between disease outbreaks, human demography, livestock (cattle and pigs), poultry (chickens), tree plantation and artificial land expansion as well as with increasing biodiversity at threat. While agricultural expansion is seen as a driver of biodiversity loss and potentially emerging infectious diseases, here we show that cropland and grassland expansion does not appear to enhance disease outbreaks directly, but indirectly and only for cropland on biodiversity loss. The links observed between infectious disease outbreaks, human demography, agriculture, livestock, urbanization and biodiversity should help rethink the global food system in ways that minimize the risk of infectious diseases while preserving biodiversity and contributing to Sustainable Development Goals.

Keywords: outbreaks, vector-borne diseases, zoonoses, biodiversity, agriculture, livestock, poultry, land-use change

Introduction

Agriculture is an essential pillar of our societies since the Neolithic and the emergence of Agrarian civilizations (Scott, 2017). Studies in environmental history, anthropology, evolution and ecology give a picture of the global history of human infectious diseases (McNeill, 1976; Diamond, 2002; Wolfe *et al.*, 2007; Morand, 2016) showing the importance of the domestication of animals and plants, which has considerably transformed the terrestrial biosphere and changed the course of human history (Diamond, 2002). The environmental impact of agricultural development has allowed infectious diseases to emerge. Vector-borne diseases such as malaria, yellow fever, trypanosomiasis or filariasis have arisen from deforestation and the extension of agricultural land and the increase in human densities (Cohen and Armelagos, 1984). The domestication of animals has also strongly affected human

*Corresponding author: serge.morand@umontpellier.fr

health by promoting the emergence of zoonotic diseases (Pearce-Duvet, 2006). The statistical test of the hypothesis of McNeill (McNeill, 1976) on the historical role of animal domestication in the burden of human pathogens confirms that the number of infectious diseases shared between domesticated mammals and humans is dependent on the time spent in proximity to humans (Morand *et al.*, 2014), that is, the number of years since the start of domestication of each animal species.

Recent agriculture expansion has been recognized as having major impacts on biodiversity along with climate change, pollution and invasive species (Alkemade *et al.*, 2013; Crist *et al.*, 2017; IPBES, 2019; Zabel *et al.*, 2019). Global cropland expansion accelerated over the past two decades, with new cropland areas often replacing natural vegetation and tree cover (Potapov *et al.*, 2022). However, during these last two decades, the global per-capita cropland area decreased by 10% due to population growth (Potapov *et al.*, 2022) associated with rapid urbanization and infrastructure growth (Sun *et al.*, 2020), which in turn favors infectious disease risk (Hassell *et al.*, 2017). Human demography and agricultural land-use activities are listed as potential drivers of infectious disease emergence (Lederberg *et al.*, 1992; Institute of Medicine (US), 2003; Olson *et al.*, 2015; Semenza *et al.*, 2016; Rohr *et al.*, 2019; Baker *et al.*, 2022), but few studies have explored globally the importance of human-induced land-use change on human infectious diseases (Lederberg *et al.*, 1992; Institute of Medicine (US), 2003; Gottdenker *et al.*, 2014; Shah *et al.*, 2019; Wegner *et al.*, 2022) including forest cover change and tree plantation expansion (Morand and Lajaunie, 2021).

The spectacular increase in livestock production over the past decades appears to be a major cause of the decline in biodiversity and the alteration of natural habitats (Steinfeld *et al.*, 2006; Reid *et al.*, 2010; Alkemade *et al.*, 2013). Livestock expansion is also recognized as a major driver for the emergence of zoonotic diseases at the interface between the environment, wildlife and humans (Cleaveland *et al.*, 2001; Jones *et al.*, 2013; Morand, 2020; Bartlett *et al.*, 2022; Bernstein *et al.*, 2022).

Several studies have highlighted both the complexity of the links between human-induced land-use change, livestock expansion and human infectious diseases (Lederberg *et al.*, 1992; Institute of Medicine (US), 2003; Murray *et al.*, 2015; Faust *et al.*, 2018) and the lack of studies investigating these links on a global scale (Morand and Lajaunie, 2021). One way around this problem is to explore the available data to help formulate hypotheses that can be tested further. For this, we used the datasets of the open databases of FAOSTAT of the Food and Agricultural Organization (FAO), the Organization for Economic Co-operation and Development (OECD), the World Bank and the database of Global Infectious Disease and Epidemiology Online Network (GIDEON). We describe the temporal and geographical patterns of infectious diseases and their likely drivers in order to infer some potential causal links using structural equation modeling that can help conduct further studies.

Review Methodology

Datasets gathered from the databases from FAOSTAT of the Food and Agricultural Organization, the Organization for Economic Co-operation and Development, the Word Bank and the Global Infectious Disease and Epidemiology Online Network helped to give a comprehensive picture of the interlinkages between human demography, agriculture, livestock, poultry, land-use changes, biodiversity and infectious diseases in humans.

Tempo and Latitudinal Trend in Outbreaks of Zoonotic and Vector-Borne Diseases

Data on human infectious diseases were obtained from the GIDEON database (GIDEON (Global Infectious Disease and Epidemiology

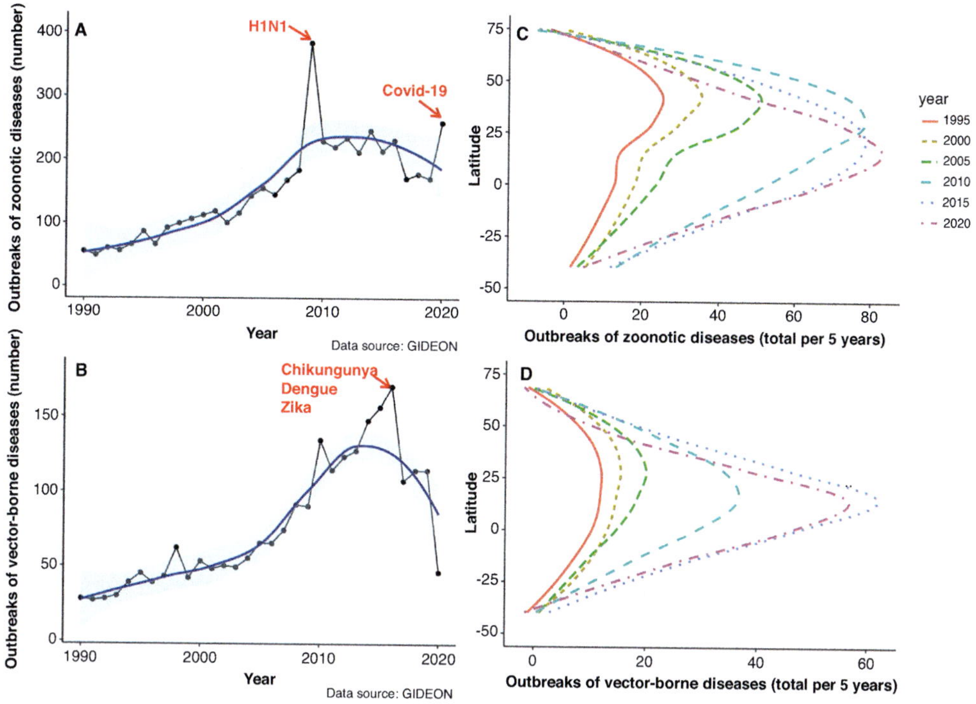

Fig. 12.1. Total number of outbreaks of (A) zoonotic diseases and (B) vector-borne diseases from 1990 to 2020. Latitudinal pattern in the number of outbreaks of (C) zoonotic diseases and (D) vector-borne diseases by period of 5 years (data from GIDEON).

Network), 2021), which contains information on the occurrence of outbreaks of human infectious diseases per year and for each nation. In the GIDEON database, an outbreak follows the general definition of the WHO as any grouping of cases, including family clusters and epidemics. We used the classification of vector-borne and zoonotic diseases for this database provided by (Smith *et al.*, 2014). The 1990–2020 extracted dataset contains 4707 outbreaks of 122 zoonotic diseases and 2375 outbreaks of 66 vector-borne infectious diseases.

Globally, the number of outbreaks of zoonotic and vector-borne diseases increased over the last decades as previously reported (Morand and Lajaunie, 2021) with the high number of outbreaks in zoonotic diseases in 2009 due to the novel influenza A(H1N1) pdm09 pandemic and in 2020 due to the Covid-19 pandemic (Fig. 12.1A), and the high number of outbreaks in vector-borne diseases in 2016 due to dengue, chikungunya and zika (Fig. 12.1B). A dramatic drop in the number of human infectious disease outbreaks other than Covid-19 occurred in 2020 due to the containment measures implemented by many countries facing Covid-19. Measures have reduced the local and global transmission of many zoonotic and vector-borne diseases. From 1990 to 2020, the increase in the number of outbreaks showed an interesting latitudinal trend, with a shift of zoonotic disease outbreaks towards the intertropical zone (Fig. 12.1C) corresponding to the pattern observed for vector-borne diseases (Fig. 12.1D). This observation should be compared with the analysis of (Dunn *et al.*, 2010) on the burden of human infectious diseases by country, which showed that the diversity of human infectious diseases is positively associated with the richness of bird and mammal species by country (Guernier et al., 2004; Vourc'h et al., 2022).

Tempo and Latitudinal Trends in Human Demography, Land Use Changes, Livestock, Poultry and Biodiversity at Threat

The use of data from the World Bank (World Bank Open Data, 2022) and FAOSTAT (FAOSTAT, 2022) allows for the exploration of the latitudinal pattern of human demography and human-induced changes in land use, livestock and threatened biodiversity from 1990 to 2020. Most of the increase in human population size occurred in the Northern temperate and tropical zones (Fig. 12.2A). In parallel, most of the artificial land expansion also occurred in the Northern temperate and tropical zones (Fig. 12.2B). The recent expansion of tree plantations occurring in the Northern hemisphere include its tropical zone (Fig. 12.2D). Cropland and grassland expansion mostly occurred in the intertropical zone (Figs 12.2E and 12.2F).

According to data from FAOSTAT, the number of cattle heads reached one billion and 587 million in 2020 while it was 992 million in 1961. The number of pigs increased from 492 million to one billion 364 million and the number of chickens from 4 billion 447 million to 37 billion 223 million in the same period. Nowadays, cattle have a higher total biomass than the biomass of all humans (Bar-On *et al.*, 2018). The total number of individual wild birds dropped from an estimation between 200 and 300 billion in 1997 (Gaston and Blackburn, 1997) to 50 billion in 2020 (Callaghan *et al.*, 2021). The current trends suggest that the total number of poultry will soon exceed the total number of wild birds. Most of these dramatic increases occurred in the inter-tropical zone for the cattle (Fig. 12.2G), at all latitudes for the pigs (Fig. 12.2H) and in the Northern hemisphere and Southern tropical region for the chickens (Fig. 12.2I).

Biodiversity loss is assessed by the Red List index of The International Union for Conservation of Nature (IUCN) (IUCN, 2022). The Red List Index measures change in extinction risk across groups of species expressed in an index ranging from 0 to 1. A value of 1 corresponds to the maximum contribution a country or region can make to global species survival, equating to all species being classified as Least Concern on the IUCN Red List, and 0 is its minimum contribution, meaning that all species in the country or region having gone or extinct. Datasets of the Red List index by year (from 2001 to 2021) and by country were obtained from the OECD database (OECD Database, 2022). The increase in biodiversity at threat (low value of the Red List index) over the last decade occurred principally in the inter-tropical zones of both the North and South hemispheres (Fig. 12.2C).

Data maps for the year 2020 visualize the differences between the West and East hemispheres for the number of outbreaks and their potential drivers (Fig. 12.3) in addition to their latitudinal representations (Fig. 12.2).

Interlinkages Between Disease Outbreaks, Human-Induced Land Use Changes, Livestock and Biodiversity

Most studies have independently explored potential drivers of infectious disease epidemics and rarely considered their interdependencies. The links between the changes in outbreaks of infectious diseases, human demography (population size), land-use changes, livestock and poultry expansion and biodiversity at threat are explored using structural equation modeling (SEM). This statistical method helps to investigate the temporal relationships between the number of outbreaks of infectious diseases, both zoonotic and vector-borne, in relation to the expansion of artificial land, tree plantation, cropland, grassland, livestock, poultry and biodiversity. SEM combines measurement models (e.g. reliability) with structural models (e.g. regression), thus testing a potential chain of causality between outbreaks of diseases and these changes. SEM is performed using the 'piecewiseSEM' package (Lefcheck, 2016).

The first set of structural equation models is tested for the period from 2001 to 2020 of the whole dataset (for which Red List index values are available) in which (1) increase in outbreaks of zoonotic or vector-borne diseases is explained by human demography, expansion of artificial land (a proxy of urban demography and wealth), cropland, grassland, tree plantation, cattle, chicken and Red list index (i.e. biodiversity

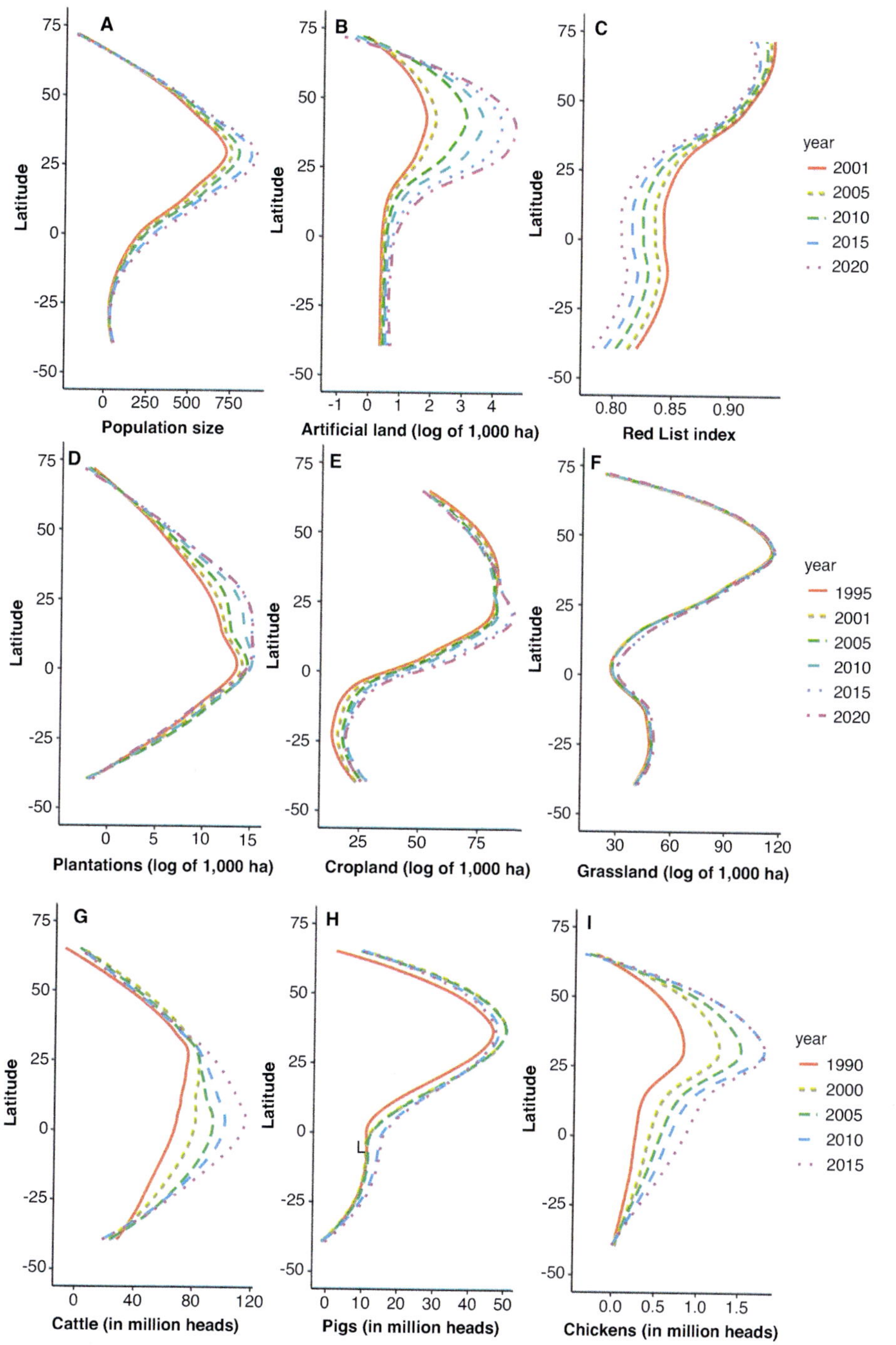

Fig. 12.2. Latitudinal pattern in human demography (population size) (A) and human-induced changes of (B) artificial land, (D) tree plantations, (E) cropland, (F) grassland, (G) number of cattle heads, (H) number of pigs and (I) number of chickens from 1992 to 2020 and (C) Red list index from 2001 to 2020 (data from World Bank, FAOSTAT and OECD for IUCN Red List).

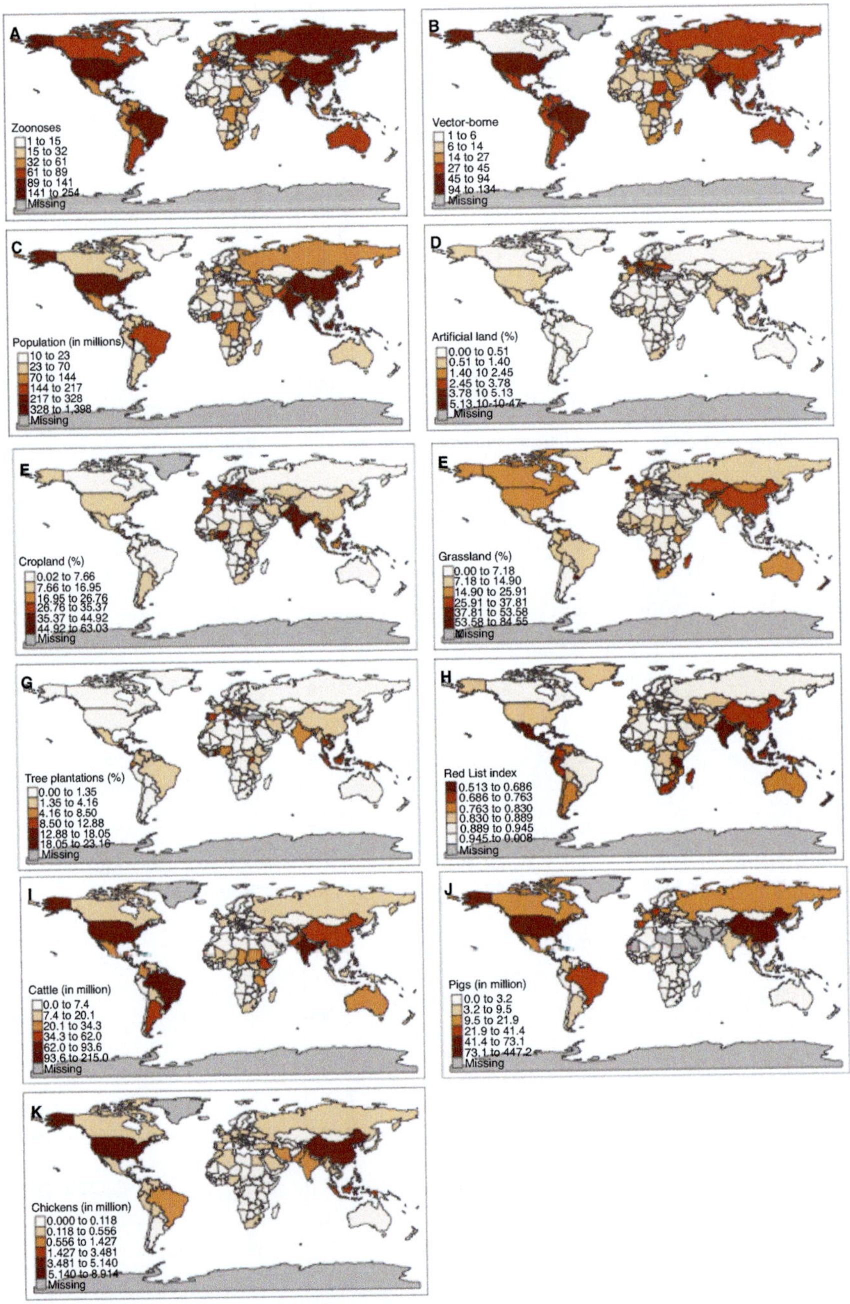

Fig. 12.3. Global maps of the total number of outbreaks of (A) zoonotic diseases and (B) vector-borne diseases from the year 1990 to the year 2020, (C) human demography (population size in million for the year 2019), (D) artificial land (in % of the total country area), (E) cropland (in % of the total country area), (F) grassland (in % of the total country area), (G) tree plantations (in % of the total country area), (H) Red List index (biodiversity at threat (in reverse color palette), (I) heads of cattle, (J) number of pigs, and (K) number of chickens for the year 2020 (data from GIDEON, Word Bank, FAOSTAT and IUCN in OECD database).

at threat) (Fig. 12.4). All these drivers are independently linked to outbreaks of infectious diseases with the exception of grassland and cropland expansion. The dependencies among the drivers are incorporated in the models with: (2) cropland expansion is explained by human demography, cattle or chicken expansion; (3) grassland expansion is explained by human demography, cattle or chicken expansion; (4) tree plantation expansion is explained by human demography; (5) cattle or chicken expansion is explained by human demography; and (6) the change in Red list index is statistically associated with all factors with the exception of grassland expansion, with cropland, tree plantation and chicken expansion increasing threatened biodiversity (i.e. decreased values of the Red list index). However, artificial land expansion and human demography are decreasing threatened biodiversity (i.e. increased values of the Red list index). This first set of models hypothesizes that artificial land expansion and population demography affect demands on living resources inducing changes in land use (Chen *et al.*, 2020), the expansion of livestock and poultry, the loss of biodiversity and the increase in outbreaks of infectious diseases (Connolly *et al.*, 2020). This first set of models also suggests that population demographics and artificial land expansion (proxy of urban demographics and wealth) do not appear to have a negative impact on biodiversity.

The results showed little difference between zoonotic diseases or vector-borne diseases in relation to the expansion of cattle or chickens (Fig. 12.4). It is important to note that all the models show a significant effect of the human population on the expansion of cropland, cattle and chickens, but also the number of outbreaks of zoonoses or vector-borne diseases. Human demography showed a negative or positive effect on grassland expansion when examining the expansion of cattle (Fig. 12.4A and 12.C) or chickens (Fig. 12.4B and 12.D) respectively, which is related to the positive effect of cattle or negative effect of chicken expansion on grassland expansion. The increase in the number of outbreaks is significantly associated with the increase in threatened biodiversity and expansion of cattle or chickens, while the impacts of grassland differ according to the type of epidemics, zoonotic or vector-borne.

To further explore the links between drivers related to the food system, the second set of models explores the expansion of cattle, pigs and chickens, cropland, grassland and threatened biodiversity on disease outbreaks, taking into account the inter-dependencies among the drivers (Fig. 12.5). Due to the number of factors included in the analyses and in order to be able to fit the models, tree plantation was not included as this factor was consistently associated with threatened biodiversity and was not found to be associated with the expansion of cropland, livestock and poultry. The results showed significant impacts of human demography, expansion of cattle, pigs and chickens, and threatened biodiversity on the number of outbreaks of zoonotic or vector-borne diseases in accordance with published studies (Cleaveland *et al.*, 2001; Morand, 2020; Morand and Lajaunie, 2021). Expansion of cropland or grassland has no effect or has a negative effect on the number of outbreaks. Interestingly, the impacts of livestock and poultry on biodiversity differ depending on the livestock animal, as well as the respective impacts of cropland or grassland. These results suggest that pastoralism and the expansion of grasslands promoted by pastoralism can have a positive impact on biodiversity (FAO, 2009), while the expansion of chickens and pigs and the expansion of croplands needed to feed animals can have a negative impact on biodiversity (Gottdenker *et al.*, 2014; Rohr *et al.*, 2019). Human demography has an indirect negative impact on biodiversity through the demand for animal protein, mainly pigs and chickens and cropland to feed these animals. However, human demography has a positive effect on biodiversity, suggesting that food consumption patterns and land use are the main drivers of biodiversity loss not demography per se. Recently, Hatfield *et al.* (Hatfield *et al.*, 2022) showed the recent recapture of local species composition over the past century in Europe, which may be amplified by ongoing rewilding.

In summary, and consistent with recent studies, significant relationships are confirmed between outbreaks of infectious diseases and the expansion of livestock (cattle, pigs, chickens) (Morand, 2020), the expansion of tree plantations (Morand and Lajaunie, 2021), human demography and the expansion of artificial land

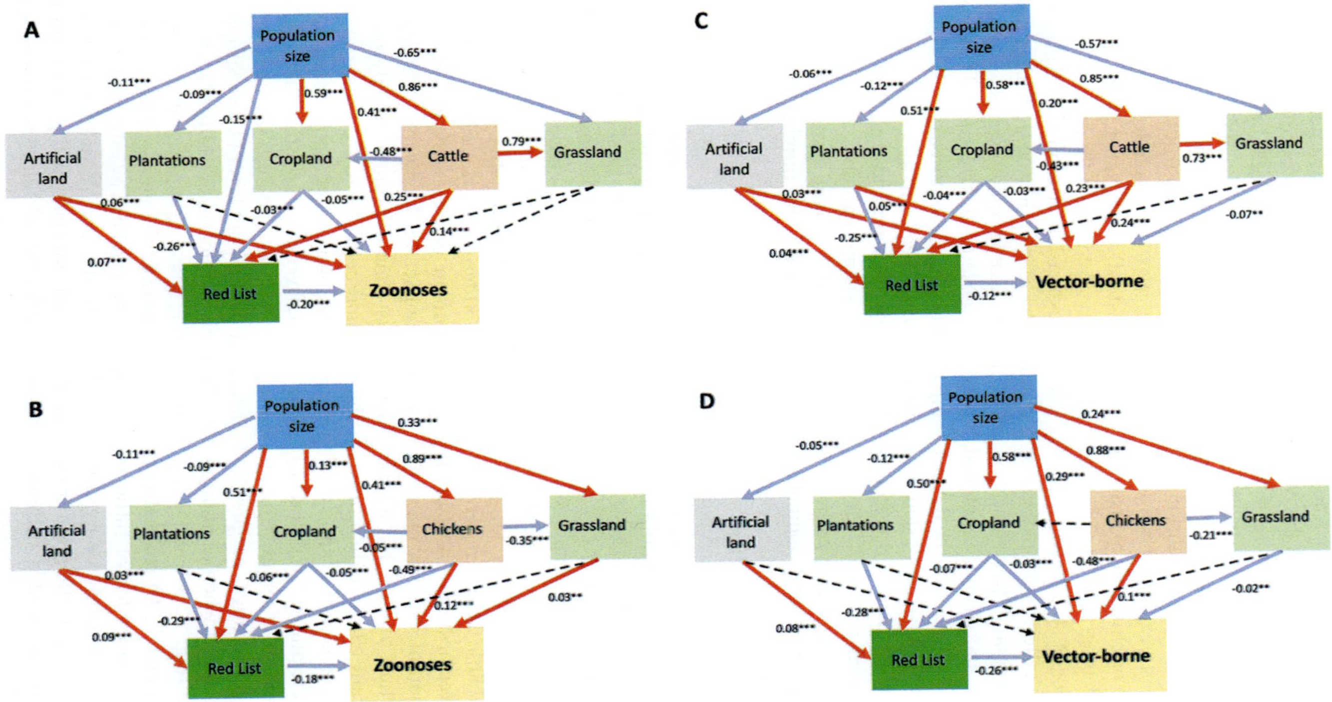

Fig. 12.4. Results of the structural equation modeling (SEM) used to investigate the temporal relationships between outbreaks of zoonoses and expansion of (A) cattle and (B) chickens, outbreaks of vector-borne diseases and expansion of (C) cattle and (D) chickens in relation to human demography, land-use changes in artificial land, tree plantation, cropland, grassland, and Red List index (biodiversity at threat) from 2001 to 2020. Significant partial correlations are presented in continuous lines (positive in red, negative in blue) with values of standardized estimates (*** = P value <0.001, ** = P value <0.01. Non-significant partial correlations are presented in dashed lines).

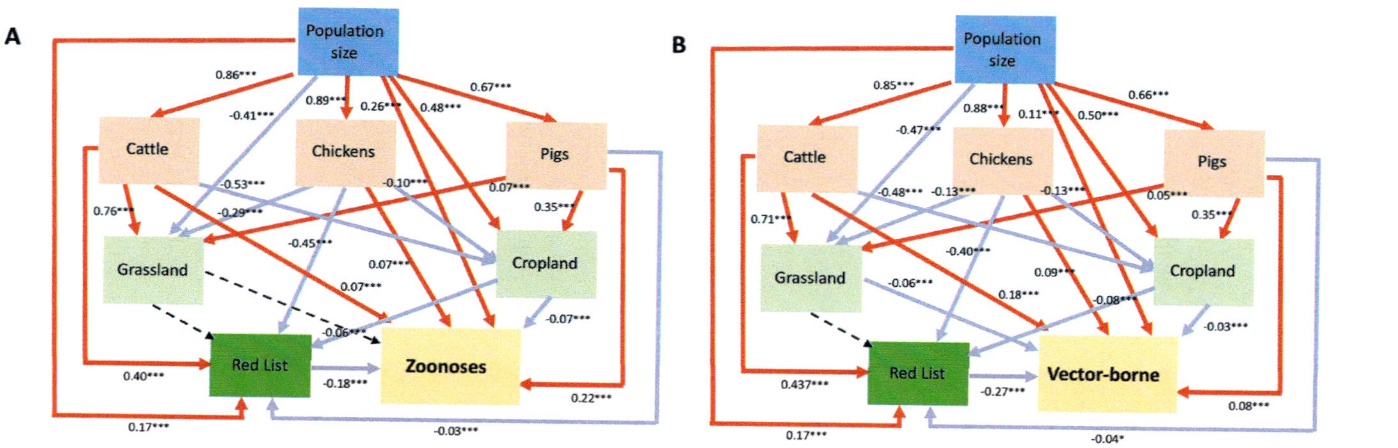

Fig. 12.5. Results of the structural equation modeling (SEM) used to investigate the temporal relationships between outbreaks of (A) zoonoses and (B) vector-borne diseases in relation to cropland, grassland, cattle, pigs, chickens and Red List index (biodiversity at threat) from 2001 to 2020. Significant partial correlations are presented in continuous lines (positive in red, negative in blue) with values of standardized estimates (*** = P value <0.001, ** = P value <0.01. Non-significant partial correlations are presented in dashed lines).

(FAO, 2009; Connolly *et al.*, 2020; Chen *et al.*, 2020; Gao *et al.*, 2021; Dobigny and Morand, 2022; Hatfield *et al.*, 2022), as well as increasing threatened biodiversity (estimated by a decreasing Red List index) (Morand, 2020). The 'negative diversity–disease' hypothesis, or 'dilution effect,' explains how biodiversity losses promote the transmission of diseases through the loss of ecological regulation, such as predation or competition, on animal reservoirs or vectors of pathogens (Morand, 2020). However, a new finding is the lack of direct effect of grassland or cropland expansion on the increase of zoonotic or vector-borne diseases, although cropland expansion has a negative impact on biodiversity.

The observed correlation between the increase in the number of outbreaks of infectious diseases with the increase in livestock confirms that economically important production animals (Thornton, 2010) strongly contribute to virus sharing between wildlife and humans (Johnson *et al.*, 2020). For instance, (Wells *et al.*, 2020) using data on 1785 DNA and RNA viruses from 725 species of mammals showed that domestic animals are central in the sharing of DNA viruses. Domestic animals promote the transmission of infectious agents from wildlife, ensure their amplification and favor zoonotic outbreaks (Thornton, 2010; Johnson *et al.*, 2020; Rulli *et al.*, 2021). For example, bats are important reservoirs of RNA viruses, but several of these viruses are also associated with domestic animals such as the Nipah virus with the domestic pig, the Hendra virus with the horse and MERS-CoV with the camel. Similarly, extensive livestock farming practices influence the increasing likelihood of influenza virus spillover from wild birds to poultry and pigs followed by amplification in domestic animals and transmission to humans (Wegner *et al.*, 2022).

Agriculture expansion is considered as a driver of biodiversity loss and the potential of emerging infectious diseases (Gottdenker *et al.*, 2014; Shah *et al.*, 2019; Zabel *et al.*, 2019; Wegner *et al.*, 2022), but here we show that grassland and cropland expansion does not appear to directly enhance disease transmission and outbreaks but indirectly, and only for cropland, through threatened biodiversity. Grassland is recognized as favoring biodiversity and contributing to ecosystem services (FAO, 2009; Thornton, 2010; Bengtsson *et al.*, 2019; Connolly *et al.*, 2020; Johnson *et al.*, 2020; Wells *et al.*, 2020; Gao *et al.*, 2021; Petermann and Buzhdygan, 2021; Rulli *et al.*, 2021; Dobigny and Morand, 2022; Hatfield *et al.*, 2022), while cropland expansion threatens biodiversity (Zabel *et al.*, 2019).

All findings presented here on the global patterns of outbreaks of infectious diseases should be used as a mere hypothesis on the potential links and interdependencies between infectious diseases, human demography, livestock, poultry, agriculture and biodiversity that needs to be further explored in depth at global and local scales.

Conclusion

Recent global changes have increased the risk of emerging and spread of infectious diseases despite improved sanitation and access to health care (Lederberg *et al.*, 1992; Institute of Medicine (US), 2003; Baker *et al.*, 2022). The global expansion of livestock farming by threatening biodiversity, land-use changes and homogenizing landscapes is increasing the epidemiological bridges between wildlife and humans (Petermann and Buzhdygan, 2021; Wegner *et al.*, 2022) particularly in the geographical hotspot of biodiversity (intertropical regions). Latitudinal trends in the global expansion of land use, livestock and threatened biodiversity highlight the importance of the different trajectories of socio-economic development between countries.

The links observed between infectious disease outbreaks, agriculture, livestock, poultry, human demography, urbanization and biodiversity should help rethink the global food system and production in ways that minimize the risk of infectious diseases while preserving biodiversity and contributing to the Sustainable Goals (Rohr *et al.*, 2019; Lajaunie and Morand, 2021; Morand and Lajaunie, 2021 Clark *et al.*, 2022). According to the OECD and FAO (OECD/FAO, 2021), growth in global meat protein consumption is projected to increase by 14% by 2030 compared to the 2018–2020 base period, particularly in low-income and middle-income countries. Changes in the global footprint of agricultural land in relation to food production may increase the divide between countries (Molotoks *et al.*, 2018; Rizvi *et al.*, 2018). Moreover, the growing meat protein consumption will enhance the international meat and animal food trade, which may also favor transboundary diseases (Beltran-Alcrudo *et al.*, 2019) and pandemics as evidenced by A(H1N1)pdm09 outbreak in North America in 2009 (Mena *et al.*, 2016). Agricultural areas dedicated to export production will continue to expand with the growing international demand (Kastner *et al.*, 2014) with an impact on biodiversity and climate (Zabel *et al.*, 2019; Kastner *et al.*, 2021; Ortiz *et al.*, 2021).

The findings presented here point to the multifaceted perspective of agriculture and livestock production when discussing the effects of international trade, land systems and health (Van Zanten *et al.*, 2018). A transformation of the global food system should be environmentally sustainable (Rockström *et al.*, 2017), prioritize health (Schneider *et al.*, 2021) and recognize the different contributions and geographical distributions of small farms that occupy 12% of all agricultural land and produce 35% of the world's food, and the 1% largest farms (larger than 50 ha) that operate more than 70% of the world's farmland (Lowder *et al.*, 2021). This transformation involves reintegrating agriculture, livestock and pastoralism into territorial development, developing agroecology and agroforestry approaches to increase resilience to climate change, while ensuring biodiversity conservation and food and health security. As Hayek recently pointed out (Hayek, 2022) the prevention of zoonotic diseases requires a comprehensive strategy to reduce the demand for animal protein as well as improved forest conservation (Morand and Lajaunie, 2021).

The Sustainable Development Goals (SDGs), including zero hunger, clean water, maintaining life on land and in water, climate action, and health are influenced by the global food system (Panel *et al.*, 2022). The One Health approach supported by the new One Health quadripartite FAO, WOAH (World Organization for Animal Health), UNEP (United Nations Environment Programme) and WHO (World Health Organization) is 'an integrated, unifying approach that aims to sustainably balance and optimize the health of people, animals, and ecosystems. It recognizes the health of humans, domestic and wild animals, plants, and the wider environment (including ecosystems) are closely linked and interdependent' (Panel *et al.*, 2022). The new One Health approach recognizes the importance of anthropogenic global stressors, including land use, climate change and biodiversity loss, through their consequences for human health. The observed patterns and interlinkages between disease outbreaks and their potential drivers presented in this study can help transform the global food system using the One Health approach to meet the SDGs.

Acknowledgements

SM is supported by the French ANR for the project funded by FutureHealth (SEA ANR-17-CE35-0003-01), and by the Thailand International Cooperation Agency (TICA) for the project 'Animal Innovative Health.'

References

Alkemade, R., Reid, R.S., Berg, M., Leeuw, J. and Jeuken, M. (2013) Assessing the impacts of livestock production on biodiversity in rangeland ecosystems. *Proceedings National Academy of Sciences USA* 110, 20900–209005.

Baker, R.E., Mahmud, A.S., Miller, I.F., Rajeev, M., Rasambainarivo, F. *et al.* (2022) Infectious disease in an era of global change. *Nature Review Microbiology* 20, 193–205.

Bar-On, Y.M., Phillips, R. and Milo, R. (2018) The biomass distribution on earth. *Proceedings National Academy of Sciences*115, 6506–6511.

Bartlett, H., Holmes, M.A., Petrovan, S.O., Williams, D.R., Wood, J.L.N. *et al.* (2022) Understanding the relative risks of zoonosis emergence under contrasting approaches to meeting livestock product demand. *Royal Society Open Science* 9, 211573.

Beltran-Alcrudo, D., Falco, J.R., Raizman, E. and Dietze, K. (2019) Transboundary spread of pig diseases: The role of international trade and travel. *BMC Veterinary Research* 15, 64.

Bengtsson, J., Bullock, J.M., Egoh, B., Everson, C., Everson, T. *et al.* (2019) Grasslands—more important for ecosystem services than you might think. *Ecosphere* 10, e02582.

Bernstein, A.S., Ando, A.W., Loch-Temzelides, T., Vale, M.M., Li, B.V. *et al.* (2022) The costs and benefits of primary prevention of zoonotic pandemics. *Scientific Advances* 8, eabl4183.

Callaghan, C.T., Nakagawa, S. and Cornwell, W.K. (2021) Global abundance estimates for 9700 bird species. *Proceedings National Academy of Sciences USA*118, *e2023170118*.

Chen, G., Li, X., Liu, X., Chen, Y., Liang, X. *et al.* (2020) Global projections of future urban land expansion under shared socioeconomic pathways. *Nature Communications* 11, 537.

Clark, M., Springmann, M., Rayner, M., Scarborough, P., Hill, J. *et al.* (2022) Estimating the environmental impacts of 57,000 food products. *Proceedings National Academy of Sciences USA*119, *e2120584119*.

Cleaveland, S., Laurenson, M.K. and Taylor, L.H. (2001) Diseases of humans and their domestic mammals: Pathogen characteristics, host range and the risk of emergence. *Philosophical Transactions Royal Society London B* 356, 991–999.

Cohen, M.N. and Armelagos, G.J. (1984) *Paleopathology at the origin of agriculture*. Academic Press, Orlando.

Connolly, C., Keil, R. and Ali, S.H. (2020) Extended urbanisation and the spatialities of infectious disease: Demographic change, infrastructure and governance. *Urban Studies* 58, 245–263.

Crist, E., Mora, C. and Engelman, R. (2017) The interaction of human population, food production, and biodiversity protection. *Science* 356, 260–264.

Diamond, J. (2002) Evolution, consequences and future of plant and animal domestication. *Nature* 418, 700–707.

Dobigny, G. and Morand, S. (2022) Zoonotic emergence at the animal-environment-human interface: The forgotten urban socio-ecosystems. *Zonodo*. DOI: 10.5281/zenodo.6444777.

Dunn, R.R., Davies, T.J., Harris, N.C. and Gavin, M.C. (2010) Global drivers of human pathogen richness and prevalence. *Proceedings Biological Sciences* 277, 2587–2595.

FAO (2009) Livestock keepers—guardians of biodiversity. Animal Production and Health Paper NO 167. Rome: FAO.

FAOSTAT (2022) FAO (Food and Agriculture Organization of the United Nations). Available at: https://www.fao.org/faostat

Faust, C.L., McCallum, H.I., Bloomfield, L.S.P., Gottdenker, N.L., Gillespie, T.R. *et al.* (2018) Pathogen spillover during land conversion. *Ecology Letters* 21, 471–483.

Gao, P., Pilot, E., Rehbock, C., Gontariuk, M., Doreleijers, S. *et al.* (2021) Land use and land cover change and its impacts on dengue dynamics in China: A systematic review. *PLoS Neglected Tropical Diseases* 15, e0009879.

Gaston, K.J. and Blackburn, T.M. (1997) How many birds are there. *Biodiversity and Conservation* 6, 615–625.

GIDEON (Global Infectious Disease and Epidemiology Network) (2021). Available at: www.gideononline.com

Gottdenker, N.L., Streicker, D.G., Faust, C.L. and Carroll, C.R. (2014) Anthropogenic land use change and infectious diseases: A review of the evidence. *EcoHealth* 11, 619–632.

Guernier, V., Hochberg, M.E. and Guégan, J.F. (2004) Ecology drives the worldwide distribution of human diseases. *PLoS Biology* 2, e141.

Hassell, J.M., Begon, M., Ward, M.J. and Fèvre, E.M. (2017) Urbanization and disease emergence: Dynamics at the wildlife-livestock-human interface. *Trends Ecology Evolution* 32, 55–67.

Hatfield, J.H., Davis, K.E. and Thomas, C.D. (2022) Lost, gained, and regained functional and phylogenetic diversity of European mammals since 8000 years ago. *Global Change Biology* 28, 5283–5293.

Hayek, M.N. (2022) The infectious disease trap of animal agriculture. *Science Advances* 8, eadd6681.

Institute of Medicine (US) (2003) Committee on emerging microbial threats to health in the 21st century. In: Smolinski, M.S., Hamburg, M.A. and Lederberg, J. (eds) *Microbial Threats to Health: Emergence, Detection, and Response*. National Academies Press, Washington, DC.

IPBES Brondizio, E.S., Settele, J., Díaz, S. and Ngo, H.T. (eds). (2019) *Global assessment report on biodiversity and ecosystem services of the intergovernmental science-policy platform on biodiversity and ecosystem services*. IPBES Secretariat, Bonn, Germany.

IUCN (2022) The IUCN red list of threatened species. Version 2022-1. Available at: https://www.iucnredlist.org

Johnson, C.K., Hitchens, P.L., Pandit, P.S., Rushmore, J., Evans, T.S. *et al.* (2020) Global shifts in mammalian population trends reveal key predictors of virus spillover risk. *Proceedings of the Royal Society of London B* 287, 20192736.

Jones, B.A., Grace, D., Kock, R., Alonso, S., Rushton, J. *et al.* (2013) Zoonosis emergence linked to agricultural intensification and environmental change. *Proceedings National Academy of Sciences USA* 110, 8399–8404.

Kastner, T., Erb, K.H. and Haberl, H. (2014) Rapid growth in agricultural trade: Effects on global area efficiency and the role of management. *Environmental Research Letters* 9, 034015.

Kastner, T., Chaudhary, A., Gingrich, S., Marques, A., Persson, U.M. *et al.* (2021) Global agricultural trade and land system sustainability: Implications for ecosystem carbon storage, biodiversity, and human nutrition. *One Earth* 4, 1425–1443.

Lajaunie, C. and Morand, S. (2021) Biodiversity targets, SDGs and health: A new turn after the coronavirus pandemic. *Sustainability* 13, 4353.

Lederberg, J., Shope, R.E. and Oaks, S.C. (1992) *Emerging Infections: Microbial Threats to Health in the United States*. National Academies Press, Washington, DC.

Lefcheck, J.S. (2016) PiecewiseSEM: Piecewise structural equation modelling in R for ecology, evolution, and systematics. *Methods Ecology Evolution* 7, 573–579.

Lowder, S.K., Sánchez, M.V. and Bertini, R. (2021) Which farms feed the world and has farmland become more concentrated? *World Development* 142, 105455.

McNeill, W.H. (1976) *Plagues and people*. Anchor Press, New York, USA.

Mena, I., Nelson, M.I., Quezada-Monroy, F., Dutta, J., Cortes-Fernández, R. *et al.* (2016) Origins of the 2009 H1N1 influenza pandemic in swine in mexico 5, e16777.

Molotoks, A., Stehfest, E., Doelman, J., Albanito, F., Fitton, N. *et al.* (2018) Global projections of future cropland expansion to 2050 and direct impacts on biodiversity and carbon storage. *Global Change Biology* 24, 5895–5908.

MorandS. (2016) *La Prochaine peste. Une histoire globale des sociétés et de leurs épidémies*. Editions Fayard, Paris, France.

Morand, S. (2020) Emerging diseases, livestock expansion and biodiversity loss are positively related at global scale. *Biological Conservation* 248, 108707.

Morand, S. and Lajaunie, C. (2021) Outbreaks of vector-borne and zoonotic diseases are associated with changes in forest cover and oil palm expansion at global scale. *Frontiers Veterinary Parasitology* 24, 661063.

Morand, S. and Lajaunie, C. (2021) Biodiversity and covid-19: A report and a long road ahead to avoid a next pandemic. *One Earth* 4, 920–923.

Morand, S., McIntyre, K.M. and Baylis, M. (2014) Domesticated animals and human infectious diseases of zoonotic origins: Domestication time matters. *Infection Genetics Evolution* 24, 76–87.

Murray, K.A., Preston, N., Allen, T., Zambrana-Torrelio, C., Hosseini, P.R. *et al.* (*2015*) Global biogeography of human infectious diseases. *Proceedings National Academy of Sciences USA*112, 12746–12751.

OECD Database (2022) Organisation for Economic Co-operation and Development. Available at: https://stats.oecd.org

OECD/FAO (2021) *OECD-FAO Agricultural Outlook 2021–2030*. OECD Publishing, Paris.

Olson, S.H., Benedum, C.M., Mekaru, S.R., Preston, N.D., Mazet, J.A. *et al.* (2015) Drivers of emerging infectious disease events as a framework for digital detection. *Emerging Infectious Diseases* 21, 1285–1292.

Ortiz, A.M.D., Outhwaite, C.L.O., Dalin, C. and Newbold, T. (2021) A review of the interactions between biodiversity, agriculture, climate change, and international trade: Research and policy priorities. *One Earth* 4, 88–101.

Panel, O.H.H.-L.E., Adisasmito, W.B., Almuhairi, S., Behravesh, C.B., Bilivogui, P. *et al.* (2022) One health: A new definition for a sustainable and healthy future. *PLoS Pathogens* 18, e1010537.

Pearce-Duvet, J.M.C. (2006) The origin of human pathogens: Evaluating the role of agriculture and domestic animals in the evolution of human disease. *Biological Review* 81, 369–382.

Petermann, J.S. and Buzhdygan, O.Y. (2021) Grassland biodiversity. *Current Biology* 31, R1195–R1201.

Potapov, P., Turubanova, S., Hansen, M.C., Tyukavina, A., Zalles, V. *et al.* (2022) Global maps of cropland extent and change show accelerated cropland expansion in the twenty-first century. *Nature Food* 3, 19–28.

Reid, R.S., Bedelian, C., Said, M.Y., Kruska, R.L., Mauricio, R.M. *et al.* Steinfeld, H., Mooney, H.A., Schneider, F. and Neville, L.E. (eds). (2010) *Global livestock impacts on biodiversity*, Livestock in a changing landscape. Drivers, consequences, and responses. Island Press, Washington, DC, pp. 111–138.

Rizvi, S., Pagnutti, C., Fraser, E., Bauch, C.T. and Anand, M. (2018) Global land use implications of dietary trends. *PLoS One* 13, e0200781.

Rockström, J., Williams, J., Daily, G., Noble, A., Matthews, N. *et al.* (2017) Sustainable intensification of agriculture for human prosperity and global sustainability. *Ambio* 46, 4–17.

Rohr, J.R., Barrett, C.B., Civitello, D.J., Craft, M.E., Delius, B. *et al.* (2019) Emerging human infectious diseases and the links to global food production. *Nature Sustainability* 2, 445–456.

Rulli, M.C., D'Odorico, P., Galli, N. and Hayman, D.T.S. (2021) Land-use change and the livestock revolution increase the risk of zoonotic coronavirus transmission from rhinolophid bats. *Nature Food* 2, 409–416.

Schneider, K.R., Fanzo, J.C., Haddad, L. and Moncayo, J.R. (2021) Global health has a stake in the upcoming UN food systems summit. *Lancet* 398, 1027–1029.

Scott, J.C. (2017) *Against the grain: A deep history of the earliest states*. Yale University Press, New Haven, USA.

Semenza, J.C., Lindgren, E., Balkanyi, L., Espinosa, L., Almqvist, M.S. *et al.* (2016) Determinants and drivers of infectious disease threat events in Europe. *Emerging Infectious Diseases* 22, 581–589.

Shah, H.A., Huxley, P., Elmes, J. and Murray, K.A. (2019) Agricultural land-uses consistently exacerbate infectious disease risks in Southeast Asia. *Nature Communications* 10, 4299.

Smith, K.F., Goldberg, M., Rosenthal, S., Carlson, L., Chen, J. *et al.* (2014) Global rise in human infectious disease outbreaks. *Journal Royal Society Interface* 11, 20140950.

Steinfeld, H., Gerber, P., Wassenaar, T.D., Castel, C., Rosales, M. *et al.* (2006) *Livestock's long shadow: Environmental issues and options*. Food and Agriculture Organization of the United Nations, Roma, Italy.

Sun, L., Chen, J., Li, Q. and Huang, D. (2020) Dramatic uneven urbanization of large cities throughout the world in recent decades. *Nature Communications* 11, 5366.

Thornton, P.K. (2010) Livestock production: Recent trends, future prospects. *Philosophical Transactions of the Royal Society B* 365, 2853–2867.

Van Zanten, H.H.E., Herrero, M., Van Hal, O., Röös, E., Muller, A. *et al.* (2018) Defining a land boundary for sustainable livestock consumption. *Global Change Biology* 24, 4185–4194.

Vourc'h, G., Moutou, F., Morand, S. and Zoonoses, J.E. (2022) *Diseases that link animals and humans*. Quae, Versailles.

Wegner, G.I., Murray, K.A., Springmann, M., Muller, A., Sokolow, S.H. *et al.* (2022) Averting wildlife-borne infectious disease epidemics requires a focus on socio-ecological drivers and a redesign of the global food system. *EClinicalMedicine* 47, 101386.

Wells, K., Morand, S., Wardeh, M. and Baylis, M. (2020) Distinct spread of DNA and RNA viruses among mammals amid prominent role of domestic species. *Global Ecology Biogeography* 29, 470–481.

Wolfe, N.D., Dunavan, C.P. and Diamond, J. (2007) Origins of major human infectious diseases. *Nature* 447, 279–283.

World Bank Open Data (2022). Available at: https://data.worldbank.org

Zabel, F., Delzeit, R., Schneider, J.M., Seppelt, R., Mauser, W. *et al.* (2019) Global impacts of future cropland expansion and intensification on agricultural markets and biodiversity. *Nature Communications* 10, 2844.

13 Man's Best Friend and Our Shared Infectious Diseases

Maxine L.A. Macpherson[1,2,3], Rhonda Pinckney[1,2], Wayne Sylvester[1,2], Satesh Bidaisee[1,3,4] and Calum N.L. Macpherson[1,3,4*]

[1]School of Graduate Studies, St. George's University, Grenada, West Indies; [2]School of Veterinary Medicine, St. George's University, Grenada, West Indies; [3]Windward Islands Research and Education Foundation, St. George's University, Grenada, West Indies; [4]School of Medicine, St. George's University, True Blue, Grenada, West Indies

Abstract

This review categorizes 62 zoonoses humans share with dogs based on their clinical, public health importance, and global distribution. Three categories were identified. Category 1 comprise the most widespread and public health important zoonoses and includes 13 zoonoses where dogs play an essential role in the maintenance and transmission of the infectious organisms. This category comprises *Rabies lyssavirus*, *Leptospirosis*, *Leishmania*, *Trypanosoma cruzi*, *Trypanosoma brucei* spp., *Clonorchis sinsensis*, *Opisthorchis viverrini*, *Paragonimus* spp., *Echinococcus granulosus*, *Echinococcus multilocularis*, *Taenia multiceps*, *Dracunculus medinensis*, *Toxocara canis*, *Ancylostoma* spp., and *Strongyloides stercoralis*. Category 2 includes 24 zoonoses of lesser public health importance in which human or dog behavior plays a major role in transmission. Category 2 includes, *Microsporum* spp., *Prevotella* spp., *Bacteroides* spp., *Porphyromonas* spp., *Bergeyella zoohelcum*, *Neisseria* spp., *Pasteurella* spp., *Capnocytophaga canimorsus*, *Staphylococcus* spp., *Streptococcus* spp., *Salmonella* spp., *Anaplasma* spp., *Ehrlichia* spp., *Borrelia* spp., *Rickettsia* spp., *Yersina pestis*, *Giardia duodenalis*, *Cryptosporidium* spp., *Toxoplasma gondii*, *Dibothriocephalus latum*, *Spirometra* spp., *Schistosoma* spp., *Echinococcus canadensis*, and *Sarcoptes scabei var canis*. Category 3 includes human infection where the zoonotic infection link is rare but has occasionally implicated dogs. This category includes SARS-CoV-2, *Bordetella bronchiseptica*, *Mycobacterium* spp., *Corynebacterium* spp., *Coxiella burnetti*, *Helicobacter* spp., *Campylobacter* spp., *Brucella canis*, *Balantioides coli*, *Blastocystis hominis*, *Bacillus anthracis*, *Dipylidium caninum*, *Taenia* spp., *Trichuris vulpis*, *Gnathostoma* spp., *Thelazia* spp., *Dirofilaria* spp., *Onchocera lupi*, *Heterophyes heterophyes*, *Metagonimus* spp., *Fasciolopsis buski*, *Ctenocephalides felis*, *Cheyletiella* spp., *Otodectes cynotis*, and *Cochliomya homnivorax*. Changes in human behavior and control of canine infection would reduce the public health importance of these zoonoses.

Keywords: zoonoses, dogs, transmission, behavior

*Corresponding author: cmacpherson@sgu.edu

Introduction

Dogs are the oldest companion animals of humans (Clutton-Brock, 1995) and of the 400 infectious diseases that dogs can carry, we share over 60 with them. Historically, the human-dog relationship has been beneficial for companionship, security, hunting, herding, sport, entertainment, space exploration, transport, food, and a source of income through breeding. In more recent decades, dogs have been trained to detect cancers, infectious diseases such as SARS-CoV-2, anthrax, and asymptomatic malaria (Kasstan *et al.*, 2019; Else, 2020; Jendrny *et al.*, 2020) and have been integral parts of border patrol, rescue teams, and translational and comparative medical research. This relationship has facilitated the sharing of zoonoses, which vary in their clinical and public health importance and transmissibility, and their existence is influenced by regional environmental and socioeconomic factors.

Climate change has played an increasing role in the transmission of zoonoses. Changing temperatures may accelerate the development of vectors, shorten environmental lifecycle stage development, influence transmission, and host susceptibility (Harvell *et al.*, 2002). Natural disasters, war, droughts, and famine, along with transhumant, nomadic, or peripatetic migrations, can result in the migration of people and their animals, including dogs, to areas endemic for zoonotic diseases that they are naïve to and they themselves may introduce zoonoses to new regions. The impact of these events on the health and behavior of owned and stray dog populations may also contribute to the zoonotic spread and public health risk. Deforestation has been incriminated in several zoonotic outbreaks in recent years (Cascio *et al.*, 2011). As urbanization steadily encroaches on wildlife habitats, the likelihood of climatic and environmental changes impacting species populations and health, pathogen lifecycles and the probability of transmission of infectious diseases increases.

Emerging and re-emerging zoonotic diseases are becoming more common and widespread, some of which have developed into pandemics, such as SARS-CoV-1 in 2002 and SARS-CoV-2 which began in 2019. The emergence and spread of these pandemics and other infectious disease outbreaks are facilitated by increasing population densities, increased international travel and trade, intensive livestock farming and agriculture, encroachment on wildlife habitats and exploitation of natural resources (The Lancet, 2020).

Expanding farmland for food production, disproportionate levels of public health surveillance of vectors and diseases, socio-economic deprivation or conflict through immigration, and spending more time in environments that house vectors of zoonoses are all human behaviors further lending to zoonotic transmission (Cascio *et al.*, 2011).

With the availability of travel and the internet, more dogs are being adopted from countries around the globe and introduced to new homelands, potentially introducing new infectious diseases. At the end of 2016, it was estimated that 38 percent of households in the USA owned at least one dog (American Veterinary Medical Association, 2018). During the SARS-CoV-2 global pandemic, the number of owned dogs around the world increased as people were quarantined and sought companionship and a sense of worth during a time of great uncertainty. There has also been a recent rise in the spread of misinformation, vaccine hesitancy among people including pet owners and reluctance to accept advice from health professionals (World Health Organization (WHO), 2019; Kogan *et al.*, 2021). The outcomes of the general public's growing distrust in scientific research and health recommendations are likely to be major factors in disease transmission and future pandemics.

This review aims to provide a comprehensive update on human:dog zoonoses and their public health importance published almost a decade ago (Macpherson, 2013; Macpherson *et al.*, 2013). To facilitate this review, all published articles and reviews were found using the keywords 'zoonoses', 'dogs', 'transmission', and 'behavior', along with the name of each organism, and were searched for in Journal/Author Name Estimator (JANE), PubMED, Veterinary Information Network (VIN), and Google Scholar. References from the source articles were also reviewed. The zoonoses covered in this review are classified into three categories viz: category one includes the most widespread and public health important zoonoses in which dogs play an essential role in the maintenance and transmission of the infectious organism to humans. Category two includes zoonoses of lesser public health importance in which human or dog behavior plays a major role in transmission. Category three includes human infections with the rare zoonotic transmission, but on occasion, dogs have been implicated to play a role in the transmission of the infectious organism. In each category, the organisms are listed in taxonomic order and do not reflect a prioritization of their public health importance.

Review Methodology

To facilitate this review, all published articles and reviews were found using the keywords 'zoonoses', 'dogs', 'transmission', and 'behavior', along with the name of each organism, and were searched for in Journal/Author Name Estimator (JANE), PubMED, Veterinary Information Network (VIN), and Google Scholar. References from the source articles were also reviewed.

Category 1: Major Human: Dog Zoonoses in Which Dogs Play an Essential Role in the Maintenance and Propagation of the Infectious Organism

Rabies lyssavirus (Virus)

Rabies lyssavirus is a neurotropic virus that is the cause of roughly 59,000 human deaths and 8.6 billion USD in economic losses globally every year (Hampson *et al.*, 2015). The virus is transmitted through infected saliva entering the body through a bite wound or injury before replicating in the nervous system. All warm-blooded animals are susceptible to rabies infection. Enzootic areas often have distinct rabies virus variants that usually adapt to one dominant reservoir host, depending on the geographical area (Greene and Dreesen, 1998).

Rabies was one of the first zoonoses ever identified. Compulsory muzzling, control of dog movement, and the culling of strays were all implemented in varying degrees from as early as the sixth century BC in India, the fourth century AD by the Talmud, second century BC in China and ancient Greece and the Roman Empire (Blancou and Meslin, 2000). Until Pasteur first utilized the rabies vaccine in 1885, there was no effective human prevention for rabies. Rabies is unique in that its pathogenesis allows for vaccination both before and after exposure (Moore, 2021). Since the twentieth century, numerous countries have had successful mass vaccination programs to eliminate enzootic canine rabies (Minghui *et al.*, 2018). In developed countries with dedicated dog and cat vaccination programs, wildlife species have become the main reservoir of rabies. Many of these countries have begun the process of eliminating rabies from wildlife species to reduce the potential for spillover into domestic species. This is done by using oral rabies vaccines in bait, along with surveillance and monitoring of vaccine effectiveness (Gilbert *et al.*, 2018; Robardet *et al.*, 2019). Rabies is a progressive, almost invariably fatal disease that is entirely preventable through measures such as canine vaccination. While it is present in most countries, rabies has the greatest public health impact on poor populations living in developing countries (Lembo *et al.*, 2013). Most human deaths occur in Asian and African countries with approximately 40 percent of cases occurring in persons below 15 years old (Gossner *et al.*, 2020). This is likely due to financial, educational, and infrastructural disparities with limited to no access to Post-Exposure Prophylaxis (PEP) in rural communities. Even where it is available, animal bite victims who are traveling or are from low socioeconomic backgrounds and rural areas often experience delays in seeking and receiving PEP at health facilities (Sambo *et al.*, 2013; Gossner *et al.*, 2020).

Clinical signs in dogs are highly variable and there is no pathognomonic feature that can be used to accurately diagnose rabies premortem. The incubation period can vary from a few days to several years, but most incubation periods observed after experimental inoculation last 3–6 weeks (Wandeler *et al.*, 2013). Prodromal symptoms such as nervousness, agitation, hyperactivity, and abnormal vocalization or sexual behavior often progress rapidly to advanced stages (Wandeler *et al.*, 2013). Depending on the manifestation of the disease, it is classified as paralytic or furious. Dogs with the paralytic form may appear dull and quiet for extended periods of time while the furious form is characterized by markedly restless and aggressive behavior. Rabies has the potential to alternate between the furious and paralytic forms in all infected individuals. The illness ultimately leads to paralysis which causes classical signs such as pseudoptyalism and uncoordinated gait, before progressing to respiratory arrest and death.

The onset of symptoms in humans depends on several factors, including the anatomical site of the bite wound, the viral quantity, and variant inoculated into the site, and how quickly PEP can be administered. The first clinical symptom is often neuropathic pain at or near the infected wound (Yousaf *et al.*, 2012). The disease is almost 100% fatal once clinical signs appear (Moore, 2021).

Although rabies is often diagnosed based on clinical presentation, the only confirmatory test is through the detection of intraneuronal inclusion bodies or Negri bodies in brain tissue. The virus remains viable in a carcass for less than 24 hours at 20°C but can last longer when refrigerated (Greene and Dreesen, 1998). Dogs suspected to be rabid are not always immediately euthanized for testing. Instead, they may be placed in ten-day isolation for observation, at the end of which the dog is assumed not to be infected if no clinical signs develop (Ma *et al.*, 2018). If clinical signs do develop, the dog is then euthanized and tested.

Direct Fluorescent Antibody (DFA) testing has historically been considered the gold standard of rabies diagnosis in animals (Beeler and Ehnert, 2020). The benefit of DFA testing is that it can detect antigens for up to five to 7 days at 25°C, at which point viable rabies particles may no longer be detectable. One of the drawbacks of DFA testing is the cost of acquiring and maintaining a fluorescent microscope, which limits access to testing, potentially resulting in underreporting of rabies in humans. Without a confirmatory test after a bite injury, the wound may be inappropriately managed and may lead to unnecessary administration of PEP, which can be scarce and expensive in some parts of the world. An alternative to DFA testing is the direct rapid immunohistochemical test, which has been shown to have the same sensitivity and specificity as the DFA test (Lembo *et al.*, 2006). It is a simple test that does not require specialized equipment and can be performed successfully on samples preserved in glycerol solution for 15 months or frozen for 2 years. This is therefore a valuable test for use in remote, rural areas, where human rabies infections are highest.

RT-PCR is not currently recommended for routine diagnosis but great strides in the development of quick and accurate PCR tests have been made in recent years (Wadhwa *et al.*, 2017; Caraballo *et al.*, 2020). The most effective way to reduce mortalities and economic losses related to rabies infection is through mass vaccination of dogs, alongside improved access to PEP (Bitek *et al.*, 2019; World Health Organization, 2013). In 2018, the UN Food and Agriculture Organization (FAO), the World Organization for Animal Health (OIE), and the Global Alliance for Rabies Control (GARC) launched a global plan to eliminate deaths from dog-transmitted rabies by 2030 (Minghui *et al.*, 2018). Substantial evidence suggests that as the reproductive number, R_0, is approximately 1.2 (Townsend *et al.*, 2013), vaccination of 70% of dogs will be adequate in eliminating canine rabies (World Health Organization, 2013). In remote and rural locations, this can be achieved through oral bait vaccination to increase coverage of dogs inaccessible for parenteral vaccination. Reproductive control measures to reduce dog population sizes are unlikely to be an effective means of controlling rabies as transmission varies only slightly with dog density (Cleaveland and Hampson, 2017). Dog population management is desirable to improve animal welfare and health, which may have positive secondary effects on rabies control and dog-human interactions. Public education on rabies, enforcement of responsible pet ownership and readily available access to routine veterinary care and vaccination should be achievable methods of control.

Leptospira spp. (Bacteria)

Leptospirosis is an increasingly important neglected public health disease that is exacerbated by the impact of climate change, particularly by the frequency of flooding (Karpagam and Ganesh, 2020). Based on published reports from 1970 to 2008, an estimated 1.03

million human cases occur annually (Costa *et al.*, 2015). Within the host, the spirochetes colonize the renal tubules, reproduce, and then are excreted in the urine. Transmission usually occurs through direct contact with urine or blood through skin lacerations, aerosol inhalation, or contact with mucosa or conjunctiva. It can also be transmitted indirectly through contact with contaminated water or soil (Pinto *et al.*, 2017). Butchers, agricultural manual laborers, sewage workers, animal handlers, and other outdoor occupations are considered an important human demographic for leptospirosis infection (Brown *et al.*, 2011). Infected dogs shed the bacteria in their urine whether they are asymptomatic or clinically ill and can infect humans through direct contact. Dogs with frequent access to outdoor rural areas and wildlife are more likely to encounter infected urine and contract leptospirosis (Hennebelle *et al.*, 2014).

Clinical signs in dogs can vary from asymptomatic to acute kidney injury, hepatic injury and icterus, pulmonary hemorrhage, uveitis, and reproductive failure (Reagan and Sykes, 2019). Thrombocytopenia, coagulopathy, proteinuria, hypoalbuminemia, and glucosuria have also been reported (Tangeman and Littman, 2013; Reagan and Sykes, 2019).

Severe leptospirosis in humans often presents with vascular endothelial damage and reportedly causes disseminated intravascular coagulation in up to 50 percent of patients (Chierakul *et al.*, 2008). Leptospirosis is also known as Weil's disease in humans. Humans are incidental hosts and can develop systemic infections but are not considered carriers and cannot transmit the infection.

Leptospirosis is a difficult disease to diagnose, and tests have varying efficacy at different stages of infection. PCR is a valuable diagnostic tool for detecting infection before the development of a serologic response (Hennebelle *et al.*, 2014). The use of two rapid tests as a screening tool for acute leptospirosis can be useful alongside suggestive clinical and laboratory results (Troìa *et al.*, 2018). Simultaneous use of Microscopic Agglutination Test (MAT) and PCR has been shown to increase the diagnostic accuracy of leptospirosis in dogs (Miotto *et al.*, 2018).

Vaccination of dogs may decrease the risk of infection but a multi-modal approach is recommended to prevent canine leptospirosis, with additional strategies being rodent control, standardized hygiene protocol, and proper management of asymptomatically infected dogs (Miotto *et al.*, 2018) and people.

***Leishmania* spp. (Protista)**

Leishmaniasis is endemic to Asia, Africa, the Americas, and the Mediterranean, with approximately 1.5–2 million new human cases occurring annually worldwide (Torres-Guerrero *et al.*, 2017). An incidence of 0.7–1.2 million cases of cutaneous leishmaniasis and 0.2–0.4 million cases of visceral leishmaniasis have been estimated from endemic regions of the world, within 87 and 75 countries (Alvar *et al.*, 2012; World Health Organization, 2021; World Health Organization, 2022), approximately 50 of which are endemic for canine leishmaniosis (Maia and Campino, 2018). *Leishmania* spp. is one of the neglected tropical diseases planned for elimination by 2030 by the WHO (World Health Organization, 2021). *L. infantum* and *L. braziliensis* are the most important canine zoonoses of the 20 *Leishmania* protozoan species that have been described to infect humans (Baneth *et al.*, 2016; Akhoundi *et al.*, 2016). Horizontal transmission via sandflies as biological vectors and, to a much lesser extent, ticks and fleas as mechanical vectors has shown to be the most common form of transmission. There have also been several reports of vertical transmission in dogs, particularly seen in North American foxhounds (da Silva *et al.*, 2009; Boggiatto *et al.*, 2011). Risk factors for human infection include malnutrition, migration of immune-naïve persons into endemic areas, and widespread deforestation (World Health Organization, 2022). Depending on the host and infecting protozoan species, the host immune response to the infection can eliminate the parasite or exacerbate the disease, especially in the case of co-infection (Rossi and Fasel, 2018).

The strength of infection depends on the genetic background of the host, their age, nutritional status, immunological status, and several other factors (Maia and Campino, 2018). Canine infections are usually asymptomatic. The most common clinical signs seen in infected dogs are atrophic myositis of the masticatory muscles, cutaneous alterations, lymphadenomegaly, onychogryphosis, and lesions due to immune-complex depositions, such as glomerulonephritis and uveitis (Maia and Campino, 2018).

There are four clinical presentations of human leishmaniasis-visceral, cutaneous, diffuse cutaneous, and mucocutaneous. Cutaneous leishmaniasis is the most common form of the disease (Alvar *et al.*, 2012). It can present as a single open sore to disseminated nodules, ulcers, or other skin lesions which may leave life-long scars accompanied by disability or stigma (World Health Organization, 2022). Diffuse cutaneous leishmaniasis is a disseminated version of cutaneous leishmaniasis that was first reported in Kenya in 1969 (Akhoundi *et al.*, 2016). Over 90% of mucocutaneous cases occur in Bolivia, Brazil, Ethiopia, and Peru (World Health Organization, 2022). Lesions mainly occur around the eyes, nose, and mouth. *L. infantum* usually causes visceral leishmaniasis in people, especially in young children or immunosuppressed persons. Visceral leishmaniasis tends to affect the spleen, liver, and bone marrow, and if left untreated is usually fatal (Akhoundi *et al.*, 2016).

Techniques for disease detection in humans and animals include cytology, biopsy or immunohistochemistry, and serological or molecular techniques (Baneth *et al.*, 2016; Duthie *et al.*, 2018; Silveria *et al.*, 2018). Surveillance in dogs and early detection of infection plays an important role in preventing the zoonotic spread of the infection (Maia and Campino, 2018). Vector control including repellant sprays, insecticide-treated nets, long-sleeved clothing, and environmental management all help to interrupt transmission cycles and reduce sandfly populations. Improved domestic sanitary conditions and housing repairs may reduce sandfly breeding and resting sites. A decline in canine cases showed a concomitant reduction in the incidence of human disease when flea collars impregnated with deltamethrin were used in dogs in Brazil (Yimam and Mohebali, 2020). While practiced in several countries, there is no scientific evidence that culling dogs to control *L. infantum* is effective and is therefore not recommended (Dantas-Torres *et al.*, 2019). Several canine *Leishmania* vaccine candidates are in development and in the interim, vector control and improved housing remain a mainstay of control of *Leishmania*.

Trypanosoma cruzi (Trematoda)

Chagas disease is endemic to the southern USA and 21 continental Latin American countries and is restricted in its distribution to the occurrence of its vectors. It is caused by the protozoan *Trypanosoma cruzi*, which is most often transmitted by triatomine species. A total of 6–7 million people were infected with *T. cruzi* in 2019 and approximately 10,000 of those infected in 2017 died from Chagas disease, which has been targeted by WHO for elimination by 2030 (World Health Organization, 2021). In many endemic countries where low socio-economic conditions occur, dogs may play a major role in *T. cruzi* transmission as they have a higher level of infectiousness to triatomines than humans (Travi, 2019). In such areas, humans maintaining dogs are more likely to be infected than households without dogs (Santos *et al.*, 2022; Travi, 2019). Thus, in such areas, dogs are important reservoir hosts for human infection and can be used as sentinel animals for local transmission in endemic regions of Central and South America (Bern *et al.*, 2011). Infection rates increase with vector stage and age as both male and female triatomines take blood meals to develop through their nymphal stages to adults. Adult females need an additional blood meal to lay eggs (Bern *et al.*, 2011). Triatomines shelter in cracks found in poor-quality housing and often feed nocturnally for up to 30 min when their hosts are sleeping. The engorgement of the stomach compresses the intestine and bugs tend to defecate during or immediately after completing a full blood meal. More rarely, iatrogenic transmission occurs through blood transfusions or organ transplants, and vertically via transplacental and lactogenic means (Grinnage-Pulley *et al.*, 2016). Occasional contamination whilst preparing meat from wild reservoir hosts has resulted in transmission (Pan-American Health Organisation, 2020).

Arrhythmias, dilated cardiomyopathy, cardiomegaly, hydropericardium, and focal, diffuse myocarditis are often seen in dogs (Barbabosa-Pliego *et al.*, 2009; Meyers *et al.*, 2020). In humans, inoculation via the conjunctiva leads to the characteristic unilateral swelling of the upper and lower eyelids known as the Romana sign or chagoma (Bern *et al.*, 2011). Persons with Chagas disease are often asymptomatic or have mild, nonspecific symptoms such as fever, myalgia, asthenia, abdominal pain, retro-orbital pain, and headaches during the acute phase of the disease (de Barros Moreira Beltrão *et al.*, 2009). The severe acute disease can present with myocarditis, pericardial effusion, and/or meningoencephalitis. This is uncommon and has increased mortality. Congenitally infected infants are usually asymptomatic but can develop clinical diseases characterized by hepatosplenomegaly, meningoencephalitis, pneumonitis, myocarditis, and anemia (Torrico *et al.*, 2004; Bern *et al.*, 2009; Howard *et al.*, 2014). Chronic disease syndromes include clinical symptoms associated with megaesophagus, megacolon, and apical aneurisms.

Motile trypomastigotes can be seen by microscopy in fresh blood or buffy coat smears during the acute phase of infection, which lasts about 4–8 weeks after the 1–2 week incubation period (Pérez-Molina and Molina, 2018). The level of parasitemia decreases within 90 days of infection and becomes undetectable by microscopy in the chronic phase. Serology is better suited for diagnosing chronic infections and can be paired with PCR when results are inconclusive (Pérez-Molina and Molina, 2018). PCR is a sensitive diagnostic tool in the acute phase and congenital infection of Chagas disease (Pérez-Molina and Molina, 2018). Other, similar tests can diagnose congenital infections, such as a newly developed IgM test (Castro-Sesquen *et al.*, 2021).

The estimated global prevalence of *T. cruzi* infection has fallen from 18 million cases in 1991 to 6–7 million in 2018 due to intensive vector control and blood bank screening (Disease WHOECotCoC, WHO, 1991; World Health Organization, 2018). Because of these control methods, transplacental transmission in humans has begun to contribute to a greater percentage of cases, as other routes of infection diminish (Bern *et al.*, 2009). A new disintegrated formulation of nifurtimox has facilitated the treatment of children since 2020: an important advancement in the prevention of the development of chronic disease (World Health Organization, 2021). A prevalence of 7.3% and 9.2% of dogs within vs outside of the established triatomine geographic range respectively, were recently found to be positive in the Southern USA, indicating an increased risk to humans and dogs (World Health Organization, 2018).

Anthropogenic deforestation and cultivation of Attalea palms, which are favored by some triatomine species in Amazonia, indicate that such areas may increase vector populations, further complicating control (Santos *et al.*, 2021). Screening, air conditioning, roofing materials, and walls not conducive to triatomine dwelling all decrease infestation and lower transmission.

Without a vaccine or specific treatment available for large-scale public health interventions, the main control strategy relies on the prevention of transmission (Pérez-Molina and Molina, 2018). The use of insecticides, insecticide-treated bed nets, improvements in housing to prevent infestation, public education, and communication on vector-borne diseases have been effective. Good hygiene practices in food preparation and serological screening of blood and organ donors are also important control measures (Pan-American Health Organisation, 2020).

Trypanosoma brucei subsp. *rhodesiense* and *gambiense* (Protista)

Human African Trypanosomiasis (HAT) or sleeping sickness is found across 37 sub-Saharan African countries, with *T. b. gambiense* found in West and Central Africa and *T. b. rhodesiense* found in East Africa (Vourchakbé *et al.*, 2020). This NTD is targeted for elimination by 2030 by the WHO through the implementation of screening, treatment, and vector control

(World Health Organization, 2021). HAT has been eliminated from Togo and Cote d'Ivoire and three other countries are under review by the WHO (Franco *et al.*, 2022). By 2021, more than 120,000 km^2 had been freed from trypanosome transmission (Franco *et al.*, 2022). Substantial progress has been made in many areas and today, greater than 80% of cases of *T. b. gambiense* are found in the Democratic Republic of Congo (World Health Organization, 2021). In West Africa, cases of *T. b. gambiense* have witnessed a 98% drop in the last 20 years, down to 565 cases in 2020 (World Health Organization, 2021). *T. b. rhodesiense* and *T. b. gambiense* are transmitted by tsetse flies, causing both human and canine African trypanosomiasis (Coleman and Welburn, 2004; Samdi *et al.*, 2008). Dogs are not considered reservoir hosts but can be used as sentinels for human infection (Umeakuana *et al.*, 2019).

Canine African trypanosomiasis often presents with corneal opacity and cachexia (Umeakuana *et al.*, 2019) and occasionally with hepatosplenomegaly, severe anemia, ascites, and collapse (Gow *et al.*, 2007).

HAT has two stages: the first is limited to the hemolymphatic system and the second involves invasion of the CNS. Without medical intervention, *T brucei* spp. will eventually cause coma and death. With *T. b. rhodesiense*, a tender, erythematous and edematous lesion called a 'chancre' is seen at the bite site in about 20% of persons infected (Malvy and Chappuis, 2011). PCR is a sensitive diagnostic tool for both species (Gibson, 2002).

Advances in control before 2020 encouraged the World Health Assembly to endorse a new road map for NTDs for 2021–2030, including HAT (Franco *et al.*, 2022). Case detection and treatment alongside tsetse fly control programs have reduced the number of reported cases over the last two decades (Büscher *et al.*, 2017). Many vector control methods have been utilized, including sterile insect technique, aerial spraying of insecticides, and use of insecticide application on cattle or wearing of deltamethrin-impregnated collars, but the most environmentally friendly technique is the use of locally made tsetse fly traps (Malele *et al.*, 2016). Traps can be locally made using local materials and no imported chemicals, but sustainability, when tsetse fly levels fall, has been a perpetual issue and tsetse populations often return after a few years to pre-control levels. Improvements to health facilities and ability to diagnose HAT have facilitated mass screening and treatment programs in many countries, helping to reduce HAT as a public health problem.

Clonorchis sinensis (Trematoda)

C. sinensis is one of the major parasitic foodborne zoonoses of East Asia and is classified as a human carcinogen (Lin *et al.*, 2011; Xu *et al.*, 2021). Along with other foodborne trematode zoonoses described below, they contribute to greater than 0.5×10^6 Daily Adjusted Life Years (DALYs) (Torgerson and Macpherson, 2011). This foodborne trematode is known to cause pathologies within the liver and bile ducts and is mainly transmitted through eating raw fish contaminated with *C. sinensis* metacercariae (Xu *et al.*, 2021). Embryonated *C. sinensis* eggs are passed in the feces of the definitive host (DH) (such as humans, dogs, pigs, and rodents), ingested by a snail intermediate host (IH) from which cercariae are released and encyst into the skin or flesh of freshwater fish as metacercariae, which are then ingested by the DH, excyst in the duodenum and ascend the biliary tract to mature. Hermaphrodite adult flukes then reproduce sexually. The practices of eating infected raw fish and building latrines over or near bodies of water where fish farming is practiced contribute to the maintenance of the parasite's life cycle (Lin et al., 2005; Tang *et al.*, 2016). Increasing population growth and the commensurate need to increase aquaculture have not seen an appropriate increase in environmental control and this parasite continues to flourish (Keiser and Utzinger, 2005). In 2016 and 2017, 405 (20.49%) out of 1997 human fecal samples from Binyang County in southern China were found to be positive for *C. sinensis* (Xu *et al.*, 2021). Seven prevalence studies of *C. sinensis* in dogs in southern China were performed from the years 1978 to 2011, with a combined prevalence in 2339 dogs of 26.4% (range: 0.8–56.4%) (Xu *et al.*, 2021). Another study found 16 (50%) out of 32 dogs in Guangxi Zhuang Autonomous Region to be infected with *C. sinensis* and 35 (40%) out of 88 fish examined were positive for metacercariae (Torgerson and Macpherson, 2011).

The literature on how *C. sinensis* infections affect dogs is limited. Adult flukes in heavy infections can cause extensive damage to the liver and other organs, leading to weight loss, icterus, and ascites (Ye *et al.*, 2013).

Adult flukes can inhabit the bile ducts for 20–25 years and persons are often asymptomatic during the early stages of infection (Torgerson and Macpherson, 2011). The most characteristic pathologies of clonorchiasis in humans are chronic inflammation and the buildup of calculi in the intrahepatic biliary passages (Rim, 2005), which can lead to cholecystolithiasis (Qiao *et al.*, 2012). Infection is also associated with cholangiocarcinoma, a primary cancer of the epithelial cells lining the biliary tree (Shin *et al.*, 2010).

Microscopic examination of fecal samples is considered the most sensitive and reliable method of screening for liver and intestinal flukes, despite egg morphologies being almost identical (Sithithaworn *et al.*, 2007). Species differentiation requires morphological identification of adult flukes or the use of molecular techniques such as PCR. Control of *C. sinensis* requires major changes to infrastructure, including the proper building of latrines and farm animal pens, public education on farming, fishing practices, proper cooking of fish, and mass treatment of infected people and other definitive animal hosts with praziquantel.

Opisthorchis viverrini (Trematoda)

Opisthorchis viverrini is endemic to Southeast Asia and estimated to infect around 10 million people (Furst *et al.*, 2012). As with *C. sinensis*, *O. viverrini* is classified as a human carcinogen and has been documented to cause cholangiocarcinoma (Petney *et al.*, 2013). Dogs act as reservoir hosts for *O. viverrini* (Hughes *et al.*, 2017). The life cycle is similar to that of *C. sinensis*, except *O. viverrini* has less snail IH species that have been documented (Sithithaworn *et al.*, 2007). Environmental alterations made for growing rice fields create new habitats for the snail and fish IHs and introduce higher human and domestic animal population densities (Sithithaworn *et al.*, 2007). Clinical features in dogs are unknown. Humans are usually asymptomatic but chronic, persistent infections and inflammation may assist in the development of cholangiocarcinoma (Khuntikeo *et al.*, 2018).

The coprological technique to find eggs in feces is the gold standard diagnosis but is not very sensitive to light infections. Worasith *et al.*, (2015) developed a urine antigen test for detecting *O. viverrini*, with a sensitivity and specificity of 81% and 70%, respectively. This test may be helpful in finding infections early and preventing the development of cholangiocarcinoma. Control is as for *C. sinensis*.

Paragonimus spp. (Trematoda)

Paragonimiasis is a global foodborne zoonosis, with different species having variable geographic distributions. Approximately one million people are infected annually by *Paragonimus* spp. (Yoshida *et al.*, 2019). *P. westermani* is distributed throughout the tropics and *Paragonimus kellicotti* is restricted to North America. Humans and dogs, especially those that hunt (Kirino *et al.*, 2009; Yoshida *et al.*, 2019), become infected by ingesting raw or undercooked freshwater crustacean IHs or raw meat of wild animal paratenic hosts (PHs). Once ingested, *Paragonimus* spp. metacercariae from secondary IHs or juvenile flukes from PHs penetrate the duodenum and travel to the thoracic pleura and lungs, where they mature into hermaphroditic pairs. Adults can self-fertilize or cross-fertilize. Unembryonated eggs are then released into bronchioles, are coughed up, swallowed, and later excreted in feces (Diaz, 2013). *Paragonimus* spp. flukes are less often found in visceral organs, the abdominal wall, mesentery, and the brain (Diaz, 2013).

Dogs may show signs associated with lung pathologies due to the nodular lesions within the lung parenchyma. Even with nodules seen on diagnostic imaging, dogs are often asymptomatic (Khuntikeo *et al.*, 2018).

Human paragonimiasis has an insidious onset, with persons presenting with a productive cough, hemoptysis, chest pain, and dyspnea (Ahn *et al.*, 2021). Occasionally, extrapulmonary paragonimiasis can occur when juvenile flukes or metacercariae invade other tissues such as the brain or cutaneous tissue (Worasith *et al.*, 2015).

Diagnosis in both humans and dogs is usually based on a thorough clinical history and presentation, detection of *Paragonimus* spp. eggs in sputum or feces, and appreciating parenchymal infiltrates on thoracic imaging (Kirino *et al.*, 2009; Yoshida *et al.*, 2019).

Hunting dogs prove to be the most important canine source of human infection, as they are often fed raw infected meat and are asymptomatic despite the development of nodular lung lesions. Regular deworming of hunting dogs and the cessation of feeding raw meat to dogs may reduce human transmission. IH crustaceans and PHs such as boar should be thoroughly cooked before human or dog consumption.

Echinococcus granulosis and *E. multilocularis* (Cestoda)

Echinococcosis occurs most frequently in rural, pastoralist regions, and communities (Gong *et al.*, 2021; Macpherson, 2005). Cystic and alveolar echinococcus are endemic in at least 111 countries and there were approximately 19,000 deaths in 2016 (World Health Organization, 2021). Cystic echinococcosis occurs worldwide. While alveolar echinococcus has only been found in the northern hemisphere, its geographical distribution is reported to be expanding southward in Europe (Lalošević *et al.*, 2016; Beck *et al.*, 2018; Massolo *et al.*, 2018). Dogs are often kept in these communities for security and herding and are the main source of human infection. Adult *Echinococcus* spp. inhabit the small intestine of the canine DH and release embryonated eggs in feces. Ungulates and small mammals such as rodents are typically the IHs for *E. granulosus* (e.g.) and *E. multilocularis* (EM), respectively (Romig *et al.*, 2015). Humans that ingest eggs become aberrant IHs. Within an IH, hooked larval oncosphere stages are released from the ingested egg in the intestine. These oncospheres penetrate the small intestinal wall and are carried passively via the mesenteric vein to the liver and over time, develop into thick-walled hydatid cysts causing Cystic Hydatid Disease (CHD) or alveolar hydatid cysts, causing Alveolar Hydatid Disease (AHD). CHD can occur in any structure or organ in the body. These larval stages develop slowly, and fertile cysts contain protoscolices. In CHD, if a cyst ruptures or if protoscolices are released during surgical intervention, they can develop into secondary hydatid disease. Dogs and other carnivore species become infected when they ingest larval stages containing viable protoscolices from IHs.

Dogs that are free roaming, used for hunting, and either scavenge or are purposefully fed condemned tissues from livestock abattoirs and home slaughter (CHD) or catch wild rodents (AHD) are important proponents in the continuation of the parasite's life cycle (Macpherson, 2005; Oba *et al.*, 2016; Toews *et al.*, 2021). A recent meta-analysis found 91% of herdsmen in China fed sheep offal to dogs, 65% of sheep have close contact with dogs, and 47% of owned dogs may interact with stray dogs (Diaz, 2013). As echinococcosis is generally lifelong in untreated animals, the most consistent risk factor for infection and cyst burden in IHs is age (Craig *et al.*, 2015). This can be particularly important in human echinococcosis infections in Buddhist communities, which believe that animals should die a natural death and the carcass be left for scavengers (Yang *et al.*, 2009). Weng *et al.* (2020) report on positive changes to dog population management, deworming, and feeding in Tibetan regions since increasing prevention awareness of echinococcosis in 2015. Infection rates in dogs were found to be similar in both agricultural and urban areas in China (Diaz, 2013). It is therefore worth focusing future studies on dogs in urban areas as they act as sentinels and environmental contaminators of *Echinococcus* spp. and zoonotic diseases tend to expand and transform in areas of development and urbanization (Liccioli *et al.*, 2015; Toews *et al.*, 2021).

In most instances, dogs are asymptomatic. Intermittent vomiting and diarrhea have been reported (Kuroki *et al.*, 2020). Echinococcosis in humans has highly variable presentations, ranging from asymptomatic to fatal infections, and a range of symptoms, which in CHD are organ dependent. Complications are often due to mass effect/compression of vessels or ducts, or through cyst rupture, causing secondary echinococcosis at new sites within the body (CHD) (Brunetti *et al.*, 2018).

Ultrasound is the most appropriate diagnostic for imaging potentially infected persons, due to its high resolution, staging and differential diagnoses, availability, repeatability, and lack of radiation (Liccioli *et al.*, 2015). Other imaging techniques such as MRI, CT, and X-Ray also play an important role in diagnosis, mostly in hospital settings. Diagnosis in ungulate IHs usually occurs during slaughter or necropsy (Craig *et al.*, 2015). Necropsy diagnosis in dogs is 100% specific if in a non-endemic region for *E. multilocularis* but should otherwise be morphologically identified by looking at the overall size of the worm and the position of the proglottid lateral pore (above mid-line in *E. multilocularis*, below mid-line in *E. granulosus* (Craig *et al.*, 2015)). Pre-mortem diagnosis of canine echinococcosis has historically been achieved with purgation using arecoline, which requires trained personnel, owner compliance, biohazard containment, a long processing time, and carries the risk of toxicity to dogs (Craig *et al.*, 2015). Coproantigen ELISA is useful in diagnosing infected animals with heavy worm burdens (Öge *et al.*, 2017). Fecal flotation is considerably less sensitive as egg shedding is intermittent and *Echinococcus* spp. eggs are indistinguishable from each other and *Taenia* spp. (Öge *et al.*, 2017).

Public health education and alterations to human behavior are paramount to reducing transmission. Halting the practice of feeding cysts to dogs, whether purposeful or not, would eliminate the life cycle of CHD. Unfortunately, this is often not practical due to a lack of alternative food options for dogs. Stricter biosecurity within abattoirs would limit dogs' access to condemned tissue. Regular mass treatment of dogs with praziquantel would quell environmental contamination for both CHD and AHD. Prophylactic treatment programs for owned pets and picking up after dogs are also recommended. Canine coproprevalence of *Echinococcus* spp. has been shown to drop significantly (29.8%) in areas where prevention programs have been implemented (Weng *et al.*, 2020). Vaccines with proteins against *E. granulosus* may be used in the future to prevent the maturation of worms in the dog (Zhang *et al.*, 2018). Improved animal welfare, particularly for stray dogs, may also help to reduce canine echinococcosis. Additional recommendations include improving hygiene practices and accessibility to clean drinking water.

Taenia multiceps (Cestoda)

Cerebral coenurosis, also known as 'gid' in livestock, is an often-fatal disease of the nervous system of ungulates, caused by the canine cestode *Taenia multiceps*. This can lead to serious economic losses and be particularly harmful in pastoralist or transhumant communities that rely heavily on their livestock for food, transport, income, and status. Human infection rates vary significantly between rural and urban areas, and approximately 100 human cases of coenurosis have been reported worldwide (Varcasia *et al.*, 2022). A recent cross-sectional survey in pastoral communities of northern Tanzania found 79.8% of households fed sheep or goat brains to dogs, including 61.3% of households that did not own dogs (Hughes *et al.*, 2019).

Eggs and gravid proglottids shed in the canid DHs' feces are immediately infective in the environment. The ungulate IH ingests the eggs on pasture, which then hatch in the intestine and release oncospheres that circulate through the blood and attach to different organs, particularly skeletal muscle, eyes, brain, and subcutaneous tissue. Over a few months, oncospheres develop into coenuri-containing protoscolices which are released into the DH after it consumes infected IH tissue. Protoscolices then attach to the DH's small intestinal wall and develop into adult cestodes.

Dogs are usually asymptomatic. Human coenurosis is uncommon. *T. multiceps* has been implicated in the cause of approximately 30 reported cases of human CNS coenurosis (Lescano and Zunt, 2013), of which five cases have been reported since 2000 (Deplazes *et al.*, 2019). Traditionally *T. multiceps* in dogs has been diagnosed similarly to *Echinococcus* spp., through arecoline purgation and necropsy. Direct and multiplex PCRs have been developed to detect *T. multiceps* eggs in dog feces more safely and effectively (Wang *et al.*, 2018; Zhu *et al.*, 2019).

The main control methods available are the anthelmintic treatment of dogs and appropriate disposal of ruminant brains. Public education on how feeding cyst-containing organs to dogs can perpetuate the parasite's life cycle and cause deaths in small ruminant herds should help begin to change the behavior of feeding cysts to dogs.

Dracunculus medinensis (Nematoda)

Historically, *Dracunculus medinensis* affected tens of millions of individuals, mostly in arid areas, but with the introduction of the safe drinking water decade in 1981 and the global eradication initiative spearheaded by the Carter Foundation, human infections today have fallen to 27 cases in 2020 (World Health Organization, 2021). A global eradication program was focused entirely on preventing human infection and little focus was placed on controlling the disease in dogs. Chad was an endemic region for *D. medinensis* for decades before a 10 year absence of cases, followed by a rediscovery of human cases in 2010 and the first canine cases being recorded in 2012 (Guagliardo *et al.*, 2020). A total of 3371 infected dogs were recorded in Chad between 2015 and 2018, of which 74% lived in fishing villages (Guagliardo *et al.*, 2020), and 1600 canine cases were recorded globally in 2020 (World Health Organization, 2021), demonstrating that dogs are important reservoir hosts for human infection. The infection in dogs will greatly hamper the declaration of eradication of the first helminth parasite to be eradicated. Five endemic countries (Angola, Chad, Ethiopia, Mali, and South Sudan) and Democratic Republic of Congo and Sudan, which are no longer reporting cases, remain to be certified for the elimination of Guinea worm (World Health Organization, 2021).

Infection occurs when people and dogs drink water contaminated with *D. medinensis* larvae in the copepod IH. From here the larvae mature and mate in the intestine, with the females surviving mating and slowly migrating to the subcutaneous tissues. After a year of infection, the female worm burrows through the host's skin, particularly around the legs and feet, which is debilitatingly painful. It is thought that this timeframe is similar in dogs (Guagliardo *et al.*, 2020). The pain is dissipated when the affected limb is submerged in water, which allows the parasite to complete its lifecycle in fresh water. In one study, the risk of infection in dogs increased with the consumption of fish, which may act as PHs, and decreased with the provision of water to dogs (McDonald *et al.*, 2020).

In both dogs and humans, a painful, vesicular-like lesion forms where the female worm begins to emerge, usually on the leg or foot (Guagliardo *et al.*, 2020). This is pathognomonic.

Prevention and control of this parasite initially relied on chemical treatment of water, killing the IH, and more recently on the provision of filters, which simply filtered out the copepod IH. Eradication in humans was close to realization in 2018 but the occurrence in larger numbers of dogs has complicated eradication efforts.

Toxocara canis (Nematoda)

Toxocariasis is one of the most widespread and economically important parasitic zoonoses that humans share with dogs. *Toxocara* spp. are intestinal ascarid nematodes that infect humans through ingestion of eggs from contaminated produce, soil, undercooked meat from PHs or directly from pets (Rostami *et al.*, 2020). Over 100 million dogs are likely to be infected with *T. canis*, shedding billions of eggs into the environment annually (Rostami *et al.*, 2020). *T. canis* is one of the very few parasites to be transmitted vertically, with 50% of puppies by 2 weeks of age being infected by *in-utero* transmission (Schwartz *et al.*, 2022). The prepatent period (PPP) varies with different modes of transmission. The PPP has been recorded to be approximately 16 days *in-utero* (Lloyd *et al.*, 1983), 28 days lactogenically (Stoye, 1976), 32–35 days after ingestion of embryonated eggs (Dubey, 1978), and 34–48 days after ingestion of a PH (Manhardt and Stoye, 1981).

Heavy prenatal infections can cause severe abdominal discomfort in nursing puppies which often adopt a straddle-legged posture or pot-belly appearance when standing. Death may result from rupture or obstruction of worms within the intestine.

Most human infections are asymptomatic (Rostami *et al.*, 2019) and there are four main syndromes. The most common syndrome is visceral larva migrans, with signs of coughing, wheezing, myalgia, and cutaneous manifestations (Ma *et al.*, 2018). Ocular larva migrans are common and mostly reported in children (Stoye, 1976). Neurotoxocariasis is rare and mainly occurs in middle-aged persons when *T. canis* larvae migrate into the CNS (Dubey, 1978). Covert/common toxocariasis has nonspecific symptoms and can be difficult to diagnose (Dubey, 1978).

Diagnosis of human toxocariasis can be performed using blood tests, histopathology, PCR, or serology (Rostami *et al.*, 2019). *T. canis* can be diagnosed in dogs on fecal flotation, PCR on feces, or an ELISA IgG antibody test (Fahrion *et al.*, 2008). Early detection of worms in puppies infected by vertical transmission is possible using abdominal ultrasound (Corda *et al.*, 2019).

It is estimated that the pooled global seroprevalence of *T. canis* in healthy populations according to WHO-epidemiological regions is 19 percent (Rostami *et al.*, 2019). A significant risk factor for seropositivity is the contamination of public places (Rostami *et al.*, 2019). As vertical transmission is a major contributor to the transmission of *T. canis* between dogs, a vertical transmission prevention program is recommended. *T. canis* larvae have been documented to begin circulating in pregnant bitches at day 42 of gestation (Overgaauw *et al.*, 1998). Treating pregnant bitches at this stage of gestation should lessen vertical transmission. An important control method is to pick up after dogs to reduce the number of *Toxocara* eggs present in the environment. Prevention is potentially best through treating the bitch before parturition to prevent vertical transmission to her offspring, as puppies are the main shedders.

Ancylostoma spp. (Nematoda)

Ancylostoma caninum, *A. ceylanicum*, *A. braziliense*, and *Uncinaria stenocephala* are the four zoonotic hookworm species of dogs. Each of these species differs in zoonotic potential, human and canine clinical presentations, means of transmission, and geographical distribution. The eggs of all hookworm species are identical, except for *U. stenocephala* eggs which are morphologically distinct, thus in the absence of necropsy to study the morphology of the adult worms, molecular differentiation of species is required. A few molecular studies have been conducted around the world, the geographical distribution of these parasites is not fully defined, ranges may overlap, and hosts may be co-infected with several species at a time. *A. caninum* has been recorded throughout the tropics, *U. stenocephala* is usually in colder climates, *A. ceylanicum* in Africa, Asia, and Oceania, and *A. brazilense* has been recorded along the southern USA down to Uruguay, and in parts of Africa, Australia, and Asia (Bowman *et al.*, 2010).

Hookworms have a direct life cycle, whereby unembryonated eggs are passed in canine DH feces. L_1 larvae develop inside the egg before hatching into the environment, where the L_1 molts to the L_2 and subsequently the infective L_3 stage. Eggs mature ideally between 15°C and 35°C (Smith and Schad, 1989). The four zoonotic canine species can all cause infection through skin penetration by the L_3 larvae and to a lesser extent, through ingestion of larvae in contaminated soil, food, or water. *A. ceylanicum* can develop patent, chronic infections in humans and is the second most common human hookworm in South-East Asia and the Pacific (Bradbury *et al.*, 2017), comprising between 6% and 23% of total patent hookworm infections in people living in endemic areas (Bradbury *et al.*, 2017). *A. caninum* eggs were recently found in feces from an infected person in South Africa, suggesting that *A. caninum* may be able to reach patency in humans (Ngcamphalala *et al.*, 2020). *A. caninum* often undergoes somatic migration in the dog, leading to the sequestration of larvae in the tissues which can be reactivated during pregnancy, with transmammary transmission and, to a less extent, transplacental transmission, providing an important means of dog-to-dog transmission and subsequently, environmental contamination (Stone and Girardeau, 1968). All four species of hookworm can cause Cutaneous Larva Migrans (CLM) (Bowman *et al.*, 2010) and *A. caninum* and *A. ceylanicum* can also cause intestinal symptoms in humans. In dogs, these hookworms, particularly *A. caninum* and *A. ceylanicum*, are a common cause of hemorrhagic diarrhea and death in puppies and chronic iron deficiency anemia in adults (Massetti *et al.*, 2020).

As the DH of these hookworm species, dogs develop pathologies associated with the parasite's blood-sucking nature. This can include iron-deficiency anemia, hypoalbuminemia and enteritis, characterized by a hemorrhagic diarrhea (Jimenez Castro *et al.*, 2019). The blood loss can be particularly severe in puppies, which can die from the anemia (Massetti *et al.*, 2020). *U. stenocephala* has been known to cause pruritic dermatitis (Chu *et al.*, 2013).

CLM is a self-limiting infection where the L_3 larvae circulate through and are limited to the cutaneous tissues. It is usually limited to the lower extremities which have increased contact with the ground. The most common hookworm to cause CLM is *A. braziliense*, which presents with highly pruritic classical creeping eruptions (Dove, 1932; Ngui *et al.*, 2012), whereas *A. caninum* causes follicular dermatitis. *A. ceylanicum*, and rarely *A. caninum*, have been known to reach patency in humans (Dove, 1932). *A caninum* is also known to cause eosinophilic enteritis and aphthous ileitis (Massetti *et al.*, 2020).

Micrometry is a useful tool in hookworm differentiation (Lucio-Forster *et al.*, 2012). In laboratories where molecular techniques are available, RT-qPCR has become the method of choice (Massetti *et al.*, 2020). Hookworm larvae have also been detected on skin scrapings or biopsies from dogs (Chu *et al.*, 2013).

Hookworms are one of the few parasites that can be vertically transmitted. A vertical transmission prevention program would likely reduce hookworm transmission in dogs and lead to significantly less environmental contamination. To further limit environmental contamination, dog owners should pick up after their dogs and it is recommended to deworm dogs at regular intervals as reinfection is common in endemic areas. Persons can wear protective clothing and footwear when spending prolonged periods in shady parts of beaches or sandboxes to prevent exposure.

Strongyloides stercoralis (Nematoda)

Strongyloides stercoralis is a soil-transmitted helminth found in tropical and subtropical regions. It is thought to infect more than 600 million people globally (Streit, 2021). Conditions for transmission are typically met where people share premises with DHs such as dogs and have substandard water and sanitation infrastructures (Jaleta *et al.*, 2017). Infective filariform or L_3 larvae penetrate the host's skin and migrate through the blood and lungs, where they are coughed up and swallowed. The larvae then develop into adult females in the small intestine, which reproduces by parthenogenesis. Progeny develops into L_1 larvae and can either progress to L_3 and autoinfect the host, female L_1 larvae can pass out of the host and develop to L_3 in the environment where they either find a new host or become free living, or the L_1 larvae can develop into males and pass out of the host to be free living in the environment (Jaleta *et al.*, 2017). Free-living adults can reproduce sexually and all progeny are females and develop into infective L_3s (Jaleta *et al.*, 2017).

Dogs are usually asymptomatic (Thamsborg *et al.*, 2017) but can occasionally present with diarrhea, vomiting, lethargy, anorexia, and a tense abdomen (Schnyder *et al.*, 2022). Human infections are often chronic and asymptomatic due to the autoinfective lifecycle this parasite sometimes undergoes (Nutman, 2017). Complicated cases can develop and potentially be deadly if not treated in a timely manner (Streit, 2021). Infection can result in various dermatological presentations, particularly larva currens, which is a creeping urticarial eruption. Pulmonary presentations have also been documented (Dogan *et al.*, 2014).

Female worms are not very fecund, producing only a few larvae per day, and therefore examining direct stool samples or using flotation and centrifugation rarely reveals active infections. To counter this, the Baermann technique, which is used to detect larvae in feces, is traditionally the diagnostic method of choice, relying on the environmental reproductive capacity of this parasite. Serology and molecular techniques are improving and are increasingly being used for diagnosis.

As with other STHs, *S. stercoralis* infections can be reduced with improved hygiene practices. This can be promoted through public health education on hand washing and teaching children not to put soil or potentially contaminated objects in their mouths.

Category 2: Human:Dog Zoonoses of Lesser Public Health Importance, but Where Human and Dog Are Important for Transmission

Microsporum spp. (Fungus)

Microsporum spp. are dermatophyte fungi, with *M. canis* being the most commonly isolated fungus from dogs (Dogan *et al.*, 2014). *Microsporum* spp. is spread through direct contact, infected hair or scale in the environment or through fomites (Foil, 1998). The fungi invade the stratum corneum of the epidermis and the keratinized tissues derived from it, such as hair, skin, and nails, causing an infection known as dermatophytosis or ringworm (Pasquetti *et al.*, 2017). Children aged 6 months to 10–12 years of age are most often infected (Hay, 2017). Most canine cases are caused by *M. canis, Trichophyton mentagrophytes, M. gypseum*, and extremely rarely, *T. tonsurans* (Mattei *et al.*, 2014). *M. gypseum* is a soil pathogen often seen in dogs that stick their noses down holes or dig in the dirt.

In dogs and humans, dermatophytosis classically presents as circular patches of alopecia and scale, with follicular papules, crusts, and epidermal collarettes. Deep masses called kerions, usually caused by *T. mentagraphytes*, may be seen in severe cases. Humans also get tinea capitis, with *M. canis* infections presenting more pruritic and inflamed than other *Microsporum* spp. (Hay, 2017).

Clinical signs are pathognomonic. Definitive diagnosis and speciation of the causative organism require molecular identification or culture. Histology can aid species identification as kerion or granulomatous ringworm are often negative on culture (Foil, 1998). In dogs, Wood's lamp can be used as a screening tool. Most *M. canis* subspecies will fluoresce bright green but *M. gypseum* and *T. mentagrophytes* do not (Foil, 1998). Hairs that fluoresce can then be plucked for trichogram and culture.

In Europe and the USA, tinea capitis was once considered a disease of poverty resulting in isolation and radiation therapy promotion. The development of griseofulvin and the ease of topical application effectively reduced infection rates in developed countries but it is still common in low socio-economic regions of the world (Hay, 2017). Veterinarians, groomers, pet owners, and carers should wear gloves to prevent transmission when dealing with infected animals. Disinfectants such as diluted chlorine bleach can be used to kill fungal spores in the environment.

Bacteria transmitted via dog bites

Dog bite wounds are often polymicrobial and reflective of the broad range of commensal bacteria found in the canine oral cavity. Some species are particularly rare and have limited literature available, such as *Bacteroides* spp., *Porphyromonas* spp., *Pasteurella* spp., *Neisseria* spp., and *Prevotella* spp. In one study, *Pasteurella canis* was the most common bacterial isolate of dog bites in humans (Talan *et al.*, 1999).

Capnocytophaga canimorsus is found in the saliva and tooth plaque of approximately 21.7% of healthy dogs and cats (Dilegge *et al.*, 2011), and is predominantly transmitted to humans through dog bites (Dilegge *et al.*, 2011). In most human cases, *C. canimorsus* causes little inflammation at the bite or access site into the body but invades the circulatory system aggressively (Dilegge *et al.*, 2011) and immunocompetent persons often develop sepsis (Mader *et al.*, 2020). One study found a 33 percent case-fatality rate, with most culture-confirmed meningitis cases surviving infection (Janda *et al.*, 2006).

Staphylococcus spp. are commensal bacteria that only cause disease when they enter and colonize a wound or there is a disturbance within the host, such as thyroid dysfunction or a dermatophytosis infection (Cox, 1998). *Staphylococcus pseudintermedius* is the most common *Staphylococcal* spp. isolated from pyoderma, otitis externa, discospondylitis, conjunctivitis, and urolithiasis in dogs (Kmieciak and Szewczyk, 2018). *Staphylococcus* spp. is usually isolated from humans in non-purulent wounds with cellulitis and lymphangitis (Talan *et al.*, 1999). While many healthy households with humans positive and dogs negative for *S. aureus*/MRSA were found in one study, 57 percent of healthy households with dogs and owners who were both positive were infected with the same pulsotype (Van Balen *et al.*, 2017). This is indicative that while infrequent, zoonotic transmission of *S. aureus*/MRSA between dogs and people may occur.

Streptococcus spp. are opportunistic bacteria that rarely infect humans (Galpérine *et al.*, 2007) and are usually seen in immunocompromised individuals. *S. canis* rarely causes human infection (Lederman *et al.*, 2020) but in dogs it is associated with dermatitis, and less often pneumonia or septicemia (Lamm *et al.*, 2010). *Streptococcus equi* subsp. *zooepidemicus* in horses is transmitted to dogs through direct contact and has been the causative agent of several accounts of acute hemorrhagic pneumonia in dogs (Priestnall and Erles, 2011). Human cases of *S. equi* subsp. *zooepidemicus* have been documented to cause significant illnesses such as meningitis, bacteremia, acute nephritis, septic arthritis, pneumonia, and death (Abbott *et al.*, 2010).

Bergeyella zoohelcum (Bacteria) is a rare canine commensal bacterium known to cause cellulitis, abscesses at inoculation sites, tenosynovitis, septicemia, pneumonia, and meningitis in people (Lin et al., 2007; Yi et al., 2016). A recent study found a 13.3 percent frequency of the bacterium in dogs that receive routine dental care compared to 90 percent in an older study without dental care (Muramatsu *et al.*, 2019). The modern habit of seeking routine dental care for dogs may limit zoonotic transmission through bites or licking.

These bacteria are typically diagnosed using culture. It is recommended to start antimicrobial treatment immediately as identification and diagnosis can take a relatively long time (Greene *et al.*, 1998). Many cases are fatal in immunocompromised people, so it is vital that veterinarians and physicians inform clients to seek medical care after an animal bite or scratch injury. Avoidance of behaviors that agitate an animal to become aggressive toward humans is the main form of prevention. This requires proper training and socialization of pet dogs and implementation of educational programs on canine communicable behavior for people with high occupational risk, such as animal control officers and postal employees (Greene *et al.*, 1998).

Salmonella spp. (Bacteria)

Salmonella infections are usually foodborne but can be transmitted through contact with contaminated feces. Raw diets are an important source of canine infection (Cantas and Suer, 2014). Dogs present subclinically or with vomiting, diarrhea, fever, lethargy, and abdominal pain (Reimschuessel *et al.*, 2017), and in humans, salmonellosis can vary from mild nausea and malaise to organ failure and paralysis (Chlebicz and Śliżewska, 2018). Zoonotic transmission is uncommon, and *Salmonella* is more often an indirect zoonosis through dog food. *Salmonella*-contaminated pet food and treats, particularly pig ears, have been implicated in several human infections (Clark *et al.*, 2001; Thomas and Feng, 2020). Thomas and Feng (Greene *et al.*, 1998) found that 78 percent of pet owners were unaware of pet food recalls or outbreaks and that less than 25 percent considered dry pet food as a potential source of foodborne pathogens. Another study isolated *Salmonella* from 20 percent of 35 commercial frozen raw meat-based diets (Van Bree *et al.*, 2018). Based on the available literature, there is a lack of public education on *Salmonella* transmission between dogs and humans, particularly through feeding.

Anaplasma spp. (Bacteria)

Anaplasma spp. are intracellular bacterium transmitted by *Ixodes* ticks and causes human granulocytic anaplasmosis (Elhamiani Khatat *et al.*, 2017). Iatrogenic transmission by blood transfusion can also occur (Sainz *et al.*, 2015). One study found the seroprevalence of *Anaplasma* spp. to be 9.4 percent and 44 percent between humans and dogs, respectively (Acosta-Jamett *et al.*, 2020). Another study performed in Morocco found a 21.9 percent prevalence of *Anaplasma* spp. antibodies among 425 dogs and 7 out of 10 owners enrolled were positive for *Anaplasma phagocytophilum* IgG antibodies

(Elhamiani Khatat *et al.*, 2017). *Anaplasma platys* is known to infect both dogs and humans but has low pathogenicity and its zoonotic potential is minor (Arraga-Alvarado *et al.*, 2014).

General signs of tickborne disease in dogs include fever, anorexia, lethargy, purpura, and lameness without orthopedic origin (Elhamiani Khatat *et al.*, 2017; Hovius *et al.*, 2018). *A. platys* is usually asymptomatic but can cause cyclic thrombocytopenia (Harvey *et al.*, 1978). Human granulocytic anaplasmosis presents as a non-specific flu-like illness about 2–3 weeks post-exposure via tick bite (Hansmann *et al.*, 2019) and can have severe complications.

A combination of PCR and serology is recommended for diagnosing human anaplasmosis (Hansmann *et al.*, 2019). *Anaplasma* spp. can be detected on a direct blood smear, but PCR is needed for species differentiation (Chlebicz and Śliżewska, 2018). An RT-PCR test for *A. phagocytophilum* and babesiosis was recently developed and would be advantageous for diagnosis (Hansmann *et al.*, 2019).

Human seroreactivity has been associated with a lower level of education and a lack of acaracide treatment for household dogs (Acosta-Jamett *et al.*, 2020). It is recommended to wear protective clothing in tick-infested areas and to use ectocide-preventative drugs on dogs when possible.

Ehrlichia spp. (Bacteria)

Ehrlichia chaffeensis is an intracellular bacterium transmitted by the *Ambylomma americanum* or 'Lone Star' tick which is maintained within the white-tailed deer population. It is the causative agent of Human Monocytic Ehrlichiosis (HME), which has been a notifiable disease in the USA since 1998 and can be life-threatening (Budachetri *et al.*, 2020). *A. americanum* has three developmental stages, all of which will feed on any mammal, including humans (Acosta-Jamett *et al.*, 2020). This and the overpopulation of deer in certain regions can lead to increased rates of *E. chaffeensis* transmission. *E. canis* has less zoonotic potential than *E. chaffeensis* but human infections have been reported (Perez *et al.*, 2006). *E. canis* is transmitted by the brown dog tick, *Rhipicephalus sanguineus*. Adult ticks can survive for up to 568 days and transmit infection for at least 155 days (Neer, 1998). One study in Egypt found that 41 percent of 500 dogs were infected with *E. canis*, with outdoor access being a major risk factor (Selim *et al.*, 2021).

E. canis and *E. chaffeensis* are clinically indistinguishable (Mylonakis and Theodorou, 2017). Ehrlichiosis in dogs may present with fever, lethargy, anorexia, stiff gait lameness, petechia, ecchymosis, or changes in eye color or appearance. Meningitis may occur in severe cases due to inflammation and hemorrhage (Neer, 1998). HME often presents as an acute, febrile illness with nausea, abdominal pain, thrombocytopenia, changes in coagulation pathways, and involvement of the liver and nervous system (Alcántara-Rodríguez *et al.*, 2020; Peng *et al.*, 2019).

PCR provides a definitive diagnosis (Franco-Zetina *et al.*, 2019). When interpreting seroprevalence results for tickborne diseases, factors such as testing and screening regularity can shift results depending on frequency, particularly in endemic regions where symptomatic dogs are probably more likely to be tested (Budachetri *et al.*, 2020; Gettings *et al.*, 2020). Tick control is likely the most efficacious control method for tickborne diseases. Prophylactic treatment is recommended for dogs, especially those living in or traveling to an endemic region. A prospective canine vaccine against *E. chaffeensis* is in development Budachetri *et al.* (2020); McGill *et al.* (2016).

Borrelia spp. (Bacteria)

Lyme disease is an emerging infectious disease in many parts of the world and is the most common vector-borne disease in Europe and northern parts of North America (Mead, 2015). *Borrelia burgdorferi* cycles between mammals and birds and is transmitted by *Ixodes* ticks (Mead, 2015), which are found in regions with moderate humidity, deciduous forest, and brushwood (Krupka and Straubinger, 2010). Hosts can be infected through bites from pre-infected nymphal stages, non-infected nymphs feeding near infected ticks, and infected adult ticks (Krupka and Straubinger, 2010).

Most seropositive dogs are asymptomatic (Littman *et al.*, 2018). Migratory arthritis, myalgia, listlessness, and shifting leg lameness are frequent in clinically infected dogs (Krupka and Straubinger, 2010; Magnarelli *et al.*, 1987). Fever, lethargy, and lymphadenopathy may also be seen (Herrin *et al.*, 2017). Renal, dermatologic, neurologic, and cardiac presentations are rare. Lyme disease in humans often involves the skin, joints, nervous system, and heart. The most common presentation is erythema migrans (Wormser *et al.*, 2006) and infections are often chronic.

The gold standard for antibody detection is ELISA followed by Western Blot (Magnarelli *et al.*, 1987). However, diagnosis in low prevalence areas does present problems for the positive predictive value of the test.

It is recommended that in endemic regions, persons and dogs should be checked for ticks daily and year-round after time outdoors and any ticks found should be removed immediately (Littman *et al.*, 2018). Passive tick surveillance can be effective in assessing the geographical risk of human Lyme disease, which relies on persons to submit their tick samples to labs for identification. Ectocides for dogs, long-sleeved clothing for humans, and clearing tall grasses and brushes around homes can improve tick control. Canine vaccination is contested, and available vaccines have variable efficacy (i.e. will not protect against infection), but may provide some assistance to a dog fighting infection in an endemic region (Littman *et al.*, 2018).

Rickettsia spp. (Bacteria)

Rickettsia rickettsii is an intracellular bacterium transmitted by *R. sanguineus* and *A. cajannense* ticks that causes Rocky Mountain Spotted Fever (RMSF), which can be fatal if left untreated. *Rickettsia conorii* causes Mediterranean Spotted Fever (MSF) and Israeli Spotted Fever (ISF) in humans, with most cases reported during the summer in the Mediterranean basin (Levin *et al.*, 2012; Solano-Gallego *et al.*, 2015). Dogs have been shown to be susceptible to *R. conorii* infection and can infect ticks experimentally, but the zoonotic potential of MSF is unknown (Levin *et al.*, 2012; Solano-Gallego *et al.*, 2015). *Rickettsia felis* is transmitted by fleas, causes human *Rickettsia* disease, and has been shown experimentally to infect dogs (Ng-Nguyen *et al.*, 2020). *Rickettsia* spp. seroprevalence can be as high as 68–81% in domestic and stray dogs in endemic regions (Levin *et al.*, 2014).

R. rickettsii in dogs presents with general signs of tickborne disease such as fever, lethargy, anorexia, and thrombocytopenia, and can be fatal if left untreated (Greene and Breitschwerdt, 1998). *R. conorri* infection presents similarly (Solano-Gallego *et al.*, 2015). *R. felis* experimentally infected dogs had mild to no symptoms (Ng-Nguyen *et al.*, 2020).

RMSF in people may mimic an upper respiratory tract infection and cause fever, headache, abdominal pain, gastrointestinal signs, and rash. RMSF is a rapidly progressive disease and can be fatal within days without early treatment (Center for Disease Control, Prevention, n.d.). MSF and ISF can present spontaneously with high fever, flu-like symptoms, a black eschar at the tick bite site, and a maculo-papular rash (Cascio and Iaria, 2006; Solano-Gallego *et al.*, 2015). Severe forms of MSF may affect several organ systems, including the nervous system (Solano-Gallego *et al.*, 2015).

A DFA test can be advantageous in confirming diagnosis within three to 4 days of infection in dogs (Greene and Breitschwerdt, 1998). Molecular techniques are also recommended.

Environmental elimination is difficult due to rodents and wildlife tick reservoirs. Human encroachment on wilderness areas has likely increased the number of annually reported human and dog cases. Tick control as described in previous tickborne infections is the most effective prevention method.

Yersinia spp. (Bacteria)

Yersinia pestis is a nonmotile bacteria most known as the causative agent of the Black Death between 1347 and 1351, during which 30 to 50% of the European population died (DeWitte, 2014), and some estimates suggest that up to 70% of inhabitants of some villages perished. It is still endemic in more than 25 countries (Demeure *et al.*, 2019). With abundant hosts, particularly in low socio-economic countries, outbreaks continue to occur. *Y. pestis* blocks the proventriculus of fleas feeding on infected rodents and so they regurgitate the bacteria as they repeatedly attempt to get a blood meal, thereby inoculating the bacterium into the host (Orloski and Lathrop, 2003). Dogs become infected by consuming infected rodents or being bitten by an infected flea. Dogs, among other mammals, seem to have developed a natural resistance to *Y. pestis* and tend to survive infection (Lewnard and Townsend, 2016; Barbieri *et al.*, 2020).

In dogs, fever, lethargy, anorexia, lymphadenopathy, vomiting, diarrhea, and abscesses have been documented (Nichols *et al.*, 2014). In humans, clinical presentation depends on transmission. An infected flea bite may cause painful lymphadenopathy followed by disseminated septicemia, whereas droplet inhalation can induce a quickly fatal pneumonic plague (Center for Disease Control, Prevention, n.d.). PCR and culture have both been used for diagnosis, but there is no gold standard test available (Riehm *et al.*, 2011).

Dogs prove to be relatively resistant to *Y. pestis* and do not pose a significant threat to human infection. Pets living in endemic areas should be supervised outdoors and owners should limit dogs' hunting activities and use ectocides on pets (Orloski and Lathrop, 2003). When housing a suspected plague-infected dog at a veterinary hospital, it should be isolated, and staff should wear appropriate PPE (Orloski and Lathrop, 2003).

Giardia duodenalis (Protista)

Giardia spp. are globally distributed intestinal protozoa, mainly transmitted by the ingestion of cysts via the fecal-oral route or by ingesting contaminated water, fruit, or vegetables. *G. duodenalis* (syn. *Giardia lamblia* and *Gasterophilus intestinalis*) is the most common intestinal parasite of humans in developed countries and companion animals pose the greatest risk of zoonotic transmission (Thompson, 2004). Young dogs are considered a reservoir for human infection (Inpankaew *et al.*, 2007), but the role of dogs in zoonotic transmission has long been debated and is still not fully understood (de Lucio *et al.*, 2017). Dogs are the hosts of *G. duodenalis* assemblages C and D but occasionally transmit the zoonotic A and B assemblages. Giardiasis mainly affects children, immune-deficient or compromised persons, and travelers to highly endemic areas (Stark et al., 2009; Muhsen and Levine, 2012). Infection is often associated with day-care centers, contaminated drinking water, swimming pools, and traveling (Dixon, 2021).

Most dogs are asymptomatic, but feces can be malodorous, pale, and steatorrheic. If the dog is febrile or emetic, there is likely co-infection as *Giardia* spp. on its own does not cause these presentations (Barr, 1998). Human infections are characterized by diarrhea, colic, headache, dehydration, and weight loss (Cotton *et al.*, 2011). The acute phase usually lasts 1–3 weeks and most infections are self-limiting, though recurrence is common (Dixon, 2021). Long-term infections through damage to the small intestinal microvilli by feeding trophozoites and secondary bacterial colonization can lead to malabsorption (Barr, 1998).

Light microscopy is used to visualize trophozoites and cysts but may lack sensitivity due to the intermittent shedding of parasites. ELISA and molecular techniques can diagnose and differentiate species (Ryan and Cacciò, 2013).

Cysts are relatively resistant to disinfectants such as chlorine, which is routinely used in water treatment, so they are difficult to eliminate. Treatment of infected dogs is recommended to reduce the risk of zoonotic transmission (Dixon, 2021). Improved sanitation and access to clean drinking water help reduce disease. Travelers should take care in peeling fruits, washing vegetables and hands when visiting highly endemic areas and campers should always use filtered water. Preferably, dogs should also be given only filtered water.

Cryptosporidium spp. (Protista)

Cryptosporidium spp. are opportunistic protozoans and the third leading cause of diarrhea-related mortality in children under 5 years (Taghipour *et al.*, 2020). Routes of transmission are zoonotic through environmental contamination or direct contact, waterborne, foodborne, and human-to-human (Khalil *et al.*, 2018). Infection does not seem to be common in dogs (Palmer *et al.*, 2008). Most human cases are due to *C. hominis* and *C. parvum*, while *C. canis* and *C. parvum* are most common in dogs (Taghipour *et al.*, 2020). *Cryptosporidium* was recently estimated to be in 6–8% of dogs worldwide (Taghipour *et al.*, 2020).

Dogs are usually asymptomatic but may show signs of diarrhea and weight loss (Ryan and Cacciò, 2013). Most immunocompetent humans are asymptomatic, but infection can be life-threatening in immunocompromised people (Khalil *et al.*, 2018). Infected children in rural, low-resource settings may be malnourished and have stunted growth (Khalil *et al.*, 2018). Clinical infections often constitute signs of explosive, offensive diarrhea, nausea, vomiting, abdominal pain, and malaise (Lucio-Forster *et al.*, 2010). A fecal smear with acid-fast staining is practical for finding oocysts as it is simple, inexpensive, and has a high positive predictive value for *Cryptosporidium* (Taghipour *et al.*, 2020).

Substandard personal hygiene and community sanitation, contaminated food and drinking water, low socioeconomic status, and close contact with infected animals all pose a risk to human infection (Taghipour *et al.*, 2020). Disposal of human and dog feces is important for limiting transmission as oocysts are shed in the environment.

Toxoplasma gondii (Protista)

Toxoplasma gondii is estimated to infect approximately 2 billion people globally, making it one of the most common parasites (Smith *et al.*, 2021). Transmission is rare between humans and dogs and occurs through the consumption of infected dog meat, which is most common in countries where dog meat is commercially sold and consumed, such as China, Vietnam, and Nigeria (Dubey *et al.*, 2020).

Ulcerative dermatitis (Dubey *et al.*, 2020), neurological and musculoskeletal signs may be seen in dogs, particularly in cases of immunosuppression or in the absence of the canine distemper vaccine (Calero-Bernal and Gennari, 2019). Vertical transmission in dogs has been reported, resulting in stillbirths (Taques *et al.*, 2016). Most immunocompetent persons are asymptomatic. Infections contracted during the first trimester are often clinical, resulting in miscarriage, chorioretinitis, hydrocephalus, or long-term learning disabilities. The frequency of infection and loss of immunity in previously asymptomatic individuals is sometimes caused by the reactivation of dormant bradyzoites, which had previously been held in check by the healthy immune system.

Molecular and immunological techniques provide excellent diagnostic capabilities. Imaging of the eye and brain can disclose the extent of space-occupying lesions.

Human behavior is an important risk factor for acquiring this disease. As previously uninfected pregnant women are at increased risk, they are an especially important target group. Properly cooking meat for consumption is important to reduce infection. Control of the increasing feral cat population would decrease environmental contamination.

Dibothriocephalus spp. (Cestoda)

Dibothriocephalus spp. are one of the longest parasites of humans, with adult worms measuring 2–25 meters long (Bazsalovicsova *et al.*, 2018). Diphyllobothriasis affects an estimated 20 million people worldwide (Conboy, 2009). *D. latum* infections occur around freshwater lakes, have extremely high fecundity, and can reach patency in numerous species (Scholz *et al.*, 2009). The practice of feeding raw fish to canine or human DHs aids in further environmental contamination (Semenas, 2013). Unembryonated eggs released in DH feces hatch in water before finding a copepod IH. Fish act as secondary IHs after ingesting infected copepods. DHs then become infected by consuming raw or undercooked infected fish. While *D. latum* is usually reported in colder regions of the world, a recent study in Ghana found 7.1% of 154 dogs to be infected with the tapeworm (Amissah-Reynolds *et al.*, 2016). *D. dendriticum* has been found in North America on rare occasions (Kuchta *et al.*, 2013).

Symptomatic canine cases are scarce in the literature. A recent report described diarrhea, inappetence, and desquamation of skin around the anus (Sasikala *et al.*, 2018). Human cases are often mild or asymptomatic (Scholz *et al.*, 2009), but diarrhea, abdominal pain, fatigue, constipation, and megaloblastic anemia have been reported with some regularity (Lee *et al.*, 2015; Sharma *et al.*, 2018). *D. latum* absorbs about 80 percent of dietary vitamin B12, with approximately 40 percent of human cases reporting a B12 deficiency (Scholz *et al.*, 2009), which can result in clinical signs associated with the nervous, respiratory, hematologic, and ocular systems (Scholz *et al.*, 2009).

Diagnosis is often based on clinical presentation and history, as well as the presence of operculated eggs or proglottids in feces, which are morphologically different from proglottids of other cestodes (Scholz *et al.*, 2009). Diagnosis and treatment of this cestode are generally straightforward and have an excellent prognosis. Reducing transmission is not as easy. This tapeworm would likely be reduced through proper cooking of fish before consumption.

Spirometra spp. (Cestoda)

Spirometra spp. is the causative agent of sparganosis, a global foodborne and waterborne disease. Over 1600 human cases have been reported, particularly in the east and southeast Asia (Liu *et al.*, 2015). Fried frog is a popular food in Guangzhou, China, and poses a risk to humans as frogs are IHs. An infection rate of 27.5% was found in 229 dogs in Guangzhou (Hong *et al.*, 2016). Adult *Spirometra* lives in the DH intestines and sheds unembryonated eggs in feces, which release coracidia when in water. Once ingested by copepod IHs, coracidia develop into procercoid larvae. Fish, reptiles, and amphibians act as secondary IHs and ingest infected copepods. The procercoids then develop into plerocercoids. PHs and DHs are infected by ingesting infected first or second IHs in drinking water, raw or uncooked meat, or by local application of infected flesh to the eye or ulcerated skin as a poultice.

Very few cases of canine sparganosis have been reported. Chronic and proliferative peritonitis, pleuritis, dyspnea, and fever have been documented (Drake *et al.*, 2008; Stief and Enge, 2011). Internal proliferative sparganosis in humans can be metastatic, particularly within bones (Kikuchi and Maruyama, 2020). Human cases are often fatal and many of those documented occurred in the early twentieth century, possibly due to a lack of early diagnosis and access to modern treatments (Liu *et al.*, 2015). Molecular techniques and clinical presentation are used in the diagnosis of sparganosis. Characteristic operculated eggs may be seen on fecal flotation and sedimentation. Food safety precautions should be adhered to when cooking meats that may harbor *Spirometra* spp. plerocercoids (Hong *et al.*, 2016).

Schistosoma spp. (esp. *japonicum*) and *Heterobilharzia americana* (Trematoda)

Schistosomiasis, or bilharzia, results from infection with more than 18 different *Schistosoma* species (Ouma and Fenwick, 1991), differing in geographical areas throughout the tropics and subtropics. Dogs serve as DHs for *S. japonicum* and *H. americana*. *S. japonicum* is found in rural, localized foci in China, the Philippines, and Indonesia (McManus *et al.*, 2018) and water buffalo are the main reservoirs. *H. americana* is endemic to North America with a raccoon and occasionally canine DH. Humans may experience symptoms when exposed to cercariae in water, but patent infections do not occur (Loker *et al.*, 2021). *Schistosoma* infection occurs when free-swimming cercariae penetrate the skin and migrate through the blood to the lungs and liver, where sexual maturation occurs. Adults travel to and mate in the mesenteric veins, where the female produces eggs that migrate into the intestine and are expelled in feces or become trapped in various organs resulting in chronic clinical manifestations.

Reports of clinical *S. japonicum* infection in dogs were not found in the literature. *H. americana* eggs can cause a granulomatous response in several organs, which often induces hypercalcemia which may lead to kidney failure (Corapi *et al.*, 2011). Dogs may present with dermatitis, bloody diarrhea, vomiting, lethargy, polyuria, and polydipsia (Hong *et al.*, 2016). The granulomatous disease also occurs in humans and may lead to anemia, hematuria, portal hypertension, impaired cognition, and stunted growth (Colley *et al.*, 2014). Acute schistosomiasis or Katayama syndrome can show myalgia, malaise, and abdominal pain (Colley *et al.*, 2014). Some larvae die within the skin after penetration and do not enter hematogenous circulation. This causes cercarial dermatitis known as 'swimmer's itch' (McManus *et al.*, 2018). *H. americana* cercariae can cause a similar dermatitis (Hong *et al.*, 2016). Diagnosis can be made with microscopy of fecal samples, PCR, ELISA, and monitoring for adult worms in ruminant reservoir hosts at slaughter.

The WHO set a roadmap toward the elimination of the public health importance of schistosomiasis by 2025 which focused on *Schistosoma mansoni* and *S. haematobium* (King and Bertsch, 2015; Deol et al., 2019; Toor *et al.*, 2020). High human prevalence is often associated with occupations that have prolonged water contact such as rice farmers, fishers, and launderers. Similarly, dogs are exposed when used for guarding crop fields, hunting, or herding. Schistosomiasis is considered a disease of poverty due to the lack of access to safe water sources and contact with snail-infested waters. Mass treatment with praziquantel has been implemented in many countries but repeat infections occur due to the parasite persisting in the snail IH and the drug does not kill immature worms in the host, resulting in the rapid reestablishment of egg-laying females. Historically, chemical molluscicides were used to control the IH but ultimately were not cost-effective, did not prevent repopulation, and had harmful environmental effects (King and Bertsch, 2015). The use of mechanized plowing equipment to replace water buffalos has helped to eliminate the disease in numerous countries (Spear *et al.*, 2017). There are currently no human or animal vaccines available, but several are in the process of development (McManus *et al.*, 2020; Molehin, 2020).

Echinococcus canadensis (Cestoda)

Echinococcus canadensis is endemic to North America, has been found in parts of Scandinavia (Thompson, 2015) and can cause human cystic echinococcosis. It has an obligate two-host life cycle, with cervid IHs and carnivorous DHs such as wild and domestic canids. As with other *Echinococcus* spp., human infection occurs following the ingestion of eggs. Dogs are subclinically infected (Jenkins, 2017). Human infections are as seen with *E. granulosus*. Molecular techniques are ideal as eggs are not shed during the PPP and only intermittently throughout patency (Jenkins, 2017). Echinococcosis due to *E. canadensis* is relatively rare in people, possibly due to its wildlife sylvatic cycles. Pets that are at high risk for infection due to their proximity to wildlife in endemic regions, particularly hunting dogs, should ideally be prophylactically treated every 6 weeks, which is the parasite's PPP (Grech-Angelini *et al.*, 2019; Jenkins, 2017).

Sarcoptes scabei var. *canis* (Arthropoda-Sarcoptiformes)

Sarcoptic mange is a highly contagious dermatitis caused by *Sarcoptes scabei* var. *canis* infestation. It causes substantial morbidity and mortality in humans and dogs (Arlian and Morgan, 2017) and intense pruritis, alopecia, excoriation, hyperkeratosis, and occasionally secondary bacterial infections and pyoderma (Hampel *et al.*, 2018). Deep skin scraping is often needed for diagnosis in dogs. Treatment with products such as afoxolaner with or without milbemycin oxime has been shown to be highly efficacious in treating canine cases (Hampel *et al.*, 2018).

Category 3: Human Infections with Rare Zoonotic Transmission, but Where Dogs Play a Minor Role in the Transmission to Humans

Rare potential zoonosis

Bacillus anthracis

Anthrax endemicity has been recategorized in countries such as Zimbabwe for anthrax surveillance (Mukarati *et al.*, 2018). Domestic dogs can be valuable for surveillance as they live in

Table 13.1. Human: Dog Zoonoses where dogs play a minor role.

Causative agent	Transmission	Risk factors	Clinical features in dogs	Clinical features in humans	Diagnosis	Control	Occurrence	References
SARS-CoV-2 (Virus)	Aerosol	Indoors, no masks, no vaccines, large groups, comorbidities	Asymptomatic	Variant-dependent, varies with phases of infection	RT-qPCR, rapid antigen tests, biodetection dogs	Masks, physical distancing, hand washing, vaccination	Global	(Hackner and Pleil, 2017; Patterson *et al.*, 2020;Sit *et al.*, 2020 ; Bosco-Lauth *et al.*, 2020; Coronaviridae Study Group of the International Committee on Taxonomy of Viruses, 2020)
Bordetella bronchiseptica (Bacteria)	Aerosol	Immunocompromised, predisposing conditions (smoking)	Canine infectious tracheobronchitis (kennel cough)	Bronchitis	Molecular techniques	Isolate infected dogs from other dogs and immunocompromised persons, well ventilated, and keep dog kennels clean and dry	Global	(Clements *et al.*, 2018; Goodnow, 1980)
Mycobacterium spp. (Bacteria)	Aerosol, handling infected carcasses	Crowding, low ventilation	Nonspecific respiratory signs	Tuberculosis. Initial infection often goes unrecognized and progresses over time	Ziehl-Neelsen acid-fast stain (cytology, histology), ID skin testing, culture	Treat or euthanize infected dogs, abstain from feeding dogs unpasteurized milk or raw offal, live Bacillus Calmette-Guerin vaccine	Global	(Greene and Gunn-Moore, 1998; Turinelli *et al.*, 2004; Une and Mori, 2007; Pérez-Lago *et al.*, 2014; Churchyard *et al.*, 2017)
Corynebacterium ulcerans (Bacteria)	Aerosol	Contact with pets	Asymptomatic, upper respiratory disease	Diphtheria-like respiratory and cutaneous illness, sepsis	Culture	Infection is rare. Recommended treatment after antimicrobial susceptibility testing is penicillin G or erythromycin and diphtheria antitoxin		(Hacker *et al.*, 2016; Otsuji *et al.*, 2017; Abbott *et al.*, 2020)

Continued

Table 13.1. Continued

Causative agent	Transmission	Risk factors	Clinical features in dogs	Clinical features in humans	Diagnosis	Control	Occurrence	References
Coxiella burnettii (Bacteria)	Aerosol, ingestion of reservoir meat, close contact with parturient animal fluids, and tick bites	Wildlife on domestic properties	Asymptomatic, abortion	Q fever: Acute: flu-like illness, pneumonia, and hepatitis Chronic: endocarditis, hepatitis, aortic aneurysms, and osteomyelitis Post-Q fever fatigue syndrome	Serology	Persons assisting in dog whelping should take precautions to limit contact with bodily fluids during parturition, vaccination available for at-risk persons (veterinarians)	Global	(Gidding *et al.*, 2009; Shapiro *et al.*, 2016; Sivabalan *et al.*, 2017; Bae *et al.*, 2019; Ni *et al.*, 2020;Ma *et al.*, 2020)
Helicobacter spp. (Bacteria)	Fecal-oral, rare	Unknown	Gastritis	Gastritis, gastric cancer	Noninvasive and invasive	N/A	Global	(Wotherspoon, 1991; Parsonnet *et al.*, 1991; Fox and Lee, 1997; Amorim *et al.*, 2015)
Campylobacter spp. (Bacteria)	Fecal-oral, rare (Sandberg *et al.*, 2002)	Unknown	Asymptomatic	Self-limiting gastroenteritis, vomiting, myalgia, headaches, watery or bloody diarrhea, and abdominal pain	Culture and molecular techniques	Keep canine shelter environments clean	Global	(Acke *et al.*, 2009; Carbonera *et al.*, 2012; Chlebicz and Śliżewska, 2018; Fox, 1998; Hald and Madsen, 1997; Iannino *et al.*, 2019; Karama *et al.*, 2019; Parsons *et al.*, 2011; Procter *et al.*, 2014)

Brucella spp. (Bacteria)	Ingestion, inhalation, or contact with aborted fetuses or reproductive fluids, rare	Assisting in canine births	Subclinical, reproductive failure, mid to late-term abortions followed by an odorless, brown to yellow vaginal discharge, discospondylitis, and lameness	Fever, chills, malaise, peripheral lymphadenomegaly, endocarditis, and peritonitis	PCR, culture	Test breeding dogs for *B. canis*, personal protective equipment (PPE) should be worn by veterinarians, animal caretakers, and laboratory personnel when working with suspect cases, biosafety level three laboratory spaces required	Global	(Boeri *et al.*, 2018;Carmichael and Kenney, 1968; Carmichael *et al.*, 1984; Cosford, 2018; Dentinger *et al.*, 2012; Dunn *et al.*, 2002; Kauffman *et al.*, 2014; Keid *et al.*, 2007; Lucero *et al.*, 2010; Mor *et al.*, 2016; Santos *et al.*, 2021; Taques *et al.*, 2016)
Balantioides coli (Protista)	Fecal-oral	Unknown	Hemorrhagic colitis	Frequent diarrhea and occult blood in stool	Fecal smear, flotation	Control disposal of pig feces	Global	(Aninagyei *et al.*, 2021; Barr, 1998; Mathison *et al.*, 2021)
Blastocystis hominis (Protista)	Fecal-oral	Unknown	Diarrhea	Asymptomatic, chronic intestinal disease, urticaria, and pruritic rash	Microscopy of stained smear or wet mount, molecular techniques	Management of canine hygiene, provision of safe drinking water	Global	(Stenzel and Boreham, 1996; Verma and Delfanian, 2013; Beyhan et al., 2015; Angelici et al., 2018; Liao et al., 2020; Hublin et al., 2021)
Dipylidium Caninum (Cestoda)	*Ctenocephalides* spp. flea vector	Contact with dogs not on preventative ectocides	Pruritis ani, flea allergy dermatitis due to flea infestation	Asymptomatic, mild diarrhea	Proglottid morphology and comprehensive history, fecal flotation	Ectocide use in dogs to control the flea IH and endocide use	Global	(Marchiondo *et al.*, 2013; García-Agudo *et al.*, 2014; Jiang *et al.*, 2017; Lahmar *et al.*, 2017)

Continued

Table 13.1. Continued

Causative agent	Transmission	Risk factors	Clinical features in dogs	Clinical features in humans	Diagnosis	Control	Occurrence	References
Taenia serialis (Cestoda)	Accidental ingestion of eggs from the environment	Wildlife reservoirs	Asymptomatic	Coenurosis	Arecoline purgation and necropsy in dogs	Endocide treatment of dogs, appropriate disposal of ruminant brains	Global	(Baneth *et al.*, 2016; Deplazes *et al.*, 2019; Yamazawa *et al.*, 2020)
Taenia brauna (Cestoda)	Rodent IH	Unknown	Asymptomatic	Coenurosis	Arecoline purgation and necropsy in dogs	Anthelmintic treatment of dogs, appropriate disposal of sheep brains	Africa	(Deplazes *et al.*, 2019)
Trichuris vulpis (Nematoda)	Accidental ingestion of eggs	Exposure to infected dogs	Asymptomatic, occasionally anemia	Asymptomatic, occasionally anemia and diarrhea	Microscopy	Anthelmintic treatment of dogs	Tropics and subtropics	(Dunn *et al.*, 2002)
Gnathostoma spp. (Nematoda)	Ingestion of raw or undercooked meat of second IH (fish, amphibians, reptiles, and birds), L_1-contaminated freshwater, or direct skin penetration by L_3 larvae	Consuming raw fish	Anorexia, vomiting, weight loss, anemia, and weakness	Four main clinical manifestations: cutaneous, visceral, neuro and ocular, eosinophilia	History, presentation, identification of adult nematode or L_3 larvae	Adequately cook and prepare meat, reduce hunting and sale of wildlife for human consumption	Southeast Asia	(Chikweto *et al.*, 2015; Diaz, 2015; Liu *et al.*, 2020)
Thelazia callipaeda (Nematoda)	Dipteran insect IH	Seasonal	Asymptomatic, bletharospasm, epiphora, keratitis, and conjunctivitis	As in dogs	Visualization of a white nematode on the conjunctiva is pathognomonic	Complete elimination in an infected host by use of an antiparasitic drug	Europe and Asia	(Beugnet *et al.*, 2018; doVale *et al.*, 2019)
Thelazia californiensis (Nematoda)	Dipteran insect IH	Seasonal	As in *T. callipaeda*	As in *T. callipaeda*	As in *T. callipaeda*	As in *T. callipaeda*	Western USA	(Beugnet *et al.*, 2018)

Dirofilaria immitis (Nematoda)	Mosquito vector	International travel, climate change	Heartworm disease, exercise intolerance, cachexia, coughing, hemoptysis, tachypnea, dyspnea, syncope, caval syndrome, and pulmonary thromboembolism	Asymptomatic, and on rare occasions, may cause pulmonary dirofilariasis, worm-induced granulomas within pulmonary arteries, chest pain, hemoptysis, and pleural effusion	SNAP 4Dx test, modified Knott's test	Monthly heartworm preventative for dogs, vector control	Tropical and increasingly to temperate regions	(American Heartworm Society, n.d.; Lee *et al.*, 2010 Kramer *et al.*, 2018; Fontes-Sousa *et al.*, 2019; Maerz, 2020; Ames and Atkins, 2020)
Dirofilaria repens (Nematoda)	Mosquitovector	International travel, climate change	Asymptomatic, skin nodules, pruritis, thinning of skin	Asymptomatic, larva migrans-like cutaneous infection	Morphologic or molecular techniques	Monthly heartworm preventative for dogs, vector control	Tropical and increasingly to temperate regions	(Ames and Atkins, 2020; Capelli *et al.*, 2018; Lee *et al.*, 2010; Maerz, 2020)
Onchocerca lupi (Nematoda)	Black fly vector	Unknown	Asymptomatic, excessive lacrimation, photophobia, conjunctivitis, exophthalmos, periorbital swelling, and subconjunctival and episcleral nodules	Conjunctival redness, pain, pruritis, and subconjunctival nodules	Morphological and molecular techniques, skin snips	Vector control	North America	(Pampiglione et al., 2001; Bergua et al., 2015; Cantey et al., 2016; Verocai et al., 2016)
Heterophyes heterophyes (Trematoda)	Ingestion of IH	Consuming raw or undercooked fish	Asymptomatic, diarrhea	Asymptomatic, mild intestinal discomfort, and mucous diarrhea	Microscopy and intradermal tests	Adequate cooking and preparation of fish	Southeast Asia, Far East, and Nile Delta of Egypt	(Ashour *et al.*, 2014; Elshazly *et al.*, 2008)

Continued

Table 13.1. Continued

Causative agent	Transmission	Risk factors	Clinical features in dogs	Clinical features in humans	Diagnosis	Control	Occurrence	References
Metagonimus spp. (Trematoda)	Ingestion of IH	Consuming raw or undercooked freshwater fish	Asymptomatic, diarrhea	Abdominal pain, diarrhea, lethargy, malabsorption, anorexia, and weight loss	Morphologic diagnosis	Adequate cooking and preparation of fish	Asia, Europe	(Chai and Jung, 2017)
Ctenocephalides felis (Arthropoda-Siphonaptera)	Flea ectoparasite	Outdoor exposure, wildlife reservoirs	Vector of *Dipylidium caninum* and cause of flea allergy dermatitis	Vector of *Dipylidium caninum* and cat-scratch fever	Gross and microscopic visualization	Regular ectocide use in dogs	Global	(Bouhsira *et al.*, 2013; Rust, 2005
Otodectes cynotis (Arthropoda-Sarcoptiformes)	Mite ectoparasite	Unknown	Otitis externa, urticaria and otodectic mange	Otitis externa	Microscopy (fecal or ear swab samples), PCR	Regular ectocide use in dogs	Global	(Salib and Baraka, 2011; Van de Heyning and Thienpont, 1977)
Cochliomya hominivorax (Arthropoda-Diptera)	Fly vector	Poor hygiene habits, cutaneous lesions and/or systemic diseases	Primary myiasis	Primary myiasis	Visualization of *C. homnivorax* larvae in fresh wounds	Sterile insect technique	South America and the Caribbean	(Costa-Junior *et al.*, 2019; Fresia *et al.*, 2011

close contact with humans and livestock, can be sampled at all ages, and provide reasonable timing of outbreak recognition (Lembo *et al.*, 2011).

Conclusion

The symbiotic relationship between dogs and humans has been incredibly beneficial throughout the history of mankind. By integrating our lives with theirs, we have gained companionship, security, work assistance, learning opportunities, and more, while providing safety, shelter, food, and companionship to dogs in return. This association has facilitated the transmission of several zoonotic infections where dogs play an essential or minor role in disease perpetuation. Many of these zoonoses are changing in geographic distribution and importance due to environmental changes and human behavior. While there are numerous diagnostics and treatments available for most of these diseases, they are not always readily available in endemic countries. Prevention through the administration of prophylactics and a greater emphasis on alterations to human behavior through appropriate education is required to minimize the public health impact of these zoonotic infections. Small steps such as hand washing after handling dogs, avoiding mouth-to-mouth contact with dogs, creating awareness about canine behavior, vaccinating, and seeking veterinary and medical care when needed and available all reduce zoonotic transmission. A One Health approach should be highlighted during veterinary and physician training and communicated to clients and patients once out in practice. With more people keeping dogs as pets every day, it is imperative to always consider the zoonotic perspective when treating a potentially infectious case. Integration of veterinary and medical fields would allow for quicker and more efficient diagnosis and treatment, reduce zoonotic transmission, and hopefully improve the livelihoods of humans and dogs through sharing of knowledge, improving infrastructure, providing access to safe water and veterinary and medical care, and creating a safer, healthier environment for all.

Conflict of interest

The authors have no conflicts of interest to declare.

References

Abbott, Y., Acke, E., Khan, S., Muldoon, E.G., Markey, B.K. *et al.* (2010) Zoonotic transmission of *Streptococcus equi* subsp. Zooepidemicus from a dog to a handler. *Journal of Medical Microbiology* 59(1), 120–123.

Abbott, Y., Efstratiou, A., Brennan, G., Hallanan, S., Leggett, B. *et al.* (2020) Toxigenic *Corynebacterium ulcerans* associated with upper respiratory infections in cats and dogs. *Journal of Small Animal Practice* 61(9), 554–560.

Acke, E., McGill, K., Golden, O., Jones, B.R., Fanning, S. *et al.* (2009) Prevalence of thermophilic *Campylobacter* species in household cats and dogs in Ireland. *Veterinary Record* 164(2), 44–47.

Acosta-Jamett G., Weitzel T., López J., Alvarado D., Abarca K. Prevalence and risk factors of antibodies to *Anaplasma* spp. in Chile: A household-based cross-sectional study in healthy adults and domestic dogs. Vector-Borne and Zoonotic Diseases 2020;20(8):572–9.

Ahn, C.-S., Shin, J.W., Kim, J.-G., Lee, W.-Y., Kang, I. *et al.* (2021) Spectrum of pleuropulmonary paragonimiasis: An analysis of 685 cases diagnosed over 22 years. *Journal of Infection* 82(1), 150–158.

Akhoundi, M., Kuhls, K., Cannet, A., Votýpka, J., Marty, P. *et al.* (2016) A historical overview of the classification, evolution, and dispersion of *Leishmania* parasites and sandflies. *PLoS Neglected Tropical Diseases* 10(3), e0004349.

Alcántara-Rodríguez, V.E., Sánchez-Montes, S., Contreras, H., Colunga-Salas, P., Fierro-Flores, L. *et al.* (2020) Human monocytic ehrlichiosis, Mexico City, Mexico. *Emerging Infectious Diseases* 26(12), 3016–3019.

Alvar, J., Vélez, I.D., Bern, C., Herrero, M., Desjeux, P. *et al.* (2012) Leishmaniasis worldwide and global estimates of its incidence. *PLoS One* 7(5), e35671.

American Heartworm Society (n.d.) Weigh the costs [infographic]. Available at: https://www.heartwormsociety.org/resources/vet/infographics/355-weigh-the-costs

American Veterinary Medical Association (2018) In: *AVMA Pet Ownership and Demographics Sourcebook [2017–2018 Edition]*.

Ames, M.K. and Atkins, C.E. (2020) Treatment of dogs with severe heartworm disease. *Veterinary Parasitology* 283, 109131.

Amissah-Reynolds, P.K., Monney, I., Adowah, L.M. and Agyemang, S.O. (2016) Prevalence of helminths in dogs and owners' awareness of zoonotic diseases in Mampong, Ashanti, Ghana. *Journal of Parasitology Research* 1–6.

Amorim, I., Smet, A., Alves, O., Teixeira, S., Saraiva, A.L. *et al.* (2015) Presence and significance of *Helicobacter* spp. in the gastric mucosa of Portuguese dogs. *Gut Pathogens* 7(1), 12.

Angelici, M.C., Nardis, C., Scarpelli, R. and Ade, P. (2018) *Blastocystis hominis* transmission by non-potable water: A case report in Italy. *New Microbiologica* 41(2), 173–177.

Aninagyei, E., Nanga, S., Acheampong, D.O., Mensah, R., Boadu, M.N. *et al.* (2021) Prevalence and risk factors of human *Balantidium coli* infection and its association with haematological and biochemical parameters in Ga West municipality, Ghana. *BMC Infectious Diseases* 21(1), 1047.

Arlian, L.G. and Morgan, M.S. (2017) A review of *Sarcoptes scabiei*: Past, present and future. *Parasites & Vectors* 10(1), 297.

Arraga-Alvarado, C.M., Parra, O.C., Hegarty, B.C., Breitschwerdt, E.B., Qurollo, B.A. *et al.* (2014) Molecular evidence of *Anaplasma platys* infection in two women from Venezuela. *The American Journal of Tropical Medicine and Hygiene* 91(6), 1161–1165.

Ashour, D.S., Othman, A.A. and Radi, D.A. (2014) Insights into regulatory molecules of intestinal epithelial cell turnover during experimental infection by Heterophyes heterophyes. *Experimental Parasitology* 143, 48–54.

Bae, M., Jin, C.E., Park, J.H., Kim, M.J., Chong, Y.P. *et al.* (2019) Diagnostic usefulness of molecular detection of *Coxiella burnetii* from blood of patients with suspected acute Q fever. *Medicine* 98(23), e15724.

Baneth, G., Thamsborg, S.M., Otranto, D., Guillot, J., Blaga, R. *et al.* (2016) Major parasitic zoonoses associated with dogs and cats in Europe. *Journal of Comparative Pathology* 155(1), S54–S74.

Barbabosa-Pliego, A., Díaz-Albiter, H.M., Ochoa-García, L., Aparicio-Burgos, E., López-Heydeck, S.M. *et al.* (2009) *Trypanosoma cruzi* circulating in the southern region of the state of Mexico (Zumpahuacan) are pathogenic: A dog model. *The American Journal of Tropical Medicine and Hygiene* 81(3), 390–395.

Barbieri, R., Signoli, M., Chevé, D., Costedoat, C., Tzortzis, S. *et al.* (2020) *Yersinia pestis*: The natural history of plague. *Clinical Microbiology Reviews* 34(1), e00044–19.

Barr, S.C. (1998) Enteric protozoal infections. In: Greene, C.E. (ed.) *Infectious Diseases of the Dog and Cat*, 2nd ed. W.B. Saunders Company, Philadelphia, pp. 482–486.

Bazsalovicsova, E., Kolenicova, A., Kralova-Hromadova, I., Minarik, G., Soltys, K. *et al.* (2018) Development of microsatellite loci in zoonotic tapeworm *Dibothriocephalus latus* (Linnaeus, 1758), Luhe, 1899 (syn. *Diphyllobothrium latum*) using microsatellite library screening. *Molecular and Biochemical Parasitology* 225, 1–3.

Beck, R., Mihaljević, Ž., Brezak, R., Bosnić, S., Janković, I.L. *et al.* (2018) First detection of *Echinococcus multilocularis* in Croatia. *Parasitology Research* 117(2), 617–621.

Beeler, E. and Ehnert, K. (2020) *Rabies in dogs and cats. Clinical small animal internal medicine*. Wiley, Hoboken, New Jersey, pp. 891–897.

Bergua, A., Hohberger, B., Held, J., Muntau, B., Tannich, E. *et al.* (2015) Human case of *Onchocerca lupi* infection, gernmany august 2014. *Eurosurveillance* 20(16), 21099.

Bern, C., Verastegui, M., Gilman Robert, H., LaFuente, C., Galdos-Cardenas, G. *et al.* (2009) Congenital *Trypanosoma cruzi* transmission in Santa cruz, Bolivia. *Clinical Infectious Diseases* 49(11), 1667–1674.

Bern, C., Kjos, S., Yabsley, M.J. and Montgomery, S.P. (2011) *Trypanosoma cruzi* and Chagas' disease in the United States. *Clinical Microbiology Reviews* 24(4), 655–681.

Beugnet, F., Halos, L. and Guillot, J. (2018) Internal non-gastrointestinal parasitoses-thelaziosis. In: *Textbook of Clinical Parasitology in Dogs and Cats*, 2nd ed. Servet, Zaragoza, Spain, pp. 200–202.

Beyhan, Y.E., Yilmaz, H., Cengiz, Z.T. and Ekici, A. (2015) Clinical significance and prevalence of *Blastocystis hominis* in Van, Turkey. *Saudi Medical Journal* 36(9), 1118–1121.

Bitek, A.O., Osoro, E., Munyua, P.M., Nanyingi, M., Muthiani, Y. *et al*. (2019) A hundred years of rabies in Kenya and the strategy for eliminating dog-mediated rabies by 2030. *AAS Open Research* 1, 23.

Blancou, J. and Meslin, F.X. (2000) Brief review of the history of zoonoses. *Revue Scientifique et Technique (International Office of Epizootics)* 19(1), 15–22.

Boeri, E.J., Wanke, M.M., Madariaga, M.J., Teijeiro, M.L., Elena, S.A. *et al*. (2018) Comparison of four polymerase chain reaction assays for the detection of *Brucella* spp. in clinical samples from dogs. *Veterinary WORLD* 11(2), 201–208.

Boggiatto, P.M., Gibson-Corley, K.N., Metz, K., Gallup, J.M., Hostetter, J.M. *et al*. (2011) Transplacental transmission of *Leishmania infantum* as a means for continued disease incidence in North America. *PLoS Neglected Tropical Diseases* 5(4), e1019.

Bosco-Lauth, A.M., Hartwig, A.E., Porter, S.M., Gordy, P.W., Nehring, M. *et al*. (2020) Experimental infection of domestic dogs and cats with SARS-CoV-2: Pathogenesis, transmission, and response to reexposure in cats. *Proceedings of the National Academy of Sciences* 117(42), 26382–26388.

Bouhsira, E., Ferrandez, Y., Liu, M., Franc, M., Boulouis, H.J. *et al*. (2013) *Ctenocephalides felis* an in vitro potential vector for five *Bartonella* species. *Comparative Immunology, Microbiology & Infectious Diseases* 36(2), 105–111.

Bowman, D.D., Montgomery, S.P., Zajac, A.M., Eberhard, M.L. and Kazacos, K.R. (2010) Hookworms of dogs and cats as agents of cutaneous larva migrans. *Trends in Parasitology* 26(4), 162–167.

Bradbury, R.S., Hii, S.F., Harrington, H., Speare, R. and Traub, R. (2017) *Ancylostoma ceylanicum* hookworm in the Solomon Islands. *Emerging Infectious Diseases* 23(2), 252–257.

Brown, P., McKenzie, M. and McGrowder, D. (2011) Environmental risk factors associated with leptospirosis among butchers and their associates in Jamaica. *International Journal of Occupational and Environmental Medicine* 2(1), 47–57.

Brunetti, E., Tamarozzi, F., Macpherson, C., Filice, C., Piontek, M. *et al*. (2018) Ultrasound and cystic echinococcosis. *Ultrasound International Open* 04(3), E70–E78.

Budachetri, K., Teymournejad, O., Lin, M., Yan, Q., Mestres-Villanueva, M. *et al*. (2020) An entry-triggering protein of *Ehrlichia* is a new vaccine candidate against tick-borne human monocytic *Ehrlichiosis*. *MBio* 11(4), e00895–20.

Büscher, P., Cecchi, G., Jamonneau, V. and Priotto, G. (2017) Human *African Trypanosomiasis*. *The Lancet* 390(10110), 2397–2409.

Calero-Bernal, R. and Gennari, S.M. (2019) Clinical toxoplasmosis in dogs and cats: An update. *Frontiers in Veterinary Science* 6, 54.

Cantas, L. and Suer, K. (2014) Review: The important bacterial zoonoses in one health concept. *Frontiers in Public Health* 2, 144.

Cantey, P.T., Weeks, J., Edwards, M., Rao, S., Ostovar, G.A. *et al*. (2016) The emergence of zoonotic *Onchocerca lupi* infection in the United States—A case-series. *Clinical Infectious Diseases* 62(6), 778–783.

Capelli, G., Genchi, C., Baneth, G., Bourdeau, P., Brianti, E. *et al*. (2018) Recent advances on *Dirofilaria repens* in dogs and humans in Europe. *Parasites & Vectors* 11(1), 663.

Caraballo, D.A., Lombardo, M.A., Becker, P., Sabio, M.S., Lema, C. *et al*. (2020) Evaluation of two real-time, taqman reverse transcription-PCR assays for detection of rabies virus in circulating variants from Argentina: Influence of sequence variation. *Viruses* 13(1), 23.

Carbonera, A., Torralbo, A., Borge, C., García-Bocanegra, I., Arenas, A. *et al*. (2012) *Campylobacter* spp., *C. jejuni and C. upsaliensis* infection-associated factors in healthy and ill dogs from clinics in Cordoba, Spain. Screening tests for antimicrobial susceptibility. *Comparative Immunology, Microbiology and Infectious Diseases* 35(6), 505–512.

Carmichael, L.E. and Kenney, R.M. (1968) Canine abortion caused by *Brucella canis*. *Journal of American Veterinary Medicine Association* 15(6), 605–616.

Carmichael, L.E., Zoha, S.J. and Flores-Castro, R. (1984) Problems in the serodiagnosis of canine brucellosis: Dog responses to cell wall and internal antigens of *Brucella canis*. *Developments in Biological Standardization* 56, 371–383.

Cascio, A. and Iaria, C. (2006) Epidemiology and clinical features of mediterranean spotted fever in Italy. *Europe PMC* 48(1–2), 131–133.

Cascio, A., Bosilkovski, M., Rodriguez-Morales, A.J. and Pappas, G. (2011) The socio-ecology of zoonotic infections. *Clinical Microbiology and Infection* 17(3), 336–342.

Castro-Sesquen, Y.E., Tinajeros, F., Bern, C., Galdos-Cardenas, G., Malaga, E.S. *et al.* (2021) The immunoglobulin M-shed acute phase antigen (SAPA)-test for the early diagnosis of congenital Chagas disease in the time of the elimination goal of mother-to-child transmission. *Clinical Infectious Diseases* 73(2), e477–e484.

Center for Disease Control, Prevention (n.d.) Rocky mountain spotted fever. CDC [Information Sheet].

Chai, J.Y. and Jung, B.K. (2017) Fishborne zoonotic heterophyid infections: An update. *Food Waterborne Parasitology* 8–9, 33–63.

Chierakul, W., Tientadakul, P., Suputtamongkol, Y., Wuthiekanun, V., Phimda, K. *et al.* (2008) Activation of the coagulation cascade in patients with *Leptospirosis*. *Clinical Infectious Diseases* 46(2), 254–260.

Chikweto, A., Bhaiyat, M., Mofya, S. and Ravindra, R. (2015) *Gnathostomiasis* in a dog in Lusaka Zambia. *International Journal of Veterinary Medicine: Research & Reports* 1–4.

Chlebicz, A. and Śliżewska, K. (2018) *Campylobacteriosis*, *Salmonellosis*, *Yersiniosis*, and *Listeriosis* as zoonotic foodborne diseases: A review. *International Journal of Environmental Research and Public Health* 15(5), 863.

Chu, S., Myers, S.L., Wagner, B. and Snead, E.C.R. (2013) Hookworm dermatitis due to *Uncinaria stenocephala* in a dog from Saskatchewan. *The Canadian Veterinary Journal (La Revue Veterinaire Canadienne)* 54(8), 743–747.

Churchyard, G., Kim, P., Shah, N.S., Rustomjee, R., Gandhi, N. *et al.* (2017) What we know about tuberculosis transmission: An overview. *The Journal of Infectious Diseases* 216(suppl_6), S629–S635.

Clark, C., Cunningham, J., Ahmed, R., Woodward, D., Fonseca, K. *et al.* (2001) Characterization of *Salmonella* associated with pig ear dog treats in Canada. *Journal of Clinical Microbiology* 39(11), 3962–3968.

Cleaveland, S. and Hampson, K. (2017) Rabies elimination research: Juxtaposing optimism, pragmatism and realism. *Proceedings of the Royal Society B: Biological Sciences* 284(1869), 20171880.

Clements, J., McGrath, C. and McAllister, C. (2018) *Bordetella bronchiseptica* pneumonia: Beware of the dog. *BMJ Case Reports* 27, e01435.

Clutton-Brock, J. (1995) Origins of the dog, domestic and early history. In: Serpell, J. (ed.) *The Domestic Dog*. Cambridge University Press, Cambridge, pp. 8–20.

Coleman, P.G. and Welburn, S.C. (2004) Are fitness costs associated with resistance to human serum in *Trypanosoma brucei rhodesiense*. *Trends in Parasitology* 20(7), 311–315.

Colley, D.G., Bustinduy, A.L., Secor, W.E. and King, C.H. (2014) Human *Schistosomiasis*. *The Lancet* 383(9936), 2253–2264.

Conboy, G. (2009) Cestodes of dogs and cats in North America. *Veterinary Clinics of North America: Small Animal Practice* 39(6), 1075–1090.

Corapi, W.V., Ajithdoss, D.K., Snowden, K.F. and Spaulding, K.A. (2011) Multi-organ involvement of *Heterobilharzia americana* infection in a dog presented for systemic mineralization. *Journal of Veterinary Diagnostic Investigation* 23(4), 826–831.

Corda, A., Tamponi, C., Meloni, R., Varcasia, A., Parpaglia, M.L.P. *et al.* (2019) Ultrasonography for early diagnosis of *Toxocara canis* infection in puppies. *Parasitology Research* 118(3), 873–880.

Coronaviridae Study Group of the International Committee on Taxonomy of Viruses (2020) The species severe acute respiratory syndrome-related coronavirus: Classifying 2019-nCoV and naming it SARS-CoV-2. *Nature Microbiology* 5(4), 536–544.

Cosford, K.L. (2018) *Brucella canis*: An update on research and clinical management. *The Canadian Veterinary Journal (La Revue Veterinaire Canadienne)* 59(1), 74–81.

Costa, F., Hagan, J.E., Calcagno, J., Kane, M., Torgerson, P. *et al.* (2015) Global morbidity and mortality of leptospirosis: A systematic review. *PLoS Neglected Tropical Diseases* 9(9), e0003898.

Costa-Junior, L.M., Chaves, D.P., Brito, D.R.B., Santos, V., Costa-Junior, H.N. *et al.* (2019) A review on the occurrence of *Cochliomyia hominivorax* (Diptera: Calliphoridae) in Brazil. *Revista Brasileira de Parasitologia Veterinária* 28(4), 548–562.

Cotton, J.A., Beatty, J.K. and Buret, A.G. (2011) Host parasite interactions and pathophysiology in *Giardia* infections. *International Journal for Parasitology* 41(9), 925–933.

Cox, H.U. (1998) Staphylococcal infections. In: Greene, C.E. (ed.) *Infectious Diseases of the Dog and Cat*, 2nd ed. Saunders Company, Philadelphia.

Craig, P., Mastin, A., van Kesteren, F. and Boufana, B. (2015) *Echinococcus granulosus* i: Epidemiology and state-of-the-art of diagnostics in animals. *Veterinary Parasitology* 213(3–4), 132–148.
da Silva, S.M., Ribeiro, V.M., Ribeiro, R.R., Tafuri, W.L., Melo, M.N. *et al.* (2009) First report of vertical transmission of *Leishmania (Leishmania) infantum* in a naturally infected bitch from Brazil. *Veterinary Parasitology* 166(1–2), 159–162.
Dantas-Torres, F., Miró, G., Baneth, G., Bourdeau, P., Breitschwerdt, E. *et al.* (2019) *Canine leishmaniasis* control in the context of one health. *Emerging Infectious Diseases* 25(12), 1–4.
de Barros Moreira Beltrão, H., de Paula Cerroni, M., de Freitas, D.R.C., das Neves Pinto, A.Y., da Costa Valente, V. *et al.* (2009) Investigation of two outbreaks of suspected oral transmission of acute Chagas disease in the Amazon region, Pará state, Brazil, in 2007. *Tropical Doctor* 39(4), 231–232.
de Lucio, A., Bailo, B., Aguilera, M., Cardona, G.A., Fernández-Crespo, J.C. *et al.* (2017) No molecular epidemiological evidence supporting household transmission of zoonotic *Giardia duodenalis* and *Cryptosporidium* spp. from pet dogs and cats in the province of Álava, Northern Spain. *Acta Tropica* 170, 48–56.
Demeure, C.E., Dussurget, O., Mas Fiol, G., Le Guern, A.-S., Savin, C. *et al.* (2019) *Yersinia pestis* and plague: An updated view on evolution, virulence determinants, immune subversion, vaccination, and diagnostics. *Genes & Immunity* 20(5), 357–370.
Dentinger, C.M., Jacob, K., Lee, L.V., Mendez, H.A., Chotikanatis, K. *et al.* (2012) Human *Brucella canis* infection and subsequent laboratory exposures associated with a puppy, New York city. *Zoonoses and Public Health* 62(5), 407–414.
Deol, A.K., Fleming, F.M., Calvo-Urbano, B., Walker, M., Bucumi, V. *et al.* (2019) *Schistosomiasis*—Assessing progress toward the 2020 and 2025 global goals. *New England Journal of Medicine* 381(26), 2519–2528.
Deplazes, P., Eichenberger, R.M. and Grimm, F. (2019) Wildlife-transmitted *Taenia* and *Versteria cysticercosis* and *coenurosis* in humans and other primates. *International Journal for Parasitology: Parasites and Wildlife* 9, 342–358.
DeWitte, S.N. (2014) Mortality risk and survival in the aftermath of the medieval black death. *PLoS One* 9(5), e96513.
Diaz, J.H. (2013) Paragonimiasis acquired in the United States: Native and nonnative species. *Clinical Microbiology Reviews* 26(3), 493–504.
Diaz, J.H. (2015) *Gnathostomiasis*: An emerging infection of raw fish consumers in gnathostoma nematode-endemic and nonendemic countries. *Journal of Travel Medicine* 22(5), 318–324.
Dilegge, S.K., Edgcomb, V.P. and Leadbetter, E.R. (2011) Presence of the oral bacterium *Capnocytophaga canimorsus* in the tooth plaque of canines. *Veterinary Microbiology* 149(3–4), 437–445.
Disease WHOECotCoC, WHO (1991) Control of Chagas disease. Technical report series 811.
Dixon, B.R. (2021) *Giardia duodenalis* in humans and animals—Transmission and disease. *Research in Veterinary Science* 135, 283–289.
Dogan, C., Gayaf, M., Ozsoz, A., Sahin, B., Aksel, N. *et al.* (2014) Pulmonary *Strongyloides stercoralis* infection. *Respiratory Medicine Case Reports* 11, 12–15.
doVale, B., Lopes, A.P., da Conceição Fontes, M., Silvestre, M., Cardoso, L. *et al.* (2019) Thelaziosis due to *Thelazia callipaeda* in Europe in the 21st century—A review. *Veterinary Parasitology* 275, 108957.
Dove, W.E. (1932) Further studies on *Ancylostoma braziliense* and the etiology of creeping eruption. *American Journal of Epidemiology* 15(3), 664–711.
Drake, D.A., Carreño, A.D., Blagburn, B.L., Little, S.E., West, M.D. *et al.* (2008) Proliferative sparganosis in a dog. *Journal of the American Veterinary Medical Association* 233(11), 1756–1760.
Dubey, J.P. (1978) Patent *Toxocara canis* infection in ascarid-naive dogs. *The Journal of Parasitology* 64(6), 1021–1023.
Dubey, J.P., Murata, F.H.A., Cerqueira-Cézar, C.K., Kwok, O.C.H., Yang, Y. *et al.* (2020) *Toxoplasma gondii* infections in dogs: 2009–2020. *Veterinary Parasitology* 287, 109223.
Dunn, J.J., Columbus, S.T., Aldeen, W.E., Davis, M. and Carroll, K.C. (2002) *Trichuris vulpis* recovered from a patient with chronic diarrhea and five dogs. *Journal of Clinical Microbiology* 40(7), 2703–2704.
Duthie, M.S., Lison, A. and Courtenay, O. (2018) Advances toward diagnostic tools for managing zoonotic visceral leishmaniasis. *Trends in Parasitology* 34(10), 881–890.
Elhamiani Khatat, S., Daminet, S., Kachani, M., Leutenegger, C.M., Duchateau, L. *et al.* (2017) *Anaplasma spp.* in dogs and owners in North-Western Morocco. *Parasites & Vectors* 10(1), 202.
Else, H. (2020) Can dogs smell COVID? Here's what the science says. *Nature* 587(7835), 530–531.

Elshazly, A.M., Elsheikha, H.M., Rahbar, M.H. and Awad, S.I. (2008) Comparison of three immunodiagnostic tests for experimental Heterophyes heterophyes infection in dogs. *Veterinary Parasitology* 151(2–4), 196–202.

Fahrion, A.S., Staebler, S. and Deplazes, P. (2008) Patent *Toxocara canis* infections in previously exposed and in helminth-free dogs after infection with low numbers of embryonated eggs. *Veterinary Parasitology* 152(1–2), 108–115.

Foil, C.S. (1998) Dermatophytosis. In: Greene, C.E. (ed.) *Infectious Diseases of the Dog and Cat*, 2nd ed. W.B. Saunders Company, Philadelphia.

Fontes-Sousa, A.P., Silvestre-Ferreira, A.C., Carretón, E., Esteves-Guimarães, J., Maia-Rocha, C. *et al.* (2019) Exposure of humans to the zoonotic nematode *Dirofilaria immitis* in Northern Portugal. *Epidemiology and Infection* 147, e282.

Fox, J.G. and Lee, A. (1997) The role of *Helicobacter* species in newly recognized gastrointestinal tract diseases of animals. *Laboratory Animal Science* 47(3), 222–255.

Fox, J.G. (1998) Campylobacter infections. In: Greene, C.E. (ed.) *Infectious Diseases of the Dog and Cat*, 2nd ed. W.B. Saunders Company, Philadelphia, pp. 226–228.

Franco, J.R., Cecchi, G., Paone, M., Diarra, A., Grout, L. *et al.* (2022) The elimination of human African *Trypanosomiasis*: Achievements in relation to WHO road map targets for 2020. *PLoS Neglected Tropical Diseases* 16(1), e0010047.

Franco-Zetina, M., Adame-Gallegos, J. and Dzul-Rosado, K. (2019) Efectividad de los métodos diagnósticos para la detección de ehrlichiosis monocítica humana y canina. *Revista Chilena de Infectología* 36(5), 650–655.

Fresia, P., Lyra, M.L., Coronado, A. and De Azeredo-Espin, A.M. (2011) Genetic structure and demographic history of new world screwworm across its current geographic range. *Journal of Medical Entomology* 48(2), 280–290.

Furst, T., Keiser, J. and Utzinger, J. (2012) Global burden of human food-borne trematodiasis: A systematic review and meta-analysis. *Lancet Infectious Diseases* 12(3), 210–221.

Galpérine, T., Cazorla, C., Blanchard, E., Boineau, F., Ragnaud, J.-M. *et al.* (2007) *Streptococcus canis* infections in humans: Retrospective study of 54 patients. *Journal of Infection* 55(1), 23–26.

García-Agudo, L., García-Martos, P., Rodríguez-Iglesias, M. (2014) *Dipylidium caninum* infection in an infant: A rare case report and literature review. *Asian Pacific Journal of Tropical Biomedicine* 4:S565–S7.

Gettings, J.R., Self, S.C.W., McMahan, C.S., Brown, D.A., Nordone, S.K. *et al.* (2020) Local and regional temporal trends (2013–2019) of canine *Ehrlichia* spp. seroprevalence in the USA. *Parasites & Vectors* 13(1), 153.

Gibson, W. (2002) Will the real *Trypanosoma brucei rhodesiense* please step forward. *Trends in Parasitology* 18(11), 486–490.

Gidding, H.F., Wallace, C., Lawrence, G.L. and McIntyre, P.B. (2009) Australia's national Q fever vaccination program. *Vaccine* 27(14), 2037–2041.

Gilbert, A., Johnson, S., Walker, N., Wickham, C., Beath, A. *et al.* (2018) Efficacy of ontario rabies vaccine baits (ONRAB) against rabies infection in raccoons. *Vaccine* 36(32), 4919–4926.

Gong, Q.-L., Ge, G.-Y., Wang, Q., Tian, T., Liu, F. *et al.* (2021) Meta-analysis of the prevalence of echinococcus in dogs in China from 2010 to 2019. *PLoS Neglected Tropical Diseases* 15(4), e0009268.

Goodnow, R.A. (1980) Biology of *Bordetella bronchiseptica*. *Microbiological Reviews* 44(4), 722–738.

Gossner, C.M., Mailles, A., Aznar, I., Dimina, E., Echevarría, J.E. *et al.* (2020) Prevention of human rabies: A challenge for the European Union and the European Economic Area. *Eurosurveillance* 25(38), 2000158.

Gow, A.G., Simpson, J.W. and Picozzi, K. (2007) First report of canine *African Trypanosomosis* in the UK. *Journal of Small Animal Practice* 48(11), 658–661.

Grech-Angelini, S., Richomme, C., Peytavin de Garam, C., Boucher, J.-M., Maestrini, O. *et al.* (2019) Identification and molecular characterization of *Echinococcus canadensis* G6/7 in dogs from Corsica, France. *Parasitology Research* 118(4), 1313–1319.

Greene, C.E. and Gunn-Moore, D.A. (1998) Tuberculous mycobacterial infections. In: *Infectiouse Diseases of the Dog and Cat*. W.B. Saunders Company, Philadelphia, pp. 313–321.

Greene, C.E. and Dreesen, D.W. (1998) Rabies. In: Greene, C.E. (ed.) *Infectious Diseases of the Dog and Cat*, 2nd ed. W.B. Saunders Company, Philadelphia.

Greene, C.E., Goldstein, E.J.C. and Wright, J.C. (1998) Bite wound infections. In: Greene, C.E. (ed.) *Infectious Diseases of the Dog and Cat*, 2nd ed. W.B. Saunders Company, Philadelphia.

Greene, C.E. and Breitschwerdt, E.B. (1998) Rocky mountain spotted fever. In: Greene, C.E. (ed.) *Infectious Diseases of the Dog and Cat*, 2nd ed. W.B. Saunders Company, Philadelphia, pp. 155–165.

Grinnage-Pulley, T., Scott, B. and Petersen, C.A. (2016) A mother's gift: Congenital transmission of *Trypanosoma* and *Leishmania* species. *PLoS Pathogens* 12(1), e1005302.

Guagliardo, S.A.J., Roy, S.L., Ruiz-Tiben, E., Zirimwabagabo, H., Romero, M. *et al.* (2020) Guinea worm in domestic dogs in Chad: A description and analysis of surveillance data. *PLoS Neglected Tropical Diseases* 14(5), e0008207.

Hacker, E., Antunes, C.A., Mattos-Guaraldi, A.L., Burkovski, A. and Tauch, A. (2016) *Corynebacterium ulcerans*, an emerging human pathogen. *Future Microbiology* 11(9), 1191–1208.

Hackner, K. and Pleil, J. (2017) Canine olfaction as an alternative to analytical instruments for disease diagnosis: Understanding 'dog personality' to achieve reproducible results. *Journal of Breath Research* 11(1), 012001.

Hald, B. and Madsen, M. (1997) Healthy puppies and kittens as carriers of *Campylobacter* spp., with special reference to *Campylobacter upsaliensis*. *Journal of Clinical Microbiology* 35(12), 3351–3352.

Hampel, V., Knaus, M., Schäfer, J., Beugnet, F., Rehbein, S. (2018) Treatment of canine sarcoptic mange with afoxolaner (NexGard®) and afoxolaner plus milbemycin oxime (NexGard Spectra®) chewable tablets: Efficacy under field conditions in Portugal and Germany. *Parasite* 25:63.

Hampson, K., Coudeville, L., Lembo, T., Sambo, M., Kieffer, A. *et al.* (2015) Estimating the global burden of endemic canine rabies. *PLoS Neglected Tropical Diseases* 9(4), e0003709.

Hansmann, Y., Jaulhac, B., Kieffer, P., Martinot, M., Wurtz, E. *et al.* (2019) Value of PCR, serology, and blood smears for human *Granulocytic anaplasmosis* diagnosis, France. *Emerging Infectious Diseases* 25(5), 996–998.

Harvell, C.D., Mitchell, C.E., Ward, J.R., Altizer, S., Dobson, A.P. *et al.* (2002) Climate warming and disease risks for terrestrial and marine biota. *Science* 296(5576), 2158–2162.

Harvey, J.W., Simpson, C.F. and Gaskin, J.M. (1978) Cyclic thrombocytopenia induced by a *Rickettsia*-like agent in dogs. *Journal of Infectious Diseases* 137(2), 182–188.

Hay, R.J. (2017) *Tinea capitis*: Current status. *Mycopathologia* 182(1–2), 87–93.

Hennebelle, J.H., Sykes, J.E. and Foley, J. (2014) Risk factors associated with *Leptospirosis* in dogs from Northern California: 2001–2010. *Vector-Borne and Zoonotic Diseases* 14(10), 733–739.

Herrin, B.H., Peregrine, A.S., Goring, J., Beall, M.J. and Little, S.E. (2017) Canine infection with *Borrelia burgdorferi*, *Dirofilaria immitis*, *Anaplasma* spp. and *Ehrlichia* spp. in Canada, 2013–2014. *Parasites & Vectors* 10(1), 244.

Hong, Q., Feng, J., Liu, H., Li, X., Gong, L. *et al.* (2016) Prevalence of *Spirometra mansoni* in dogs, cats, and frogs and its medical relevance in Guangzhou, China. *International Journal of Infectious Diseases* 53, 41–45.

Hovius, E., de Bruin, A., Schouls, L., Hovius, J., Dekker, N. *et al.* (2018) A lifelong study of a pack rhodesian ridgeback dogs reveals subclinical and clinical tick-borne *Anaplasma phagocytophilum* infections with possible reinfection or persistence. *Parasites & Vectors* 11(1), 238.

Howard, E.J., Xiong, X., Carlier, Y., Sosa-Estani, S. and Buekens, P. (2014) Frequency of the congenital transmission of *Trypanosoma cruzi*: A systematic review and meta-analysis. *BJOG: An International Journal of Obstetrics & Gynaecology* 121(1), 22–33.

Hublin, J.S.Y., Maloney, J.G. and Santin, M. (2021) *Blastocystis* in domesticated and wild mammals and birds. *Research in Veterinary Science* 135, 260–282.

Hughes, E.C., Kibona, T.K., de Glanville, W.A., Lankester, F., Davis, A. *et al.* (2019) Taenia multiceps coenurosis in Tanzania: A major and under-recognised livestock disease problem in pastoral communities. *Veterinary Record* 184(6), 191.

Hughes, T., O'Connor, T., Techasen, A., Namwat, N., Loilome, W. *et al.* (2017) *Opisthorchiasis* and *Cholangiocarcinoma* in Southeast Asia: An unresolved problem. *International Journal of General Medicine* 10, 227–237.

Iannino, F., Salucci, S., Di Donato, G. and Badagliacca, P. (2019) Campylobacter and antimicrobial resistance in dogs and humans: "One Health" in practice. *Veterinria Italiana* 55(3), 203–220.

Inpankaew, T., Traub, R., Thompson, A.R.C. and Sukthana, Y. (2007) Canine parasitic zoonoses in Bangkok temples. *Southeast Asian Journal of Tropical Medicine and Public Health* 38(2), 247–255.

Jaleta, T.G., Zhou, S., Bemm, F.M., Schär, F., Khieu, V. *et al.* (2017) Different but overlapping populations of *Strongyloides stercoralis* in dogs and humans—Dogs as a possible source for zoonotic strongyloidiasis. *PLoS Neglected Tropical Diseases* 11(8), e0005752.

Janda, J.M., Graves, M.H., Lindquist, D. and Probert, W.S. (2006) Diagnosing *Capnocytophaga canimorsus* infections. *Emerging Infectious Diseases* 12(2), 340–342.

Jendrny, P., Schulz, C., Twele, F., Meller, S., Köckritz-Blickwede, M. *et al.* (2020) Scent dog identification of samples from COVID-19 patients—A pilot study. *BMC Infectious Diseases* 20(1), 536.

Jenkins, E. (2017) *Echinococcus* spp. tapeworms in dogs and cats. *Clinician's Brief*. Available at: https://www.cliniciansbrief.com/article/echinococcus-spp-tapeworms-dogs-cats

Jiang, P., Zhang, X., Liu, R.D., Wang, Z.Q. and Cui, J. (2017) A human case of zoonotic dog tapeworm, *Dipylidium caninum* (Eucestoda: Dilepidiidae), in China. *The Korean Journal of Parasitology* 55(1), 61–64.

Jimenez Castro, P.D., Howell, S.B., Schaefer, J.J., Avramenko, R.W., Gilleard, J.S. *et al.* (2019) Multiple drug resistance in the canine hookworm *Ancylostoma caninum*: An emerging threat. *Parasites & Vectors* 12(1), 576.

Karama, M., Cenci-Goga, B.T., Prosperi, A., Etter, E., El-Ashram, S. *et al.* (2019) Prevalence and risk factors associated with *Campylobacter* spp. occurrence in healthy dogs visiting four rural community veterinary clinics in South Africa. *Onderstepoort Journal of Veterinary Research* 86(1), 1673.

Karpagam, K.B. and Ganesh, B. (2020) *Leptospirosis*: A neglected tropical zoonotic infection of public health importance—An updated review. *European Journal of Clinical Microbiology & Infectious Diseases* 39(5), 835–846.

Kasstan, B., Hampshire, K., Guest, C., Logan, J.G., Pinder, M. *et al.* (2019) Sniff and tell: The feasibility of using bio-detection dogs as a mobile diagnostic intervention for asymptomatic malaria in sub-Saharan Africa. *Journal of Biosocial Science* 51(3), 436–443.

Kauffman, L.K., Bjork, J.K., Gallup, J.M., Boggiatto, P.M., Bellaire, B.H. *et al.* (2014) Early detection of brucella canis via quantitative polymerase chain reaction analysis. *Zoonoses and Public Health* 61(1), 48–54.

Keid, L.B., Soares, R.M., Vasconcellos, S.A., Chiebao, D.P., Salgado, V.R. *et al.* (2007) A polymerase chain reaction for detection of *Brucella canis* in vaginal swabs of naturally infected bitches. *Theriogenology* 68(9), 1260–1270.

Keiser, J. and Utzinger J. Emerging foodborne trematodiasis. *Emerging Infectious Diseases* 2005;11(10): 1507–14.

Khalil, I.A., Troeger, C., Rao, P.C., Blacker, B.F., Brown, A. *et al.* (2018) Morbidity, mortality, and long-term consequences associated with diarrhoea from *Cryptosporidium* infection in children younger than 5 years: A meta-analyses study. *The Lancet Global Health* 6(7), e758–e768.

Khuntikeo, N., Titapun, A., Loilome, W., Yongvanit, P., Thinkhamrop, B. *et al.* (2018) Current perspectives on opisthorchiasis control and cholangiocarcinoma detection in Southeast Asia. *Frontiers in Medicine* 5, 117.

Kikuchi, T. and Maruyama, H. (2020) Human proliferative sparganosis update. *Parasitology International* 75, 102036.

King, C.H. and Bertsch, D. (2015) Historical perspective: Snail control to prevent *Schistosomiasis*. *PLoS Neglected Tropical Diseases* 9(4), e0003657.

Kirino, Y., Nakano, N., Doanh, P.N., Nawa, Y. and Horii, Y. (2009) A seroepidemiological survey for paragonimosis among boar-hunting dogs in central and southern Kyushu, Japan. *Veterinary Parasitology* 161(3–4), 335–338.

Kmieciak, W. and Szewczyk, E.M. (2018) Are zoonotic *Staphylococcus pseudintermedius* strains a growing threat for humans? *Folia Microbiologica* 63(6), 743–747.

Kogan, L.R., Hellyer, P.W. and Rishniw, M. (2021) American and Canadian veterinarians' perceptions on dog and cat core vaccination rates and the impact of the human medicine anti-vaxx movement on veterinary medicine. *The Canadian Veterinary Journal (La Revue Veterinaire Canadienne)* 62(3), 247–252.

Kramer, L., Crosara, S., Gnudi, G., Genchi, M., Mangia, C. *et al.* (2018) Wolbachia, doxycycline and macrocyclic lactones: New prospects in the treatment of canine heartworm disease. *Veterinary Parasitology* 254, 95–97.

Krupka, I. and Straubinger, R.K. (2010) *Lyme borreliosis* in dogs and cats: Background, diagnosis, treatment and prevention of infections with *Borrelia burgdorferi* sensu stricto. *Veterinary Clinics of North America: Small Animal Practice* 40(6), 1103–1119.

Kuchta, R., Brabec, J., Kubáčková, P. and Scholz, T. (2013) Tapeworm *Diphyllobothrium dendriticum* (Cestoda)—neglected or emerging human parasite? *PLoS Neglected Tropical Diseases* 7(12), e2535.

Kuroki, K., Morishima, Y., Neil, J., Beerntsen, B.T., Matsumoto, J. *et al.* (2020) Intestinal echinococcosis in a dog from Missouri. *Journal of the American Veterinary Medical Association* 256(9), 1041–1046.

Lahmar, S., Arfa, I., Ben Othmen, S., Jguirim, W., Saïd, Y. *et al.* (2017) Intestinal helminths of stray dogs from Tunisia with special reference to zoonotic infections. *Parasitology Open* 3, e18.

Lalošević, D., Lalošević, V., Simin, V., Miljević, M., Čabrilo, B. *et al.* (2016) Spreading of multilocular *Echinococcosis* in Southern Europe: The first record in foxes and jackals in Serbia, Vojvodina province. *European Journal of Wildlife Research* 62(6), 793–796.

Lamm, C.G., Ferguson, A.C., Lehenbauer, T.W. and Love, B.C. (2010) Streptococcal infection in dogs. *Veterinary Pathology* 47(3), 387–395.

Lederman, Z., Leskes, H. and Brosh-Nissimov, T. (2020) One health and *Streptococcus canis* in the emergency department: A case of cellulitis and bacteremia in an immunocompromised patient treated with etanercept. *The Journal of Emergency Medicine* 58(3), e129–e132.

Lee, A.C.Y., Montgomery, S.P., Theis, J.H., Blagburn, B.L. and Eberhard, M.L. (2010) Public health issues concerning the widespread distribution of canine heartworm disease. *Trends in Parasitology* 26(4), 168–173.

Lee, S.H., Park, H. and Yu, S.T. (2015) *Diphyllobothrium latum* infection in a child with recurrent abdominal pain. *Korean Journal of Pediatrics* 58(11), 451.

Lembo, T., Niezgoda, M., Velasco-Villa, A., Cleaveland, S., Ernest, E. *et al.* (2006) Evaluation of a direct, rapid immunohistochemical test for rabies diagnosis. *Emerging Infectious Diseases* 12(2), 310–313.

Lembo, T., Hampson, K., Auty, H., Beesley, C.A., Bessell, P. *et al.* (2011) Serologic surveillance of anthrax in the Serengeti ecosystem, Tanzania, 1996–2009. *Emerging Infectious Diseases* 17(3), 387–394.

Lembo, T., Craig, P.S., Miles, M.A., Hampson, K.R. and Meslin, F.X. (2013) Zoonoses prevention, control and elimination in dogs. In: Macpherson, C.N.L., Meslin, F.X. and Wandeler, A.I. (eds) *Dogs, Zoonoses and Public Health*, 2nd ed. CAB International, CPI Group (K) Ltd, Croydon, pp. 205–258.

Lescano, A.G. and Zunt, J. (2013) Chapter 27—other cestodes: *Sparganosis*, *Coenurosis* and *Taenia crassiceps* cysticercosis. In: Garcia, H.H., Tanowitz, H.B. and Del Brutto, O.H. (eds) *Handbook of Clinical Neurology*, Vol. 114. pp. 335–345.

Levin, M.L., Killmaster, L.F. and Zemtsova, G.E. (2012) Domestic dogs (*Canis familiaris*) as reservoir hosts for *Rickettsia conorii*. *Vector-Borne and Zoonotic Diseases* 12(1), 28–33.

Levin, M.L., Killmaster, L.F., Zemtsova, G.E., Ritter, J.M. and Langham, G. (2014) Clinical presentation, convalescence, and relapse of rocky mountain spotted fever in dogs experimentally infected via tick bite. *PLoS One* 9(12), e115105.

Lewnard, J.A. and Townsend, J.P. (2016) Climatic and evolutionary drivers of phase shifts in the plague epidemics of colonial India. *Proceedings of the National Academy of Sciences* 113(51), 14601–14608.

Liao, S., Lin, X., Sun, Y., Qi, N., Lv, M. *et al.* (2020) Occurrence and genotypes of *Cryptosporidium* spp., *Giardia duodenalis*, and *Blastocystis* sp. in household, shelter, breeding, and pet market dogs in Guangzhou, Southern China. *Scientific Reports* 10(1), 17736.

Liccioli, S., Giraudoux, P., Deplazes, P. and Massolo, A. (2015) Wilderness in the 'city' revisited: Different urbes shape transmission of *Echinococcus multilocularis* by altering predator and prey communities. *Trends in Parasitology* 31(7), 297–305.

Lin, R., Li, X., Lan, C., Yu, S. and Kawanaka, M. (2005) Investigation on the epidemiological factors of *Clonorchis sinensis* infection in an area of South China. *Southeast Asian Journal of Trop Med Public Health* 36, 1114–1117.

Lin, R.-Q., Tang, J.-D., Zhou, D.-H., Song, H.-Q., Huang, S.-Y. *et al.* (2011) Prevalence of infection in dogs and cats in subtropical Southern China. *Parasites & Vectors* 4(1), 180.

Lin, W.-R., Chen, Y.-S. and Liu, Y.-C. (2007) Cellulitis and bacteremia caused by *Bergeyella zoohelcum*. *Journal of the Formosan Medical Association* 106(7), 573–576.

Littman, M.P., Gerber, B., Goldstein, R.E., Labato, M.A., Lappin, M.R. *et al.* (2018) ACVIM consensus update on *Lyme borreliosis* in dogs and cats. *Journal of Veterinary Internal Medicine* 32(3), 887–903.

Liu, G.-H., Sun, M.-M., Elsheikha, H.M., Fu, Y.-T., Sugiyama, H. *et al.* (2020) Human *Gnathostomiasis*: A neglected food-borne zoonosis. *Parasites & Vectors* 13(1), 616.

Liu, Q., Li, M.-W., Wang, Z.-D., Zhao, G.-H. and Zhu, X.-Q. (2015) Human sparganosis, a neglected food borne zoonosis. *The Lancet Infectious Diseases* 15(10), 1226–1235.

Lloyd, S., Amerasinghe, P.H. and Soulsby, E.J.L. (1983) Periparturient immunosuppression in the bitch and its influence on infection with *Toxocara canis*. *Journal of Small Animal Practice* 24(4), 237–247.

Loker, E.S., Dolginow, S.Z., Pape, S., Topper, C.D., Alda, P. *et al.* (2021) An outbreak of canine schistosomiasis in utah: Acquisition of a new snail host (*Galba humilis*) by *Heterobilharzia americana*, a pathogenic parasite on the move. *One Health* 13, 100280.

Lucero, N.E., Corazza, R., Almuzara, M.N., Reynes, E., Escobar, G.I. *et al.* (2010) Human *Brucella canis* outbreak linked to infection in dogs. *Epidemiology and Infection* 138(2), 280–285.

Lucio-Forster, A., Griffiths, J.K., Cama, V.A., Xiao, L. and Bowman, D.D. (2010) Minimal zoonotic risk of cryptosporidiosis from pet dogs and cats. *Trends in Parasitology* 26(4), 174–179.

Lucio-Forster, A., Liotta, J.L., Yaros, J.P., Briggs, K.R., Mohammed, H.O. *et al.* (2012) Morphological differentiation of eggs of *Ancylostoma caninum*, *Ancylostoma tubaeforme*, and *Ancylostoma braziliense* from dogs and cats in the United States. *Journal of Parasitology* 98(5), 1041–1044.

Ma, G., Holland, C.V., Wang, T., Hofmann, A., Fan, C.-K. *et al.* (2018) Human toxocariasis. *The Lancet Infectious Diseases* 18(1), e14–e24.

Ma, G.C., Norris, J.M., Mathews, K.O., Chandra, S., Šlapeta, J. *et al.* (2020) New insights on the epidemiology of *Coxiella burnetii* in pet dogs and cats from New South Wales, Australia. *Acta Tropica* 205, 105416.

Ma, X., Monroe, B.P., Cleaton, J.M., Orciari, L.A., Li, Y. *et al.* (2018) Rabies surveillance in the United States during 2017. *Journal of the American Veterinary Medical Association* 253(12), 1555–1568.

Macpherson, C.N.L. (2005) Human behaviour and the epidemiology of parasitic zoonoses. *International Journal for Parasitology* 35(11–12), 1319–1331.

Macpherson, C.N.L. (2013) Dog zoonoses and human health: A global perspective—mini review. *CAB Reviews: Perspectives in Agriculture, Veterinary Science, Nutrition and Natural Resources* 8(2).

Macpherson, C.N.L., Meslin, F.X. and Dogs, W.A.I. (2013) *Zoonoses and Public Health*, 2nd ed. CAB International, Washington, DC.

Mader, N., Lührs, F., Langenbeck, M. and Herget-Rosenthal, S. (2020) *Capnocytophaga canimorsus*—A potent pathogen in immunocompetent humans—systematic review and retrospective observational study of case reports. *Infectious Diseases* 52(2), 65–74.

Maerz, I. (2020) Clinical and diagnostic imaging findings in 37 rescued dogs with heartworm disease in Germany. *Veterinary Parasitology* 283, 109156.

Magnarelli, L.A., Anderson, J.F., Schreier, A.B. and Ficke, C.M. (1987) Clinical and serologic studies of *Canine borreliosis*. *Journal of American Veterinary Medicine Association* 191, 1089–1094.

Maia, C. and Campino, L. (2018) Biomarkers associated with *Leishmania infantum* exposure, infection, and disease in dogs. *Frontiers in Cellular and Infection Microbiology* 8, 302.

Malele, I.I., Nyingilili, H.S., Malulu, D.J., Ouma, J.O., Kitwika, W.A. *et al.* (2016) Comparative performance of traps in catching tsetse flies (Diptera: Glossinidae) in Tanzania: Original research. *Onderstepoort Journal of Veterinary Research* 83(1), 1057.

Malvy, D. and Chappuis, F. (2011) Sleeping sickness. *Clinical Microbiology and Infection* 17(7), 986–995.

Manhardt, J. and Stoye, M. (1981) Behavior of *Toxocara canis* werner 1782 (*Anisakidae*) larvae during and following lung migration in the definitive host (Beagle). *Zentralblatt Fur Veterinarmedizin Reihe B (Journal of Veterinary Medicine Series B)* 28(5), 386–406.

Marchiondo, A.A., Holdsworth, P.A., Fourie, L.J., Rugg, D., Hellmann, K. *et al.* (2013) World Association for the Advancement of Veterinary Parasitology (W.A.A.V.P.) second edition: Guidelines for evaluating the efficacy of parasiticides for the treatment, prevention and control of flea and tick infestations on dogs and cats. *Veterinary Parasitology* 194(1), 84–97.

Massetti, L., Colella, V., Zendejas, P.A., Ng-Nguyen, D., Harriott, L. *et al.* (2020) High-throughput multiplex qPCRs for the surveillance of zoonotic species of canine hookworms. *PLoS Neglected Tropical Diseases* 14(6), e0008392.

Massolo, A., Valli, D., Wassermann, M., Cavallero, S., D'Amelio, S. *et al.* (2018) Unexpected *Echinococcus multilocularis* infections in shepherd dogs and wolves in south-western Italian alps: A new endemic area. *International Journal for Parasitology: Parasites and Wildlife* 7(3), 309–316.

Mathison, B.A., Bradbury, R.S. and Pritt, B.S. (2021) Medical parasitology taxonomy update january 2018 to may 2020. *Journal of Clinical Microbiology* 59(2), e01308–20.

Mattei, A.S., Beber, M.A. and Madrid, I.M. (2014) Dermatophytosis in small animals. *SOJ Microbiology & Infectious Diseases* 2(3), 1–6.

McDonald, R.A., Wilson-Aggarwal, J.K., Swan, G.J.F., Goodwin, C.E.D., Moundai, T. *et al.* (2020) Ecology of domestic dogs *Canis familiaris* as an emerging reservoir of Guinea worm *Dracunculus medinensis* infection. *PLoS Neglected Tropical Diseases* 14(4), e0008170.

McGill, J.L., Nair, A.D.S., Cheng, C., Rusk, R.A., Jaworski, D.C. *et al.* (2016) Vaccination with an attenuated mutant of *Ehrlichia chaffeensis* induces pathogen-specific CD4+ t cell immunity and protection from tick-transmitted wild-type challenge in the canine host. *PLoS One* 11(2), e0148229.

McManus, D.P., Dunne, D.W., Sacko, M., Utzinger, J., Vennervald, B.J. *et al.* (2018) *Schistosomiasis. Nature Reviews Disease Primers* 4(1), 13.

McManus, D.P., Bergquist, R., Cai, P., Ranasinghe, S., Tebeje, B.M. *et al.* (2020) *Schistosomiasis*—From immunopathology to vaccines. *Seminars in Immunopathology* 42(3), 355–371.

Mead, P.S. (2015) Epidemiology of lyme disease. *Infectious Disease Clinics of North America* 29(2), 187–210.

Meyers, A.C., Ellis, M.M., Purnell, J.C., Auckland, L.D., Meinders, M. *et al.* (2020) Selected cardiac abnormalities in *Trypanosoma cruzi* serologically positive, discordant, and negative working dogs along the Texas-Mexico border. *BMC Veterinary Research* 16(1), 101.

Minghui, R., Stone, M., Semedo, M.H. and Nel, L. (2018) New global strategic plan to eliminate dog-mediated rabies by 2030. *The Lancet Global Health* 6(8), e828–e829.

Miotto, B.A., Guilloux, A.G.A., Tozzi, B.F., Moreno, L.Z., da Hora, A.S. *et al.* (2018) Prospective study of canine leptospirosis in shelter and stray dog populations: Identification of chronic carriers and different *Leptospira* species infecting dogs. *PLoS One* 13(7), e0200384.

Molehin, A.J. (2020) *Schistosomiasis* vaccine development: Update on human clinical trials. *Journal of Biomedical Science* 27(1), 28.

Moore, S.M. (2021) Challenges of rabies serology: Defining context of interpretation. *Viruses* 13(8), 1516.

Mor, S.M., Wiethoelter, A.K., Lee, A., Moloney, B., James, D.R. *et al.* (2016) Emergence of *Brucella suis* in dogs in new South Wales, Australia: Clinical findings and implications for zoonotic transmission. *BMC Veterinary Research* 12(1), 199.

Muhsen, K. and Levine, M.M. (2012) A systematic review and meta-analysis of the association between *Giardia lamblia* and endemic pediatric diarrhea in developing countries. *Clinical Infectious Diseases* 55(suppl_4), S271–S293.

Mukarati, N.L., Ndumnego, O., van Heerden, H., Ndhlovu, D.N., Matope, G. *et al.* (2018) A serological survey of anthrax in domestic dogs in Zimbabwe: A potential tool for anthrax surveillance. *Epidemiology and Infection* 146(12), 1526–1532.

Muramatsu, Y., Haraya, N., Horie, K., Uchida, L., Kooriyama, T. *et al.* (2019) Bergeyella zoohelcum isolated from oral cavities of therapy dogs. *Zoonoses and Public Health* 66(8), 936–942.

Mylonakis, M.E. and Theodorou, K.N. (2017) Canine monocytic ehrlichiosis: An update on diagnosis and treatment. *Acta Veterinaria* 67(3), 299–317.

Neer, T.M. (1998) Canine monocytic and granulocytic ehrlichiosis. In: Greene, C.E. (ed.) *Infectious Diseases of the Dog and Cat*, 2nd ed. W.B. Saunders Company, Philadelphia, pp. 139–147.

Ngcamphalala, P.I., Lamb, J. and Mukaratirwa, S. (2020) Molecular identification of hookworm isolates from stray dogs, humans and selected wildlife from South Africa. *Journal of Helminthology* 94, e39.

Ng-Nguyen, D., Hii, S.F., Hoang, M.T.T., Nguyen, V.A.T., Rees, R. *et al.* (2020) Domestic dogs are mammalian reservoirs for the emerging zoonosis flea-borne spotted fever, caused by *Rickettsia felis*. *Scientific Reports* 10(1), 4151.

Ngui, R., Lim, Y.A.L., Traub, R., Mahmud, R. and Mistam, M.S. (2012) Epidemiological and genetic data supporting the transmission of *Ancylostoma ceylanicum* among human and domestic animals. *PLoS Neglected Tropical Diseases* 6(2), e1522.

Ni, J., Lin, H., Xu, X., Ren, Q., Aizezi, M. *et al.* (2020) *Coxiella burnetii* is widespread in ticks (ixodidae) in the Xinjiang areas of China. *BMC Veterinary Research* 16(1), 317.

Nichols, M.C., Ettestad, P.J., VinHatton, E.S., Melman, S.D., Onischuk, L. *et al.* (2014) *Yersinia pestis* infection in dogs: 62 cases (2003– 2011). *Journal of the American Veterinary Medical Association* 244(10), 1176–1180.

Nutman, T.B. (2017) Human infection with *Strongyloides stercoralis* and other related strongyloides species. *Parasitology* 144(3), 263–273.

Oba, P., Ejobi, F., Omadang, L., Chamai, M., Okwi, A.L. *et al.* (2016) Prevalence and risk factors of *Echinococcus granulosus* infection in dogs in Moroto and Bukedea districts in Uganda. *Tropical Animal Health and Production* 48(2), 249–254.

Öge, H., Öge, S., Gönenç, B., Sarımehmetoğlu, O. and Özbakış, G. (2017) Coprodiagnosis of *Echinococcus granulosus* infection in dogs from Ankara, Turkey. *Veterinary Parasitology* 242, 44–46.

Orloski, K.A. and Lathrop, S.L. (2003) Plague: A veterinary perspective. *Journal of the American Veterinary Medical Association* 222(4), 444–448.

Otsuji, K., Fukuda, K., Endo, T., Shimizu, S., Harayama, N. *et al.* (2017) The first fatal case of *Corynebacterium ulcerans* infection in Japan. *JMM Case Reports* 4(8), e005106.

Ouma, J.H. and Fenwick, A. (1991) Animal reservoirs of *Schistosomiasis*. In: Macpherson, C.N.L. and Craig, P.S. (eds) *Parasitic Helminths and Zoonoses in Africa*. Unwin Hyman Ltd, London, pp. 224–233.

Overgaauw, P.A.M., Okkens, A.C., Bevers, M.M. and Kortbeek, L.M. (1998) Incidence of patent *Toxocara canis* infection in bitches during the oestrous cycle. *Veterinary Quarterly* 20(3), 104–107.

Palmer, C.S., Traub, R.J., Robertson, I.D., Devlin, G., Rees, R. *et al.* (2008) Determining the zoonotic significance of *Giardia* and *Cryptosporidium* in Australian dogs and cats. *Veterinary Parasitology* 154(1–2), 142–147.

Pampiglione, S., Vakalis, N., Lyssimachou, A., Kouppari, G. and Orihel, T.C. (2001) Subconjunctival zoonotic *Onchocerca* in an Albanian man. *Annals of Tropical Medicine and Parasitology* 95(8), 827–832.

Pan-American Health Organisation (2020) Chagas disease, Fact Sheets. Available at: https://www.paho.org/en/topics/chagas-disease

Parsonnet, J., Friedman, G.D., Vandersteen, D.P., Chang, Y., Vogelman, J.H. *et al.* (1991) *Helicobacter pylori* infection and the risk of gastric carcinoma. *New England Journal of Medicine* 325(16), 1127–1131.

Parsons, B.N., Williams, N.J., Pinchbeck, G.L., Christley, R.M., Hart, C.A. *et al.* (2011) Prevalence and shedding patterns of *Campylobacter* spp. in longitudinal studies of kennelled dogs. *The Veterinary Journal* 190(2), 249–254.

Pasquetti, M., Min, A., Scacchetti, S., Dogliero, A. and Peano, A. (2017) Infection by *Microsporum canis* in paediatric patients: A veterinary perspective. *Veterinary Sciences* 4(4), 46.

Patterson, E.I., Elia, G., Grassi, A., Giordano, A., Desario, C. *et al.* (2020) Evidence of exposure to SARS-cov-2 in cats and dogs from households in Italy. *Nature Communications* 11(1), 6231.

Peng, S.H., Yang, S.L., Ho, Y.N., Chen, H.F. and Shu, P.Y. (2019) Human case of *Ehrlichia chaffeensis* infection, Taiwan. *Emerging Infectious Diseases* 25(11), 2141–2143.

Perez, M., Bodor, M., Zhang, C., Xiong, Q. and Rikihisa, Y. (2006) Human infection with *Ehrlichia canis* accompanied by clinical signs in Venezuela. *Annals of the New York Academy of Sciences* 1078(1), 110–117.

Pérez-Lago, L., Navarro, Y. and García-de-Viedma, D. (2014) Current knowledge and pending challenges in zoonosis caused by *Mycobacterium bovis*: A review. *Research in Veterinary Science* 97, S94–S100.

Pérez-Molina, J.A. and Molina, I. (2018) Chagas disease. *The Lancet* 391(10115), 82–94.

Petney, T.N., Andrews, R.H., Saijuntha, W., Wenz-Mücke, A. and Sithithaworn, P. (2013) The zoonotic, fish-borne liver flukes *Clonorchis sinensis*, *Opisthorchis felineus* and *Opisthorchis viverrini*. *International Journal for Parasitology* 43(12–13), 1031–1046.

Pinto, P.S., Libonati, H. and Lilenbaum, W. (2017) A systematic review of leptospirosis on dogs, pigs, and horses in Latin America. *Tropical Animal Health and Production* 49(2), 231–238.

Priestnall, S. and Erles, K. (2011) *Streptococcus zooepidemicus*: An emerging canine pathogen. *The Veterinary Journal* 188(2), 142–148.

Procter, T.D., Pearl, D.L., Finley, R.L., Leonard, E.K., Janecko, N. *et al.* (2014) A cross-sectional study examining campylobacter and other zoonotic enteric pathogens in dogs that frequent dog parks in three cities in South-western Ontario and risk factors for shedding of *Campylobacter* spp. *Zoonoses and Public Health* 61(3), 208–218.

Qiao, T., Ma, R.H., Luo, X.B., Luo, Z.L. and Zheng, P.M. (2012) *Cholecystolithiasis* is associated with *Clonorchis sinensis* infection. *PLoS One* 7(8), e42471.

Reagan, K.L. and Sykes, J.E. (2019) Diagnosis of canine *leptospirosis*. *Veterinary Clinics of North America: Small Animal Practice* 49(4), 719–731.

Reimschuessel, R., Grabenstein, M., Guag, J., Nemser, S.M., Song, K. *et al.* (2017) Multilaboratory survey to evaluate *Salmonella* prevalence in diarrheic and nondiarrheic dogs and cats in the United States between 2012 and 2014. *Journal of Clinical Microbiology* 55(5), 1350–1368.

Riehm, J.M., Rahalison, L., Scholz, H.C., Thoma, B., Pfeffer, M. *et al.* (2011) Detection of *Yersinia pestis* using real-time PCR in patients with suspected bubonic plague. *Molecular and Cellular Probes* 25(1), 8–12.
Rim, H.J. (2005) *Clonorchiasis*: An update. *Journal of Helminthology* 79(3), 269–281.
Robardet, E., Bosnjak, D., Englund, L., Demetriou, P., Martín, P.R. *et al.* (2019) Zero endemic cases of wildlife rabies (classical rabies virus, RABV) in the European Union by 2020: An achievable goal. *Tropical Medicine and Infectious Disease* 4(4), 124.
Romig, T., Ebi, D. and Wassermann, M. (2015) Taxonomy and molecular epidemiology of *Echinococcus granulosus* sensu lato. *Veterinary Parasitology* 213(3–4), 76–84.
Rossi, M. and Fasel, N. (2018) How to master the host immune system? *Leishmania* parasites have the solutions! *International Immunology* 30(3), 103–111.
Rostami, A., Riahi, S.M., Holland, C.V., Taghipour, A., Khalili-Fomeshi, M. *et al.* (2019) Seroprevalence estimates for *Toxocariasis* in people worldwide: A systematic review and meta-analysis. *PLoS Neglected Tropical Diseases* 13(12), e0007809.
Rostami, A., Riahi, S.M., Hofmann, A., Ma, G., Wang, T. *et al.* (2020) Global prevalence of *Toxocara* infection in dogs. *Advanced Parasitology* 109, 561–583.
Rust, M.K. (2005) Advances in the control of *Ctenocephalides felis* (cat flea) on cats and dogs. *Trends in Parasitology* 21(5), 232–236.
Ryan, U. and Cacciò, S.M. (2013) Zoonotic potential of *Giardia*. *International Journal for Parasitology* 43(12–13), 943–956.
Sainz, Á., Roura, X., Miró, G., Estrada-Peña, A., Kohn, B. *et al.* (2015) Guideline for veterinary practitioners on *Canine ehrlichiosis* and *Anaplasmosis* in Europe. *Parasites & Vectors* 8(1), 75.
Salib, F.A. and Baraka, T.A. (2011) Epidemiology, genetic divergence and acaricides of *Otodectes cynotis* in cats and dogs. *Veterinary World* 4(3), 109–112.
Sambo, M., Cleaveland, S., Ferguson, H., Lembo, T., Simon, C. *et al.* (2013) The burden of rabies in Tanzania and its impact on local communities. *PLoS Neglected Tropical Diseases* 7(11), e2510.
Samdi, S.M., Abenga, J.N. and Kalgo, A.M. (2008) Trypanosomosis in hunting dogs in Kaduna, north Central Nigeria: Implications on the disease in humans. *Journal of Biomedical Investigation* 4(1), 15–18.
Sandberg, M., Bergsjø, B., Hofshagen, M., Skjerve, E. and Kruse, H. (2002) Risk factors for *Campylobacter* infection in Norwegian cats and dogs. *Preventive Veterinary Medicine* 55(4), 241–253.
Santos, F., Magalhães-Junior, J.T., IdO, C., Santos, F.L.N., Silva, Â.A.O. *et al.* (2022) Eco-epidemiology of vectorial *Trypanosoma cruzi* transmission in a region of northeast Brazil. *Acta Tropica* 225, 106184.
Santos, R.L., Souza, T.D., Mol, J.P.S., Eckstein, C. and Paíxão, T.A. (2021) *Canine brucellosis*: an update. *Frontiers in Veterinary Science* 8, 594291.
Santos, W.S., Gurgel-Gonçalves, R., Garcez, L.M. and Abad-Franch, F. (2021) Deforestation effects on attalea palms and their resident *Rhodnius*, vectors of Chagas disease, in Eastern Amazonia. *PLoS One* 16(5), e0252071.
Sasikala, M., Yogespriya, R., Jayalakshmi, K., Dhivya, B. and Arulkumar, T. (2018) Rare incidence of diphyllobothriosis in a dog. *Indian Veterinary Journal* 95(3), 74–75.
Schnyder, M., Reichler, I.M., Eichenberger, R.M., Hofer-Inteeworn, N., Kümmerle-Fraune, C. *et al.* (2022) *Strongyloides stercoralis* in Swiss dogs—A retrospective study suggests an increasing occurrence of this potentially zoonotic parasite as a consequence of dog imports. *Schweizer Archiv Für Tierheilkunde* 164(1), 89–104.
Scholz, T., Garcia, H.H., Kuchta, R. and Wicht, B. (2009) Update on the human broad tapeworm (genus *Diphyllobothrium*), including clinical relevance. *Clinical Microbiology Reviews* 22(1), 146–160.
Schwartz, R., Bidaisee, S., Fields, P.J., Macpherson, M.L.A. and Macpherson, C.N.L. (2022) The epidemiology and control of *Toxocara canis* in puppies. *Parasite Epidemiology and Control* 16, e00232.
Selim, A., Alanazi, A.D., Sazmand, A. and Otranto, D. (2021) Seroprevalence and associated risk factors for vector-borne pathogens in dogs from Egypt. *Parasites & Vectors* 14(1), 175.
Semenas, L. (2013) Sushi y ceviche: ¿Peligrosamente ricos? *Desde La Patagonia: Difundiendo Saberes* 10, 26–33.
Shapiro, A.J., Norris, J.M., Heller, J., Brown, G., Malik, R. *et al.* (2016) Seroprevalence of *Coxiella burnetii* in Australian dogs. *Zoonoses and Public Health* 63(6), 458–466.
Sharma, K., Wijarnpreecha, K. and Merrell, N. (2018) *Diphyllobothrium latum* mimicking subacute appendicitis. *Gastroenterology Research* 11(3), 235–237.

Shin, H.R., Oh, J.K., Masuyer, E., Curado, M.P., Bouvard, V. *et al.* (2010) Epidemiology of cholangiocarcinoma: An update focusing on risk factors. *Cancer Science* 101(3), 579–585.

Silveria, A.P.S.D, Vieira, V.B.D., Batalini, L.S., SBd, C., Friozi, E. *et al.* (2018) PCR sensitivity of peripheral blood of dogs co-infected with *Leishmania* spp. and *Ehrlichia* spp. in endemic area of Brazil. *Revista Da Sociedade Brasileira de Medicina Tropical* 51(6), 843–847.

Sithithaworn, P., Yongvanit, P., Tesana, S. and Pairojkul, C. (2007) Liver flukes. In: Murrell, K.D. and Fried, B. (eds) *Food Borne Parasitic Zoonoses: Fish and Plant-Borne Parasites*. Springer, New York, pp. 3–52.

Sit, T.H.C., Brackman, C.J., Ip, S.M., Tam, K.W.S., Law, P.Y.T. *et al.* (2020) Infection of dogs with SARS-CoV-2. *Nature* 586(7831), 776–778.

Sivabalan, P., Saboo, A., Yew, J. and Norton, R. (2017) Q fever in an endemic region of north Queensland, Australia: A 10 year review. *One Health* 3, 51–55.

Smith, G. and Schad, G.A. (1989) *Ancylostoma duodenale* and *Necator americanus*: Effect of temperature on egg development and mortality. *Parasitology* 99(Pt 1), 127–132.

Smith, N.C., Goulart, C., Hayward, J.A., Kupz, A., Miller, C.M. *et al.* (2021) Control of human toxoplasmosis. *International Journal for Parasitology* 51(2–3), 95–121.

Solano-Gallego, L., Caprì, A., Pennisi, M.G., Caldin, M., Furlanello, T. *et al.* (2015) Acute febrile illness is associated with *Rickettsia* spp infection in dogs. *Parasites & Vectors* 8(1), 216.

Spear, R., Zhong, B. and Liang, S. (2017) Low transmission to elimination: Rural development as a key determinant of the end-game dynamics of *Schistosoma japonicum* in China. *Tropical Medicine and Infectious Disease* 2(3), 35.

Stark, D., Barratt, J.L.N., van Hal, S., Marriott, D., Harkness, J. *et al.* (2009) Clinical significance of enteric protozoa in the immuno suppressed human population. *Clinical Microbiology Reviews* 22(4), 634–650.

Stenzel, D.J. and Boreham, P.F. (1996) Blastocystis hominis revisited. *Clinical Microbiology Reviews* 9(4), 563–584.

Stief, B. and Enge, A. (2011) Proliferative peritonitis with larval and cystic parasitic stages in a dog. *Veterinary Pathology* 48(4), 911–914.

Stone, W.M. and Girardeau, M. (1968) Transmammary passage of *Ancylostoma caninum* larvae in dogs. *The Journal of Parasitology* 54(3), 426.

Stoye, M. (1976) Galactogenic and prenatal *Toxocara canis* infections in dogs (Beagle). (Brief communication), *Deutsche Tierärztliche Wochenschrift*.

Streit, A. (2021) Strongyloidiasis: Really a zoonosis? In: Strube, C. and Mehlhorn, H. (eds) *Dog Parasites Endangering Human Health*. Springer Cham, Manhattan, New York City, pp. 195–226.

Taghipour, A., Olfatifar, M., Bahadory, S., Godfrey, S.S., Abdoli, A. *et al.* (2020) The global prevalence of *Cryptosporidium* infection in dogs: A systematic review and meta-analysis. *Veterinary Parasitology* 281, 109093.

Talan, D.A., Citron, D.M., Abrahamian, F.M., Moran, G.J. and Goldstein, E.J.C. (1999) Bacteriologic analysis of infected dog and cat bites. *New England Journal of Medicine* 340(2), 85–92.

Tangeman, L.E. and Littman, M.P. (2013) Clinicopathologic and atypical features of naturally occurring leptospirosis in dogs: 51 cases (2000–2010). *Journal of the American Veterinary Medical Association* 243(9), 1316–1322.

Tang, Z.-L., Huang, Y. and Yu, X.-B. (2016) Current status and perspectives of *Clonorchis sinensis* and *clonorchiasis*: Epidemiology, pathogenesis, omics, prevention and control. *Infectious Diseases of Poverty* 5(1), 71.

Taques, I., Barbosa, T.R., Martini, A., Pitchenin, L.C., Braga, Í.A. *et al.* (2016) Molecular assessment of the transplacental transmission of *Toxoplasma gondii*, *Neospora caninum*, *Brucella canis* and *Ehrlichia canis* in dogs. *Comparative Immunology, Microbiology and Infectious Diseases* 49, 47–50.

Thamsborg, S.M., Ketzis, J., Horii, Y. and Matthews, J.B. (2017) *Strongyloides* spp. infections of veterinary importance. *Parasitology* 144(3), 274–284.

The Lancet (2020) Zoonoses: Beyond the human–animal–environment interface. *The Lancet* 396(10243), 1.

Thomas, M. and Feng, Y. (2020) Risk of foodborne illness from pet food: Assessing pet owners' knowledge, behavior, and risk perception. *Journal of Food Protection* 83(11), 1998–2007.

Thompson, R.C.A. (2004) The zoonotic significance and molecular epidemiology of *Giardia* and giardiasis. *Veterinary Parasitology* 126(1–2), 15–35.

Thompson, R.C.A. (2015) Neglected zoonotic helminths: *Hymenolepis nana*, *Echinococcus canadensis* and *Ancylostoma ceylanicum*. *Clinical Microbiology and Infection* 21(5), 426–432.

Toews, E., Musiani, M., Checkley, S., Visscher, D. and Massolo, A. (2021) A global assessment of *Echinococcus multilocularis* infections in domestic dogs: Proposing a framework to overcome past methodological heterogeneity. *International Journal for Parasitology* 51(5), 379–392.

Toor, J., Rollinson, D., Turner, H.C., Gouvras, A., King, C.H. *et al.* (2020) Achieving elimination as a public health problem for *Schistosoma mansoni* and *S. haematobium*: When is community-wide treatment required? *The Journal of Infectious Diseases* 221(Supplement_5), S525–S530.

Torgerson, P.R. and Macpherson, C.N.L. (2011) The socioeconomic burden of parasitic zoonoses: Global trends. *Veterinary Parasitology* 182(1):79–95.

Torres-Guerrero, E., Quintanilla-Cedillo, M.R., Ruiz-Esmenjaud, J. and Arenas, R. (2017) *Leishmaniasis*: A review. *F1000 Research 2017* 6, 750.

Torrico, F., Alonso-Vega, C., Suarez, E., Rodriguez, P., Torrico, M.-C. *et al.* (2004) Maternal *Trypanosoma cruzi* infection, pregnancy outcome, morbidity, and mortality of congenitally infected and non-infected newborns in Bolivia. *The American Journal of Tropical Medicine and Hygiene* 70(2), 201–209.

Townsend, S.E., Sumantra, I.P., Pudijiatmoko, Bagus, G.N., Brum, E. *et al.* (2013) Designing programs for eliminating canine rabies from islands: Bali, Indonesia as a case study. *PLoS Neglected Tropical Diseases* 7(8), e2372.

Travi, B.L. (2019) Considering dogs as complementary targets of chagas disease control. *Vector-Borne and Zoonotic Diseases* 19(2), 90–94.

Troìa, R., Balboni, A., Zamagni, S., Frigo, S., Magna, L. *et al.* (2018) Prospective evaluation of rapid point-of-care tests for the diagnosis of acute leptospirosis in dogs. *The Veterinary Journal* 237, 37–42.

Turinelli, V., Ledieu, D., Guilbaud, L., Marchal, T., Magnol, J.P. *et al.* (2004) Mycobacterium tuberculosis infection in a dog from Africa. *Veterinary Clinical Pathology* 33(3), 177–181.

Umeakuana, P.U., Gibson, W., Ezeokonkwo, R.C. and Anene, B.M. (2019) Identification of *Trypanosoma brucei gambiense* in naturally infected dogs in Nigeria. *Parasites & Vectors* 12(1), 420.

Une, Y. and Mori, T. (2007) Tuberculosis as a zoonosis from a veterinary perspective. *Comparative Immunology, Microbiology and Infectious Diseases* 30(5–6), 415–425.

Van Balen, J.C., Landers, T., Nutt, E., Dent, A. and Hoet, A.E. (2017) Molecular epidemiological analysis to assess the influence of pet-ownership in the biodiversity of *Staphylococcus aureus* and MRSA in dog- and non-dog-owning healthy households. *Epidemiology and Infection* 145(6), 1135–1147.

Van Bree, F.P.J., Bokken, G., Mineur, R., Franssen, F., Opsteegh, M. *et al.* (2018) Zoonotic bacteria and parasites found in raw meat-based diets for cats and dogs. *The Veterinary Record* 182(2), 50.

Van de Heyning, J. and Thienpont, D. (1977) Otitis externa in man caused by the mite *Otodectes cynotis*. *Laryngoscope* 87(11), 1938–1941.

Varcasia, A., Tamponi, C., Ahmed, F., Cappai, M.G., Porcu, F. *et al.* (2022) Taenia multiceps coenurosis: A review. *Parasites & Vectors* 15(1), 84.

Verma, R. and Delfanian, K. (2013) *Blastocystis hominis* associated acute urticaria. *The American Journal of the Medical Sciences* 346(1), 80–81.

Verocai, G.G., Conboy, G., Lejeune, M., Marron, F., Hanna, P. *et al.* (2016) *Onchocerca lupi* nematodes in dogs exported from the United States into Canada. *Emerging Infectious Diseases* 22(8), 1477–1479.

Vourchakbé, J., Tiofack, Z.A.A., Kante, T.S., Mpoame, M. and Simo, G. (2020) Molecular identification of *Trypanosoma brucei gambiense* in naturally infected pigs, dogs and small ruminants confirms domestic animals as potential reservoirs for sleeping sickness in Chad. *Parasite* 27, 63.

Wadhwa, A., Wilkins, K., Gao, J., Condori Condori, R.E., Gigante, C.M. *et al.* (2017) A pan-lyssavirus taqman real-time RT-PCR assay for the detection of highly variable rabies virus and other lyssaviruses. *PLoS Neglected Tropical Diseases* 11(1), e0005258.

Wandeler, A.I., Bingham, J. and Meslin, F.X. (2013) Dogs and rabies. In: Macpherson, C.N.L., Meslin, F.X. and Wandeler, A.I. (eds) *Dogs, Zoonoses and Public Health*, 2nd ed. CAB International, CPI Group (K) Ltd, Croydon, pp. 43–66.

Wang, N., Wang, Y., Ye, Q., Yang, Y., Wan, J. *et al.* (2018) Development of a direct PCR assay to detect Taenia multiceps eggs isolated from dog feces. *Veterinary Parasitology* 251, 7–11.

Weng, X., Mu, Z., Wei, X., Wang, X., Zuo, Q. *et al.* (2020) The effects of dog management on *Echinococcus* spp. prevalence in villages on the Eastern Tibetan plateau, China. *Parasites & Vectors* 13(1), 207.

Worasith, C., Kamamia, C., Yakovleva, A., Duenngai, K., Wangboon, C. *et al.* (2015) Advances in the diagnosis of human opisthorchiasis: development of *Opisthorchis viverrini* antigen detection in urine. *PLoS Neglected Tropical Diseases* 9(10), e0004157.

World Health Organization (WHO) (2019) Ten threats to global health in 2019, fact sheets. Available at: https://www.who.int/news-room/spotlight/ten-threats-to-global-health-in-2019

World Health Organization. (2013) WHO expert consultation on rabies: Second report. Available at: https://apps.who.int/iris/bitstream/handle/10665/85346/9789240690943_eng

World Health Organization (2018) Chagas disease (American *Trypanosomiasis*), Fact Sheets. Available at: https://www.who.int/health-topics/chagas-disease#tab=tab_1

World Health Organization (2021) Ending the neglect to attain the Sustainable Development Goals: A road map for neglected tropical diseases 2021-2030. Available at: https://www.who.int/publications/i/item/9789240010352

World Health Organization (2021) WHO and Bayer renew longstanding collaboration to accelerate control and elimination of neglected tropical diseases, Fact sheets. 2021. Available at: news/item/15-11-2021-who-and-bayer-renew-longstanding-collaboration-to-accelerate-control-and-elimination-of-neglected-tropical-diseases

World Health Organization (2022) Leishmaniasis, Fact Sheets. Available at: https://www.who.int/news-room/fact-sheets/detail/leishmaniasis

Wormser, G.P., Dattwyler, R.J., Shapiro, E.D., Halperin, J.J., Steere, A.C. *et al.* (2006) The clinical assessment, treatment, and prevention of Lyme disease, human granulocytic *Anaplasmosis*, and *Babesiosis*: Clinical practice guidelines by the infectious diseases society of America. *Clinical Infectious Diseases* 43(9), 1089–1134.

Wotherspoon, A. (1991) *Helicobacter pylori*-Associated gastritis and primary B-cell gastric lymphoma. *The Lancet* 338(8776), 1175–1176.

Xu, M., Jiang, Y., Yin, J., Cao, S., Shen, Y. *et al.* (2021) Risk factors for *Clonorchis sinensis* infection in residents of Binyang, Guangxi: A cross-sectional and logistic analysis study. *Frontiers in Public Health* 9, 588325.

Yamazawa, E., Ohno, M., Satomi, K., Yoshida, A., Miyakita, Y. *et al.* (2020) First case of human neuro-coenurosis caused by *Taenia serialis*: A case report. *International Journal of Infectious Diseases* 92, 171–174.

Yang, Y.R., McManus, D.P., Huang, Y. and Heath, D.D. (2009) *Echinococcus granulosus* infection and options for control of cystic *Echinococcosis* in Tibetan communities of Western Sichuan province, China. *PLoS Neglected Tropical Diseases* 3(4), e426.

Ye, C.-Y., Yang, Z.-D. and Zheng, H.-L. (2013) Fatal multi-organ *Clonorchis sinensis* infection in dog: A case report. *Veterinary Parasitology* 195(1–2), 173–176.

Yi, J., Humphries, R., Doerr, L., Jerris, R.C. and Westblade, L.F. (2016) *Bergeyella zoohelcum* associated with abscess and cellulitis after a dog bite. *Pediatric Infectious Disease Journal* 35(2), 214–216.

Yimam, Y. and Mohebali, M. (2020) Effectiveness of insecticide-impregnated dog collars in reducing incidence rate of canine visceral leishmaniasis: A systematic review and meta-analysis. *PLoS One* 15(9), e0238601.

Yoshida, A., Doanh, P.N. and Maruyama, H. (2019) *Paragonimus* and *Paragonimiasis* in Asia: An update. *Acta Tropica* 199, 105074.

Yousaf, M.Z., Qasim, M., Zia, S., Mu, R.K., Ashfaq, U.A. *et al.* (2012) Rabies molecular virology, diagnosis, prevention and treatment. *Virology Journal* 9(1), 50.

Zhang, Z.-Z., Guo, G., Li, J., Shi, B.-X., Zhao, L. *et al.* (2018) Dog vaccination with EgM proteins against *Echinococcus granulosus*. *Infectious Diseases of Poverty* 7(1), 61.

Zhu, G.Q., Li, L., Ohiolei, J.A., Wu, Y.T., Li, W.H. *et al.* (2019) A multiplex PCR assay for the simultaneous detection of *Taenia hydatigena*. *BMC Infectious Diseases* 19(1), 854.

14 Food Systems During the COVID-19 Pandemic: Vulnerabilities, Adaptations, and Resilience

Jill E. Hobbs*

Department of Agricultural and Resource Economics, University of Saskatchewan, 51 Campus Drive (3D34.1), Saskatoon, S7N 5A8, Canada

Abstract

This paper reviews the emerging literature on food systems and food supply chains during the COVID-19 pandemic. Four themes are explored: consumer demand and retail market effects; supply-side shocks; food system and supply chain resilience; and developing countries and food insecurity. The effect of demand-side shocks is explored, including the sudden shift in expenditures from food service to food retail. Longer-run structural changes in the food retailing landscape include the expansion of online food delivery. The effect of supply-side shocks is examined extensively in the literature, including short-run adaptations as supply chains pivoted from the food service sector to food retail, along with supply-side disruptions due to labour force outbreaks of COVID-19. Resilience is a common theme in the literature, at both food system and food supply chain levels. While a variety of perspectives are offered, most assessments point to a surprising degree of resilience and adaptability, while identifying the points of vulnerability. The pandemic increased food insecurity through the effect on household incomes from reduced labour mobility, lockdowns, and a contraction in economic activity.These effects were particularly prominent among vulnerable populations in developing countries. Significant attention has been paid to the short- and medium-run effects of the pandemic on food systems, with further research needed to understand any longer-term structural changes that may arise.The COVID-19 pandemic offers lessons for the robustness of food systems and the importance of timely, well-informed policy responses in preparation for future global shocks.

Keywords: COVID-19, pandemic, food supply chains, resilience, food security

Review Methodology

The following databases and search engines were searched: CAB Reviews, ABI/Inform, Web of Science, Econlit, Google Scholar. Searches were also conducted through journals relevant to the topic, several of which featured special issues or special sections dedicated to the COVID-19 pandemic, including Agribusiness, Agricultural Systems, Agriculture and Human Values, Ambio, American Journal of Agricultural Economics, Applied Economic Perspectives and Policy, Canadian Journal of Agricultural Economics, Food Policy, Food Security, Global Food Security, World Development. Additional literature was identified using references from the articles located through these methods.

*Corresponding author: jill.hobbs@usask.ca

The date range for publications included in the search criteria was January 2020–September 2021. Search terms included COVID, pandemic, food supply chain, resilience.

Introduction

COVID-19 is caused by severe acute respiratory syndrome coronavirus-2 (SARS-CoV-2). The virus emerged at the end of 2019, spreading rapidly worldwide. The World Health Organization declared the COVID-19 outbreak a global pandemic on 11 March 2020. By March 2022, COVID-19 had caused over 6 million deaths worldwide, with rates of serious illness and death slowing as effective vaccinations emerged.[1] First and foremost a global health crisis, the COVID-19 pandemic has also been the source of unprecedented and widespread economic disruption, as countries moved to limit the spread of the disease through lockdowns, social distancing, movement and travel restrictions, self-isolation and quarantine requirements, and other containment measures. Potential disruptions to food systems, and the (sometimes surprising) abilities of those systems to adjust to exogenous shocks, have garnered significant attention, both in the public domain and among the research community. A large and rapidly expanding body of literature has arisen examining food systems during the COVID-19 pandemic. This review provides an overview of key themes emerging in this literature.

Four themes serve as the basis for organizing this review: consumer demand and retail market effects; (ii) supply-side shocks; (iii) food system and supply chain resilience; and (iv) developing countries and food insecurity. These themes are by no means mutually exclusive, with cross-cutting issues across themes, for example supply-side shocks and food system resilience, and supply chain resilience in developing country contexts. Following a short summary of the review methodology, the following sections provide an overview of the literature across the four themes, identifying cross-cutting issues where relevant.

Methodological Approach

The review is necessarily selective given the scope and pace with which new literature in this area is emerging but aims to provide a wide-ranging overview of the core set of issues and primary insights in the literature. Literature was drawn from a range of disciplines in the social sciences, but primarily agricultural economics, development, and business management. Primary search engines included CAB Reviews, ABI/Inform, Web of Science, Econlit, and Google Scholar, along with key journals in agricultural economics, development, food security, and food policy. Key search terms included combinations of 'COVID, pandemic, food supply chain, resilience'.

The review is limited to academic, peer-reviewed literature and publications in the English language. Approximately two-thirds of papers considered for inclusion in the review focus on developed countries, with the remainder focusing on supply chains in developing countries and emerging economies. Countries and regions encompassed by the review include the United States (U.S.), Canada, the European Union (EU), UK, Australia, New Zealand, South Pacific, Asia, Africa, and Latin America. The review includes papers utilizing a range of methodologies including discussions, conceptual analyses, case studies, empirical analysis of survey data, and simulation/scenario analysis. Papers were categorized according to key content, including developing countries/humanitarian, food insecurity/vulnerable populations, consumers, trade, sectors (meat, fruit and vegetables), resilience/supply chains/firms, logistics, food systems, local, early assessments/first wave/lockdowns, other pandemics. Cross-cutting themes were identified from this key content, and the literature further categorized into the four broad themes outlined above.

Consumer Demand and Retail Market Effects

The early stages of the pandemic, particularly in developed countries, were characterized by sudden shifts in consumer expenditures from food service to food retail (grocery), driven by fears of the virus, closure of restaurants, cafés and other food service outlets during lockdowns, and a widespread shift to working from home.The significance of this demand shift was widely recognized at an early stage in the literature, with inevitable disruptions as supply chains realigned in response to the surge in demand from food retail and the collapse in demand from food service (Hobbs, 2020; Weersink *et al.*, 2021; Malone *et al.*, 2021; Hobbs, 2021). Prior to the pandemic, food-away-from-home (food service) expenditures comprised a growing proportion of consumer food expenditures, for example over 50% in the U.S. and over 30% in Canada and some European countries (Goddard, 2020; Hobbs, 2021; Luckstead *et al.*, 2021).The sudden shift in these expenditures to food retail outlets generated a demand shock,requiring the realignment of supply chains previously focused on supplying the food service sector.

An additional (although less sustained) demand-side shock during the early stages of the pandemic was caused by panic-buying and hoarding behaviors as consumers stocked up on staples and non-perishable items (flour, pasta, rice, canned goods). The motivations for panic buying and stockpiling behaviors are complex, including self-insurance due to supply uncertainties, loss aversion, and herd mentality (people responding to what they perceive others are doing). Nevertheless, these were short-run effects (Melo, 2020; Hobbs, 2020; Béné, 2020; Montanari *et al.*, 2020; Norwood and Peel, 2021; Santeramo and Perez-Dominguez, 2021).

The pandemic focused consumers' attention on the food system and food supply chains, with a variety of complex behavioral outcomes related to risk perceptions, food values, and interest in local foods. Consumer surveys conducted during the early stage of the pandemic (spring to summer 2020) in the United States point to concerns over the potential temporary relaxation of environmental and food safety regulations (Kecinski *et al.*, 2020), concerns about transmission of COVID-19 while grocery shopping along with misperceptions about the risk of transmission from consuming food (McFadden *et al.*, 2021), and generally higher risk perceptions due to the pervasive climate of uncertainty during the first phase of the pandemic (Mexiner and Katt, 2020).

Food values are an intermediary set of human values related to food preferences (Lusk and Briggeman, 2009). Food safety, nutrition, taste, and price are found consistently to be the most important set of core values in various studies across time and across countries, with the importance of food values related to credence attributes such as origin, traceability, or sustainability the source of considerable heterogeneity among consumers (Hobbs, 2021). Ellison *et al.* (2021) examine changes in food expenditures, shopping behaviors, and food values among U.S. consumers during the early stages of the pandemic (mid-March to late April 2020). Their analysis suggests that although food values remained relatively stable, price and nutrition decreased in importance as households shifted their food purchase patterns. In contrast, Malone *et al.* (2021) find that the pandemic significantly reduced premiums for credence attributes in the U.S. egg market (e.g. cage-free, vegetarian-fed hens, and organic eggs). Price premiums for these credence attributes had not fully recovered once markets returned to more normal patterns later in 2020, suggesting some softening in consumers' willingness to pay for these attributes.

To what extent did the pandemic result in higher retail prices for food or a widening of the retail-wholesale-farm price spread due to anticompetitive behavior in food supply chains? Compelling evidence in the literature supporting this assertion is sparse. Disruptions to food supply chains, such as the temporary closure of food processing plants due to COVID-19 outbreaks or new regulatory measures, cause a widening of the retail-farm price spread as a natural outcome of the forces of supply and demand in a vertically linked market (Lusk *et al.*, 2021; Hayes *et al.*, 2021). Determining whether a change in food prices can be attributed to pandemic-induced disruptions and/or anticompetitive behavior requires empirical analysis controlling for other factors simultaneously affecting food prices. Despite fears to the contrary, initial evidence suggests that the pandemic did not lead to a sustained increase in food prices in developed economies e.g. table eggs (Malone *et al.*, 2021); online grocery prices (Hillen, 2021); U.S. dairy markets (Liu and Rabinowitz, 2021).

Two additional consumer and retail market trends emerging from the COVID-19 pandemic include an increased interest in local foods and the growth in online grocery shopping. The interest in 'local' foods is not new but gained additional traction amidst pervasive uncertainty at the onset of the pandemic (Hobbs, 2020; Goddard, 2021; Thilmany *et al.*, 2021; Chang and Meyerhoefer, 2021). Goddard (2021) reports a significant increase in online searches for information about local food in 2020 in Canada, in addition to a 45% increase in newspaper articles about local food. Regional policy initiatives arose facilitating the ability of farmers to supply local markets through the development of online farmers' markets and direct sales initiatives (Goddard, 2021). The initial uptick in interest in local foods eventually settled back, particularly as mainstream food supply chains proved to be robust. Local food marketing channels are generally seen as complements to rather than substitutes for mainstream food supply chains.

The pandemic generated a strong and sustained upswing in online grocery shopping in many countries as consumers sought to reduce their risk of exposure to the virus (Hobbs, 2020; Goddard, 2021; Chang and Meyerhoefer, 2021). Retailers and third-party providers moved quickly to expand their online grocery shopping infrastructure. While many consumers returned to in-person grocery shopping as vaccinations became more widely available, the pandemic has initiated a permanent restructuring towards multiple channel retailing where companies offer a combined in-store and online shopping experience, including click and collect and contactless delivery (Hobbs, 2021; Goddard, 2021).

The pandemic caused unprecedented disruptions to the food service sector, and to the supply chains tied to this sector. Restaurants rapidly adopted app-based online meal delivery services during initial and subsequent lockdown periods often using third-party delivery services, including the development of so-called ghost kitchens (delivery-only restaurants) (Goddard, 2021). As with the grocery retail sector, investments in online delivery infrastructure (websites, apps, transportation), either directly or through third party providers, are likely to be a permanent change even as consumers return to in-restaurant dining experiences.

Supply-Side Shocks

With the sudden switch in food demand from food service to food retail outlets, supply chains specializing in supplying food service needed time to adapt. Product requirements often differ between these two channels; for example, in the U.S., whole bird, deboned, and cut-up chicken markets have different bird size specifications, and supply chains (processing plants, growers) are often specialized in supplying a specific channel (Hobbs, 2021; Maples *et al.*, 2021). In the egg sector, breaker eggs are destined for the food service market, while table eggs tend to be sold *via* food retail (Weersink *et al.*, 2021; Malone *et al.*, 2021). Specialized supply chains in the fresh fruit and vegetable sector faced challenges in diverting excess supply from the food service sector to other channels (Çakir *et al.*, 2021). Food packaging and labelling regulations, as well as food package sizes, differ between food service and food retail, creating some rigidity in reallocating supplies between these two channels in response to sudden exogenous shocks. Given the biological nature of agri-food production, the extent of disruption and the ability for food production to adjust varied across agricultural commodities. For the most part, however, disruptions to food supply chains in developed economies in North America, Europe, and Asia proved to be a relatively short-run phenomenon (Montanari *et al.*, 2020; Fan *et al.*, 2021; Orden, 2021; Weersink *et al.*, 2021).

Supply-side vulnerabilities due to labour force and community outbreaks of COVID-19 in and around food processing establishments have garnered significant attention in the literature, with a particular focus on the meat sector (see e.g. (Luckstead *et al.*, 2021; Hobbs, 2021; Lusk *et al.*, 2021; Hayes *et al.*, 2021; Rude, 2021; Martinez *et al.*, 2021; Saitone *et al.*, 2021)). Labour shortages due to illness or worker availability, temporary plant closures due to workforce outbreaks, as well as slower processing line speeds to accommodate social distancing disrupted livestock/meat supply chains, particularly during the early stages of the pandemic. The cold, humid environmental conditions within food processing facilities, along with a crowded noisy workplace (workers in close proximity along meat-cutting lines), proved conducive to the spread of the respiratory virus.

While the U.S. meat packing sector was particularly badly affected, disruptions were also reported at meat processing plants in several countries, including Canada, Brazil, and Europe (Hobbs, 2020; Aday and Aday, 2020; Weersink *et al.*, 2021). Daily processing volumes for beef and pork in the U.S. were about 40% below 2019 levels from late April through early May 2020, with similar declines in Canada over the same time period (Weersink *et al.*, 2021; Lusk *et al.*, 2021). The magnitude of these short-run effects was exacerbated by the concentrated nature of the meat packing sector in these countries, with the temporary closure of one large packing plant having a significant effect on slaughter volumes within the sector. For example, in the U.S., the largest 22 beef packing plants represent only 3.3% of all packing plants but are responsible for almost 72% of federally inspected cattle processing (Ma and Lusk, 2021). In Canada, the three largest beef packing plants account for 85% of slaughter capacity (Hobbs, 2021).

The temporary closure of a large meat packing plant causes the demand for livestock to fall, while simultaneously reducing the supply of meat to wholesale and retail markets, widening the farm to retail price spread (Lusk *et al.*, 2021). Nevertheless, these effects were relatively short-lived, with price effects in the U.S. and Canadian livestock markets settling out by late summer 2020 (Weersink *et al.*, 2021; Orden, 2021; Rude, 2021).

Agricultural sectors dependent on seasonal labour, such as the fruit, vegetable, and horticultural sector, were vulnerable to the imposition of movement restrictions and border closures. Disruptions to the supply of agricultural labour were reported during the first few weeks of the pandemic, for example in the U.S. and Canadian fresh produce sectors and in Europe (Richards and Rickard, 2020; Coluccia *et al.*, 2021). Recognizing the importance of cross-border labour flows and cross-border food supply chains, governments moved quickly to introduce essential worker designations encompassing workers involved in the production and distribution of food. Chenarides *et al.* (2021) track the effect of the pandemic on the U.S. fruit and vegetable sector using labour market and shipments data from the first year of the pandemic, finding that the fruit and vegetable sector adjusted relatively quickly. The feared labour shortages did not materialize or were isolated in nature (Chenarides *et al.*, 2021).

Several studies document a link between a higher incidence of community-level COVID-19 infections in regions dominated by labour-intensive agricultural production (e.g. fruit, vegetable, and horticulture production) or meat packing plants (Saitone *et al.*, 2021; Charlton, 2021). Saitone *et al.* (2021) compare per capita infection rates in the U.S. counties with and without large meat processing facilities. Within 150 days of the emergence of COVID-19 in a given U.S. county, the presence of a large meat processing plant resulted in community infection rates 110% higher (relative to counties without a plant) for beef packing, 160% for pork processing, and 20% for chicken processing. Over time, however, the difference between meat packing and non-meat packing counties converges (Saitone *et al.*, 2021). Charlton (2021) also finds a positive relationship between the presence of fruit, vegetable, and horticultural production within a U.S. county and higher rates of COVID-19.

A potential longer-run response to workforce outbreaks of COVID-19 in meat processing establishments and labour-intensive agricultural sectors is increased adoption of robotics and automation to reduce dependence on labour (Aday and Aday, 2020; Charlton, 2021; Hobbs, 2021). The extent to which these technologies are adopted at an increased pace following the COVID-19 pandemic will depend on both technological feasibility and economic feasibility. Adoption of robotics in beef packing plants is challenged by the wide variation in carcass shapes and sizes (Weersink *et al.*, 2021), which may be addressed with advancements in machine learning. The economic feasibility of increased automation will depend on the benefits of increased automation (increased productivity, improved quality control, reduced vulnerability to pandemic-related labour force risks) vs the costs (Hobbs, 2021).

Food System and Supply Chain Resilience

The resilience of food supply chains and food systems has garnered a great deal of attention in the aftermath of the COVID-19 pandemic. Ponomarov and Holcomb (Ponomarov and Holcomb, 2009) define supply chain resilience as 'the adaptive capability of the supply chain to prepare for unexpected events, respond to disruptions, and recover from them by maintaining continuity of operations at the desire level of connectedness and control over structure and function' (p. 131).

Food system resilience is a broader concept, related to the capacity of the system as a whole to withstand and/or adapt to disturbances (both predictable and unpredictable) over time (Tendall *et al.*, 2015). Tendall *et al.* (2015) offer the following definition of food system resilience: 'capacity over time of a food system and its units at multiple levels, to provide sufficient, appropriate and accessible food to all, in the face of various and even unforeseen circumstances' (p. 19). Food system resilience is discussed in the context of an action cycle framework where a food system absorbs a disruption, reacts, restore, learns, and builds robustness to future events (Tendall *et al.*, 2015; Love *et al.*, 2021).

In the wake of the COVID-19 pandemic, the literature is divided on the extent to which food supply chains or food systems are perceived to have been resilient in response to the exogenous shocks imposed by the pandemic. The dichotomy arises from different conceptions of 'resilience', different time frames of analysis, as well as different disciplinary approaches. Some authors point to challenges arising from increased supply chain and logistics costs (Rejeb *et al.*, 2021), or highlight as evidence of 'fragility' the short-run disruptions and adaptations within supply chains and food markets (Boyacı-Gündüz *et al.*, 2021). Others argue that disruptions to food systems entrenched social inequalities (Sanderson Bellmay *et al.*, 2021). Nevertheless, many studies find a surprising degree of resilience in food systems and their ability to adapt to the unprecedented shocks caused by the pandemic (Montanari *et al.*, 2020; Ker and Cardwell, 2021; Hobbs, 2021; Weersink *et al.*, 2021). Lusk *et al.* (2021) make a useful distinction between a food system that provides efficiency and affordable food to consumers during 'normal' times, and the costs associated with adding capacity, flexibility, and resiliency to a sector for 'abnormal' times.

Drilling down to a firm-level analysis, Norwood and Peel (2021) discuss the merits of supply chain mapping as a management tool for firms to identify supply chain vulnerabilities and disruption risks. While not specific to food supply chains per se, Black and Glaser-Segura (2020) draw insights from the supply chain management literature on the management and control of risks to develop a strategic mitigation model in the context of pandemic risks, including the elements of leadership, preparedness, digitalization, resilience, and pivoting. As Hobbs (2021) points out, agri-food supply chains differ from manufacturing goods supply chains in a number of important facets with respect to resilience, including the biological nature of production, perishability (time specificity), structure, and political sensitivity (food as a necessity).

Adaptability and flexibility are common themes in the literature on supply chain resilience. Chenarides *et al.* (2021) discuss a real option approach to decision-making at a firm-level, where there may be value in investing in alternative supplier and distribution networks to provide flexibility and adaptability in the event of disruptions. The sudden closure or scaling back of the food service sector created significant uncertainty for upstream supply chains specialized in supplying the sector. These firms needed to adapt to supplying retail outlets as well as the expanding home meal kit delivery sector (Hobbs, 2021; Chenarides *et al.*, 2021).

At a food system level, some authors point to the perceived flexibility of local and regional food system actors during the early stages of the pandemic, with shorter supply chains based on strong interpersonal networks allowing firms to pivot to alternative marketing channels (Thilmany *et al.*, 2021). The widespread consensus within the agricultural economics literature, however, is that mainstream food systems and food supply chains in developed economies performed remarkably well during the COVID-19 pandemic given the unprecedented nature of the demand and supply shocks occurring in these food systems. Consumers continued to enjoy access to a wide variety of safe, nutritious foodstuffs, with disruptions proving relatively short-run in nature.

The use of an appropriate counterfactual is critical in assessing supply chain (or food system) resilience: would a different type of food system (smaller scale, more diffused) have performed any better or worse during the pandemic? (Hobbs, 2021; Ker and Cardwell, 2021). While a more dispersed, smaller-scale food system might be less susceptible to losing one large food processing (meat packing) plant due to an exogenous shock, localized food systems would still be vulnerable to localized shocks (e.g. climate events). There is widespread acknowledgement of the economies of scale and economies of scope advantages of larger-scale commercial food systems that yield efficiency and cost (and therefore price) advantages (Rude, 2020; Ma and Lusk, 2021; Orden, 2021; Lusk *et al.*, 2021; Hobbs, 2021; Weersink *et al.*, 2021). The potential trade-off between resilience and efficiency has been identified as a fruitful area for future research (Balagtas and Cooper, 2021).

Developing Countries and Food Insecurity

The effects of the COVID-19 pandemic on food systems in developing countries, where food systems supply vulnerable populations who may already be food insecure, have been examined in a variety of contexts. Disentangling the effects of direct pandemic-related (health) disruptions to food systems from the broader economic impact of the pandemic on incomes is a strong theme within this literature.

Early assessments of the impacts of the pandemic on food and nutrition security (January through June 2020) identified widespread economic effects arising directly from the pandemic itself, and from the lockdowns and reductions in economic activity accompanying the pandemic (see e.g. Béné, 2020; Love *et al.*, 2021; Davila *et al.*, 2021; Adjognon *et al.*, 2021; Amare *et al.*, 2021; Kansiime *et al.*, 2021). Love *et al.* (Love *et al.*, 2021) examine the effects of the pandemic on the global seafood sector in January–June 2020. Using the food system resilience action cycle framework (Tendall *et al.*, 2015), Love *et al.* (2021) suggest that while some supply chains, market segments, and firms showed initial signs of resilience, the pandemic had a disproportionate effect on groups in low-income countries who work in or are dependent upon the seafood sector. For example, migrant fish workers were unable to leave fishing boats in some ports, while the closure of fish markets resulted in unemployment among fish workers. A nationwide lockdown in India forced the closure of firms throughout the aquaculture sector (hatcheries, feed mills, processing plants), while the near closure of the food service sector in high-income countries severely impacted the global demand for seafood. Developing countries that are heavily dependent on seafood exports (e.g. Bangladesh, Myanmar) suffered severe disruption to their seafood sectors.

As Béné (2020) notes, the main and immediate impact of the pandemic arose from lockdown and mobility restrictions imposed by local and national governments in a bid to protect public health. The subsequent loss of income and purchasing power had a direct and immediate impact on food security, particularly among the poor. These effects are exacerbated in countries with under-developed, poorly functioning, or under-resourced social safety net polices.

Davila *et al.* (2021) examine the early impacts of the pandemic (February–July 2020) on small island developing nations in the Pacific, arguing that these countries are particularly vulnerable to the conflation of risks from COVID-19 (health), economic downturns, and underlying climate vulnerabilities. Unemployment and economic contraction were compounded by precipitous drops in tourism revenue, restrictions on labour migration, and a significant drop in remittances. While short-run disruptions to the distributions and marketing of food occurred in Small Island Developing States due to lockdowns, local food economies were fairly quick to stabilize and cross-border international food supply chains continued to function effectively, reducing the risk of food insecurity in import-dependent nations (Davila *et al.*, 2021).

Household-level survey data collected in Nigeria in April–May 2020 show a clear relationship between households exposed to higher levels of COVID-19 case rates or mobility lockdowns and an increase in food insecurity (Amare *et al.*, 2021). Non-farm and urban households tended to have worse food security outcomes during the early stages of the pandemic, an effect reported from household survey data in Nigeria (Amare *et al.*, 2021) and Mali (Adjognon *et al.*, 2021), although Adjognon *et al.* (2021) find that the rural–urban gap in food insecurity in Mali dissipated after 3 months.

Household survey data from Kenya (April 2020) reveal significant income shocks at the outset of the pandemic (Kansiime *et al.*, 2021). Two-thirds of surveyed respondents experienced an immediate income shock as the pandemic hit, with a decline in food security and diet quality (a reduced consumption of nutritionally rich foods). Loss of income, reduced access to markets due to travel restrictions, and lower purchasing power contributed to rising rates of food insecurity. Suggested policy responses to mitigate the effects of future pandemic-like shocks include strategies to stabilize incomes through improved social safety nets (Kansiime *et al.*, 2021).

While the effects on food insecurity are the most striking in developing country contexts given the higher proportion of vulnerable low-income households, food insecurity also rose in developed countries due to loss of income from unemployment and reduced hours of work (e.g. in the U.S. (Fang *et al.*, 2022) and Canada (Deaton and Deaton, 2021). Indeed, Deaton and Deaton (2021) warn against rhetoric that conflates food insecurity with a failure of the food system, emphasizing that household income (along with food prices) is a central part of the story.

While much of the literature on food supply chains during the pandemic focuses on developed countries, Liverpool-Tasie *et al.* (2021) argue that food supply chains (as opposed to subsistence agriculture) are also extremely important for food access and livelihoods in developing economies. This role is often overlooked, leading to ineffective policy responses to protect food security. A conceptual model linking vertical food supply chains (from farmer to consumer) to lateral supply chains illustrates the important role of logistics services (trucking, distribution), migrant labour, raw material supplies, and financial services to the continued smooth operation of vertical supply chains during a pandemic. The authors contend that the classification of essential vs non-essential businesses during the early period of lockdown in Nigeria failed to recognize the importance of lateral supply chain actors, including logistics and transportation services, wholesale markets, and banking, as core contributors for smooth functioning of food supply chains (Liverpool-Tasie *et al.*, 2021).

The need for a nuanced understanding of the nature of food supply chains and the food system when crafting policy responses to pandemic-like shocks is a recurring theme in the literature. Wegerif (2020) argues that initial policy responses to the pandemic in South Africa failed to take into consideration the substantial role of informal traders in the food system, including street traders, and other small retailers and food enterprises.

The rapid growth of e-commerce in developing countries prior to the pandemic is well documented, particularly in Asia and Latin America and more gradually in Africa (Reardon *et al.*, 2021). Using examples from Asia and Latin America, Reardon *et al.* discuss how firms in developing regions 'pivoted' to e-commerce to reach downstream consumers and to e-procurement to reach upstream processors and farmers. Delivery intermediaries played a significant role in facilitating these rapid adjustments in distribution and input supply. Food supply chains in many developing countries proved to have a surprisingly high degree of resilience and adaptability (Reardon *et al.*, 2021; Fang *et al.*, 2022). Nevertheless, the degree of vulnerability is different for different food systems, making broad generalizations difficult (Rivera-Ferre *et al.*, 2021).

Conclusions

Context matters, and the complex, multifaceted nature of food systems and food supply chains worldwide resulted in a wide range of outcomes; nevertheless, the review points to several key themes. The COVID-19 pandemic caused unprecedented shocks to the global economy, challenging the resilience of food systems and food supply chains. In disentangling the effects of the pandemic on food systems, it is important to distinguish between short-run and long-run effects, as well as disruptions to food systems directly vs indirect effects on incomes and economic well-being. Given the global health crisis and economic disruption caused by the pandemic, it is no surprise that a large and rapidly growing literature has emerged evaluating the short- and medium-, and longer- term impacts of the pandemic on food systems in both developed and developing countries. The pandemic highlighted areas of vulnerability in food supply chains, particularly at the onset of the pandemic with the introduction of lockdowns and other containment methods necessary to protect public health prior to the availability of vaccines. Nevertheless, a common theme in the literature is the adaptability and versatility of food supply chain actors in responding to sudden exogenous demand and supply shocks. Another common theme is the importance of crafting policy responses with a well-informed understanding of the nature of food supply chains in a given country context. Policy responses that address the root causes of increased food insecurity during the pandemic in developing and developed countries—loss of household income exacerbated by weak social safety nets—are a recurring recommendation in the literature.

Looking ahead, key learnings that arise from this review are as follows:

1. The concept of resilience needs further refinement, and the trade-off between inherent resilience (during 'normal times') vs adaptive resilience (during 'abnormal times') deserves explicit recognition in attempts to measure the degree of resilience of food systems and food supply chains.
2. The pandemic had a disproportionately larger impact on vulnerable populations, in both developed and developing country contexts. In many cases, these impacts arose from the broader economic disruption caused by the pandemic (unemployment, reduced hours of work, lockdowns), rather than signalling a problem with the food system itself. Disentangling these effects remains important in on-going analyses of the longer-term impacts of the pandemic and in devising policy responses to address the root cause of vulnerabilities.
3. Short-run disruptions to food supply chains were ameliorated through timely policy interventions, including essential worker designations and efforts to ensure cross-border supply chains continued to function effectively. Robust existing policy frameworks and good inter-governmental communication facilitated these adaptations, while jurisdictions with weaker governance experienced more sustained disruptions. Future research could evaluate the effectiveness of specific policy interventions in different jurisdictions to better understand which interventions were effective (or ineffective) at different stages of the pandemic, and why.
4. Adaptations at the level of individual firms and individual supply chains were substantial, including pivoting to new delivery modes, new methods of sourcing inputs, and new ways of managing the workforce. The existence of robust communications networks (Internet, mobile phone), logistics, and financial services helped facilitate these adaptations. Nevertheless, the ability to 'pivot' differs across sectors, commodities, and stages of the supply chain. Further case study analyses at the level of individual firms and specific supply chains can provide insights into successes and failures in managerial strategies to enhance resilience in the face of uncertainty.

A large body of literature addressing many dimensions of COVID-19 and food systems has emerged in a very short period of time, necessitating limitations to the scope and scale of literature encompassed by this review. While the review is necessarily selected in coverage, the aim was to capture main over-arching themes in the literature. At the time of conducting this review, most published work focused on impacts during the first 12–18 months of the pandemic. Thus, while significant attention has been paid to the short- and medium-run effects of the pandemic on food systems, the longer-run effects and any longer-term structural changes that may arise from the pandemic are on-going topics of research. In preparation for future global shocks, be it another pandemic or the effects of climate change, the COVID-19 pandemic offers lessons for the robustness of food systems, the importance of timely, well-informed policy responses both nationally and internationally, and the need to develop better metrics by which we can assess the drivers and outcomes of resilience.

Note

[1] https://www.statista.com/statistics/1093256/novel-coronavirus-2019ncov-deaths-worldwide-by-country/

References

Aday, S. and Aday, M.S. (2020) Impact of COVID-19 on the food supply chain. *Food Quality and Safety* 4, 167–180.

Adjognon, G.S., Bloem, J.R. and Sanoh, A. (2021) The coronavirus pandemic and food security. *Evidence from Mali. Food Policy* 101, 102050.

Amare, M., Abay, K.A., Tiberti, L. and Chamberlin, J. (2021) COVID-19 and food security: Panel data evidence from Nigeria. *Food Policy* 101, 102099.

Balagtas, J.V. and Cooper, J. (2021) The impact of COVID-19 on United States meat and livestock markets. Theme issue: Agricultural Market Responses to COVID-19, *Choices* 36(3). Available at: choicesmagazine/theme-articles/agricultural-market-response-tocovid-19/the-impact-of-covid-19-on-united-states-meat-and-livestockmarkets

Béné, C. (2020) Resilience of local food systems and links to food security—A review of some important concepts in the context of COVID-19 and other shocks. *Food Security* 12, 805–822.

Black, S. and Glaser-Segura, D. (2020) Supply chain resilience in a pandemic: The need for contingency planning. *Management Dynamics in the Knowledge Economy* 8(4), 325–343.

Boyacı-Gündüz, C., Ibrahim, S.A., Wei, O.C. and Galanakis, C.M. (2021) Transformation of the food sector: Security and resilience during the COVID-19 pandemic. *Foods* 10, 497.

Çakir, M., Li, Q. and Yang, X. (2021) COVID-19 and fresh produce markets in the United States and China. *Applied Economic Perspectives and Policy* 43(1), 341–354.

Chang, H.-H. and Meyerhoefer, C.D. (2021) COVID-19 and the demand for online food shopping services: Empirical evidence from Taiwan. *American Journal of Agricultural Economics* 103(2), 448–465.

Charlton, D. (2021) Seasonal farm labor and COVID-19 spread. *Applied Economic Perspectives and Policy* forthcoming. DOI: 10.1002/aepp.13190.

Chenarides, L., Richards, T.J. and Rickard, B. (2021) COVID-19 impact on fruit and vegetable markets: One year later. *Canadian Journal of Agricultural Economics* 69(2), 203–214.

Chenarides, L., Manfredo, M. and Richards, T.J. (2021) COVID-19 and food supply chains. *Applied Economic Perspectives and Policy* 41(1), 270–279.

Coluccia, B., Agnusdei, G.P., Miglietta, P.P. and Leo, F. (2021) Effects of COVID-19 on the Italian agri-food supply and value chains. *Food Control* 123, 107839.

Davila, F., Bourke, R.M., McWilliam, A., Crimp, S., Robins, L. *et al.* (2021) COVID-19 and food systems in Pacific Island Countries, Papua New Guinea, and Timor-Leste: Opportunities for actions towards sustainable development goals. *Agricultural Systems* 191, 103137.

Deaton, B.J. and Deaton, B.J. (2021) Food security and canada's agricultural system challenged by COVID-19: One year later. *Canadian Journal of Agricultural Economics* 69(2), 161–166.

Ellison, B., McFadden, B., Rickard, B.J. and Wilson, N.L.W. (2021) Examining food purchase behavior and food values during the COVID-19 pandemic. *Applied Economic Perspectives and Policy* 43(1), 58–72.

Fan, S., Teng, P., Chew, P., Smith, G. and Copeland, L. (2021) Food system resilience and COVID-19—lessons from the Asian experience. *Global Food Security* 28, 100501.

Fang, D., Thomsen, M.R., Nayga, R.M., Jr and Yang, W. (2022) Food insecurity during the COVID-19 pandemic: Evidence from a survey of low-income americans. *Food Security* 14, 165–183. DOI: 10.1007/s12571-021-01189-1.

Goddard, E. (2020) The impact of covid-19 on food retail and food service in Canada: Preliminary assessment. *Canadian Journal of Agricultural Economics* 68(2), 157–161.

Goddard, E. (2021) The impact of COVID-19 on food retail and food service in Canada: A second assessment. *Canadian Journal of Agricultural Economics* 69, 167–175.

Hayes, D.J., Schulz, L.L., Hart, C.E. and Jacobs, K.L. (2021) A descriptive analysis of the COVID-19 impacts on U.S. pork, turkey, and egg markets. *Agribusiness* 37, 122–141.

Hillen, J. (2021) Online food prices during the COVID-19 pandemic. *Agribusiness* 37, 91–107.

Hobbs, J.E. (2020) Food supply chains during the COVID-19 pandemic. *Canadian Journal of Agricultural Economics* 68, 171–176.

Hobbs, J.E. (2021) Food supply chain resilience and the COVID-19 pandemic: What have we learned? *Canadian Journal of Agricultural Economics* 69(2), 189–196.

Hobbs, J.E. (2021) The covid-19 pandemic and meat supply chains. *Meat Science* 181, 108459.

Kansiime, M.K., Tambo, J.A., Mugambi, I., Bundi, M., Kara, A. *et al.* (2021) COVID-19 implications on household income and food security in Kenya and Uganda: Findings from a rapid assessment. *World Development* 137, 105199.

Kecinski, M., Messer, K.D., McFadden, B.R. and Malone, T. (2020) Environmental and regulatory concerns during the COVID-19 pandemic: Results from the pandemic food and stigma survey. *Environmental and Resource Economics* 76, 1139–1148.

Ker, A.P. and Cardwell, C. (2021) Introduction to the special issue on COVID-19 and the Canadian agriculture and food sectors: Thoughts one year into the pandemic. *Canadian Journal of Agricultural Economics* 69, 155–159.

Liu, Y. and Rabinowitz, A.N. (2021) The impact of the COVID-19 pandemic on retail dairy prices. *Agribusiness* 37, 108–121.

Love, D.C., Allison, E.H., Asche, F., Belton, B., Cottrell, R.S. *et al.* (2021) Emerging COVID-19 impacts, responses, and lessons for building resilience in the seafood system. *Global Food Security* 28, 100494.

Luckstead, J., Nayga, R.M., Jr. and Snell, H.A. (2021) Labor issues in the food supply chain amid the COVID-19 pandemic. *Applied Economic Perspectives and Policy* 43(1), 382–400.

Lusk, J.L. and Briggeman, B.C. (2009) Food values. *American Journal of Agricultural Economics* 91(1), 184–196.

Lusk, J.L., Tonsor, G.T. and Schultz, L.L. (2021) Beef and pork marketing margins and price spreads during COVID-19. *Applied Economic Perspectives and Policy* 43(1), 4.

Ma, M. and Lusk, J.L. (2021) Concentration and resilience in the U.S. meat supply chains. Working paper no. 29103, *National Bureau of Economic Research*. Available at: https://www.nber.org/papers/w29103

Malone, T., Schaefer, K.A. and Lusk, J.L. (2021) Unscrambling U.S. egg supply chains amid COVID-19. *Food Policy* 101(May), 102046.

Maples, J.G., Thompson, J.M., Anderson, J.D. and Anderson, D.P. (2021) Estimating COVID-19 impacts on the broiler industry. *Applied Economic Perspectives and Policy* 43(1), 315–328.

Martinez, C.C., Maples, J.G. and Benavidez, J. (2021) Beef cattle markets and COVID-19. *Applied Economic Perspectives and Policy* 31(1), 304–314.

McFadden, B.R., Malone, T., Kecinski, M. and Messer, K.D. (2021) COVID-19 induced stigma in U.S. consumers: Evidence and implications. *American Journal of Agricultural Economics* 103(2), 486–497.

Melo, G. (2020) The path forward: U.S. consumer and food retail responses to COVID-19. *Choices* 35(3). Available at: https://www.choicesmagazine.org/choices-magazine/theme-articles/covid-19-and-the-agriculture-industry-laborsupply-chains-and-consumer-behavior/the-path-forward-us-consumer-and-food-retail-responses-to-covid-19

Mexiner, O. and Katt, F. (2020) Assessing the impact of COVID-19 on consumer food safety perceptions—A choice-based willingness to pay study. *Sustainability* 12, 7270.

Montanari, F., Arayess, S., Toma, B., Clavarino, A., Ferreira, I.M. *et al.* (2020) The response of the EU agri-food chain to the COVID-29 pandemic: Chronicles from the EU and selected member states. *European Food and Feed Law Review: EFFL* 15(4), 336–356.

Norwood, F.B. and Peel, D. (2021) Supply chain mapping to prepare for future pandemics. *Applied Economic Perspectives and Policy* 43(1), 412–429.

Orden, D. (2021) Agrifood markets and support in the United States after 1 year of COVID-19 pandemic. *Canadian Journal of Agricultural Economics* 69(2), 243–249.

Ponomarov, S.Y. and Holcomb, M.C. (2009) Understanding the concept of supply chain resilience. *The International Journal of Logistics Management* 20(1), 124–143.

Reardon, T., Belton, B., Saweda, O., Liverpool-Tasie, L., Lu, L. *et al.* (2021) E-commerce's fast-tracking diffusion and adaptation in developing countries. *Applied Economic Perspectives and Policy* 43, 1243–1259. DOI: 10.1002/aepp.13160.

Reardon, T., Heiman, A., Lu, L., Nuthalapati, C.S.R., Vos, R. *et al.* (2021) "Pivoting" by food industry firms to cope with COVID-19 in developing regions: E-commerce and "copivoting" delivery intermediaries. *Agricultural Economics* 52(3), 459–475.

Rejeb, A., Rejeb, K. and Keogh, J.G. (2021) COVID-19 and the food chain. *Impacts and Future Research Trends Logforum* 16(4), 475–485.

Richards, T. and Rickard, B. (2020) COVID-19 impact on fruit and vegetable markets. *Canadian Journal of Agricultural Economics* 68, 189–194.

Rivera-Ferre, M.G., López-i-Gelats, F., Ravera, F., Oteros-Rozas, E., Masso, M. *et al.* (2021) The two-way relationship between food systems and the COVID19 pandemic: Causes and consequences. *Agricultural Systems* 191, 103134.

Rude, J. (2020) *Resilience versus efficiency: The feasibility of small local meatpacking plants in Canada.* The Canadian Agri-Food Policy Institute (CAPI), Ottawa, Canada. Available at: https://capi-icpa.ca/wp-content/uploads/2021/03/2020-11-23-The-Feasibility-of-Small-Local-Meat-Packing-Plants-in-Canada-James-Rude.pdf

Rude, J. (2021) COVID-19 and the Canadian cattle/beef sector: A second look. *Canadian Journal of Agricultural Economics* 69(2), 233–241.

Saitone, T.L., Schaefer, K.A. and Scheitrum, D.P. (2021) COVID-19 morbidity and mortality in U.S. meat-packing counties. *Food Policy* 101, 102072.

Sanderson Bellmay, A., Furness, E., Nicol, P., Pitt, H. and Taherzadeh, A. (2021) Shaping more resilient and just food systems: Lessons from the COVID-19 pandemic. *Ambio* 50, 782–793.

Santeramo, F.G. and Perez-Dominguez, I. (2021) On the effects of the COVID epidemic on global and local food access and availability of strategic sectors: Role of trade and implications for policymakers. *International Agricultural Trade Research Consortium Commissioned Paper* 25, 49 .

Saweda O. Liverpool-Tasie, L., Reardon, T. and Belton, B. (2021) "Essential non-essentials": COVID-19 policy missteps in Nigeria rooted in persistent myths about african supply chains. *Applied Economic Perspectives and Policy* 43(1), 205–224.

Tendall, D.M., Joerin, J., Kopainsky, B., Edwards, P., Shreck, A. *et al.* (2015) Food system resilience: Defining the concept. *Global Food Security* 6, 17–23.

Thilmany, D., Canales, E., Low, S.A. and Boys, K. (2021) Local food supply chain dynamics and resilience during COVID-19. *Applied Economic Perspectives and Policy* 43(1), 86–104.

Weersink, A., Massow, M., Bannon, N., Ifft, J., Maples, J. *et al.* (2021) COVID-19 and the agri-food system in the United States and Canada. *Agricultural Systems* 188(March), Article no. 103039.

Wegerif, M.C.A. (2020) "Informal" food traders and food security: Experiences from the covid-19 response in South Africa. *Food Security* 12, 797–800.

15 Constraints to Using Livestock to Meet Dietary Needs in Developing Countries: Role of Vaccines

Cynthia L. Baldwin[1,2*] **and Samuel J. Black**[1,2]
[1]Department of Veterinary & Animal Sciences, 661 North Pleasant Street, University of Massachusetts, Amherst, MA 01003, United States; [2]Program in Molecular & Cellular Biology, University of Massachusetts, Amherst, MA 01003, United States

Abstract
Animal agriculture and animal-source foods (ASF) play a critical role in food security, childhood nutrient sufficiency, and economic development in sub-Saharan Africa. Here, we consider constraints to production of ASF in Africa with a focus on infectious animal diseases and climate stress and their control, by vaccines and selective breeding, respectively. This is not a meta-analysis but rather is meant to act as an overview or primer for discussing the value of livestock in developing countries, constraints to this, possible solutions, and finally some roadblocks to accomplishing this. The material provided is based on our own knowledge gained through careers in this field as well as discussions with colleagues.

Keywords: livestock, trypanosomiasis, East Coast fever, contagious bovine pleuropneumonia, African swine fever, vaccines

Review Methodology

This is an invited review that acts as a primer for discussing the value of livestock in developing countries, constraints to this focused on the role of infectious diseases in sub-Saharan Africa, possible solutions, and finally some roadblocks to accomplishing this. The material provided is based on our own knowledge gained through careers in this field as well as discussions with colleagues. This is not a comprehensive literature review nor was it intended to be so. You might consider it to be an opinion piece.

Introduction

Over the last decade there has been a growing trend in industrialized countries to move away from or reduce intake of animal-source foods (ASF) for health, esthetic, and ethical reasons. Some of the practical concerns include the amount of water and cost of feeds, particularly grains, needed to raise ASF. It has been suggested that roughly 10 times more water per pound of hamburger is required than per pound of maize. Similarly, the conversion of grain to meat is considered inefficient despite the greater nutrient density in meat compared to grains as summarized in the following quote: 'chickens

*Corresponding author: cbaldwin@umass.edu

and pigs convert grain into meat at ratios of two or three to one ... (while) ... the ratio for lamb is between four and more than six to one and that for beef starts at five to one and goes as high as 20 to one' (The Economist, Feast and Famine, Dec 31, 2013). In both industrialized and developing countries there is also a concern about destruction of the environment and wildlife habitat by over-grazing of livestock and by growing vast acreage of corn for cattle fodder for example. Furthermore, while food safety is a concern for animal-based as well as plant-based food, there is an added risk associated with growing ASF due to zoonotic disease. Indeed, when zoonotic outbreaks occur, some feel the appropriate way to address this is by slaughter of animals (swine in Egypt in response to H1N1 influenza outbreak) and adoption of veganism (Abdelwhab and Hafez, 2011; Seef and Jeppsson, 2013; Leach and Tadros, 2014).

Despite the current concern in industrialized countries regarding the many costs of ASF (Fig. 15.1), it is recognized that livestock offer a powerful pathway out of poverty for hundreds of millions of poor farmers in South Asia and Africa by providing nutritional and economic security (Fig. 15.2). 'Globally, two billion people suffer from micronutrient deficiencies, 151 million children under five suffer from stunting, and millions more have impaired cognitive development related to poor nutrition. This is partly due to insufficient consumption of ASF, which supply multiple bioavailable nutrients that are lacking in the cereal-based diets of the poor' (Neumann *et al.*, 2003, 2004; Adesogan *et al.*, 2020), although other factors are involved (Akombi *et al.*, 2017).

DETRIMENTS	BENEFITS
Water usage	Nutrition (meat, milk, eggs, blood)
Grain consumption	Micronutrients
Land erosion	Fertilizer
Habitat limiting	Hides & fiber
Zoonotic diseases	Construction material
Over consumption potentially detrimental to health	Traction
Aesthetics	Transport
Ethical considerations	Banking & social status
	Food source in environment where crops cannot survive

FACTORS IMPACTING PRODUCTIVITY

- Infectious diseases
- Climate stress
- Ectoparasites
- Genetics
- Epigenetics

Fig. 15.1. Comparison chart of the detractors and benefits of livestock farming. Some factors may be more prevalent in the developed world than the developing world and vice versa.

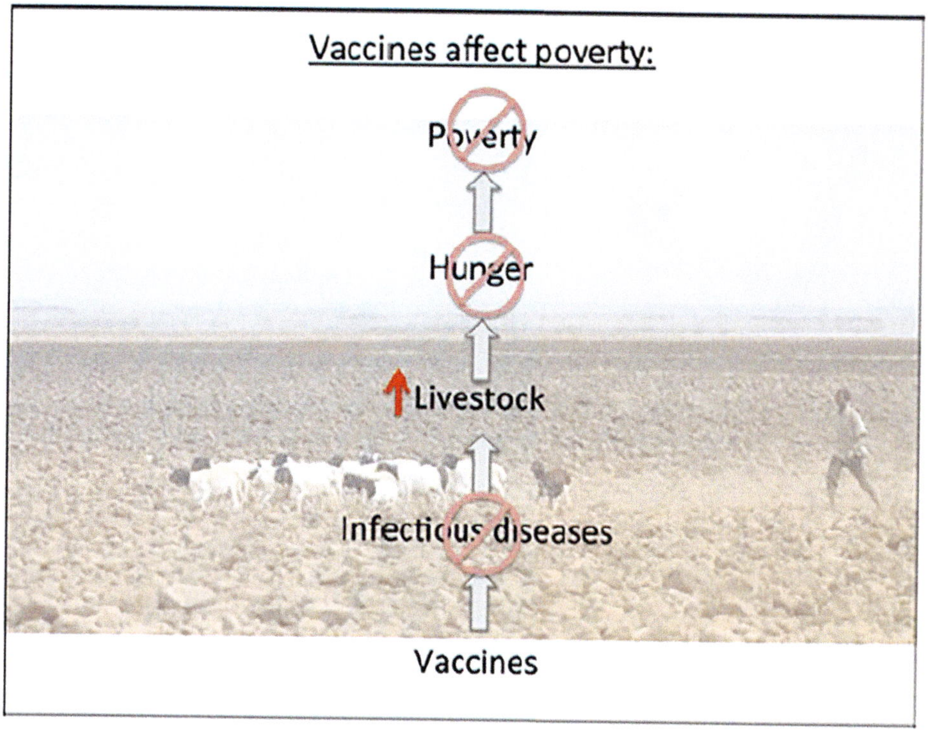

Fig. 15.2. The potential impact of vaccine development. This impact is focused on neglected tropical diseases regarding livestock farming and human well-being for the world's poorest who reside in marginal landscapes. Background photograph is courtesy of the International Livestock Research Institute (ILRI), Nairobi, Kenya.

Supplementation of diets with ASF has been shown to increase childhood cognitive development in nutritional studies conducted in Africa and to prevent stunting of growth, thus supporting individual and societal development, reviewed in Murphy and Neumann, 2014. However, attention needs to be paid to level of consumption to avoid the health issues associated with overconsumption of ASF in the industrialized world (Salter, 2018). With respect to the contribution of animal agriculture to rural economies, it is also important to recognize that meat is only a portion of the economic value of livestock and poultry; eggs, milk, blood, hides, wool, feathers, manure for fertilizer as well as fuel and construction materials for homes, traction, transportation, banking, social status, and warmth are all valuable by-products of animal-based agriculture (Baltenweck *et al.*, 2020) (Fig. 15.1). Beyond the farm, during the last two decades urbanization and expanding populations have created expanding markets for livestock products, making them the fastest growing sector of the agricultural market and an engine for growth of rural economies. In this regard, in sub-Saharan Africa, agriculture of which animal-based agriculture is a critical component accounts for about 30% of regional GDP, 20% of exports and 60% of employment (FAO Pro-Poor Livestock Policy Initiative, RR Nr. 05–09 Nov 2005).

While livestock is a high-growth, high-value agricultural sub-sector and sustainable integration of livestock production into the smallholder farmer's portfolio is a route to decreasing poverty and improving nutrition, the impediments cannot be ignored. Disease, climatic stress, and environmental fragility contribute to constrain the goal of increasing livestock production. To decrease these constraints, there is a need to both develop disease-resistant and climatic stress-tolerant livestock (and plants) that thrive in the smallholder production unit (Fig. 15.3)

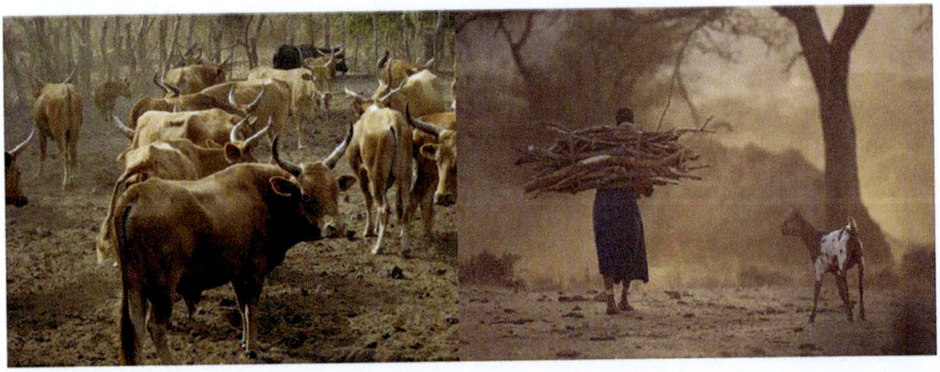

Fig. 15.3. Marginal landscapes for raising ruminants in Africa. Photos courtesy of ILRI, Nairobi, Kenya.

and to protect against food contamination during production and in post-harvest processing. Some of these issues are discussed here.

Livestock and Infectious Diseases

Infectious diseases remain one of the key constraints to animal-based agriculture in sub-Saharan Africa. Some of those with profound effects are listed in (Fig. 15.4). Creating stress-tolerant, including disease-tolerant, livestock necessarily requires breeding, and development of such animals may contribute to resistance to infectious diseases. However, overall, it is generally agreed that control of infectious diseases is most effectively done though vaccination. Vaccines can in some cases prevent disease, while in other cases they decrease pathogenicity and accelerate cure. This has become highly apparent during the current pandemic with SARS-CoV2. Nevertheless, a vaccine must have specificity for the infectious agent and stimulate vaccine antigen-specific lymphocytes with functions that protect the host and that have immunological memory capable of effecting recall responses to future disease challenges. Thus, development of vaccines against high-impact infectious disease has high potential for improving livestock meat and milk yields in sub-Saharan Africa through maintenance of animal health, which in turn is predicted to reduce poverty and support human health as noted above.

Vaccine development and testing, as well as investigation of mechanisms of infectious disease pathology in cattle and other livestock species, is facilitated by the capacity to conduct in-depth analysis of the ensuing immune responses following vaccination and challenge with virulent strains of the pathogens. However, it is critical to note that a large and sustained investment in research is needed to be able to accomplish this. As an example, the study of bovine immunology over the last 50 years has resulted in the development of reagents for identification of immune system cells, that is, leukocyte populations and sub-populations, their receptors for antigen-specific, inflammatory, and other signals, and their roles in protection against infectious diseases. Much of the original reagent development for cattle originated in Africa at the International Laboratory for Research on Animal Diseases (ILRAD) and subsequently its successor the International Livestock Research Institute (ILRI).This has been recently reviewed (Black and Baldwin, 2021).

Overall, progress in vaccinology includes high-resolution mapping of vaccine antigens, integration of pathogen genome mining and vaccine antigen selection, and the design of novel adjuvants (agents that expedite development of the appropriate immune responses). Tackling the most challenging diseases, including those highlighted below, requires networks of academic, national, regional, and international organizations, including the public, private, and development sectors that collectively work toward this goal. While most modern research facilities are in the developed world, the location of research facilities in disease-endemic regions

Disease or pathogen	Relative economic impact (US$ billions)	Species affected	Type of pathogen
Peste des Petit Ruminants	4.80	Goats	Virus
Endoparasites	4.45	All	Helminths
Contagious Bovine Pleural Pneumonia	4.25	Cattle	Mycoplasma bacteria
Contagious Caprine Pleural Pneumonia	3.75	Goats	Mycoplasm bacteria
Ectoparasites	2.50	All	Arthropods
Trypanosomiasis	1.75	Cattle & goats	Protozoa
Foot & Mouth Disease	1.25	Cattle	Virus
Shoat pox	0.75	Sheep & goats	Virus
Lumpy Skin Disease	0.75	Cattle	Virus
Rift Valley Fever	0.75	Cattle	Virus
Brucellosis	0.40	All	Bacteria
East Coast Fever (Theileriosis)	0.40	Cattle	Protozoa
Bovine Tuberculosis	0.33	Cattle	Bacteria
Bovine Viral Diarrhea	0.10	Cattle	Virus

Fig. 15.4. Relative economic impact on ruminant health in sub-Saharan Africa. These are relative estimates provided by Dr Delia Grace, Program Leader, ILRI, July 2015. Currently, a more comprehensive study is underway to attempt to obtain more accurate and comprehensive values. 'All' means cattle, goats, and sheep.

with access to diverse pathogen strains and indigenous livestock breeds and wildlife, some of which have genetically acquired resistance to particular diseases, is an advantage and a necessary part of the disease research network. This allows ready access to and thus potentially rapid characterization of regionally prevalent pathogen strains or components of these pathogens as well as the ability to identify potentially protective host immune responses in indigenous breeds and species to the relevant pathogens.

In the past before the advent of molecular tools, most livestock vaccines were developed using an empirical approach based on observation and experience rather than one based on theory, logic, and rationale. This includes most vaccines that are in use today. That approach is changing or has changed. The smallpox vaccine for humans is an example of one of the first empirically developed vaccines (Riedel, 2005), while the current highly effective SARS-CoV2 (COVID-19) vaccines are based on the latter (Calina *et al.*, 2020). Some of the aspects of the basic approach to development of vaccines for addressing livestock disease constraints in the developing world include the following:

- Prioritizing target diseases and developing vaccine product profiles based on prevalence, economic impact, zoonotic potential and, finally, those with a lack of research investment toward their control in developed countries thereby indicating it is a neglected tropical disease (Fig. 15.4).
- Developing or identifying pathogen strain and/or species-specific recombinant vaccine antigens, DNA or RNA vaccine counterparts, and/or attenuated vaccine strains.
- Testing candidate vaccines for improved protection of livestock against disease in conventional as well as in selected disease-tolerant and climatic stress-tolerant livestock, thereby potentially increasing productivity as well as production range.

Accurate and inexpensive productivity sensing devices, point-of-care diagnostics, centralized reporting of infectious diseases, and large-scale data processing have important roles in monitoring disease progression and control. Thus, consideration should also be given to the need for development of these quantitative tools as components of strategies to improve livestock productivity in addition to vaccine development.

Case study: rinderpest vaccination campaign and eradication of disease

One decade ago, the ability of a vaccine to control infectious disease in livestock was unequivocally demonstrated by the eradication of rinderpest. After centuries of effort, on June 28, 2011, the United Nations officially declared the eradication of rinderpest (https://www.unmultimedia.org/radio/english/2011/06/cattle-killer-disease-rinderpest-eradicated/rinderpest-eradication1/). This disease of cattle is also known as 'cattle plague' because of its devastating effects on livestock and the dread it evoked in producers and consumer populations. Rinderpest caused widespread famine when introduced into sub-Saharan Africa in the late 1800s, spreading through and from Europe and Asia to Africa (Mack, 1970; Barrett and Rossiter, 1999). Caused by a virus, it is only the second infectious disease to be wiped out by human efforts, smallpox being the first. It has been suggested that this is probably the greatest achievement in veterinary medicine.

The last strongholds of the rinderpest virus in Africa were remote pastoral areas where transporting vaccine required ice to maintain the vaccine at refrigerator temperatures. Requiring this temperature-controlled supply chain, known as a 'cold chain,' was particularly problematic. A similar problem has been associated with some of the vaccines against SARS CoV2 in developed countries during current days. Developing a thermostable rinderpest vaccine that could survive for 20 weeks at body temperature (37°C) (Mariner *et al.*, 1990) meant the vaccine could be transported and stored at the remote locations where the disease persisted.

The vaccine used in the eradication of rinderpest was a modification of the Plowright vaccine and was commercially produced at large scale by 1992. It was first tested in Niger where it saved the country more than $3 million annually because of the lack of need to maintain a cold chain for vaccination. Subsequently, in the remote regions in other parts of Africa, vaccination programs were implemented by trained pastoral livestock owners guided by veterinarians. This represents a milestone in the history of veterinary medicine not only because of the disease eradication but because of the development of service delivery models where community animal health workers transported and administered the vaccine in remote and insecure areas. Thus, there was an important and crucial sociological aspect to the success of this campaign. Finally, it is important to note that although not used in the eradication campaign, recombinant rinderpest vaccines were also developed and shown to be efficacious demonstrating the principal of vaccine design using molecular approaches early during the advent of molecular biology (Yilma *et al.*, 1988; Giavedoni *et al.*, 1991).

Livestock and Climate Change

Livestock can be the main food source in marginal areas since they convert grass and shrubs, often the only available 'crops,' to protein. In addition to specific infectious diseases, temperature extremes, drought, general disease prevalence, and other forms of climatic-induced challenges can result in slower growth rates of livestock, reduced production performance, and reproductive inefficiencies (Okagawa *et al.*, 2012; Konnai *et al.*, 2017; Morenikeji *et al.*, 2019; Jiang *et al.*, 2020; Godde *et al.*, 2021). Since most livestock in the developing world are raised outside, there are limited means available to livestock keepers to modify or mitigate the effects of climate change. It is also difficult to predict or model how climate change will affect infectious diseases of humans and livestock due to the complexity of the systems involved. Changes in moisture, temperature, and wind will no doubt affect the animal hosts of infectious diseases, the pathogens themselves and the vectors that transmit them, as well as the environment of humans and their livestock that serves as the pathogen habitat. In turn, animal and human movement and their distribution upon the land will be likely to change and thus, disease transmission patterns will change (McMichael, 2015; Zinsstag *et al.*, 2018; Caminade *et al.*, 2019) adding to the complexity of predicting future impacts. Nevertheless, given the increased demand for animal products in the developing world there is a need to develop productive livestock that are more resilient to climate change and the associated issues that accompany it.

Despite the uncertainty regarding how change will be wrought, reasonable generalized predictions include (i) increased rate of eukaryotic and prokaryotic pathogen development in areas with the modest temperature increases, (ii) decreased parasite/pathogen/vector survival in areas with more severe rises in temperature and decreased moisture (especially for pathogens that are not vector-transmitted and require survival outside the host for maintenance), and, finally, (iii) changes in winds will affect the direction or rate of spreading of pathogens, particularly viruses that survive outside the host. The conclusion is that increased pressure on the world food supply due to infectious diseases could occur as a result of the effects that climate change has on the fitness of livestock in general especially in areas where temperatures rise and water becomes scarce. As a documented example, Newcastle Disease (Ganar *et al.*, 2014; Dimitrov *et al.*, 2017) and other diseases of poultry have become more frequent in West Africa with extended dry seasons over the last 10 years. They are now recurrent epidemics on some poultry farms. A decrease in the nutritional value of animal feeds may also result from higher temperatures and/or drought, which then, in turn, may affect the immune status of the livestock and thus disease resistance in addition to affecting their overall growth.

The impact of climate change and environmental stress on plants and animals may be partially mitigated by genetic selection through reproductive fitness and survival. Fitness and adaptation traits are in part controlled by the genetic makeup of the animal and this genetic makeup determines an animal's tolerance to stress and climatic shocks. Particular breeds of cattle (Carroll *et al.*, 2013; Davis *et al.*, 2017; Kim *et al.*, 2017), goats (Devendra, 2013; Rout *et al.*, 2016; Aleena *et al.*, 2018), and chickens (Nawab *et al.*, 2018; Wang *et al.*, 2018; Zhuang *et al.*, 2020) demonstrate considerable heat tolerance making them better adapted to the hot and water-stressed regions of the globe, which gives them an advantage in the face of climate change. Identification of the underlying genes associated with the ability to adapt to climate challenges could facilitate selective breeding and genomic selection of adapted infectious disease-resistant breeds of livestock with increased production potential. One such approach is the method referred to as landscape genomics, which is the combination of population genetics, modern genomics, and landscape ecology (Lowry, 2010; McManus *et al.*, 2020).

Landscape genomics analysis is the simultaneous study of thousands of single-nucleotide polymorphism (SNP) markers, ideally including markers in candidate genes for adaptive change. These may have been under natural or artificial selection and can be accessed through global information system (GIS)-referenced samples of animal or plant species collected across landscapes that vary in their climatic conditions. The goal is to find different genome spatial patterns within a species that are associated with regional climatic differences. These genomic reflections of natural and artificial selection are labeled 'signatures of selection.' Examples may include genomic regions for improved performance that are associated with specific types of environments from particular geographic regions. Others might include increased parasite resistance in livestock within a geographic region and its association with specific chromosomes and genes. Landscape genomics may also help define differences in the fitness of livestock from certain geographic regions in general but especially in areas where temperatures are rising, and water is becoming increasingly scarce.

It is envisioned that confirmation of individual signatures of selection for their ability to increase disease or parasite resistance and/or adapt to climate challenges would be achieved by breeding schemes. Ultimately, the goal is genomic selection of adapted breeds of livestock with increased production potential. However, in recent years it has become apparent that epigenetics plays a role in disease susceptibility and resistance that could thwart the best breeding intention. Epigenetic modifications have been shown to explain the heritability of a trait that is not a result of germline encoding. This includes DNA methylation and chromatin accessibility. As a result of these, there may be a difference in expression of transcription factors and other DNA-binding molecules such as siRNA and their ability to affect gene expression. The epigenome has been explored for different tissues of cattle and goats although results are not yet linked to disease susceptibility (Zhang *et al.*, 2017; Zhou *et al.*, 2020; Zhang *et al.* 2020).

Mitigating Infectious Diseases: Designing Vaccines and Targeted Genetic Modification

While advanced breeding schemes based on genomic signatures of disease and climatic stress tolerance may improve livestock productivity over the long term, control of animal diseases by vaccination is likely to have a more immediate impact. When taking the rational approach to vaccine development, it is necessary to first understand what type of immune response is needed for protection. One source of information is to evaluate the immune response of recovered individuals or animals determining which classes of antibodies were developed and which type of T cell responses were prevalent among the responding population. A second approach is to adoptively transfer cells or serum-containing antibodies from protected individuals into naïve individuals and then challenge those individuals with the infectious agent to determine which cells or antibodies correlate with protection. Finally, when working with model animals, such as mice, knocking out cell populations or immune cell functions by gene deletion or blocking specific immune system molecules with antibodies has facilitated identification of the cellular and molecular basis of effective immune responses. Deletion of leukocyte populations by administration of specific monoclonal antibodies has been achieved in cattle (Naessens *et al.*, 1998) but requires a large quantity of antibody and is thus costly compared to rodent models. Thus, the dearth or complications of approaches to evaluate immune responses in target animals other than rodent models hampers our understanding of what is required of a protective immune response and thus what type of immune response the vaccine should be stimulating.

It has been difficult to develop vaccines to some infectious disease organisms that can evade protective immune responses, for example, by varying their antigens or by misdirecting immune responses. The latter includes eliciting pathogenic as opposed to protective immune responses. The mammalian immune system is tremendously complex and there are many possible outcomes when it is 'activated.' For example, activation of macrophages, which are phagocytic cells of the innate immune system, may have different outcomes (Murray *et al.*, 2014; Juhas *et al.*, 2015; Hussen and Schuberth, 2017) depending upon which receptors they use to detect the presence of the infectious pathogen and which cytokines and chemokines (soluble meditators of the immune system that allow cell communication) they are exposed to. This is because the receptors transduce distinct signals to the macrophage, and thus, the gene expression patterns that are elicited differ depending on the receptor array that is engaged. The response by the innate immune cells can in turn influence the type of response expressed by the lymphocytic cells of the adaptive immune system. Different pathogens have various structures known as pathogen-associated molecular patterns (PAMPs) that interact with the innate system cells through receptors known as pattern recognition receptors (PRR). A well-known example of PRRs is the toll-like receptor (TLR) family. Viruses and bacteria interact with different TLRs. Pathogen components that interact with the TLR family include viral and bacterial nucleic acids, cell wall lipids of Gram-positive and Gram-negative bacteria, carbohydrates and proteins. These interactions may aid the host in control of the infection or they may misdirect the immune response.

Some T lymphocytes use a combination of the antigen-specific T cell receptors (TCR) as well as PRR (i.e. used by innate-like T cells), while others rely essentially exclusively on the TCR interaction with pathogen components (i.e. used by adaptive T cells). In turn, these cells can make different responses including production of distinct sets of cytokines as a result of the combination of cells' receptors stimulated and the response by the innate immune cells in their milieu.The most simplistic example is the Th1 vs Th2 vs Th17 paradigm (Butcher and Zhu, 2021; Stockinger, 2021) where CD4T cells known as Th1-responding cells principally make the cytokine interferon-γ (IFNγ) that activates macrophages for a cellular pro-inflammatory response. In contrast, Th2-responding CD4T cells release a cytokine, IL-4, that is important in B lymphocyte activation and development of antibody responses, and finally, Th17-responding CD4T cells release a cytokine, IL-17, that attracts neutrophils. Depending upon the lifestyle of the pathogen, one of these responding cells and its cytokines may be more effective than the others in controlling the infection.

The types of vaccines used differ in their ability to stimulate various components of the immune system. Considerations are modified live vaccines for viruses and live attenuated for bacteria vs a variety of killed or subunit vaccines. Recent advances such as viral vector vaccines, DNA vaccines, and most recently RNA vaccines (Brisse *et al.*, 2020; Lundstrom, 2020) are able to mimic the results of live vaccines with fewer of the side effects or inherent risks of live modified or attenuated pathogens such as the pathogen undergoing genetic mutations that could result in reverting to the wild-type virulent pathogen.

Some of the more recent considerations in vaccine design have been to include stimulation of non-conventional cell types that may be acting upstream of the response by conventional adaptive αβ T cells or B2B cells. An example is NKT cells that are innate-like and that are stimulated by lipid molecules such as α-gal-cer. In pigs (Artiaga *et al.*, 2016; Yang *et al.*, 2017), this approach has been shown to vastly increase B cell antibody production and decrease viral titers. γIV T cells, another innate-like T cell type, in cattle have been stimulated by amphotericin B that results in increased IFNγ production and protection against *Salmonella*. A commercial vaccine against *Leptospira* also stimulates cattle γIV T cells in the first month following vaccination prior to reception of the second vaccine dose, resulting in IFNγ production as shown in *in vitro* recall responses; this presumably contribute to a protective immune response (Naiman *et al.*, 2002; Baldwin *et al.*, 2014).

Finally, it is important to consider control of responses to vaccines. As in other inflammatory responses, following vaccination the immune system may undergo T cell exhaustion or suppression of responses. This can be the result of cytokines produced by regulatory T cells including IL-10 and TGFβ or as a result of signaling T cells through molecules that inhibit T cell responses such as CTLA-4, PD-1, and Tim3. Finally, microRNAs can result in post-transcriptional regulation of transcription factors such as Eomesodermin and thus decreased effector molecule production (perforin and granzyme B) (Okagawa *et al.*, 2012; Konnai *et al.*, 2017; Morenikeji *et al.*, 2019; Jiang *et al.*, 2020).

In addition to vaccines, modern techniques may allow a targeted development of disease resistant livestock. This is a much newer field than vaccinology but some encouraging examples of its power nevertheless are already available. Affordable targeted gene deletion in ruminants and pigs through genetic engineering can be achieved by application of new technologies such as CRISPR. Use of these technologies in livestock has been recently reviewed (Islam *et al.*, 2020) in the context of engineering disease resistant animals. As examples, the molecule CD163 involved in infection of swine by the porcine respiratory and reproductive syndrome (PRRS) virus was genetically modified, rendering the cells expressing CD163 and thus the host animals to be resistant to PRRS virus infection, while in a second example, resistance to African swine fever virus was achieved by disrupting the *Rosa26* locus (Whitworth *et al.*, 2014; Xie *et al.*, 2018; Guo *et al.*, 2019).

Challenges of Vaccine Development for Select Diseases of Livestock

Peste des Petits Ruminants (PPR)

Peste des Petits Ruminants (PPR) (Parida *et al.*, 2015; Dundon *et al.*, 2020) was first reported in 1942 in Ivory Coast and is now found in Central and West Africa as well as Central, South and East Asia. PPR is caused by a Morbillivirus of the family Paramyxoviridae. The virus is highly contagious in goats, sheep, and wild ruminants where it causes a disease that is clinically similar to rinderpest in cattle and measles in humans. Cattle and camelids can also be infected by the PPRV but do not develop signs of disease and may be dead end hosts.The PPR virus spreads by close contact between infected and naïve animals, infecting lymphoid tissue as well as gastrointestinal and respiratory tracts. Spread of the virus is rapid in susceptible animals at high-grazing density or when kept in close contact during confinement. This can result in devastating loses. For example, during the 2006–2008 PPR outbreak in Turkana, Kenya, over 1 million animals perished, and during the 2017 PPR outbreak in Mongolia 80% of saiga antelope, which are an endangered species, were lost as well as large numbers of domesticated small ruminants.

There is only one serotype of PPRV but various PPRV strains which can be grouped into four lineages based on N and F gene sequences. Lineages I and II are mostly but not exclusively found in Africa, Lineage III in the Arabian peninsula and Lineage IV in Asia. Rinderpest vaccines were initially used to control PPRV but a live-attenuated PPRV vaccine was developed in 1989 (Diallo *et al.*, 1989). Two attenuated strains are now used in Africa, Middle Eastern, and Asian countries to induce broad protective immunity. These are PPRV Nigeria 75/1 and Sungri 96. These two attenuated vaccines induce protective immunity against all four lineages of PPRV when challenged subcutaneously or intranasally (Sarkar *et al.*, 2003; Sen *et al.*, 2010; Hodgson *et al.*, 2018; Mahapatra *et al.*, 2020). Vaccine distribution has been expedited by development of thermostabilizers to circumvent a need for a cold chain. Optimization of this process is ongoing. For example, Mariner and colleagues used the rinderpest freeze drying method together with hydrolyzed lactoprotein sucrose as a stabilizer to preserve the Nigeria 75/1 PPRV strain. This resulted in vaccine shelf lives of 105 and 13.7 days respectively at 37 and 56°C (Mariner *et al.*, 2017). PPRV subunit vaccines have also been developed but so far are less effective at inducing long-lived immunity than the attenuated vaccine strains.

In April 2015, the Food and Agriculture Organization and the World Organization for Animal Health launched the PPR Global Control and Eradication Strategy with the vision of eradication by 2030. A multi-stage, multi-country approach incorporating assessment, control, eradication and maintenance of PPRV free status is envisaged, reviewed in (Njeumi *et al.*, 2020). Success will be expedited by tracking of effective vaccination, which requires the development of tests that distinguish vaccinated from infected animals. To that end, it has recently been reported that two recombinant live-attenuated PPR DIVA (**D**ifferentiating **I**nfected from **V**accinated **A**nimals) vaccines have been developed at the Purbright Institute, UK. These were tested in goats and provided similar immune responses to their parent Nigeria 75/1 and Sungri 96 live-attenuated vaccine strains, reviewed in (Zhao *et al.*, 2021). These or similar DIVA will be needed for disease eradication.

Contagious bovine pleuropneumonia (CBPP)

Contagious bovine pleuropneumonia (CBPP) (Muuka *et al.*, 2013; Di Teodoro *et al.*, 2020; Alhaji *et al.*, 2020) is a respiratory disease of livestock caused by the bacterium *Mycoplasma mycoides* (MCC). Under natural conditions, the wall-less bacterium infects ruminants of the *Bos* genus, but it has also been isolated from sheep and goats in Africa, Portugal, and India. CBPP had a worldwide distribution by the middle to late 1800s but was thought to be eliminated from most of the world's continents by the mid-1900s. CBPP was previously prevalent in the US, Australia, and Europe but controlled through culling although this had a severe economic impact. Since then, there has been a dramatic resurgence of the disease. Currently, CBPP is considered to be one of the most important bacterial livestock diseases in sub-Saharan Africa by African Union-Inter-Africa Bureau of Animal Resources (AU-IBAR) affecting greater than 20 countries in Africa. It restricts trading of cattle products to disease-free countries. While only a small percentage of infected animals die, survivors show greatly decreased productivity including for dairy cattle with severe lactation loss.

CBPP control measures currently used in African and other areas of the world include restriction of animal movement, test and slaughter, and quarantine of infected or suspect animals. Both *M. mycoides mycoides* and *M. mycoides capri* (the equivalent disease in goats known as CCPP) are killed by treatment of the host with antibiotics and this treatment decreases transmission, but the regime may create antibiotic-resistant bacteria with subsequent adverse effects on human and animal health and hence should be prohibited according to OIE. A live vaccine for CBPP currently exists but requires a cold chain, elicits short-lived immunity (March, 2004) (8 months), and causes severe reactions at the inoculation site (Muuka *et al.*, 2014). Creation of an efficient subunit vaccine against different *M. mycoides* infections in ruminants using cutting edge technologies is a current goal of researchers (Jores *et al.*, 2020). A subunit vaccine will not require a cold chain; it could be designed for greater efficacy, longer immunity, and fewer side effects than a live-attenuated vaccine. Construction of a protein subunit vaccine or an RNA vaccine that elicits production of protective antigens is likely now that there are available innovative technologies to manipulate the genes of these bacteria through synthetic biology approaches.

African Swine Fever Virus (ASFV)

African Swine Fever Virus (ASFV) (Dixon *et al.*, 2019; Teklue *et al.*, 2020) is a contagious hemorrhagic viral disease of pigs. ASFV is an OIE-listed disease, which affects trans-boundary trade and poses a serious threat to the global pig industry. It is present in the continents of Africa, Europe, and Asia and disease outbreaks have occurred in South America and Spain, and are spreading through Europe as well as China currently. In Africa, it was first described in Kenya but is now present in most of sub-Saharan Africa and outbreaks are frequent due to spread of the virus into naïve pig populations, with mortality rates as high as 100%. The disease situation is further complicated by reservoirs of ASFV in some tick species as well as warthog and bush pig, differential sensitivity to disease by different pig breeds and because the reference diagnostic tests may not function on all viral genotypes. In Europe, there is endemic transmission of ASFV in countries north of the Black Sea following ASFV outbreaks from viral contamination of ship garbage containing pig products originating in southeastern Africa. ASFV has now reached the Caribbean threatening North America. Infections with virulent strains are lethal within days of infection, while those with less virulent strains can survive and impart a degree of immunity to subsequent challenge with the more virulent strains. Currently, the disease is generally controlled by slaughter. In China alone, it is estimated that 6 million pigs were culled between 2018 and 2020 as a result of ASFV (OEI Bulletin, #2020–1).

Pigs are among the most profitable livestock species for poor farmers, enabling them to earn cash income for education and health. This activity is affordable for resource-poor smallholders since pigs convert food wastes and agricultural by-products into protein, and have a short reproductive cycle, large litter sizes, and mature quickly. Better incomes and urbanization have increased global demand for pork; especially in Africa, for example, in Uganda, the swine industry is growing rapidly, and pork consumption is almost equal to that of beef and is the highest in Africa. However, the frequent outbreaks of ASF are a significant constraint to pig production in sub-Saharan Africa. Backyard and free-ranging swine production are particularly vulnerable thereby impacting poor farmers. Escape of the virus from endemic regions also poses an increasing threat to the global pork industry given that pork products are frequently illegally imported by travelers and the virus can survive for long periods of times in pork products. Therefore, development of a vaccine is anticipated to transform the lives of pig farmers in sub-Saharan Africa as well as reduce the risk posed by ASFV to the global swine industry.

The genome of ASFV is large and complex and shows obvious genetic diversity. This is reflected in recognition of 24 genotypes based on the sequence of the gene encoding the major capsid protein p72 and 8 serotypes of the viral hemagglutinin CD2-like protein (Wu *et al.*, 2020). There are no drugs or vaccines for the control of ASFV. Evidence indicates that pigs can develop immunity to ASFV especially following infection with viral strains of lower virulence, providing a rationale for the development of a vaccine as a sustainable control option. Ongoing investigations explore gene deletion to generate modified live-attenuated virus vaccines, and development of a subunit vaccine through identification of immunoprotective antigens (Gaudreault and Richt, 2019; Sang *et al.*, 2020). The former approach has so far suffered from a poor safety profile of the putative attenuated viruses. With respect to the latter approach, it has recently been reported that immunization with a pool of eight viral-vectored ASFV genes induced cellular and humoral immune responses that protected pigs against infection with a lethal dose of a virulent genotype 1 strain of ASFV (Goatley *et al.*, 2020). In addition, a complex DNA vaccine has been developed, which is comprised of 15 plasmids encoding individual peptide-bearing ASFV ORFs selected on their ability to stimulate CD8T cells. Priming with this DNA vaccine improved protection afforded by a suboptimal dose of the BA71ΔCD2 live-attenuated vaccine against a lethal dose of Georgia2007/1 (Bosch-Camos *et al.*, 2021).

Application of these approaches to other genotypes of ASFV may lead to improved control of the disease through vaccination.

African trypanosomiasis

Animal African trypanosomiasis (AAT) (Maudlin, 2006; Morrison *et al.*, 2016; Odeniran *et al.*, 2018) is endemic in tsetse-infested areas of Africa that are primarily grazed by livestock, and epidemic in regions where livestock meet trypanosomes-transmitting tsetse flies (*Glossina* spp.) from the wildlife reservoir. Three species of African trypanosomes, *Trypanosoma brucei*, *T. congolense* and *T. vivax*, are responsible for AAT. These protozoan parasites are transmitted to mammals in tsetse saliva during blood feeding and inhabit host blood, and in the case of *T. brucei* also lymph and tissue fluids. Tsetse flies infest 10 million square kilometers of over 40 African countries, thereby excluding cattle ranching from all but the fringes of this habitat where trypanosome challenge is low to moderate. Where cattle ranching is possible, it has been estimated that 48,000,000 cattle are at risk for AAT and 3,000,000 cattle die annually because of it. Thus, AAT is a major obstacle to economic development in sub-Saharan Africa since it is prevalent in the humid and semi-humid regions of sub-Saharan Africa, which encompasses vast areas highly suited to rain-fed agriculture.

AAT control involves three strategies: vector control, use of trypanocides, and farming of trypanotolerant cattle. Tsetse chemoattractants have been identified (Rayaisse *et al.*, 2010) and included in traps, which, with diligent use and maintenance, remain a useful way to reduce infection risk. A good deal of data has been collected showing that the West African *Bos taurus* N'dama breed can be productive at low-to-medium levels of tsetse and trypanosome challenge without use of trypanocides or tsetse control (Yaro *et al.*, 2016; Black, 2021). However, their small size, feisty nature, and low suitability for traction have prevented their widespread adoption by small holder farmers throughout Africa. Crosses and backcrosses between N'dama and Boran, a trypanosomiasis-susceptible East Africa *Bos indicus* breed, show the involvement of numerous quantitative trait loci in trypanotolerance.

Control of AAT by vaccination has been a goal of veterinary immunologists for the past century but so far has not met with success. The main reason for this is antigenic variation of the immunodominant and immunoprotective variable surface glycoprotein (VSG) that coats all three species of AAT parasites. *T. brucei* variable surface glycoprotein antigenic variation occurs at telomeric expression sites (Saha *et al.*, 2020) and involves a process of segmented gene conversion through recombination (McCulloch *et al.*,

2015; Sima et al., 2019), which results in huge VSG antigenic diversity. In contrast, *T. vivax* coat antigenic variation does not involve segmented gene conversion, and its VSG repertoire is broadly conserved across clinical isolates (Pereira *et al.*, 2020). Irrespective of differences in mechanisms of VSG antigenic variation among pathogenic African trypanosome species its practical outcome is the same. Each parasite expresses a single VSG gene at a time encoding a single species of variable surface glycoprotein, the expressed VSG gene changes at a rate that exceeds immune clearance of progenitor trypanosomes. This results in recurring waves of parasitemia and chronic infection. The repertoire of VSGs in all three species of AAT parasites is large and precludes their assembly into an effective composite vaccine.

An intact VSG coat prevents antibodies from reacting with underlying parasite plasma membrane antigens. Although receptors for essential macronutrients, for example, iron-loaded transferrin, breach the VSG barrier and are accessible to serum antibodies, they do not serve as targets for immune attack because of receptor diversification (Trevor *et al.*, 2019) and endocytosis in association with their cognate ligands, which results in clearance from the cell surface. These findings have led to the idea that it is not possible to generate an effective vaccine against any of the African trypanosomes, but this conclusion may be unwarranted. Investigations carried out by the Wright group using a systematic genome-led vaccinology approach and a murine model of *T. vivax* AAT identified several invariant protective antigens. Vaccination of mice with one of these comprising the extracellular region of a conserved cell surface protein localized to the flagellar membrane induced long-lasting immunity mediated by antibody and complement (Autheman *et al.*, 2021). This immunity could be passively transferred between hosts by immune serum or invariant flagellar antigen-specific monoclonal antibodies. Studies are underway to investigate whether the *T. vivax* invariant flagellar antigen will induce protective immunity in cattle.

East Coast Fever (ECF)

East Coast Fever (Irvin and Mwamachi, 1983; Dolan, 1999) or theileriosis is a tick-borne protozoan disease of cattle in Africa caused by *Theileria parva*. It is found in 11 countries in eastern, central, and southern Africa where it is endemic, thereby estimated to affect approximately 20 million smallholder farmers with approximately 28 million cattle at risk. A subunit vaccine directed at the parasite, the tick carrier, or a combination would be a cheaper and a safer option than the current use of anti-tick chemicals. A *Theileria*-specific subunit vaccine would overcome the need for a cold chain for delivery of the live vaccine currently used and would prevent the risk of spreading disease that the live vaccine poses. Development of such a vaccine is expected to result in annual on-farm yield gains of hundreds of million liters of milk and tens of thousands of tons of meat. It would also result in savings by reducing cost of tick control, which would additionally reduce environmental pollution.

Theileria parva parasites are transmitted to cattle and Cape buffalo hosts in the saliva of *Rhipicephalus appendiculatus* (brown ear tick) during feeding. Infections of cattle are typically lethal, while those of Cape buffalo are benign. In cattle, it is a progressive and very aggressive lymphoproliferative disease, which is fatal within 3–4 weeks after infection. Ticks become infected with *T. parva* when they take up infected red blood cells during feeding. The replicative stage of *T. parva* is intracellular; therefore, immune protection at this stage of infection requires killing of infected cells. This has been shown to be mediated by CD8T cells that arise during infection (Morrison, 2007; Morrison *et al.*, 2015). However, in naïve cattle replication of *T. parva*-infected cells far exceeds the capacity of parasite specific CD8T cells to control the infection.

ECF provides a well-characterized disease model with a clear challenge model to evaluate vaccine efficacy. Cattle can be immunized against *T. parva* by administration of the parasite sporozoites together with long-acting tetracycline, which slows the rate of infected cell replication allowing the development of a robust and parasite-specific cytotoxic CD8T cell response. This is the basis of the *T. parva* infection and treatment regime, established about 45 years ago to generate ECF immune cattle, and which has been improved during ensuing decades (Bishop *et al.*, 2020). *T. parva*-infected bovine lymphocytes can be cultured as cell lines *in vitro*. These cell lines can be generated from a lymphocyte infected with a single sporozite providing tools to dissect the *T. parva* strain specificity of host protective cytotoxic CD8T cells (Morrison *et al.*, 2015). Empirical studies using infection and treatment combined with homologous or heterologous *T. parva* strain challenge, *in vitro* killing assays, and DNA sequencing show that there is a good deal of *T. parva* strain molecular and antigenic diversity, and that this is particularly broad in strains of *T. parva* transmitted *via* ticks from Cape buffalo to cattle (Bishop *et al.*, 2020; Morrison et al., 2020). Despite the challenge of strain-specific antigenic diversity, a cocktail of three *T. parva* strains called the Muguga cocktail has been developed; when used for infection and treatment, it induces immunity against ECF in many regions of Africa although not against infections transmitted from Cape buffalo-derived *T. parva* strains (Nene and Morrison, 2016; Nene *et al.*, 2016; Bishop *et al.*, 2020). Development of other strain cocktails could be achieved by propagation of local *T. parva* strains allowing the development of region-specific infection and treatment regimes. However, infection and treatment-type immunization require reproducible production of the parasite in ticks, careful titration of these to determine an appropriate infective dose, a cold chain for transport of the parasites, and co-administration of long-acting tetracycline and veterinary oversight to make sure that ensuing infection is controlled by the antibiotic in the vaccinated cattle.

Progress has been made during the past 40 years in identifying schizont proteins that induce protective immunity and which might be included in a subunit vaccine, similarly, neutralizing monoclonal antibodies for the infective stage of the parasite have been generated, and a conserved coat protein, p67, identified as a putative vaccine antigen, although field trials suggest that administration of this protein alone does not ensure sterile immunity (Nene and Morrison, 2016). Recent advances in designing a highly immunogenic and effective vaccine against the malarial parasite sporozoite coat antigen (Wadman, 2021) may be applicable to the *Theileria* p67 protein and increase its vaccine efficacy. It will also be of interest to see if application of RNA vaccine technology, which has been critical to control of the COVID-19 pandemic, to the ECF field accelerates the development of effective schizont protein vaccines. Overall, new technologies may revitalize the goal of developing an effective ECF subunit vaccine.

Conclusion/summary

Despite climate stress, a plethora of animal diseases, rural poverty, and an overall low global investment for the development of vaccines against pathogens of livestock prevalent in sub-Saharan Africa, smallholder farmers, pastoralists, large-scale ranchers, and integrated agriculture practices in the region support a vigorous animal agriculture industry. It is hoped that scientists, agriculturalists, development agencies, and governments worldwide join in rolling back constraints to ASF production and integrated agriculture. Growth of animal-based agriculture in sub-Saharan Africa will improve child nutrition, decrease rural poverty, and help sub-Saharan Africa achieve food security.

Abbreviations

AAT	animal African trypanosomiasis
ASF	animal source food
ASFV	African swine fever virus
AU-IBAR	African Union Inter-African Bureau for Animal Resources
CBPP	contagious bovine pleuropneumonia
CCPP	contagious caprine pleuropneumonia
CD	cluster of differentiation
CRISPR	clustered regularly interspaced short palindromic repeats

CTLA-4	cytotoxic T lymphocyte associated protein-4
DIVA	differentiating infected from vaccinated animals
ECF	East coast fever
GIS	global information system
IFN	interferon
ILRAD	International laboratory for research on animal diseases
ILRI	International livestock research institute
NKT	natural killer T
OIE	Office International des Epizooties
PAMP	pathogen associated molecular pattern
PD	programmed cell death protein
PPR	Peste des petits ruminants
PRR	pattern recognition receptor
PRRS	porcine respiratory and reproduction syndrome
SNP	single-nucleotide polymorphism
SSA	sub-Saharan Africa
TCR	T cell receptor
TGF	transforming growth factor
TLR	toll-like receptor
VSG	variable surface glycoprotein

References

Abdelwhab, E.M. and Hafez, H.M. (2011) An overview of the epidemic of highly pathogenic H5N1 avian influenza virus in Egypt: Epidemiology and control challenges. *Epidemiology and Infection* 139(5), 647–657.

Adesogan, A.T., Havelaar, A.H., McKune, S.L., Eilittä, M. and Dahl, G.E. (2020) Animal source foods: Sustainability problem or malnutrition and sustainability solution? *Perspective Matters Global Food Security* 25(2020), 100325.

Akombi, B.J., Agho, K.E., Hall, J.J., Wali, N., Renzaho, A. *et al.* (2017) Stunting, wasting and underweight in Sub-Saharan Africa: A systematic review. *International Journal of Environmental Research and Public Health* 14(8), 863.

Aleena, J., Sejian, V., Bagath, M., Krishnan, G., Beena, V. *et al.* (2018) Resilience of three indigenous goat breeds to heat stress based on phenotypic traits and PBMC HSP70 expression. *International Journal of Biometeorology* 62(11), 1995–2005.

Alhaji, N.B., Ankeli, P.I., Ikpa, L.T. and Babalobi, O.O. (2020) Contagious bovine *Pleuropneumonia*: Challenges and prospects regarding diagnosis and control strategies in Africa. *Veterinary Medicine: Research and Reports* 11, 71–85.

Artiaga, B.L., Yang, G., Hutchinson, T.E., Loeb, J.C., Richt, J.A. *et al.* (2016) Rapid control of pandemic H1N1 influenza by targeting NKT-cells. *Scientific Reports* 6, 37999.

Autheman, D., Crosnier, C., Clare, S., Goulding, D.A., Brandt, C. *et al.* (2021) An invariant *Trypanosoma vivax* vaccine antigen induces protective immunity. *Nature* 595, 96–100.

Baldwin, C.L., Hsu, H., Chen, C., Palmer, M., McGill, J. *et al.* (2014) The role of bovine γδ t cells and their WC1 co-receptor in response to bacterial pathogens and promoting vaccine efficacy: A model for cattle and humans. *Veterinary Immunology and Immunopathology* 159(3–4), 144–155.

Baltenweck, I., Enahoro, D., Frija, A. and Tarawali, S. (2020) Why is production of animal source foods important for economic development in Africa and Asia? *Animal Frontiers* 10(4), 22–29.

Barrett, T. and Rossiter, P.B. (1999) Rinderpest: The disease and its impact on humans and animals. *Advances in Virus Research* 53, 89–110.

Bishop, R.P., Odongo, D., Ahmed, J., Mwamuye, M., Fry, L.M. *et al.* (2020) A review of recent research on *Theileria parva*: Implications for the infection and treatment vaccination method for control of East Coast fever. *Transboundary and Emerging Diseases* 67(Suppl 1), 56–67.

Black, S.J. and Baldwin, C.L. (2021) Impact assessment of immunology and immunoparasitology at ILRAD, ILCA and ILRI. In: McIntire, J. and Grace, D. (eds) *The Impact of the International Livestock Research Institute,Nairobi, Kenya*. ILRI and Wallingford, UK: CABI, pp. 103–147.

Black, S.J. (2021) Control of pathogenesis in animal African trypanosomiasis: A search for answers at ILRAD, ILCA and ILRI 1975–1978. In: McGuire, J. and Grace, D. (eds) *The Impact of the International Livestock Reserach Institute Nairobi, Kenya*. ILRI and Wallingford: Cabi, pp. 164–207.

Bosch-Camos, L., López, E., Collado, J., Navas, M.J., Blanco-Fuertes, M. *et al*. (2021) M448R and MGF505-7R: Two African swine fever virus antigens commonly recognized by ASFV-specific T-cells and with protective potential. *Vaccines (Basel)* 9(5), 508.

Brisse, M., Vrba, S.M., Kirk, N., Liang, Y. and Ly, H. (2020) Emerging concepts and technologies in vaccine development. *Frontiers in Immunology* 11, 583077.

Butcher, M.J. and Zhu, J. (2021) Recent advances in understanding the Th1/Th2 effector choice. *Faculty Reviews* 10, 30.

Calina, D., Sarkar, C., Arsene, A.L., Salehi, B., Docea, A.O. *et al*. (2020) Recent advances, approaches and challenges in targeting pathways for potential COVID-19 vaccines development. *Immunologic Research* 68(6), 315–324.

Caminade, C., McIntyre, K.M. and Jones, A.E. (2019) Impact of recent and future climate change on vector-borne diseases. *Annals of the New York Academy of Sciences* 1436(1), 157–173.

Carroll, J.A., Sanchez, N.B., Chaffin, R., Chase Jr, C.C., Coleman, S.W. *et al*. (2013) Heat-tolerant versus heat-sensitive bos taurus cattle: Influence of air temperature and breed on the acute phase response to a provocative immune challenge. *Domestic Animal Endocrinology* 45(3), 163–169.

Davis, S.R., Spelman, R.J. and Littlejohn, M.D. (2017) Breeding and genetics symposium: Breeding heat tolerant dairy cattle: The case for introgression of the "slick" prolactin receptor variant into dairy breeds. *Journal of Animal Science* 95(4), 1788–1800.

Devendra, C. (2013) Investments on pro-poor development projects on goats: Ensuring success for improved livelihoods. *Asian-Australasian Journal of Animal Sciences* 26(1), 1–18.

Di Teodoro, G., Marruchella, G., Di Provvido, A., D'Angelo, A.R., Orsini, G. *et al*. (2020) Contagious bovine pleuropneumonia: A comprehensive overview. *Veterinary Pathology* 57(4), 476–489.

Diallo, A., Taylor, W.P., Lefevre, P.C. and Provost, A. (1989) Attenuation of a strain of rinderpest virus: Potential homologous live vaccine. *Revue d'élevage et de Médecine Vétérinaire Des Pays Tropicaux* 42(3), 311–319.

Dimitrov, K.M., Afonso, C.L., Yu, Q. and Miller, P.J. (2017) Newcastle disease vaccines—a solved problem or a continuous challenge? *Veterinary Microbiology* 206, 126–136.

Dixon, L.K., Sun, H. and Roberts, H. (2019) African swine fever. *Antiviral Research* 165, 34–41.

Dolan, T.T. (1999) Dogmas and misunderstandings in East Coast fever. *Tropical Medicine and International Health* 4(9), A3–11.

Dundon, W.G., Diallo, A. and Cattoli, G. (2020) Peste des petits ruminants in Africa: A review of currently available molecular epidemiological data, 2020. *Archives of Virology* 165(10), 2147–2163.

Ganar, K., Das, M., Sinha, S. and Kumar, S. (2014) Newcastle disease virus: Current status and our understanding. *Virus Research* 184, 71–81.

Gaudreault, N.N. and Richt, J.A. (2019) Subunit vaccine approaches for African swine fever virus. *Vaccines (Basel)* 7(2), 56.

Giavedoni, L., Jones, L., Mebus, C. and Yilma, T. (1991) A vaccinia virus double recombinant expressing the F and H genes of rinderpest virus protects cattle against rinderpest and causes no pock lesions. *Proceedings of the National Academy of Sciences of the United States of America* 88(18), 8011–8015.

Goatley, L.C., Reis, A.L., Portugal, R., Goldswain, H., Shimmon, G.L. *et al*. (2020) A pool of eight virally vectored African swine fever antigens protect pigs against fatal disease. *Vaccines (Basel)* 8(2), 234.

Godde, C.M., Mason-D'Croz, D., Mayberry, D.E., Thornton, P.K. and Herrero, M. (2021) Impacts of climate change on the livestock food supply chain; A review of the evidence. *Global Food Security* 28, 100488.

Guo, C., Wang, M., Zhu, Z., He, S., Liu, H. *et al*. (2019) Highly efficient generation of pigs harboring a partial deletion of the CD163 SRCR5 domain, which are fully resistant to porcine reproductive and respiratory syndrome virus 2 infection. *Frontiers in Immunology* 10, 1846.

Hodgson, S., Moffat, K., Hill, H., Flannery, J.T., Graham, S.P. *et al.* (2018) Comparison of the immunogenicities and cross-lineage efficacies of live attenuated peste des petits ruminants virus vaccines PPRV/Nigeria/75/1 and PPRV/ Sungri/96. *Journal of Virology* 92(24).

Hussen, J. and Schuberth, H.J. (2017) Heterogeneity of bovine peripheral blood monocytes. *Frontiers in Immunology* 8, 1875.

Irvin, A.D. and Mwamachi, D.M. (1983) Clinical and diagnostic features of East Coast fever (*Theileria parva*) infection of cattle. *Veterinary Record* 113(9), 192–198.

Islam, M.A., Rony, S.A., Rahman, M.B., Cinar, M.U., Villena, J. *et al.* (2020) Improvement of disease resistance in livestock: Application of immunogenomics and CRISPR/Cas9 technology. *Animals (Basel)* 10(12), 2236.

Jiang, K., Yang, J., Yang, C., Zhang, T., Shaukat, A. *et al.* (2020) miR-148a suppresses inflammation in lipopolysaccharide-induced endometritis. *Journal of Cellular and Molecular Medicine* 24(1), 405–417.

Jores, J., Baldwin, C., Blanchard, A., Browning, G.F., Colston, A. *et al.* (2020) Contagious bovine and caprine pleuropneumonia: A research community's recommendations for the development of better vaccines. *NPJ Vaccines* 5, 66.

Juhas, U., Ryba-Stanisławowska, M., Szargiej, P. and Myśliwska, J. (2015) Different pathways of macrophage activation and polarization. *Advances in Hygiene & Experimental Medicine/Postepy Higieny i Medycyny Doswiadczalnej* 69, 496–502.

Kim, J., Hanotte, O., Mwai, O.A., Dessie, T., Bashir, S. *et al.* (2017) The genome landscape of indigenous African cattle. *Genome Biology* 18(1), 34.

Konnai, S., Murata, S. and Ohashi, K. (2017) Immune exhaustion during chronic infections in cattle. *The Journal of Veterinary Medical Science* 79(1), 1–5.

Leach, M. and Tadros, M. (2014) Epidemics and the politics of knowledge: Contested narratives in Egypt's H1N1 response. *Medical Anthropology* 33(3), 240–254.

Lowry, D.B. (2010) Landscape evolutionary genomics. *Biology Letters* 6(4), 502–504.

Lundstrom, K. (2020) Self-amplifying RNA viruses as RNA vaccines. *International Journal of Molecular Sciences* 21(14), 5130.

Mack, R. (1970) The great African cattle plague epidemic of the 1890s. *Tropical Animal Health and Production* 2, 210–219.

Mahapatra, M., Selvaraj, M. and Parida, S. (2020) Comparison of immunogenicity and protective efficacy of PPR live attenuated vaccines (Nigeria 75/1 and Sungri 96) administered by intranasal and subcutaneous routes. *Vaccines (Basel)* 8(2), 168.

March, J.B. (2004) Improved formulations for existing CBPP vaccines—Recommendations for change. *Vaccine* 22(31–32), 4358–4364.

Mariner, J.C., House, J.A., Sollod, A.E., Stem, C., Van de Ende, M. *et al.* (1990) Comparison of the effect of various chemical stabilizers and lyophilization cycles on the thermostability of a Vero cell-adapted rinderpest vaccine. *Veterinary Microbiology* 21(3), 195–209.

Mariner, J.C., Gachanja, J., Tindih, S.H. and Toye, P. (2017) A thermostable presentation of the live, attenuated peste des petits ruminants vaccine in use in Africa and Asia. *Vaccine* 35(30), 3773–3779.

Maudlin, I. (2006) African trypanosomiasis. *Annals of Tropical Medicine and Parasitology* 100(8), 679–701.

McCulloch, R., Morrison, L.J. and Hall, J.P.J. (2015) DNA recombination strategies during antigenic variation in the African trypanosome. *Microbiology Spectrum* 3(2), Mdna3-0016-2014.

McManus, C.M., Rezende Paiva, S. and Faria, D. (2020) Genomics and climate change. *Scientific and Technical Review* 39(2), 481–490.

McMichael, C. (2015) Climate change-related migration and infectious disease. *Virulence* 6(6), 548–553.

Morenikeji, O.B., Hawkes, M.E., Hudson, A.O. and Thomas, B.N. (2019) Computational network analysis identifies evolutionarily conserved miRNA gene interactions potentially regulating immune response in bovine trypanosomosis. *Frontiers in Microbiology* 10, 2010.

Morrison, W.I. (2007) The biological and practical significance of antigenic variability in protective T cell responses against *Theileria parva*. *Veterinary Parasitology* 148(1), 21–30.

Morrison, L.J., Vezza, L., Rowan, T. and Hope, J.C. (2016) Animal african trypanosomiasis: Time to increase focus on clinically relevant parasite and host species. *Trends in Parasitology* 32(8), 599–607.

Morrison, W.I., Connelley, T., Hemmink, J.D. and MacHugh, N.D. (2015) Understanding the basis of parasite strain-restricted immunity to *Theileria parva*. *Annual Review of Animal Biosciences* 3, 397–418.

Morrison, W.I., Hemmink, J.D. and Toye, P.G. (2020) *Theileria parva*: A parasite of African buffalo, which has adapted to infect and undergo transmission in cattle. *International Journal for Parasitology* 50(5), 403–412.

Murphy, S.P. and Neumann, C.G. (2014) Dietary approaches to diet quality improvement: Introduction. *Food and Nutrition Bulletin* 35(4 Suppl), S171–S173.

Murray, P.J., Allen, J.E., Biswas, S.K., Fisher, E.A., Gilroy, D.W. *et al*. (2014) Macrophage activation and polarization: Nomenclature and experimental guidelines. *Immunity* 41(1), 14–20.

Muuka, G., Songolo, N., Kabilika, S., Hang'ombe, B.M., Nalubamba, K.S. *et al*. (2013) Challenges of controlling contagious bovine pleuropneumonia in sub-Saharan Africa: A Zambian perspective. *Tropical Animal Health and Production* 45(1), 9–15.

Muuka, G.M., Chikampa, W., Mundia, C., Bounavoglia, D., Pini, A. *et al*. (2014) Recent observations on site reactions in cattle to vaccination against contagious bovine pleuropneumonia (CBPP) using T1/44 vaccine in Zambia. *Tropical Animal Health and Production* 46(2), 481–483.

Naessens, J., Scheerlinck, J.P., Buysscher, E.V., Kennedy, D. and Sileghem, M. (1998) Effective *in vivo* depletion of t cell subpopulations and loss of memory cells in cattle using mouse monoclonal antibodies. *Veterinary Immunology and Immunopathology* 64(3), 219–234.

Naiman, B.M., Blumerman, S., Alt, D., Bolin, C.A., Brown, R. *et al*. (2002) Evaluation of type 1 immune response in naïve and vaccinated animals following challenge with *Leptospira borgpetersenii* serovar hardjo: Involvement of WC1(+) gammadelta and CD4 T cells. *Infection and Immunity* 70(11), 6147–6157.

Nawab, A., Ibtisham, F., Li, G., Kieser, B., Wu, J. *et al*. (2018) Heat stress in poultry production: Mitigation strategies to overcome the future challenges facing the global poultry industry. *Journal of Thermal Biology* 78, 131–139.

Nene, V. and Morrison, W.I. (2016) Approaches to vaccination against *Theileria parva* and *Theileria annulata*. *Parasite Immunology* 38(12), 724–734.

Nene, V., Kiara, H., Lacasta, A., Pelle, R., Svitek, N. *et al*. (2016) The biology of *Theileria parva* and control of East Coast fever—Current status and future trends. *Ticks and Tick-Borne Diseases* 7(4), 549–564.

Neumann, C.G., Bwibo, N.O., Murphy, S.P., Sigman, M., Whaley, S. *et al*. (2003) Animal source foods improve dietary quality, micronutrient status, growth and cognitive function in Kenyan school children: Background, study design and baseline findings. *Journal of Nutrition* 133(11 Suppl 2), 3941S.

Neumann, C.G., Gewa, C. and Bwibo, N.O. (2004) Child nutrition in developing countries. *Pediatric Annals* 33(10), 658–674.

Njeumi, F., Bailey, D., Soula, J., Diop, B. and Tekola, B.G. (2020) Eradicating the scourge of peste des petits ruminants from the world. *Viruses* 12(3), 313.

Odeniran, P.O., Ademola, I.O., Macleod, E.T. and Welburn, S.C. (2018) Bovine and small ruminant African animal trypanosomiasis in Nigeria—A review. *Veterinary Parasitology: Regional Studies and Reports* 13, 5–13.

Okagawa, T., Konnai, S., Ikebuchi, R., Suzuki, S., Shirai, T. *et al*. (2012) Increased bovine Tim-3 and its ligand expressions during bovine leukemia virus infection. *Veterinary Research* 43(1), 45.

Parida, S., Muniraju, M., Mahapatra, M., Muthuchelvan, D., Buczkowski, H. *et al*. (2015) Peste des petits ruminants. *Veterinary Microbiology* 181(1–2), 90–106.

Pereira, S.S., Neto, K.J., Duffy, C.W., Richards, P., Noyes, H. *et al*. (2020) Variant antigen diversity in trypanosoma vivax is not driven by recombination. *Nature Communications* 11(1), 844.

Rayaisse, J.B., Tirados, I., Kaba, D., Dewhirst, S.Y., Logan, J.G. *et al*. (2010) Prospects for the development of odour baits to control the tsetse flies glossina tachinoides and G *Palpalis* s.l. *PLoS Neglected Tropical Disease* 4(3), e632.

Riedel, S. (2005) Edward jenner and the history of smallpox and vaccination. *Proceedings (Baylor University Medical Center)* 18(1), 21–25.

Rout, P.K., Kaushik, R. and Ramachandran, N. (2016) Differential expression pattern of heat shock protein 70 gene in tissues and heat stress phenotypes in goats during peak heat stress period. *Cell Stress and Chaperones* 21(4), 645–651.

Saha, A., Nanavaty, V.P. and Li, B. (2020) Telomere and subtelomere R-loops and antigenic variation in trypanosomes. *Journal of Molecular Biology* 432(15), 4167–4185.

Salter, A.M. (2018) The effects of meat consumption on global health. *Scientific and Technical Review* 37(1), 47–55.

Sang, H., Miller, G., Lokhandwala, S., Sangewar, N., Waghela, S.D. *et al*. (2020) Progress toward development of effective and safe African swine fever virus vaccines. *Frontiers in Veterinary Science* 7, 84.

Sarkar, J., Sreenivasa, B.P., Singh, R.P., Dhar, P. and Bandyopadhyay, S.K. (2003) Comparative efficacy of various chemical stabilizers on the thermostability of a live-attenuated peste des petits ruminants (PPR) vaccine. *Vaccine* 21(32), 4728–4735.

Seef, S. and Jeppsson, A. (2013) Is it a policy crisis or it is a health crisis? The Egyptian context—Analysis of the Egyptian health policy for the H1N1 flu pandemic control. *Pan African Medical Journal* 14, 59.

Sen, A., Saravanan, P., Balamurugan, V., Rajak, K.K., Sudhakar, S.B. *et al*. (2010) Vaccines against peste des petits ruminants virus. *Expert Review of Vaccines* 9(7), 785–796.

Sima, N., McLaughlin, E.J., Hutchinson, S. and Glover, L. (2019) Escaping the immune system by DNA repair and recombination in african trypanosomes. *Open Biology* 9(11), 190182.

Stockinger, B. (2021) Lumpers and splitters: Birth of Th17 cells. *Journal of Experimental Medicine* 218(5), e20210645.

Teklue, T., Sun, Y., Abid, M., Luo, Y. and Qiu, H.J. (2020) Current status and evolving approaches to African swine fever vaccine development. *Transboundary and Emerging Diseases* 67(2), 529–542.

Trevor, C.E., Gonzalez-Munoz, A.L., Macleod, O.J., Woodcock, P.G., Rust, S. *et al*. (2019) Structure of the trypanosome transferrin receptor reveals mechanisms of ligand recognition and immune evasion. *Nature Microbiology* 4(12), 2074–2081.

Wadman, M. (2021) Malaria vaccine achieves striking early success. *Science* 372(6541).

Wang, Y., Saelao, P., Chanthavixay, K., Gallardo, R., Bunn, D. *et al*. (2018) Physiological responses to heat stress in two genetically distinct chicken inbred lines. *Poultry Science* 97(3), 770–780.

Whitworth, K.M., Lee, K., Benne, J.A., Beaton, B.P., Spate, L.D. *et al*. (2014) Use of the CRISPR/Cas9 system to produce genetically engineered pigs from in vitro-derived oocytes and embryos. *Biology of Reproduction* 91(3), 78.

Wu, K., Liu, J., Wang, L., Fan, S., Li, Z. *et al*. (2020) Current state of global African wwine fever vaccine development under the prevalence and transmission of ASF in China. *Vaccines (Basel)* 8(3), 531.

Xie, Z., Pang, D., Yuan, H., Jiao, H., Lu, C. *et al*. (2018) Genetically modified pigs are protected from classical swine fever virus. *PLoS Pathogens* 14(12), e1007193.

Yang, G., Richt, J.A. and Driver, J.P. (2017) Harnessing invariant NKT cells to improve influenza vaccines: A pig perspective. *International Journal of Molecular Sciences* 19(1), 68.

Yaro, M., Munyard, K.A., Stear, M.J. and Groth, D.M. (2016) Combatting african animal trypanosomiasis (AAT) in livestock: The potential role of trypanotolerance. *Veterinary Parasitology* 225, 43–52.

Yilma, T., Hsu, D., Jones, L., Owens, S., Grubman, M. *et al*. (1988) Protection of cattle against rinderpest with vaccinia virus recombinants expressing the HA or F gene. *Science* 242(4881), 1058–1061.

Zhang, K., Lenstra, J.A., Zhang, S., Liu, W. and Liu, J. (2020) Evolution and domestication of the Bovini species. *Animal Genetics* 51(5), 637–657.

Zhang, X., Zhang, S., Ma, L., Jiang, E., Xu, H. *et al*. (2017) Reduced representation bisulfite sequencing (RRBS) of dairy goat mammary glands reveals DNA methylation profiles of integrated genome-wide and critical milk-related genes. *Oncotarget* 8(70), 115326–115344.

Zhao, H., Njeumi, F., Parida, S. and Benfield, C.T. (2021) Progress towards eradication of peste des petits ruminants through vaccination. *Viruses* 13(1), 59.

Zhou, Y., Liu, S., Hu, Y., Fang, L., Gao, Y. *et al*. (2020) Comparative whole genome DNA methylation profiling across cattle tissues reveals global and tissue-specific methylation patterns. *BMC Biology* 18(1), 85.

Zhuang, Z.X., Chen, S.E., Chen, C.F., Lin, E.C. and Huang, S.Y. (2020) Genomic regions and pathways associated with thermotolerance in layer-type strain Taiwan indigenous chickens. *Journal of Thermal Biology* 88, 102486.

Zinsstag, J., Crump, L., Schelling, E., Hattendorf, J., Maidane, Y.O. *et al*. (2018) Climate change and one health. *FEMS Microbiology Letters* 365(11).

16 Cattle Tick Control in Africa: Potential of Ethnoveterinary Plants

Brighton M. Mvumi[1*], Emmanuel T. Nyahangare[2], Jacobus N. Eloff[3], Steven R. Belmain[4] and Philip C. Stevenson[4,5]

[1]Department of Agricultural and Biosystems Engineering, Faculty of Agriculture, Environment and Food Systems, University of Zimbabwe, P.O. Box MP167, Mt. Pleasant, Harare, Zimbabwe; [2]Department of Livestock Sciences Faculty of Agriculture, Environment and Food Systems, University of Zimbabwe, P.O. Box MP167, Mt. Pleasant, Harare, Zimbabwe; [3]Phytomedicine Programme Faculty of Veterinary Science, University of Pretoria, Private Bag X04, Onderstepoort 0110, Pretoria, South Africa; [4]Natural Resources Institute, University of Greenwich, Chatham Maritime, Chatham, Kent ME4 4TB, United Kingdom; [5]Royal Botanic Gardens, Kew, Surrey TW9 3AB, United Kingdom

Abstract

Cattle are a livelihood asset to smallholder farmers in Africa yet remain threatened by the effects of ticks and tick-borne diseases during production because they cause morbidity and premature death. The use of indigenous plants in tick control is a worldwide practice spanning thousands of years. Changes in the agricultural and socio–cultural landscape over time have, however, led to neglect of indigenous pesticidal plants in favour of synthetic products. The benefits of synthetic acaricides are well-recognized, but emerging observation indicates that they cannot solve all livestock health problems across production systems, farmer circumstances and agro-ecologies. Concerns associated with commercial acaricides have revived research interest in alternative or complementary remedies. Past research has focused on documenting ethnoveterinary practices, scientific validation of the practices and optimization of these practices. Here, we review the challenges of synthetic acaricides and progress made in ethnoveterinary plant research and development in Africa. The review highlights challenges of access, affordability and availability of commercial acaricides to resource-poor communities; synthetic acaricide resistance development; disposal of obsolete acaricides and environmental pollution; reduced water supply and implications on conventional use of acaricide-treated dipping facilities; and plant bioprospecting and downstream development of products in Africa.This information contributes towards shaping the ethnoveterinary plant research agenda and policy, and investment interventions in Africa.

Keywords: anti-tick plants, acaricidal plants, plant bioprospecting, ethnobotanical IPR, primary animal health care, botanical acaricides

*Corresponding author: mvumibm@agric.uz.ac.zw; mvumibm@hotmail.com

Review Methodology

Information screening was conducted to identify relevant literature and studies, published and unpublished (grey literature), that included either in the title or abstract the terms:

1. 'Cattle tick control' plus:
   a. Synthetic acaricides, acaricides resistance, challenges, alternatives,
   b. Ethnoveterinary science, ethnoveterinary plants, ethnobotanical pesticides, botanical pesticides, botanical acaricides, anti-tick plants, pesticidal plants, acaricidal plants;
2. 'Botanical pesticides or acaricides' plus:
   a. Commercialisation,
   b. Intellectual property rights,
   c. Bio-prospecting,
   d. Policy and regulatory,
   e. Optimisation,
   f. Bioassays, and
   g. Phytochemistry.

The following online databases of renowned peer-reviewed publications were sequentially searched: CAB Abstracts, Web of Science Core Collection and Scopus. The search engines used to access online published and unpublished literature also included Research Gate, Google scholar, and Google.

The following inclusion or exclusion criteria were applied to the title and abstract and the full-text review stages:

- Animals: study included cattle as one of the study animals.
- Geographical area: study included the geographical area of SSA or Africa.
- Study type: study was a review or original research and *in vitro* or *in vivo*.
- Date: no date restrictions were applied.
- Language: the search terms were done only in English.

Finally, the literature that met the criteria was synthesized to generate an analytical and critical review report categorised into thematic areas guided by the search terms.

Introduction

Livestock play a crucial role for 70% of the world's resource-poor population mainly living in rural areas (Herrero and Thornton, 2023; Randolph *et al.*, 2007). The role of livestock, particularly cattle, is especially important in drier agroecological zones where crop production is restricted by low and irregular rainfall coupled with recurring droughts. Productivity of animals in these regions is, however, often hampered by animal diseases and poor animal health service provision (Adenubi *et al.*, 2018). One of the major health concerns affecting cattle is ticks and tick-borne diseases (TTBD). Ticks are vectors of fatal diseases, for example, babesiosis and theileriosis, which have serious economic impacts to farmers (Jabbar *et al.*, 2015; Luseba *et al.*, 2016; Madison-Antenucci *et al.*, 2020). The challenges posed by ticks have a major impact on the livelihoods of smallholder farmers in Low and Middle Income Countries (LMIC) across the world (Jabbar *et al.*, 2015). In Africa, TTBD remain one of the biggest challenges to animal health (Manjunathachar *et al.*, 2014; Mapholi *et al.*, 2014), and the solution of the situation has no end in sight. Although considerable efforts have been made to control ticks, it is apparent that their eradication is not feasible but they can be managed and their effects on cattle reduced (Mapholi *et al.*, 2014). Conventionally, intensive use of commercial chemical acaricides has been the main control method of ticks, but several associated negative effects are emerging (Adenubi *et al.*, 2016). Some of the issues include widespread development of acaricidal resistance, ever-increasing cost of acaricides, high toxicity of chemicals, chemical residues in meat and milk and negative impacts on non-target organisms (Willadsen, 2006; Fuente *et al.*, 2007; Adehan *et al.*, 2016). It has also been realized that the current tick control methods are not well-suited for marginalised smallholder farmers in LMICs, thereby creating many challenges in the control of ticks. This is because most of the foci in the management of ticks and synthetic acaricide development have been largely targeting vulnerable exotic and commercial cattle breeds and not so much on the smallholder sector and indigenous cattle breeds where the challenges are somewhat different (Nyahangare *et al.*, 2015). All these factors have made intensive dipping and spraying using commercial acaricides less suitable for smallholder farmers. Several options have been postulated, including the use of vaccines, genomics and integration of several systems with various degrees of adoption and success (Godfray *et al.*, 2010; Merino *et al.*, 2013; Mapholi *et al.*, 2014).

One innovative approach that has received wide approval from many stakeholders is integration of existing conventional methods of animal health management with age-old ethnoveterinary practices and products (Isman, 1997; Moyo and Masika, 2009; Madzimure *et al.*, 2011; Madzimure *et al.*, 2013). There is renewed interest in them due to the aforementioned challenges with commercial products. Available evidence suggests that pesticidal plants have considerable potential in ecto-parasite control programs, particularly for resource-poor smallholder farmers (Isman, 1997; Kiss *et al.*, 2012). An important challenge now is to identify the plants that are effective against target pests and parasites and how to optimise their use. Bioprospecting is the systematic process of discovery, development and commercialisation of new sources of chemical compounds, genes, micro-organisms, macro-organisms, and other valuable products from natural resources (Harvey and Gericke, 2011). However it must be acknowledged that most discoveries of new compounds have happened in companies in the high-income countries, yet the biodiverse resources are in LMICs. Strategies are required that are mutually beneficial. To regulate collection of samples, the United Nations developed a framework for preserving the world's biodiversity while encouraging the sustainable use of biodiversity (Harvey and Gericke, 2011).

One of the challenges with using ethnoveterinary technologies based on acaricidal and tick-repellent plants is that most of them have not been subjected to rigorous efficacy and safety testing as is required with conventional synthetic acaricides. Consequently, these technologies are often regarded as backward, less effective and generally not applicable in serious farming operations (Wanzala *et al.*, 2005). It is no wonder that there are few registered commercial botanical pesticides worldwide despite mention of many plants with reported pesticidal properties (Pavela, 2016; Adenubi *et al.*, 2018). Unless issues like efficacy (in laboratory bioassays and on-farm trials), phytochemistry, safety and toxicity of these ethnobotanical plants are scientifically established, their value to the widespread primary health care of livestock remains limited.

The comprehensive study of characteristics of ethnoveterinary plants used for controlling ticks may offer a good opportunity for the development of alternative tick control remedies that can improve smallholder livestock productivity and reduce over-reliance on the use of chemical acaricides in conventional tick control programmes. Here we critically appraise the status of pesticidal plants used for controlling cattle ticks with a particular emphasis on LMICs in Africa. We argue that safe and effective tick control products can be developed from locally available traditionally used acaricidal and tick-repellent plants.

Economic Implications of Ticks and Tick-Borne Diseases

The threat of ticks and tick-borne diseases (TTBD) to the productivity of cattle globally is not a new phenomenon but well-documented (Pegram *et al.*, 1993; Ghosh *et al.*, 2007; Simuunza *et al.*, 2011; Jabbar *et al.*, 2015; Atif *et al.*, 2016). It is also clear that effective management and control of ticks continues to be costly. In response to these challenges, governments of LMICs including Zimbabwe and Zambia assumed the responsibility of controlling ticks by heavily subsidizing acaricides required for communal cattle-dipping (Pegram *et al.*, 1993; Moyo and Masika, 2009). This somewhat prevented and cushioned smallholder farmers from loss of their animals and, in the process, enhanced food security and livelihoods. At a global level, many countries are spending large amounts of money in tick control programmes estimated to be in the range of approximately US$13.9 – US$18.7 billion annually (Jongejan and Uilenberg, 2004; Ghosh *et al.*, 2007) while Africa is estimated to use approximately US$720 million annually (Adenubi *et al.*, 2016), which in most cases is not sustainable for most LMICs. These high figures exemplify the financial burden of using conventional acaricides for tick control and the need to strengthen research efforts into alternative effective and environmentally benign plant-based methods of tick control. However, accurate and current data on economic losses associated with TTBD are scarce.

In Africa, the most economically important ticks are from the *Ambylomma, Hyalomma* and *Rhipicephalus* genera and the subgenus *Boophilus* (Frans, 2000). *Ambylomma variegatum* is ubiquitous on the continent (over 30 countries) causing heartwater disease in cattle, sheep and goats. It is regarded as the second most invasive tick species after *R. (B.) microplus* and distributed as shown in Fig. 16.1 (Nyangiwe *et al.*, 2018). It must be noted, however, that distributional changes in ticks in the tropics and subtropics is occurring and is a concern for livestock stakeholders. The native tick species are being displaced by invasive species like what has happened in West Africa, South Africa and Namibia where *R. (B.) microplus* has invaded these areas (Nyangiwe *et al.*, 2018).

Synthetic Chemical Control of Ticks

Overview

The different types of synthetic acaricides like dichlorodiphenyltrichloroethane (DDT), carbaryl and amitraz that have been used to control ticks since the early 1890s to date is a clear indication that the development of acaricides has been on-going in response to the different challenges that are faced with developed products on the market, chief amongst them being the development of tick resistance and banning of certain chemicals deemed environmentally harmful or toxic to target animals.

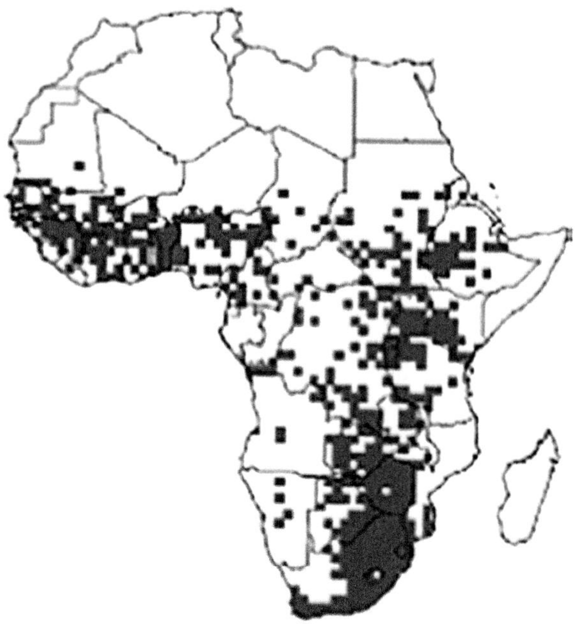

Fig. 16.1. Distribution of the *Rhipicephalus (Boophilus) microplus* tick in Africa (Nyangiwe *et al.*, 2018).

There are other negative issues associated with the use of these products that include high costs, residual contamination of animal products and availability of the chemicals when required especially for resource-poor farmers in remote areas (Graf *et al.*, 2004; Abbas *et al.*, 2014; Grzywacz *et al.*, 2014). Most of these concerns are increasingly becoming pertinent and requiring considerable efforts to identify effective alternative products.

Development of acaricide resistance by ticks

Tick resistance to acaricides is a critical issue for the livestock sector because this could lead to an unprecedented threat to livestock productivity. Abbas *et al.* (Abbas *et al.*, 2014) reviewed how ticks develop resistance, corroborating earlier work reported in (George *et al.*, 2004). Tick populations develop resistance because most acaricides are developed from single compounds. This, together with frequent applications, and often at lower than prescribed concentrations, exacerbates the situation. Consequently, it has not been possible to eradicate ticks using synthetic products. Malaria has been eradicated in parts of the world, but at a high environmental cost. The environmental cost of eradicating ticks using a synthetic product may be too high. Attention has therefore shifted to focus on investigating alternative strategies for managing the ticks rather than eliminating them (Ntondini *et al.*, 2008; Madzimure *et al.*, 2011; Madzimure *et al.*, 2013; Abbas *et al.*, 2014; Nyahangare *et al.*, 2017). While natural resistance development is probably inevitable, more can be done to address resistance that is caused by incorrect and inconsistent use of acaricides. There are several factors that can contribute to tick resistance development including adulteration, failure by users to adhere to acaricide manufacturer's instructions, illiteracy, and failure to interpret and implement label instructions (Okello-Onen *et al.*, 2003; Sola *et al.*, 2014; Grzywacz *et al.*, 2014). This is perhaps mainly because most acaricides come with instructions given in foreign languages and not in the vernacular African languages. We also observed that the acaricide packaging often comes with a small font on the label that makes it difficult for especially the elderly to read.

In the use of acaricidal plant extracts, farmers are in more control of products leading to fewer problems with adulteration. If a plant extract contains more than one acaricidal compound and the compounds have different modes of action, it may delay the development of resistance in contrast to synthetic products, which typically contain one or two active ingredients (Shyma *et al.*, 2014; Adenubi *et al.*, 2016). In any case, at any given time there are several plant alternatives that can be used, therefore reducing the likelihood of ticks developing tolerance or resistance.

The language barrier is a disadvantage because the majority of cattle (and generally livestock) producers are smallholder farmers with low literacy levels (Isman, 1997). Geographical location also plays an important role because some farmers cannot access veterinary extension services because of where they live. It is not uncommon for some farmers in these circumstances to think that they can save their acaricides by using less than recommended concentrations, thereby unwittingly contributing to development of acaricide resistance Okello-Onen *et al.*, 2003; Grzywacz *et al.*, 2014). Unfortunately, the performance of acaricides is generally dependent on quality and quantity administered to the animal, and inadequate or excessive applications can lead to the development of resistance. There should be more programmes that educate farmers on the importance of following application instructions and the potential for the development of tick strains with resistance to acaricides.

Disposal of obsolete acaricides and environmental pollution

Despite acaricides playing a critical role in animal health programmes, they pose dangers to the environment and people through persistence in water, soil and air pollution and reducing beneficial populations of insect species (Karstensen *et al.*, 2006; Shah and Devkota, 2009; Damalas and Eleftherohorinos, 2011). Regarding human health, it is estimated that at least 1 million people are victims of pesticide poisoning globally, with the bulk of these people being in Africa (Isman, 1997; Damalas and Eleftherohorinos, 2011). Active ingredients used to make synthetic pesticides formulations degrade over time, producing toxic by-products that can be more toxic than the original pesticides (Shah and Devkota, 2009). This has informed the argument put forth by proponents of plant-based acaricides that they are probably easily degradable because they are natural and so are non-persistent (Isman, 2006; Lengai *et al.*, 2020). Increasing evidence from biorational pest management in field crops reports that pesticidal plants are effective at controlling pests but have reduced effects on non-target organisms (Mkenda *et al.*, 2015; Mkindi *et al.*, 2017; Tembo *et al.*, 2018). This could also be the case with ethnoveterinary plants.

Many of the obsolete pesticides are persistent organic pollutants (POPs), which have toxic properties and can be transferred across international boundaries, officially becoming '*everybody's problem*' (Karstensen *et al.*, 2006). In many countries there are stockpiles of these obsolete pesticides that need to be disposed of safely. Where chemicals are banned because of the negative effects on animal and human health that come to light after their commercialisation and widespread distribution, large stockpiles can occur. A good example was the global ban on the use of DDT in agriculture through the Stockholm Convention on Persistent Organic Pollutants in 2001. Prior to its ban, DDT was a multipurpose pesticide that was used globally and boosted agricultural productivity, but studies linking the chemical to health problems, particularly cancer, prompted its ban (Richardson, 1998). Despite this development, some LMICs still have stockpiles of DDT today because they lack the capacity and expertise to dispose of them, thereby predisposing the environment to pollution. Disposal in developing countries often involves repackaging and transportation to Europe for incineration in appropriate facilities at very high costs, estimated at US$3000–US$5000 per ton of waste (Richardson, 1998). It is estimated that the continent requires at least US$100 million to expedite the discarding of these obsolete pesticides. As it is, Africa is a net importer of active ingredients of agricultural pesticides but is the least prepared continent to deal with the growing stockpiles of decommissioned pesticides.

High cost and inaccessibility of synthetic acaricides

The pesticide industry is a multi-billion dollar business based on research and development programmes that require scientific expertise and substantial resource investment. These investments should be realized with a profit from sales of the chemical products. This is the reason why these products come at high costs that may be beyond the reach of resource-poor farmers. As a mitigation measure, some governments heavily subsidize acaricides for communal dipping of animals, but, as anticipated, this has not been a sustainable approach (Ntondini *et al.*, 2008; Moyo and Masika, 2009; Madzimure *et al.*, 2011). In most southern African countries, for example South Africa, Namibia, Zambia and Zimbabwe, authorities have already started revising this approach, imposing the full costs of tick control onto farmers (Chamboko *et al.*, 1999; Makala *et al.*, 2003; Moyo and Masika, 2009). Apart from the high costs, the products may not always be available in the veterinary shops. This was the case in Zimbabwe during the economic slump between 2004 and 2010 (Moyo and Masika, 2009). Even if someone had money to buy the products, they were not available on the market and the cattle industry relied on acaricides imported from South Africa, Namibia, Botswana and inexpensive imitations from Asia. Because some areas are remote, smallholder cattle farmers may not have regular access to synthetic acaricides on the local market resulting in the farmers resorting to incurring high cattle mortalities while others turn to alternative control options such as ethnoveterinary products and methods.

Inadequate water supply

In the past, African governments made significant investment in the construction of community dipping and spraying infrastructure for the purposes of tick and other ectoparasite control. However, maintaining these facilities is increasingly becoming a challenge as water availability is declining because of persistent droughts due to climate change in some areas. Most farmers are concerned that it is becoming increasingly drier and the frequency of droughts is on the increase in the tropics and subtropics (Collier *et al.*, 2008; Dantas-Torres, 2015), making cattle dipping costly and difficult to implement. Communities that have been using communal dip tanks are now faced with another challenge since dip tanks require large volumes of water to dilute the chemical acaricides (Muhammad *et al.*, 2008; Sungirai *et al.*, 2016). Adequate water is important for effective full body immersion and spraying of the animals and also prevention of fracture injuries as the animals plunge into the dip tank. This is perhaps the reason why most dip tanks were conveniently sited close to reliable perennial water sources. Recent trends however show that even those reliable water sources are now compromised as the water-table continues to recede. In a recent survey (Nyahangare *et al.*, 2015), farmers in Zimbabwe stated that water was a limiting factor in normal dipping programmes because of its unavailability due to recurrent droughts and prolonged dry spells. As a result, cattle may go for months on end without dipping, predisposing the animals to TTBD (Maroyi, 2012; Nyahangare *et al.*, 2015; Sungirai *et al.*, 2016). Most farmers have now abandoned community dipping to using smaller knapsack sprayers that use less water and are better suited for fewer animals and targeted applications, and which are better suited to dispensing locally collected and prepared acaricidal plant extracts.

Alternatives to Synthetic Chemical Tick Control

It is clear that no single method is adequate to deal with the complexities of tick control (Estrada-Peña and Salman, 2013). Over the years, plunge dipping programmes have been replaced by newer methods for application of acaricides that involve the use of ear tags, neck bands and pour-ons (Makala *et al.*, 2003; Willadsen, 2006; Moyo and Masika, 2009). The different methods used therefore support the view that it is not one but an integration of pest management approaches that present the most effective tick control programmes going forward (Magadum *et al.*, 2009). Studies have shown that cattle have been immunized with vaccines to prevent TTBD (Rajput *et al.*, 2006; Nene *et al.*, 2016); pheromones combined with toxicants have also been used (Sonenshine, 2004; Benelli *et al.*, 2016), while other methods based on the disruption of the tick's life cycle have been tried (Estrada-Peña and De La Fuente, 2014). There is another report on pheromones being used to attract ticks combined with entomopathogenic fungi, which have been used with some success (Nchu *et al.*, 2009). Correct management of pastures and the purposive breeding for animals that are TTBD-resistant are also very important measures that are being used in non-chemical control of ticks (George *et al.*, 2004; Ghosh *et al.*, 2007; Ravindran *et al.*, 2011; Shyma *et al.*, 2013; Van Zyl *et al.*, 2017).

The use of newer technologies is not without its challenges to particular production systems. Synthetic acaricides and most of the technologies used in the control of ticks are biased towards tick control programmes for exotic breeds of cattle in commercial cattle farming enterprises (Chamboko *et al.*, 1999). Under these systems in Africa and other developing countries, farmers raise exotic specialized breeds (*Bos taurus*), which have low resistance to TTBD. Under these circumstances these modern technologies give optimum productivity, but the same cannot be said for poorly resourced smallholder farmers who produce the bulk of cattle on the market in developing countries and whose farms are located in remote and rainfall-marginal areas that may be geographically and logistically less accessible (Mapiye *et al.*, 2009).The road networks are often poor and the areas may not have access to amenities like electricity. These places may also have very limited access to conventional veterinary services (Hlatshwayo and Mbati, 2005; Moyo and Masika, 2009; Gumbochuma *et al.*, 2013).

Use of Acaricidal Plants

The global context

Plants have been used to control agricultural pests and parasites for centuries, but this practice had been overtaken in recent decades by the use of formulated synthetic acaricides and pesticides (Isman and Machial, 2006; Dubey *et al.*, 2010). Terrestrial plants are a diverse reservoir of natural secondary metabolites that have evolved as defensive adaptations in plants to herbivory and pathogenic attack (Isman and Machial, 2006; McGaw and Eloff, 2008; Sultana *et al.*, 2009; Baetz and Martinoia, 2014; Grzywacz *et al.*, 2014). It is estimated that there are over 100,000 different secondary plant metabolites of which hundreds have been shown to have bioactivity against internal and external parasites (Isman and Machial, 2006; Koul *et al.*, 2008; Adenubi et al., 2018). There are renewed efforts to develop the botanical pesticide industry as a primary health care alternative for animals because of the challenges associated with using commercial synthetic acaricides (George *et al.*, 2004; Bissinger and Roe, 2010; Ghosh *et al.*, 2015).Already, the demonstration of efficacy and other bioactivity characteristics of plant chemicals is a growing industry that has attracted many professional scientists including botanists, biochemists, ecologists, pest management experts, toxicologists and social scientists (Isman and Grieneisen, 2014). In the period between 1980 and 2011, a total of 4997 and 2180 journal paper articles on neem and essential oils of different plants have been published the world over showing the growing interest in botanical pesticides (Isman and Machial, 2006; Isman and Grieneisen, 2014).

Most of the issues around the research and development of pesticidal botanical products, including acaricidal ones, have already been extensively reviewed by many authors (Mkindi *et al.*, n.d.; Miresmailli and Isman, 2014; Benelli *et al.*, 2016; Isman, 2020). Recently, a global review of published articles on plants used for tick control showed more than 200 species that have acaricidal properties (Adenubi *et al.*, 2016). Other reviews also showed that researchers in different laboratories use different *in vitro* bioassay techniques, extractants and tick species in determining efficacy (Adenubi *et al.*, 2018) The high acaricidal activity found in using acetone (a solvent not available to rural farmers) instead of water indicates that random screening of plants may deliver useful extracts or compounds. The focus may therefore have to be wider than plants used in ethnoveterinary medicine (Adenubi *et al.*, 2018). The absence of standardised procedures, however, does not overshadow the important critical data that are being generated on the plants that have acaricidal activity. However, using standard procedures is essential to be able to compare activity of different extracts under similar conditions.

Commercial botanical pesticides developed for the agricultural industry

Despite the high number of plant secondary metabolites that have been identified,there has not been a corresponding high number of commercialised botanical products on the market (Koul *et al.*, 2008; Isman and Grieneisen, 2014; Pavela, 2016). The earliest known botanical pesticide products include pyrethrum, rotenone and nicotine. Currently, neem and essential oils from different plant species form the bulk of botanical insecticides that are popular today (Isman and Machial, 2006). Pyrethrum *Tanacetum (Chrysanthemum) cinerariifolium* is a commonly used plant in Kenya, Tanzania and Australia (Tasmania). It is a contact acaricide whose effect is through pyrethrum esters found in it. Rotenone is also a natural chemical mainly found from the subtropical and tropical species of Leguminosae plants for example *Derris elliptica* and *Lonchocarpus* sp. (Ott KC. Rotenone, 2008). The botanical pesticide has been isolated from *Tephrosia vogelii* in Malawi (Belmain *et al.*, 2012; Stevenson *et al.*, 2012). Nicotine mainly occurs on the tobacco plant *Nicotiana tabacum* and other *Nicotiana* and *Anabasis* species. The use of nicotine and rotenone has come under strong criticism as they are highly toxic and therefore no longer used in industrialised countries (Isman and Machial, 2006; Ott KC. Rotenone, 2008). Recent work has, however, shown that in fact rotenone is not as toxic to humans and birds as earlier suspected, but fish are highly susceptible. It is the possible link to Parkinson's disease in humans popularized by the media that led to its acceptability challenges on the market and the subsequent ban, but natural levels of exposure in plant-based applications is too low to present an acute risk to people (Belmain *et al.*, 2012). Nevertheless, these examples demonstrate that using plant extracts is not without their challenges.

Products from *Azadirachta indica* (neem) are probably the most well-known biological insecticides today. Neem is found mainly in India, Australia, Central America and East and West Africa. It has anti-feedant properties and also acts as a growth regulator, mainly due to the presence of limonoids and azadirachtin (Webb and David, 2002). Apart from neem, essential oils also significantly contribute to botanical pesticides and are found worldwide in the flavouring and fragrance industries (Isman, 1997). Most essential oils have contact toxicity, fumigant, deterrent and repellent activities and are most effective against sucking pests (Bissinger and Roe, 2010).

Besides neem and essential oils from plant species, there are also other plant species that have been tested and shown to have acaricidal activity, for example *Stylosanthes scabra* (Khudrathulla and Jagannath, 2000); *Solanum dasypyllum* (Kaposhi, 1992); *Gynandropsis gynandra* (Malonza *et al.*, 1992) and *Melinis minutiflora* (Fernandez-Ruvalcaba *et al.*, 2004). *Melinis minutiflora*, *Stylosanthes* sp. and *Cassia absus* have also been used as repellents in the control of ticks (Ghosh *et al.*, 2007). The challenge, however, is still that despite experimental evidence suggesting efficacy, there are not as many products commercially produced for the market. The private sector with the financial ability to drive this process has not been very keen to explore this route, and the reasons have not been very explicit though regulatory hurdles is one of them (Sola *et al.*, 2014). There are many other plants that have been used by communities or tribes in Africa and this cultural, empirical knowledge of tick control may be valuable, must be tested scientifically and developed into commercial products. This justifies the need to continue engaging knowledgeable people in communities so that this important information is not lost across generations.

Research on anti-tick plants and product development

It is evident that research on botanicals differs across the world. If publications are used as a measure of progress in acaricidal research, then India, China and Brazil are the biggest players, accounting for 40.9% of the 1207 botanical insecticide articles published in 2012 (Isman and Grieneisen, 2014). In Africa, Egypt and Nigeria are the leading countries (Isman and Grieneisen, 2014; Miresmailli and Isman, 2014). However, it does not necessarily follow that areas with fewer publications do not use acaricidal plants and traditional methods for pest and parasite control, but this could be an issue of poor documentation and unavailability of resources for formal scientific testing.The World Health Organization (WHO) estimates that 80% of the people in Africa rely on traditional medicines, mainly plants, either alone or in conjunction with conventional medicine, to meet their health care needs (World Health Organization, 2002). A similar percentage may rely on using plants for pest control including in the livestock sub-sector.

Generally, scientific research on, and commercial production of, anti-tick products in Africa is still limited in scope and scale (Sola *et al.*, 2014). Perhaps the industry can take a leaf from South Africa, which has managed to commercially produce several products ranging from herbal teas and medicines, and some food products through companies like PhytoNova,

Thebe Medicare and Afriplex (Brendler *et al.*, 2010; Van Wyk, 2011). While these examples are not tick management products, the product development framework used for these products could be adapted for anti-tick commercial plant product development.

Scientists are good at determining and providing evidence of efficacy, but the development of products for the market requires other skills on product development and marketing, necessitating the participation of other players in the value chain. The net result is that research and commercialisation on botanical pesticides is relatively low and often uncoordinated nationally, regionally and even globally. There are few isolated efforts to identify potentially useful plants from ethnobotanical surveys and other indigenous knowledge sources to produce marketable commercial products (Kaposhi, 1992; Matekaire and Bwakura, 2004; Ndhlovu and Masika, 2012; Gumbochuma *et al.*, 2013; Chinsembu *et al.*, 2014; Nyahangare *et al.*, 2015; Marandure, 2016; Kamanula *et al.*, 2017). It must be noted, however, that there are still many plant uses to be 'discovered' with a high priority because of the richness of Africa's biodiversity and there are risks of biopiracy (McGaw and Eloff, 2008; Dubey *et al.*, 2010).

Recent and current research on botanical acaricides

Literature focusing on plants that are effective against cattle ticks is available but still sparse compared to those used in human medicine and field crops pest management. It therefore remains a significant gap and major opportunity considering the cultural and biodiversity in Africa. In comparison with other aspects of botanical acaricides development, ethnobotanical surveys dominate what has been done already, but scientific evaluation for efficacy, phytochemistry, and toxicity is still limited. This limitation is good because surveys are a foundation for screening for efficacy of plants. There are also various opportunities for different stakeholders in plant-based products value chain to take up ethnoveterinary medicine a notch higher. On the other hand, a lack of critical information delays the development of a commercial product and stalled informed policy-making on acaricidal plant products. Overall, the biggest beneficiaries of these products will continue to have losses incurred from sub-optimal livestock productivity; a fact well illustrated in (Isman, 1997) who observed that it is the LMICs that can benefit more from these technologies compared to high-income countries. In Table 16.1 we catalogue plants from different parts of the African continent that have been scientifically tested against ticks. While the list is not exhaustive, it suggests that much research has been undertaken but more is required in order to develop the botanical acaricides industry in Africa. Most of the studies are *in vitro* and need to be verified under field conditions *in vivo* (Table 16.1). The latter is critical and the ultimate evidence of efficacy of plant-based acaricidal products.

Chemical analysis and identification of active fractions in plants is also a key component missing in many of the studies, even at global level (Isman and Grieneisen, 2014), and can help better understand approaches to optimising the use of pesticidal plant plants (Belmain *et al.*, 2012; Stevenson *et al.*, 2012). This limits the potential to optimise the performance of the plant materials for use by smallholder farmers or to understand the human and environmental safety of the plant extracts.

Bio-Prospecting Challenges of Anti-Tick Plants

It is not surprising that field identification of anti-tick plants dominates many publications in Africa because this is arguably the '*easier*' component of anti-tick plant product research (Adenubi *et al.*, 2016). Several authors have given accounts from surveys that show different plant materials with potential anti-tick properties (Kaposhi, 1992; Chamboko *et al.*, 1999; Hlatshwayo and Mbati, 2005; McGaw and Eloff, 2008; Moyo and Masika, 2009; Matlebyane *et al.*, 2010; Chinsembu *et al.*, 2014; Nyahangare *et al.*, 2015). This is not to say that there are no challenges, but it appears that Africa does have enough human capital to address this kind of

Table 16.1. Some anti-tick plants that have been studied scientifically in Africa.

Family	Plant species	Plant part(s)	Focal country	Key findings	Reference
Asteraceae	*Tagetes minuta* *Tagetes multiflora*	Essential oils	Kenya	Repellent against *R. appendiculatus*	(Wanzala *et al.*, 2014)
	Vernonia amygdalina	Leaves	Western Ethiopia	Tested *in vitro* showing high effectiveness ranging between 30 and 100%	(Regassa, 2000)
	Schkuria pinnata	Whole plant	South Africa	Extracts effective against *R. turanicus* ticks *in vitro*	(Fouche *et al.*, 2017)
Brassicaceae	*Lepidium sativum*	Seeds	Western Ethiopia	Tested *in vitro* showing high effectiveness ranging between 30 and 100%	(Regassa, 2000)
Burseraceae	*Commiphora holtiziana*	Exudate	South Africa	Effective against cattle ticks in laboratory bioassays	(Birkett *et al.*, 2008)
Capparaceae	*Cleome monophylla*	Leaves	Kenya	Repelled ticks in a climbing assay	(Ndungu *et al.*, 1995)
	Gynandropsis gyandra	Leaves	Kenya	Excellent repellent effects against ticks *in vitro*	(Lwande *et al.*, 1999)
	G. gyandra	Leaves	Kenya	*In vivo* repellent activity against ticks	(Malonza *et al.*, 1992)
	Maerua edulis	Leaves	Zimbabwe	Hot water and methanol extracted *M. edulis* caused high mortality of tick larvae in efficacy laboratory bioassays. Extracts did not cause any mortality in mice in toxicological experiments suggesting apparent safety to non-target organisms	(Nyahangare *et al.*, 2016)

Continued

Table 16.1. Continued

Family	Plant species	Plant part(s)	Focal country	Key findings	Reference
	M. edulis	Tubers	Zimbabwe	On station trials showed a marked increase in acaricidal activity of the plant extracts after using hot water and surfactant for extraction	(Nyahangare *et al.*, 2017)
	M. edulis	Leaves and tuber	Zimbabwe	Addition of a surfactant to *M. edulis* tuber water extracts increased efficacy against ticks *in vitro*	(Nyahangare *et al.*, 2019)
Fabaceae	*Bobgunnia madagascariensis*	Pods	Zambia	Methanol extracts toxic to ticks causing high mortalities	(Muyobela *et al.*, 2016)
	Calpurnia aurea	Leaves	Ethiopia	*In vitro* studies show that the extract is effective by attracting and killing ticks	(Zorloni *et al.*, 2010)
	C. aurea	Leaves	South Africa	Potent activity against ticks in laboratory tests	(Wellington *et al.*, 2017)
	C. aurea	Leaves	South Africa	Extracts effective against *R. turanicus* ticks *in vitro*	(Fouche *et al.*, 2017)
	Cassia adenocucaulius	Leaves	Uganda	Showed excellent repellent activity to ticks in a laboratory bioassay	(Opiro *et al.*, 2013)
	Neorautanenia mitis	Roots	Rwanda	Effective against female *R. appendiculatus in vitro*	(Van Puyvelde *et al.*, 1985)
	N. mitis	Roots	Nigeria		(Lasisia and Adesomoju, 2015)
	Senna italica	Root extracts	South Africa	Effective *in vitro* against adult *Hyalomma marginatum rufipes*	(Thembo *et al.*, 2010)
	Sphenostylis erecta	Leaves	Zimbabwe	*In vitro* efficacy of the aqueous root extracts caused 96% mortality of ticks	(Chikwanda *et al.*, 2013)

Continued

Table 16.1. Continued

Family	Plant species	Plant part(s)	Focal country	Key findings	Reference
	Tephrosia vogelii	Leaves	Zambia	Methanol extracts toxic to ticks causing high mortalities	(Muyobela *et al.*, 2016)
	T. vogelii	Leaves	Zimbabwe	Water extracts of *T. vogelii* leaves reduced ticks on dairy cows as effectively as commercial acaricide (Triatix) at 5% v/v	(Gadzirayi *et al.*, 2009)
Lamiaceae	*Hyptis suaveolens*	Leaves	Nigeria	Effective against the dog tick	(Ohimain *et al.*, 2015)
	Lavandula angustifolia	Leaves	South Africa	Effective against dog ticks *in vitro*	(Mkolo and Magano, 2007)
	Ocimum suave	Leaves	Kenya	Effective against *R. decoloratus*	(Mwangi *et al.*, 1995)
	O. suave	Leaves	Namibia	Effective against cattle ticks *in vitro*	(Kaaya, 2003)
	Nepeta cataria	Leaves	Kenya	Effective repellent of ticks	(Birkett *et al.*, 2011)
Loganiaceae	*Strychnos spinosa*	Unripe fruits	Zimbabwe	Water extracts of unripe *S. spinosa* fruits caused mortality in mice in acute oral toxicity studies suggesting that they have toxic effects on non-target organisms	(Nyahangare *et al.*, 2012)
	S. spinosa	Unripe fruits	Zimbabwe	On station efficacy trials showed acaricidal activity against cattle ticks in on station trials. Laboratory bioassays against tick larvae also confirmed the activity	(Madzimure *et al.*, 2013)
Meliaceae	*Azadirachta indica*	Leaves	Namibia	Organic solvent extracts effective against different life cycles of the ticks *in vitro*	(Kaaya *et al.*, 2007)
	A. indica	Leaves	Namibia	Effective against cattle ticks *in vitro*	(Kaaya, 2003)

Continued

Table 16.1. Continued

Family	Plant species	Plant part(s)	Focal country	Key findings	Reference
Moraceae	*Ficus brachypoda*	Seeds	Western Ethiopia	Tested *in vitro* showing high effectiveness ranging between 30 and 100%	(Regassa, 2000)
Myrtaceae	*Eucalyptus globoidea*	Whole plant	South Africa	Very high repellent activity against *Hyalomma marginatum*	(Magano *et al.*, 2011)
Phyllanthaceae	*Margaritaria discoidea*	Dry wood	Namibia	Induced high mortality in the nymphs and adult ticks	(Kaaya *et al.*, 1995)
Solanaceae	*Solanum diphyllum*	Fruits	Rwanda	Effective against female *R. appendiculatus in vitro*	(Van Puyvelde *et al.*, 1985)
	Solanum incanum	Ripe fruits	Zimbabwe	On station efficacy trials showed acaricidal activity against cattle ticks in on station trials. Laboratory bioassays against tick larvae also confirmed the activity	(Madzimure *et al.*, 2013)
	S. incanum	Seeds	Western Ethiopia	Tested *in vitro* showing high effectiveness ranging between 30 and 100%	(Regassa, 2000)
Verbenaceae	*Lippia javanica*	Leaves	Zimbabwe	Crude water extracts of L. javanica were effective against cattle ticks in efficacy on station trials at 10% w/v	(Muyobela *et al.*, 2016)
Vitaceae	*Cissus quadrangularis*	Stems	South Africa	Ethanol extracts effective against ticks *in vitro*	(Fouche *et al.*, 2016)
	C. quadrangularis	Stems	South Africa	Potent activity against ticks in laboratory tests	(Wellington *et al.*, 2017)

research. Bio-prospecting, on the other hand, offers bigger challenges in achieving sufficient quantitative and qualitative data required for anti-tick product formulation.Issues like toxicity, efficacy and characterization of active components require adequate financial investment, enabling infrastructure and laboratory equipment supported by scientific expertise capital to be adequately addressed (Isman and Grieneisen, 2014). Unfortunately, many countries in Africa fall short of these requirements, but there is need for concerted efforts to make sure that this happens sooner than later because it is in the best interest of the region that this happens and improves livelihoods of low-income farmers.

Challenges to Development of Anti-Tick Products From Plants

While pesticidal plants are proving to be useful in controlling agricultural pests and there is scope to increase their use, this field is not without its own challenges. There are some grey areas, which include limited finances, inadequate human capital, inadequate infrastructure and lack of enabling policies, which limit full exploitation of the pesticidal plants (Sola *et al.*, 2014).

Research finances

Production of plant-based acaricides requires a good financial support base. Bio-prospecting experiments are generally very expensive, and it is estimated that producing a novel pesticidal plant product requires at least US$100 million and in a period of no less than 10 years (Graf *et al.*, 2004; Njoroge and Bussmann, 2006). Most of the recorded studies available therefore are not conclusive and limited to efficacy of extracts *in vitro*. There is need to identify the active ingredients in the formulations, understand their mode of action and determine the residual period and the effective application interval of the extracts (Isman and Grieneisen, 2014; Miresmailli and Isman, 2014). Ultimately, the plant extracts must demonstrate efficacy under field conditions because *in vitro* data by themselves are not sufficient (Nyahangare *et al.*, 2017). All this requires strong research and development investment, which unfortunately may not be available in most developing countries and research institutions.

Research expertise and entrepreneurship

Research finances must always be complemented by expertise to design and execute robust experiments along the product development value chain. Isman and Grieneisen (Isman and Grieneisen, 2014) reported that there were too many inconsistencies in bio-prospecting procedures leading to accumulation of many manuscripts but unfortunately with practically unusable data. The same review also noted that most papers published did not have chemical composition data, thus further limiting the usefulness of these manuscripts. Botanical pesticides development, just like synthetic drug/pesticides value chains, requires biochemists, toxicologists, chemists, botanists, ecologists, pharmacologists, economists, lawyers and many other relevant experts. Unfortunately, such complementarity of expertise is often not readily available, which hampers the bio-prospecting and product development processes. In addition, the culture of research in African research institutions needs to change as most findings remain 'academic' and the conversion of innovations into social and economic use remains incomplete. The business element is often missing, and hence many research outputs remain on the shelves, uncommercialized.

Infrastructure

Bio-prospecting requires fully furnished laboratories. The reason why LMICs have lagged behind is because, even if they wanted to test material, they do not have adequately equipped laboratories. As a result, there is a risk of biopiracy as researchers expose themselves by seeking collaboration with scientists from other countries. Many laboratories in Africa do not have even basic equipment for phytochemical analysis even in institutes of higher learning and universities. The private sector is encouraged to invest in infrastructural development, but it seems that they are not sure of the return on investment on bio-pesticidal products (Sola *et al.*, 2014).

Policy and regulatory challenges

Existing policy and resultant regulatory frameworks on the use of bio-pesticides have been formulated to guide synthetic pesticide use the world over for many years (Isman, 1997). As a result, because most bio-pesticides do not comply with these regulations, they are therefore illegally produced, informally traded and used, and as such do not influence policy much (Sola *et al.*, 2014). It is perhaps time policy-makers deliberately create conducive policies and legislature for the growth of the botanical pesticide industry including anti-tick plants. There is no doubt that the botanical pesticide industry has a very important role to play in agricultural production because there is overwhelming scientific evidence that some are efficacious, safe, environmentally benign and relatively cheap compared to synthetic products on the market. There are a few countries in the world that exempt botanical products from being regulated like the United States of America, but the majority of countries use the same legislation for synthetics to apply to botanical pesticides (Koul *et al.*, 2008). This gives an unfair advantage to synthetics and downplays the many advantages that botanical pesticides may have over synthetic products. As a way forward (Sola *et al.*, 2014), put the challenge to private and public research institutions to invest in more comprehensive research that should nudge policy-makers to believe that botanicals are potentially safe and effective products that can be used in the market. Funding for research in these areas is limited because investors are sceptical about the returns that can come out of this industry (Isman, 1997; Sola *et al.*, 2014).

Intellectual property rights

Patent rights have always been a contentious issue associated with plant-based product development, largely because information about use of these plants is based on indigenous knowledge largely from the traditional healers, farmers and rural communities (Wanzala *et al.*, 2005; Nyahangare et al., 2015). However, without support, communities normally have no capacity to develop and produce a competitive product for formal markets. These bottlenecks to local community commercial production can be overcome with sustainable collaborations among farmers, researchers and development organisations. Community networking with researchers has been shown to be effective when promoting relatively unrefined plant pesticide products and spraying services as part of research and development programmes. Enabling farmers to make money by selling botanical spraying services to other local farmers as well as pre-ground plant materials has incentivised the use of botanical pesticides and encouraged community investment in scaling-up botanical pesticide production and use as part of ongoing research and development programmes in Tanzania and Malawi (https://www.ccrp.org/grants/botanical-pesticides/). Such schemes could be scaled-up further as sustainable local business development opportunities that generally avoid intellectual property and regulatory issues. However, in formalised markets the prospects of developing a botanical product can be held back by legal issues around access, benefit-sharing and patent rights among the farmers/communities, the scientists and the private sector developers. The private sector has been hesitant to invest in these ventures because of these uncertainties (Isman *et al.*, 2006). There is also growing mistrust between researchers and farmers, mostly from the farmers' side, because of the perception that researchers conduct surveys to extract information, which they use to develop commercial interests without due recognition to the farmers (Nyahangare *et al.*, 2015). This is despite the fact that the application of very few plant materials actually passes the rigorous quality assurance required for the development of a new product and that large investments are needed to produce a new botanical pesticide product (Graf *et al.*, 2004).

The Future of Anti-Tick Plants

Development of anti-tick plant products is complex with many factors to consider. There is still more that can be done to fully understand properties of plants and associated phytochemicals that can facilitate the development of safe, effective and sustainable products. The following are specific aspects of future research and development that could be prioritised:

- Comprehensive chemical analysis of anti-tick plants (bioassay guided isolation and identification of the active chemical compounds) and test them against ticks, individually and in blends found in the plants, which can lead to the identification of new products.
- Conducting anti-microbial tests on the acaricidal plants to determine if they are effective against microbes present in abscesses and lesions caused by ticks. Investment in propagation and cultivation of anti-tick plants to service niche plant processing industries (Pauw and Eloff, 2014).
- Carrying out more surveys in other areas to build a comprehensive anti-tick plant database as there are likely to be many yet undiscovered plants.

Integration and development of collaborative research groups

Given the current status of fragmented uncoordinated research in ethnoveterinary plants and practices in Africa, there are steps that the scientific community can take to improve visibility and uptake of these technologies. One of the ways is the deliberate working together of different groups involved in plant use research. Already there are a number of research groups interested in plant products research and working together on various facets of ethnobotany and developing useful plant based products (http://www.nri.org/projects/sapp/; http://www.nri.org/projects/adappt/; http://www.nri.org/projects/options/; https://naprecanetwork.net; http://www.up.ac.za/phyto).

Some of the benefits coming from collaborations with these different bodies are the development of peer-reviewed scientific protocols used to test efficacy, toxicity, safety and chemistry of plant extracts. With the creation of a critical mass of experts, research groups can lobby for the recognition of ethnoveterinary products with national governments to eventually facilitate formulation of a clear policy on ethnoveterinary research and development if not yet in place. There is need for policy-makers in the agricultural sector, particularly in countries that do not support traditional anti-tick plant technologies, to reconsider and facilitate promotion and integration of traditional practices that can be used in tick control. Formalisation and promotion of known remedies can help ease this challenge. Industrialists should also take advantage of this generated body of knowledge and facilitate designing anti-tick plant packages that can be used by different types of farmers.

Inter-disciplinary collaborations also attract funding from both national and international institutions. All research requires resources and collaboration for the development of stronger competitive proposals and capacity development. What is absent is the participation of the private sector. There is a need to engage this sector to facilitate development of products and the social and economic use of the product(s). Future research also needs to embrace the marketing and institutional components rather than just the traditional natural science approach. In other words, the value chain approach as articulated by Sola *et al.*, 2014 should be used to bring all facets of ethnoveterinary research into perspective.

Developing low-cost optimisation strategies

The evidence of efficacy in most of the tested plants should be a platform to convert 'village science' into robust evidence-based decision-making science. The information from farmers on how to prepare the medicines and acaricides is very simple. Mostly water is used in various extraction programmes. However, it is known that water only is not an optimum solvent (Eloff, 1998; Kotzé and Eloff, 2002; Belmain *et al.*, 2012). It is, therefore, imperative that exploratory work continue to search for low-cost methods of improving extraction and improve efficacy. In some areas, the use of hot water for extraction, use of a surfactant, use of pure compounds and mixing different plant materials have been explored. While the results have not been very conclusive, there is sufficient evidence to suggest that use of hot water and use of a surfactant are low-cost measures that can be used to increase efficacy of plant products (Nyahangare *et al.*, 2016). There is also need to fully understand the stage of plant growth and growth conditions that yield effective active compounds in appreciable concentrations. It is known that the concentration of plant chemicals does vary with stage of growth of the plant, geography and other environmental factors (Sarasan *et al.*, 2011; Stevenson et al., 2012). Further work should also be carried out that looks at residual effects, effect of storage of the plant material and also a cost benefit analysis of using the plant products. For example, Amoabeng *et al.* (Amoabeng *et al.*, 2014) showed that pesticidal plants are cost-effective in controlling cabbage pests. The same approach could be adapted for ethnoveterinary plants especially for tick control. This body of information will be crucial for optimal use. There are also a lot more plant materials reported in surveys that still need to have their perceived medicinal, acaricidal and pesticidal properties scientifically verified.

Further screening experiments

It is a possibility that an even bigger database of useful ethno-veterinary plants can be realized if all the different agro-ecological zones, cultures and experiences in different parts of Africa are factored in. The challenge, however, for scientists is to be able to screen the useful plants from those with no medicinal or acaricidal properties. The screening should inevitably include the following:

Laboratory bioassays with cattle ticks

Quick laboratory experiments should be able to give an indication of the efficacy of the plants in question and also serve as a quick screening procedure. This preliminary information should help focus research resources on plants with appreciable activity. Not all the plants that farmers claim to have pesticidal or medicinal activity are proven so under rigorous experimental investigations (Sarasan *et al.*, 2011). However, it must be noted that good *in vitro* bioassay results from the laboratory with ticks do not necessarily translate to good results when ticks on actual animals are treated *in vivo*. It is therefore not advisable to simply use information generated from *in vitro* trials and apply it to live animals without further experimentation.

Bioassays of acaricides with ticks placed on animals

Live animal trials on station and on farm should be the ultimate determinants of whether a plant product does have acaricidal/medicinal effects (Stevenson *et al.*, 2012). Sometimes rats and mice models are used in laboratory bioassays but eventually the actual affected animals should be used to cater for species differences and different dosage requirements. It is also very important to have farmers participating in the trials since they are the most likely beneficiaries of the innovations. Technology adoption is always better under a co-learning and co-innovating environment necessitated by farmer participation. Despite *in vivo* trials being necessary, they are often affected by cost, expertise, labour, availability of facilities and sufficient animal numbers for statistically sound trials (Githiori *et al.*, 2005). In comparison, on-station trials can be easily carried out compared to on-farm trials mainly because of lack of adequate negative controls in on-farm trials and also convincing farmers to use their animals especially for a negative control treatment. Projects may need to consider providing insurance services (treatment of animals or replacing) to cater for any unlikely event of animals succumbing to lack of treatments during exposure to diseases or heavy parasite infestation.

Phytochemical analyses

The chemical composition of acaricidal plants is a major knowledge gap in the development of plant-based tick control but is essential if the value of pesticidal plants is to be optimized (Sarasan *et al.*, 2011; Stevenson *et al.*, 2012). For example, it is a requirement for the active compounds to be identified and evaluated for efficacy and toxicity before a product is registered and patented (Sola *et al.*, 2014). Even though there have not been many commercialised ethnoveterinary plant products, it is anticipated that as research continues, some will lead to commercial products. It is an opportunity for communities to realise some financial benefit from their indigenous knowledge and resources. Closely associated with labelling is also the issue of non-target toxicity. Many plant-based acaricides are regarded as safe, but many plants also produce toxic compounds and so may be hazardous (Nyahangare *et al.*, 2012). Chemical analysis can therefore serve as an indicator of harm and efficacy. Phytochemical profiles are also required in the optimisation of extraction, formulation and application of the plant-based acaricides (Stevenson *et al.*, 2018).

Working with communities

One of the concerns that communities raised in a recently published survey was that scientists never return to communities with results of how the plants that they provided performed under scientific scrutiny (Nyahangare *et al.*, 2015). It is recommended that the findings and benefits be shared equitably with smallholder farmers alongside training sessions on effective use of plants to control ticks and the information also be transferred to field agricultural extension workers. Unfortunately, elements of packaging the results and communicating them back to communities as well as capacity building of value chain actors is not often built in to research and development projects limiting the impact of research findings. For example the use of surfactants and the use of boiling water are easy and affordable ways of increasing extraction efficiency and activity of local remedies. This information should be made readily available to beneficiaries of these plant-based technologies. Users should also be trained on sustainable harvesting of the plant materials from nature but as demand for such products increases, scientific methods of propagating and cultivating the plants should be pursued.

Conclusion

While still lacking in Africa, a botanical acaricide industry is growing globally, and is supported by a need for alternative and complementary tick-control measures, necessitated by the numerous challenges presented by the use of synthetic acaricides. The challenges Africa faces include lack of research and development finances, standardization of protocols, conducive and supportive policies and regulations, expertise and equipment, all of which hamper commercialisation of the products. There are also performance variations in both bioassays with ticks in laboratory vs bioassays with ticks placed on animals for the same plant species. Because of these bottlenecks, there is apparently a lot of information on acaricidal plants but some of it is incomplete, resulting in very few products actually available on the market. The scope for identifying potentially useful plants and screening them through efficacy and toxicity experiments and potentially making commercial products is still promising and should be explored further. One strategy to circumvent regulatory and patent issues is to facilitate establishment of cottage industries of the crude botanical acaricides based on scientific screening of the pesticidal plants.

Acknowledgements

This work was funded by the European Commission's European Development Fund ACP Science and Technology Programme grants FED/2009/217064 (ADAPPT) and FED /2013/329272 (OPTIONs).

Conflict of Interest

The authors declare no conflict of interest whatsoever in publishing this research.

References

Abbas, R.Z., Zaman, M.A., Colwell, D.D., Gilleard, J. and Iqbal, Z. (2014) Acaricide resistance in cattle ticks and approaches to its management: The state of play. *Veterinary Parasitology [Internet]* 203(1–2), 6–20. DOI: 10.1016/j.vetpar.2014.03.006.

Adehan, S.B., Biguezoton, A., Adakal, H., Assogba, M.N., Zoungrana, S.S. *et al.* (2016) Acaricide resistance of *Rhipicephalus microplus* ticks in Benin. *African Journal of Agricultural Research [Internet]* 11(14), 1199–1208. Available at: http://www.academicjournals.org/journal/AJAR/article-abstract/31AC1495 7918%5Cnhttp://www.academicjournals.org/journal/AJAR/article-full-text-pdf/31AC14957918

Adenubi, O.T., Fasina, F.O., McGaw, L.J., Eloff, J.N. and Naidoo, V. (2016) Plant extracts to control ticks of veterinary and medical importance: A review. *South African Journal of Botany* 105, 178–193.

Adenubi, O.T., Ahmed, A.S., Fasina, F.O., McGaw, L.J., Eloff, J.N. *et al.* (2018) Pesticidal plants as a possible alternative to synthetic acaricides in tick control: A systematic review and meta-analysis. *Industrial Crops and Products* 123, 779–806.

Amoabeng, B.W., Gurr, G.M., Gitau, C.W. and Stevenson, P.C. (2014) Cost: Benefit analysis of botanical insecticide use in cabbage: Implications for smallholder farmers in developing countries. *Crop Protection* 57, 71–76.

Atif, F.A., Khan, M.S., Iqbal, H.J., Ali, Z. and Ullah, S. (2016) Prevalence of cattle tick infestation in three districts of the Punjab, Pakistan. *Pakistan Journal of Science* 64(1), 49–53.

Baetz, U. and Martinoia, E. (2014) Root exudates: The hidden part of plant defense. *Trends in Plant Science* 19(2), 90–98.

Belmain, S.R., Amoah, B.A., Nyirenda, S.P., Kamanula, J.F. and Stevenson, P.C. (2012) Highly variable insect control efficacy of *Tephrosia vogelii* chemotypes. *Journal of Agricultural and Food Chemistry* 60, 10055–10063.

Benelli, G., Pavela, R., Canale, A. and Mehlhorn, H. (2016) Tick repellents and acaricides of botanical origin: A green roadmap to control tick-borne diseases? *Parasitology Research* 115(7), 2545–2560.

Birkett, M.A., Al Abassi, S., Kröber, T., Chamberlain, K., Hooper, A.M. *et al.* (2008) Antiectoparasitic activity of the gum resin, gum haggar, from the East African plant, *Commiphora holtziana*. *Phytochemistry* 69(8), 1710–1715.

Birkett, M.A., Hassanali, A., Hoglund, S., Pettersson, J. and Pickett, J.A. (2011) Repellent activity of catmint, nepeta cataria, and iridoid nepetalactone isomers against afro-tropical mosquitoes, ixodid ticks and red poultry mites. *Phytochemistry* 72(1), 109–114.

Bissinger, B.W. and Roe, R.M. (2010) Tick repellents: Past, present, and future. *Pesticide Biochemistry and Physiology [Internet]* 96(2), 63–79. DOI: 10.1016/j.pestbp.2009.09.010.

Brendler, T., Eloff, J.N., Gurib-Fakim, A. and Phillips, L.D. (2010) In: *African Herbal Pharmacopoeia. Port Louis*. Association for African Medicinal Plants Standards (AAMPS) Publishing, Mauritius, p. 289.

Chamboko, T., Mukhebi, A.W., Callaghan, C.J.O., Peter, T.F., Kruska, R.L. *et al.* (1999) The control of heartwater on large-scale commercial and smallholder farms in Zimbabwe. *Preventive Veterinary Medicine* 39(3), 191–210.

Chikwanda, D., Mapanda, T., Chikosi, V.E. and Chikwanda, A.T. (2013) The efficacy of *Sphenostylis erecta* root extracts in controlling blue tick, *Boophilus decoloratus* infestation. *Biopesticides International* 9(2), 195–203.

Chinsembu, K.C., Negumbo, J., Likando, M. and Mbangu, A. (2014) An ethnobotanical study of medicinal plants used to treat livestock diseases in Onayena and Katima Mulilo, Namibia. *South African Journal of Botany* 94, 101–107.

Collier, P., Conway, G. and Venables, T. (2008) Climate change and Africa. *Oxford Review of Economic Policy* 24(2), 337–353.

Damalas, C.A. and Eleftherohorinos, I.G. (2011) Pesticide exposure, safety issues, and risk assessment indicators. *International Journal of Environmental Research and Public Health* 8, 1402–1419.

Dantas-Torres, F. (2015) Climate change, biodiversity, ticks and tick-borne diseases: The butterfly effect. *International Journal for Parasitology: Parasites and Wildlife* 4(3), 452–461.

Dubey, N.K., Shukla, R., Kumar, A., Singh, P. and Prakash, B. (2010) Prospects of botanical pesticides in sustainable agriculture. *Current Science* 98(4), 479–480.

Eloff, J.N. (1998) Which extractant should be used for the screening and isolation of antimicrobial components from plants? *Journal of Ethnopharmacology* 60, 1–8.

Estrada-Peña, A. and Salman, M. (2013) Current limitations in the control and spread of ticks that affect livestock: A review. *Agriculture [Internet]* 3, 221–235. Available at: www.mdpi.com/journal/agriculture

Estrada-Peña, A. and De La Fuente, J. (2014) The ecology of ticks and epidemiology of tick-borne viral diseases. *Antiviral Research* 108, 104–128.

Fernandez-Ruvalcaba, M., Torre, P. and Cruz-Vazquez, C. (2004) Anti-tick effects of *Melinis minutiflora* and *Andropogon gayanus* grasses on plots experimentally infested with *Boophilus microplus* larvae. *Experimental and Applied Acarology* 32, 293–299.

Fouche, G., Ramafuthula, M., Maselela, V., Mokoena, M., Senabe, J. *et al.* (2016) Acaricidal activity of the organic extracts of thirteen South African plants against *Rhipicephalus* (Boophilus) decoloratus (Acari: Ixodidae). *Veterinary Parasitology* 224, 39–43.

Fouche, G., Sakong, B.M., Adenubi, O.T., Dzoyem, J.P., Naidoo, V. *et al.* (2017) Investigation of the acaricidal activity of the acetone and ethanol extracts of 12 South African plants against the adult ticks of *Rhipicephalus turanicus*. *The Onderstepoort Journal of Veterinary Research* 84(1), a1523. DOI: 10.4102/ojvr.v84i1.1523.

Frans, J. (2000) Final report, integrated control of ticks and tick-borne diseases (ICTTD).p. 4. Available at: http://www.uu.nl/tropical.ticks

Fuente, D., Almaza, C., Canales, M., Pe, M., Lastra, D. *et al.* (2007) A ten-year review of commercial vaccine performance for control of tick infestations on cattle. *Animal Health Research Reviews* 8(1), 23–28.

Gadzirayi, C.T., Mutandwa, E. and Mwale, M. (2009) Utilization of *Tephrosia vogelii* in controlling ticks in dairy cows by small-scale commercial farmers in Zimbabwe. *African Journal of Biotechnology* 8(17), 4134–4136.

George, J.E., Pound, J.M. and Davey, R.B. (2004) Chemical control of ticks on cattle and the resistance of these parasites to acaricides. *Parasitology* 129, S353–S366.

Ghosh, S., Azhahianambi, P. and Yadav, M.P. (2007) Upcoming and future strategies of tick control: A review. *Journal of Vector Borne Diseases* 44(2), 79–89.

Ghosh, S., Tiwari, S.S., Kumar, B., Srivastava, S., Sharma, A.K. *et al.* (2015) Identification of potential plant extracts for anti-tick activity against acaricide resistant cattle ticks, *Rhipicephalus* (Boophilus) microplus (Acari: Ixodidae). *Experimental and Applied Acarology [Internet]* 66(1), 159–171. DOI: 10.1007/s10493-015-9890-7.

Githiori, J.B., Ho, J. and Waller, P.J. (2005) Ethnoveterinary plant preparations as livestock dewormers: Practices, popular beliefs, pitfalls and prospects for the future. *Animal Health Research Reviews* 6(1), 91–103.

Godfray, H., Beddington, J.R., Crute, I.R., Haddard, L., Lawrence, D. *et al.* (2010) The challenge of food security. *Science [Internet]* 327(February), 812–819. Available at: http://www.elgaronline.com/view/9780857939371.xml

Graf, J.F., Gogolewski, R., Leach-Bing, N., Sabatini, G.A., Molento, M.B. *et al.* (2004) Tick control: An industry point of view. *Parasitology* 129 Suppl(2), S427–42.

Grzywacz, D., Stevenson, P.C., Mushobozi, W.L., Belmain, S. and Wilson, K. (2014) The use of indigenous ecological resources for pest control in Africa. *Food Security* 6, 71–86.

Gumbochuma, G., Hamandishe, V.R., Nyahangare, E.T., Imbayarwo-Chikosi, V.E. and Ncube, S. (2013) Ethno veterinary practices for poultry and cattle in Zimbabwe: A case study of Takavarasha village. *Scientific Journal of Animal Science* 2(212), 355–359.

Harvey, A.L. and Gericke, N. (2011) Bioprospecting: Creating a value for biodiversity. In: Pavlinov, I.Y. (ed.) *Research in Biodiversity-Models and Applications*. pp. 323–338.

Herrero, M. and Thornton, P.K. (2013, December 24) Livestock and global change: Emerging issues for sustainable food systems. *Proceedings of the National Academy of Sciences* 110(52), 20878–20881.

Hlatshwayo, M. and Mbati, P.A. (2005) A survey of tick control methods used by resource-poor farmers in the Qwa-Qwa area of the Eastern free state province, South Africa. *The Onderstepoort Journal of Veterinary Research* 72(3), 245–249.

Isman, M.B. (1997) Neem and other botanical insecticides: Barriers to commercialization. *Phytoparasitica* 25(4), 339–344.

Isman, M.B. (2020) Botanical insecticides in the twenty-first century— fulfilling their promise? *Annual Review of Entomology* 65, 1–17.

Isman, M.B. (2006) Botanical insecticides, deterrents, and repellents in modern agriculture and an increasingly regulated world. *Annual Review of Entomology* 51(1), 45–66.

Isman, M.B. and Machial, C.M. (2006) Pesticides based on plant essential oils: From traditional practice to commercialization. *Advances in Phytomedicine* 3(1), 29–44.

Isman, M.B., Machial, C.M., and Rai (2006) Pesticides based on plant essential oils: From traditional practice to commercialization. In: *Naturally Occuring Bioactive Compounds*. Elsevier, pp. 29–44.

Isman, M.B. and Grieneisen, M.L. (2014) Botanical insecticide research: Many publications, limited useful data. *Trends in Plant Science* 19(3), 140–145.

Jabbar, A., Abbas, T., Saddiqi, H.A., Qamar, M.F. and Gasser, R.B. (2015) Tick-borne diseases of bovines in Pakistan: Major scope for future research and improved control. *Parasites & Vectors* 8(1), 283.

Jongejan, F. and Uilenberg, G. (2004) The global importance of ticks. *Parasitology* 129(7), S3.

Kaaya, G.P. (2003) Prospects for innovative tick control methods in Africa. *Insect Science and Application* 23(1), 59–67.

Kaaya, G.P., Mwangi, E.N. and Malonza, M.M. (1995) Acaricidal activity of *Margaritaria discoidea* (Euphorbiaceae) plant extracts against the ticks *Rhipicephalus appendiculatus* and *Amblyomma variegatum* (Ixodidae). *International Journal of Acarology* 21(2), 123–129.

Kaaya, G.P., Saxena, R.C. and Gebre, S. (2007) The potential of neem products for control of economically-important African ticks. *Biosciences, Biotechnology Research Asia* 4, 95–104.

Kamanula, J.F., Belmain, S.R., Hall, D.R., Farman, D., Goyder, D.J. *et al.* (2017) Chemical variation and insecticidal activity of *Lippia javanica* (Burm. f) Spreng essential oil against *Sitophilus zeamais* Motschulsky. *Industrial Crops & Products* 110, 75–82.

Kaposhi, C. (1992) The role of natural products in integrated tick management in Africa. *Insect Science and Application* 13(4), 595–598.

Karstensen, K.H., Kinh, N.K., Thang, L.B., Viet, P.H., Tuan, N.D. *et al.* (2006) Environmentally sound destruction of obsolete pesticides in developing countries using cement kilns. *Environmental Science and Policy* 9(6), 577–586.

Khudrathulla, M. and Jagannath, M.S. (2000) In vitro efficacy of aqueous extracts of *Stylosanthes scabra* against ixodid ticks. *Journal of Veterinary and Animal Sciences* 31, 17–21.

Kiss, T., Cadar, D. and Spînu, M. (2012) Tick prevention at a crossroad: New and renewed solutions. *Veterinary Parasitology* 187(3–4), 357–366.

Kotzé, M. and Eloff, J.N. (2002) Extraction of antibacterial compounds from *Combretum microphyllum* (Combretaceae). *South African Journal of Botany [Internet]* 68(1), 62–67. Available at: http://linkinghub.elsevier.com/retrieve/pii/ S025462991530442

Koul, O., Walia, S. and Dhaliwal, G.S. (2008) Essential oils as green pesticides: Potential and constraints. *Biopesticides International* 4(1), 63–84.

Lasisia, A.A. and Adesomoju, A. (2015) Neoraudiol, a new isoflavonoid and other antimicrobial constituents from the tuberous root of *Neorautanenia mitis* (A. Rich) Verdcourt. *Journal of Saudi Chemical Society* 19, 404–409.

Lengai, G.M., Muthomi, J.W. and Mbega, E.R. (2020) Phytochemical activity and role of botanical pesticides in pest management for sustainable agricultural crop production. *Scientific African* 7, e00239.

Luseba, D., Putuka, N., Katerere, D. and Mwanza, M. (2016) Evaluation of repellent properties of some plants used in Venda and tsonga ethnoveterinary medicine. *Journal of Human Ecology* 56, 166–170.

Lwande, W., Ndakala, A.J., Hassanali, A., Moreka, L., Nyandat, E. *et al.* (1999) *Gynandropsis gynandra* essential oil and its constituents as tick (*Rhipicephalus appendiculatus*) repellents. *Phytochemistry* 50(3), 401–405.

Madison-Antenucci, S., Kramer, L.D., Gebhardt, L.L. and Kauffman, E. (2020) Crossm. *Clinical Microbiology Reviews* 33(2), 1–34.

Madzimure, J., Nyahangare, E.T., Hamudikuwanda, H., Hove, T., Stevenson, P.C. *et al.* (2011) Acaricidal efficacy against cattle ticks and acute oral toxicity of *Lippia javanica* (Burm F.) Spreng. *Tropical Animal Health and Production* 43(2), 481–489.

Madzimure, J., Nyahangare, E.T., Hamudikuwanda, H., Hove, T., Belmain, S.R. *et al.* (2013) Efficacy of *Strychnos spinosa* (Lam.) and *Solanum incanum* L. aqueous fruit extracts against cattle ticks. *Tropical Animal Health and Production* 45(6), 1341–1347.

Magadum, S., Mondal, D.B. and Ghosh, S. (2009) Comparative efficacy of *Annona squamosa* and *Azadirachta indica* extracts against *Boophilus microplus* Izatnagar isolate. *Parasitology Research* 105(4), 1085–1091.

Magano, S.R., Nchu, F. and Elof, J.N. (2011) In-vitro investigation of the repellent effects of the essential oil of *Lippia javanica* on adults of *Hyalomma marginatum* rufipes. *African Journal of Biotechnology* 10(44), 8970–8975.

Makala, L., Mangani, P., Fujisaki, K. and Nagasawa, H. (2003) The current status of major tick borne diseases in Zambia. *Veterinary Research* 34(1), 27–45.

Malonza, M.M., Dipeolu, O.O., Amoo, A.O. and Hassan, S.M. (1992) Properties of the plant *Gynandropsis gynandra. Veterinary Parasitology* 42, 123–136.

Manjunathachar, H.V., Saravanan, B.C., Kesavan, M., Karthik, K., Rathod, P. *et al.* (2014) Economic importance of ticks and their effective control strategies. *Asian Pacific Journal of Tropical Disease* 4, S770–9.

Mapholi, N.O., Marufu, M.C., Maiwashe, A., Banga, C.B., Muchenje, V. *et al.* (2014) Towards a genomics approach to tick (Acari: Ixodidae) control in cattle: A review. *Ticks and Tick-Borne Diseases [Internet]*5(5), 475–483. DOI: 10.1016/j.ttbdis.2014.04.006.

Mapiye, C., Chimonyo, M., Dzama, K., Raats, J.G. and Mapekula, M. (2009) Opportunities for improving nguni cattle production in the smallholder farming systems of South Africa. *Livestock Science [Internet]* 124(1–3), 196–204. DOI: 10.1016/j.livsci.2009.01.013.

Marandure, T. (2016) Concepts and key issues of ethnoveterinary medicine in Africa: A review of its application in Zimbabwe. *African Journal of Agricultural Research [Internet]* 11(20), 1836–1841. Available at: http://academicjournals.org/journal/AJAR/article-abstract/009EC0858567

Maroyi, A. (2012) Use of traditional veterinary medicine in Nhema communal area of the midlands province, Zimbabwe. *African Journal of Traditional, Complementary and Alternative Medicines* 9(3), 315–322.

Matekaire, T. and Bwakura, T.M. (2004) Ethnoveterinary medicine: A potential alternative to orthodox animal health delivery in Zimbabwe. *International Journal of Applied Research in Veterinary Medicine* 2(4), 269–273.

Matlebyane, M.M., Ng'ambi, J.W. and Aregheore, E.M. (2010) Indigenous knowledge (IK) ranking of available browse and grass species and some shrubs used in medicinal and ethno-veterinary practices in ruminant livestock production in Limpopo province, South Africa. *Livestock Research for Rural Development* 22(3), 54.

McGaw, L.J. and Eloff, J.N. (2008) Ethnoveterinary use of Southern African plants and scientific evaluation of their medicinal properties. *Journal of Ethnopharmacology [Internet]* 119(3), 559–574. Available at: http://www.ncbi.nlm.nih.gov/pubmed/18620038

Merino, O., Alberdi, P., Lastra, J.M. and Fuente, J. (2013) Tick vaccines and the control of tick-borne pathogens. *Frontiers in Cellular and Infection Microbiology* 3, 30.

Miresmailli, S. and Isman, M.B. (2014) Botanical insecticides inspired by plant-herbivore chemical interactions. *Trends in Plant Science [Internet]* 19(1), 29–35. DOI: 10.1016/j.tplants.2013.10.002.

Mkenda, P., Mwanauta, R., Stevenson, P.C., Ndakidemi, P., Mtei, K. *et al.* (2015) Field margin weeds provide economically viable and environmentally benign pest control compared to synthetic pesticides. *PLoS One* 10, e0143530.

Mkindi, A., Mpumi, N., Tembo, Y., Stevenson, P.C., Ndakidemi, P.A. *et al.* (2017) Invasive weeds with pesticidal properties as potential new crops. *Industrial Crops and Products* 110, 113–122.

Mkindi, A.G., Mtei, K.M., Njau, K.N. and Ndakidemi, P.A. (n.d.) The potential of using indigenous pesticidal plants for insect pest control to small scale farmers in Africa. *American Journal of Plant Sciences* 06(19), 3164–3174.

Mkolo, M.N. and Magano, S.R. (2007) Repellent effects of the essential oil of *Lavendula angustifolia* against adults of *Hyalomma marginatum* rufipes. *Journal of the South African Veterinary Association* 78(3), 149–152.

Moyo, B. and Masika, P.J. (2009) Tick control methods used by resource-limited farmers and the effect of ticks on cattle in rural areas of the Eastern Cape Province, South Africa. *Tropical Animal Health and Production* 41(4), 517–523.

Muhammad, G., Naureen, A., Firyal, S. and Saqib, M. (2008) Tick control strategies in dairy production medicine. *Pakistan Veterinary Journal* 28(1), 43–50.

Muyobela, J., Nkunika, P.O. and Mwase, E.T. (2016) *In vitro* acaricidal activity of *Bobgunnia madagascariensis* desv. against *Amblyomma variegatum* (Fabricius)(Acari: Ixodidae). *Tropical Animal Health and Production* 48(3), 625–631.

Mwangi, E.N., Hassanali, A., Essuman, S., Myandat, E., Moreka, L. *et al.* (1995) Repellent and acaricidal properties of *Ocimum suave* against *Rhipicephalus appendiculatus* ticks. *Experimental & Applied Acarology* 19(1), 11–18.

Nchu, F., Maniania, N.K., Touré, A., Hassanali, A. and Eloff, J. (2009) The use of a semiochemical bait to enhance exposure of *Amblyomma variegatum* (Acari: Ixodidae) to *Metarhizium anisopliae* (Ascomycota: Hypocreales). *Veterinary Parasitology* 160(3–4), 279–284.

Ndhlovu, D.N. and Masika, P.J. (2012) Ethno-veterinary control of bovine dermatophilosis and ticks in Zhombe, Njelele and Shamrock resettlement in Zimbabwe. *Tropical Animal Health and Production* 45(1), 525–532.

Ndungu, M., Lwande, W., Hassanali, A., Moreka, L. and Chhabra, S.C. (1995) *Cleome monophylla* essential oil and its constituents as tick (*Rhipicephalus appendiculatus*) and maize weevil (*Sitophilus zeamais*) repellents. *Entomologia Experimentalis et Applicata* 76(3), 217–222.

Nene, V., Kiara, H., Lacasta, A., Pelle, R., Svitek, N. *et al.* (2016) The biology of *Theileria parva* and control of east coast fever– Current status and future trends. *Ticks and Tick-Borne Diseases* 7(4), 549–564.

Njoroge, G.N. and Bussmann, R.W. (2006) Diversity and utilization of antimalarial ethnophytotherapeutic remedies among the Kikuyus (Central Kenya). *Journal of Ethnobiology and Ethnomedicine* 2(1), 8.

Ntondini, Z., Dalen, E., Horak, I.G. and Dalen, E.M.S.P. (2008) The extent of acaricide resistance in 1-, 2- and 3-host ticks on communally grazed cattle in the Eastern region of the eastern cape province, South Africa. *Journal of the South African Veterinary Association [Internet]* 79(3), 130–135. Available at: http://www.ncbi.nlm.nih.gov/pubmed/19244821

Nyahangare, E.T., Mvumi, B.M. and Maramba, T. (2016) Acute oral mammalian toxicity and effect of solvents on efficacy of *Maerua edulis* (Gilg. & Ben.) de wolf against *Rhipicephalus* (*Boophilus*) *decoloratus* Koch, 1844 (Acarina: Ixodidae), tick larvae. *BioMed Research International [Internet]* 1–8. DOI: 10.1155/2016/7078029.

Nyahangare, E.T., Mvumi, B.M. and Mutibvu, T. (2015) Ethnoveterinary plants and practices used for ecto-parasite control in semi-arid smallholder farming areas of Zimbabwe. *Journal of Ethnobiology and Ethnomedicine [Internet]* 11(1), 30. Available at: http://www.scopus.com/inward/record.url?eid=2-s2.0-84930666291&partnerID=tZOtx3y1

Nyahangare, E.T., Mvumi, B.M., Mcgaw, L.J. and Eloff, J.N. (2019) Addition of a surfactant to water increases the acaricidal activity of extracts of some plant species used to control ticks by Zimbabwean smallholder farmers. *Journal Title Is BMC Veterinary Research* 3, 3–9.

Nyahangare, E.T., Hove, T., Mvumi, B.M., Hamudikuwanda, H., Belmain, S.R. *et al.* (2012) Acute mammalian toxicity of four pesticidal plants. *Journal of Medicinal Plants Research [Internet]* 13, 2674–2680. Available at: http://dx.doi.org/10.1155/2016/7078029

Nyahangare, E.T., Mvumi, B.M., Magona, C. and Eloff, J.N. (2017) An aqueous extract of *Maerua edulis* (Gilg & Ben) DeWolf tuber is as effective as a commercial synthetic acaricide in controlling ticks on cattle *in vivo*. *Industrial Crops and Products* 110, 88–93.

Nyangiwe, N., Yawa, M. and Muchenje, V. (2018) Driving forces for changes in geographic range of cattle ticks (Acari: Ixodidae) in Africa: A review. *South African Journal of Animal Science* 48(5), 829–841.

Ohimain, E.I., Angaye, T.C., Bassey, S.E. and Izah, S.C. (2015) Acaricidal activities of *Hyptis suaveolens* and *Ocimum sanctum* against African dog tick (*Rhipicephalus sanguinneus*). *European Journal of Medicinal Plants* 30, 149–156.

Okello-Onen, J., Ssekitto, C.M. and Mwayi, W. (2003) Some factors affecting the sustainability of tick and tick-borne disease control in Uganda. 1. Malpractice associated with acaricide use. *Uganda Journal of Agricultural Sciences* 8, 30–33.

Opiro, R., Osinde, C., Okello-Onen, J. and Akol, A.M. (2013) Tick-repellent properties of four plant species against *Rhipicephalus appendiculatus* Neumann (Acarina: Ixodidae) tick species. *Journal of Agricultural Research and Development* 3(2), 17–21.

Ott, K.C. Rotenone (2008) A brief review of its chemistry, environmental fate, and the toxicity of rotenone formulations. Santa Fe: New Mexico Council of Trout Unlimited. Available at: http://www.newmexicotu.org/Rotenonesummary.pdf

Pauw, E. and Eloff, J.N. (2014) Which tree orders in Southern Africa have the highest antimicrobial activity and selectivity against bacterial and fungal pathogens of animals. *BMC Complementary and Alternative Medicine* 14(317), 1–12.

Pavela, R. (2016) History, presence and perspective of using plant extracts as commercial botanical insecticides and farm products for protection against insects—A review. *Plant Protection Science* 52(4), 229–241.

Pegram, R.G., Tatchell, R.J., De, C.J., Chizyuka, H.G.B., Creek, M.J. *et al.* (1993) *Tick control: New concepts*. FAO, Rome.

Rajput, Z.I., Hu, S., Chen, W., Arijo, A.G. and Xiao, C. (2006) Importance of ticks and their chemical and immunological control in livestock. *Journal of Zhejiang University Science B [Internet]* 7(11), 912–921. Available at: http://www.pubmedcentral.nih.gov/articlerender.fcgi?artid=1635821&tool=pmcentrez&rendertype=abstract

Randolph, T.F., Schelling, E., Grace, D., Nicholson, C.F., Leroy, J.L. *et al.* (2007) Invited review: Role of livestock in human nutrition and health for poverty reduction in developing countries. *Journal of Animal Science* 85(11), 2788–2800.

Ravindran, R., Juliet, S., Kumar, K.G.A., Sunil, A.R., Nair, S.N. *et al.* (2011) Toxic effects of various solvents against *Rhipicephalus* (*Boophilus*) *annulatus*. *Ticks and Tick-Borne Diseases [Internet]* 2(3), 160–162. DOI: 10.1016/j.ttbdis.2011.04.001.

Regassa, A. (2000) The use of herbal preparations for tick control in Western Ethiopia. *Journal of the South African Veterinary Association* 71(4), 240–243.

Richardson, M. (1998) Pesticides—friend or foe? Water science and technology. *Internet* 37(8), 19–25. DOI: 10.1016/S0273-1223(98)00257-1.

Sarasan, V., Kite, G.C., Sileshi, G.W. and Stevenson, P.C. (2011) Applications of phytochemical and *in vitro* techniques for reducing over-harvesting of medicinal and pesticidal plants and generating income for the rural poor. *Plant Cell Reports* 30(7), 1163–1172.

Shah, B. and Devkota, B. (2009) Obsolete pesticides: Their environmental and human health hazards. *The Journal of Agriculture and Environment* 10, 51–56.

Shyma, K.P., Gupta, J.P. and Singh, V. (2013) Breeding strategies for tick resistance in tropical cattle: A sustainable approach for tick control. *Journal of Parasitic Diseases* 39(1), 1–6.

Shyma, K.P., Gupta, J.P., Ghosh, S., Patel, K.K. and Singh, V. (2014) Acaricidal effect of herbal extracts against cattle tick *Rhipicephalus (Boophilus) microplus* using *in vitro* studies. *Parasitology Research* 113(5), 1919–1926.

Simuunza, M., Weir, W., Courcier, E., Tait, A. and Shiels, B. (2011) Epidemiological analysis of tick-borne diseases in Zambia. *Veterinary Parasitology* 175, 331–342.

Sola, P., Mvumi, B.M., Ogendo, J.O., Mponda, O., Kamanula, J.F. *et al.* (2014) Botanical pesticide production, trade and regulatory mechanisms in Sub-Saharan Africa: Making a case for plant-based pesticidal products. *Food Security* 6(3), 369–384.

Sonenshine, D.E. (2004) Pheromones and other semiochemicals of ticks and their use in tick control. *Parasitology* 129(April 2005), S405–S425.

Stevenson, P.C., Nyirenda, S.P., Mvumi, B.M., Sola, P., Kamanula, J.F. *et al.* (2012) Pesticidal plants: A viable alternative insect pest management approach for resource poor farming in Africa. In: *Biopesticdes in Environment and Food Security*. Scientific Publishers, Jodhpur, pp. 212–238.

Stevenson, P.C., Green, P.W.C., Farrell, I.W., Brankin, A., Mvumi, B.M. *et al.* (2018) Novel agmatine derivatives in *Maerua edulis* with bioactivity against *Callosobruchus maculatus*, a cosmopolitan storage insect pest. *Frontiers in Plant Science* 9(October), 1506.

Sultana, B., Anwar, F. and Ashraf, M. (2009) Effect of extraction solvent/ technique on the antioxidant activity of selected medicinal plant extracts. *Molecules (Basel, Switzerland) [Internet]* 14(6), 2167–2180. Available at: http://www.ncbi.nlm.nih.gov/pubmed/19553890

Sungirai, M., Moyo, D.Z., Clercq, P. and Madder, M. (2016) Communal farmers' perceptions of tick-borne diseases affecting cattle and investigation of tick control methods practiced in Zimbabwe. *Ticks and Tick-Borne Diseases [Internet]* 7(1), 1–9. DOI: 10.1016/j.ttbdis.2015.07.015.

Tembo, Y., Mkindi, A., Mkenda, P., Mpumi, Mwanauta, R. and Stevenson, P.C. (2018) Pesticidal plant extracts improve yield and reduce insect pests on legume crops without harming beneficial arthropods. *Frontiers in Plant Science* 9, 1425.

Thembo, K.M., Vismer, H.F., Nyazema, N.Z., Gelderblom, W.C. and Katerere, D.R. (2010) Antifungal activity of four weedy plant extracts against selected mycotoxigenic fungi. *Journal of Applied Microbiology* 109(4), 1479–1486.

Van Puyvelde, L., Geysen, D., Ayobangira, F.X., Hakizamungu, E., Nshimiyimana, A. *et al.* (1985) Screening of medicinal plants of Rwanda for acaricidal activity. *Journal of Ethnopharmacology* 13(2), 209–215.

Van Wyk, B.E. (2011) The potential of South African plants in the development of new medicinal products. *South African Journal of Botany* 77(4), 812–829.

Van Zyl, E.A., Botha, F.S., Eloff, K.J.N., Msuntsha, P.P., Oosthuizen, P.A. *et al*. (2017) The use of *lespedeza cuneata* for natural control of gastrointestinal nematodes in merino sheep. *Onderstepoort Journal of Veterinary Research* 84(1), 1–7.

Wanzala, W., Hassanali, A., Mukabana, W.R. and Takken, W. (2014) Repellent activities of essential oils of some plants used traditionally to control the brown ear tick, *Rhipicephalus appendiculatus*. *Journal of Parasitology Research* 434506, 10. DOI: 10.1155/%202014/4345061–10.

Wanzala, W., Zessin, K.H., Kyule, N.M., Baumann, M.P.O., Mathias, E. *et al*. (2005) Ethnoveterinary medicine: A critical review of its evolution, perception, understanding and the way forward. *Livestock Research for Rural Development* 17(11).

Webb, E.C. and David, M. (2002) The efficacy of neem seed extract (*Azadirachta indica*) to control tick infestation in Tswana, Simmentaler and Brahman Cattle. *South African Journal of Animal Sciences* 32(1), 1–6.

Wellington, K.W., Leboho, T., Sakong, B.M., Adenubi, O.T., Eloff, J.N. *et al*. (2017) *Further studies on South African plants: Acaricidal activity of organic plant extracts against* Rhipicephalus (Boophilus) microplus *(Acari: Ixodidae)*, Vol. 234. Veterinary Parasitology, Acari, pp. 10–12.

Willadsen, P. (2006) Tick control: Thoughts on a research agenda. *Veterinary Parasitology* 138(1–2), 161–168.

World Health Organization (2002) Programme on traditional medicine. WHO traditional medicine strategy 2002–2005. Geneva: World Health Organization. Available at: https://apps.who.int/iris/handle/10665/67163

Zorloni, A., Penzhorn, B.L. and Eloff, J.N. (2010) Extracts of *Calpurnia aurea* leaves from Southern Ethiopia attract and immobilise or kill ticks. *Veterinary Parasitology* 168(1–2), 160–164.

17 Zoonotic Diseases: A One Health Perspective

Assadullah Samadi[1]* and Nabil Hailat[2]

[1]Paraclinic Department, Faculty of Veterinary Science, Kabul University, Jamal Mina, Kabul, Kabul 1006, Afghanistan; [2]Pathology and Public Health Department, Faculty of Veterinary Medicine, Jordan University of Science and Technology (JUST), P.O. Box 3030, Irbid, Irbid 22110, Jordan

Abstract

The emergence and re-emergence of infectious diseases including zoonoses and persistence of neglected zoonotic diseases threaten the global health and economy of rural societies now more than any time in the history of humanity. Animals are the main reservoirs of zoonotic disease agents, and zoonotic pathogens are transmitted to humans by direct contacts with infected animals or indirectly through animal products and the environment. A range of factors contribute in persistence and emergence of zoonoses, and globalization, climate change, and lack of proper coordination among the governmental organization responsible for human and animal health are the key indicators. Given the shared nature of zoonotic diseases and the spread, emergence, and re-emergence of zoonotic diseases in human and animal populations, integrated One Health is the only effective approach to solve this most important health issue. In this article, different aspects of zoonotic diseases, their role in incremental poverty, and the needs for integrated activities for their control and management are reviewed and discussed in detail.

Keywords: zoonoses, poverty, One Health approach

Review Methodology

Medical and veterinary databases were searched frequently during Jan to Aug 2020 to find articles published about zoonoses and One Health approach. For this purpose, Google Scholar, PubMed, NCBI, CAB Abstracts, Scopus, and Science Citation Index databases were searched for English articles and studies without any time restriction. The keyword terms utilized were 'zoonoses/zoonotic diseases' OR 'food borne disease' OR 'emerging diseases' and then combined with 'One Health' OR 'economic impacts' OR 'poverty'. Meanwhile, we used the references from the articles obtained by this method to check for additional relevant materials about the subjects. The websites of international organizations including WHO, OIE, FAO, and CDC were also explored to review and include all relevant published reports and guidelines about zoonoses and a One Health integrated approach.

Introduction

Human and animal health and diseases and their interconnection and interaction with their environments are gaining national, regional,

*Corresponding author: assad.samadi@gmail.com

and international attention. Human and animal diseases including zoonoses are widespread and caused by different microbial agents (bacteria, chlamydia, rickettsia, fungi, viruses, prions, and parasites) (İnci *et al.*, 2018). About 75% of human infectious diseases originated from animals and their environments (Bidaisee and Macpherson, 2014; Maxwell *et al.*, 2017). It was not so long ago that infectious diseases were killing over 17 million people a year, and nearly 50,000 men, women, and children were dying every day from infectious diseases (https://www.who.int/whr/1996/media_centre/press_release/en/). Although the burden of infectious diseases has decreased in the last few years, recent data indicate that infectious diseases represented 12 million deaths (23%) in 2000 and 9.5 million deaths (17%) in 2012, of all causes of global mortality in humans (Mattar *et al.*, 2016). Of the 56.9 million deaths worldwide in 2016, more than half (54%) were from the top 10 causes, which again include infectious diseases (e.g. lower respiratory infections and tuberculosis) and these remain the top 10 leading causes of deaths worldwide. The situation of infectious disease–related deaths is worse in low- and middle-income countries (LMICs) (https://www.who.int/news-room/fact-sheets/detail/the-top-10-causes-of-death), because it has been estimated that 25% of the total annual deaths that have occurred globally are caused by pathogenic microorganisms, of which a large proportion have happened in developing countries (Asokan *et al.*, 2011). It has been estimated that 20% of human sickness and deaths are due to zoonotic diseases in the least-developed countries, and based on their impacts on animal and human health and the economy of poor rural communities, zoonotic gastrointestinal disease, zoonotic tuberculosis, rabies, leishmaniasis, brucellosis, echinococcosis, toxoplasmosis, Q fever, zoonotic trypanosomiasis, and anthrax are the most important diseases in these settings (ILRI, 2012). Globalization, urbanization, rapid communication, transportation, free trade, and fast movement of people have facilitated the spread of infectious diseases very rapidly, and the presence of new environments has facilitated the emergence and re-emergence of infectious diseases, which have added to the global health burden (Shallcross and Davies, 2014; Ahmed *et al.*, 2019). The pandemic occurrence of severe acute respiratory syndrome (SARS) in 2002–2003, which rapidly spread over the world, and many pandemics of influenza A virus subtypes, especially H1N1, are clear examples of such conditions, which facilitate rapid spread and expansion of disease to almost all continents during very limited time periods (Yang, 2020; Widdowson *et al.*, 2017). Based on the current global food chain system, the transmission of pathogens, especially antibiotic-resistant food-borne microorganisms that threaten global health, will be very fast, because about 15% of emerging infectious disease events have been associated with food-borne transmission. For example, contaminated poultry meat and eggs are the important vehicles of *Salmonella enterica* serovar enteritidis and *Campylobacter jejuni* infections for humans, which cause millions of cases and hundreds of thousands of deaths annually in the world (Foley *et al.*, 2011; Melo *et al.*, 2013; WHO FERG, 2015; Lammie and Hughes, 2016).

The current burden of zoonotic diseases issue can only be tackled by an integrated One Health approach, where all relevant sectors including public health, animal health, and environmental health professions work together in a coordinated manner for the same goal. Animal health, human health, and more broadly the ecosystem health are interdependent issues in which each element affects the others (Bonilla-Aldana *et al.*, 2020). In this scope, WHO has proposed the *Healthier Livestock and Wealthier People in a Reliable Ecosystem* slogan to all professionals to enhance the livelihood of all living organisms present in the ecosystem. In addition, WHO, OIE, and FAO have established a network named 'Global Early Warning System (GLEWS)' for combating infectious diseases, including zoonoses. This network is also linked with national stakeholders to assist in early warning, prevention, and control of animal diseases and their zoonotic threats, and the International Food Safety Authorities Network to ensure food safety (İnci *et al.*, 2018). In the meantime, attention should also be given to reverse zoonosis, where humans can act as the reservoirs and transmit the pathogens to animals; influenza A viruses, methicillin-resistant *Staphylococcus aureus*, *Mycobacterium tuberculosis*, *Helicobacter pylori*, and *Cryptosporidium parvum* are the clear examples of such zoonoses that are transmitted from infected humans to animals (Messenger *et al.*, 2014).

What Is a Zoonotic Disease?

Zoonotic infections and diseases are those transmitted from animals to humans and vice versa, or any disease transmitted between vertebrate animals and humans is known as zoonosis. But, reverse zoonoses are a specific category of diseases where humans are the primary source of infection for animals. Zoonoses are classified as food-borne, water-borne, and vector-borne and can be transmitted directly through contact with animals, or indirectly by fomites or contaminated environment (Messenger *et al.*, 2014; FAO, OIE, WHO, 2019). Zoonotic diseases, which constitute more than 60% of all known infectious diseases, are identified as a major pandemic threat by World Health Organization (Roycea and Fu, 2019). To be specific, more than 200 zoonotic diseases have been described and occur in sporadic, endemic, epidemic, and pandemic forms with different rates of morbidity and mortality among humans, domestic animals, and wildlife (İnci *et al.*, 2018). Such zoonotic pathogens cause a global human health burden of about one billion cases annually (Roycea and Fu, 2019) and the global increase in zoonotic diseases was reported as 22% in 1990–2000 and 21% in 2000–2010 (İnci *et al.*, 2018). Most of the known infectious diseases, epidemic or pandemic, occurring in human populations throughout history, including several influenza A virus pandemics, SARS, Ebola, Nipah, Hendra, rabies, CCHF and so many others have animal origin (Roycea and Fu, 2019), and it has been proposed that COVID-19, the ongoing viral pandemic, has a zoonotic nature (Bonilla-Aldana *et al.*, 2020; Contini *et al.*, 2020; Ye *et al.*, 2020). An almost old database showed that there are more than 1415 species of pathogens causing diseases in humans, of which 868 (68%) of them have zoonotic potential, and animals constitute the primary source of infection in 97% of conditions (Taylor *et al.*, 2001). Meanwhile, a great proportion of notifiable human diseases are zoonoses.

Zoonotic Disease Transmission Routes

Zoonoses are transmitted and spread by different routes. Generally, zoonotic pathogens are transmitted to humans through direct contact with domestic or wild animals or exposure to animal products, contaminated vegetables, water, and environment, or through vector bites. Loh *et al.* (Loh *et al.*, 2015) conducted a systematic literature search to identify the most important transmission routes of pathogens from animals to humans. They found the following five broad but distinct transmission pathways of zoonotic pathogens transmission from animals to humans: '(i) direct contact (skin-to-skin contact; scratches; animal bites; contact with body fluids, organs, and tissues; direct large droplet exposure); (ii) air-borne transmission (via dust particles and airborne small droplets); (iii) vector-borne (by biting or mechanical transfer by arthropods); (iv) oral transmission (consumption of contaminated food or water); and (v) contaminated environment or fomite (indirect contact with soil or vegetation, contact with water, indirect transmission by contaminated inanimate objects)'. In the meantime, an increasing trend of human population growth with a combination of economic development has resulted in an increased demand for food products of animal origin, and their process, trade, and finally consumption. This food chain also increases the pathways of zoonotic pathogen transmission and likelihood of human exposure to such agents (Häsler *et al.*, 2012).

Although Taylor *et al.* (Taylor *et al.*, 2001) stated that most of the zoonotic diseases are transmitted by vectors or indirect contact, Loh *et al.* (Loh *et al.*, 2015) found that '42% of all zoonotic pathogens were transmitted through oral transmission, 42% via vector-borne, 36% by air-borne transmission, 29% by direct contact, and 24% via contact with a contaminated environment or fomite'. In addition, they clarify that vector-borne, air-borne, and direct animal contact were the most common transmission modes of viral zoonoses, respectively. But, food-borne disease, contaminated environment, and direct contact were the most likely transmission pathways for bacterial zoonoses.

Classification of Zoonoses

Based on the epidemiology and public health and economic impacts of zoonoses, the International Livestock Research Institute (ILRI, 2012) categorized all zoonotic diseases in three main groups: endemic, epidemic, and emerging zoonoses.

- Endemic zoonoses are present in many places and affect many people and animals. It has been estimated that endemic zoonoses cause 99.9% of cases and 96% of deaths due to zoonotic diseases in human populations and have the greatest reduction in livestock production. Examples are bovine tuberculosis, brucellosis, leptospirosis, food-borne zoonoses, and cysticercosis.
- Outbreaks of epidemic zoonoses are sporadic in temporal and spatial distribution. They may be more feared because of their unpredictability and, in some cases, severity. They are often present in neglected populations with poor health services and infrastructure. Examples are Rift Valley fever, rabies, anthrax, and leishmaniasis.
- Emerging zoonoses newly appear in a population or have existed previously but are rapidly increasing in incidence or geographical range. Many of these categories occur as outbreaks. They are relatively rare, with around 300 events in the last 70 years. Historically, most of the emerging diseases have been responsible for massive impacts. Examples are high-threat and high-impact diseases such as severe acute respiratory syndrome (SARS), Nipah virus, influenza virus, Ebola, CCHF, and recently COVID-19 (Bonilla-Aldana *et al.*, 2020; Contini *et al.*, 2020; Goneau *et al.*, 2018; Nickol and Kindrachuk, 2019; Samadi *et al.*, 2021; Tiwari *et al.*, 2020).

The fourth category of zoonoses, which are termed old zoonoses, is also present. They were originally zoonotic but now spread mainly or entirely by human-to-human transmission, although some of them have animal reservoirs. Examples are HIV-AIDS, influenza, malaria, measles, dengue, and cutaneous leishmaniasis (Ready, 2010; ILRI, 2012).

Food-borne zoonoses

Among zoonotic agents, food-borne pathogens are a big health issue in both high-income and low- and middle-income countries (İnci et al., 2018). Forty percent of food-borne disease occurs in children ≤ 5 years of age, which represents 9% of the global population (WHO FERG, 2015). According to recent estimates of WHO FERG (WHO FERG, 2015), food-borne diseases caused 600 million illnesses, 420,000 deaths, and 33 million Disability-Adjusted Life Years just in 2010. Worldwide, nontyphoid *Salmonella* incidence has increased and its cases are estimated to be 94 million, with approximately 155,000 deaths (Lammie and Hughes, 2016), and just in 2010, 80 million infections and 60,000 deaths were caused by these pathogens (WHO FERG, 2015). Meantime, overuse of antibiotic in food animals has resulted in the emergence of resistant *Campylobacter* strains that can spread to humans (Lammie and Hughes, 2016), and these strains caused 95 million infections and 21,000 deaths in 2010, for which food-producing animals are the predominant source of these and so many other food-borne pathogens. These estimates do not include the human health burden of antimicrobial-resistant food-borne diseases, which might be very much higher than the recorded data (WHO FERG, 2015). Resistant *Clostridium difficile* isolate is another global concern, causing infections that are particularly difficult to treat and its emerging strains causing severe epidemic disease. About 250,000 hospitalized cases and approximately 14,000 deaths due to *C. difficile* occur in the USA annually, which costs at least $1 billion. The role of food in transmission of *C. difficile* is not well described and could be considered a priority for future research (Lammie and Hughes, 2016). All of these food-borne agents are contaminants of animal origin. Although it has been suggested that SARS-CoV-2 could probably be a food-borne infection (Tiwari *et al.*, 2020), recently, the experts in the International Commission for Microbiological Specification of Foods (ICMSF) concluded that '*it is highly unlikely that*

SARS-Cov-2 is a food safety risk' (https://www.foodsafetynews.com/2020/09/experts-affirm-that-coronavirus-is-highly-unlikely-to-be-food-risk/).

Emerging zoonoses and their risk factors and determinants

Emerging diseases are those that are caused by novel pathogens or existing pathogens that expanded their host range or geographic distribution (Mattar *et al.*, 2016). It has been estimated that 75% of emerging diseases are caused by zoonotic pathogens (Maxwell *et al.*, 2017). Different factors contributed to the wide spread of zoonotic diseases in human populations. Mattar *et al.* (Mattar *et al.*, 2016) describe six main factors facilitating the spread of emerging disease including zoonoses: 1) growth of human population and increased mobility due to such diseases as cholera and influenza A virus; 2) widespread food-borne pathogens such as *Escherichia coli* and *Salmonella enterica* through intensive agriculture and livestock farming and food production; 3) legal or illegal wildlife trade (e.g. influenza virus); 4) influence of land use and climate change on loss of biodiversity (e.g. malaria and leishmaniasis); 5) poor biosafety and biosecurity measures and unintentional or intentional release of laboratory agents (e.g. anthrax and brucellosis); and 6) poor infrastructure and leadership across public and private sectors (cholera and tuberculosis). We also think that weak and lack of proper coordination among the governmental organizations responsible for human and animal health, different priorities, lack of accountability, and sometimes responsibility could worsen and magnify the impacts of these six factors. Meanwhile, regional civil wars and poverty, modern farming practices especially in developing countries to complete the needed food resources, microbial adaptation/change, change in human lifestyle, and breakdown in public health measures are considered the most important predisposing factors that impact the emergence and worldwide distribution of zoonotic diseases (Sanyaolu *et al.*, 2016; Bao *et al.*, 2017; Maxwell *et al.*, 2017; İnci *et al.*, 2018). Interestingly, Loh *et al.* (2015) found that most of the emerging zoonotic diseases are caused by viral and bacterial pathogens; helminths, fungi, and prions constitute a very small portion of all zoonotic diseases.

As proposed, different priorities and geographical variations could also influence the emergence and re-emergence of zoonotic diseases and their control strategies. To find the most important factors contributing to the emergence and re-emergence of zoonotic diseases in India, Dhiman and Tiwari (Dhiman and Tiwari, 2018) conducted a Systematic Review. They found that occupational risk (e.g. being a veterinarian, farmer, or worker in slaughterhouses and labs, expansion of agriculture or livestock farming and the resultant disturbing of the natural ecosystem of wild animals), natural migration of wild animals, deforestation and urban expansion, travel and tourism, climate change and disaster, poverty, and political conflicts were the major factors in emerging and re-emerging of zoonoses in different parts of India. In addition, the Pan American Health Organization (PAHO) conducted a survey of priority emerging and endemic zoonoses in 33 Latin American and Caribbean (LAC) countries. It has been found that leptospirosis, rabies, and brucellosis were the three priority endemic zoonoses for the Ministries of Health (MoHs), while brucellosis, rabies, and tuberculosis were the three priority diseases for the Ministries of Agriculture (MoAgs) of these countries. Meantime, the Ebola virus disease, avian influenza, and chikungunya were considered the three priority emerging zoonoses for the MoHs, whereas avian influenza, bovine spongiform encephalopathy, and West Nile virus were priority emerging diseases for the MoAgs (Maxwell *et al.*, 2017). These examples clarify the shared nature of diseases between animal and human populations and emphasize the need for One Health integrated activities to prevent and control zoonotic diseases, because infectious diseases including zoonoses do not respect the borders and they should be considered as common threats to national, regional, and international health security (Maxwell *et al.*, 2017). Therefore, cooperative and coordinated approaches among countries in the region are required to control zoonotic and transboundary animal diseases (TADs) through shared approaches, strategies, action plans, and financial resourcing.

Animal species have also a potential role in the emergence of zoonotic diseases. Many factors such as the prevalence of particular microorganisms within a given animal population, the number of microorganisms in a species, the number of host species shared by the same microorganism, and the frequency of contact within animal species and with humans are considered influential in this regard. Among domestic animals, poultry and pigs play the key role in emergence of new zoonotic diseases. Although the number of people working with these animals and exposure rates of human are much lower than other species (e.g. companion animals), keeping large number of animals with high turnover rates facilitates continuous circulation, genetic material transmission, and reassortment of new strains, and as consequence, the emergence of new virulent pathogens with high host range (Häsler *et al.*, 2012).

The number of households keeping companion animals has increased in developed and even in developing countries and it is considered a health threat for companion animal-borne zoonoses in these settings. This type of animal ownership increases close contact with carriers and reservoirs of zoonotic pathogens, which may lead to increased risk of zoonosis outbreaks in human populations (Takahashi-Omoe and Omoe, 2012).

It has been shown that the most important and dangerous zoonotic diseases have important wildlife reservoirs. These include gastro-intestinal zoonoses, leptospirosis, anthrax, Q fever, psittacosis, leishmaniasis, toxoplasmosis, echinococcosis, trypanosomiasis, rabies, Chagas, chikungunya, Ebola, Hanta disease, avian influenza, and Rift Valley fever (ILRI, 2012). Among wild animals, nonhuman primates, rodents, and bats are considered the main reservoirs of zoonotic pathogens and potential sources of new zoonotic disease agents; leptospirosis, plague, typhus, SARS, lyssaviruses, Ebola, Hendra, and Nipah viruses (Häsler *et al.*, 2012) and now COVID-19 (Contini *et al.*, 2020; Tiwari *et al.*, 2020) are just a few to name.

It has been concluded that behavioral changes in humans and increased interaction of humans with domestic animals and wildlife, mainly due to urbanization, which facilitates increased movement of people and animals and their products, accelerating human travel and global trade are linked to the emergence of new zoonoses and spread of such diseases in areas previously considered free of diseases (Ahmed *et al.*, 2019; Roycea and Fu, 2019). Based on the mentioned transmission pathways, farmers, livestock handlers, abattoir workers, butchers, shearers, hunters, knackery workers, veterinarians, and health facility staff are considered high-risk occupational groups for contracting zoonotic diseases (Sharifi-Mood *et al.*, 2014; Champour *et al.*, 2016; Morwal and Sharma, 2017; Moradi *et al.*, 2019).

Historical Perspective of One Health Approach in Human and Animal Medicines

Domestication of animals facilitates close contact of animals and their products with humans and enables the transmission of diseases, mainly from animals to humans. Ancient medical practitioners including Egyptian, Chinese, and Indian healers often diagnosed and treated the diseases in animals and humans simultaneously through anatomical and pathological skills from slaughtering sacrificial animals. Typically, they were specialized in certain problem or treatment types, for example bonesetters and herbalists, respectively. Veterinary medicine as a distinct discipline established during the Zhou Dynasty in China (11–13th century), which had one of the earliest integrated public health system organized by medical doctors and veterinarians. An ancient Chinese text states that '*The foundations of veterinary medicine are as comprehensive and subtle as those of human medicine and it is not possible to place one above the other*' (Thrusfield, 2007; Zinsstag *et al.*, 2011; Mersha and Tewodros, 2012).

The concept of epidemiologic triangle that human health is influenced by animal health and the environment is relatively new, but the One Health concept has been recognized since 1800s. Hippocrates' ideas about how public health is connected to the environment are the earliest written evidence of what we now call One Health, a concept apparent even in ancient times. As veterinary medicine and education continue progressing into the future, and embrace this interdisciplinary approach, it's exciting to trace the history of veterinary medicine back to the roots of civilization (Narins, 2003). In addition, the 224 and 225 Codes of Hammurabi (1795–1750 BC) also indicate the shared nature of human and veterinary medicines (Halwani and Takrouri, 2006).

Later in nineteenth and twentieth centuries, researchers embraced the concept that human and animal health is inextricably linked (Kahn *et al.*, 2008; Mattar *et al.*, 2016). Although the term 'zoonosis' was coined by Virchow in 1880s, which facilitated meat inspections by veterinarians in Europe and eventually in the USA, it was William Osler, the student of Virchow in nineteenth century and finally Dr Calvin W. Schwabe, a veterinary epidemiologist, who invented and introduced the term 'One Medicine' in 1960s, which integrated medical and veterinary approaches against zoonotic disease. Rudolf Virchow said '... *between animal and human medicine there are no dividing lines—nor should there be*'. Later in 1959, zoonoses were defined by WHO as '*those diseases and infections which are naturally transmitted between vertebrate animals and man*'. Subsequently, the concept of 'One Medicine' changed to 'One Health' to consider a broader approach to health and well-being of societies. It argued that there is no difference between the principles of human and veterinary medicine and both can jointly work for the development of each other (Kahn *et al.*, 2008; Zinsstag *et al.*, 2011; Lammie and Hughes, 2016; Morwal and Sharma, 2017; Bonilla-Aldana *et al.*, 2020).

One Health has been described as the collaborative effort of multiple health sector professions to obtain optimal health for people, domestic animals, wildlife, plants, and the environment (Yang, 2020), or the approach where multiple sectors including human, veterinary, and environmental health discipline authorities design and implement programs, policies, legislations, and researches to achieve better health outcomes (McEwen and Collignon, 2018; Collignon and McEwen, 2019; Kamenshchikova *et al.*, 2019). International organizations such WHO, the OIE, and Food and Agriculture Organization (FAO) of United Nations identified the One Health approach as an accepted method in combating zoonotic pathogens and antimicrobial resistance, because conventional separated sector activities are not able to tackle these global threat emergencies effectively (Zinsstag *et al.*, 2011).

Collaborative Education and Research in Human and Animal Medicines

Human and veterinary medicines share many commonalities in principle disciplines including physiology, anatomy, pathology, and ecology and pathogeneses of infectious diseases (especially zoonosis), diagnostic methodologies, treatment and preventive measures (Zinsstag *et al.*, 2011; Mersha and Tewodros, 2012). One of the shared areas where veterinary and medical researchers can work collaboratively with each other is comparative medicine. This field, which exemplified the One Medicine concept, involves the study of interactions between pathogenic microorganisms and hosts in infectious diseases' (especially zoonosis) pathogenesis. Successful examples are the team work of a physician and veterinarian, Theobald Smith and F. L. Kilbourne, respectively, in the discovery of arthropod (tick) transmission of *Babesia bigemina*; and the discovery of immune system function in distinguishing normal cells from virus-infected cells by Rolf Zinkernagel and Peter C. Doherty, a physician and veterinarian, respectively, who received the Nobel Prize in 1996 (Kahn *et al.*, 2008). Additionally, veterinary services have many other responsibilities for human health, including preventing and controlling emerging zoonotic diseases and protecting the environment and ecosystems (Thrusfield, 2007). Meanwhile, different animal species are used as models to study human diseases, of which feline immunodeficiency virus 'FIV' is a clear example in the development of a vaccine against human immunodeficiency virus 'HIV' (Mazzetti *et al.*, 1999; Yamamoto *et al.*, 2010; Scherk, 2013).

Historically, the collaborations between veterinary and human health professionals at different levels including education and research activities were very pronounced in late nineteenth and early twentieth centuries, but this collaboration declined in late twentieth century (Kahn *et al.*, 2008). Emerging and re-emerging of deadly zoonotic diseases, especially Rift Valley fever, Dengue fever, Ebola hemorrhagic fever, Nipah virus, human acquired immunodeficiency virus, West Nile virus, severe acute respiratory syndrome, different subtypes of influenza A virus, rabies, new cholera strain O:139, brucellosis, the ongoing COVID-19 pandemic, and emergence of antimicrobial resistance, enforced these professions to renew and increase their collaborations and use a One Health approach to combating these problems (Kahn *et al.*, 2008; Samadi *et al.*, 2010; Sachan and Singh, 2010; Lavan *et al.*, 2017; Hailat *et al.*, 2018; Matar *et al.*, 2019; Bagheri *et al.*, 2020; Chen *et al.*, 2020; Contini *et al.*, 2020). Additionally, it has been identified that collaborations between medical and veterinary schools remain limited, which raises the problem of control of zoonotic diseases. It has been shown that medical schools do not emphasize zoonotic disease ecology in comparison to veterinary medicine schools, so collaborative efforts by veterinarians and medical doctors are the only approach in combating against zoonotic diseases including public awareness campaigns (Kahn *et al.*, 2008).

Based on the points mentioned, One Health is an accepted strategy to control zoonoses and related health issues through coordinated collaboration and communication within, between, and among all sectors that take care of human, animal, and environmental health at national, regional, and international levels (Asokan *et al.*, 2011). This could be achieved through introducing new codes and regulations to ensure proper collaboration, and synergizing and synchronizing resources for the same goal.

The Burden of Zoonotic Diseases

It is obvious that zoonoses have high impacts on human health, livelihoods, animal health, and production and ecosystem (ILRI, 2012), and the economic burden of zoonoses is severe, especially in LMICs that include trade restriction, loss of market due to decreased consumer confidence, cost of control programs, and compensation to the farmers (Sachan and Singh, 2010; Asokan *et al.*, 2011). To mention the historic reality, early developments of veterinary medicine as an independent discipline were governed largely by economic motives, associated with the importance of domestic animals as a source of food, working and transport animals, and still the economic reasons are critical drivers in combating against diseases in animal populations (Thrusfield, 2007); even in human medicine, development of medicines, vaccines, diagnostic tools, and other related items are largely due to economic benefits.

Zoonoses could be considered one of the key factors in poverty increment. Poverty is identified as a pronounced deprivation of well-being, and factors contributing to the situation vary in different populations. The people whose incomes are <\$1.25 per day are considered poor, of which most of them are living in Asia and Africa (ILRI, 2012). Occurrence of infectious diseases including zoonoses has high socio-economic impacts on any nation, but the burden of such impacts is much more severe in poor and marginalized populations (Molyneux *et al.*, 2011; Seimenis, 2012). It has been estimated that around 70% of the rural poor and 10% of the urban poor, who constitute about 1 billion people, are livestock dependent. India, Nigeria, Ethiopia, and Bangladesh have 44% of the worlds' poor livestock keepers, and livestock provide 6–36% of protein intake in poor countries. These communities are deprived of health care, education, communication, and political process, which exacerbate the problem of public awareness and health service delivery in these populations (Molyneux *et al.*, 2011; ILRI, 2012). Animal diseases can worsen their economic situation and increase poverty. A very good example is bovine brucellosis, which poses not only a significant threat to human health due to its zoonotic nature but also can cause a huge economic constraint for livestock-dependent rural societies through abortion, infertility, calf death, carpal hygromas, and a 20% reduction in milk yield in affected cattle populations (Makita *et al.*, 2011).

It has been shown that poor livestock production practices are the main reasons for zoonoses significantly impacting the livelihood of people in Africa (Bidaisee and Macpherson, 2014). Zoonotic diseases have very severe devastating impact on the already weakened economic conditions of developing countries and are considered one of the predisposing factors in poverty. It has been estimated that the direct and indirect global economic losses of zoonotic diseases in the last decade were $200 and $20 billion, respectively (İnci *et al.*, 2018). Meanwhile, estimation showed that an outbreak of bovine encephalopathy can cost about $6.3 billion annually, and totally food-borne zoonotic disease costs about $1.3 billion annually (Sanyaolu *et al.*, 2016). To consider just the total economic losses due to rabies (a well-known endemic zoonosis in most LMICs) in human and animal populations as an example, it has been estimated that the total annual global cost of human deaths from canine rabies, post-exposure vaccination, diagnostic testing, dog vaccination, and livestock losses is in the tens of billions of dollars (Shwiff *et al.*, 2013), and most of the rabies cases are in third-world countries with low income. A recent USDA estimate shows that global economic losses due to canine rabies and its related conditions in most endemic regions (Asia, Africa, and Latin America) could be approximately $124 billion per year (Lavan *et al.*, 2017). Another example is zoonotic tuberculosis due to *Mycobacterium bovis*, which has a high impact on human health, food safety, food security, international trade, and huge economic loses for farmers and rural families (Bennett, 2009; Butler *et al.*, 2010; Kwaghe and Ameh, 2015; Samadi, 2016).

To conclude, a strong association between poverty, hunger, livestock keeping, and zoonoses exist. So, the most important zoonotic diseases that have high health and socioeconomic impacts on poor livestock keepers are zoonotic gastrointestinal diseases, leptospirosis, cysticercosis, zoonotic tuberculosis, rabies, leishmaniasis, brucellosis, echinococcosis, toxoplasmosis, Q fever, zoonotic trypanosomiasis, hepatitis E, and anthrax, respectively. These diseases are causing millions of cases and deaths in humans each year (ILRI, 2012). While those human populations that are dependent on livestock are at increased risk of zoonotic diseases, animal production decrease and food security due to zoonotic pathogens exacerbate the poverty cycle in these settings (Molyneux *et al.*, 2011).

The Needs for One Health Approach in Zoonotic Diseases Battle

Zoonoses are continuous health threats to human and animal populations, and in order to control and decrease the global burden of infectious diseases especially those with a potential zoonotic nature, an integrated One Health approach involving the human health, veterinary, agricultural, educational, wildlife and environment, and sanitation sectors is needed (Sachan and Singh, 2010; Asokan *et al.*, 2011; Mattar *et al.*, 2016; Sanyaolu *et al.*, 2016). But coordinating the activities of these multifaceted sectors in response to zoonoses is still a challenging issue especially in LMICs (Molyneux *et al.*, 2011), because approaching any issue from a One Health perspective necessitates looking at the interactions of people, domestic animals, wildlife, plants, and our environment (Matar *et al.*, 2019).

Although a One Health approach framework has been introduced and adopted by WHO, OIE, and FAO and other international organization in 2007, real cooperation had been started in 2008 combating avian influenza. This strategy is now increasingly applied in many health issues such as antimicrobial resistance (AMR), food safety, and zoonoses (Kamenshchikova *et al.*, 2019). So in order to implement this venue efficiently, increased One Health instruction, integrated training, and increased venues of discussions are needed among veterinarians, physicians, and other health professionals, which facilitate improved communication between those treating members of the same household (Lammie and Hughes, 2016).

The integrated One Health approach in the surveillance of zoonotic diseases between human and veterinary medicines in most developing countries has not established yet, where diagnostic capacity and health infrastructure are also not sufficient (İnci *et al.*, 2018). It has been shown that applying One Health approach in zoonotic disease control and eradication is much more effective and provides long term cost savings than those attained by either group working alone. This practice was useful in canine rabies eradication in Texas, where public health and veterinary health professionals worked together in a coordinated manner in an oral rabies vaccination program (Shwiff *et al.*, 2013). It is worth mentioning that community engagement and increased public education, which are neglected in developing countries, are required for successful infectious diseases control programs (Berrian *et al.*, 2018).

The cost–benefit analysis would be more valuable when considering a One Health approach in combating zoonoses. One of the clear advantages of this approach in response to zoonoses is that interventions in one sector can result in health and socioeconomic benefits more efficiently than just doing so in any sector alone. For example, mass vaccination of domestic dog reservoirs can prevent cost-effectively the human rabies cases that place a significant burden on health budgets. Another example is the control and prevention of human brucellosis, a bacterial disease, through animal vaccinations with Rev-1, S19, and RB51 vaccines of sheep, goats, and cattle enforced by some governmental authorities (Molyneux *et al.*, 2011; Takahashi-Omoe and Omoe, 2012; Hailat *et al.*, 2018; Bagheri *et al.*, 2020). In addition, mass chemotherapy treatment of the cattle reservoir and insecticidal treatment to control tsetse populations were very effective in the control of sleeping sickness caused by *Trypanosoma rhodesiense*, which also reduces tick populations (Molyneux *et al.*, 2011). In the meantime, investment in laboratory infrastructures and enhancing diagnostic capacity in human health or animal health sectors can jointly be used in any sectors without the need to spend large amount of money and human resources in both sectors.

International Movement and Tripartite (FAO/OIE/WHO) Initiative

Responses to issues such as food safety, zoonoses, and antimicrobial resistance, which have shared nature in animal-human-environmental interface, need collaborative efforts of all related sectors at different levels. To tackle these One Health–related issues, different networks have been established nationally, regionally, and globally. The International Food SafetyAuthorities Network (INFOSAN) is one such network that has been launched in 2004 at global level, consisting of more than 600 members from a broad range of relevant sectors including human-animal-environmental health, tourism, trade, and industry, jointly managed by FAO and WHO. The main goal of INFOSAN is to prevent food-borne diseases and strength food safety systems globally through a One Health approach. Then, the collaborative Tripartite Concept Note of FAO, OIE, and WHO addressing risks at human-animal-ecosystems and focusing mainly on multisectoral collaboration was formally declared in 2010 and was further reiterated in 2017. In 2011, the Tripartite determined three main topics including antimicrobial resistance, rabies, and zoonotic influenza to indicate the effective collaboration in all relevant sectors. Since then, considerable efforts and results have been achieved in antimicrobial resistance surveillance and management (e.g. publish global action plan on AMR surveillance system (GLASS) in 2015), zoonotic influenza outbreak detection (from months to days and even hours) and rabies control, and prevention and elimination (e.g. Global Conference in December 2015 and World Rabies Day, 2016), in animal and human populations. In addition, WHO, OIE, and FAO developed *Zoonotic diseases: a guide to establishing collaboration between animal and human health sectors at the country level* in 2008 which further developed to *Taking a multisectoral One Health approach: a tripartite guide to addressing zoonotic diseases in countries* in 2019 (FAO, OIE and WHO, October 2017; FAO, OIE, WHO, 2019; Gongal *et al.*, 2020). To consider a sustainable multisectoral One Health approach in effective implementation of zoonotic disease control activities, the following points have been prioritized by FAO, OIE, and WHO (FAO, OIE, WHO, 2019): (i) high level political will and commitment, (ii) sufficient financial domestic resources, (iii) designing programs based on national infrastructure and circumstances, (iv) common goals, (v) strong national governance, (vi) effective routine coordination and communication, and (vii) evidence-based improved outcome. Besides zoonoses, AMR threatens the health of human and animal populations more than at any time, and it has been stated by Thakur and Gray (Thakur and Gray, 2019) that '*surveillance must become a global 'One Health' effort if we are to solve one of today's most significant threats to human, animal, and environmental health*' which is AMR. At the present time, more than 700,000 people die of resistant infections every year, and it has been estimated that 10 million lives a year and a cumulative of 100 trillion USD of economic output are at risk due to the rise of drug-resistant infections by 2050 (O'Neill, 2016; Queenan *et al.*, 2016; AMF, 2017).

Discussion

As stated, emerging and re-emerging infectious diseases including zoonoses threaten global health now more than at any time in the history of humanity. As is obvious, all living organisms including humans and animals are part of a larger ecosystem where activities and conditions of each member affect the others. This condition necessitates all sectors including human, animal, and environmental health professionals to work together for better health of each member of our continent. These interconnected activities are assessed under the umbrella of the One Health approach (Mersha and Tewodros, 2012), the only strategy that can tackle today's most challenging health issues including zoonoses.

Although neglected zoonotic diseases cause a severe health and socioeconomic burden mainly in LMICs (Munyua *et al.*, 2016), emerging zoonoses can cause widespread epidemic or pandemic diseases in different human and animal populations, which are of great concern. Endemic zoonoses such as rabies, brucellosis, tuberculosis, and so many others have a greater socioeconomic effect mainly in LMIC where public health services are already weakened (Maxwell *et al.*, 2017). Generally speaking, due to insufficient laboratory infrastructure, misdiagnosis,and low awareness among health professionals and public, and underreporting, the real situation of most zoonotic diseases is not known in most LMICs (Sachan and Singh, 2010). For example, the emergence of Rift Valley fever (RVF) in Kenya in 2006–2007 was well characterized and its economic loses were estimated at US$32 million, but other neglected endemic zoonoses like rabies and anthrax with great socioeconomic impacts were largely undetermined (Munyua *et al.*, 2016). In addition, rabies, a prevalent endemic zoonotic disease mostly in LMICs, causes more than 55,000 deaths per year, with 99% of them occurring in Asia and Africa. It has been estimated that 3,529,000 and 802,100 animal bites per year occurred in Asia and Africa, respectively, mostly from dogs which account for more than 99% of all human cases worldwide (Lavan *et al.*, 2017). In India alone, 15 million people are bitten by animals and about 30,000 people die of rabies every year (Kumar *et al.*, 2015). These factors indicate the burden of neglected zoonotic diseases, mostly in poor societies where the health and economic situations are already weakened.

Although a wide range of infectious agents including viruses, prions, bacteria, fungi, and helminthes can cause emerging zoonoses, given their ability to exchange genetic information and change gene expression in response to environmental factors, viruses and bacteria are at the top of the list for the emerging zoonotic diseases burden worldwide (Häsler *et al.*, 2012). Among two mentioned agents, RNA viruses, due to their high mutation rates, and drug-resistant bacterial strains are more likely to cause emerging zoonoses (Häsler *et al.*, 2012). Just to review the epidemics or pandemics of zoonoses in the history, several influenza A virus subtypes, SARS, Ebola, Nipah, Hendra, rabies, CCHF (Roycea and Fu, 2019), and COVID-19 (Ye *et al.*, 2020; Tiwari *et al.*, 2020) are all viral agents, and most importantly they have animal origin.

The threat of zoonotic diseases is almost the same for human and animals, but the ways and aims combating this threat in human and animal sectors may vary. The human health sector focuses more on maximizing healthy lives and well-being, but animal health sector especially regarding food-producing animals may focus more on food production and economic concern, although for companion animals, it may have the same goals as human health (Kamenshchikova *et al.*, 2019). Lack of joint preparation and integrated activities in zoonotic disease events and emergencies or endemic conditions can result in confusion and delay responses and can lead to poorer health outcomes or obstruct and complicate the implementation of effective disease control programs. So, effective collaboration under the umbrella of One Health among the animal health, public health, and environment sectors is essential to tackle zoonotic diseases issues (FAO, OIE, WHO, 2019). For example, rabies is endemic in Indonesia and 99% of bite cases were reported and managed by the human health system. Due to the zoonotic nature of diseases, they have started an integrated bite case management (IBCM) involving four ministries (Public Health, Agriculture, Environment and Forestry, and Human Development and Cultural Affairs) and conducted training on a One Health approach in this regard. Integrated bite case management reports increased from 1% before training to 44% posttraining (74), which cost-effectively manages the cases and reduces the burden of disease in animal and human populations. This highlights the role of One Health approach tackling complex health issues such as zoonoses.

The other issue, which can misguide the proper detection and control of zoonoses, is the lack of efficient surveillance systems in many countries. Unfortunately, most of the zoonotic disease surveillance and control programs have a reactive nature, tackling diseases after they have already emerged. However, an important approach is to discover potential zoonoses in a proactive manner mostly in wildlife, the main reservoir and carrier of a wide range of zoonotic pathogens in nature (Loh *et al.*, 2015). (Meslin, 2010) proposed a biphasic approach to respond to zoonoses outbreak: (1) a short- to intermediate-term response to detect cases and outbreaks of diseases, and (2) a long-term response to study the ecology of zoonotic pathogens comprehensively. Generally, they propose vaccination, prophylactic use of antiparasitic drugs (e.g. antitrypanosomals or coccidiostats), application of biosecurity measures and quarantine, eradication programs for specific diseases, and herd health programs and enhanced disease surveillance as practical methods in response to zoonoses. As mentioned, most endemic zoonoses affect marginalized poor communities, so increased awareness and empowerment of rural families and communities to participate in zoonoses control and even eradication programs will be a cost-effective strategy in this regard (Molyneux *et al.*, 2011).

Conclusion

Zoonotic diseases pose continuous health threats to human and animal populations. Given their shared nature, separated activities to tackle this global health threat are not effective, and need to be corrected towards a One Health approach. Although not functionalized in most LMICs, integrated One Health involving human medicine, veterinary medicine, and the environmental profession is the only approach to effectively solve today's most critical health burden globally. This needs to be coupled with enhancing and revising our educational systems, policy making, and improving governance and regulations in all sectors involved.

References

Ahmed, S., Dávila, J.D., Allen, A., Haklay, M., Tacoli, C. *et al.* (2019) Does urbanization make emergence of zoonosis more likely? Evidence, myths and gaps. *Environment and Urbanization* 31(2), 443–460.

AMF (2017) Antimicrobial resistance benchmark 2018, Methodology report. Amsterdam, The Netherlands: Access to Medicine Foundation.

Asokan, G.V., Asokan, V. and Tharyan, P. (2011) One health national programme across species on zoonoses: A call to the developing world. *Infection Ecology and Epidemiology* 1, 8293. DOI: 10.3402/iee.v1i0.8293.

Bagheri, N.R., Krecek, R.C., Khalaf, O.H., Hailat, N. and Arenas-Gamboa, A.M. (2020) Brucellosis in the Middle East: Current situation and a pathway forward. *PLoS Neglected Tropical Diseases* 14(5), e0008071.

Bao, M., Pierce, G.J., Pascual, S., González-Muñoz, M., Mattiucci, S. *et al.* (2017) Assessing the risk of an emerging zoonosis of worldwide concern: Anisakiasis. *Scientific Reports* 7, 43699. DOI: 10.1038/srep43699.

Bennett, R.M. (2009) Farm costs associated with premovement testing for bovine tuberculosis. *Veterinary Record* 164, 77–79.

Berrian, A.M., Smith, M.H., Rooyen, J., Martínez-Lópeze, B., Plank, M.N. *et al*. (2018) A community-based One Health education program for disease risk mitigation at the human-animal interface. *One Health* 5, 9–20.

Bidaisee, S. and Macpherson, C.N.L. (2014) Zoonoses and One Health: A review of the literature, review article. *Journal of Parasitology Research, Hindawi Publishing Corporation* Article ID 874345(8). DOI: 10.1155/2014/874345.

Bonilla-Aldana, D.K., Dhama, K. and Rodriguez-Morales, A.J. (2020) Revisiting the One Health approach in the context of COVID-19: A look into the ecology of this emerging disease. *Advances in Animal and Veterinary Sciences* 8(3), 234–237.

Butler, A., Lobley, M. and Winter, M. (2010). Exeter: CRPR Research Paper. Available at: www.centres.ex.ac.uk/crpr/publications/

Champour, M., Chinikar, S., Mohammadi, G., Razmi, G., Mostafavi, E. *et al*. (2016) Crimean-congo hemorrhagic fever in the one-humped camel (*Camelus dromedarius*) in East and Northeast of Iran. *Journal of Arthropod-Borne Diseases* 10(2), 168–177.

Chen, N., Zhou, M., Dong, X., Qu, J., Gong, F. *et al*. (2020) Epidemiological and clinical characteristics of 99 cases of 2019 novel coronavirus pneumonia in Wuhan, China: a descriptive study. Available at: www.thelancet.com

Collignon, P.J. and McEwen, S.A. (2019) One health—its importance in helping to better control antimicrobial resistance. *Tropical Medicine and Infectious Disease* 4(22), 1–22. DOI: 10.3390/tropicalmed4010022.

Contini, C., Nuzzo, D.M., Barp, N., Bonazza, A., Giorgio, D.R. *et al*. (2020) The novel zoonotic COVID-19 pandemic: an expected global health concern. *Journal of Infection in Developing Countries* 14(3), 254–264.

Dhiman, R.C. and Tiwari, A. (2018) Emergence of zoonotic diseases in India: A systematic review. *Medical Reports and Case Studies* 3, 163. DOI: 10.4172/2572-5130.1000163.

FAO, OIE and WHO (October 2017) The Tripartite's commitment providing multi-sectoral, collaborative leadership in addressing health challenges. Available at: www.who.int›zoonoses›tripartite_oct2017

FAO, OIE, WHO (2019) In: *Taking A Multisectoral, One Health Approach: A Tripartite Guide to Addressing Zoonotic Diseases in Countries*. World Health Organization (WHO), Food and Agriculture Organization of the United Nations (FAO) and World Organisation for Animal Health (OIE), Geneva, Switzerland, pp. 978–992. 978-92-4-151493-4 (WHO) 978-92-5-131236-0 (FAO) 978-92-9-511504-0 (OIE)

Foley, L.S., Nayak, R., Hanning, B.I., Johnson, J.T., Han, J. *et al*. (2011) Population dynamics of *Salmonella enterica* serotypes in commercial egg and poultry production. *Applied and Environmental Microbiology* 77(13), 4273–4279.

Goneau, L.W., Mehta, K., Wong, J., L'Huillier, A.G. and Gubbay, J.B. (2018) Zoonotic influenza and human health—Part 1: Virology and epidemiology of zoonotic influenzas. *Current Infectious Disease Reports* 20, 37. DOI: 10.1007/s11908-018-0642-9.

Gongal, G., Ofrin, R.H., Balogh, K.D., Oh, Y., Kugita, H. *et al*. (2020) Operationalization of One Health and tripartite collaboration in the Asia-Pacific region. *WHO South-East Asia Journal of Public Health* 9(1), 21–25.

Hailat, N., Khlouf, S., Ababneh, M. and Brown, C. (2018) Pathological, immunological and molecular diagnosis of abortions in small ruminants in Jordan with reference to *Chlamydia abortus* and *Brucella melitensis*. *Pakistan Veterinary Journal* 38(1), 109–112.

Halwani, T. and Takrouri, M. (2006) Medical laws and ethics of Babylon as read in Hammurabi's code (History). *The Internet Journal of Law, Healthcare and Ethics* 4(2), 1–8.

Häsler, B., Gilbert, W., Jones, B.A., Pfeiffer, D.U., Rushton, J. *et al*. (2012) The economic value of One Health in relation to the mitigation of zoonotic disease risks. In: *Current Topics in Microbiology and Immunology*. Springer-Verlag, Berlin Heidelberg. DOI: 10.1007/82_2012_239.

ILRI (2012) *Mapping of poverty and likely zoonoses hotspots zoonoses, Project 4, Report to Department for International Development, UK*. International Livestock Research Institute, UK, p. 119.

İnci, A., Doğanay, M., Ozdarendeli, A., Duzlu, O. and Yıldırım, A. (2018) Overview of zoonotic diseases in Turkey: The One Health concept and future threats. *Türkiye Parazitolojii Dergisi* 42, 39–80.

Kahn, H.L., Kaplan, B., Monath, P.T. and Steele, H.J. (2008) Teaching "one medicine, one health." *The American Journal of Medicine* 121(3), 169–170.

Kamenshchikova, A., Wolffs, P.F.G., Hoebe, C. and Horstman, K. (2019) *Anthropocentric framings of One Health: An analysis of international antimicrobial resistance policy documents. Critical Public Health*. Taylor & Francis, UK. DOI: 10.1080/09581596.2019.1684442.

Kumar, R., Singh, S.P. and Savalia, C.V. (2015) Overview of emerging zoonoses in India: Areas of concern. *International Journal of Tropical Diseases* 3, 165. DOI: 10.4172/2329891X.1000165.

Kwaghe, A.V. and Ameh, A.J. (2015) Prevalence and economic losses from bovine tuberculosis in Maiduguri, Borno State, Nigeria. *International Journal of Life Sciences* 4(4), 283–287.

Lammie, L.S. and Hughes, M.J. (2016) Antimicrobial resistance, food safety, and One Health: The need for convergence. *Annual Review of Food Science and Technology* 7, 287–312.

Lavan, P.R., King, A.I., Mac, G., Sutton, J.D. and Tunceli, K. (2017) Rationale and support for a One Health program for canine vaccination as the most cost-effective means of controlling zoonotic rabies in endemic settings. *Vaccine* 35, 1668–1674.

Loh, E.H., Zambrana-Torrelio, C., Olival, K.J., Bogich, T.L., Johnson, C.K. *et al.* (2015) Targeting transmission pathways for emerging zoonotic disease surveillance and control. *Vector Borne and Zoonotic Diseases* 15(7), 432–437.

Makita, K., Fèvre, E.M., Waiswa, C., Eisler, M.C., Thrusfield, M. *et al.* (2011) Welburn SC. Herd prevalence of bovine brucellosis and analysis of risk factors in cattle in urban and peri-urban areas of the Kampala economic zone, Uganda. *BMC Veterinary Research* 7(60), 1–8.

Matar, G.M., Andremont, A. and Bazzi, W. (2019) Editorial: combating antimicrobial resistance - a one health approach. *Frontiers in Cellular and Infection Microbiology* 9, 458. DOI: 10.3389/fcimb.2019.00458.

Mattar, C., Ore, A.S., Fagerberg, S.K. *et al.* (2016) One Health and antimicrobial resistance. *World Medical Journal* 108–111.

Maxwell, M.J., Carvalho, M.H., Hoet, A.E., Vigilato, M.A.N., Pompei, J.C. *et al.* (2017) Building the road to a regional zoonoses strategy: A survey of zoonoses programmes in the Americas. *PLoS One* 12(3), e0174175. DOI: 10.1371.journal.pone.0174175.

Mazzetti, P., Giannecchini, S., Mauro, D.D. *et al.* (1999) AIDS vaccination studies using an ex vivo feline immunodeficiency virus model: Detailed analysis of the humoral immune response to a protective vaccine. *Journal of Virology* 73(1), 1–10.

McEwen, S.A. and Collignon, P.J. (2018) Antimicrobial resistance: A one health perspective. *Microbiology Spectrum* 6(2), 0009–2017. DOI: 10.1128/microbiolspec.ARBA-0009-2017.

Melo, R.T., Nalevaiko, P.C., Mendonça, E.P. *et al.* (2013) *Campylobacter jejuni* strains isolated from chicken meat harbor several virulence factors and represent a potential risk to humans. *Food Control* 33.

Mersha, C. and Tewodros, F. (2012) One health one medicine one world: Co-joint of animal and human medicine with perspectives, a review. *Veterinary World* 5(4), 238–243.

Meslin, F.X. (2010) Public health impact of zoonoses and international approaches for their detection and containment. *Veterinaria Italiana* 44(4), 583–590.

Messenger, A.M., Barnes, A.N. and Gray, G.C. (2014) Reverse zoonotic disease transmission (*Zooanthroponosis*): A systematic review of seldom-documented human biological threats to animals. *PLoS One* 9(2), e89055. DOI: 10.1371/journal.pone.0089055.

Molyneux, D., Hallaj, Z., Keusch, G.T., McManus, D.P., Ngowi, H. *et al.* (2011) Zoonoses and marginalised infectious diseases of poverty: Where do we stand. *Parasites & Vectors* 4, 106.

Moradi, G., Piroozi, B., Alinia, C., Safari, H., Nabavi, M. *et al.* (2019) Incidence, mortality, and burden of Crimean Congo hemorrhagic fever and its geographical distribution in Iran during 2009-2015. *Iranian Journal of Public Health* 48(1), 44–52.

Morwal, S. and Sharma, S.K. (2017) Bacterial zoonosis - A public health importance. *Journal of Dairy, Veterinary & Animal Research* 5(2), 56–59. DOI: 10.15406/jdvar.2017.05.00135.

Munyua, P., Bitek, A., Osoro, E., Pieracci, E.G., Muema, J. *et al.* (2016) Prioritization of zoonotic diseases in Kenya, 2015. *PLoS One* 11(8), e0161576. DOI: 10.1371/journal.pone.0161576.

Narins, B. (2003) World of microbiology and immunology. In: *And 2 A-Z*, Vol. Volumes 1. Gale, USA. 0-7876-6540-1

Nickol, E.M. and Kindrachuk, J. (2019) A year of terror and a century of reflection: Perspectives on the great influenza pandemic of 1918–1919. *BMC Infectious Diseases* 19, 117.

O'Neill, J. (2016) *Tackling drug-resistant infections globally: Final report and recommendations, the review on Antimicrobial resistance*. Welcome Trust, UK.

Queenan, K., Häsler, B. and Rushton, J. (2016) A One Health approach to antimicrobial resistance surveillance: Is there a business case for it. *International Journal of Antimicrobial Agents*. DOI: 10.1016/j.ijantimicag.2016.06.014.

Ready, P.D. (2010) Leishmaniasis emergence in Europe. *Eurosurveillance* 15(10), pii=19505. DOI: 10.2807/ese.15.10.19505-en.

Roycea, P.K. and Fu, F. (2019) Mathematically modeling spillover dynamics of emerging zoonoses with intermediate hosts. *Journal of Theoretical Biology*.

Samadi, A. (2016) The effects of bovine tuberculosis on socio-economic situation of farmers in developing countries. *Scientific Research Journal of Kabul University* 4, 195–202.

Sachan, N. and Singh, V.P. (2010) Effect of climatic changes on the prevalence of zoonotic diseases. *Veterinary World* 3(11), 519–522.

Samadi, A., Ababneh, M.M.K., Giadinis, N.D. and Lafi, S.Q. (2010) Ovine and caprine brucellosis (*Brucella melitensis*). *CAB Reviews: Perspectives in Agriculture, Veterinary Science, Nutrition and Natural Resources* 5(42).

Samadi, A., Esmati, A.B., Ababneh, M.M.K., Amiri, M. and Ahmadi, M.S. (2021) Descriptive epidemiology of Crimean – Congo hemorrhagic fever cases admitted to Kabul main hospitals during 2015 to 2018. *Veterinary Medicine and Public Health Journal* 2(1), 1–7.

Sanyaolu, A., Okorie, C., Mehraban, N., Ayodele, O., Tshitenge, S.K. *et al*. (2016) Epidemiology of zoonotic diseases in the United States: A comprehensive review. *Journal of Infectious Diseases and Epidemiology* 2, 021.

Scherk, A.M. (2013) Feline immunodeficiency virus, disease information fact sheet, AAFP Feline Vaccination Advisory Panel Report. *Journal of Feline Medicine and Surgery* 15, 785–808.

Samadi, A., Ababneh, M.M.K., Giadinis, N.D. and Lafi, S.Q. (2010) Ovine and caprine brucellosis (*Brucella melitensis*) in aborted animals in Jordanian sheep and goat flocks. *Veterinary Medicine International* 2010, 1–7. DOI: 10.4061/2010/458695.

Seimenis, A. (2012) Zoonoses and poverty – a long read to the alleviation of suffering. *Veterinaria Italiana* 48(1), 5–13.

Shallcross, L.J. and Davies, S.C. (2014) The World Health Assembly resolution on antimicrobial resistance. *The Journal of Antimicrobial Chemotherapy* 69, 2883–2885.

Sharifi-Mood, B., Metanat, M. and Alavi-Naini, R. (2014) Prevalence of Crimean-Congo hemorrhagic fever among high risk human groups. *International Journal of High Risk Behaviors & Addiction* 3(1), e11520.

Shwiff, S.A., Hampson, K. and Anderson, A.M. (2013) Potential economic benefits of eliminating canine rabies. USDA National Wildlife Research Center - Staff Publications, p. 1243. Available at: https://digitalcommons.unl.edu/icwdm_usdanwrc/1243

Suseno, P.P., Jatikusumah, A., Husein, W.F., Wicaksono, A., Gozali, A. *et al*. Building sustainable multi-sectoral One Health emerging infectious disease and zoonosis surveillance and response capacity in Indonesia: key components and results.

Takahashi-Omoe, H. and Omoe, K. (2012) Social environment and control status of companion animal-borne zoonoses in Japan. *Animals* 2, 38–54. DOI: 10.3390/ani2010038.

Taylor, L.H., Latham, S.M. and Woolhouse, M.E.J. (2001) Risk factors for human disease emergence. *Philosophical Transactions of the Royal Society B: Biological Sciences* 356, 983–989.

Thakur, S. and Gray, G.C. (2019) The Mandate for a Global "One Health" Approach to Antimicrobial Resistance Surveillance. *The American Journal of Tropical Medicine and Hygiene* 100(2), 227–228.

Thrusfield, M. (2007) *Veterinary epidemiology*, 3rd ed. Blackwell Science, UK.

Tiwari, R., Dhama, K., Sharun, K., Yatoo, M.I., Malik, Y.S. *et al*. (2020) COVID-19: Animals, veterinary and zoonotic links. *Veterinary Quarterly* 40(1), 169–182.

WHO FERG (2015) WHO estimates of the global burden of food-borne diseases: Food-borne Disease Burden Epidemiology Reference Group 2007–2015. Geneva: World Health Organization. Available at: http://apps.who.int/iris/bitstream/10665/199350/1/9789241565165_eng.pdf?ua=1 (accessed 6 September 2017).

Widdowson, M.A., Bresee, S.J. and Jernigan, B.D. (2017) The global threat of animal influenza viruses of zoonotic concern: Then and now. *The Journal of Infectious Diseases* 216(S4), S493–8.

Yamamoto, K.J., Sanou, P.M., Abbott, R.J. and Coleman, K.J. (2010) Feline immunodeficiency virus model for designing HIV/AIDS vaccines. *Current HIV Research* 8(1), 14–25.

Yang, Y. *et al*. (2020) The deadly coronaviruses: The 2003 SARS pandemic and the 2020 novel coronavirus epidemic in China. *Journal of Autoimmunity*. DOI: 10.1016/j.jaut.2020.102434.

Ye, Z.W., Yuan, S., Yuen, K.S., Fung, S.Y., Chi-Ping Chan, C.P. *et al*. (2020) Zoonotic origins of human coronaviruses. *International Journal of Biological Sciences, Review* 16(10), 1686–1697. DOI: 10.7150/ijbs.45472.

Zinsstag, J., Schellinga, E., Waltner-Toews, D. and Tanner, M. (2011) From "one medicine" to "one health" and systemic approaches to health and well-being. *Preventive Veterinary Medicine* 101(3–4), 148–156.

18 Pursuing Effective Vaccines Against Cattle Diseases Caused by Apicomplexan Protozoa

Monica Florin-Christensen[1,2], Leonhard Schnittger[1,2], Reginaldo G. Bastos[3], Vignesh A. Rathinasamy[4], Brian M. Cooke[4], Heba F. Alzan[3,5] and Carlos E. Suarez[3,6*]

[1]Instituto de Patobiologia Veterinaria, Centro de Investigaciones en Ciencias Veterinarias y Agronomicas (CICVyA), Instituto Nacional de Tecnologia Agropecuaria (INTA), Hurlingham 1686, Argentina; [2]Consejo Nacional de Investigaciones Cientificas y Tecnologicas (CONICET), C1425FQB Buenos Aires, Argentina; [3]Department of Veterinary Microbiology and Pathology, Washington State University, P.O. Box 647040, Pullman, WA, 991664-7040, United States; [4]Australian Institute of Tropical Health and Medicine, James Cook University, Cairns, Queensland, 4870, Australia; [5]Parasitology and Animal Diseases Department, National Research Center, Giza, 12622, Egypt; [6]Animal Disease Research Unit, Agricultural Research Service, USDA, WSU, P.O. Box 646630, Pullman, WA, 99164-6630, United States

Abstract

Apicomplexan parasites are responsible for important livestock diseases that affect the production of much needed protein resources, and those transmissible to humans pose a public health risk. Vaccines, recognized as a cost-effective and environmentally friendly method for the prevention of infectious diseases in livestock, can avert losses in food production and decrease the exposure of humans to zoonotic pathogens. This review focuses on the need for and advances in vaccine development against the apicomplexan parasites Theileria spp., Babesia spp., Toxoplasma gondii, Neospora caninum, Eimeria spp., Besnoitia spp., Sarcocystis spp., and Cryptosporidium parvum. Together, the effect of these parasites on the cattle industry worldwide causes an enormous burden, yet they remain poorly controlled and very few effective and practical vaccines against them are available. Vaccine development is hampered by our scarce and limited knowledge of the biology and mechanisms of pathogenesis of these microorganisms, and the absence of correlates of host immune protection. More studies focused on these aspects as well as on the identification of parasite vulnerabilities that can be exploited for vaccine design are needed. Novel 'omics' and gene editing approaches in understanding complex parasite biology together with advances in vaccinology will facilitate the development of effective, sustainable, and practical vaccines against cattle diseases caused by apicomplexan parasites. Such vaccines will help prevent animal and human diseases and allow production of enough animal protein to feed the growing human population in the twenty-first century and beyond.

*Corresponding author: carlos.suarez@usda.gov

Keywords: cattle, vaccination, animal production, apicomplexan protozoa, *Theileria*, *Babesia*, *Toxoplasma*, *Eimeria*, *Sarcocystis*, *Besnoitia*, *Cryptosporidium*

Review Methodology

For this review study, we performed systematic searches of scientific manuscripts focused on vaccines against cattle diseases caused by apicomplexan protozoa. We searched academic databases, such as PubMed, Scopus, and Web of Science. We searched for terms, such as cattle, *Babesia*, *Theileria*, *Toxoplasma*, *Neospora*, *Eimeria*, *Besnoitia*, and *Cryptosporidium*, among others. We also used as reference the chapters on *Neospora* and *Eimeria* of the book 'Parasitic Protozoa of Farm Animals and Pets' (M. Florin-Christensen & L. Schnittger, eds.), Springer, Cham, Switzerland, 2018 (ISBN 978-3-319-70131-8). Timeframe of our search covered scientific manuscripts from early 1970s to 2021. In addition, institutional websites, such as the European Food Safety Authority and the USDA Animal Research Service, were also consulted in order to gather information on the studied subject.

Introduction

Protozoa are a highly diversified group of single-celled eukaryotic organisms of the kingdom Protista. They can be free-living or parasitic and are distinctive by their animal-like behaviors, including predation and motility. Some protozoa play beneficial roles to their ruminant hosts while living in symbiotic association with their digestive systems. However, some species of parasitic protozoa can be responsible for important and mostly neglected or emerging diseases in livestock, and some of them have potential for zoonotic transmission (Schnittger and Florin-Christensen, 2018). Depending on their motility and cell structure, protozoa can be classified as amoebas, flagellates, ciliates, and Sporozoa (syn. Apicomplexa). As the classical name Sporozoa for Apicomplexa suggests, sporozoan parasites have the ability to form sporozoites, a motile form that invades cells in the vertebrate host at some point in their life cycles, initiating an asexual reproductive cycle in their respective vertebrate hosts. In addition, Apicomplexa, as their name in effect implies, are equipped with a set of secretory organelles that form the apical complex and are required for host cell invasion (Harding and Frischknecht, 2020).

Some apicomplexan parasites are responsible for diseases of human importance, including malaria, while others have a high global impact on livestock productive systems. Apicomplexan parasites that are responsible for cattle diseases that are addressed in this review belong to the Piroplasmida, Coccidia, and Cryptogregarina taxa (Schnittger and Florin-Christensen, 2018).

Piroplasmida, such as *Theileria* and *Babesia*, require Ixodid ticks as arthropod vectors that, while feeding, directly inoculate sporozoites into a vertebrate host (inoculative transmission). The dixenous coccidian parasites *Toxoplasma*, *Neospora*, and *Sarcocystis* are transmitted to a ruminant host by ingestion of infective oocysts present in the feces of the infected definitive carnivore host. In turn, the carnivore acquires the parasite after consumption of the infected prey animal (consumptive transmission). The coccidium *Besnoitia* is believed to have a dixenous life cycle, but its mode of transmission is still to be unraveled. In the case of the monoxenous apicomplexans, the coccidium *Eimeria* and the Cryptogregarina *C. parvum*, oocysts excreted with the feces are later taken up orally by the same host species (fecal-oral transmission) (Florin-Christensen and Schnittger, 2018). Moreover, transplacental transmission from mother to fetus (vertical transmission) is a main route of infection in the case of the coccidians *Toxoplasma* and *Neospora* and has been also reported for piroplasmids (Yeruham *et al.*, 2003; Sudan *et al.*, 2015; Sant *et al.*, 2016; Mekata *et al.*, 2018; Lindsay and Dubey, 2020).

Vaccines are preventive tools aimed at decreasing the severity of illnesses and remain the most cost-effective and environmentally friendly approach to the control of infectious diseases, yet only a few vaccines are currently available to prevent diseases caused by apicomplexan parasites in livestock. There are many reasons for this, including the complexity of their life cycles and their relationships with their hosts, and our incomplete knowledge on the biology of these parasites, mechanisms of pathogenesis, and the nature of the protective immune responses that they elicit. Importantly, parasitic diseases remain essentially neglected and are rarely the focus of investment of large research funds. This might be partly because many parasitic diseases occur in less wealthy and less developed regions of the world. However, the changing dynamics of some of these diseases due, in part, to worldwide climate change and globalization is modifying these perceptions.

This review focuses on the state of the art of vaccines and vaccine development against apicomplexan protozoan parasites responsible for major diseases of cattle. Endemic regions of many of these parasites are quickly expanding, and some, such as *Cryptosporidium* and *Toxoplasma*, have an important direct impact on human health, posing additional public health risks that need to be addressed immediately.

Phylogenetic Relationships and Basic Biology of Apicomplexan Protozoa

Among apicomplexans of veterinary relevance that cause important diseases in livestock, coccidians (*Toxoplasma*, *Neospora*, *Eimeria*, *Sarcocystis*, and *Besnoitia*) are able to form cysts, and some have a vertebrate carnivore as a definitive host (such as dogs or cats) and are transmitted via feces. Piroplasmids (*Babesia* and *Theileria*) belong, together with *Plasmodium* spp., to Haemosporidia, characterized for infecting erythrocytes as part of their life cycle and the use of an Ixodid tick, as their definitive host (Schnittger *et al.*, 2012). Finally, *Cryptosporidium parvum* is a zoonotic parasite that has recently been reclassified within the Cryptogregarina since it is more closely related to apicomplexan gregarines than to Coccidia and Piroplasmida (Tomazic *et al.*, 2018). The phylogenetic relationships of these parasites are depicted in Fig. 18.1. It can be observed that the monoxenous *Eimeria* is a sister taxon of dixenous coccidians, whereas *Cryptosporidium* is a sister taxon to all other taxons included in the tree, suggesting a more ancient evolutionary origin.

As members of the phylum Alveolata, apicomplexans are characterized for having flattened vesicles or sacks known as alveoli underlying their cell membrane. They display an obligate parasitic lifestyle and have a great ability to manipulate their hosts. Characteristically, they are equipped with an apical complex, and most contain a unique plastid, known as the apicoplast. The apical complex, which defined and gave the name to this group of parasites, plays a fundamental role in the process of host cell invasion and contains a set of secretory organelles, such as rhoptries, micronemes, and dense granules or spherical bodies, as well as a polar ring and, except for Haemosporidia, a conoid (Harding and Frischknecht, 2020). The apicoplast is a relic of a photosynthetic organelle structure, which originated from a secondary endosymbiotic event involving a red alga and contains a genome of about 30–40 kb. Importantly, plastids are involved in the biosynthesis of fatty acids, isoprenoids, and heme and can be targeted by pharmacological interventions (Salomaki and Kolisko, 2019). In contrast to coccidians and piroplasmids, *Cryptosporidium* lacks an apicoplast and mitochondria and can complete its life cycle in host cell–free *in vitro* cultures, which questions its classification as an obligate intracellular apicomplexan (Hijjawi *et al.*, 2004; Tomazic *et al.*, 2018).

Apicomplexan parasites typically have complex life cycles that alternate sexual and asexual reproduction. Parasites adopt distinct morphologies and their life cycle stages and multiple antigenic variants move around diverse body or tissue environments in their hosts, including the infectious sporozoite stage, intracellular trophozoites and schizonts, invasive merozoites and ookinetes, and gametes, among others. With the exception of the gametes of some species, apicomplexans do not possess cilia or flagella and move by

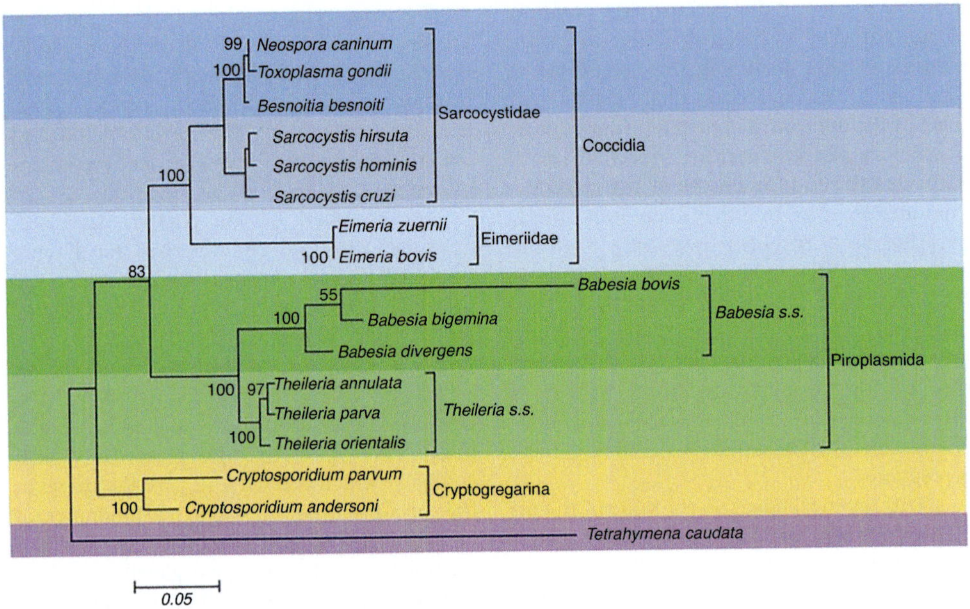

Fig. 18.1. Molecular phylogenetic tree based on 18S rRNA gene sequences of bovine apicomplexan protozoa that infect cattle. After alignment of sequences, the tree was inferred by maximum likelihood, using *Tetrahymena caudata* as outgroup. Accession numbers of sequences are *Neospora caninum*, L24380; *Toxoplasma gondii*, U00458; *Besnoitia besnoiti*, KJ746531; *Sarcocystis cruzi*, KT901167; *Sarcocystis hirsuta*, AF017122; *Sarcocystis hominis*, JX679470; *Eimeria zuernii*, KT184356; *Ei-meria bovis*, KT184336; *Babesia divergens*, FJ944825; *Babesia bigemina*, X59604; *Babesia bovis*, HQ264112; *Theileria parva*, L02366; *Theileria annulata*,AY524666; *Theileria orientalis*,AB520954; *Cryptosporidium parvum*, AF164102; and *Cryptosporidium andersoni*, AY954885.The length of the bar corresponds to the number of amino acid substitutions at any given site.

gliding motility (Frénal *et al.*, 2017). Except for *Cryptosporidium* and the coccidian *Eimeria*, which have a monoxenic life cycle, all other apicomplexans discussed are dixenous and, thus, require one definitive host where they undergo their sexual mode of replication and at least one nondefinitive or intermediate host where the parasites reproduce asexually. For piroplasmids, the definitive host is an invertebrate, the tick, whereas the intermediate host is a vertebrate, including livestock. On the other hand, the dixenous coccidian parasites addressed in this review use a vertebrate carnivore as a definitive host (Fig. 18.2). In the case of dixenous coccidia and piroplasmids, sexual meiotic reproduction happens in the definitive host and asexual mitotic propagation in the intermediate vertebrate hosts.In monoxenic apicomplexans, the sexual phase and several cycles of massive asexual propagation happen in a single vertebrate host. With the host feces, either from the only host in monoxenous or from the definitive host in dixenous parasites, an environment-resistant oocyst is excreted in massive quantities, which significantly increases the probability of parasite transmission (Florin-Christensen and Schnittger, 2018).

For vaccine design purposes, it is of great importance to take into account the characteristics of the biology and life cycle of these parasites, including their antigenic composition, which may differ drastically within a species. Thus, strategies toward developing new vaccines include defining which parasite stage would be more efficiently targeted by a protective immune response. Alternatively, novel vaccines might need to be directed against several distinct life cycle stages in order to be effective.

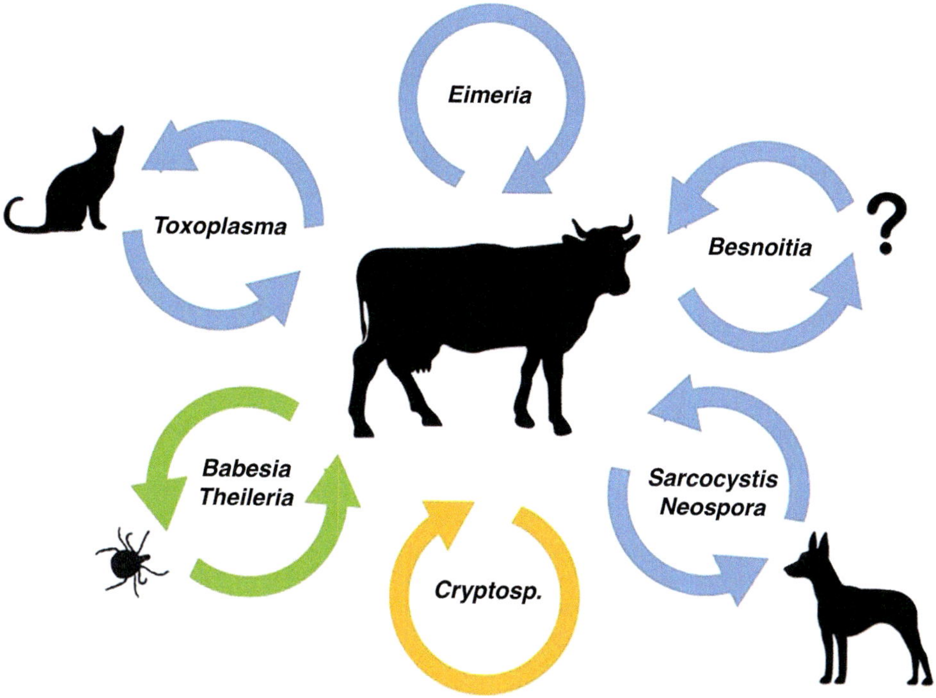

Fig. 18.2. Schematic representation of the life cycles of apicomplexan protozoa that infect cattle.The cycles of monoxenous parasites are depicted with closed arrows, and those of dixenous parasites with open arrows. The respective definitive hosts are represented inside the circles. *Sarcocystis* spp. are exemplified with *S. cruzi*, for which canids are the definitive hosts. The definitive host of *Besnoitia* spp. remains currently unknown.The color of the arrow corresponds to the different phylogenetic groups depicted in Fig. 18.1.

Current Options for the Control of Cattle Diseases

Nowadays, we witness a dramatic expansion of diseases caused by apicomplexan parasites in cattle. This has a direct effect on the production of very much needed protein resources worldwide. In addition to their effects on current animal stock, these diseases also impose a severe limit to the introduction of susceptible animals, which is needed to increase milk and meat production in areas where persistent infections occur.This poses an increased risk, as this is becoming common practice in many countries in order to improve animal production. In general, some of the apicomplexan parasites that cause disease in cattle can be controlled using a variety of drugs (Mosqueda *et al.*, 2012; Noack *et al.*, 2019). However, these treatments are usually costly, may be environmentally toxic, and have the potential to generate undesirable residues that are not allowed in the food chain. In addition, excessive and indiscriminate drug usage often leads to the selection of drug-resistant populations. Other methods of control may rely on the management of cattle, preventive measures, manipulation of the definitive host, and, in the case of piroplasmids, eradication of the tick vector (Pérez de León AA, Mitchell RD, 3rd, Watson DW, 2020).

Vaccines to prevent infections are an environmentally friendly option, but for most of these pathogens, they are yet not available. Reasons for the current lack of vaccines are multiple. In some cases, the diseases are neglected, and little research efforts have been invested. As a result, there are considerable knowledge gaps on the biology of most of these parasites, their relationship with hosts, and the immune mechanisms leading to protection, among others. On the other hand, the development of vaccines is usually difficult due to the complexity of the parasite-host relationships and our inability to culture and genetically manipulate some of these parasites and to decipher the immune mechanisms involved in protection. Furthermore, studies of the immune defense, parasite cultures, and vaccine trials in cattle are expensive and require extensive and costly infrastructure and reagents, for which reason they are out of the reach of the majority of research groups (Florin-Christensen *et al.*, 2014). Importantly, it is recognized that apicomplexan parasites have a particularly long history of coevolutionary interactions with their definitive and intermediate hosts resulting in the development of a large repertoire of mechanisms that allow them to evade the hosts' immune systems. As a result, these parasites can establish persistent infections in the absence of obvious clinical signs, suggesting a compromise of 'peaceful coexistence' between the parasite and host. However, these compromises, which lead to inapparent and usually chronic infections and ensure transmission of the parasite to other hosts, are sometimes precarious and may lead to serious disease or other consequences, such as decrease in milk and protein production and abortions. Parasite adaptations due to the long-term parasite-host coevolution, coupled with a large parasite genetic diversity, complicate the development of effective vaccines. During evolution, the parasites already infected, survived, and were selected upon exposure to a large number of possible scenarios presented by their hosts and the environment in their long struggle for survival. In addition, parasite populations are usually complex and genetically diverse and may be composed of several subpopulations with distinct fitness and geno-/phenotypes, some of which can eventually emerge upon selective pressures. Thus, successful parasites may find redundant pathways to overcome the constraints imposed by the host immune responses and/or may develop different strategies to escape or regulate the host immune system. These realities imply the need of adopting vaccine development strategies that take into account the challenges posed by these complex parasites. On one hand, antibodies against highly antigenic variable antigens might be effective in blocking the parasites, but they may not be effective as vaccine components, whereas on the other hand, conserved functionally relevant antigens might be antigenically subdominant and/or poorly exposed to the immune system effectors. In summary, apicomplexan parasites are master manipulators, may have genomic plasticity, and are adaptable and efficient cell invaders. Therefore, identifying parasite vulnerabilities and life cycle bottlenecks is of great importance for developing efficient methods of control, including vaccines. However, the above-mentioned characteristics of these parasites pose a considerable challenge to vaccine development and can only be overcome by adequate internationally concerted and focused, often multidisciplinary, research efforts.

Effective control methods should be based on parasite-specific targets. The quest for such targets is complicated since parasites and hosts are coevolved eukaryotes and thus share a large number of essential metabolic pathways. On the other hand, reduction of some biochemical pathways has occurred during parasite evolution, with replacement by mechanisms that scavenge metabolites from the host, which has resulted in a reduced number of potential molecular targets. Once a target has been identified, it is highly desirable that parasites are not equipped to circumvent it, that is, the target needs to remain as such in the short and long term.This may be a daunting, but not an impossible, task that requires a deeper knowledge of the biology of the parasites to identify potential 'Achilles heels.' Another possible risk is the possibility of applying control measures that may result in the selection of parasite variants that may be able to infect novel hosts, where they would be, at least in theory, more pathogenic. On a positive note, the quest for improved drugs and vaccines against apicomplexan parasites will be facilitated by the application of a new arsenal of research strategies that have been recently developed and are now available to researchers, including genomics, proteomics, and other 'omics,' in conjunction with advances in vaccinology, immunology, and novel genetic manipulation techniques, such as CRISPR/Cas9 and stable transfection (Suarez *et al.*, 2018).

In the following sections, we will address the state of the art on the development of vaccines against the above introduced apicomplexan parasites of cattle.

Current Status of Available Vaccines and Vaccine Development

Vaccines against *Theileria* spp. of importance to cattle

Tick-borne apicomplexan parasites of the genus *Theileria* cause some of the most economically important diseases that impact the cattle industry worldwide. Here, we focus on relevant studies on vaccine development against *Theileria annulata*, *T. parva*, and *T. orientalis*, three major parasites of this genus and the etiological agents of tropical theileriosis, East Coast fever (ECF), and oriental theileriosis, respectively. During a tick bite, infective sporozoites are transmitted to the cattle host. Clinical disease caused by *T. annulata* and *T. parva* occurs when sporozoites infect leukocytes and develop into macroschizonts, which induces uncontrolled leukocyte proliferation (Agina *et al.*, 2020). By contrast, it is the *T. orientalis* piroplasm stage, which infects the host red blood cells, causing anemia that is ultimately associated with the clinical signs of acute oriental theileriosis (Kawamoto *et al.*, 1990). Improvement of the currently available vaccines and development of novel, efficient strategies to control *Theileria* parasites are critical to ensure elevated standards of animal health and supply the human population access to high-quality animal protein.

T. annulata infects wild and domestic animals in Southern Europe, Northern Africa, and the Middle East. In addition, India, China, and some southern locations in Russia are also affected by the parasite (Yin *et al.*, 2008; El Hussein *et al.*, 2012; Gharbi *et al.*, 2020). It is estimated that more than 250 million cattle are currently at risk of developing an infection with *T. annulata*, which poses a dramatic risk to animal production and food safety in affected areas. The prevalence of tropical theileriosis is difficult to assess in part due to intrinsic differences in susceptibility to the disease of *Bos taurus*, *Bos indicus*, and indigenous breeds of cattle. *T. annulata* and *Theileria* parasites in general present a complex life cycle with development of sexual stages, kinetes and sporozoites in the tick vectors, and schizonts and piroplasms in their vertebrate hosts. *T. annulata* sporozoites are transmitted to cattle by infected ticks upon feeding and rapidly invade MHC class II–expressing cells, mainly monocytes and B cells, which leads to the formation of schizonts and uncontrolled proliferation of the parasite-infected host cells (Ahmed and Mehlhorn, 1999; Morrison *et al.*, 2015). A percentage of schizonts form merozoites that parasitize erythrocytes and develop to piroplasms, which are eventually acquired by ticks during feeding on an infected host and later transmit the parasite to a naïve bovine. Clinical signs of acute *T. annulata* infection are mainly associated with malignant uncontrolled proliferation of infected leukocytes and, to a lesser extent, to hemolytic anemia caused by the replication of piroplasms in red blood cells (Ahmed and Mehlhorn, 1999).

Historically, strategies to control tropical theileriosis have relied on approaches to decrease tick infestation, the use of anti-theilerial drugs, and in some areas the use of indigenous and cross breeds of cattle that are more resistant to the parasite. In addition, the use of attenuated macroschizont cell lines as vaccines has been successfully utilized to control the clinical signs associated with acute *T. annulata* infection (Pipano and Shkap, 2000; Morrison and McKeever, 2006). Despite the fact that attenuated cell lines induce protection, concerns remain regarding this strategy. Specifically, vaccination with attenuated cell lines can potentially lead to the development of parasite piroplasms that may be acquired by ticks in the field, which can result in the spread of the infection and, eventually, to an increase in parasite diversity (Morrison, 2009; Nene and Morrison, 2016). Considering these limitations, efforts have been concentrated on the discovery of novel antigens associated with different stages of the parasite for the development of approaches to prevent infection and/or the clinical signs of acute disease. Consequently, several *T. annulata* antigens have been identified, and specifically, two of them, the surface sporozoite antigen 1 (SPAG-1) and the merozoite surface antigen 1 (TAMS-1), have received special attention as potential vaccine antigens (Williamson *et al.*, 1989; Kawazu *et al.*, 1992). Vaccines based on SPAG-1 and TAMS-1 have been tested using numerous immunization regimes and delivery systems (d'Oliveira *et al.*, 1997; Boulter *et al.*, 1998; Boulter and Hall, 1999; Darghouth *et al.*, 2006). In addition to showing significant levels of protection, results indicate a potential synergistic effect of SPAG-1 and TAMS-1 in inducing protection against *T. annulata* (Gharbi *et al.*, 2011). Despite the promising results, definitive evidence of the efficacy of SPAG-1– and TAMS-1–based vaccines in context with the development of protective cellular immune responses to *T. annulata* remains to be established.

Immunological approaches have also been used as a strategy for the discovery of novel *T. annulata* vaccine antigens. As a result, *T. annulata* antigens 5 (Ta5) and 9 (Ta9) have been identified in context with CD8 +T cells (MacHugh *et al.*, 2011; Nene and Morrison, 2016). Interestingly, these studies have shown that the role of cytotoxic cells is less evident in the protection against *T. annulata* than *T. parva*, as *ex vivo* studies using CD8 +T cells from immune cattle have identified only a few schizont antigens (MacHugh *et al.*, 2011). This suggests that alternative and more efficient strategies are needed to reveal additional, previously unknown, vaccine targets of *T. annulata*. In this context, a recent study proposed the use of a mouse-tick infection model to investigate mechanisms used by *T. orientalis* sporozoites to invade the host leukocytes (Hayashida *et al.*, 2018). However, it remains to be determined if the mouse model represents an improved approach compared to *in vitro* and *in vivo* strategies using bovines for the development of efficient vaccines to control tropical theileriosis.

Another recent study used *in silico* analysis combined with gene expression in tick stages of the parasite to identify *T. annulata* candidate antigens for a transmission-blocking vaccine. By searching the *T. annulata* genome for amino acid domains on similar transmission-blocking sexual-stage targets from *Plasmodium* and *Babesia* parasites, this study identified candidates encoding the 6-cys and cysteine-rich domain protein families (Lempereur *et al.*, 2017). Vaccine trials in cattle are needed to test these newly identified vaccine candidates in their efficiency to block *T. annulata* transmission. Overall, despite recent progress, no subunit vaccine is currently available against *T. annulata*. Therefore, it is important to investigate the profile of antibody and cell immune responses in naturally infected, immune, as well as in vaccinated, animals to identify novel vaccine antigens and biomarkers of protection. In addition, detailed investigation of the parasite life cycle may also reveal bottleneck steps, such as the molecular mechanisms of sexual reproduction that can be potentially exploited for vaccine development.

T. parva causes an acute and usually fatal condition named ECF that affects bovines in Eastern and Southern Africa. The disease poses a tremendous economic impact, especially on pastoralist and small farmers in the affected regions. Following transmission to cattle by infected ticks, parasite sporozoites enter and develop within the cytoplasm of lymphocytes, primarily CD4+ and CD8+ cells. Inside these lymphocytes, sporozoites transform into schizonts that induce uncontrolled proliferation of the infected cells, which, in turn, promotes parasite growth (Palmer *et al.*, 1997). In addition to the lymphoproliferative aspects of the disease, dysregulation of the host immune responses to *T. parva* has also been associated with the acute signs of ECF (Fry *et al.*, 2016; Bastos *et al.*, 2019). The development of persistent infection in animals that survive the acute phase of the disease and the presence of asymptomatic reservoir animals in affected regions, such as water buffaloes, demonstrate the complexity of the disease epidemiology. In addition, the widespread tick vectors, mainly *Rhipicephalus* ticks, in endemic areas poses an extra challenge for the development of control strategies.

The infection and treatment method (ITM) has been historically the primary choice to prevent the dramatic effects of ECF. This method consists of inoculating animals with a cocktail of *T. parva* strains following administration of long-acting oxytetracycline (Di Giulio *et al.*, 2009; Nene and Morrison, 2016). Despite inducing a protective immune response, ITM presents several constraints, such as high cost and complexity of the production of vaccine batches and need for a cold chain for distribution. Another downside of ITM is the establishment of persistent infection in vaccinated animals and the potential risk for tick transmission, even though recent studies showed that ITM parasites do not replace the local parasite population, which, at least in part, favors the use of ITM to mitigate acute ECF (Bishop *et al.*, 2020; Gwakisa *et al.*, 2020). In addition, ITM relies on the use of oxytetracycline, which raises concerns on the spread of antibiotic resistance and contamination of food and dairy products. Altogether, these factors indicate that novel and more sustainable vaccines are needed to control ECF. The polymorphic immunodominant molecule (PIM) is a well-characterized protein expressed by both the sporozoite and schizont stages of *T. parva* and has been evaluated as a vaccine antigen using different delivery platforms (Ververken *et al.*, 2008; Fry *et al.*, 2019). Despite eliciting strong humoral and cellular immune responses, PIM vaccination induced no protection. This finding is in agreement with similar observations in vaccine trials using comparable immunodominant antigens in distinct apicomplexan hemoparasites, such as *Babesia* spp. (Norimine *et al.*, 2003). The *T. parva* p67 is another well-studied antigen expressed on the surface of sporozoites that has been evaluated in subunit and virus-vectored vaccines to control ECF (Kaba *et al.*, 2003; Musoke *et al.*, 2005). Although vaccination with p67 induces the development of *in vitro* neutralizing antibodies, variable levels of protection in field trials have been observed following challenge with parasite sporozoites (Nene *et al.*, 1999; Nyagwange *et al.*, 2018). Explanations for this finding may rely on the fact that other immune mechanisms, besides antibodies, may be involved in protection induced by p67 and that novel antigen delivery systems may need to be utilized to improve the efficacy of p67-based vaccines (Obara *et al.*, 2015; Mukolwe *et al.*, 2020). In that context, a recent study reported the use of novel nanotechnologies to present a polypeptide derived from p67 C-terminal to the immune system of cattle (Lacasta *et al.*, 2021). Despite the variation among animals, results showed significant protection by comparing vaccinated and control animals, which encourages further evaluation of this vaccination approach.

It has been established that the development of cell-mediated immune response is associated with protection against ECF (McKeever *et al.*, 1994; Morrison, 2015). In this regard, a seminal study used adoptive transfer immunity to demonstrate that CD8+ cytotoxic T cells are implicated in controlling the spread of schizont-infected cells and, ultimately, responsible for protection against ECF (McKeever *et al.*, 1994). In addition, it has been demonstrated that genomic polymorphisms of parasite strains and isolates and MHC haplotype diversity of the vertebrate hosts also influence ECF pathogenesis and immunity (Taracha *et al.*, 1995; Shaw *et al.*, 1995; MacHugh *et al.*, 2009; Svitek *et al.*, 2018). Altogether, these aspects have set the rationale to identify novel *T. parva* antigen candidates for vaccines. Recent studies screening CD8+ T cell lines from *T. parva*–immune cattle have identified promising vaccine candidate antigens, named Tp1-10 and Tp12 (Graham *et al.*, 2006; Hemmink *et al.*, 2016; Bastos *et al.*, 2019). In a recent subsequent study, Tp1 antigen expressed in human adenovirus and vaccinia virus induced specific cellular immune response in vaccinated animals (Svitek *et al.*, 2018). However, only 36% of the Tp1-vaccinated cattle survived a lethal challenge with *T. parva*, suggesting that additional antigens and delivery systems are needed to have an efficient vaccine to elicit protection against ECF. Considering current progress and shortcomings, further studies are needed to evaluate the potential of these novel Tp antigens in vaccine formulations. Collectively, these studies that used CD8+ T cells to identify novel *T. parva* antigens represent a breakthrough in reverse vaccinology that can be applied to other apicomplexans. Altogether, regarding the availability of ITM as a control strategy to ECF, this method presents several logistical, economic, and scientific drawbacks, and therefore, the development of efficient and more sustainable alternative vaccines is required. We propose the use of the available data on the immune ITM cattle coupled with genomic targets from *T. parva* and transcriptomic analyses of the mammalian host response as a combined strategy to reveal novel antigens and protective biomarkers that can be used to develop improved vaccines against ECF (Nene *et al.*, 2000; Nyagwange *et al.*, 2018; Tonui *et al.*, 2018). Such vaccines will likely be multicomponent formulations, targeting both sporozoite and schizont stages of *T. parva* and incorporating state-of-the-art adjuvants to drive elicitation of specific protective immune responses. Also, success of this strategy might require the evaluation of alternative antigen delivery systems capable of activating bovine MHC class I–restricted cells, and subsequent induction of CD8+ cytotoxic responses associated with protection against ECF.

T. orientalis, also historically known as *T. sergenti* and *T. buffeli*, is considered an emerging parasitic pathogen that poses a severe threat to the cattle industry in Japan, Australia, and New Zealand, among other countries (Uilenberg *et al.*, 1985). Anemia is the major clinical sign associated with *T. orientalis* infection, which is detected by pale mucosae, pyrexia, and elevated heart and respiratory rates. These signs are typically associated with a history of cattle being moved into an endemic area for *T. orientalis*. The Chitose and Ikeda types of the parasite are associated with marked anemia, whereas the Buffeli type seems to be less virulent (Eamens *et al.*, 2013). Interestingly, considering that anemia is the most pronounced sign of oriental theileriosis, it makes this disease more similar to bovine babesiosis than to ECF or tropical theileriosis, and this fact needs to be taken in consideration for clinical differential diagnosis. The recent identification of the *T. orientalis* Ikeda genotype in animals showing anemia in Virginia, US, combined with the presence of competent *Haemaphysalis longicornis* vector ticks in the region, has brought major concerns to the country's cattle industry (Oakes *et al.*, 2019; Thompson *et al.*, 2020). Over the years, attempts have been made in Japan and Australia to treat bovine theileriosis with several compounds, such as imidocarb, buparvaquone, and pamaquine, among others. However, the use of these drugs is impractical for large herds considering their questionable efficacy in field conditions, toxicity, and high costs (Minami *et al.*, 1985; Watts *et al.*, 2016). Altogether, variation in pathogenicity of parasite genotypes, widespread distribution of competent tick vectors, and impracticality of available treatments pose a real challenge for the development of efficient strategies to control the disease.

No commercial vaccines are currently available to control *T. orientalis*. Early attempts were made to produce a live vaccine using piroplasm parasites; however, this strategy was discontinued due to low efficacy of the approach and concerns on the potential risk of transmitting blood pathogens during vaccination. Therefore, efforts have been concentrated on the identification of novel antigens for subunit vaccines against *T. orientalis*. In that context, partial protection and reduction of clinical signs of acute disease were demonstrated by using subunit vaccines generated from full-length or immunogenic segments of the *T. orientalis* major piroplasm surface protein (MPSP) (Onuma *et al.*, 1998). However, MPSP is highly diverse, which may affect its wide use as a vaccine antigen. In addition, considering the MPSP diversity, this target has been used to classify *T. orientalis* into several distinct genotypes worldwide (Khukhuu *et al.*, 2011; Sivakumar *et al.*, 2014; Agina *et al.*, 2020). Recent studies on the *T. orientalis* draft genome have revealed interesting features among the Ikeda, Chitose, and Buffeli genotypes that can be explored for vaccine development. As a result, newly identified proteins predicted to be expressed on the surface of *T. orientalis* piroplasms can potentially be evaluated as vaccine antigens (Bogema *et al.*, 2018). Collectively, recurrent outbreaks of oriental bovine theileriosis in Japan, Australia, and New Zealand in the last decades have demonstrated the complexity of this disease (Agina *et al.*, 2020). In general, considering that no vaccines are available to control the disease, outbreaks of *T. orientalis* are generally managed by the use of acaricides to decrease the population of competent tick vectors in a target, affected region. However, this is a risky strategy considering that ticks can develop resistance to acaricides and the use of such drugs can have environmental implications. More studies on the interactions among *T. orientalis*, tick vectors, and cattle are needed to develop sustainable control measures to oriental theileriosis. The ultimate goal is to develop a vaccine, probably containing a cocktail of antigens, to induce a protective immune response in cattle.

In conclusion, the main current strategy to decrease the devastating effects of acute infection with *T. annulata*, *T. parva*, and *T. orientalis* is the use of acaricides to control their respective tick vectors and, to a lesser extent, anti-*Theileria* drugs. Despite the availability of ITM and cell line vaccines to control ECF and tropical theileriosis, respectively, these are far from optimal strategies. Considering the similarities among these *Theileria* parasites,we propose the development of a systemic and multifactorial approach to discover immune mechanisms associated with protection and novel parasite antigens for vaccines. We predict that by focusing on the host aspects of protection, such as diversity of MHC haplotypes and additional genetic factors of the immune response, disappointing results in field trials of antigens identified by T-cell approaches, especially for *T. parva* and *T. annulata*, might be reevaluated. Also, special attention should focus on mechanisms involved in sexual reproduction of these parasites inside the tick midgut that could potentially be explored for the development of transmission-blocking vaccines. In addition, detailed investigation of host-parasite interactions (i.e. protective immune responses and parasite antigens that are targets of such immune responses) in immune animals that survived acute infection, especially for ECF and tropical theileriosis, can potentially provide additional insights for the discovery of novel vaccine antigens and biomarkers of protection. Evaluation of innovative and practical alternative vaccine delivery systems, such as liposomes, virus-like particles (VLP), immune-stimulating complexes (ISCOMS), and nanoparticles, is also crucial for the development of efficient control strategies against tropical theileriosis, ECF, and oriental theileriosis.

Vaccines against bovine babesiosis

Bovine babesiosis is a tick-borne disease caused mainly by the apicomplexan parasites *Babesia bovis*, *B. bigemina*, and *B. divergens*. While *B. bovis* and *B. bigemina* may have worldwide impact, *B. divergens* is found mainly in Europe. Other parasites that can cause bovine babesiosis include *B. major* and *B. ovata*. In contrast to *Theileria* parasites, *Babesia* spp. only invade erythrocytes in their vertebrate hosts, where they reproduce asexually. The definitive hosts of *Babesia* parasites are Ixodid ticks, mainly *Rhipicephalus* spp. for *B. bovis* and *B. bigemina* (such as *R. microplus*) and *Ixodes ricinus* for *B. divergens*. *Babesia* undergoes sexual reproduction in the midgut of the tick hosts and can be transmitted transovarially after invasion of the eggs in the female ticks by kinete stages of the parasites circulating in the hemolymph, a defining feature of *sensu stricto Babesia* spp. (Schnittger *et al.*, 2012).

Bovine babesiosis is characterized by fever, anemia, and hemoglobinuria. However, the clinical signs are variable depending on the *Babesia* spp. involved and other factors, such as the age and general condition of the animals. Massive hemolysis and hematuria are typical signs of *B. bigemina* infection. In addition to anemia, *B. bovis* infection causes sequestration of infected erythrocytes in the microvasculature of the host, including those of the brain and lungs, leading to cerebral babesiosis and respiratory distress syndrome, respectively (Cooke *et al.*, 2005; Gohil *et al.*, 2010). During acute infection in naïve animals, parasites expand essentially unchecked by the adaptive immune system, which may lead to death when adult cattle are infected. However, young animals are more resistant to acute infections than adult cattle (> 1 year old).The innate immune system of younger animals plays an important role in controlling the disease, especially through clearance of infected erythrocytes in the spleen (Ganzinelli *et al.*, 2018). Interestingly, IL-12 and IFNγ are released earlier in younger *B. bovis*–infected animals. In addition, they are also more efficient at producing high levels of inducible nitric oxide synthase (iNOS), an effector that is essential for the destruction of the parasite. In fact, the activity of the innate immune system is critical for the survival of infected animals, and it needs to be considered for the development of novel control measures. By contrast, older cattle infected with *Babesia* usually quickly succumb to acute disease, in general about 10–12 days after the onset of infection. However, animals that survive acute babesiosis develop a strong protective adaptive immunity, although they cannot fully eliminate the parasite and become persistently infected (Goff *et al.*, 2010). Herds in endemic areas develop a condition known as endemic stability, where few clinical cases are evident, despite high levels of *Babesia* infection in the population (>75%).The occurrence of endemic stability is facilitated by the increased resistance of young calves to infection, combined with maternal antibodies in the colostrum in lactating calves. However, naïve animals, especially adult individuals, cannot be incorporated in to these herds in regions with endemic stability without a high risk of succumbing to acute disease (Jonsson *et al.*, 2012). These scenarios require the application of distinct strategies, such as vaccination, tick control using acaricides, and chemotherapeutic treatments in endemic areas. Because of this and other limitations, including the effect of climate change, endemic stability approaches are not considered effective for the long-term control of bovine babesiosis (Pérez de León *et al.*, 2012; Morel *et al.*, 2019). A tick control strategy based on acaricides is also a frequent approach, especially when eradication of ticks and *Babesia* is attempted, but it is also problematic because of the emergence of drug-resistant ticks and the negative environmental impact of current available acaricide compounds. Antitick vaccines are, however, an interesting alternative for the control of ticks and bovine babesiosis. A tick vaccine based on the concealed Bm86 antigen showed promising results initially, but there were important drawbacks when applied to control ticks in some countries and their production was essentially discontinued (de la Fuente *et al.*, 2007). More effective alternative tick vaccines based on other tick antigens and antigen cocktails are currently under development (Ndawula and Tabor, 2020).

Babesia live vaccines based on attenuated parasites are also available for the prevention of *B. bigemina* and *B. bovis* infections, but not for *B. divergens*. These live vaccine strategies evolved from the common practice of 'premunition,' consisting of the inoculation of blood of an infected animal into naïve recipients, a procedure that resulted in the cotransmission of other blood-circulating pathogens. *B. bovis*–attenuated parasites used in live vaccines are usually prepared by serial rapid passages of a virulent strain in splenectomized calves, and normally 22–25 passages are required. By contrast, the *B. bigemina*–attenuated strains are generated by 'slow' similar passages but using spleen-intact calves (Bock *et al.*, 2004).The attenuated strains obtained by these procedures are usually poorly virulent for young calves, but they still can cause severe acute babesiosis and high mortality rates when applied to adult animals (> 1 year old). However, vaccinated animals remain persistently infected with the vaccine strains and develop a solid humoral and cell immunity that usually protects them against homologous and heterologous strain challenge (Florin-Christensen *et al.*, 2014).

The correlates of protection using live vaccines remain unclear, but several lines of research suggest that protective immunity requires the production of a Th-1 type of response with production of IFNγ, IL-12, and antibodies of the IgG2a subtype (Rodriguez *et al.*, 2012). The mechanisms involved in the process of attenuation by serial passages also remain unknown, but it is possible that it involves the selection of preexisting attenuated parasite populations present in the virulent isolates (Baravalle *et al.*, 2012). *Babesia* parasites can also be attenuated by exposure to low doses of radiation, and this is the source of parasites in the vaccines used in Mexico (Rojas *et al.*, 2006). Once an attenuated *Babesia* strain is obtained, it can be amplified for vaccine production using different approaches. Thus, the *Babesia* vaccines currently available in Australia and South Africa are produced by expansion of the attenuated strain in highly controlled, pathogen-free calves. Live vaccines are also produced by expanding the parasites in *in vitro* cultures, in some countries such as Argentina and Israel (Florin-Christensen *et al.*, 2014).

While live *Babesia* vaccines are quite effective to prevent the devastating effects of the acute disease, they present several drawbacks. These limitations include the need to maintain the vaccines in a cold chain, which may be difficult in some endemic areas located in tropical and semitropical regions of the globe, the risk of coinfection with contaminating coinfecting agents, and the possibility for parasite reversion to virulence. In addition, the decision of using attenuated vaccines implies the maintenance of *Babesia* parasites in the herds, which may become problematic if vaccines are based on tick-transmissible parasites. Currently, it is difficult, if not impossible, to differentiate vaccinated from naturally infected animals using serology, and it might be desirable to incorporate markers into the vaccine parasite strain,or to develop a differentiating infected from vaccinated animals (DIVA) vaccine. Taking all these aspects together, future options consist of improving live vaccines by using nontransmissible strains, DIVA markers, or genetically manipulated strains unable to revert to virulence (Suarez *et al.*, 2018).

Alternative options to live vaccines include developing subunit or inactivated vaccines. Evidence for the feasibility of subunit vaccines was collected initially by testing inactivated vaccines based on protein fractions obtained from merozoites or infected erythrocytes, or secreted parasite antigens (SPA) derived from *in vitro* culture of *Babesia* parasites, successfully employed to develop inactivated vaccines against *B. canis* (Schetters *et al.*, 2009). These vaccines, based on a mix of antigens that were 'secreted' by cultured *B. bovis* parasites, showed promising results, but overall, they appeared to be more effective against homologous parasite challenge (Schetters and Montenegro-James, 1995). Although vaccines based on such antigens are not currently available, they provide a strong rationale for using recombinant versions of antigens in vaccine formulations. As described below in more detail, none of the recombinant antigens so far tested, either alone or in association, proved effective for subunit vaccines against *B. bovis* or *B. bigemina*. However, effective experimental vaccines using recombinant forms of antigens identified in culture supernatants have been developed for *B. divergens* and *B. canis* (Hadj-Kaddour *et al.*, 2007; Moubri *et al.*, 2018).

Among the abundant vaccine candidates for *B. bovis*, only a few have so far been tested in vaccination-challenge experiments (Florin-Christensen *et al.*, 2014). These include, among a few others, the rhoptry-associated protein-1 (RAP-1), two members of the variable major surface antigens (VMSA), the merozoite surface antigen-1 (MSA-1), and MSA-2c, the 12D3 antigen, and the heat-shock protein 20, either as whole recombinant proteins or selected B-and/or T-cell epitopes from them. Unfortunately, none of the formulations based on these antigens were able to elicit effective and strong protective immunity comparable to live vaccines in animal trials (Hines *et al.*, 1995; Norimine *et al.*, 2003; Alvarez *et al.*, 2010; Jaramillo-Ortiz *et al.*, 2019). The perceived collective experience indicates that the issues involved in vaccine development against bovine *Babesia* spp. are complex and more research is needed. The lessons so far learned suggest that more knowledge is required on establishing the mechanisms of disease and the correlates of protection in animals resistant to *Babesia* infection, either due to natural processes or due to vaccination with live vaccines. The identification of correlates of protection could help develop screens to identify protective antigens. Combined, the identification of the correlates of protection and protective antigens may lead to the rational design of efficient subunit vaccines.

While protection against acute babesiosis may be difficult to achieve, novel alternative vaccine approaches have also been emerging (Gohil *et al.*, 2013; Rathinasamy *et al.*, 2019). This includes the development of vaccines that can block transmission of the parasites. Several transmission-blocking vaccine (TBV) candidates have been identified and characterized recently in *B. bovis* and *B. bigemina*, including members of the CCp and 6Cys families, and HAP2 (Bastos *et al.*, 2013; Hussein *et al.*, 2017; Camacho-Nuez *et al.*, 2017; Bohaliga GAR *et al.*, 2018; Alzan *et al.*, 2019). Most of these antigens are also conserved in related parasites such as *Plasmodium* spp. and *Theileria* spp. (Bastos *et al.*, 2013; Liu *et al.*, 2015; Lempereur *et al.*, 2017; Feng *et al.*, 2018) and have been shown to be effective in reducing transmission upon vaccination in different models (Duffy and Gorres, 2020). Antigens differentially expressed in kinete stages are also possible candidates for developing TBV. These include the *B. bovis* protein BboKSP, encoded by the gene identified as BBOV_I002220 (Johnson *et al.*, 2017), and its *B. bigemina* homologous, BbiKSP, encoded by the BBBOND_0206730 gene (Bohaliga GAR *et al.*, 2018). Such TBV candidates are exclusively expressed in tick stages and this unique expression profile could be the result of an evolutionary adaptation to escape the vertebrate host immune responses, in addition to adapting for functional requirements. Furthermore, vaccination with such concealed antigens that have not been exposed to the pressure of the bovine host immune system may be restricted in their ability to vary antigenically.This is clearly an example of confronting the parasite with a challenge that it did not face during its long coevolutionary history between the arthropod and vertebrate hosts. An advantage of this approach is that these antigens are widely conserved and not exposed to the selection pressure of the vertebrate host immune system, since they are only expressed in tick stages, which makes these parasite targets reasonable for intervention to block transmission. However, it is likely that frequent revaccinations will be required in order to maintain high antibody titers against such tick-stage–specific antigens, since natural boosts will not occur due to their differential expression in tick-stages. A realistic approach, based on the current state of the art, would be to generate a vaccine containing blood-stage antigens and tick-stage antigens in which blood-stage antigens elicit an immune response that alleviates the devastating effects of acute babesiosis and allows time for the animals to develop a strong adaptive immune response, and tick-stage antigens to prevent parasite transmission between hosts. This combination of recombinant vaccine including both blood-stage and tick-stage antigens could be the most promising approach to control bovine babesiosis in the future. Combining a blood-stage vaccine capable of controlling clinical disease with a TBV would improve animal production and keep the parasite numbers low in the vaccinated areas.

Vaccines against bovine coccidiosis caused by *Eimeria*

The genus *Eimeria* comprises about 200 species that infect a large variety of vertebrates around the world.While these parasites are strictly host specific and their distribution follows that of their hosts, one host can be infected by several species at the same time. *Eimeria* has a monoxenic life cycle with endogenous and exogenous developmental stages. The endogenous phase generally takes place at species-dependent predilection sites of the digestive tract, where intracellular asexual and sexual multiplication occurs.

The latter results in the generation of a zygote around which a resistant protective oocyst wall develops. When oocysts are mature, they rupture their host cells, are released to the intestine lumen, and shed with the feces. Shed oocysts need to sporulate outside the host to become infective, which takes one to 4 days under ideal temperature, moisture, and oxygen levels, or up to several weeks, under less favorable conditions. Upon ingestion of sporulated oocysts by the host, parasites excyst in the intestine and invade mucosal intestinal cells, where new cycles of multiplication begin (Bangoura and Daugschies, 2018).

Oocysts are very resistant and last for months in the environment. They are also highly infective, and a few oocysts can establish an infection in a susceptible host that will yield millions of oocysts in the next life cycle. These features make *Eimeria* spp. extremely successful parasites, especially in areas where animals congregate or are crowded, and feces are more concentrated on the ground (Keeton and Navarre, 2018).

Thirteen *Eimeria* species are known to infect cattle, three of which, *E. zuernii*, *E. bovis*, and *E. alabamensis*, are pathogenic, and have also been detected in water buffaloes (Morgoglione *et al.*, 2020). Clinical signs, mainly diarrhea and anorexia, are present in young calves, between 6 and 12 months old, while adult cattle are normally asymptomatic, unless immunosuppressed due to stress or other diseases. Depending on the level of exposure, general condition, genetic susceptibility, and other factors, clinical signs can vary from self-limiting, in which animals recover without treatment, to fast deterioration and death. Heavy infections of calves with *E. zuernii* can lead to nervous coccidiosis with tremors, convulsions, and other central nervous system signs,resulting in high mortality rates (Keeton and Navarre, 2018).

Production losses are associated with increased calf mortality, as well as delayed fertility caused by a retarded weight gain and lower final weight (Lassen and Ostergaard, 2012). Prevention is considered preferable than treatment from economic and animal welfare points of view and is carried out by avoiding overcrowding, improving nutrition, and increasing hygiene of feeding and watering equipment (Keeton and Navarre, 2018). Additionally, anticoccidial drugs that inhibit parasite growth have proved useful not only to treat clinical disease but also as a metaphylactic treatment to improve productive parameters in herds naturally exposed to *Eimeria* spp.,as well as to decrease environmental contamination with oocysts (Veronesi *et al.*, 2011; Veronesi *et al.*, 2013).

Bovine coccidiosis is an extremely under-researched parasitic disease, reflected by the scarcity of published reports on vaccine development. The available evidence supports the potential of the approach of using *Eimeria* sp. oocysts as immunogen in vaccine formulations against bovine coccidiosis. Thus, inoculation of calves with *E. alabamensis* oocysts induced protection upon field exposure to the parasite (Svensson *et al.*, 1996). Also, a vaccine based on sonicated formalin-inactivated *E. bovis* sporulated oocysts elicited high levels of specific antibodies and protection upon challenge in calves (Sultana *et al.*, 2014). Finally, UV inactivation of *Eimeria* sp. oocysts was applied to produce an experimental protective immunogen against coccidiosis in lambs (Ramadan *et al.*, 2018). However, further exploration of this and related lines of research have remained essentially neglected. Conversely, successful vaccines against poultry coccidiosis have been used for 70 years, based on oocysts of wildtype and, more recently, attenuated avian *Eimeria* strains (Shirley *et al.*, 2005). Also, important research efforts devoted to whole-genome sequencing, transcriptomic analysis, characterization of vaccine candidate antigens for subunit vaccines, and gene editing have been so far exclusively concentrated on avian *Eimeria* species (Fan *et al.*, 2020; Soutter *et al.*, 2020). Importantly, as in the case of avian coccidiosis vaccines, a desirable vaccine against bovine coccidiosis should be based on parasite antigens that are accessible to the host intestinal immune system and that elicit an immune response that can decrease parasite proliferation, as well as a strong memory response to protect animals from reinfection (Wang and Suo, 2020). Considering the current research status, a vaccine against bovine coccidiosis does not seem to be an achievable goal in the near future, but this area of research will eventually benefit from the far more rapid advances in avian coccidiosis vaccines.

Vaccines against bovine toxoplasmosis and neosporosis

Toxoplasmosis is a very common zoonotic disease caused by *Toxoplasma gondii*.This coccidian is an obligate intracellular parasite that is very apt to infect nearly all warm-blooded animals and can invade many different types of cells. In fact, it was estimated that 92% of the world cattle population harbors antibodies against *T. gondii* (Hosein *et al.*, 2016). As it is such an important global zoonosis, it was the target of 'one health approaches' for vaccine development (Innes *et al.*, 2019). Although toxoplasmosis is not generally considered a high-risk disease for immunocompetent human populations, it can cause abortions in pregnant women and acute disease in immunocompromised individuals. In addition, it was found that the parasite may alter brain chemistry by affecting the production of dopamine (Skallová *et al.*, 2006). The usual treatment for toxoplasmosis in humans consists of a combination of pyrimethamine with sulfadiazine. Felines are the key and definitive hosts for *T. gondii*. Cats can acquire the parasite by predating on rodents, birds, and other species and are the only definitive host, where the sexual life cycle of the parasite can occur in their guts, resulting in the shedding of *T. gondii* oocysts in feces. Transmission of *T. gondii* may occur through consumption of sporulated parasites derived from oocysts deposited by cats in contaminated food, such as vegetables or water (Jones and Dubey, 2010), or raw or undercooked meats containing *T. gondii* tissue cysts (Hussain *et al.*, 2017).

Toxoplasmosis is also considered a mild disease in bovines, which are usually able to mount strong immunity against the parasite, and the development of vaccines for this species is not considered a priority (Dubey, 1983; Burrells *et al.*, 2018). However, whether infection of cattle with *T. gondii* constitutes a relevant risk factor to humans remains to be established. While toxoplasmosis is not usually regarded as a risky disease for cattle, it is known to be an important cause of abortion in sheep, and a live vaccine for this species is available (Buxton *et al.*, 2007). In addition, swine meat contaminated with *T. gondii* is also an important human health risk.Therefore, addressing *T. gondii* control in pig herds may be of relevance (Mateus-Pinilla *et al.*, 1999; Suijkerbuijk *et al.*, 2018).

A One Health approach for toxoplasmosis is based on the development of livestock vaccines that reduce infection in the cat and therefore shedding into the environment, which, in turn, can help reduce the burden of this potentially dangerous disease in immunocompromised patients and pregnant women. Also, the strategic application of vaccination of food animals was suggested as a means of preventing/ reducing viable tissue cysts in meat, making it safer for human and animal consumption (EFSA, 2010). Numerous *T. gondii* vaccine candidate antigens have been identified, and an attenuated genetically manipulated KO strain was also tested, as recently reviewed in (Innes *et al.*, 2019). An important factor for developing a *T. gondii* vaccine is selecting the most appropriate life stage of this parasite as an effective target. Despite intensive research, no subunit or killed parasite vaccines are currently available, but studies on protective immune mechanisms suggest that a successful subunit or inactivated vaccine candidate should be able to stimulate key protective immune responses involving the production of IFNγ and activated CD4+ T cells and then activated CD8+ T cells, followed by the detection of specific antibodies (Innes *et al.*, 1995). In addition, interventions aimed at interfering with production and/or sporulation of oocysts may help limit spreading of *T. gondii* in the environment, resulting in turn in a reduction of the incidence of toxoplasmosis in humans and livestock. Recent work identified genes encoding for proteins involved in the formation of sexual stages and oocyte walls that can be candidates for transmission-blocking vaccines against *T. gondii*. Furthermore, it was demonstrated that a genetically engineered nontransmissible mutant *T. gondii* strain lacking expression of the HAP2 sexual stage gene was able to generate immune responses that prevent transmission of *T. gondii* by cats (the only known definitive host of the parasite), thus demonstrating the feasibility of developing TBVs against *T. gondii* (Ramakrishnan *et al.*, 2019).

The causative agent of bovine neosporosis is *Neospora caninum*, an apicomplexan protozoon belonging to the Sarcocystidae family, which is highly related to *T. gondii*. This parasite was first described in the 1980s as an agent of neuromuscular disease in dogs and only later recognized as a major agent of abortion and neonatal mortality of cattle worldwide. Cattle producers experience annual losses of millions of dollars due to *N. caninum*–associated abortions in dairy and beef cows and other indirect costs (Reichel *et al.*, 2013; O'Doherty *et al.*, 2015).

As other members of the Sarcocystidae family, *N. caninum* displays a two-host, predator-prey life cycle. The sexual stage is completed in the digestive tract of dogs and other canids that excrete unsporulated oocysts with their feces. Under adequate environmental conditions, oocysts undergo sporulation and become infective. Ingestion of oocyst-contaminated water or food leads to infection of a large variety of intermediary hosts, including cattle, sheep, deer, bison, water buffalo, and even wolves and dogs. Tachyzoites formed in the intermediary host gut disseminate by moving between tissues or through the bloodstream, invade different tissues, and reproduce intracellularly, inside a parasitophorous vacuole. Eventually, responding to a host signal, they undergo stage conversion into bradyzoites, which form a dormant thick-walled tissue cyst stage and slowly divide, until reaching approximately 100 parasites per cyst. The parasite life cycle is completed when a canid ingests meat infected with tissue cysts. Most importantly, *N. caninum* tachyzoites are efficiently transmitted through the placenta in several intermediary hosts and, indeed, vertical infection is the main transmission route in cattle. An infected dam produces 90% infected fetuses. Depending on factors such as the time of infection and their immunological status, infected fetuses can die *in utero* or can be resorbed, mummified, autolyzed, stillborn, or born alive. Infected born calves show occasionally neurological signs, weakness, and/or underweight but are generally asymptomatic. They remain chronical carriers and females are able to transmit vertically the parasite to the next generation. Transplacental transmission can take place upon a primary infection of a pregnant dam after oocyst ingestion, but more commonly, upon recrudescence of a preexistent infection during pregnancy. Abortions can be epidemic or endemic and are caused by parasite-provoked placental necrosis that hampers fetal survival, primary tissue damage due to parasite multiplication in the fetus and/or placental inflammation, and release of maternal proinflammatory cytokines that provoke maternal expulsion of the fetus (Dubey *et al.*, 2006; Lindsay and Dubey, 2020).

There are no commercially available drugs to protect against bovine neosporosis, albeit a considerable number of compounds have been tested in animal models or in cattle under controlled conditions with some promising results. Drug therapies would be useful to prevent abortions due to primary infections or recrudescence of preexistent ones and to avoid the establishment of chronic infections in calves born to infected dams (Sánchez-Sánchez *et al.*, 2018). However, the need for prolonged preventive treatments would make drug therapies uneconomical, with the additional risk of generating unacceptable residues in meat and milk. Currently recommended control measures include selective culling of infected cattle, embryo transfer, limitation of the access of canids and their feces to water and food destined for cattle consumption, and preventing canids from eating tissues resulting from abortions. However, these measures are either highly costly or only partially effective due to the existence of a sylvatic cycle of the parasite in birds, rodents, and other mammals. Vaccination to limit vertical transmission and abortion is considered the most cost-effective measure to control neosporosis (Reichel and Ellis, 2006).

A vaccine (Bovilis Neoguard) based on killed tachyzoites was commercialized for a few years and shown to induce anti–*N. caninum* antibodies, be safe, and not to affect meat quality in feedlot steers (Barling *et al.*, 2003). However, it only yielded partial reduction in abortion rates and has been removed from the market (Romero *et al.*, 2004; Weston *et al.*, 2012).

As in the case of sheep and human toxoplasmosis, natural exposure to the parasite before pregnancy is the most efficient way to prevent abortions in cattle; hence, a live vaccine appears as a simple and attractive tool for the control of bovine neosporosis (Reichel *et al.*, 2015). Indeed, vaccination of pregnant dams with an attenuated strain, isolated from an asymptomatic *N. caninum*–infected calf from Australia, prevented abortion upon challenge with a virulent parasite strain. This effect was not observed in cows vaccinated with a lysate of the attenuated strain. Interestingly, while both live and lysate preparations elicited a strong antibody response, only live vaccination induced proliferation of CD4+ T cells and production of IFNγ, suggesting that a cellular response is needed for protection (Miller *et al.*, 2002; Williams *et al.*, 2007). The production of live attenuated vaccines can benefit from the availability of *in vitro* culture protocols for *N. caninum* and is considered to have a high chance of success; however, such vaccines have not yet reached the market (Reichel *et al.*, 2015).

Importantly, some disadvantages of live vaccines, such as maintenance of the parasite in immunized herds with potential for pathogenicity reversion, costly production and distribution, and short storage life, render a subunit vaccine an attractive alternative. An important amount of research has been carried out to identify *N. caninum* proteins and parasite fractions with a role in host cell invasion and/or differentiation from the tachyzoite to the bradyzoite stage and to develop vaccine formulations that generate humoral and cellular immunity against these components. The majority of vaccination/challenge experiments have been carried out in a mouse model, either using nonpregnant mice to evaluate acute disease and infection of the central nervous system or pregnant mice to assess transplacental transmission and female/offspring health. However, immunological differences between mice and cattle restrict the validity of the results to preliminary indications of potential protective effects. On the other hand, while experiments in cattle are constrained by their high costs, sheep have emerged as a cost-efficient small ruminant model for neosporosis, since they can also experience abortions due to *N. caninum* infections. So far, only live attenuated vaccines have conferred convincing protection; thus, further efforts are needed to produce an efficient subunit vaccine (Reichel and Ellis, 2006; Hemphill *et al.*, 2016; Horcajo *et al.*, 2016).

Unraveling new targets for vaccine development using molecular biology tools is not as advanced in *N. caninum* as in other more extensively studied apicomplexan parasites. Genomic sequencing of geographic isolates has thrown light on interesting aspects of the parasite population structure (Khan *et al.*, 2019). Conversely, the application of other advanced methodologies, such as 'omics' approaches to antigen discovery, has been hampered by the incomplete annotation of the *N. caninum* genome, where a large number of functionally significant proteins were annotated as 'hypothetical' and have thus remained unnoticed (Calarco and Ellis, 2020). Bioinformatics tools have shown that some of these previously uncharacterized proteins are likely involved in essential biological processes such as parasite motility, adhesion, invasion, signaling, and interaction with host cells and thus constitute attractive vaccine and drug targets (Calarco and Ellis, 2019).

Validation of the functional relevance of these and other antigens could be carried out by knock-out experiments using available gene-editing tools,including stable transfection and CRISPR/Cas9 technology (Zhang *et al.*, 2010; Arranz-Solís *et al.*, 2018). Gene editing could also be applied to produce attenuated vaccine strains in which genes encoding major virulence factors have been deleted, and/or with introduced markers to be used as DIVA vaccines.

Progress in the advancement of bovine neosporosis control strategies has been hampered by the status of *N. caninum* as a nonmodel organism. This disease will continue to pose a burden for cattle producers around the world and generate substantial reproductive and productive losses until consistent financial support is granted for the production of safe and efficacious vaccines that limit *N. caninum* proliferation and dissemination.

Vaccines against besnoitiosis and sarcosporidiosis

Bovine besnoitiosis (elephant skin disease) is an emerging acute and chronic disease caused by the apicomplexan intracellular protozoan *Besnoitia besnoiti*, a cystogenic coccidium. Illness begins with fever, followed by warm, painful swellings ventrally (anasarca). *B. besnoiti* merozoites invade and proliferate in macrophages, endothelial cells, and fibroblasts producing characteristic large, thick-walled cysts filled with bradyzoites, causing vasculitis and thrombosis. These stages, together with the oocyte and the tachyzoite, are the infectious parasite forms. The subsequent cellular destruction and immune response lead to the characteristic acute signs of anorexia, lethargy, generalized skin edema, and the chronic signs of alopecia and scleroderma. Other signs, such as swollen lymph nodes, diarrhea, photophobia, rhinitis, and orchitis, among others, can also occur. The parasite affects cattle production in several European, Asian, and African countries. Although mortality is considered low (less than 10% of the cases), convalescence is slow in severe cases. Therefore, this parasite may be responsible for important economic losses for the cattle industry (Besnoitiosis, 2018).

Cattle are known to be intermediate hosts; however, definitive hosts and mode of transmission remain unknown, and there are substantial knowledge gaps on the life cycle and biology of this parasite. Although the route of transmission remains unclear, cattle are usually isolated and protected from biting insects and ticks and then treated symptomatically. Chemotherapy remains very limited and is only minimally effective. Both antimony and sulfanilamide complexes prevented cyst development by *B. besnoiti* in rabbits, and oxytetracycline may have some therapeutic value if given early in the disease course (Shkap *et al.*, 1985). However, there is still no effective drug available for the control of besnoitiosis in cattle.

South Africa and Israel have used a live attenuated vaccine against bovine besnoitiosis (Basson *et al.*, 1970). An extensive field trial that was carried out in South African farms, where the disease was severe, found that 100% of the cattle inoculated with a blue wildebeest strain of *B. besnoiti* vaccine were protected from the clinical form of the disease over an observation period of 1–4 years (Bigalke *et al.*, 1974). In Europe, at present, only reliable diagnosis together with herd-management measures are available to avoid that noninfected herds acquire the infection due to trade with infected animals (EFSA, 2010). These data suggest that developing a safer live or subunit vaccine is an achievable goal. However, the nature of protective immune responses remains unknown and the identification of novel targets for chemotherapeutic or immunological interventions remains severely limited by the lack of genomic and transcriptomic data (Cortes *et al.*, 2014). Bradyzoite-specific antigens that could be candidates for vaccine development were also identified, but little progress has been documented on the development of subunit vaccines against this parasite (Fernández-García *et al.*, 2009). Altogether, this indicates that additional research is needed in order to generate effective subunit or killed vaccines that can ameliorate the impact of this parasite in bovine populations at risk.

Sarcosporidiosis is another disease in livestock with zoonotic potential. The disease, caused by apicomplexan parasites of the genus *Sarcocystis*, is characterized by the formation of sarcocysts containing infective bradyzoites that range in size from micrometers to a few centimeters, in the muscle or nervous tissue of their hosts. *Sarcocystis* spp. infections are quite prevalent in farm animals; however, there have been few reported outbreaks of clinical disease. Most animals are asymptomatic, and the parasite is discovered only upon slaughter.

The genus *Sarcocystis* contains more than 100 species that may differ in host specificity and pathogenicity but have a typical coccidian life cycle involving merogony, gametogony, and sporogony. The identification of different species is achieved by molecular studies and cyst wall morphology. *Sarcocystis* spp. normally develop in obligatory two-host cycles consisting of an intermediate host (prey) and the final host (predator). Usually, the herbivore is the intermediary host, while a carnivore (i.e. dog, cat, human, etc.) is the definitive one. Species-specific prey-predator life cycles have been demonstrated for cattle-dog (*S. cruzi*), cattle-cat (*S. hirsuta*), cattle-human (*S. hominis*), pig-human (*S. suihominis*), and others. Human ingestion of sarcocysts of *S. suihominis* or *S. hominis* in uncooked pork or beef, respectively, may cause nausea, abdominal pain, loss of appetite, vomiting, and diarrhea lasting as long as 48 hours (Decker *et al.*, 2018; Lindsay and Dubey, 2020).

As stated above, *Sarcocystis* spp. infections are generally considered highly prevalent worldwide, but of low pathogenicity. However, induced infection with *S. cruzi* sporocysts from canine feces may cause acute disease in calves, microscopic cysts in myocardium, as well as eosinophilic myositis in cattle, and abortions, stillbirths, and deaths in pregnant cows. Similar pathogenicity has been demonstrated for *S. tenella* in lambs and ewes and for *S. miescheriana* in pigs. The manifestation of clinical disease may depend on the immune status of the host and the dose of sporocysts. A procedure involving preventive immunization using small doses of sporocysts appears to prevent the development or reduce severity of clinical disease in sheep when challenged later with large doses (premunitive immunity). Pigs can also have persistent acquired immunity after immunization infections. Importantly, cattle and llama meat containing visible cysts are usually condemned upon inspection after slaughter, with consequent economic losses (Franco *et al.*, 2020).

No vaccines to control *Sarcocystis* spp. infections are currently available for any livestock species, and little research has been performed in the identification of vaccine candidate antigens. Importantly, methods to initiate cultures from sporocysts and merozoites and for cryopreservation of various *Sarcocystis* spp. are now emerging (Verma *et al.*, 2017). This will facilitate our understanding of the antigenic composition of the parasites and the identification of novel vaccine candidates. A study by Howe *et al.* (Howe *et al.*, 2008) demonstrated the expression of surface antigens of the SAG family that could constitute attractive vaccine candidates in *S. neurona*, a species that infects and causes encephalitis in horses. SAG antigen genes were also recently shown to be transcribed in bradyzoites of *S. aucheniae*, a *Sarcocystis* species that produces macroscopic cysts in South American camelids (Franco *et al.*, 2020). However, it should be assessed whether vaccines are needed, for which species, and which life stages of the parasite should be targeted.

Livestock become infected by sporocysts from the feces of carnivores.The main strategy to control sarcocystosis is based on interrupting the parasite life cycle. Thus, simple preventive measure can be taken to control this disease. For instance, dogs and other carnivores should be precluded from eating raw meat, offal, or dead animals. There is no specific therapeutic method for sarcocystosis,but anticoccidial drugs are an option for prophylactic or curative chemotherapy, though the efficiency of drugs on different life stages may vary (Chhabra and Samantaray, 2013). Noteworthy, it has been shown that infected pork and beef could be made safe for consumption by cooking at 70°C or freezing. In summary, *Sarcocystis* spp.can be considered as neglected understudied parasites. Many research gaps remain, and there is a scarcity of options for the prevention and treatment of this disease.

Vaccines against bovine cryptosporidiosis

Bovine cryptosporidiosis is caused by infection of preweaned calves with *Cryptosporidium parvum*, leading to gastroenteritis and profuse diarrhea. The disease is occasionally fatal and animals surviving the infection do not entirely compensate growth retardation, resulting in considerable production losses. The parasite is ubiquitous in all cattle farms but is of particular importance in intensive management systems, such as dairy farms. In addition to *C. parvum*, the species *C. bovis* and *C. ryanae* may be detected in weaned calves but have not been found associated with clinical disease (Santín, 2013). A fourth species, *C. andersoni*, is occasionally detected in the abomasum of adult cattle and considered to be asymptomatic, though reduced weight gain and milk production associated with this infection have been reported (Ralston *et al.*, 2010). In neonatal sheep and especially goats, cryptosporidiosis can lead to high morbidity (100%) and mortality (50%), and the species most frequently detected is *C. parvum*. In pigs, infection with *C. parvum* leads to diarrhea of 3–5 days duration and is most frequently observed in piglets or starter pigs (Santín, 2013; Tonui *et al.*, 2018).

Cryptosporidium displays a monoxenous life cycle. The sporulated oocyst stage is excreted with the feces into the environment where it remains infective for a prolonged period and is resistant against a large variety of environmental conditions. Transmission of oocysts occurs via the fecal-oral route either directly through contact with feces of infected hosts or indirectly by uptake of contaminated water or food. After ingestion of oocysts, excystation takes place and results in the release of four sporozoites that infect endothelial cells of the gastrointestinal tract. There they develop into type I meronts, where asexual propagation into eight merozoites takes place. Merozoites either autoinfect neighboring endothelial cells spreading the infection to other sites of the intestine or develop into type II meronts starting sexual reproduction. The latter finally results in the production of thin-wall and thick-wall oocysts. Thin-wall oocysts release sporozoites that autoinfect intestine cells, further promoting parasite multiplication in the host individual, whereas thick-wall oocysts are excreted and infect other host individuals, promoting dissemination of the parasite in the population (Tomazic *et al.*, 2018).

The completion of the life cycle of the parasite is facilitated by three factors. First, multiple consecutive propagation cycles, including two autoinfection loops, result in massive parasite multiplication and an enormous parasite load in the host. This, in turn, ensures efficient oocyst excretion and dissemination into the environment. Thus, it has been reported that a single calf excretes up to about 600 million oocysts per day (Nydam *et al.*, 2001). Second, oocyst persistence under a wide range of environmental conditions is ensured by a thick wall formed by four layers composed of acidic polysaccharides, glycoproteins, and lipids. In addition, oocysts are resistant to chlorine-based disinfectants commonly used to sanitize drinking water and swimming pools. Third, a very low infective dose of only 17 oocysts secures establishment of infection in calves after parasite ingestion (Zambriski *et al.*, 2013). On the one hand, these characteristics ensure completion of the life cycle and parasite survival, while, on the other hand, they result in massive environmental contamination with oocysts. As *C. parvum* is zoonotic, the study of oocyst viability and environmental transmission routes is essential for a one health approach to tackle animal and human cryptosporidiosis (Innes *et al.*, 2019).

Calves can be infected immediately after birth. Oocyst excretion may be observed as early as 2 days after ingestion (prepatent time) and excretion may extend from 1 to 14 days (patent time). A dose dependency has been suggested, as the number of oocysts ingested has been observed to correlate with those excreted. Furthermore, the younger the age of the calf at oocyst intake, the longer the excretion period and severity of disease (Zambriski *et al.*, 2013). Importantly, in artificial rearing, all calves become infected at some point during the preweaning phase. Besides liquid diarrhea, clinical signs include dehydration, loss of appetite, lethargy, and abdominal pain and may be fatal. In severe cases, recovery of calves may take up to three to 4 weeks during which restoration of intestine absorption of nutrients occurs (Klein *et al.*, 2008). Currently, the treatment of cryptosporidiosis of calves is palliative as curative drugs are not available. The only licensed drug is halofuginone, which is used for preventive treatment reducing oocyst excretion and severity and duration of diarrhea (Trotz-Williams *et al.*, 2011).

C. parvum is a zoonotic parasite that also causes human cryptosporidiosis, characterized by profuse and prolonged watery diarrhea, abdominal pain, malabsorption, fever, nausea, and vomiting. Besides the zoonotic *C. parvum*, the disease is also caused by the anthroponotic *C. hominis*, which is confined to humans. Recent reports suggest that the majority of waterborne outbreaks, which include recreational and drinking water, are caused by *C. hominis*, whereas food-borne outbreaks are mostly caused by *C. parvum* (Zahedi and Ryan, 2020). The disease in humans is self-limiting and may last up to 2 weeks in healthy immunocompetent individuals. By contrast, in immunocompromised patients, such as HIV patients, young children, and the elderly, the disease may be difficult to control and often leads to death. In industrialized countries, regular outbreaks are reported and result in considerable economic costs. In developing countries, the largest disease burden of cryptosporidiosis is carried by young children. About 1.2 million children under 5 years of age worldwide die due to diarrhea (Liu *et al.*, 2012). It has been reported that in global outbreaks between 2004 and 2010, in 60% of cases, the responsible etiological agent was *Cryptosporidium* spp. (Baldursson and Karanis, 2011).

Research on *Cryptosporidium* lags behind in a number of aspects with regard to other apicomplexan protozoans of veterinary or human importance. This is because only recently methods for *in vitro* cultivation of *C. parvum*, an animal model to reproduce its life cycle, and a genome-editing tool based on the CRISPR/Cas9 system have been established (Vinayak *et al.*, 2015; Morada *et al.*, 2016). It can be foreseen that these developments will greatly facilitate a rational approach to vaccine development. Thus, genome editing and the established animal model will allow functional studies of parasite proteins and antigens to assess their suitability as vaccine candidates. Furthermore, the development of stem-cell–derived epithelial organoids has recently been reported in which the parasite propagates and completes its life cycle (Heo *et al.*, 2018). The availability of such *in vitro* cultivation systems will allow testing parasite neutralization by antisera raised against vaccine candidates before their use in vaccination trials (Jossé *et al.*, 2019).

For the above-mentioned reason, whole-genome sequencing (WGS) has been likewise hampered, as the relatively low numbers of oocysts usually isolated from feces could, due to lack of an *in vitro* culturing system, not be propagated to numbers suitable for genome sequencing. However, recently, protocols that allow the purification of large numbers of oocysts and the amplification of the recovered genome to quantities suitable forWGS sequencing have been established (Robinson and Chalmers, 2020). This allowed the sequencing of an increasing number of diverse *Cryptosporidium* isolates, revealing exciting novel insights with respect to gene duplications, genetic recombination, population genetics, and the existence of 'cryptic species' within *C. parvum* and other *Cryptosporidium* spp. (Fan *et al.*, 2019).

Currently, no vaccine to protect against cryptosporidiosis in calves or humans is available. A vaccine against bovine cryptosporidiosis would be highly desirable to prevent disease thereby favoring animal health and to decrease dissemination of oocysts into the environment, reducing the risk to public health (Innes *et al.*, 2019). A considerable number of potential parasite antigens have been identified by traditional molecular approaches through screening of expression libraries for immunodominant antigens, using sera of infected hosts (Boulter-Bitzer *et al.*, 2007). As *in vitro* culturing will likely be restricted to some laboratories, a convenient approach for the identification of additional vaccine candidates without parasite cultivation is reverse vaccinology. Indeed, by focusing onto the GPI-anchored proteome, this approach has allowed identification of a number of hitherto unknown vaccine candidates for subsequent use in vaccination trials (Manque *et al.*, 2011; Tomazic *et al.*, 2018). Interestingly, an exclusive immunoinformatics approach to design a multisubunit vaccine against *C. parvum* has been recently reported (Dhal *et al.*, 2019).

When conceiving a vaccination strategy that imparts protection to neonatal calves, the following considerations are imperative. Like many farm animals, bovines possess a syndesmochorial placenta, and the fetus does not receive immunoglobulins through transplacental transmission. Instead, passive transfer of immunoglobulins to calves is achieved by feeding of the first milking colostrum. Considering this, a strategy of active immunization of calves is unlikely to be successful. This is so, first, because the immune system of calves is still immature and, second, calves are already exposed to the infection directly after birth leaving insufficient time to mount an immune response that will protect within the first 3 weeks at which infection typically occurs (Mead, 2014). Notwithstanding, immunization of calves shortly after birth with gamma-irradiated oocysts has been done. Irradiation prevented development of inoculated oocysts and no clinical signs were observed following immunization. After challenge at day 21, calves were shown to be protected against subsequent oocyst excretion and clinical cryptosporidiosis (Jenkins *et al.*, 2004). However, as calves are infected directly after birth and predominantly excrete oocysts during their first 3 weeks of age, the protection generated after this period is unsuitable to prevent calf cryptosporidiosis in the field.

Active immunization of pregnant cows is considered a more promising approach. Immunized cows generate protective antibodies in hyperimmune colostrum, which, when taken up by calves, results in their immediate passive immunization. In two independent studies, immunization of pregnant cows was done using the vaccine candidate p23. After ingestion of hyperimmune colostrum and subsequent challenge of calves, a substantial reduction in the number of excreted oocysts of 98% and 90% was observed (Perryman *et al.*, 1999; Askari *et al.*, 2016). Importantly, no diarrhea or other clinical signs were determined as compared to control groups. Vaccination of pregnant cows with the oocyst surface antigen Cp15/60 resulted in a high titer of specific antibodies in sera and hyperimmune colostrum. After hyperimmune colostrum ingestion, anti-CP15/60 antibodies in sera of calves were found to correlate with the titer of anti-CP15/60 antibodies in colostrum (Burton *et al.*, 2011). However, in this study, no subsequent challenge was carried out to test the protection of calves. Oral application of protective antibodies as a strategy of passive immunization has been studied extensively in a mouse model. It has been shown that passive immunotherapy is effective in reducing the number of intestinal infective oocysts in mice. In this study, experimentally infected neonatal mice were treated with the whole whey or purified specific immunoglobulin isotypes IgG1 and IgA from hyperimmune colostrum of a cow immunized with *C. parvum* oocysts. Oocyst shedding and occurrence of diarrhea were significantly decreased, compared with mice that had received the corresponding immunoglobulin isotypes of control colostrum (Fayer *et al.*, 1990).

Egg yolk antibody IgY can be generated in large quantities and low costs with relative ease and has been extensively used for the treatment and prevention of various infections in animals and humans (Mine and Kovacs-Nolan, 2002). Anti-*Cryptosporidium* IgY antibodies may be generated by immunization of chickens, harvested from eggs, and later fed as supplement to newborn calves. This strategy has been successfully applied to viral and bacterial enteric pathogens (Vega *et al.*, 2020). In contrast to immunization of pregnant cows, the advantage of this strategy is that it can be applied not only as an immunoprophylaxis to prevent disease but also as an immunotherapeutic measure. In two independent studies, anti-*Cryptosporidium* sporozoite IgY antibodies were orally applied to SCID and C57BL/6 mice, respectively, and in both, a significant reduction of oocyst shedding was observed (Kobayashi *et al.*, 2004; Omidian *et al.*, 2014). However, this vaccination strategy has not yet been tested in cattle.

There is a consensus that a vaccine against bovine cryptosporidiosis is feasible and will bring significant benefits with respect to animal production, animal welfare, and public health. Research on *C. parvum* has made a significant jump in the last few years, and thus, it can be expected that this is an achievable goal in the near future.

Conclusions

Apicomplexan parasites affect cattle globally, posing an important threat for the production of much needed animal-based food resources. It is widely recognized that vaccination approaches are the most effective methods for the control of infectious diseases, including apicomplexan parasites. Some of these parasites are also zoonotic, and a 'one health' vaccination approach is required in most cases. Thus, an important remaining goal is diminishing the risk imposed by these parasites to humans by reducing the level of parasite burden/contamination in the herds, the environment, and in the food chain through vaccination.

In general, parasitic diseases caused by apicomplexan parasites have so far remained neglected, and greater awareness about the greater challenges posed by these parasites needs to be promoted through research, education, and outreach activities. This will likely enhance the interest among policy makers and attract the next generation of researchers to work in this area resulting in enhanced capacity to manage these parasitic infections. Furthermore, efforts to increase awareness of these parasites should result in increasing funding for research aimed at finding new and improved prevention and/or control methods. As research efforts into a number of these parasites and parasitic diseases remain in their infancy, adequate and feasible vaccine approaches and strategies should be first identified for each of these parasites. For instance, while infections may require transmission-blocking strategies, others may require prevention of acute disease, or a combination of both approaches.

Regardless of the strategy used, vaccine development essentially requires the identification of antigens that can elicit protective responses and effective methods for delivery. In order to be practical, vaccines also need to be affordable, stable under reasonable environmental conditions, nontoxic to the host, environmentally friendly, and easily available. However, basic knowledge of the biology of apicomplexan parasites and the nature of the protective immune mechanisms is lacking in most cases. Addressing the control of these parasitic diseases requires epidemiological assessments, predictive disease modeling, novel diagnostic systems, and new vaccines and effective drugs. The roadmap for the development of novel vaccines should also include the definition of immune correlates of protection and application of full genome sequencing coupled with novel 'omics' approaches. These methods, integrated with genetic analysis using state-of-the-art gene-editing approaches, should result in the identification of novel vaccine candidates.Vaccine delivery regimens and adequate adjuvants also need to be defined for each case, and a pipeline of candidate antigens and their priority for testing should be established. Appropriate vaccine testing models should also be developed to expedite vaccine development and minimize costs.

Altogether, despite the high impact and neglected status of most diseases caused by apicomplexan parasites, the goal of developing effective vaccines against these parasites remains feasible in the light of recent progress in the fields of vaccinology, immunology, molecular biology, and bioinformatics. Enhanced awareness, improved research funding, higher researcher numbers, and enhanced global collaboration will no doubt lead to the development of effective and sustainable control measures against these important parasitic diseases of cattle in the future.

Funding

We acknowledge financial support from the National Research Center and Ministry of High Education and Scientific Research of Egypt, the International Development Research Center (IDRC) (Livestock Vaccine Innovation Fund (Grant 108525), funded by the Canadian Government and the Bill and Melinda Gates Foundation), the United States Department of Agriculture (ARS-USDA CRIS 2090-32000-039-00-D), the Australian Research Council (DP180102584), the National Institute of Agricultural Technology (INTA, 2019-PD-E5-I102 and 2019-PD-E5-I109) and Ministry of Science and Technology (PICT2018-03314), Argentina, and the USDA National Institute of Food and Agriculture (NIFA) (Award Number: 2020-67015-31809; Proposal Number:2019–05375,Accession Number:1022541).

Competing Interests

The authors declare that they have no competing interests.

Authors' Contributions

CES conceived and drafted the manuscript; MFC, LS, RGB, HFA, and CES contributed sections of the manuscript; MFC, LS, RGB, VR, BMC, and CES provided intellectual input and revised the work.

References

Agina, O.A., Shaari, M.R., Isa, N.M.M., Ajat, M., Zamri-Saad, M. *et al.* (2020) Clinical pathology, immunopathology and advanced vaccine technology in Bovine Theileriosis: A review. *Pathogens (Basel, Switzerland) 2020* 9, 697.

Ahmed, J.S. and Mehlhorn, H. (1999) Review: The cellular basis of the immunity to and immunopathogenesis of tropical theileriosis. *Parasitology Research* 85, 539–549.

Alvarez, A.J., Lopez, U., Rojas, C., Borgonio, V.M., Sanchez, V. *et al.* (2010) Immunization of *Bos taurus* steers with *Babesia bovis* recombinant antigens MSA-1, MSA-2c and 12D3. *Transboundary and Emerging Diseases* 57, 87–90.

Alzan, H.F., Cooke, B.M. and Suarez, C.E. (2019) Transgenic Babesia bovis lacking 6-Cys sexual-stage genes as the foundation for non-transmissible live vaccines against bovine babesiosis. *Ticks and Tick-Borne Diseases* 10, 722–728.

Arranz-Solís, D., Regidor-Cerrillo, J., Lourido, S., Ortega-Mora, L.M. and Saeij, J.P.J. (2018) Toxoplasma CRISPR/Cas9 constructs are functional for gene disruption in *Neospora caninum*. *International Journal for Parasitology* 48, 597–600.

Askari, N., Shayan, P., Mokhber-Dezfouli, M.R., Ebrahimzadeh, E., Lotfollahzadeh, S. *et al.* (2016) Evaluation of recombinant P23 protein as a vaccine for passive immunization of newborn calves against *Cryptosporidium parvum*. *Parasite Immunology* 38, 282–289.

Baldursson, S. and Karanis, P. (2011) Waterborne transmission of protozoan parasites: Review of worldwide outbreaks - an update 2004-2010. *Water Research* 45, 6603–6614.

Bangoura, B. and Daugschies, A. (2018) Eimeria. In: Florin-Christensen, M. and Schnittger, L. (eds) *Parasitic Protozoa of Farm Animals and Pets*. Springer International Publishing, New York City, NY, USA, pp. 55–102.

Baravalle, M.E., Thompson, C., Valentini, B., Ferreira, M., Torioni de Echaide, S. *et al.* (2012) Babesia bovis biological clones and the inter-strain allelic diversity of the Bv80 gene support subpopulation selection as a mechanism involved in the attenuation of two virulent isolates. *Veterinary Parasitology* 190, 391–400.

Barling, K.S., Lunt, D.K., Graham, S.L. and Choromanski, L.J. (2003) Evaluation of an inactivated *Neospora caninum* vaccine in beef feedlot steers. *Journal of the American Veterinary Medical Association* 222, 624–627.

Basson, P.A., McCully, R.M. and Bigalke, R.D. (1970) Observations on the pathogenesis of bovine and antelope strains of *Besnoitia besnoiti* (Marotel, 1912) infection in cattle and rabbits. *The Onderstepoort Journal of Veterinary Research* 37, 105–126.

Bastos, R.G., Suarez, C.E., Laughery, J.M., Johnson, W.C., Ueti, M.W. *et al.* (2013) Differential expression of three members of the multidomain adhesion CCp family in *Babesia bigemina*, *Babesia Bovis* and *Theileria Equi*. *PLOS ONE* 8, e67765.

Bastos, R.G., Sears, K., Dinkel, K.D., Knowles, D.P. and Fry, L.M. (2019) Changes in the molecular and functional phenotype of bovine monocytes during *T. parva* infection. *Infection and Immunity* e00703–19.

Bastos, R.G., Franceschi, V., Tebaldi, G., Connelley, T., Morrison, W.I. *et al.* (2019) Molecular and antigenic properties of mammalian cell-expressed *Theileria parva* antigen Tp9. *Frontiers in Immunology* 10, 897.

Besnoitiosis, M.H. (2018) In *Babesia* in domestic ruminants. In: Florin-Christensen, M. and Schnittger, L. (eds) *Parasitic Protozoa of Farm Animals and Pets*. Springer International Publishing, New York City, NY, USA, pp. 169–186.

Bigalke, R.D., Schoeman, J.H. and McCully, R.M. (1974) Immunization against bovine besnoitiosis with a live vaccine prepared from a blue wildebeest strain of *Besnoitia besnoiti* grown in cell cultures. 1. studies on rabbits. *The Onderstepoort Journal of Veterinary Research* 41, 1–5.

Bishop, R.P., Odongo, D., Ahmed, J., Mwamuye, M., Fry, L.M. *et al.* (2020) A review of recent research on *Theileria parva*: Implications for the infection and treatment vaccination method for control of East Coast fever. *Transboundary and Emerging Diseases* 67(Suppl 1), 56–67.

Bock, R., Jackson, L., de Vos, A. and Jorgensen, W. (2004) Babesiosis of cattle. *Parasitology* 129(Suppl), S247–69.

Bogema, D.R., Micallef, M.L., Liu, M., Padula, M.P., Djordjevic, S.P. *et al.* (2018) Analysis of *Theileria orientalis* draft genome sequences reveals potential species-level divergence of the Ikeda, Chitose and Buffeli genotypes. *BMC Genomics* 19, 298.

Bohaliga GAR, J.W., Taus, N.S., Hussein, H.E., Bastos, R.G., Suarez, C.E. *et al.* (2018) Identification of a putative methyltransferase gene of *Babesia bigemina* as a novel molecular biomarker uniquely expressed in parasite tick stages. *Parasit Vectors*.

Boulter, N. and Hall, R. (1999) Immunity and vaccine development in the bovine theilerioses. *Advances in Parasitology* 44, 41–97.

Boulter, N.R., Brown, C.G., Kirvar, E., Glass, E., Campbell, J. *et al.* (1998) Different vaccine strategies used to protect against *Theileria annulata*. *Annals of the New York Academy of Sciences* 849, 234–246.

Boulter-Bitzer, J.I., Lee, H. and Trevors, J.T. (2007) Molecular targets for detection and immunotherapy in *Cryptosporidium parvum*. *Biotechnology Advances* 25, 13–44.

Burrells, A., Taroda, A., Opsteegh, M., Schares, G., Benavides, J. *et al.* (2018) Detection and dissemination of *Toxoplasma gondii* in experimentally infected calves, a single test does not tell the whole story. *Parasites & Vectors* 11, 45.

Burton, A.J., Nydam, D.V., Jones, G., Zambriski, J.A., Linden, T.C. *et al.* (2011) Antibody responses following administration of a *Cryptosporidium parvum* rCP15/60 vaccine to pregnant cattle. *Veterinary Parasitology* 175, 178–181.

Buxton, D., Maley, S.W., Wright, S.E., Rodger, S., Bartley, P. *et al.* (2007) *Toxoplasma gondii* and ovine toxoplasmosis: New aspects of an old story. *Veterinary Parasitology* 149, 25–28.

Calarco, L. and Ellis, J. (2019) Annotating the “hypothetical” in hypothetical proteins: In-silico analysis of uncharacterised proteins for the apicomplexan parasite, *Neospora caninum*. *Veterinary Parasitology* 265, 29–37.

Calarco, L. and Ellis, J. (2020) Species diversity and genome evolution of the pathogenic protozoan parasite, *Neospora Caninum*. *Infection, Genetics and Evolution* 84, 104444.

Camacho-Nuez, M., Hernandez-Silva, D.J., Castaneda-Ortiz, E.J., Paredes-Martinez, M.E., Rocha-Martinez, M.K. *et al.* (2017) Hap2, a novel gene in *Babesia bigemina* is expressed in tick stages, and specific antibodies block zygote formation. *Parasites & Vectors* 10, 568.

Chhabra, M.B. and Samantaray, S. (2013) *Sarcocystis* and sarcocystosis in India: Status and emerging perspectives. *Journal of Parasitic Diseases* 37, 1–10.

Cooke, B.M., Mohandas, N., Cowman, A.F. and Coppel, R.L. (2005) Cellular adhesive phenomena in apicomplexan parasites of red blood cells. *Veterinary Parasitology* 132, 273–295.

Cortes, H., Leitão, A., Gottstein, B. and Hemphill, A. (2014) A review on bovine besnoitiosis: A disease with economic impact in herd health management, caused by *Besnoitia besnoiti* (Franco and Borges). *Parasitology* 141, 1406–1417.

Darghouth, M.A., Boulter, N.R., Gharbi, M., Sassi, L., Tait, A. *et al.* (2006) Vaccination of calves with an attenuated cell line of *Theileria annulata* and the sporozoite antigen SPAG-1 produces a synergistic effect. *Veterinary Parasitology* 142, 54–62.

de la Fuente, J., Almazán, C., Canales, M., Pérez de la Lastra, J.M. *et al.* (2007) A ten-year review of commercial vaccine performance for control of tick infestations on cattle. *Animal Health Research Reviews* 8, 23–28.

Decker, F.C., Schnittger, L. and Florin-Christensen, M. (2018) Sarcocystis. In: Florin-Christensen, M. and Schnittger, L. (eds) *Parasitic Protozoa of Farm Animals and Pets*. Springer International Publishing, pp. 103–124.

Dhal, A.K., Pani, A., Mahapatra, R.K. and Yun, S.I. (2019) An immunoinformatics approach for design and validation of multi-subunit vaccine against *Cryptosporidium parvum*. *Immunobiology* 224, 747–757.

Di Giulio, G., Lynen, G., Morzaria, S., Oura, C. and Bishop, R. (2009) Live immunization against East Coast fever - current status. *Trends in Parasitology* 25, 85–92.

d'Oliveira, C., Feenstra, A., Vos, H., Osterhaus, A.D., Shiels, B.R. *et al.* (1997) Induction of protective immunity to *Theileria annulata* using two major merozoite surface antigens presented by different delivery systems. *Vaccine* 15, 1796–1804.

Dubey, J.P. (1983) Distribution of cysts and tachyzoites in calves and pregnant cows inoculated with *Toxoplasma gondii* oocysts. *Veterinary Parasitology* 13, 199–211.

Dubey, J.P., Buxton, D. and Wouda, W. (2006) Pathogenesis of bovine neosporosis. *Journal of Comparative Pathology* 134, 267–289.

Duffy, P.E. and Gorres, J.P. (2020) Malaria vaccines since 2000: Progress, priorities, products. *NPJ Vaccines* 5, 48.

Eamens, G.J., Bailey, G., Gonsalves, J.R. and Jenkins, C. (2013) Distribution and temporal prevalence of *Theileria orientalis* major piroplasm surface protein types in eastern Australian cattle herds. *Australian Veterinary Journal* 91, 332–340.

EFSA (2010) *Bovine besnoitiosis*: An emerging disease in Europe, p. 15. Available at: www.efsa.europa.eu

El Hussein, A.M., Hassan, S.M. and Salih, D.A. (2012) Current situation of tropical theileriosis in the Sudan. *Parasitology Research* 111, 503–508.

Fan, X.C., Liu, T.L., Wang, Y., Wu, X.M., Wang, Y.X. *et al.* (2020) Genome-wide analysis of differentially expressed profiles of mRNAs, lncRNAs and circRNAs in chickens during *Eimeria necatrix* infection. *Parasites & Vectors* 13, 167.

Fan, Y., Feng, Y. and Xiao, L. (2019) Comparative genomics: How has it advanced our knowledge of cryptosporidiosis epidemiology? *Parasitology Research* 118, 3195–3204.

Fayer, R., Guidry, A. and Blagburn, B.L. (1990) Immunotherapeutic efficacy of bovine colostral immunoglobulins from a hyperimmunized cow against cryptosporidiosis in neonatal mice. *Infection and Immunity* 58, 2962–2965.

Feng, J., Dong, X., Pinello, J., Zhang, J., Lu, C. *et al.* (2018) Fusion surface structure, function, and dynamics of gamete fusogen HAP2. *eLife* 7e39772. DOI: 10.7554/eLife.39772.

Fernández-García, A., Alvarez-García, G., Risco-Castillo, V., Aguado-Martínez, A., Marugán-Hernández, V. *et al.* (2009) Pattern of recognition of *Besnoitia besnoiti* tachyzoite and bradyzoite antigens by naturally infected cattle. *Veterinary Parasitology* 164, 104–110.

Florin-Christensen, M., Suarez, C.E., Rodriguez, A.E., Flores, D.A. and Schnittger, L. (2014) Vaccines against bovine babesiosis: Where we are now and possible roads ahead. *Parasitology* 1–30.

Florin-Christensen, M. and Schnittger, L. (eds) (2018) *Parasitic protozoa of farm animals and pets*. Springer International Publishing, New York City, NY, USA.

Franco, C.D., Wieser, S.N., Soria, M., de Alba, P., Florin-Christensen, M. *et al.* (2020) In silico identification of immunotherapeutic and diagnostic targets in the glycosylphosphatidylinositol metabolism of the coccidian *Sarcocystis aucheniae*. *Transboundary and Emerging Diseases* 67(Suppl 2), 165–174.

Frénal, K., Dubremetz, J.F., Lebrun, M. and Soldati-Favre, D. (2017) Gliding motility powers invasion and egress in apicomplexa. *Nature Reviews. Microbiology* 15, 645–660.

Fry, L.M., Schneider, D.A., Frevert, C.W., Nelson, D.D., Morrison, W.I. *et al.* (2016) East coast fever caused by *Theileria parva* is characterized by macrophage activation associated with vasculitis and respiratory failure. *PLoS One* 11, 1–20.

Fry, L.M., Bastos, R.G., Stone, B.C., Williams, L.B., Knowles, D.P. *et al.* (2019) Gene gun DNA immunization of cattle induces humoral and CD4 t-cell-mediated immune responses against the *Theileria parva* polymorphic immunodominant molecule. *Vaccine* 37(12), 1546–1553. Epub 2019 Feb 16. DOI: 10.1016/j.vaccine.2019.02.009.

Ganzinelli, S., Rodriguez, A.E., Schnittger, L. and Florin-Christensen, M. (2018) *Babesia* in domestic ruminants. In: Florin-Christensen, M. and Schnittger, L. (eds) *Parasitic Protozoa of Farm Animals and Pets*. Springer International Publishing, New York City, NY, USA, pp. 215–240.

Gharbi, M., Darghouth, M.A., Weir, W., Katzer, F., Boulter, N. *et al.* (2011) Prime-boost immunisation against tropical theileriosis with two parasite surface antigens: Evidence for protection and antigen synergy. *Vaccine* 29, 6620–6628.

Gharbi, M., Darghouth, M.A., Elati, K., Al-Hosary, A.A.T., Ayadi, O. *et al.* (2020) Current status of tropical theileriosis in Northern Africa: A review of recent epidemiological investigations and implications for control. *Transboundary and Emerging Diseases* 67(Suppl 1), 8–25.

Goff, W.L., Bastos, R.G., Brown, W.C., Johnson, W.C. and Schneider, D.A. (2010) The bovine spleen: Interactions among splenic cell populations in the innate immunologic control of hemoparasitic infections. *Veterinary Immunology and Immunopathology* 138, 1–14.

Gohil, S., Kats, L.M., Sturm, A. and Cooke, B.M. (2010) Recent insights into alteration of red blood cells by *Babesia bovis*: Moovin' forward. *Trends in Parasitology* 26, 591–599.

Gohil, S., Herrmann, S., Günther, S. and Cooke, B.M. (2013) Bovine babesiosis in the 21st century: Advances in biology and functional genomics. *International Journal for Parasitology* 43, 125–132.

Graham, S.P., Pellé, R., Honda, Y., Mwangi, D.M., Tonukari, N.J. *et al.* (2006) *Theileria parva* candidate vaccine antigens recognized by immune bovine cytotoxic T lymphocytes. In: *Proceedings of the National Academy of Sciences of the United States of America*, pp. 3286–3291 (Vol. 103).

Gwakisa, P., Kindoro, F., Mwega, E., Kimera, S., Obara, I. *et al.* (2020) Monitoring vaccinated cattle for induction and longevity of persistent tick-transmissible infection: Implications for wider deployment of live vaccination against East Coast fever in Tanzania. *Transboundary and Emerging Diseases* 67(Suppl 1), 79–87.

Hadj-Kaddour, K., Carcy, B., Vallet, A., Randazzo, S., Delbecq, S. *et al.* (2007) Recombinant protein Bd37 protected gerbils against heterologous challenges with isolates of *Babesia divergens* polymorphic for the Bd37 gene. *Parasitology* 134, 187–196.

Harding, C.R. and Frischknecht, F. (2020) The riveting cellular structures of apicomplexan parasites. *Trends in Parasitology* S1471-4922, 30241–30245.

Hayashida, K., Umemiya-Shirafuji, R., Sivakumar, T., Yamagishi, J., Suzuki, Y. *et al.* (2018) Establishment of a mouse-tick infection model for *Theileria orientalis* and analysis of its transcriptome. *International Journal for Parasitology* 48, 915–924.

Hemmink, J.D., Weir, W., MacHugh, N.D., Graham, S.P., Patel, E. *et al.* (2016) Limited genetic and antigenic diversity within parasite isolates used in a live vaccine against *Theileria parva*. *International Journal for Parasitology* 46, 495–506.

Hemphill, A., Aguado-Martínez, A. and Müller, J. (2016) Approaches for the vaccination and treatment of *Neospora caninum* infections in mice and ruminant models. *Parasitology* 143, 245–259.

Heo, I., Dutta, D., Schaefer, D.A., Iakobachvili, N., Artegiani, B. *et al.* (2018) Modelling Cryptosporidium infection in human small intestinal and lung organoids. *Nature Microbiology* 3, 814–823.

Hijjawi, N.S., Meloni, B.P., Ng'anzo, M., Ryan, U.M., Olson, M.E. *et al.* (2004) Complete development of *Cryptosporidium parvum* in host cell-free culture. *International Journal for Parasitology* 34, 769–777.

Hines, S.A., Palmer, G.H., Jasmer, D.P., Goff, W.L. and McElwain, T.F. (1995) Immunization of cattle with recombinant Babesia bovis merozoite surface antigen-1. *Infection and Immunity* 63, 349–352.

Horcajo, P., Regidor-Cerrillo, J., Aguado-Martínez, A., Hemphill, A. and Ortega-Mora, L.M. (2016) Vaccines for bovine neosporosis: Current status and key aspects for development. *Parasite Immunology* 38, 709–723.

Hosein, S., Limon, G., Dadios, N., Guitian, J. and Blake, D.P. (2016) *Toxoplasma gondii* detection in cattle: A slaughterhouse survey. *Veterinary Parasitology* 228, 126–129.

Howe, D.K., Gaji, R.Y., Marsh, A.E., Patil, B.A., Saville, W.J. *et al.* (2008) Strains of *Sarcocystis neurona* exhibit differences in their surface antigens, including the absence of the major surface antigen SnSAG1. *International Journal for Parasitology* 38, 623–631.

Hussain, M.A., Stitt, V., Szabo, E.A. and Nelan, B. (2017) *Toxoplasma gondii* in the food supply. *Pathogens (Basel, Switzerland)* 6.

Hussein, H.E., Bastos, R.G., Schneider, D.A., Johnson, W.C., Adham, F.K. *et al.* (2017) The *Babesia bovis* hap2 gene is not required for blood stage replication, but expressed upon *in vitro* sexual stage induction. *PLoS Neglected Tropical Diseases* 11, e0005965.

Innes, E.A., Panton, W.R., Sanderson, A., Thomson, K.M., Wastling, J.M. *et al.* (1995) Induction of CD4+ and CD8+ T cell responses in efferent lymph responding to *Toxoplasma gondii* infection: Analysis of phenotype and function. *Parasite Immunology* 17, 151–160.

Innes, E.A., Hamilton, C., Garcia, J.L., Chryssafidis, A. and Smith, D. (2019) A one health approach to vaccines against *Toxoplasma gondii*. *Food Waterborne Parasitol* 15, e00053.

Jaramillo-Ortiz, J.M., Paoletta, M.S., Gravisaco, M.J., López Arias, L.S., Montenegro, V.N. *et al.* (2019) Immunisation of cattle against *Babesia bovis* combining a multi-epitope modified vaccinia Ankara virus and a recombinant protein induce strong Th1 cell responses but fails to trigger neutralising antibodies required for protection. *Ticks and Tick-Borne Diseases* 10, 101270.

Jenkins, M., Higgins, J., Kniel, K., Trout, J. and Fayer, R. (2004) Protection of calves against cryptosporiosis by oral inoculation with gamma-irradiated *Cryptosporidium parvum* oocysts. *The Journal of Parasitology* 90, 1178–1180.

Johnson, W.C., Taus, N.S., Reif, K.E., Bohaliga, G.A., Kappmeyer, L.S. *et al.* (2017) Analysis of stage-specific protein expression uring *Babesia bovis* development within female *Rhipicephalus microplus*. *Journal of Proteome Research* 16, 1327–1338.

Jones, J.L. and Dubey, J.P. (2010) Waterborne toxoplasmosis--recent developments. *Experimental Parasitology* 124, 10–25.

Jonsson, N.N., Bock, R.E., Jorgensen, W.K., Morton, J.M. and Stear, M.J. (2012) Is endemic stability of tick-borne disease in cattle a useful concept? *Trends in Parasitology* 28, 85–89.

Jossé, L., Bones, A.J., Purton, T., Michaelis, M. and Tsaousis, A.D. (2019) A cell culture platform for the cultivation of *Cryptosporidium parvum*. *Current Protocols in Microbiology* 53, e80.

Kaba, S.A., Hemmes, J.C., van Lent, J.W., Vlak, J.M., Nene, V. *et al.* (2003) Baculovirus surface display of *Theileria parva* p67 antigen preserves the conformation of sporozoite-neutralizing epitopes. *Protein Engineering* 16, 73–78.

Kawamoto, S., Takahashi, K., Kurosawa, T., Sonoda, M. and Onuma, M. (1990) Intraerythrocytic schizogony of *Theileria sergenti* in cattle. *Nihon Juigaku Zasshi* 52, 1251–1259.

Kawazu, S., Sugimoto, C., Kamio, T. and Fujisaki, K. (1992) Molecular cloning and immunological analysis of immunodominant piroplasm surface proteins of *Theileria sergenti* and *T. Buffeli*. *The Journal of Veterinary Medical Science* 54, 305–311.

Keeton, S.T.N. and Navarre, C.B. (2018) Coccidiosis in large and small ruminants. *The Veterinary Clinics of North America. Food Animal Practice* 34, 201–208.

Khan, A., Fujita, A.W., Randle, N., Regidor-Cerrillo, J., Shaik, J.S. *et al.* (2019) Global selective sweep of a highly inbred genome of the cattle parasite *Neospora caninum*. In: *Proceedings of the National Academy of Sciences of the United States of America*, pp. 22764–22773 (Vol. 116).

Khukhuu, A., Lan, D.T., Long, P.T., Ueno, A., Li, Y. *et al.* (2011) Molecular epidemiological survey of *Theileria orientalis* in Thua Thien Hue Province, Vietnam. *The Journal of Veterinary Medical Science* 73, 701–705.

Klein, P., Kleinová, T., Volek, Z. and Simůnek, J. (2008) Effect of *Cryptosporidium parvum* infection on the absorptive capacity and paracellular permeability of the small intestine in neonatal calves. *Veterinary Parasitology* 152, 53–59.

Kobayashi, C., Yokoyama, H., Nguyen, S.V., Kodama, Y., Kimata, T. *et al.* (2004) Effect of egg yolk antibody on experimental *Cryptosporidium parvum* infection in scid mice. *Vaccine* 23, 232–235.

Lacasta, A., Mody, K.T., De, I., Yu, C., Zhang, J. *et al.* (2021) Synergistic effect of two nanotechnologies enhances the protective capacity of the *Theileria parva* sporozoite p67C antigen in cattle. *Journal of Immunology* 1950(206), 686–699.

Lassen, B. and Ostergaard, S. (2012) Estimation of the economical effects of *Eimeria* infections in Estonian dairy herds using a stochastic model. *Preventive Veterinary Medicine* 106, 258–265.

Lempereur, L., Larcombe, S.D., Durrani, Z., Karagenc, T., Bilgic, H.B. *et al.* (2017) Identification of candidate transmission-blocking antigen genes in *Theileria annulata* and related vector-borne apicomplexan parasites. *BMC Genomics* 18, 438.

Lindsay, D.S. and Dubey, J.P. (2020) Neosporosis, toxoplasmosis, and sarcocystosis in ruminants: An update. *The Veterinary Clinics of North America. Food Animal Practice* 36, 205–222.

Liu, L., Johnson, H.L., Cousens, S., Perin, J., Scott, S. *et al.* (2012) Global, regional, and national causes of child mortality: An updated systematic analysis for 2010 with time trends since 2000. *Lancet* 379, 2151–2161.

Liu, Y., Pei, J., Grishin, N. and Snell, W.J. (2015) The cytoplasmic domain of the gamete membrane fusion protein HAP2 targets the protein to the fusion site in *Chlamydomonas* and regulates the fusion reaction. *Development* 142, 962–971.

MacHugh, N.D., Connelley, T., Graham, S.P., Pelle, R., Formisano, P. *et al.* (2009) CD8+ T-cell responses to *Theileria parva* are preferentially directed to a single dominant antigen: Implications for parasite strain-specific immunity. *European Journal of Immunology* 39, 2459–2469.

MacHugh, N.D., Weir, W., Burrells, A., Lizundia, R., Graham, S.P. *et al.* (2011) Extensive polymorphism and evidence of immune selection in a highly dominant antigen recognized by bovine CD8 T cells specific for *Theileria annulata*. *Infection and Immunity* 79, 2059–2069.

Manque, P.A., Tenjo, F., Woehlbier, U., Lara, A.M., Serrano, M.G. *et al.* (2011) Identification and immunological characterization of three potential vaccinogens against *Cryptosporidium* species. *Clinical and Vaccine Immunology* 18, 1796–1802.

Mateus-Pinilla, N.E., Dubey, J.P., Choromanski, L. and Weigel, R.M. (1999) A field trial of the effectiveness of a feline *Toxoplasma gondii* vaccine in reducing *T. gondii* exposure for swine. *The Journal of Parasitology* 85, 855–860.

McKeever, D.J., Taracha, E.L., Innes, E.L., MacHugh, N.D., Awino, E. *et al.* (1994) Adoptive transfer of immunity to *Theileria parva* in the CD8+ fraction of responding efferent lymph. In: *Proceedings of the National Academy of Sciences of the United States of America*, pp. 1959–1963 (Vol. 91).

Mead, J.R. (2014) Prospects for immunotherapy and vaccines against *Cryptosporidium*. *Human Vaccines & Immunotherapeutics* 10, 1505–1513.

Mekata, H., Minamino, T., Mikurino, Y., Yamamoto, M., Yoshida, A. *et al.* (2018) Evaluation of the natural vertical transmission of *Theileria orientalis*. *Veterinary Parasitology* 263, 1–4.

Miller, C.M., Quinn, H.E., Windsor, P.A. and Ellis, J.T. (2002) Characterisation of the first Australian isolate of *Neospora caninum* from cattle. *Australian Veterinary Journal* 80, 620–625.

Minami, T., Nakano, T., Shimizu, S., Shimura, K., Fujinaga, T. *et al.* (1985) Efficacy of naphthoquinones and imidocarb dipropionate on *Theileria sergenti* infections in splenectomized calves. *Nihon Juigaku Zasshi* 47, 297–300.

Mine, Y. and Kovacs-Nolan, J. (2002) Chicken egg yolk antibodies as therapeutics in enteric infectious disease: A review. *Journal of Medicinal Food* 5, 159–169.

Morada, M., Lee, S., Gunther-Cummins, L., Weiss, L.M., Widmer, G. *et al.* (2016) Continuous culture of *Cryptosporidium parvum* using hollow fiber technology. *International Journal for Parasitology* 46, 21–29.

Morel, N., Mastropaolo, M., de Echaide, S.T., Signorini, M.L. and Mangold, A.J. (2019) Risks of cattle babesiosis (*Babesia bovis*) outbreaks in a semi-arid region of Argentina. *Preventive Veterinary Medicine* 170, 104747.

Morgoglione, M.E., Bosco, A., Maurelli, M.P., Alves, L.C., Saralli, G. *et al.* (2020) A 10-year surveillance of *Eimeria* spp. in cattle and buffaloes in a Mediterranean area. *Frontiers in Veterinary Science* 7, 410.

Morrison, W.I. (2009) Progress towards understanding the immunobiology of *Theileria* parasites. *Parasitology* 136, 1415–1426.

Morrison, W.I. (2015) The aetiology, pathogenesis and control of theileriosis in domestic animals. *Revue Scientifique et Technique* 34, 599–611.

Morrison, W.I. and McKeever, D.J. (2006) Current status of vaccine development against *Theileria* parasites. *Parasitology* 133(Suppl), S169–87.

Morrison, W.I., Connelley, T., Hemmink, J.D. and MacHugh, N.D. (2015) Understanding the basis of parasite strain-restricted immunity to *Theileria parva*. *Annual Review of Animal Biosciences* 3, 397–418.

Mosqueda, J., Olvera-Ramirez, A., Aguilar-Tipacamu, G. and Canto, G.J. (2012) Current advances in detection and treatment of babesiosis. *Current Medicinal Chemistry* 19, 1504–1518.

Moubri, K., Kleuskens, J., Van de Crommert, J., Scholtes, N., Van Kasteren, T. *et al.* (2018) Discovery of a recombinant *Babesia canis* supernatant antigen that protects dogs against virulent challenge infection. *Veterinary Parasitology* 249, 21–29.

Mukolwe, L.D., Odongo, D.O., Byaruhanga, C., Snyman, L.P. and Sibeko-Matjila, K.P. (2020) Analysis of p67 allelic sequences reveals a subtype of allele type 1 unique to buffalo-derived *Theileria parva* parasites from Southern Africa. *PLoS One* 15, e0231434.

Musoke, A., Rowlands, J., Nene, V., Nyanjui, J., Katende, J. *et al.* (2005) Subunit vaccine based on the p67 major surface protein of *Theileria parva* sporozoites reduces severity of infection derived from field tick challenge. *Vaccine* 23, 3084–3095.

Ndawula, C., Jr and Tabor, A.E. (2020) Cocktail anti-tick vaccines: The unforeseen constraints and approaches toward enhanced efficacies. *Vaccines (Basel)* 8, 457.

Nene, V. and Morrison, W.I. (2016) Approaches to vaccination against *Theileria parva* and *Theileria annulata*. *Parasite Immunology* 38, 724–734.

Nene, V., Gobright, E., Bishop, R. and Musoke, A. (1999) Linear peptide specificity of bovine antibody responses to p67 of *Theileria parva* and sequence diversity of implications for a vaccine linear peptide specificity of bovine antibody responses to p67 of *Theileria parva* and sequence diversity of sporozoite. *Infection and Immunity* 67, 1261–1266.

Nene, V., Bishop, R., Morzaria, S., Gardner, M.J., Sugimoto, C. *et al.* (2000) *Theileria parva* genomics reveals an atypical apicomplexan genome. *International Journal for Parasitology* 30, 465–474.

Noack, S., Chapman, H.D. and Selzer, P.M. (2019) Anticoccidial drugs of the livestock industry. *Parasitology Research* 118, 2009–2026.

Norimine, J., Mosqueda, J., Suarez, C., Palmer, G.H., McElwain, T.F. *et al.* (2003) Stimulation of T-helper cell gamma interferon and immunoglobulin G responses specific for *Babesia bovis* rhoptry-associated protein 1 (RAP-1) or a RAP-1 protein lacking the carboxy-terminal repeat region is insufficient to provide protective immunity against virulent *B. bovis* challenge. *Infection and Immunity* 71, 5021–5032.

Nyagwange, J., Nene, V., Mwalimu, S., Henson, S., Steinaa, L. *et al.* (2018) Antibodies to in silico selected GPI-anchored *Theileria parva* proteins neutralize sporozoite infection *in vitro*. *Veterinary Immunology and Immunopathology* 199, 8–14.

Nyagwange, J., Tijhaar, E., Ternette, N., Mobegi, F., Tretina, K. *et al.* (2018) Characterization of the *Theileria parva* sporozoite proteome. *International Journal for Parasitology* 48, 265–273.

Nydam, D.V., Wade, S.E., Schaaf, S.L. and Mohammed, H.O. (2001) Number of *Cryptosporidium parvum* oocysts or *Giardia* spp. cysts shed by dairy calves after natural infection. *American Journal of Veterinary Research* 62, 1612–1615.

Oakes, V.J., Yabsley, M.J., Schwartz, D., LeRoith, T., Bissett, C. *et al.* (2019) *Theileria orientalis* ikeda genotype in cattle virginia, USA. *Emerging Infectious Diseases* 25, 1653–1659.

Obara, I., Ulrike, S., Musoke, T., Spooner, P.R., Jabbar, A. *et al.* (2015) Molecular evolution of a central region containing B cell epitopes in the gene encoding the p67 sporozoite antigen within a field population of *Theileria parva*. *Parasitology Research* 114, 1729–1737.

O'Doherty, E., Sayers, R., O'Grady, L. and Shalloo, L. (2015) Effect of exposure to *Neospora caninum*, *Salmonella*, and *Leptospira interrogans* serovar Hardjo on the economic performance of Irish dairy herds. *Journal of Dairy Science* 98, 2789–2800.

Omidian, Z., Ebrahimzadeh, E., Shahbazi, P., Asghari, Z. and Shayan, P. (2014) Application of recombinant *Cryptosporidium parvum* P23 for isolation and prevention. *Parasitology Research* 113, 229–237.

Onuma, M., Kakuda, T. and Sugimoto, C. (1998) *Theileria* parasite infection in East Asia and control of the disease. *Comparative Immunology, Microbiology and Infectious Diseases* 21, 165–177.

Palmer, G.H., Machado, J., Jr., Fernandez, P., Heussler, V., Perinat, T. *et al.* (1997) Parasite-mediated nuclear factor kappaB regulation in lymphoproliferation caused by *Theileria parva* infection. In: *Proceedings of the National Academy of Sciences of the United States of America*, pp. 12527–12532 (Vol. 94).

Pérez de León, A.A., Teel, P.D., Auclair, A.N., Messenger, M.T., Guerrero, F.D. *et al.* (2012) Integrated strategy for sustainable cattle fever tick eradication in USA is required to mitigate the impact of global change. *Frontiers in Physiology* 3, 195.

Pérez de León, A.A., Mitchell R.D., 3rd, Watson, D.W. (2020) Ectoparasites of cattle. *The Veterinary Clinics of North America. Food Animal Practice* 36, 173–185.

Perryman, L.E., Kapil, S.J., Jones, M.L. and Hunt, E.L. (1999) Protection of calves against cryptosporidiosis with immune bovine colostrum induced by a *Cryptosporidium parvum* recombinant protein. *Vaccine* 17, 2142–2149.

Pipano, E. and Shkap, V. (2000) Vaccination against tropical theileriosis. In: *Annals of the New York Academy of Sciences*, Vol. 916. pp. 484–500.

Ralston, B., Thompson, R.C., Pethick, D., McAllister, T.A. and Olson, M.E. (2010) *Cryptosporidium andersoni* in Western Australian feedlot cattle. *Australian Veterinary Journal* 88, 458–460.

Ramadan, M.Y., Elmadway, R.S., Lashin, A. and Eldiarby, A. (2018) Immunization of lambs against coccidiosis by using ultraviolet irradiated *Eimeria* oocysts for the first time. *Benha Veterinary Medical Journal* 34, 246–258.

Ramakrishnan, C., Maier, S., Walker, R.A., Rehrauer, H., Joekel, D.E. *et al.* (2019) An experimental genetically attenuated live vaccine to prevent transmission of *Toxoplasma gondii* by cats. *Scientific Reports* 9, 1474.

Rathinasamy, V., Poole, W.A., Bastos, R.G., Suarez, C.E. and Cooke, B.M. (2019) Babesiosis vaccines: Lessons learned, challenges ahead, and future glimpses. *Trends in Parasitology* 35, 622–635.

Reichel, M.P. and Ellis, J.T. (2006) If control of *Neospora caninum* infection is technically feasible does it make economic sense? *Veterinary Parasitology* 142, 23–34.

Reichel, M.P., Alejandra Ayanegui-Alcérreca, M., Gondim, L.F. and Ellis, J.T. (2013) What is the global economic impact of *Neospora caninum* in cattle - the billion dollar question. *International Journal for Parasitology* 43, 133–142.

Reichel, M.P., Moore, D.P., Hemphill, A., Ortega-Mora, L.M., Dubey, J.P. *et al.* (2015) A live vaccine against *Neospora caninum* abortions in cattle. *Vaccine* 33, 1299–1301.

Robinson, G. and Chalmers, R.M. (2020) Preparation of *Cryptosporidium* DNA for whole genome sequencing. *Methods in Molecular Biology* 2052, 129–138.

Rodriguez, A.E., Schnittger, L., Tomazic, M.L. and Florin-Christensen, M. (2012) Current and prospective tools for the control of cattle-infecting *Babesia* parasites. In: Castillo, V. and Harris, R. (eds) *Protozoa: Biology, Classification and Role in Disease*. Nova Publishers, New York City, NY, USA, pp. 1–44.

Rojas, C., Figueroa, J.V., Alvarado, A., Mejia, P., Mosqueda, J.J. *et al.* (2006) Bovine babesiosis live vaccine production: Use of gamma irradiation on the substrate. *Annals of the New York Academy of Sciences* 1081, 405–416.

Romero, J.J., Pérez, E. and Frankena, K. (2004) Effect of a killed whole *Neospora caninum* tachyzoite vaccine on the crude abortion rate of Costa Rican dairy cows under field conditions. *Veterinary Parasitology* 123, 149–159.

Salomaki, E.D. and Kolisko, M. (2019) There is treasure everywhere: Reductive plastid evolution in apicomplexa in light of their close relatives. *Biomolecules* 9(8): 378. DOI: 10.3390/biom9080378.

Sánchez-Sánchez, R., Vázquez, P., Ferre, I. and Ortega-Mora, L.M. (2018) Treatment of toxoplasmosis and neosporosis in farm ruminants: State of knowledge and future trends. *Current Topics in Medicinal Chemistry* 18, 1304–1323.

Sant, C., d'Abadie, R., Pargass, I., Basu, A.K., Asgarali, Z. *et al.* (2016) Prospective study investigating transplacental transmission of equine piroplasmosis in thoroughbred foals in Trinidad. *Veterinary Parasitology* 226, 132–137.

Santín, M. (2013) Clinical and subclinical infections with *Cryptosporidium* in animals. *New Zealand Veterinary Journal* 61, 1–10.

Schetters, T.P. and Montenegro-James, S. (1995) Vaccines against babesiosis using soluble parasite antigens. *Parasitology Today* 11, 456–462.

Schetters, T.P., Moubri, K. and Cooke, B.M. (2009) Comparison of *Babesia rossi* and *Babesia canis* isolates with emphasis on effects of vaccination with soluble parasite antigens: A review. *Journal of the South African Veterinary Association* 80, 75–78.

Schnittger, L. and Florin-Christensen, M. (2018) Introduction into parasitic protozoa. In: *Parasitic protozoa of farm animals and pets*. Springer International Publishing, New York City, NY, USA, p. 438.

Schnittger, L., Rodriguez, A.E., Florin-Christensen, M. and Morrison, D.A. (2012) Babesia: A world emerging. *Infection, Genetics and Evolution* 12, 1788–09.

Shaw, M.K., Tilney, L.G., Musoke, A.J. and Teale, A.J. (1995) MHC class I molecules are an essential cell surface component involved in *Theileria parva* sporozoite binding to bovine lymphocytes. *Journal of Cell Science* 108(Pt 4), 1587–1596.

Shirley, M.W., Smith, A.L. and Tomley, F.M. (2005) The biology of avian *Eimeria* with an emphasis on their control by vaccination. *Advances in Parasitology* 60, 285–330.

Shkap, V., Ungar-Waron, H., Pipano, E. and Greenblatt, C. (1985) Specific antibodies to *Besnoitia besnoiti* precipitated from serum of cattle by live parasites and by soluble antigen. *Veterinary Immunology and Immunopathology* 9, 53–57.

Sivakumar, T., Hayashida, K., Sugimoto, C. and Yokoyama, N. (2014) Evolution and genetic diversity of *Theileria*. *Infection, Genetics and Evolution* 27, 250–263.

Skallová, A., Kodym, P., Frynta, D. and Flegr, J. (2006) The role of dopamine in Toxoplasma-induced behavioural alterations in mice: An ethological and ethopharmacological study. *Parasitology* 133(5), 525–535. DOI: 10.1017/S0031182006000886.

Soutter, F., Werling, D., Tomley, F.M. and Blake, D.P. (2020) Poultry Coccidiosis: Design and interpretation of vaccine studies. *Frontiers in Veterinary Science* 7, 101.

Suarez, C.E., Alzan, H.F. and Cooke, B.M. Florin-Christensen, M. and Schnittger, L. (eds). (2018) *Genomics and genetic manipulation of protozoan parasites affecting farm animals*. Springer International Publishing, New York City, NY, USA, pp. 413–438.

Sudan, V., Singh, S.K., Jaiswal, A.K., Parashar, R. and Shanker, D. (2015) First molecular evidence of the transplacental transmission of *Theileria annulata*. *Tropical Animal Health and Production* 47, 1213–1215.

Suijkerbuijk, A.W.M., van Gils, P.F., Bonačić Marinović, A.A., Feenstra, T.L., Kortbeek, L.M. *et al.* (2018) The design of a social cost-benefit analysis of preventive interventions for *Toxoplasmosis*: An example of the one health approach. *Zoonoses and Public Health* 65, 185–194.

Sultana, R., Maqbool, A., Ahmad, M.-U.-D., Anjum, A.A., Ch, S.I. *et al.* (2014) Control of Coccidiosis in calves by vaccination. *Journal of Bacteriology and Parsitology* 5, 4. DOI: 10.4172/2155-9597.1000197.

Svensson, C., Olofsson, H. and Uggla, A. (1996) Immunisation of calves against *Eimeria alabamensis* coccidiosis. *Applied Parasitology* 37, 209–216.

Svitek, N., Saya, R., Awino, E., Munyao, S., Muriuki, R. *et al.* (2018) An ad/MVA vectored *Theileria parva* antigen induces schizont-specific CD8(+) central memory T cells and confers partial protection against a lethal challenge. *NPJ Vaccines* 3, 35.

Taracha, E.L., Goddeeris, B.M., Morzaria, S.P. and Morrison, W.I. (1995) Parasite strain specificity of precursor cytotoxic T cells in individual animals correlates with cross-protection in cattle challenged with *Theileria parva*. *Infection and Immunity* 63, 1258–1262.

Thompson, A.T., White, S., Shaw, D., Egizi, A., Lahmers, K. *et al.* (2020) *Theileria orientalis* Ikeda in host-seeking *Haemaphysalis longicornis* in Virginia, U.S.A.Ticks and Tick-Borne Diseases 11:101450.

Tomazic, M.L., Garro, C.J. and Schnittger, L. Florin-Christensen, M. and Schnittger, L. (eds). (2018) *Cryptosporidium*. Springer International Publishing, New York City, NY, USA, pp. 11–54.

Tomazic, M.L., Rodriguez, A.E., Lombardelli, J., Poklepovich, T., Garro, C. *et al.* (2018) Identification of novel vaccine candidates against cryptosporidiosis of neonatal bovines by reverse vaccinology. *Veterinary Parasitology* 264, 74–78.

Tonui, T., Corredor-Moreno, P., Kanduma, E., Njuguna, J., Njahira, M.N. *et al.* (2018) Transcriptomics reveal potential vaccine antigens and a drastic increase of upregulated genes during *Theileria parva* development from arthropod to bovine infective stages. *PLoS One* 13, e0204047.

Trotz-Williams, L.A., Jarvie, B.D., Peregrine, A.S., Duffield, T.F. and Leslie, K.E. (2011) Efficacy of halofuginone lactate in the prevention of cryptosporidiosis in dairy calves. *The Veterinary Record* 168, 509.

Uilenberg, G., Perié, N.M., Spanjer, A.A. and Franssen, F.F. (1985) *Theileria orientalis*, a cosmopolitan blood parasite of cattle: Demonstration of the schizont stage. *Research in Veterinary Science* 38, 352–360.

Vega, C.G., Bok, M., Ebinger, M., Rocha, L.A., Rivolta, A.A. *et al.* (2020) A new passive immune strategy based on IgY antibodies as a key element to control neonatal calf diarrhea in dairy farms. *BMC Veterinary Research* 16, 264.

Verma, S.K., Lindsay, D.S., Grigg, M.E. and Dubey, J.P. (2017) Isolation, culture and cryopreservation of *Sarcocystis* species. *Current Protocols in Microbiology* 45(20d.21), 21–27.

Veronesi, F., Diaferia, M., Viola, O. and Fioretti, D.P. (2011) Long-term effect of toltrazuril on growth performances of dairy heifers and beef calves exposed to natural *Eimeria zuernii* and *Eimeria bovis* infections. *Veterinary Journal* 190, 296–299.

Veronesi, F., Nisoli, L., Diaferia, M., Falcini, R., Ficola, E. *et al.* (2013) Influence of a metaphylactic treatment with Baycox(®) Bovis on the reproductive performances of *Fresian heifers*: A preliminary study. *Parasitology Research* 112, 2137–2142.

Ververken, C., Geysen, D., Loots, K., Janssens, M.E., Guisez, Y. *et al.* (2008) Orientation of bovine CTL responses towards PIM, an antibody-inducing surface molecule of *Theileria parva*, by DNA subunit immunization. *Veterinary Immunology and Immunopathology* 124, 253–263.

Vinayak, S., Pawlowic, M.C., Sateriale, A., Brooks, C.F., Studstill, C.J. *et al.* (2015) Genetic modification of the diarrhoeal pathogen *Cryptosporidium parvum*. *Nature* 523, 477–480.

Wang, S. and Suo, X. (2020) Still naïve or primed: Anticoccidial vaccines call for memory. *Experimental Parasitology* 216, 107945.

Watts, J.G., Playford, M.C. and Hickey, K.L. (2016) *Theileria orientalis*: A review. *New Zealand Veterinary Journal* 64, 3–9.

Weston, J.F., Heuer, C. and Williamson, N.B. (2012) Efficacy of a *Neospora caninum* killed tachyzoite vaccine in preventing abortion and vertical transmission in dairy cattle. *Preventive Veterinary Medicine* 103, 136–144.

Williams, D.J., Guy, C.S., Smith, R.F., Ellis, J., Björkman, C. *et al.* (2007) Immunization of cattle with live tachyzoites of *Neospora caninum* confers protection against fetal death. *Infection and Immunity* 75, 1343–1348.

Williamson, S., Tait, A., Brown, D., Walker, A., Beck, P. *et al.* (1989) *Theileria annulata* sporozoite surface antigen expressed in *Escherichia coli* elicits neutralizing antibody. In: *Proceedings of the National Academy of Sciences of the United States of America*, pp. 4639–4643 (Vol. 86).

Yeruham, I., Avidar, Y., Aroch, I. and Hadani, A. (2003) Intra-uterine infection with *Babesia bovis* in a 2-day-old Calf. *Journal of Veterinary Medicine. B, Infectious Diseases and Veterinary Public Health* 50, 60–62.

Yin, H., Luo, J. and Lu, W. (2008) Control of tropical *Theileriosis* with attenuated schizont vaccine in China. *Vaccine* 26(Suppl 6), G11–3.

Zahedi, A. and Ryan, U. (2020) *Cryptosporidium* - an update with an emphasis on foodborne and waterborne transmission. *Research in Veterinary Science* 132, 500–512.

Zambriski, J.A., Nydam, D.V., Bowman, D.D., Bellosa, M.L., Burton, A.J. *et al.* (2013) Description of fecal shedding of *Cryptosporidium parvum* oocysts in experimentally challenged dairy calves. *Parasitology Research* 112, 1247–1254.

Zambriski, J.A., Nydam, D.V., Wilcox, Z.J., Bowman, D.D., Mohammed, H.O. *et al.* (2013) *Cryptosporidium parvum*: Determination of ID_{50} and the dose-response relationship in experimentally challenged dairy calves. *Veterinary Parasitology* 197, 104–112.

Zhang, Z.-X., Ma, Y., Wang, H., Arp, J., Jiang, J. *et al.* (2010) This information is current as of October 7, 2010. *The Journal of Immunology*.

19 Impacts of COVID-19 on Agriculture and Food Security in Developing Countries: Potential Mitigation Strategies

Kehinde O. Erinle[1*], Matthew C. Ogwu[2,3], Smith E. Evivie[4,5,6], Muhammad S. Zaheer[7,8], Solabomi O. Ogunyemi[9] and Samson O. Adeniran[10]

[1]School of Agriculture, Food and Wine, The University of Adelaide, Australia, South Austrialia, Urrbrae SA 5064; [2]Department of Plant Biology and Biotechnology, Faculty of Life Sciences, University of Benin, Ugbowo, Benin City, PMB 1154, Edo State, Nigeria; [3]School of Biosciences and Veterinary Medicine, University of Camerino – Center for Floristic Research of the Apennine, 67021, L'Aquila, Italy; [4]Key Laboratory of Dairy Science, Ministry of Education, College of Food Science, Northeast Agricultural University, Harbin, 150030, China; [5]Department of Animal Science, Faculty of Agriculture, University of Benin, Benin City, 300001, Nigeria; [6]Department of Food Science and Human Nutrition, Faculty of Agriculture, University of Benin, Benin City, 300001, Edo State, Nigeria; [7]Department of Agricultural Engineering, Khwaja Fareed University of Engineering and Information Technology, Rahim Yar Khan, 64200, Pakistan; [8]Department of Agronomy, University College of Agriculture and Environmental Sciences, Islamia University of Bahawalpur, 63100, Pakistan; [9]State Key Laboratory of Rice Biology, Ministry of Agriculture Key Lab of Molecular Biology of Crop Pathogens and Insects, Institute of Biotechnology, Zhejiang University, Hangzhou, 310058, China; [10]Department of Animal Genetics, Breeding and Reproduction, College of Animal Science and Technology, Northeast Agricultural University, Harbin, 150030, China

Abstract

Despite efforts to reduce global food insecurity, success has been limited in many developing countries due to numerous inherent problems. The challenges and vulnerabilities associated with food security in these countries have been exacerbated by the current coronavirus (COVID-19) pandemic. As a rapid response strategy to minimize the coronavirus' spread, countries have put in place different forms of movement restrictions, locally and globally, which have therefore affected agricultural production, food availability, and accessibility. Focusing on the four pillars of food security, this paper provides an overview of the pandemic's impacts on food availability, accessibility, utilization, and stability drawing examples from different developing countries. The report also suggests some response strategies that could be adopted or (where already in existence) strengthened to promote food security in developing countries, during and after a pandemic/crisis. The strategies of major concern to ensure continued availability and accessibility of food during and after a pandemic/crisis include (i) establishment of

*Corresponding author: kehinde.erinle@adelaide.edu.au

community-based food networks, (ii) food and agriculture data collection and maintenance, (iii) stabilizing food prices, (iv) infrastructural development for food security, (v) increasing investment in agricultural research and policies, (vi) adopting modern farming practices, and (vii) reduction and management of agricultural and food waste.

Keywords: agricultural facilities, COVID-19, developing countries, food security, food system protection, social distancing

Review Methodology

Academic search engines and databases such as Google Scholar, Scopus, ProQuest, Web of Science, and CAB Abstracts were utilized to discover a broad range of literature cited.

Introduction

More than 80% of the world's population is resident in underdeveloped and developing countries with long-term incidences of food insecurity (Alvaredo and Gasparini, 2015). Most of these countries are part of the 'Global South' characterized by developing economic and political systems (Mitlin and Satterthwaite, 2013; Wolvers *et al.*, 2015). As opined by Drazen (2008), key political and economic mechanisms, issues, features, and models differ in developed and developing countries. According to the World Bank classification (World Bank, 2020), countries with gross national income (GNI) per capita below the threshold of $ 12,535 are described as 'developing.' These countries are mostly those from the six geographical regions of East Asia and the Pacific, South Asia, Latin America and the Caribbean, Sub-Saharan Africa, Middle East and North Africa, and Eastern Europe and Central Asia. Therefore, by *developing countries*, the emphasis is placed on countries from these regions identified by the World Bank and characterized by an industrially underdeveloped and developing base with a low Human Development Index (HDI) relative to other countries (O'Sullivan and Sheffrin, 2003). Food insecurity is a global problem, but the effects are more evident in developing countries. According to a global survey (Smith and Meade, 2019), heightened food insecurity was noted among developing countries of Sub-Saharan Africa, Latin America and the Caribbean, and South Asia, compared to countries from other regions (Table 19.1). Food insecurity in most developing countries may be caused by the incidence of natural disaster, war and civil conflict, poor health, dysfunctional food markets, inequality, partial or permanent unemployment, changes in social and economic factors, hike in food prices, and poor allocation of food resources (Smith *et al.*, 2000; Kah, 2017; Firdaus *et al.*, 2019). As suggested by Smith *et al.* (2000), these causes may be summarized

Table 19.1. Food insecurity and severe food insecurity rates in 2017 by regions (%) (source: USDA, Economic Research Service using data from the 2017 Gallup World Poll) (Smith and Meade, 2019).

Region	Food insecurity	Severe food insecurity
Sub-Saharan Africa	55	28
Latin America and Caribbean	32	12
South Asia	30	13
Middle East and North Africa	20	7
East Asia and Pacific	13	4
North America	12	3
Europe and Central Asia	11	2
Worldwide	26	11

as insufficient availability and accessibility to food by households and individuals. Fukuda-Parr and Orr (2014) opined that food insecurity is a food distribution problem but not of production, of accessibility but not of supply. Although strategies to increase food availability are being explored in developing countries, food availability does not always guarantee accessibility. Despite attempts by different initiatives, such as the United Nations Millennium Development Goals (UN-MDGs) and the Sustainable Development Goals (SDGs) to eradicate poverty, hunger, and food insecurity, particularly in developing countries, success has been marginal at best. For example, at the end of the 15 year UN-MDGs plan of September 2000, the report observed only about 8.1% poverty reduction in Africa from 1990 to 2013 (D'Alessandro and Zulu, 2017). Moreover, funding for longer-term food security programs has declined, concurrent with a significant increase in emergency food aid (Fukuda-Parr and Orr, 2014). According to an FAO final report appraising the success of the MDG Target 1, only a few regions have been able to halve the population of undernourished individuals (Fig. 19.1). As a successor to the MDGs, the SDGs aim to promote sustainable agriculture by 2030 (FAO, 2015; Pérez-Escamilla, 2017). This, however, offers new opportunities but also challenges to developing nations (Otekunrin *et al.*, 2020). More importantly, the overreliance on external aid for food security and improvement of agricultural systems in developing countries will continue to expose them to external forces beyond their control, especially in times of crisis (such as COVID-19) when major donor countries choose to prioritize their internal food security and agricultural systems.

Food security exists when there is physical and economic access to sufficient, safe, and nutritious food to meet an individual/household's dietary needs for an active and healthy

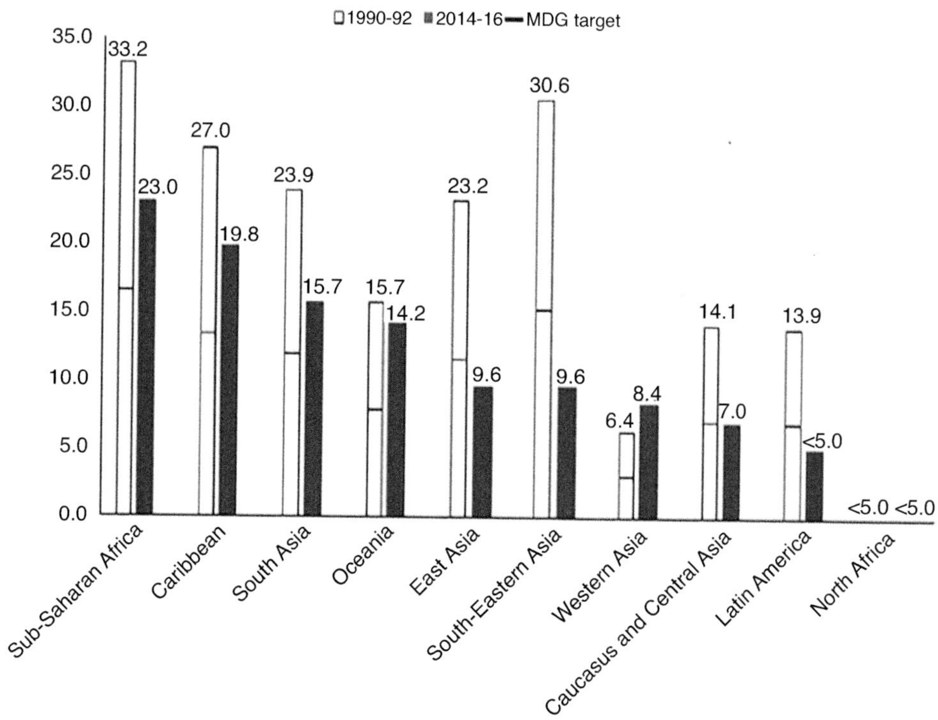

Fig. 19.1. Undernourishment by regions (%) (source: FAO 2016, Asia Pacific Commission on Agricultural Statistics, Agenda Item 6.4).

life (IFPRI, 2020). Food security is based on four pillars: availability, accessibility, utilization, and stability (Charlton, 2016).

Food availability is concerned with the amount of safe and nutritious food, which is a function of production, stock, and net trade (Gross *et al.*, 2000; Gregory *et al.*, 2005; FAO, 2008). Food distribution is a crucial factor for availability, as the majority of agricultural products are produced in rural areas by smallholder and low-income farmers and will need to be transported to other regions. Food availability may not always translate to accessibility. Food accessibility refers to the affordability, allocation, and preferences for good-quality and nutritious food in sufficient quantity (Schmidhuber and Tubiello, 2007; Gebremariam *et al.*, 2017). It is a measure of the capability to secure food entitlements, which are defined as the set of resources (including legal, political, economic, and social) needed to obtain access to good-quality and nutritious food (Kayser *et al.*, 2014; Sage, 2014). Poor households are often unable to access food, even at a lower cost, and these households constitute the majority in developing countries. Food utilization entails the biological capability to make use of food for a productive and healthy life (FAO, 2006; FAO, 2008). Food utilization also depends on the benefits derivable from the consumption of food and may be correlated with its nutritional status. Proper food utilization can result in improved health and well-being of an individual or a household. Individuals with health challenges may find it difficult to utilize certain food, thus limiting the ability of the body to absorb nutrients, resulting in further health problems or malnutrition (Portier *et al.*, 2013; Jones, 2018).

Food stability, which is the continued access to adequate food at all times (FAO, 2006), is intricately linked to the availability, accessibility, and utilization dimensions of food security. Therefore, food instability involves inadequate availability and accessibility to adequate food (FAO, 2008; Schleifer and Sun, 2020). Instability in agri- and food markets that may arise from civil conflicts, economic crises, natural or human-made disasters, and health-related pandemics (such as the current incidence of the coronavirus disease) can cause increase in food prices resulting in temporary food instability (Ecker and Breisinger, 2012; FAO, 2019). In the later section discussing the exacerbating influence of COVID-19 on food insecurity in developing countries, the effect of the pandemic on food stability is discussed in the light of the other three dimensions of food security.

Methods and Organization

This paper is written as a narrative assessment of the impacts of the coronavirus (COVID-19) pandemic on food security and agricultural production in developing countries. The literature reviewed was published between 2000 and 2020, with only a few works preceding this period, carefully selected as the foundation for this review. Academic search engines and databases such as Google Scholar, Scopus, ProQuest, Web of Science, and CAB Abstracts were utilized to discover a broad range of literature cited. Some of the key terms that were used to obtain research data, among others, were 'COVID-19', 'Food Security Developing Countries,' and 'COVID-19 Food Security'. Based on these data, the work discusses several points that relate to the impacts of COVID-19 on agricultural systems and food security, emphasizing developing countries. The work is divided into three sections, with each section reviewing critical thematic areas.

The first section summarizes an up-to-date incidence of COVID-19 in some regions of developing countries and informs on strategies put in place to curtail the spread of the virus. The second section addresses the exacerbating influence of the COVID-19 pandemic on food insecurity in developing countries, using the known factors of food security (availability, accessibility, and utilization) as determinants. The review climaxes with some possible actions that can be taken by the government, stakeholders, and individuals to mitigate food insecurity as well as to improve the agricultural systems in developing countries post-COVID-19 pandemic. The paper considers the prevailing pandemic situation and suggests possible mitigating strategies in the case of a near-future occurrence of a pandemic or global crisis.

Incidence and Prevalence of COVID-19 in Developing Countries

The coronavirus disease (COVID-19) was first discovered in Wuhan, the capital and major trade city of Hubei province, China, in December 2019 (Luo *et al.*, 2020; Guo *et al.*, 2020; Rothan and Byrareddy, 2020). On March 11, 2020, the World Health Organization (WHO) declared COVID-19 a pandemic, having met the epidemiological criteria of infecting more than 100,000 people in more than 100 countries with a remarkable infection speed (Ohia *et al.*, 2020; Kakodkar and Kaka, 2020). To date, there have been cases of the disease in about 218 countries and independent territories around the world. At the subregional level, countries of the Middle East and North Africa recorded the first occurrence of COVID-19 in late February in Iran, and as of May 6, 2020, all of the 22 countries of the region had reported cases of infection (Sharifi *et al.*, n.d.). Fortunately, these countries have received support from the United Nations and other international agencies in the form of capacity building and hospital equipment and preparedness (Karamouzian and Madani, 2020). In addition, they have also received financial aid of about 247 million USD from the WHO to combat the coronavirus disease (WHO, 2020). Among the countries in South Asia, Pakistan confirmed the first two cases of COVID-19 on February 26, 2020, in Karachi and Islamabad (Ali, 2020). As of November 22, 2020, there were 371,508 confirmed cases in the country, with about 7603 deaths (Luo *et al.*, 2020). As a response strategy, the Pakistani Ministry of Health declared new guidelines for its control following the WHO recommendations (Khan *et al.*, 2020; Waris *et al.*, 2020). In India, the first reported case of COVID-19 was on January 30, 2020, in Kerala (Kotwal *et al.*, 2020). By November 22, 2020, they had recorded about 9,095,806 confirmed cases with about 133,227 deaths (Handley, 2020). Given the large population of over 1.3 billion, the government's first response to limit the spread of the coronavirus disease was to declare a lockdown across the country (Nair *et al.*, 2020), and a ban was placed on nonessential traveling. Africa recorded the first case on February 14, 2020; in Egypt, and as of November 22, 2020, the number of confirmed cases had risen to 1,446,041, with 32,538 deaths across the continent (Abdul Rahman, 2020). In response to the pandemic, the Africa Centre for Disease Control and Prevention established the Africa Task Force for Novel Coronavirus in order to strengthen the communication and establishment of trust and unity of purpose with the African governments (WHO, 2020). The first case of COVID-19 in the Latin America and the Caribbean was reported in late February in Brazil, and since then, reported cases in the region had continued to increase. However, as a means to suppress the further spreading of the disease, the Brazilian Society for Infectious Diseases has developed technical recommendations (da Cunha *et al.*, 2020; Rodriguez-Morales *et al.*, 2020).

Children and young adults aged below 40 years have been suggested to have a relatively lower risk of death from COVID-19, compared to older (>50 years) individuals whose higher mortality rate is attributed to their compromised immune systems (Akbar and Gilroy, 2020; Lewnard and Lo, 2020; Sariol and Perlman, 2020; Stein, 2020). Given the initial absence of pharmaceutical mediations for COVID-19, all countries, including the developing ones, have implemented a social distancing method and the use of personal protective equipment to limit the spread of the disease. COVID-19 has led to the shutdown of major places of gathering, such as religious places of worship, restaurants, public markets and squares, and, in some places, schools. Also, the complete or partial restriction of movement (lockdown) was imposed in different countries. However, such measures have disrupted the internal food supply chains, halted food production, and destabilized food prices.

How COVID-19 Exacerbates Food Insecurity in Developing Countries

Impacts on food availability

Globalization has resulted in greater availability and diversity of food. This was made possible through increased urbanization, wages/incomes, market liberalization, and foreign direct investment. Globalization has also brought significant changes to food availability by influencing production, processing, and distribution/marketing. In developing countries, the larger parts of the food supply chains are coordinated by Small and Medium Enterprises (SMEs) and local manufacturers (Kot, 2018). For example, in Nigeria, processed foods contributed to about 50–90% of the total nutrient intake of individuals between 20 and 40 years of age (Reardon *et al.*, 2003; Olayiwola *et al.*, 2004). In most developing countries, phenomenal growth has been observed in supermarket sales and the number of fast-food restaurants in the last 30 years (Reardon and Hopkins, 2006), highlighting their importance in the food supply chain.

However, crises, such as COVID-19 that destabilize food supply chains and therefore food availability, have created a food crisis for many households and individuals. Since the incidence of COVID-19, (food) movement and importation have been halted due to territorial border closures, consequently resulting in the reduction of food exportation by industrial (George, 2020; Hailu, 2020; Udmale *et al.*, 2020) and developing countries. Locally, COVID-19 has disrupted the food supply chains, particularly in developing countries. In India, about 80% of food consumed is purchased, and about 90% of purchases are from SMEs (Reardon *et al.*, 2020). However, the lockdown and restriction of movement in the country have left many households and individuals with no food or to consume low-quality foods (Harris *et al.*, 2020). In Pakistan, a survey of the impact of the COVID-19 pandemic on activities of SMEs showed that over 83% of businesses were negatively affected by the pandemic. More than two-thirds of the respondents indicated that they could not survive if the coronavirus-induced lockdown persisted (Shafi *et al.*, 2020). In many developing countries, COVID-19 has limited farmers' access to markets to buy and/or sell products, as well as restrained the supply of farm inputs. For example in Ethiopia, vegetable farmers recorded an increase in farm losses together with a shortage of inputs and labor (Tamru *et al.*, 2020). Also in India, there was a reduction in produce demand, an increase in retail prices of vegetables, and difficulty in finding harvest labor and transportation to the market (Harris *et al.*, 2020; Pothan *et al.*, 2020).

The COVID-19 pandemic has significantly negated food availability efforts in developing countries that are just recovering from a natural disaster. An example is the recent locust infestation on farms in East Africa, where COVID-19–imposed movement restrictions frustrated efforts to eliminate the pests. According to FAO (2020), at least 10 million people in this region were already food insecure. Further, in the middle of the COVID-19–imposed movement restrictions, Kenya suffered a severe flash flood that caused the displacement of over 500 families (Kibet, 2020). Also, many countries in Southern Africa are currently struggling with poor corn production due to drought and pests (USDA, 2020). India, with yearly recurring incidences of hydrometeorological disasters (flood, cyclone, and landslide) resulting in the displacement of villages and destruction of farmlands, coupled with the present COVID-19 pandemic, is currently experiencing operational difficulties and unable to cope with food security (Saibal, 2020).

Effects on food accessibility

There is the potential for a 'crisis within a crisis' in which a hunger crisis could further complicate the ongoing health crises due to the COVID-19 pandemic and further complicate post–COVID-19 recovery efforts (Otekunrin and Otekunrin, 2020). Already, the UN has declared the incidence of COVID-19 in food insecure nations a 'crisis within a crisis' because these countries were already at the end of the hunger spectrum and are less well equipped to fend off the disease (Bennett *et al.*, 2020; UN News, 2020). This is worrisome as food-insecure households and individuals are more likely to be less immune to the virus (Hossain, 2020; Jayawardena and Misra, 2020; Jayawardena *et al.*, 2020; Naja and Hamadeh, 2020).

At the beginning of the COVID-19 pandemic, foodstuffs were fast disappearing from supermarket shelves due to panic buying and fear that these items may not be available or may increase in price when available (Taras, 2005; Ke and Ford-Jones, 2015; Kathiresan *et al.*, 2020; Glauber *et al.*, 2020; Competitive Commission, 2020; Hossain, 2020; Hirvonen *et al.*, 2021). This exacerbated challenges linked to food accessibility, particularly for households with insufficient financial power in developing countries. Moreover, in response to the pandemic, many countries around the world enacted measures to maintain internal stock. These measures are already having negative impacts on the supply of fruits and vegetables to developing countries (Naja and Hamadeh, 2020; Glauber *et al.*, 2020; Glauber *et al.*, 2020). To ease their financial burden during this pandemic, many agriculture and food processing industries, particularly in developing countries, have opted to reduce their workforce (Hossain, 2020), further increasing the number of unemployed persons.

Unemployment has been a major challenge faced by countries, including developing countries. This has been worsened by the ongoing coronavirus disease (Blustein, 2020; Woolhandler and Himmelstein, 2020). Unemployment will result in a significant reduction in food accessibility due to lost purchasing power (Barua, 2020). For example, before the incidence of COVID-19, Nigeria's total unemployment rate in 2018 increased by 4.3%, with a forecasted 33.5% unemployment rate by 2020 (NBS, 2020). However, with the incidence of coronavirus disease in Nigeria, the situation has gotten worse with an anticipated 39.4 million job losses by December 2020 and a 3.4% economic contraction (The World Bank, 2020). In November 2020, the Nigerian economy slumped into recession based on cumulative GDP figures for the first nine months of the year (Nairametrics, 2021). This had earlier been forecasted by the World Bank Nigeria Development and is the second recession in 5 years and the worst since the 1980s (The World Bank Nigeria Development Update, 2020).

Instability in food prices has resulted in market disruptions and negatively impacted on food accessibility. During a crisis, major factors that are likely to (directly or indirectly) induce a hike in food prices, as experienced during this COVID-19 pandemic, include reduction in supply where demand is ever increasing, hoarding where food is available and accessible, fluctuation in the dollar exchange rate resulting in increased prices of imported foods, and lower oil prices due to crisis-induced drop in mobility and industrial activity (Mogues, 2020). The effects of unstable food prices in some developing countries have been documented by Robles and Torero (2010) to include economic, social, and health dimensions. Prolonged denial of access to good-quality and nutritious food and a shift to cheaper, less nutritious food could lead to malnutrition and further exacerbate disease incidences (Reardon *et al.*, 2021).

Effects on food utilization

Malnutrition, caused by the consumption of diets deficient in micronutrients, macronutrients, or both, is a major public health problem throughout developing countries (FAO, 2002; Millward and Jackson, 2004; FAO, 2004; Müller and Krawinkel, 2005). It is also the most important contributor to poor health, disease prevalence, and even higher child mortality in developing countries (Nemer *et al.*, 2001; Müller *et al.*, 2003; FAO, 2004). Significant contributors to malnutrition in developing countries include poor economic conditions, poor public health infrastructure, and the absence of social welfare programs (Bhagat *et al.*, 2020; Ozili, 2020). According to Tebeje and Bikes (Tebeje *et al.*, 2017), individuals or households that experience instability in food availability, accessibility, and utilization are more vulnerable to malnutrition. The incidence of COVID-19 has only compounded the problems of malnutrition. For example, recent evidence examining adults infected with COVID-19 has indicated a significant impact of malnutrition on health outcomes (Bencivenga *et al.*, 2020; Handu *et al.*, 2020; Li *et al.*, 2020).

While the impact of the coronavirus disease is significant in individuals with compromised immune systems, the consumption of vitamin-rich, trace elements, and fermented foods could help to boost the immune system to resist viral and other infectious diseases (Gibson, 2012; Zabetakis *et al.*, 2020; Calder, 2020; Arshad *et al.*, 2020; Jayawardena *et al.*, 2020). According to the WHO dietary recommendations to optimize the nutritional requirements during the COVID-19 pandemic, individuals and households have been advised to take four servings of fruits and five servings of vegetables per day, in addition to a combination of whole-grain cereals (180 g), meat, and beans (160 g) (WHO, 2020). However, for poor households and individuals in developing countries, consumption of such healthy diet as suggested by the WHO during this period of lockdown could be a tremendous challenge. Poor families and individuals are more likely to consume low-quality diets, particularly during this period. Butler and Barrientos (2020) pointed out that the consumption of high saturated fatty foods and 'Western diets' (containing high amounts of refined carbohydrates and sugars, unsaturated fats, and low fiber content) increased macrophage infiltration to the alveoli. This is important to patients of the coronavirus disease since the virus also contributes to the inflammation of lung tissues and alveolar damage (Xu *et al.*, 2020). Among an African and Latino population, obese individuals and those with type two diabetes were observed to be most affected by the coronavirus disease due to an already compromised immune system (Cai *et al.*, 2020; Dietz and Santos-Burgoa, 2020). Also, Lighter *et al.* (2020) found an increased risk of COVID-19 susceptibility in obese patients under 60 years of age. As the food insecurity status of poor families worsens, these families may find it increasingly difficult to eat well and stay healthy as the pandemic lingers.

A healthy lifestyle framework has been proposed to enhance individual physical and mental health during the COVID-19 pandemic by stressing the interplay between healthy personal activities, proactive community campaigns, and aggressive national policies to ensure food security at all levels (Fig. 19.2).

Potential Strategies to Mitigate Food Insecurity During and After a Crisis

The incidence of a global or national crisis affects access to agricultural resources, food products, farmlands, and farming activities, particularly in developing countries where

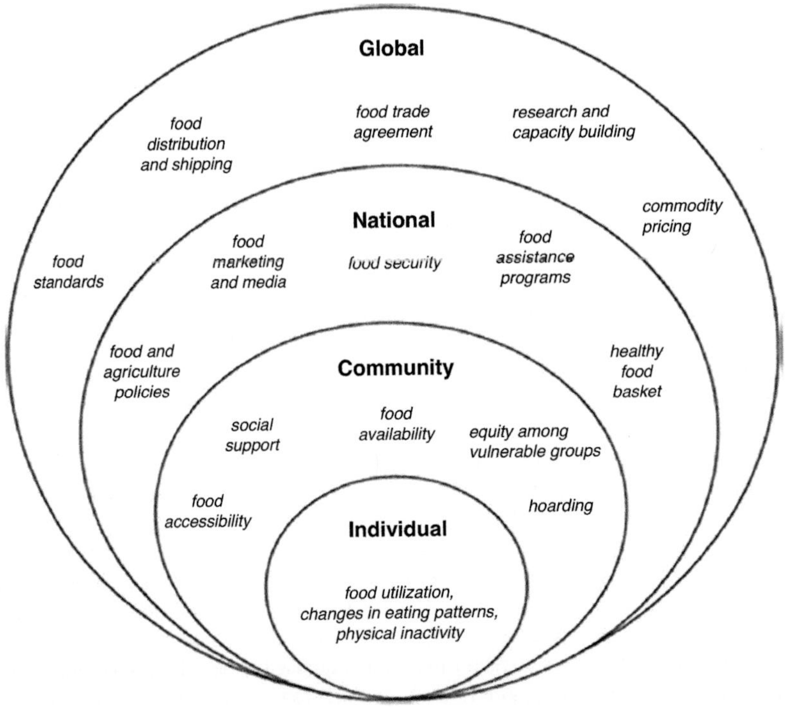

Fig. 19.2. A multilevel framework to support nutrition and food security during the COVID-19 pandemic, using the various levels of the ecological health model: individual, community, national and global (Jayawardena and Misra, 2020).

agriculture and food production are controlled primarily by SMEs (NEPAD, 2013; IFAD, 2013; Borsellino *et al.*, 2020). It is important to note that the availability and accessibility of food during and after a crisis do not rely solely on factors that directly impact agriculture and food production (Mengoud, 2020). Lessons from previous global food, energy, and economic crises suggest the need for greater cooperation (including knowledge sharing) by all countries to bridge research and policy response (Torero, 2020). Addressing postcrisis food insecurities in developing countries might require a critical examination of the nature and magnitude of the impact on the different dimensions of food security and agricultural systems through a critical analysis of existing policies to pinpoint areas for trade-offs, which often require multiple dimensions and simultaneous exploration (Staatz *et al.*, 2009). For example, in response to the 2014 Ebola virus outbreak, the World Bank (2014) proposed a pronged approach to address the resulting challenges involving direct and indirect financial and human costs. These approaches may be applied to address food security and agricultural challenges during and postcrisis in developing countries, COVID-19 inclusive.The most crucial strategy is advanced preparation by improving the resilience of all the dimensions of food security in developing countries. We herein present and discuss selected response strategies to promote food security in developing countries, during and postcrisis. These strategies are selected by the authors based on their paramount importance and appropriateness to the needs at hand and are not intended to be exhaustive. It is noteworthy to point out that COVID-19 has added urgency to long-standing development needs, thus the solutions proposed below are not necessarily 'new.'

Establishment of community-based food networks

The value of culture in developing countries cannot be overstated, and it is often evident by the coming together and staying together of people with similar norms, values, or blood ties, particularly during and immediately after a crisis. It is one of the main pillars of development and sustenance of communities, without which no society can progress (Wiktor-Mach, 2020). A community-based food and agricultural governing system should be established and maintained to link producers with consumers. Such a system could also be used to gather local reports and advise external networks on how best to address local food challenges. Perdana *et al.* (2020) suggested the development of regional food hubs for handling the impact of COVID-19 on food supply. They noted that such food hubs could help to connect food producers and customers/consumers within a community. Similar to this is the Public Food and Nutrition Security Program established in the state of Rio Grande do Norte, Brazil, for combating problems of food insecurity (Araújo and Calazans, 2020). This program has been instrumental in combating food crisis particularly during this COVID-19 pandemic. These food networks could also be used to monitor food production chains and commercialization at local and national levels. These strategies could be combined with tracing and monitoring jobs and income losses and to ensure the continuity of the food systems during and after a crisis. The establishment of community-based food networks is in line with the FAO (2010) recommendation that identified the need for broader relief-oriented social protection measures that can act as safety nets, insurance, and representative voices during a protracted crisis in developing countries.

Food and agriculture data collection and maintenance

Many developing countries lack primary food and agriculture data that may be instrumental in tackling issues of food insecurity (Kelly and Donovan, 2008). However, in order to acquire agricultural data for solving the problems of food insecurity (in developing countries), the FAO has proposed the use of the food balance sheets (FBSs) concept (Kelly *et al.*, 1991; FAO, 2001). The FBSs provide information on a country's food system over a period of time through (i) locally available food (through production, imports, and stock exchanges), (ii) locally utilized food (food converted into other forms such as animal feed, seeds, processing, waste, export, etc.), and (iii) food available per person (Kelly *et al.*, 1991; FAO, 2001). Although the accuracy of the FBSs depends on the reliability of basic data, they provide an approximate picture of the overall food situation in a country and can be a useful instrument for economic and nutritional studies, for preparing development plans and for formulating related projects (Jacobs and Sumner, 2002; Sheehy and Sharma, 2011; Arsenault *et al.*, 2015; Thar *et al.*, 2020). Maintaining up-to-date and accurate FBSs can help developing countries through conditions of crisis, such as the current COVID-19. For example, in the early periods of the COVID-19 outbreak, India (Saroj *et al.*, 2020) and Kenya Food Balance Sheet (2020) updated their FBSs to 2020 by assessing essential commodities and considering all broad aspects of the FBSs including stock, production, export, import, and consumption. Based on these updates, India was in a comfortable position for food crops such as rice, wheat, onions, sugar, potatoes, and milk and was in a propitious position to export a fraction of its surplus to neighboring countries. Other developing countries could similarly move to ensure stability in food dimensions at the national level. In order to develop accurate and useful FBSs, developing countries should recruit and train data scientists who will work alongside extension officers, agricultural scientists, and social scientists to minimize tendencies of inaccuracy and ensure quality assurance of data collected. Also, developing countries should have comprehensive statistical systems that record all current information relating to each component of the FBS (starting from on-farm/producers to consumers). Calicioglu *et al.* (2019) posited that the analyses of data on the dimensions of food security would improve nutrition outcomes in developing countries and expose systemic flaws and future challenges in the agriculture and food systems by highlighting root cause and trends, as well as social interlinkages and networks.

Stabilizing food prices

Fluctuating food prices will result in greater socioeconomic challenges due to food insecurity. A slight fluctuation in food prices, particularly during a crisis, would render millions of poor families in developing countries hungry. In order to stabilize food prices during and postcrisis situations, a suite of approaches are suggested, lending from those witnessed in other developing countries.

As a rapid response strategy in preventing food insecurity and hike in food prices due to COVID-19, food provisions through direct distribution, distribution of food vouchers, and cash transfers were among strategies adopted by governments of different developing countries (Arndt *et al.*, 2020; Crush and Si, 2020; Mengoub, 2020; Mussell *et al.*, 2020; Una *et al.*, 2020). Although direct food distribution may bear a greater risk of disease transference, particularly in the outbreak of a disease pandemic, the use of innovative technologies in food distribution has been developed in some developing countries. For example, Malaysia, Vietnam, and Indonesia initiated the 'rice ATMs' for grain distribution in order to minimize physical contacts and maintain social distancing (IMF, 2008; Muneeza, 2019).

During the 2007–2008 food crisis, the International Monetary Fund (IMF) advised the removal of export bans and taxes as a mitigating strategy for hikes in food prices (IMF, 2008)). In the wake of the COVID-19 pandemic, a similar strategy has been advised among suites of measures to mitigate hikes in food prices (IMF, 2020). Removal of export bans and taxes may be applied to promote cross-border trade among developing countries within a specific region, thereby minimizing crisis-induced hikes in food prices and mitigating food insecurity. Establishment and maintenance of national (or regional) grain reserves (termed 'strategic grain reserves', SGRs) could be another useful tool in price stabilization during and postcrisis situations.The SGRs contain grains that are utilized in situations of emergency and targeted toward food-insecure communities, particularly during a crisis (Kalkuhl *et al.*, 2016). In order to build a more robust grain reserve, there may be the need for cross-national cooperation to establish regional grain reserves, such as the Association of Southeast Asian Nations (ASEAN) emergency rice reserve, the East Asia Emergency Rice Reserve (Daño, 2006), and the Regional Food Security Reserve meant to serve ECOWAS countries (ECOWAS, 2020; FAO, 2020). In order to ensure dietary diversity, the grain reserves may be complemented with provisions of fruits, vegetables, and animal-sourced foods. In addition to the aforementioned approaches, there is the need to initiate a close public-private partnership and multistakeholder collaboration in developing countries to purchase agricultural products directly from farmers for redistribution and to ensure a continuous flow to the market in order to maintain fair prices for both farmers and consumers (Poulton and Macartney, 2012; Soullier and Moustier, 2020; Ray *et al.*, 2020; Fei *et al.*, 2020; Lencucha *et al.*, 2020). China established the 'Green Channels' as a means to allow free flow of farm inputs and farm produce during COVID-19 (Pu and Zhong, 2020). Similarly, Kenya, using the public-private partnerships in buying and selling farm produce, had an estimated surplus of grains and dairy food products during this pandemic (Agriculture KMo, 2020).

Infrastructural development for food security

Developing countries seem to be plagued with the inadequacy of agricultural infrastructure to ensure food security. Where agricultural activities and production are greatly incentivized, lack of or inadequate physical infrastructure could jeopardize the supply of raw and finished food products to the final end users. Therefore, the development of physical infrastructure in developing countries is of utmost importance in order to combat food insecurity. Various physical infrastructures that are necessary for mitigating problems of agricultural production and food insecurity in developing countries include proper transport, communication, storage, and marketing infrastructure. Agricultural producers, including farmworkers and workers in food processing facilities, have also been classified as 'essential critical infrastructure workers' (Ramos *et al.*, 2020; US Department of Homeland Security, 2020). In most developing countries, there is a shortfall or near absence of proper storage and transportation facilities for fresh agricultural produce. Provision or upgrading of storage infrastructure for perishable farm products signifies an additional action that could help to avoid wastage of agricultural products. Efficient and improved transport infrastructure will reduce the time taken for rural farmers to travel to urban settlements or marketplaces to sell their produce, also minimizing food loss. Although the development of agricultural infrastructure may be a long-term solution to mitigating problems of food security in developing countries, the governments and stakeholders have a significant role to play in ensuring that these infrastructures are adequately put in place and properly maintained to achieve their objectives.

Sometimes, particularly in low-income developing countries, external help could be sought to improve infrastructural development targeted at mitigating food insecurity. For example in Nepal, the World Bank– supported construction of road networks helped set the course for post–COVID-19 economic recovery through greater cross-border trade, creation of more jobs particularly for women, and better road safety (World Bank, 2020). By partnering with local digital technology start-ups in Kenya, efforts are being made to improve producer-consumer communications, delivery of agricultural inputs, soil testing, and market linkages (World Bank, 2020).

Decentralization of food manufacture might also be a means of improving food security in developing countries (Aday and Aday, 2020; Crawford, 2020). Establishment of low-scale food processing facilities near consumers could help reduce the problems and costs of storage and transportation. This would also ensure that consumers get fresh products periodically. Also, with the increase in population growth and urbanization, home gardening and urban agriculture have been suggested as strategies for advancing food and nutritional security during and after the COVID-19 pandemic (Altieri *et al.*, 2020; Kumar A. Padhee and Kumar, 2020; Lal, 2020; Lal *et al.*, 2020; Profiroiu *et al.*, 2020). The UN has projected that 68% of the world population will live in urban areas by 2050 (UN, 2018). It has also been projected that by 2030, 80% of megacities will be in developing countries (Crawford, 2020). However, cities in these countries are ill-equipped to provide sustainable sources of adequate food and nutrition for their population, even in the absence of a crisis, such as the COVID-19 pandemic. Therefore, there is the need for governments and stakeholders in developing countries to critically consider the option of decentralizing food manufacture and the role of home gardening and urban agriculture in ensuring food security.

Increasing investment in agricultural research and policies

Globally, science, agricultural research, and technology development play important roles in achieving significant increases in food and agricultural production and in reducing food insecurity. In most developing countries, research and development on agriculture are mainly carried out by government-funded institutions and laboratories as well as nonprofit institutions. Unfortunately, the majority of government-funded institutions and laboratories in developing countries suffer from low or lack of financial investment, thus limiting their contribution to improving agricultural production and food security. For example, the Comprehensive Africa Agriculture Development Programme (CAADP), launched in 2003 by African heads of state, proposed the allocation of 10% of total annual budgets to agricultural productivity (African Union, 2003). In the 2020 review of CAADP's achievement in Africa, only 4 out of 49 reporting countries were found to be on track (Benin, 2020; IFPRI, 2020). Of these four reporting countries, Rwanda that has the best performance has allocated only about 7.24% of the nation's annual budget to achieving CAADP's objective. In 2019, Nigeria earmarked about 40 billion naira for various national agricultural research agencies. However, of this amount, almost 50% was spent on offsetting personnel costs and overheads (PWC, 2020). Incidence of COVID-19 has been suggested to exacerbate problems of agricultural development in Africa (Vos *et al.*, 2020) making it more difficult to achieve any agricultural developmental objective. As a means to end hunger and food insecurity, there is the need for African leaders and stakeholders to show commitment to policies and ideas, such as those proposed by CAADP and other agriculture development–targeted causes, and follow relevant processes.

In Asia and the Pacific region, despite great progress in reducing food insecurity, an estimated 490 million people still experience hunger and are undernourished (FAO, 2020). Increasing investment in agricultural research, policies, and development is absolutely necessary to achieving food security in the region. According to the Asian Development Bank (ADB), the region needs a total annual agricultural investment of 78.6 billion USD to reduce hunger by 2030 (IFPRI *et al.*, 2019). Much of the funding will be allocated to investments in agricultural research and development, irrigation, and rural infrastructure. Also, the investments will be aimed at combating the effects of climate change that will reduce yields and production.

It is therefore evident that in order to achieve the goal of improving agricultural production and to increase national resilience against future crisis-induced food insecurity, governments and stakeholders in developing countries need to put in place evidence-based policies, supportive institutions, and corresponding human resources. Emphasis is needed to be placed on increasing public investments in agriculture by revamping existing or establishing new agricultural research institutions, genetic improvement of local food cultivars, and enhancing access to and the use of financial services by smallholder farmers. Involvement of the youths and empowering of rural women in agriculture should also be considered in order to reduce unemployment and poverty.

Adopting modern farming practices

Modern agricultural practices involve less use of human input, and this could be a viable option to address agricultural production and, indirectly, food security during and postcrisis. Most developing countries rely heavily on foreign aid, and during crisis, donor countries redirect resources to address pertinent issues in their own countries. Moreover, a recurrent challenge is that agriculture only accounts for four of the humanitarian official development assistance (FAO, 2010). Therefore, modernizing agriculture in developing countries will help improve their self-reliance to produce sufficient food during a crisis. Human capital resources in developing countries have historically been plagued with health challenges. The associated difficulties that come with agriculture and farming in most developing countries do not arouse the interest of the youths to venture into agricultural production. Modernized agriculture will fill the gap in the workforce and ensure improved output through efficiency and quality. However, the modernization of agriculture in developing countries is not without potential challenges such as financial and technical requirements. Agriculture is mostly labor intensive in most developing countries, which makes them more vulnerable to health-related crises. A shift toward adopting innovative mechanized farming can make the agriculture systems of developing countries more resilient.

Reduction and management of agricultural and food waste

According to FAO (2019, 2020), about 1.3 billion tons per year (equivalent to 3300 Mtn of CO_2 emission per year) of food produced globally is wasted. As human population is on the increase, further increases in food waste could result in a new food crisis similar to the one of 2007–2008 (Galanakis, 2020). Ironically, developing countries are significant contributors to global food and agricultural waste. During the COVID-19 pandemic, a crucial factor that may have contributed to increase in food loss and waste in developing countries is the lack of technologies, storage infrastructure, and transport system (FAO, 2020). In addition, disruption in feeding habits during this COVID-19 pandemic has also been noted to contribute significantly to food loss and waste. For example, in Spain, Aldaco *et al.* (2020) noted that COVID-19 induced a more than 12% food loss and waste with a concomitant rise in economic and environmental impact, and significant decrease in food nutritional quality.There is a need to adopt strategies that seek to reduce food loss and waste (Galanakis, 2012; Thi *et al.*, 2015; Mourad, 2016; Cristóbal *et al.*, 2018; Pleissner, 2018), thus improving the sustainability of food systems and mitigating food insecurity in developing countries.

As a strategic measure to reduce food loss and waste, the European Union established the Farm to Fork Strategy, which aims at making food systems fair, healthy, and environmentally friendly (EC, 2020). Similar initiatives could be replicated across developing countries to mitigate problems of food loss and waste and to minimize environmental impacts.The FAO has also recommended a suite of strategic measures and interventions to reducing food loss and waste in developing countries (FAO, 2020). These include prioritizing a focus on individual health, management of harvest glut in traditional local supply chains and scaling up food loss reduction initiatives, purchasing of agricultural produce and products from smallholder farmers for establishment of strategic emergency reserves, investment in postharvest technologies and mechanization, and establishment of food processing communities in close proximity to rural smallholder farmers, among others. Kumar *et al.* (2017) posited that food waste contains active compounds that can be harvested and reprocessed to produce essential products. Such active compounds include polysaccharides, fibers, proteins, secondary phytochemicals, nutrients, and microorganisms. Understanding the composition of waste is key to reusing it, and this is possible through culture-independent, high-throughput sequencing technologies called *wastomics*, a branch of *foodomics* (Ogwu, 2019). The combination of this novel approach and existing methods of extracting chemical compounds from organic waste is capable of creating a paradigm shift in food and agricultural waste management. Moreover, with policy support, waste can be perceived as an essential resource for creating wealth.

Conclusion

While the occurrence of the coronavirus pandemic was unplanned, it has given us the opportunity to assess the agricultural and food production capabilities of various countries, developing ones inclusive. Before now, the weak agricultural systems in developing countries, caused by a number of inherent and environmental factors, had exposed the population to food insecurity. The occurrence of COVID-19 has only further exacerbated the problem of food insecurity in these countries.

Many of the problems of food insecurity in developing countries can be solved internally with minimal external assistance. As the pandemic lingers, with a second wave of infection already being experienced in various countries, there is the need for governments and stakeholders in these countries to urgently and sincerely commit to policies and ideas that can help eradicate, or reduce, food insecurity, during and after the pandemic.

The importance of food security in times of crisis is evident in their consideration as part of essential services. The occurrence of new health crises causes a decline in demand for agricultural products and food production globally, but a greater impact is felt by developing countries where contagion might have been hit hardest. In this review, the timelines of COVID-19 activities in developing countries were highlighted by citing examples from specific countries such as Iran, Pakistan, India, Nigeria, and Egypt.

The observations noted in this review highlight the strategies and interventions put in place by the governments of respective developing countries in mitigating impacts of the pandemic-induced food insecurity.

In conclusion, we propose a staged food and agricultural system response in line with a specific health crisis. For example, in the case of COVID-19, we have three stages: early phase, rapid spread, and declining phase. It is important to emphasize that the recommendations (plausibly at a national level) proposed in this review do not support actions that contribute to hoarding or widespread trade disruptions.

1. *The early phase* is characterized by the entry or detection of the disease in a developing country. Food security and agricultural system response should be defined by stockpiling and fortifying agricultural warehouses—rapid production of agricultural raw materials and an efficient system of information dissemination. However, stockpiling needs to stop short of hoarding and does not need to act as a widespread trade disruption.
2. *The rapid spread* stage is characterized by a higher number of infections within the society. Food security and agricultural system response may involve ensuring the health and fitness of farmworkers and production systems. Efficient rationing of available food, increasing food access, and distribution will help ensure food resources do not run out.
3. *The declining phase* is characterized by the rapid decline in infection (and/or death). Food security and agricultural system response should target slow and strategic resumption of normal food production processes.

Acknowledgments

This research did not receive any grant from funding agencies in the public, commercial, or not-for-profit sectors.

Declaration of competing interest

There is no conflict of interest among authors. All authors contributed equally.

References

Abdul Rahman, A.S. (2020) Coronavirus in Africa. Available at: https://www.africanews.com/2020/06/21/coronavirus-in-africa-breakdown-of-infected-virus-free-countries/

Aday, S. and Aday, M.S. (2020) Impact of COVID-19 on the food supply chain. *Food Quality and Safety* 4(4), 167–180. DOI: 10.1093/fqsafe/fyaa024.

African Union (2003) Comprehensive Africa agriculture development programme. NEPAD. Available at: http://www.fao.org/nr/water/aquastat/sirte2008/NEPAD-CAADP%202003.pdf

Agriculture KMo (2020) Kenya Ministry of Agriculture, livestock, fisheries and cooperatives: Key staple food balance sheet as at end of June 2020. Available at: https://www.kilimo.go.ke/wp-content/uploads/2020/04/KENYA-KEY-STAPLES-FOOD-BALANCE-SHEET-TO-END-OF-JUNE-2020.pdf

Akbar, A.N. and Gilroy, D.W. (2020) Aging immunity may exacerbate COVID-19. *Science* 369(6501), 256–257.

Aldaco, R., Hoehn, D., Laso, J., Margallo, M., Ruiz-Salmón, J. *et al.* (2020) Food waste management during the COVID-19 outbreak: A holistic climate, economic and nutritional approach. *Science of the Total Environment* 742, 140524.

Ali, I. (2020) Pakistan prepared for the COVID-19 epidemic? A questionnaire-based survey. Available at: https://www.dawn.com/news/amp/1536792

Altieri, M.A., Padhee, A.K. and Kumar, S. (2020) Indian agriculture should change after COVID-19. *Food Security* 4(7), 837–840.

Alvaredo, F. and Gasparini, L. (2015) Recent trends in inequality and poverty in developing countries. *Handbook of Income Distribution* 2, 697–805. DOI: 10.1016/B978-0-444-59428-0.00010-2.

Araújo, F.R.d and Calazans, D.L.M. (2020) Management of food security actions during the COVID-19 pandemic. *Revista de Administração Pública* 54(4), 1123–1133.

Arndt, C., Davies, R., Gabriel, S., Harris, L., Makrelov, K. *et al.* (2020) Covid-19 lockdowns, income distribution, and food security: An analysis for South Africa. *Global Food Security* 26, 100410.

Arsenault, J.E., Hijmans, R.J. and Brown, K.H. (2015) Improving nutrition security through agriculture: An analytical framework based on national food balance sheets to estimate nutritional adequacy of food supplies. *Food Security* 7(3), 693–707.

Arshad, M.S., Khan, U., Sadiq, A., Khalid, W., Hussain, M. *et al.* (2020) Coronavirus disease (COVID-19) and immunity booster green foods: A mini review. *Food Science and Nutrition* 8(8), 3971–3976.

Barua, S. (2020) Understanding coronanomics: The economic implications of the coronavirus (COVID-19) pandemic. *SSRN Newsletter* 44p. DOI: 10.2139/ssrn.3566477.

Bencivenga, L., Rengo, G. and Varricchi, G. (2020) Elderly at time of coronavirus disease 2019 (COVID-19): Possible role of immunosenescence and malnutrition. *GeroScience* 42(4), 1089–1092.

Benin, S. (2020) Impact of COVID-19 on the CAADP Biennial Reviews. Available at: https://wca.ifpri.info/2020/05/10/ impact-of-covid-19-on-the-caadp-biennial-reviews/

Bennett, N.J., Finkbeiner, E.M., Ban, N.C., Belhabib, D., Jupiter, S.D. *et al.* (2020) The COVID-19 pandemic, small-scale fisheries and coastal fishing communities. *Coastal Management* 48(4), 336–347. DOI: 10.1080/08920753.202.

Bhagat, R., Reshmi, R., Sahoo, H., Roy, A.K. and Govil, D. (2020) The COVID-19, migration and livelihood in India: Challenges and policy issues. *Migration Letters* 17(5), 705–718. DOI: 10.33182/ml.v17i5.1048.

Blustein, K. (2020) International Labor Organization. Almost 25 million jobs could be lost worldwide as a result of COVID-19, says ILO 2020. Available at: https://www.ilo.org/global/about-the-ilo/newsroom/news/WCMS_738742/lang--en/index.htm

Borsellino, V., Schimmenti, E. and El Bilali, H. (2020) Agri-food markets towards sustainable patterns. *Sustainability* 12(6), 2193.

Butler, M.J. and Barrientos, R.M. (2020) The impact of nutrition on COVID-19 susceptibility and long-term consequences. *Brain, Behavior, and Immunity* 87, 53–54. DOI: 10.1016/j.bbi.2020.04.040.

Cai, Q., Chen, F., Wang, T., Luo, F., Liu, X. *et al.* (2020) Obesity and COVID-19 severity in a designated hospital in Shenzhen, China. *Diabetes Care* 43(7), 1392–1398.

Calder, P.C. (2020) Nutrition, immunity and covid-19. *BMJ Nutrition, Prevention and Health*. DOI: bmjnph-2020-000085.

Calicioglu, O., Flammini, A., Bracco, S., Bellù, L. and Sims, R. (2019) The future challenges of food and agriculture: An integrated analysis of trends and solutions. *Sustainability* 11(1), 222.

Charlton, K.E. (2016) Food security, food systems and food sovereignty in the 21st century: A new paradigm required to meet sustainable development goals. *Nutrition and Dietetics* 73(1), 3–12.

Competitive Commission (2020) Joint briefing to the portfolio committee on trade and industry and select committee on economic development, small business development, tourism, employment and labour: 19 May 2020. South Africa: Competition Commission. Available at: http://www.thedtic.gov.za/wp-content/uploads/Competition-Commission19-May-2020.pdf

Crawford, E. (2020) Decentralized production & enhanced biodiversity, bioavailability are key for a 'perfect food system'. Available at: https://www.foodnavigator-usa.com/Article/2020/09/22/Decentralized-production-enhanced-biodiversity-bioavailability-are-key-for-a-perfect-food-system?utm_source=copyright&utm_medium=OnSite&utm_campaign=copyright

Cristóbal, J., Castellani, V., Manfredi, S. and Sala, S. (2018) Prioritizing and optimizing sustainable measures for food waste prevention and management. *Waste Management* 72, 3–16.

Crush, J. and Si, Z. (2020) COVID-19 containment and food security in the Global South. *Journal of Agriculture, Food Systems, and Community Development* 9(4), 1–3.

da Cunha, C.A., Cimerman, S., Weissmann, L., Chebabo, A. and Bellei, N.C.J. (2020) Sociedade brasileira de infectologia. Sao Paulo, Brasil: Informativo da Sociedade Brasileira de Infectologia: Primeiro caso confirmado de doença pelo novo Coronavírus (COVID-19) no Brasil – 26/02/2020.

D'Alessandro, C. and Zulu, L.C. (2017) From the millennium development goals (MDGs) to the sustainable development goals (SDGs): Africa in the post-2015 development agenda. A geographical perspective. *African Geographical Review* 36(1), 1–18.

Daño, E. (2006) ASEAN's emergency rice reserve schemes: Current developments and prospects for engagement. *Women in Action* 3(35–45). Available at: https://www.isiswomen.org/downloads/wia/wia-2006-3/03wia06_04aDano.pdf

Dietz, W. and Santos-Burgoa, C. (2020) Obesity and its implications for COVID-19 mortality. *Obesity* 28(6), 1005–1006. DOI: 10.1002/oby.22818.

Drazen, A. (2008) Is there a different political economy for developing countries? Issues, perspectives and methodology. *Journal of African Economies* 17(1). DOI: 10.1093/jae/ejm035.

EC (2020) Communication from the Commission to the EuropeanParliament, the Council, the European Economic and Social Committee and the Committee of the Regions. A Farm to Fork Strategy for a Fair, Healthy and Environmentally-Friendly Food System. COM(2020) 381 Final 2020. Available at: https://ec.europa.eu/food/farm2fork_en

Ecker, O. and Breisinger, C. (2012) The food security system: A new conceptual framework. IFPRI Discussion paper 1166. Washington, D.C: International Food Policy Research Institute (IFPRI). Available at: http://ebrary.ifpri.org/cdm/ref/collection/p15738coll2/id/126837

ECOWAS (2020) COVID – 19: ECOWAS in solidarity donates food to the most vulnerable households in Nigeria. Available at: https://www.ecowas.int/covid-19-ecowas-in-solidarity-donates-food-to-the-most-vulnerable-households-in-nigeria/

FAO (2001) The state of food insecurity in the world: The multiple dimensions of food insecurity. Available at: http://www.fao.org/docrep/018/i3434e/i3434e.pdf

FAO (2002) *World Health Organization. World health report*. The Organization, Geneva.

FAO (2004) Food and agriculture organization of the united nations. Undernourishment around the world. In: *The State of Food Insecurity in the World*. The Organization, Rome.

FAO (2006) Policy brief: Food security. *FAO* 2, 1–4. Available at: http://www.fao.org/fileadmin/templates/faoitaly/documents/pdf/pdf_Food_Security_Cocept_Note.pdf

FAO (2008) *An introduction to the basic concepts of food security*. FAO, Rome, p. 3.

FAO (2010) *The state of food insecurity in the world: Addressing food insecurity in protracted crisis*. FAO, Rome, p. 62.

FAO (2015) FAO and the 17 sustainable development goals. Available at: http://www.fao.org/3/a-i4997.epdf

FAO (2019) *The state of food security and nutrition in the world 2019: Safeguarding against economic slowdowns and downturns*. FAO, IFAD, UNICEF, WFP and WHO, Italy, Rome.

FAO (2019) The State of Food and Agriculture 2019: Moving forward on food loss and waste reduction. Rome: Food and Agriculture Organization of the United Nations. Licenc: CCBY-NC-SA 3.0. Available at: http://www.fao.org/3/ca6030en/ca6030en.pdf

FAO (2020) Desert locust. Available at: http://www.fao.org/locusts

FAO (2020) National agrifood systems and COVID-19 in ECOWAS: Effects, policy responses, and long-term implications. Available at: http://www.fao.org/3/cb1336en/CB1336EN.pdf

FAO (2020) Food and agriculture organization of the United Nations: State of food and agriculture in Asia and the Pacific region, including future prospects and emerging issues. In: *The 34th Session of the FAO Regional Conference for Asia and the Pacific*, Thimphu, Bhutan, p. 19. Available at: http://www.fao.org/3/nb840en/nb840en.pdf

FAO (2020) Global food losses and food waste 2020. Available at: http://www.fao.org/3/mb060e/mb060e00.htm

FAO (2020) Mitigating risks to food systems during COVID-19: Reducing food loss and waste. Available at: http://www.fao.org/3/ca9056en/ca9056en.pdf

Fei, S., Ni, J. and Santini, G. (2020) Local food systems and COVID-19: An insight from China. *Resources, Conservation and Recycling* 162, 105022.

Firdaus, R.R., Senevi Gunaratne, M., Rahmat, S.R. and Kamsi, N.S. (2019) Does climate change only affect food availability? What else matters. *Cogent Food & Agriculture* 5, 1. DOI: 10.1080/23311932.2019.1707607.

Fukuda-Parr, S. and Orr, A. (2014) The MDG hunger target and the competing frameworks of food security. *Journal of Human Development and Capabilities* 15(2–3), 147–160.

Galanakis, C.M. (2012) Recovery of high added-value components from food wastes: Conventional, emerging technologies and commercialized applications. *Trends in Food Science & Technology* 26(2), 68–87.

Galanakis, C.M. (2020) The food systems in the era of the coronavirus (COVID-19) pandemic crisis. *Food* 9(4), 523.

Gebremariam, M.K., Vaqué-Crusellas, C., Andersen, L.F., Stok, F.M., Stelmach-Mardas, M. *et al.* (2017) Measurement of availability and accessibility of food among youth: A systematic review of methodological studies. *International Journal of Behavioral Nutrition and Physical Activity* 14(1), 22.

George, L. (2020) COVID-19 is exacerbating food shortages in Africa. The world economic forum COVID action platform. *World Economic Forum*. Available at: https://www.weforum.org/agenda/2020/04/africa-coronavirus-covid19-imports-exports-food-supply-chains

Gibson, M. (2012) Food security-a commentary: What is it and why is it so complicated? *Food* 1(1), 18–27.

Glauber, J., Laborde, D., Martin, W. and Vos, R. (2020) COVID-19: Trade restrictions are worst possible response to safeguard food security. *Issue Post March* 27(2020).

Glauber, J., Laborde, D., Martin, W. and Vos, R. (2020) COVID-19: Trade restrictions are worst possible response to safeguard food security. Washington, D.C: International Food Policy Research Institute. Available at: https://www.ifpri.org/blog/covid-19-trade-restrictions-are-worst-possible-response-safeguard-food-security

Gregory, P.J., Ingram, J.S. and Brklacich, M. (2005) Climate change and food security. *Philosophical Transactions of the Royal Society B: Biological Sciences* 360(1463), 2139–2148.

Gross, R., Schoeneberger, H., Pfeifer, H. and Preuss, H.-J. (2000) The four dimensions of food and nutrition security: Definitions and concepts. *SCN News* 20(20), 20–25.

Guo, Y.R., Cao, Q.D., Hong, Z.S., Tan, Y.Y., Chen, S.D. *et al.* (2020) The origin, transmission and clinical therapies on coronavirus disease 2019 (COVID-19) outbreak-An update on the status. *Military Medical Research* 7(1), 11.

Hailu, G. (2020) Economic thoughts on COVID-19 for Canadian food processors. *Canadian Journal of Agricultural Economics/ Revue Canadienne d'agroeconomie* 68(2), 163–169.

Handley, E. (2020) India has the fourth-highest number of COVID-19 cases, but the Government denies community transmission. Available at: https://www.abc.net.au/news/2020-06-21/india-coronavirus-fourth-highest-covid19-community-transmission/12365738

Handu, D., Moloney, L., Rozga, M. and Cheng, F.W. (2020) Malnutrition care during the COVID-19 pandemic: Considerations for registered dietitian nutritionists. *Journal of the Academy of Nutrition and Dietetics*. DOI: 10.1016/j.jand.2020.05.012.

Harris, J., Depenbusch, L., Pal, A.A., Nair, R.M. and Ramasamy, S. (2020) Food system disruption: Initial livelihood and dietary effects of COVID-19 on vegetable producers in India. *Food Security* 12(4), 841–851.

Hirvonen, K., Mohammed, B., Minten, B. and Tamru, S. (2021) Food marketing margins during the COVID-19 pandemic: Evidence from vegetables in Ethiopia. ESSP Working Paper 150. Washington, D.C: International Food Policy Research Institute. DOI: 10.2499/p15738coll2.133931.

Hossain, S.T. (2020) Impacts of COVID-19 on the agri-food sctor: Food scurity plicies of Asian poductivity oganization mmbers. *Journal of Agricultural Science-Sri Lanka* 15(2), 116–132.

IFAD (2013) Smallholders, food security, and the environment. IFAD and UNEP Press. Available at: http://www.fao.org/family-farming/detail/en/c/285693

IFPRI (2020) Food security. Available at: https://www.ifpri.org/topic/food-security

IFPRI (2020) International Food Policy Research Institute: Second Biennial Review report highlights urgent need to accelerate progress toward achieving Malabo Declaration goals by 2025. Available at: https://www.ifpri.org/blog/second-biennial-review-report-highlights-urgent-need-accelerate-progress-toward-achieving

IFPRI, ADB, International Food Policy Research Institute (IFPRI), and Asian Development Bank (ADB) (2019) *Ending Hunger in Asia and the Pacific by 2030: An assessment of investment requirements in agriculture*. Asian Development Bank (ADB), Manila, Philippines. DOI: 10.22617/TCS190499-2.

IMF (2008) International monetary fund. Food and fuel prices— Recent developments, macroeconomic impact, and policy responses. *Fiscal Affairs, Strategy, Policy, and Review, and Research Departments*. Available at: https://www.imf.org/-/media/Websites/IMF/imported-full-text-pdf/external/np/pp/eng/2008/_091908.ashx

IMF (2020) International Monetary Fund. WTO and IMF heads call for lifting trade restrictions on medical supplies and food. Available at: https://www.imf.org/en/News/Articles/2020/04/24/pr20187-wto-and-imf-joint-statement-on-trade-and-the-covid-19-response

Jacobs, K. and Sumner, D.A. (2002) *The food balance sheets of the food and agriculture organization: A review of potential ways to broaden the appropriate uses of the data*. Department of Agricultural Economics, University of California, Berkeley, CL.

Jayawardena, R. and Misra, A. (2020) Balanced diet is a major casualty in COVID-19. *Diabetes and Metabolic Syndrome* 14(5), 1085–1086.

Jayawardena, R., Sooriyaarachchi, P., Chourdakis, M., Jeewandara, C. and Ranasinghe, P. (2020) Enhancing immunity in viral infections, with special emphasis on COVID-19: A review. *Diabetes and Metabolic Syndrome* 14(4), 367–382.

Jones, A. (2018) Malnutrition, poverty, and climate change are also human rights issues in child labor. *Health and Human Rights* 20(2), 249–251.

Kah, H.K. (2017) Boko Haram is losing, but so is food production: Conflict and food insecurity in Nigeria and Cameroon. *Africa Development* Available from(3), 177–196. Available at: http://www.jstor.org/stable/90018140

Kakodkar, P. and Kaka, N. (2020) Comprehensive literature review on the clinical presentation, and management of the pandemic coronavirus disease 2019 (COVID-19). *Cureus* 12(4), e7560–e.

Kalkuhl, M., Braun, J. and Torero, M. (2016) *Food price volatility and its implications for food security and policy*. Springer Nature.

Karamouzian, M. and Madani, N. (2020) COVID-19 response in the middle East and North Africa: Challenges and paths forward. *The Lancet Global Health* 8(7), S2214–109X. DOI: 10.1016/S2214-109X(20)30233-3.

Kathiresan, A., Nagai, T. and Haneishi, Y. (2020) Policy options for galvanizing Africa's rice sector against impacts of COVID-19. *World Development* 136, 105126.

Kayser, O., Klarsfeld, L. and Brossard, S. (2014) *Marketing nutrition for the base of the Pyramid-Introducing successful practices for improved access to nutritious complementary foods: Key lessons from case studies*. Hystra Hybrid Strategy Consulting, Paris. Available at: https://www.susana.org/_resources/documents/default/3-2178-7-1424861514.pdf

Ke, J. and Ford-Jones, E.L. (2015) Food insecurity and hunger: A review of the effects on children's health and behaviour. *The Journal of Paediatrics and Child Health* 20(2), 89–91.

Kelly, A., Becker, W. and Helsing, E. (1991) Food balance sheets. In: *Food and Health Data: Their Use in Nutrition Policy-Making*. WHO Regional Office for Europe, Copenhagen, pp. 39–47.

Kelly, V. and Donovan, C. (2008) Agricultural statistics in sub-saharan Africa: Differences in institutional arrangements and their impacts on agricultural statistics systems. A synthesis of four country case studies. In: *Food Security International Development Working Papers, Department of Agricultural, Food, and Resource Economics*. Michigan State University. DOI: 10.22004/ag.econ.54558.

Kenya Food Balance Sheet (2020) Kenya Food Balance Sheet during COVID-19 pandemic. Available at: https://www.kilimo.go.ke/covid-19/food-balance-sheet/

Khan, S., Khan, M., Maqsood, K., Hussain, T. and Zeeshan, M. (2020) Is Pakistan prepared for the COVID-19 epidemic? A questionnaire-based survey. *Journal of Medical Virology* 92(7), 824–832. DOI: 10.1002/jmv.25814.

Kibet, R. (2020) Floods in East Africa threaten the fight against COVID-19. Available at: http://climatetracker.org/floods-in-east-africa-threaten-fight-against-covid-19/ (accessed 5 December 2020).

Kot, S. (2018) Sustainable supply chain management in small and medium enterprises. *Sustainability* 10(4), 1143.

Kotwal, A., Yadav, A.K., Yadav, J., Kotwal, J. and Khune, S. (2020) Predictive models of COVID-19 in India: A rapid review. *Medical Journal Armed Forces India* 76(4), 377–386. DOI: 10.1016/j.mjafi.2020.06.001.

Kumar, K., Yadav, A.N., Kumar, V., Vyas, P. and Dhaliwal, H.S. (2017) Food waste: A potential bioresource for extraction of nutraceuticals and bioactive compounds. *Bioresources and Bioprocessing* 4(1), 18.

Kumar A. Padhee, A.K. and Kumar, S. (2020) How Indian agriculture should change after COVID-19. *Food Security* 12(4), 837–840.
Lal, R. (2020) Home gardening and urban agriculture for advancing food and nutritional security in response to the COVID-19 pandemic. *Food Security* 12(871–876), s12571–020. DOI: 10.1007/s12571-020-01058-3.
Lal, R., Brevik, E.C., Dawson, L., Field, D., Glaser, B. *et al.* (2020) Managing soils for recovering from the COVID-19 pandemic. *Soil Systems* 4(3), 46.
Lencucha, R., Pal, N.E., Appau, A., Thow, A.-M. and Drope, J. (2020) Government policy and agricultural production: A scoping review to inform research and policy on healthy agricultural commodities. *Globalization and Health* 16(1), 11.
Lewnard, J.A. and Lo, N.C. (2020) Scientific and ethical basis for social-distancing interventions against COVID-19. *The Lancet: Infectious Diseases* 20(6), 631.
Li, T., Zhang, Y., Gong, C., Wang, J., Liu, B. *et al.* (2020) Prevalence of malnutrition and analysis of related factors in elderly patients with COVID-19 in Wuhan, China. *European Journal of Clinical Nutrition* 74(6), s41430–020. DOI: 10.1038/s41430-020-0642-3.
Lighter, J., Phillips, M., Hochman, S., Sterling, S., Johnson, D. *et al.* (2020) Obesity in patients younger than 60 years is a risk factor for covid-19 hospital admission. *Clinical Infectious Diseases*.
Luo, Y., Trevathan, E., Qian, Z., Li, Y., Li, J. *et al.* (2020) Asymptomatic SARS-CoV-2 infection in household contacts of a healthcare provider, Wuhan, China. *Emerging Infectious Diseases* 26(8), 1930–1933. DOI: 10.3201/eid2608.201016.
Mengoub, F.E. (2020) *Ensuring food security during the COVID-19 pandemic: Review of short-term responses in selected countries. Rabat, Morocco*. p. 9.
Mengoud, F.E. (2020) *Ensuring food security during the COVID-19 pandemic: Review of short-term responses in selected countries*. Policy Center of the New South, Rabat, Morocco, p. 9.
Millward, D.J. and Jackson, A.A. (2004) Protein/energy ratios of current diets in developed and developing countries compared with a safe protein/energy ratio: Implications for recommended protein and amino acid intakes. *Public Health Nutrition* 7(3), 387–405.
Mitlin, D. and Satterthwaite, D. (2013) *Urban poverty in the global south: Scale and nature*. Taylor and Francis Group/Routledge, London/New York.
Mogues, T. (2020) Food markets during COVID-19 2020. Available at: www.imf.org
Mourad, M. (2016) Recycling, recovering and preventing "food waste": Competing solutions for food systems sustainability in the United States and France. *Journal of Cleaner Production* 126, 461–477.
Müller, O. and Krawinkel, M. (2005) Malnutrition and health in developing countries. *Canadian Medical Association Journal* 173(3), 279–286.
Müller, O., Garenne, M., Kouyaté, B. and Becher, H. (2003) The association between protein–energy malnutrition, malaria morbidity and all-cause mortality in West African children. *Tropical Medicine & International Health* 8(6), 507–511.
Muneeza, A. (2019) Rice ATMs: Technology based innovations for enhancement of Zakat. *IF Hub* 2, 8–15.
Mussell, A., Bilyea, T. and Hedley, D. (2020) *Agri-food supply chains and Covid-19: Balancing resilience and vulnerability*. Agri-Food Economic Systems, Ontario, Canada, p. 6.
Nair, A.G., Gandhi, R.A. and Natarajan, S. (2020) Effect of COVID-19 related lockdown on ophthalmic practice and patient care in India: Results of a survey. *Indian Journal of Ophthalmology* 68(5), 725.
Nairametrics (2021) Nigeria to exit recession by first quarter of 2021. Available at: https://nairametrics.com/2020/11/23/nigeria-to-exit-recession-by-first-quarter-of-2021/ (accessed 29 November 2020).
Naja, F. and Hamadeh, R. (2020) Nutrition amid the COVID-19 pandemic: A multi-level framework for action. *European Journal of Clinical Nutrition* 1–5.
NBS (2020) National Bureau of Statistics, Nigeria 2020. Available at: https://tradingeconomics.com/nigeria/unemployment-rate
Nemer, L., Gelband, H. and Jha, P. (2001) The evidence base for interventions to reduce malnutrition in children under five and school-age children in low- and middle-income countries. CMH working paper no. WG5: 11. Geneva: World Health Organization.
NEPAD (2013) Agriculture in Africa: Transformation and outlook. Midrand Johannesburg. South Africa: New Partnership for African Development. Available at: https://www.nepad.org/file-download/download/public/15582
Ogwu, M.C. (2019) Understanding the composition of food waste: An "-Omics" approach to food waste management. In: Gunjal, A.B. (ed.) *Global Initiatives for Waste Reduction and Cutting Food Loss*. IGI Global, Pennsylvania, USA, pp. 212–236. DOI: 10.4018/978-1-5225-7706-5.ch011.

Ohia, C., Bakarey, A.S. and Ahmad, T. (2020) COVID-19 and Nigeria: Putting the realities in context. *International Journal of Infectious Diseases*.

Olayiwola, K., Soyibo, A. and Atinmo, T. (2004) Impact of globalization on food consumption, health and nutrition in Nigeria: Impact on food security and nutrition. *Globalization of Food Systems in Developing Countries* 83, 99.

O'Sullivan, A. and Sheffrin, S.M. (2003) *Economics: Principles in action. Upper Saddle River*. Pearson Prentice Hall, New Jersey 07458, p. 57.

Otekunrin, O.A. and Otekunrin, O.A. (2020) COVID-19 and Hunger in Africa: A crisis within a crisis. In: *Archives in Food and Nutrition. 6th International Conference on Food Science and Food Safety*, Vienna, Austria; October 16–17.

Otekunrin, O.A., Otekunrin, O.A., Fasina, F.O., Omotayo, A.O. and Akram, M. (2020) Assessing the zero hunger target readiness in Africa in the face of COVID-19 pandemic. *Caraka Tani: Journal of Sustainable Agriculture* 35(2), 213–227.

Ozili, P.K. (2020) Covid-19 pandemic and economic crisis: The Nigerian experience and structural causes. *SSRN Newsletter* 29. DOI: 10.2139/ssrn.3567419.

Perdana, T., Chaerani, D., Achmad, A.L.H. and Hermiatin, F.R. (2020) Scenarios for handling the impact of COVID-19 based on food supply network through regional food hubs under uncertainty. *Heliyon* 6(10), e05128.

Pérez-Escamilla, R. (2017) Food security and the 2015-2030 sustainable development goals: From human to planetary health: Perspectives and opinions. *Current Developments in Nutrition* 1(7), e000513–e.

Pleissner, D. (2018) Recycling and reuse of food waste. *Current Opinion in Green and Sustainable Chemistry* 13, 39–43.

Portier, C.J., Tart, K.T., Carter, S.R., Dilworth, C.H., Grambsch, A.E. *et al*. (2013) A human health perspective on climate change: A report outlining the research needs on the human health effects of climate change. *Journal of Current Issues in Globalization* 6(4), 621.

Pothan, P.E., Taguchi, M. and Santini, G. (2020) *Local food systems and COVID-19: A glimpse on India's responses*. FAO, Rome. Available at: http://www.fao.org/uploads/pics/COVID-19_and_Indian_food_systems-edited_draft-17-04-2020mt_pepcopy1_.pdf

Poulton, C. and Macartney, J. (2012) Can public–private partnerships leverage private investment in agricultural value chains in Africa? A preliminary review. *World Development* 40(1), 96–109.

Profiroiu, C.M., Bodislav, D.A., Burlacu, S. and Rădulescu, C.V. (2020) Challenges of sustainable urban development in the context of population growth. *European Journal of Sustainable Development* 9(3), 51.

Pu, M. and Zhong, Y. (2020) Rising concerns over agricultural production as COVID-19 spreads: Lessons from China. *Global Food Security* 26, 100409.

PWC (2020) Price Waterhouse Coopers. Responding to the impact of COVID-19 on food security and agriculture in Nigeria. Available at: https://www.pwc.com/ng/en/assets/pdf/impact-covid19-food-security-nigeria.pdf

Ramos, A.K., Lowe, A.E., Herstein, J.J., Schwedhelm, S., Dineen, K.K. *et al*. (2020) Invisible no more: The impact of COVID-19 on essential food production workers. *Journal of Agromedicine* 1–5.

Ray, P., Acharya, K.K. and Thakur, A. (2020) COVID-19 impact and implication to agriculture and food security. *Food and Scientific Reports* 1(7), 24–26.

Reardon, T. and Hopkins, R. (2006) The supermarket revolution in developing countries: Policies to address emerging tensions among supermarkets, suppliers and traditional retailers. *The European Journal of Development Research* 18(4), 522–545.

Reardon, T., Timmer, C.P. and Berdegue, J.A. Regmi, A. and Gehlhar, M. (eds). (2003) *The rise of supermarkets in Latin America and Asia: implications for international markets for fruits and vegetables*. Agricultural Information, Washington, D.C.

Reardon, T., Mishra, A., Nuthalapati, C.S., Bellemare, M.F. and Zilberman, D. (2020) Covid-19's disruption of India's transformed food supply chains. *Economic and Political Weekly* 55(18), 18–22.

Reardon, T., Tschirley, D., Liverpool-Tasie, L.S.O., Awokuse, T., Fanzo, J. *et al*. (2021) The processed food revolution in African Food systems and the double burden of malnutrition. *Global Food Security* 28, 100466.

Robles, M. and Torero, M. (2010) Understanding the impacts of high food prices in Latin America. *Economia* 10(2), 117–164.

Rodriguez-Morales, A.J., Gallego, V., Escalera-Antezana, J.P., Méndez, C.A., Zambrano, L.I. *et al.* (2020) COVID-19 in Latin America: The implications of the first confirmed case in Brazil. *Travel Medicine and Infectious Disease* 35, 101613. DOI: 10.1016/j.tmaid.2020.101613.

Rothan, H.A. and Byrareddy, S.N. (2020) The epidemiology and pathogenesis of coronavirus disease (COVID-19) outbreak. *Journal of Autoimmun* 109, 102433.

Sage, C. (2014) Impacts of climate change on food accessibility. In: Freedman, B. (ed.) *Handbook of Global Environmental Change*. Springer Science+Business Media, Dordrecht, pp. 709–715.

Saibal, G. (2020) How India should be prepared for natural disasters in light of the current pandemic situation of Covid-19. Available at: https://www.financialexpress.com/lifestyle/science/how-the-nation-should-be-prepared-for-natural-disasters-in-light-of-the-current-pandemic-situation-of-covid-19/1957664/

Sariol, A. and Perlman, S. (2020) Lessons for COVID-19 immunity from other coronavirus infections. *Immunity* 53(2), 248–263.

Saroj, S., Pradhan, M. and Roy, D. (2020) Assessing India's food supply situation using a food balance sheet and COVID-19 sensitive markers. Available at: http://southasia.ifpri.info/2020/08/06/assessing-indias-food-supply-situation-using-a-food-balance-sheet-and-covid-19-sensitive-markers/

Schleifer, P. and Sun, Y. (2020) Reviewing the impact of sustainability certification on food security in developing countries. *Global Food Security* 24, 100337.

Schmidhuber, J. and Tubiello, F.N. (2007) Global food security under climate change. *Proceedings of the National Academy of Sciences* 104(50), 19703–19708.

Shafi, M., Liu, J. and Ren, W. (2020) Impact of COVID-19 pandemic on micro, small, and medium-sized enterprises operating in Pakistan. *Research in Globalization* 2, 100018.

Sharifi, H., Jahani, Y., Mirzazadeh, A., Gohari, M.A., Nakhaeizadeh, M. *et al.* (n.d.) Estimating the number of COVID-19-related infections, deaths and hospitalizations in Iran under different physical distancing and isolation scenarios. *International Journal of Health Policy and Management*. DOI: 10.34172/ijhpm.2020.134.

Sheehy, T. and Sharma, S. (2011) The nutrition transition in the republic of Ireland: Trends in energy and nutrient supply from 1961 to 2007 using food and agriculture organization food balance sheets. *British Journal of Nutrition* 106(7), 1078–1089.

Smith, M.D. and Meade, B. (2019) Who are the world's food insecure? Identifying the risk factors of food insecurity around the world. Amber waves: The economics of food, farming. *Natural Resources, and Rural America*. Available at: https://www.ers.usda.gov/amber-waves/2019/june/who-are-the-world-s-food-insecure-identifying-the-risk-factors-of-food-insecurity-around-the-world

Smith, L.C., El Obeid, A.E. and Jensen, H.H. (2000) The geography and causes of food insecurity in developing countries. *Agricultural Economics* 22(2), 199–215.

Soullier, G. and Moustier, P. (2020) The modernization of the rice value chain in Senegal: A move towards the Asian quiet revolution. *Development Policy Review* 00, 1–21. DOI: 10.1111/dpr.12459.

Staatz, J.M., Boughton, D.H. and Donovan, C. (2009) *Food Security in developing countries*. Department of Agricultural, Food and Resource Economics, Michigan State University, East Lansing, Michigan 48824, p. 39.

Stein, R.A. (2020) COVID-19 and rationally layered social distancing. *International Journal of Clinical Practice* 74(7), e13501. DOI: 10.1111/ijcp.13501.

Tamru, S., Hirvonen, K. and Minten, B. (2020) Impacts of the COVID-19 crisis on vegetable value chains in Ethiopia. IFPRI COVID-blog. Available at: https://www.ifpri.org/blog/impacts-covid-19-crisis-vegetable-value-chains-ethiopia

Taras, H. (2005) Nutrition and student performance at school. *Journal of School Health* 75(6), 199–213.

Tebeje, N., Bikes, G., Abebe, S. and Yesuf, M. (2017) Prevalence and major contributors of child malnutrition in developing countries: Systematic review and meta-analysis. *Journal of Childhood Obesity* 2(4).

Thar, C.-M., Jackson, R., Swinburn, B. and Mhurchu, C.N. (2020) A review of the uses and reliability of food balance sheets in health research. *Nutrition Reviews* 78(12), 989–1000.

The World Bank (2020) Unemployment, total (% of total labor force) (modelled ILO estimate). Available at: https://data.worldbank.org/indicator/SL.UEM.TOTL.ZS (accessed 1 March 2020).

The World Bank Nigeria Development Update (2020) Nigeria's economy faces worst recession in four decades, says new World Bank Report. Available at: https://www.worldbank.org/en/news/press-release/2020/06/25/nigerias-economy-faces-worst-recession-in-four-decades-says-new-world-bank-report (accessed 29 November 2020).

Thi, N.B.D., Kumar, G. and Lin, C.-Y. (2015) An overview of food waste management in developing countries: Current status and future perspective. *Journal of Environmental Management* 157, 220–229.

Torero, M. (2020) Without food, there can be no exit from the pandemic. *Nature* 580, 588–589.

Udmale, P., Pal, I., Szabo, S., Pramanik, M. and Large, A. (2020) Global food security in the context of COVID-19: A scenario-based exploratory analysis. *Progress in Disaster Science* 7, 100120.

UN News (2020) UN working to avert dual crises as COVID-19 hits Hunger hotspots. Italy: United Nations. Available at: https://www.un.org/en/un-coronavirus-communicationssteam/un-working-avert-dual-crises-covid-19-hits-hungerhotspots

UN (2018) United Nations, Department of Economic and Social Affairs. 68% of the world population projected to live in urban areas by 2050. Available at: https://www.un.org/development/desa/en/news/population/2018-revision-of-world-urbanization-prospects.html

Una, G., Richard, A., Sailendra, P. and Gwenaelle, S. (2020) *Digital solutions for direct cash transfers in emergencies. Special series on fiscal policies to respond to COVID-19*. International Monetary Fund, Washington, pp. 1–9.

USDA (2020) South Africa continues corn exports amidst COVID-19. South Africa: Global Agricultural Information Network: United State Department of Agriculture-Foreign Agricultural Service Pretoria.

US Department of Homeland Security (2020) Advisory memorandum on identification of essential critical infrastructure workers during COVID-19 response. Available at: https://www.cisa.gov/sites/default/files/publications/Version_3.0_CISA_Guidance_on_Essential_Critical_Infrastructure_Workers_1.pdf

Vos, R., Martin, W. and Laborde, D. (2020) How much will global poverty increase because of COVID-19? *IFPRI Blog Research Post*. Available at: https://www.ifpri.org/blog/how-much-will-global-poverty-increase-because-covid-19

Waris, A., Khan, A.U., Ali, M., Ali, A. and Baset, A. (2020) COVID-19 outbreak: Current scenario of Pakistan. *New Microbes and New Infections* 35, 100681. DOI: 10.1016/j.nmni.2020.100681.

WHO (2020) WHO Regional Office for the Eastern Mediterranean Coronavirus disease 2019 (COVID-19) weekly situation report 06. Available at: http://www.emro.who.int/images/stories/coronavirus/covid-19-sitrep-6.pdf?ua=1

WHO (2020) Emergency ministerial meeting on COVID-19 organized by the African union and the Africa centres for disease control and prevention. Available at: https://www.who.int/dg/speeches/detail/emergency-ministerial-meeting-on-covid-19-organized-by-the-african-union-and-the-africa-centres-for-disease-controland-prevention

WHO (2020) World Health Organization Nutrition advice for adults during the COVID-19 outbreak 2020. Available at: http://www.emro.who.int/nutrition/nutrition-infocus/nutrition (accessed 19 June 2020).

Wiktor-Mach, D. (2020) What role for culture in the age of sustainable development? UNESCO's advocacy in the 2030 agenda negotiations. *International Journal of Cultural Policy* 26(3), 312–327.

Wolvers, A., Tappe, O., Salverda, T. and Schwarz, T. (2015) Voices from around the world: Concepts of the global south. Global South Studies Center Cologne, Cologne, Cologne, Germany. Available at: http://kups.ub.uni-koeln.de/6399/1/voices012015_concepts_of_the_global_south.pdf

Woolhandler, S. and Himmelstein, D.U. (2020) Intersecting U.S. epidemics: COVID-19 and lack of health insurance. *Annals of Internal Medicine* 173(1), 63–64.

World Bank (2014) *The economic impact of the 2014 Ebola epidemic: Short and medium term estimates for Guinea, Liberia, and Sierra Leone*. World Bank, Washington D.C., USA.

World Bank (2020). Available at: https://datahelpdesk.worldbank.org/knowledgebase/articles/906519-world-bank-country-and-lending-groups

World Bank (2020) World Bank's $450 million road support in Nepal to spur COVID-19 recovery. Available at: https://www.worldbank.org/en/news/press-release/2020/06/09/new-world-bank-strategic-roads-project-to-aid-economic-recovery-post-covid-19-in-nepal

World Bank (2020) World Bank's response to COVID-19 (coronavirus) in Africa. Available at: https://www.worldbank.org/en/news/factsheet/2020/06/02/world-banks-response-to-covid-19-coronavirusin-africa

Xu, Z., Shi, L., Wang, Y., Zhang, J., Huang, L. *et al.* (2020) Pathological findings of COVID-19 associated with acute respiratory distress syndrome. *The Lancet Respiratory Medicine* 8(4), 420–422.

Zabetakis, I., Lordan, R., Norton, C. and Tsoupras, A. (2020) COVID-19: The inflammation link and the role of nutrition in potential mitigation. *Nutrients* 12(5), 1466.

20 Emotional Contagion and its Implications for Animal Welfare

Sandra Düpjan, Annika Krause, Liza R. Moscovice and Christian Nawroth*
Institute of Behavioural Physiology, Leibniz Institute for Farm Animal Biology (FBN), 18196 Dummerstorf, Germany

Abstract

Altering one's emotional state in response to the emotional expressions of others, called emotional contagion, is a well-studied phenomenon in humans and many nonhuman animals. Here we describe the methods that are typically used to assess changes in the emotional state in demonstrators and the transmission of emotions to naïve observers.We then review the evidence for the transmission of positive and negative emotions in farm animals. We conclude by highlighting examples of how a better understanding of emotional contagion in farm animals can lead to novel and innovative interventions to improve their welfare.

Keywords: affective state, arousal, cognition, emotions, empathy, farm animals, livestock, mood, valence

Review Methodology

We searched Web of Science for relevant articles using the search terms '(TS = ('emotional contagion') AND TS = ('farm animal' OR 'farm animals' OR pig OR pigs OR piglet OR piglets OR sow OR sows OR gilt OR gilts OR boar OR boars OR swine OR 'Sus scrofa' OR cow OR cows OR calve OR calves OR cattle OR dairy OR 'Bos taurus' OR 'Bos indicus' OR chicken OR chickens OR hen OR hens OR chick OR chicks OR poultry OR goat OR goats OR capra OR sheep OR ewe OR ovis) NOT TS = ('guinea pig' OR 'guinea-pig')) AND DOCUMENT TYPES: (Article).' We also used references from these articles for additional relevant material.

Definition and Descriptions

Affective states, referring to short-term emotions and long-term moods, are inherently 'personal' experiences of individuals. However, individuals often live in social groups, and there is increasing evidence that social partners are highly sensitive to indicators of affective states in others, whether these are expressed as signals in a voluntary act of communication or as involuntary cues. This sensitivity to others' emotional states can lead to emotional contagion, which is defined as the tendency to alter one's behavioral (e.g. postures, vocalizations) and physiological (e.g. heart rate, hormone levels) states in response to the emotional expressions of others (reviewed

*Corresponding author: nawroth.christian@gmail.com

by Prochazkova and Kret, 2017), reflecting changes in the observer's affective state. Emotional contagion is suggested to have its evolutionary origins in the subconscious, automatic mimicry of behavioral expressions, including emotional ones, and has been described by two conceptually distinct and empirically separable components, namely socially-mediated arousal, referring to an observer's heightened sensitivity in response to changes in a demonstrator, and behavioral/physiological contagion, referring to the matching of the demonstrator's behavioral or physiological state (Edgar and Nicol, 2018). It is a highly efficient way for fitness-relevant information to spread through a social group, and is widely considered the most basic form of empathic responses (Panksepp and Panksepp, 2013). While emotional contagion does not involve all of the cognitive and emotional systems that we associate with human empathy, it is highly relevant given that it is widespread in animals (Špinka, 2012) and has applied value for animal welfare, especially under captive conditions (Baciadonna *et al.*, 2018). Emotional contagion implies that it is not only important to consider the effect of a treatment on an individual, but also the extent to which its group members may be affected by its response, even if they were not subjected to the treatment themselves.

State of the Art

Research into emotional contagion in animals integrates multiple behavioral, autonomic, and/or physiological measures to provide evidence for the transmission not only of arousal but also of valence (i.e. the positive or negative perception of a situation (Edgar *et al.*, 2012)). In typical paradigms, a naïve individual directly observes a conspecific demonstrator during a situation that induces a change in the demonstrator's emotional state.The observer has access to visual, olfactory, and/or auditory cues, but usually is not allowed to directly interact with the demonstrator (Goumon and Špinka, 2016). Measuring the transmission of emotions requires methods to assess changes in emotional states in demonstrators, as well as evaluating whether observers exhibit corresponding changes that indicate a similarly valenced (e.g. pleasant vs unpleasant) emotional response. Indicators of emotions that have been studied in the context of emotional contagion include functionally relevant behaviors that accompany emotional states, such as approach and avoidance, freezing, vocalizations, tail wagging, ear postures, or facial expressions (Goumon and Špinka, 2016; Reimert *et al.*, 2017). Autonomic indicators such as changes in heart rate (HR) and its variability (HRV) and surface eye temperature are also commonly used (Edgar *et al.*, 2011; Edgar and Nicol, 2018). In addition, concentrations of neuroendocrine hormones such as cortisol and oxytocin can change rapidly in blood, saliva, or urine in response to positive or negative stimuli (e.g. Burkett *et al.*, 2016). The integration of multiple behavioral and physiological measures can provide insights into both the arousal and valence aspects of emotional contagion.

Evidence for emotional contagion is widespread across animal taxa, but primarily restricted to the transmission of negative emotional states such as fear, pain, or distress (Edgar and Nicol, 2018; Goumon and Špinka, 2016; Edgar *et al.*, 2011), see Table 20.1. This may be in part because negative emotional states are easier to detect, due to their more direct link to survival and fitness, but it also may reflect the more well-developed methods for identifying negative emotional states in animals (reviewed in Baciadonna *et al.*, 2018).While studies of emotional contagion in farm animals have lagged behind other species (see Fig. 20.1), the available evidence suggests that farm animals may also transmit both negative and positive emotions (Reimert *et al.*, 2017), see also Table 20.1. Modifications to standard paradigms suggest that emotions can even be transmitted to naïve individuals who do not directly observe demonstrators receiving a positive or negative treatment, but merely interact with them beforehand when they are anticipating the stimulus (Reimert *et al.*, 2013; Reimert *et al.*, 2015), or afterward when they are returned to their social groups (Colditz *et al.*, 2012; Reimert *et al.*, 2017). For example, naïve pigs responded differently to being reunited with group mates who had experienced a negative or positive treatment. They exhibited decreased activity and exploration when group mates received a negative treatment, and increased

Table 20.1. Overview of behavioral and physiological responses* of demonstrators and observers in different testing paradigms for emotional contagion in farm animals.

Reference	Species	Test paradigm	Treatments	Measures	Test	Statistics (effect of...)	Reaction of the demonstrator/ treated individual	Reaction of the observer/naïve individual
Edgar *et al.* (2011)	Chicken	During experience of a negative treatment	Negative: aversive air puff Control: no treatment Control with noise	Eye temperature, comb temperature, heart rate, heart rate variability, behavior: standing alert, preening, vocalizations, maternal clucking	During a negative treatment: air puff to hen itself (vs pre-treatment)	Interaction of treatment* period	Standing alert ↑, preening ↓, eye temperature ↓, comb temperature ↓, total vocalizations ↑	Data not shown
					During a negative treatment: air puff to chicks (vs pre-treatment)	Interaction of treatment* period	No interaction effect between treatment and period concerning chick distress vocalization	Standing alert ↑, preening ↓, heart rate ↑, eye temperature ↓, total vocalizations ↑, maternal clucking ↑
Edgar and Nicol (2018)	Chicken	During experience of a negative treatment	Negative: aversive air puff to conspecifics Control: air puff was directed away	Eye temperature, behavior: ground pecking, standing, sitting, preening, freezing, walking	During a negative treatment (vs pre-treatment)	Interaction of treatment* period	Freezing ↑, preening ↓, ground pecking ↓, eye temperature ↓	Freezing ↑, preening ↓, ground pecking ↓, eye temperature ↓
					During control treatment (vs pre-treatment)	Interaction of treatment* period	No statistical differences	No statistical differences
					During a negative treatment (vs control)	Pearson/ Spearman correlation	Highly correlated demonstrator-observer behavior (ground pecking, standing, freezing) and eye temperature	

Continued

Table 20.1. Continued

Reference	Species	Test paradigm	Treatments	Measures	Test	Statistics (effect of...)	Reaction of the demonstrator/ treated individual	Reaction of the observer/naïve individual
Goumon and Špinka (2016)	Pig	During experience of a negative treatment	Negative: restrained behind a movable wall Control: wall moves, but no restraint	Heart rate, heart rate variability, behavior: locomotion, proximity, escape attempts, freezing, defecating, urinating, lying, looking at/nosing pair mate, ears back, tail low/ wag, vocalization	Phase 1: naïve observers			
					During a negative treatment (vs control)	Treatment (negative vs control)	Ears back ↑, looking at pen mate ↑, walking ↓, escape attempts ↑, snout contact ↓, lying ↓, grunts (of the pair) ↓, squeals (of the pair) ↑	Looking at pen mate ↑, proximity to pen mate ↑, snout contact ↑, walking ↓, freezing ↑, lying ↓, grunts (of the pair) ↓, squeals (of the pair) ↑
					Phase 2: experienced observers			
					During a negative treatment (vs control)	Treatment (negative vs control)	No significant differences	Proximity to pen mate ↑, looking at pen mate ↑, walking ↓, freezing ↑
Reimert *et al.* (2013)	Pig	During anticipation and experience of a negative/positive treatment	Negative: social isolation with negative handling Positive: access to a compartment with straw and food reward	Cortisol, behavior: freezing, escape attempts, play, defecating, urinating, ears back, ear posture changes, tail curled/wag/low, vocalization	During anticipation of a negative (vs positive) treatment	Treatment (negative vs positive)	Ears back ↑, ear posture change ↑, nosing of start box ↓, orienting head toward start box ↓	No statistical differences

					During a negative (vs positive) treatment	Treatment (negative vs positive)	Urinating ↑, defecating ↑, tail curled ↑, play ↓, tail wagging ↓, tail posture changes ↓	Nosing aversive door ↑, low-pitch vocalization ↑, play ↓, nosing the rewarding door ↓
Reimert *et al.* (2015)	Pig	During anticipa- tion and experience of a negative/ positive treatment Effect of intranasal administration of oxytocin in observers	Negative: social isolation with negative handling Positive: access to a compartment with straw and food reward	Behavior: standing alert, escape attempts, play, urinating, defecating, exploring doors, ear postures, head postures, head orientation, vocalization	During anticipation of a negative (vs positive) treatment	Treatment (negative vs positive)	No statistical analysis, descrip- tive reporting only	No statistical analysis, descriptive reporting only
					Without intranasal administration of oxytocin:			
					During a negative (vs positive) treatment	Treatment (negative vs positive)	Standing alert ↑, escape attempts ↑, urinating ↑, defecating ↑, exploring treatment door ↑, ears back ↑, tail in curl ↑, tail wag ↓, play ↓ low- and high-pitched vocaliza- tions ↑, barks ↓	Negative treatment vs positive treatment vs without pen mates present: standing alert ↑, exploring door to positive compart- ment ↓, exploring door to demonstrator ↑
					During a treatment with (vs without) pen mates present	Situation	Standing alert ↑, ears back ↓	

Continued

Table 20.1. Continued

Reference	Species	Test paradigm	Treatments	Measures	Test	Statistics (effect of...)	Reaction of the demonstrator/ treated individual	Reaction of the observer/naïve individual
					During a negative/ positive treatment with/without pen mates present	Interaction of treatment* situation	Standing alert	
					With intranasal administration of oxytocin or placebo in observer/naïve individuals:			
					During a negative (vs positive) treatment	Treatment (negative vs positive)	Standing alert ↑, play ↓, urinating ↑, defecating ↑, tail in curl ↑, tail wag ↓, low-pitched vocalization ↑	Standing alert ↑, exploring door to positive compartment ↓
					During a negative/ positive treatment with admin. of oxytocin (vs placebo)	Intranasal administration	Defecating ↓	Low-pitched vocalizations ↑
					During a negative/ positive treatment with admin. of oxytocin/placebo	Interaction of treatment* administration	Defecating, exploring treatment door, tail low	Exploring neutral door
Reimert *et al.* (2017)	Pig	During reunion after exposure to a negative/ positive treatment	Negative: social isolation with negative handling Positive: access to a compartment with straw and food reward	Behavior: standing, standing alert, sitting, lying, walking, play, drinking, eating, comfort behavior, nosing (nose/ body of pen mate), manipu-late pen mate, aggressive behavior,	Day 2 (at the beginning of the experiment)			

		exploring chain/ substrate/pen, tail postures (in curl, wagging, low, between legs), initiator/ receiver of social interaction behaviors (nosing nose/body of pen mate)				
			After a negative (vs positive) treatment	Treatment (negative vs positive)	Lying ↑, walking ↓, exploring pen ↓ nosing the nose of the observer ↓	Lying ↑, walking ↓, standing ↓, exploring pen ↓, nosing behavior (nose-nose, nose-body) ↓
			After a treatment being the observer (vs demonstrator)	Type (only in the context of social behaviors)	Nosing the nose of the demonstrator ↑	
			Day 18 (at the end of the experiment)			
			After a negative (vs positive) treatment	Treatment (negative vs positive)	Eating ↑, nosing the nose and body of the demonstrator ↓	Lying ↑, walking ↓, standing ↓, nosing behavior (nose-nose, nose-body) ↓, tail low ↑
			After a treatment being the observer (vs demonstrator)	Type (only in the context of social behaviors)	Nosing the nose and body of the demonstrator ↑	

Continued

Table 20.1. Continued

Reference	Species	Test paradigm	Treatments	Measures	Test	Statistics (effect of...)	Reaction of the demonstrator/ treated individual	Reaction of the observer/naïve individual
Colditz *et al.* (2012)	Sheep	After the experience of a negative treatment	Negative: ring/ knife castration Control: sham castration	Cortisol, rectal temperature, pain avoidance behavior: restlessness, kicking/ foot stamping, rolling, jumping, licking wound, easing quarters, teat seeking, postural behavior: normal ventral lying, abnormal ventral lying, ventral lying other, lateral lying, abnormal lying, total lying, normal standing, statue standing, abnormal standing, standing other, normal walking, abnormal walking, walking other, total standing, total abnormal behaviors, synchrony of behavior	After a negative (knife castration) treatment vs ring vs sham castration	Treatment (negative1 vs negative2 vs control)	Cortisol ↑, rectal temperature ↑, normal ventral lying ↓, statue standing ↑, abnor- mal standing ↑, total standing ↑, total abnormal behaviors ↑	

After a negative treatment in homogenous (vs heterogeneous) social groupings	Social grouping	Cortisol ↑, restless behavior ↑, normal ventral lying ↑, normal standing ↓, total standing ↓, walking ↑, total abnormal behavior ↓
After a negative/ control treatment in homogenous/ heterogeneous social groupings	Interaction of treatment* social grouping	Lateral lying
At three different time periods after a negative/control treatment	Interaction of treatment* period	Statue standing, total abnormal behaviors
After a treatment in homogenous (vs heterogeneous) social groupings	Behavioral synchrony (K coefficient of synchroniza- tion)	Heterogeneous groups: synchronization of walking homogeneous groups: synchronization of feeding at the trough (sham + ring castration) negative synchronization of lying and standing (ring + knife castration)

Increases (↑) and decreases (↓) in the response of demonstrators and observers between the respective treatments and/or periods are indicated by arrows.
[a]Behavioral and physiological responses with statistical differences ($p < 0.05$) are illustrated

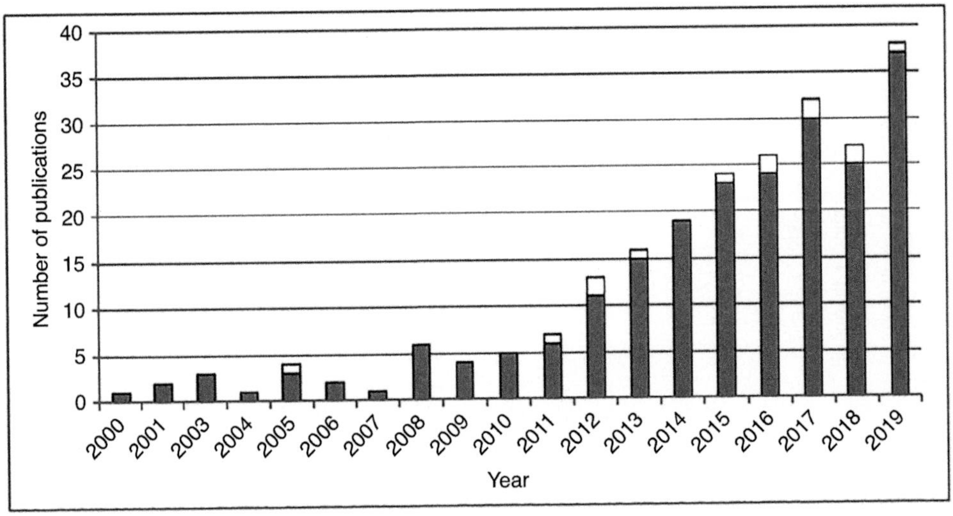

Fig. 20.1. Number of publications covering emotional contagion in humans and animal species other than farm animals (gray bars) and in farm animals (white bars) over the last 20 years (according to WoS).

social contact and exploration when group mates received a positive treatment (Reimert *et al.*, 2017), see also Table 20.1. This suggests that the impact of a specific treatment on an individuals' emotional state can last well beyond the treatment itself, and can also affect the emotional state of group members.

Implications for Farm Animals and Outlook for Future Studies

Emotions, both positive and negative, have the potential to spread across a group of individuals via emotional contagion.This phenomenon is especially important from a farm animal welfare perspective, since it suggests that even brief husbandry interventions can have positive or negative impacts on the affective states of individuals who anticipate and experience them, as well as on the rest of their social group. Although research on transmission of emotions in applied ethology is still in its infancy (see Fig. 20.1), the available literature is a promising indicator of what we might expect to find across a range of farm animals (Baciadonna *et al.*, 2018).

Future research should aim at increasing our knowledge of emotional contagion in farm animals to design husbandry environments that improve their welfare, that is, by decreasing the spread of negative emotions or promoting the spread of positive ones (Baciadonna *et al.*, 2018). This could be achieved through modifications to the husbandry and management environment. For example, selective noise-canceling of high-pitched distress calls, while allowing low-pitched non-distress calls that might provide social support, is one possibility to reduce the spread of negative emotions through groups. In addition to noise-canceling speaker systems, technical innovations such as visual or acoustic displays of demonstrators in positive states also have potential.To this end, we need to investigate the sensory modalities (including visual, acoustic, or olfactory cues) that make individuals of a specific species most susceptible to emotional contagion. Several studies have also shown that previous experience of the observer with the same positive or negative event as the demonstrator (Goumon and Špinka, 2016), or the strength of social relationships between the observer and demonstrator (Edgar *et al.*, 2011) can influence the likelihood of emotional contagion and these areas deserve further research. The development and integration of a broader range of indicators, including non-invasive physiological parameters, to validate emotional states in demonstrators and track changes in emotional states in observers, are also needed. Lastly, future research should take into account that emotional contagion does not require exact matching of every aspect of the demonstrator's response. It can also lead to a more generalized synchronization of behavioral and physiological parameters resulting in varied responses that still match the valence aspect of the observed emotional state.

In the long term, an increased understanding of when and how emotional contagion occurs will provide novel insights into the emotional experiences of animals, and is thus key to improving their welfare.

Acknowledgments

This work was supported by a grant from the Deutsche Forschungsgemeinschaft (DFG, LA 1187/6–1) to CN. The publication of this article was funded by the Open Access Fund of the Leibniz Association and the Open Access Fund of the Leibniz Institute for Farm Animal Biology (FBN).

References

Baciadonna, L., Düpjan, S., Briefer, E.F., Torre, M. and Nawroth, C. (2018) Looking on the bright side of livestock emotions—the potential of their transmission to promote positive welfare. *Frontiers in Veterinary Science* 5, 218.

Burkett, J.P., Andari, E., Curry, D.C., De Waal, F.B.M. and Young, L.J. (2016) Oxytocin-dependent consolation behavior in rodents. *Science* 351(6271), 375–378.

Colditz, I.G., Paull, D.R. and Lee, C. (2012) Social transmission of physiological and behavioural responses to castration in suckling Merino lambs. *Applied Animal Behaviour Science* 136(2–4), 136–145.

Edgar, J.L. and Nicol, C.J. (2018) Socially-mediated arousal and contagion within domestic chick broods. *Scientific Reports* 8(1), 1–10.

Edgar, J.L., Lowe, J.C., Paul, E.S. and Nicol, C.J. (2011) Avian maternal response to chick distress. *Proceedings of the Royal Society B* 278(1721), 3129–3134.

Edgar, J.L., Nicol, C.J., Clark, C.C. and Paul, E.S. (2012) Measuring empathic responses in animals. *Applied Animal Behaviour Science* 138(3–4), 182–193.

Goumon, S. and Špinka, M. (2016) Emotional contagion of distress in young pigs is potentiated by previous exposure to the same stressor. *Animal Cognition* 19(3), 501–511.

Panksepp, J. and Panksepp, J.B. (2013) Toward a cross-species understanding of empathy. *Trends in Neurosciences* 36(8), 489–496.

Prochazkova, E. and Kret, M.E. (2017) Connecting minds and sharing emotions through mimicry: A neurocognitive model of emotional contagion. *Neuroscience and Biobehavioral Reviews* 80, 99–114.

Reimert, I., Bolhuis, J.E., Kemp, B. and Rodenburg, T.B. (2013) Indicators of positive and negative emotions and emotional contagion in pigs. *Physiology & Behavior* 109, 42–50.

Reimert, I., Bolhuis, J.E., Kemp, B. and Rodenburg, T.B. (2015) Emotions on the loose: Emotional contagion and the role of oxytocin in pigs. *Animal Cognition* 18(2), 517–532.

Reimert, I., Fong, S., Rodenburg, T.B. and Bolhuis, J.E. (2017) Emotional states and emotional contagion in pigs after exposure to a positive and negative treatment. *Applied Animal Behaviour Science* 193, 37–42.

Špinka, M. (2012) Social dimension of emotions and its implication for animal welfare. *Applied Animal Behaviour Science* 138(3–4), 170–181.

21 Direct and Indirect Threats Imposed by Plant Pathogenic and Saprophytic Fungi on Humans and Animals

Elham Ahmed Kazerooni[1], Rethinasamy Velazhahan[1], Musthafa Mohamed Essa[2] and Abdullah Mohammed Al-Sadi[1*]

[1]Department of Crop Sciences, College of Agricultural and Marine Sciences, College of Agricultural and Marine Sciences Sultan Qaboos University, Muscat, 123, Sultanate of Oman; [2]Department of Food Science and Nutrition, Sultan Qaboos University, Muscat, 123, Sultanate of Oman

Abstract

Fungi play an important role in our life. Several species of fungi act as biocontrol agents, antibiotic producers, and waste material decomposers. On the other hand, several harmful fungi cause problems by attacking plants, humans, and animals, while others can spoil our food. Fungi attacking plants result in various diseases in the roots, stems, leaves, flowers, and fruits, which could result in either mild reduction in the yield or complete loss of a crop. There are also some fungal species that reside inside the plant tissues without causing diseases (endophytes) and others that survive as saprophytes on plant leaves, stems, or roots without causing damage to plants. Considerable knowledge and reviews have been generated on the effects of plant pathogenic fungi on plants' survival and yield. Although some studies indicated the possible effects of plant fungi on humans and animals, there is a lack of a comprehensive review on this aspect. This review paper discusses the direct and indirect effects of plant pathogenic and saprophytic fungal species on humans and animals.

Keywords: toxins, asthma, allergy, oomycetes, plant disease

Review Methodology

A survey was done via Scopus (www.scopus.com) and Google Scholar (https://scholar.google.com). The survey targeted most available publications that dealt with fungi infecting or residing in/on plants and at the same time having direct or indirect effects on humans. The direct ways included the various types of infections and allergies caused by plant saprophytic and pathogenic fungi on humans, while the indirect ways include the effects of these fungi on food security, safety, and quality. Due to the lack of previous reviews on this aspect, the focus was mainly on recent and previous publications. The search terms included, but were not limited

*Corresponding author: alsadi@squ.edu.om

to, saprophytic, pathogenic, endophytic, fungi, humans, plants, and food.

Introduction

Fungi are a heterogeneous, heterotrophic, and eukaryotic group of organisms that can be found almost in every ecological niche. Environmental requirements for the survival of fungi vary among different species, and some of them may be so specific, while others may survive under a broad range of environments (Sharon and Shlezinger, 2013). This large and diverse group of organisms produces exoenzymes and absorbs nutrients through their hyphal network and reproduces mostly by spores (Kendrick, 2000). They can play major positive or negative roles in our ecosystems and life. Their positive roles include their use as biocontrol agents for insects and diseases, production of antibiotics, promotion of plant growth and development, and decomposition of waste material (Suman et al., 2016; Yao *et al.*, 2017; Kashyap *et al.*, 2017; Halo *et al.*, 2018). Many fungi on the other hand play negative and detrimental roles as pathogens of plants, animals, and humans (Rodríguez-Gálvez *et al.*, 2017; Naseri and Ansari Hamadani, 2017; Esmaeili Taheri *et al.*, 2017; Al-Balushi *et al.*, 2018).

Plant disease is an abnormal condition and a physiological process that affect plants and alters their function and appearance over time. Moreover, it reduces yield and quality of plant products. Plants are invaded by various pathogens such as fungi, bacteria, and viruses. Fungi are the largest group of microorganisms that can cause diseases in plants. For example, among fungal species, more than 250 species of them can cause diseases on rice, while only 12 bacterial species may cause diseases on rice (McBeath and McBeath, 2010). Favorable environmental conditions such as temperature, moisture, light, soil structure, nutrient, and wind or rain splash are highly important in the dissemination of microbes and disease development (Schumann and D'Arcy, 2006).

Previous data and outbreaks support the idea that fungi cause threat to plant diversity, and they also cause greater threat to biodiversity loss in the ecosystem than other taxonomic classes of pathogens (Fisher *et al.*, 2012). The resilient dispersal and long-lived stages and their ability to survive as saprophytes or durable spores are some features of fungi (Mitchell *et al.*, 2008). For example, fungi belonging to *Ascomycota* phylum are common residents of soil and can tolerate environmental conditions such as salinity. Some fungi, such as *Fusarium solani*, can cause infection on the nests of loggerhead turtles when they enter into the marine system (Rypien *et al.*, 2008; Sarmiento-Ramírez *et al.*, 2010). In addition, some fungi have a wide host range, which helps them survive and maintain infectious stages on susceptible hosts (Holdich *et al.*, 2009).

Some fungal species reside inside the plants without causing symptoms (endophytes) (Kotilínek *et al.*, 2017; Perera *et al.*, 2017; Yuan *et al.*, 2017), and some of these endophytes may be beneficial to plant's growth and development. Other fungal species survive on the organic products released by plants without causing direct effects on plants (saprophytes) (Kazerooni *et al.*, 2017).

Fungi infecting or residing in/on plants are usually restricted to plants and are not commonly known to cause direct effects on humans or animals. *Corynespora cassiicola*, a pathogen of several plant species (Lopez *et al.*, 2018), has been isolated recently from a 74-year-old man suffering from mycotic keratitis (Chung *et al.*, 2018). However, infecting or residing fungi in plants may affect humans and animals by various indirect ways that include their effects on the available food for humans or feed for animals, by producing toxic secondary metabolites to humans and or animals, or by causing effects on human and animal respiratory systems after inhalation.

Effects of Plant Pathogenic Fungi on Food Security

Some plant diseases can pose a serious threat to food security and national economy (Asibi *et al.*, 2019; Rajaram and Dubin, 2019). Some factors, including climate change, drought, salinity, and flooding, may alter the distribution of disease organisms (Váry *et al.*, 2015; Launay *et al.*, 2020). Similarly, globalization and movement of goods could also lead to the spread of disease organisms (James Downer *et al.*, 2009).

Studies suggest that these diseases and several thousands of other plant diseases limit food and feed available to humans and animals, respectively. This results in indirect effects on humans and animals by exposing them to food shortage or hunger. Some of the examples of fungal diseases and their effect on humans are delineated below.

Invasive fungal and fungal-like diseases have caused many outbreaks during the past decades. These worldwide outbreaks have affected ecosystems, plants, animals, and humans very seriously (Fisher *et al.*, 2012; Bjelke *et al.*, 2016). One of the serious diseases in history is potato late blight caused by the pseudo-fungus (oomycete) *Phytophthora infestans*. This disease caused widespread epidemics and failure of potato crops in the 1840s, which led to the great Irish famine.This famine led to death of approximately 1 million Irish people and immigration of 1.5 million people to the USA, Canada, and other countries. *Phytophthora* can spread in all parts of the infected plant quickly (McBeath and McBeath, 2010).

Rice is one of the two most important cereal crops in the world in terms of production and consumption. Around 3.5 billion consumers are dependent on this universal crop as their staple food. The importance of rice in food security could be due to the fact that this crop contributes 23% of the calories consumed by humans. Rice is considered as the most important food product in Asia, and around 92% of rice is cultivated and consumed mainly in this continent (Wilson and Talbot, 2009).

Rice blast disease is the most widely distributed and serious disease that affects cultivated rice. Rice blast has been found in 85 countries where rice is cultivated for commercial purpose. Rice blast epidemics have been reported in various countries including China, the USA, Korea, Vietnam, and Japan and caused destruction of 5.7 million hectares of rice between 2001 and 2005 (Wilson and Talbot, 2009). This disease is caused by a filamentous ascomycete fungus called *Magnaporthe oryzae* (He *et al.*, 2019). Rice blast spores are capable of surviving and overwintering and reappearing in the following year.

Wheat (*Triticum aestivum*) is the most important stable food of humans nowadays. Rust fungi are a destructive group of fungi parasitizing wheat and causing significant losses in grain yield and quality (Al-Sadi, 2017). Rust diseases are categorized as one of the oldest diseases in the world.The earliest rust epidemic was recorded in 700 BC (McBeath and McBeath, 2010). Rusts are well known for their long-distance dispersal through wind.The rust pathogen species that cause strip rust, stem rust, and leaf rust are *Puccinia striiformis* f. sp. *tritici*, *Puccinia graminis* f. sp. *tritici*, and *Puccinia triticina*, respectively (Tang *et al.*, 2018). Wheat rusts can cause yield losses up to 100%.

Mycotoxins and Their Effects on Food Safety

Microscopic fungi are capable of producing secondary metabolites to enhance their fitness in nature (Nielsen, 2003). However, some of these compounds that can be detrimental or toxic in higher vertebrates and evoke pathological changes in them are called mycotoxins (Nielsen, 2003). It has been estimated that the number of these toxic metabolites could be in the thousands (CATS, 2003). Kendrick (Kendrick, 2000) reported species of 46 fungal genera as mycotoxin producers. Diseases caused by mycotoxins are called mycotoxicoses, and the symptoms depend on mycotoxin type and amount, exposure length, organism age, and sex and interaction with the other physiological factors (Zain, 2011; da Rocha *et al.*, 2014; Sarma *et al.*, 2017). Mycotoxins may interfere with various mechanisms. For instance, fumonisin inhibits the biosynthesis of sphingolipid, while protein synthesis is interfered by with trichothecens (Eaton and Groopman, 1994; DeVries *et al.*, 2002).

The production of mycotoxins in cereal grains and forages occurs under various environmental conditions during plant growth and after or during harvesting, storage, or processing (Nonzom and Sumbali, 2017). Temperature, moisture, humidity, soil tillage, irrigation practices, and pathogens involved are some of the environmental and biological factors that affect mycotoxin production (Nonzom and

Sumbali, 2017). These secondary metabolites cause severe pathological changes in humans and animals, and their toxic properties could stay stable without eradication and remain camouflaged in foodstuffs. Mycotoxin producing fungi have affected 25% of the world's food production, and higher levels of contamination have been reported in cereal grains (CATS, 2003). Various species belonging to *Aspergillus, Penicillium*, and *Fusarium* are the main producers of these mycotoxins. Desjardins (Desjardins, 2006) indicated the immunocompromising ability of some mycotoxins, which lead to reduction of resistance to infectious diseases.

Mycotoxin-producing fungi are divided into two groups known as field fungi and storage fungi. *Aspergillus flavus* and *Fusarium* species are known as preharvest or field toxin producers, which produce mycotoxins such as aflatoxins and invade the growing plants. Ochratoxins, patulin, and citrinin are postharvest or storage toxins, which are produced after harvesting or during storage and marketing (Nonzom and Sumbali, 2017).

Maize is one of the most susceptible crops in the field, where its quality and yield get influenced by various fungal species such as *Fusarium* species and their toxins (Kommendahl and Windels, 1981; Logrieco *et al.*, 2002; Dorn *et al.*, 2009; Scauflaire *et al.*, 2011). Fumonisins, trichothecenes, and zearalenone are some of the mycotoxins produced by *Fusarium* species in infected maize.

Rice can lose its yield due to various fungal and bacterial diseases. Various *Fusarium* species were found to be responsible for 40% and 60% of rice yield loss in Nepal and Korea, respectively (Desjardins *et al.*, 2000; Park *et al.*, 2005). Wulff *et al.* (Wulff *et al.*, 2010) indicated the production of mycotoxins such as fumonisin B and moniliformin by some *Fusarium* species that are casual agents of rice sheath rot.The outer part of the rice grain is commonly occupied with mycotoxins, and the concentration of mycotoxins is reduced to about 75%–80% after hulling.

Rice false smut is a destructive worldwide disease, which is caused by *Ustilaginoidea virens* (Rani and Sharma, 2018; Yong *et al.*, 2018). Rice false smut is one of the most serious diseases of rice found in warm and humid rice cultivation areas, which could affect the yield and quality of rice grains. This disease attacks at the flowering stage, and it transforms the panicle grains to greenish false smut balls. This fungus contaminates rice seeds and produces antimitotic peptides, which are toxic for humans, animals, and plants (Koiso *et al.*, 1998).

Fusarium head blight is a common and worldwide disease of wheat that significantly reduces quality and yield of wheat (Windels, 2000). *Fusarium* species associated with this disease have various toxigenic abilities. For instance, beauvericin is produced by *F. poae*, while *F. avenaceum* is capable of producing enniatins, moniliformin, and beauvericin (Xu and Berrie, 2005).

Gibberella zeae-vomitoxin/Fusarium graminearum could cause wheat scab or head blight, a major and devastating head disease affecting wheat yield, grain quality, and edibility. This disease emerged as a major threat for human health and global food security over three decades ago (Del Ponte *et al.*, 2017). The grains produced from contaminated fields may contain a mycotoxin called vomitoxin (Clifford *et al.*, 2003; Pei-Sheng *et al.*, 2011; Jia *et al.*, 2017). This toxin can induce muscle spasms and vomiting in humans and can stay stable for years in stored grain.

Claviceps species are common pathogens of diverse groups of grass species. Based on historical records, ergotism is probably the first recognized mycotoxicosis (Nonzom and Sumbali, 2017). Consumption of cereals contaminated with ergot sclerotia (*Claviceps purpurea*) could result in ergotism in humans, which mutilated and killed thousands of people in Europe. The ingestion could be by direct intake of grain or by eating bread made with ergot contaminated flour (Bennett and Klich, 2003). This mycotoxin can cause gastrointestinal symptoms such as nausea and vomiting, and nervous symptoms including paralysis, drowsiness, and blindness (Peraica *et al.*, 1999).

Another important crop, which is known for its use in brewing and malting, is barley. Similarly, Fusarium head blight can affect barley and cause decline in crop yield and quality. Considerable amounts of mycotoxins such as nivalenol, zearalenone, and deoxynivalenol have been detected in barley grains (Prom *et al.*, 1999).

The most important indoor toxicogenic fungi with detrimental health impacts are *Aspergillus* species, *Penicillium* species, *Trichoderma* species, *Fusarium* species, *Paecilomyces* species, and *Stachybotrys chartarum* (Croft *et al.*, 1967; Flannigan *et al.*, 1991; Johanning *et al.*, 1993). Disease coming from exposure to mycotoxins is defined as mycotoxicosis, which can be acute or chronic (CATS, 2003). Human exposure to these nonvolatile or low volatile, toxic, immunogenic secondary metabolites of fungi could be through dermal absorption, inhalation, or diet (Croft *et al.*, 1967; Matossian, 1989; Miller, 1992; Smoragiewicz *et al.*, 1993; Johanning *et al.*, 1993; Singh, 1994; Dill *et al.*, 1997; Andersson *et al.*, 1997; Nielsen, 2003; CATS, 2003; Boonen *et al.*, 2012; Bennett and Inamdar, 2015). Based on historical records, exposure of humans to mycotoxins mainly happens through ingestion of food products containing or contaminated with these compounds (CATS, 2003). However, because of health effects of indoor fungi, the inhalation of fungal spores containing mycotoxins plays a primary role in the indoor environment and has become a major public health concern. Schiefer (Schiefer, 1990) believed that the inhalation of mycotoxins is not very likely due to their low volatility nature. Two mycotoxins including deoxynivalenol and T-2 toxin have been detected in the conidia of *Fusarium graminearum* and *F. sporotrichioides* (Miller, 1992). Aflatoxins, trichothecens, fumonisins, gliotoxin, zearalenone, and ochratoxins are considered as the most well documented mycotoxins in indoor environments (Kilburn, 2004; Zain, 2011).

Aflatoxin is one of the most studied and potent carcinogenic mycotoxins on humans and animals, which is produced by *Aspergillus flavus* and *Aspergillus parasiticus* (Thacker, 2004). Some of the mycotoxin effects on human health include mucous membrane irritation, skin rash, nausea, acute or chronic liver damage, inhibition of protein and DNA synthesis, endocrine effects and cancer, excessive fatigue, joint ache, and respiratory problems (Olsen *et al.*, 1988; CATS, 2003; Gottschalk *et al.*, 2008; Bonetta *et al.*, 2010; Karunasena *et al.*, 2010). The disease severity depends on the level and type of aflatoxin in diet, the extent of exposure, age, and nutritional status of the individual (Peraica *et al.*, 1999).

In Western India, an outbreak of aflatoxicoses was reported in 1974, which caused 106 deaths and 397 cases (Krishnamachari *et al.*, 1975). In Kenya, aflatoxicosis outbreaks occurred in 2004 due to consumption of aflatoxin-contaminated maize, which resulted in 125 deaths and 317 cases (Azziz-Baumgartner *et al.*, 2005). In Malaysia, in 1995, consumption of rice spaghetti contaminated with aflatoxins caused brain damage, encephalopathy, and acute damage in the livers of children (Munn Sann *et al.*, 1995).

The prevalence of high incidence of liver cancer has been linked with food contaminated with aflatoxins (Bababunmi *et al.*, 1978). Li *et al.* (Li *et al.*, 2001) reported that the content of Aflatoxins B1, B2, and G1 was significantly higher in corn samples collected from the high incidence areas for human hepatocellular carcinoma. The presence of aflatoxins in children with Reye syndrome has been reported from Czechoslovakia (Dvorackova, 1976), New Zealand (Becroft and Webster, 1972), Thailand (Shank *et al.*, 1971), and the USA (Hogan *et al.*, 1978; Ryan *et al.*, 1979). Aflatoxins have been reported to be present in the blood of pregnant women and in breast milk in African countries (Coulter *et al.*, 1984; Maxwell *et al.*, 1989; Gatwiri *et al.*, 2017).

Studies conducted in Ghana, Kenya, Liberia, Sudan, Transkei, Zimbabwe, and Nigeria revealed the presence of high concentrations of aflatoxins in liver specimens from children with kwashiorkor symptoms (Hendrickse *et al.*, 1982; Apeagyei *et al.*, 1986; Hendrickse and Maxwell, 1989; de Vries *et al.*, 1990; Oyelami *et al.*, 1997).

Infection of Humans and Animals by Plant Pathogenic and Saprophytic Fungi

Fungi infecting plants may also result in serious problems to humans and animals. *Fusarium oxysporum* f. sp. *lycopersici* causes wilt disease in tomatoes. Studies have also shown that immuno-depressed mice could be killed by this type of fungus (Ortoneda *et al.*, 2004). *Fusarium solani*, a widely distributed soil-borne saprophyte, is usually isolated from soil and plant debris (Sarmiento-Ramírez *et al.*, 2010), and this fungus is capable of causing serious plant diseases under conducive conditions and also poses diseases in immunocompromised animals (Booth, 1971; Summerbell, 2003). Rebell (Rebell, 1981) reported *Fusarium solani* as a causal agent of infection on marine turtle's skin and shells. This fungus has been isolated from the dead eggs of various sea turtle species from different locations (Phillott and Parmenter, 2001; Marco *et al.*, 2006; Abella *et al.*, 2008). It has led to 100% morbidity and mortality of the turtle eggs.

Many fungi are decomposers or saprophytes and can be found in indoor or outdoor environments. *Schizophyllum commune* is considered as a wood decomposing fungus. However, some reports indicated that it causes human infection, meningitis, and lung disorders (Kern and Uecker, 1986). Since it is a facultative parasite and does not depend on a living organism or a particular host, it attacks its host belligerently, and it can kill its host. It should be noted that this fungus normally affects humans whose immune system has become compromised.

Scedosporium apiospermum is a fungus found in parks, playgrounds, gardens, potting or feces-enriched soil, sewers, and saltwater habitats. It can cause trauma-related infections, systemic invasive disease, and pneumonia or brain abscess (de Hoog *et al.*, 1994; Rainer and Hoog, 2006; Chen *et al.*, 2011). *Cryptococcus gattii* is a fungus belonging to the phylum Basidiomycota and is transmitted through inhalation (Miller *et al.*, 2002). Virulent strains of *C. gattii* can infect immuno-competent humans, animals and marine organisms, wildlife and cause illness and death (Byrnes *et al.*, 2010). It has been isolated from trees, soil, air, and water in human and animal vicinity (Fraser *et al.*, 2005; Kidd *et al.*, 2005). Moreover, this species has been isolated from the flowers and bark of eucalyptus trees (Gugnani *et al.*, 2005). Another study done by Davies *et al.* (Davies *et al.*, 1988) demonstrated asthma symptoms among workforce who were working in a tomato greenhouse contaminated with *Verticillium albo-atrum*.

Induction of Allergy by Plant Pathogenic and Saprophytic Fungi

The most common human reaction to airborne fungi is probably allergy. It has been proven that more than 80 genera of major fungi, belonging to Ascomycetes and Basidiomycetes, are associated with respiratory disorders (Levetin, 1995; Bush and Portnoy, 2001). Fungal spores were recognized as one of the main allergens in indoor environment (Baxi *et al.*, 2016; Reddy and Srinivas, 2017). Sources of fungal spores in indoor environment could be flowers, groceries, dust, and carpet. For instance, *Aspergillus* spores are often present in the soil of pot plants (Gąska-Jedruch and Dudzinska, 2009; Żukiewicz-Sobczak *et al.*, 2012). In the external environment, various fungi such as *Cladosporium, Alternaria, Botrytis, Epicoccum*, and *Penicillium* have been categorized as allergenic fungi. Some of them are specialized pathogens of economically important crops, fruits, and vegetables (Zukiewicz-Sobczak, 2013). Many studies have demonstrated the relationship between increasing the fungal spore counts, fungal antigen levels, and allergic symptoms (Bush and Portnoy, 2001). *Alternaria* and *Penicillium* spores and spore extracts produce immediate and late asthma symptoms, and *Aspergillus* can cause atopic diseases (Sakamoto *et al.*, 1990; Knutsen *et al.*, 2012).

Spores of fungi especially *Alternaria* and *Aspergillus* are the most common allergens causing severe asthma and respiratory infections (Denning *et al.*, 2006; Żukiewicz-Sobczak *et al.*, 2012). Malling (Malling, 1990) reported *Cladosporium herbarum* as a potential cause of allergic asthma and rhinitis. Garrett *et al.* (Garrett *et al.*, 1998) found that *Penicillium* and *Cladosporium* were the most common fungal allergies among children in winter or musty odor. Previous studies indicated *Alternaria alternata* and closely related genera such as *Stemphylium* and *Ulocladium* as the most important mold allergens in the USA (Hoffman, 1984; Reed, 1985; O'Hollaren *et al.*, 1991; Knutsen *et al.*, 2012). Ascospores are considered as important airborne allergens and unique antigens (Eversmeyer and Kramer, 1987). Among Ascomycetes, *Chaetomium* species are commonly found in indoor environments on wood products or water damaged papers (Li and Yang, 2004). Basidiospores of fungi including *Agaricus campestris, Coprinus micaceus*, and *Ustilago maydis* can cause rhinitis, asthma, and immediate skin reactivity in sensitive patients (Santilli and Rockwell, 2003). Inhaling the spores of mushrooms such as edible mushroom (*Pholiota nameko*) can pose hypersensitivity pneumonitis (Nakazawa and Tochigi, 1989). *Pleurotus ostreatus* was characterized as allergens and can cause allergic alveolitis (Cox, 1988; Elliot Horner *et al.*, 1988). It should be noted that fungal allergy symptoms are usually indistinguishable from the other types of allergy, which happen by inhalation of dust, pollen, and so on (Savilahti *et al.*, 2010). Krzysztofik (Krzysztofik, 1992) believed that fungal allergens cause more severe respiratory system symptoms than the other environmental allergens, which could be due to the additional capacity of fungi to multiply and colonize the respiratory system and infect the skin.

Plant Fungi and Skin Diseases

Besides allergies, fungi can cause infectious diseases on skin or other body organs, which are called mycoses. Inhalation of airborne fungal spores in regions with high frequency of spores can cause endemic mycosis (Pitt, 1979; Lacey, 1991). Immunocompromised patients (such as HIV or organ transplant) might be at an increased risk of opportunistic fungal pathogens if these fungi become airborne and their concentration elevates in indoor environments. *Aspergillus fumigatus*, *A. flavus*, and *A. niger* are categorized as significant concern fungi. One of the most important airborne pathogenic fungi is *Aspergillus fumigatus* because of its thermophilic and small size spores (Klich and Pitt, 1988; Brakhage and Langfelder, 2002). These fungi might originate from various sources including houseplants, soil, organic waste, water damaged materials, and bird droppings (Benenson, 1990; Burge, 1990; Larsen and Frisvad, 1995).

Health Effects of Volatile Fungal Metabolites

To date, around 300 fungal volatile organic compounds have been categorized (Chiron and Michelot, 2005). Blends of volatile organic compounds (VOCs) are emitted by fungi, and the quantity and quality of them depend on the fungal species and environmental condition (Bennett and Inamdar, 2015). Volatile fungal metabolites (VFMs) are correlated with fungal growth, and they could be used as indicators of fungal growth or as environmental signaling compounds (Bennett and Inamdar, 2015). Fungi release them as low molecular weight secondary metabolites during their metabolic processes. These compounds have low molecular weight and can disseminate easily through air, causing harmful effects in enclosed environments (Bennett and Inamdar, 2015). These compounds may have a distinctive musty, earthy, or moldy odor with low odor threshold (Flannigan *et al.*, 1991; Magan and Evans, 2000). Chemical structures of these compounds are diverse and include alcohols, alkenes, ketones, and aldehydes (Wilkins *et al.*, 2003; Bornehag *et al.*, 2004). Previous studies of household fungi showed that their VFM composition stays stable over a range of conditions and growth media (Nilsson *et al.*, 2004; Moularat *et al.*, 2008). Bennett and Inamdar (Bennett and Inamdar, 2015) suggested the term volatoxin for fungal volatile organic compounds with toxic properties and toxigenic effects. Some evidence proposed that exposure to low concentrations of volatile fungal metabolites might pose respiratory irritation (Weinhold, 2007). Edmondson *et al.* (Edmondson *et al.*, 2005) mentioned VOCs as potential asthma triggers. Moreover, it has been shown that there is a link between some symptoms such as headache, dizziness, fatigue, nasal irritation, feeling stuffiness, nausea, and exposure to volatile organic compounds (Flannigan and Miller, 1994; Burton *et al.*, 2008). For example, odor complaints and irritation symptoms have been reported due to the volatile contaminants from composting plants (Müller *et al.*, 2004). A study done by Kreja and Seidel (Kreja and Seidel, 2002) concluded less toxicity of microbial volatile organic compounds for humans than mycotoxins.

Conclusion

To summarize, fungi infecting plants or residing in/on plants could cause indirect effects on humans and animals. Flexibility and ability of fungi to undergo genetic recombination, hybridization, or horizontal gene transfer, allow them to produce new races with different characteristics (Fraser *et al.*, 2005; Stukenbrock and McDonald, 2008; Richards *et al.*, 2011). Consequently, phenotypic leaps can be obtained and lead to a rise in virulence, host jumps, and new pathotype formation in plant pathogens (Mallet, 2007; Giraud *et al.*, 2010). The toxins from fungi including aflatoxins and mycotoxins are causing severe health effects in humans and animals. The possibility of overcoming or bringing novel methods to find and remove the affected crops could play a major role in reducing the disease impact of fungi to humans and animals. More studies are required in the future on the relationship between plant pathogenic and saprophytic fungi and human health.

Acknowledgments

The authors would like to thank Sultan Qaboos University and Oman Animal and Plant Genetic Resources Center.

References

Abella, E., Marco, A., Di'eguez-Uribeondo, J. and López-Jurado, L. (2008) Pathogenic effect of microorganisms on loggerhead eggs. In: *28th Sea Turtle Symposium, International Sea Turtle Society*, National Marine Fisheries Service.

Al-Balushi, Z.M., Agrama, H., Al-Mahmooli, I.H., Maharachchikumbura, S.S.N. and Al-Sadi, A.M. (2018) Development of resistance to hymexazol among *Pythium* species in cucumber greenhouses in Oman. *Plant Disease* 102, 202–208.

Al-Sadi, A.M. (2017) Epidemiology and management of fungal diseases in dry environments. In: Farooq, M. and Siddique, K. (eds) *Innovations in Dryland Agriculture*. Springer International Publishing, Cham, Switzerland, pp. 187–209.

Andersson, M.A., Nikulin, M., Köljalg, U., Andersson, M.C., Rainey, F. *et al.* (1997) Bacteria, molds, and toxins in water-damaged building materials. *Applied and Environmental Microbiology* 63, 387–393.

Apeagyei, F., Lamplugh, S.M., Hendrickse, R.G., Affram, K. and Lucas, S. (1986) Aflatoxins in the livers of children with kwashiorkor in Ghana. *Tropical and Geographical Medicine* 38, 273–276.

Asibi, A.E., Chai, Q. and Coulter, J.A. (2019) Rice blast: A disease with implications for global food security. *Agronomy* 9, 451.

Azziz-Baumgartner, E., Lindblade, K., Gieseker, K., Rogers, H.S., Kieszak, S. *et al.* (2005) Case-control study of an acute aflatoxicosis outbreak, Kenyam 2004. *Environmental Health Perspectives* 113, 1779–1783.

Bababunmi, E.A., Uwaifo, A.O. and Bassir, O. (1978) Hepatocarcinogens in nigerian foodstuffs. In: Bourne, G.H. (ed.) *Some Aspects of Human and Veterinary Nutrition*. Karger Publishers, Basel, Switzerland, pp. 188–209.

Baxi, S.N., Portnoy, J.M., Larenas-Linnemann, D., Phipatanakul, W., Barnes, C. *et al.* (2016) Exposure and health effects of fungi on humans. *The Journal of Allergy and Clinical Immunology. In Practice* 4, 396–404.

Becroft, D.M. and Webster, D.R. (1972) Aflatoxins and Reye's disease. *British Medical Journal* 4, 117.

Benenson, A.S. (1990) *Control of communicable disease in man*. American Public Health Association, Washington (DC).

Bennett, J.W. and Klich, M. (2003) Mycotoxins. *Clinical Microbiology Reviews* 16, 497–516.

Bennett, J.W. and Inamdar, A.A. (2015) Are some fungal volatile organic compounds (vocs) mycotoxins? *Toxins* 7, 3785–3804.

Bjelke, U., Boberg, J., Oliva, J., Tattersdill, K. and McKie, B.G. (2016) Dieback of riparian alder caused by the *Phytophthora alni* complex: Projected consequences for stream ecosystems. *Freshwater Biology* 61, 565–579.

Bonetta, S., Bonetta, S., Mosso, S., Sampò, S. and Carraro, E. (2010) Assessment of microbiological indoor air quality in an Italian office building equipped with an HVAC system. *Environmental Monitoring and Assessment* 161, 473–483.

Boonen, J., Malysheva, S.V., Taevernier, L., Mavungu, J., Saeger, S. *et al.* (2012) Human skin penetration of selected model mycotoxins. *Toxicology* 301, 21–32.

Booth, C. (1971) *The genus Fusarium*. CABI, Kew, UK.

Bornehag, C.G., Sundell, J. and Sigsgaard, T. (2004) Dampness in buildings and health (DBH): Report from an ongoing epidemiological investigation on the association between indoor environmental factors and health effects among children in Sweden. *Indoor Air* 14, 59–66.

Brakhage, A.A. and Langfelder, K. (2002) Menacing mold: The molecular biology of *Aspergillus fumigatus*. *Annual Review of Microbiology* 56, 433–455.

Burge, H.A. Morey, P., Feeley, J. and Otten, J. (eds). (1990) *Biological Contaminants in Indoor Environments*. American Society for Testing and Materials, Philadelphia, pp. 136–162.

Burton, N.C., Adhikari, A., Iossifova, Y., Grinshpun, S.A. and Reponen, T. (2008) Effect of gaseous chlorine dioxide on indoor microbial contaminants. *Journal of the Air and Waste Management Association* 58, 647–656.

Bush, R.K. and Portnoy, J.M. (2001) The role and abatement of fungal allergens in allergic diseases. *Journal of Allergy and Clinical Immunology* 107, S430–40.

Byrnes, I.E.J., Li, W., Lewit, Y., Ma, H., Voel, K. *et al.* (2010) Emergence and pathogenicity of highly virulent *Cryptococcus gattii* genotypes in the Northwest United States. *PLoS Pathogens* 6, 1–16.

CATS (2003) Mycotoxins: Risks in plant, animal, and human systems. Task force report. Ames, Iowa: Council for Agricultural Science and Technology.

Chen, S.C.A., Blyth, C.C., Sorrell, T.C. and Slavin, M.A. (2011) Pneumonia and lung infections due to emerging and unusual fungal pathogens. *Seminars in Respiratory and Critical Care Medicine* 32, 703–716.

Chiron, N. and Michelot, D. (2005) Mushrooms odors, chemistry and role in the biotic interactions – a review. *Cryptogamie Mycologie* 26, 299–364.

Chung, R.S., Lee, H.S. and You, I.C. (2018) Fungal keratitis caused by *Corynespora cassiicola*, a plant pathogen. *Journal of Mycology and Infection* 23, 24–26.

Clifford, L.J., Jia, Q. and Pestka, J.J. (2003) An improved method for the purification of the trichothecene deoxynivalenol (Vomitoxin) from *Fusarium graminearum* culture. *Journal of Agricultural and Food Chemistry* 51, 521–523.

Coulter, J.B.S., Lamplugh, S.M., Suliman, G.I., Omer, M.I. and Hendrickse, R.G. (1984) Aflatoxins in human breast milk. *Annals of Tropical Paediatrics* 4, 61–66.

Cox, A. (1988) Extrinsic allergic alveolitis caused by spores of the oyster mushroom *Pleurotus ostreatus*. *European Respiratory Journal* 1, 466–468.

Croft, W.A., Jarvis, B.B. and Yatawara, C.S. (1967) Airborne outbreak of *Trichothecene toxicosis*. *Atmospheric Environment* 20, 549–552.

da Rocha, M.E.B., Freire, F.D.C.O., Maia, F.E.F., Guedes, M.I.F. and Rondina, D. (2014) Mycotoxins and their effects on human and animal health. *Food Control* 36, 159–165.

Davies, P.D.O., Jacobs, R., Mullins, J. and Davies, B.H. (1988) Occupational asthma in tomato growers following an outbreak of the fungus *Verticillium albo-atrum* in the crop. *The Journal of the Society of Occupational Medicine* 38, 13–17.

de Vries, H.R., Maxwell, S.M. and Hendrickse, R.G. (1990) Aflatoxin excretion in children with Kwashiorkor or marasmic kwashiorkor – a clinical investigation. *Mycopathologia* 110, 1–9.

de Hoog, G.S., Marvin-Sikkema, F.D., Lahpoor, G.A., Gottschall, J.C., Prins, R.A. *et al.* (1994) Ecology and physiology of the emerging opportunistic fungi *Pseudallescheria boydii* and *Scedosporium prolificans*. *Mycoses* 37, 71–78.

Del Ponte, E.M., Valent, B. and Bergstrom, G.C. (2017) A special issue on *Fusarium* head blight and wheat blast. *Tropical Plant Pathology* 42, 143–145.

Denning, D.W., O'Driscoll, B.R., Hogaboam, C.M., Bowyer, P. and Niven, R.M. (2006) The link between fungi and severe asthma: A summary of the evidence. *European Respiratory Journal* 27, 615–626.

Desjardins, A., Manandhar, H., Plattner, R., Manandhar, G., Poling, S. *et al.* (2000) *Fusarium* species from Nepalese rice and production of mycotoxins and gibberellic acid by selected species. *Applied and Environmental Microbiology* 66, 1020–1025.

Desjardins, A. (2006) *Fusarium mycotoxins: Chemistry, genetics and biology*. American Phytopathological Society Press, Minnesota, USA.

DeVries, J.W., Trucksess, M.W. and Jackson, L.S. (2002) *Mycotoxins and food safety*. Academic/Plenum Publications, New York (NY).

Dill, I., Trautmann, C. and Szcwzyk, R. (1997) Mass development of *Stachybotrys chartarum* on decomposable plant-pots made of recycling paper. *Mycoses, Supplement* 40, 110–114.
Dorn, B., Forrer, H., Schurch, S. and Vogelgsang, S. (2009) Fusarium species complex on maize in Switzerland: Occurrence, prevalence, impact and mycotoxins in commercial hybrids under natural infection. *European Journal of Plant Pathology* 125, 51–61.
Dvorackova, I. (1976) Aflatoxin inhalation and alveolar cell carcinoma. *British Medical Journal* 1, 691.
Eaton, D. and Groopman, J. (1994) *The toxicology of aflatoxins*. San Diego (CA): Academic Press.
Edmondson, D.A., Nordness, M.E., Zacharisen, M.C., Kurup, V.P. and Fink, J.N. (2005) Allergy and "toxic mold syndrome." In: *Annals of Allergy, Asthma and Immunology: Official Publication of the American College of Allergy, Asthma, and Immunology*, Vol. 94. pp. 234–239.
Elliot Horner, W., Ibanez, M.D., Liengswangwong, V., Salvaggio, J.E. and Lehrer, S.B. (1988) Characterization of allergens from spores of the oyster mushroom, *Pleurotus ostreatus*. *The Journal of Allergy and Clinical Immunology* 82, 978–986.
Esmaeili Taheri, A., Chatterton, S., Foroud, N.A., Gossen, B.D. and McLaren, D.L. (2017) Identification and community dynamics of fungi associated with root, crown, and foot rot of field pea in western Canada. *European Journal of Plant Pathology* 147, 489–500.
Eversmeyer, M.G. and Kramer, C.L. (1987) Single versus multiple sampler comparisons. *Grana* 26, 109–112.
Fisher, M.C., Henk, D.A., Briggs, C.J., Brownstein, J.S., Madoff, L.C. *et al.* (2012) Emerging fungal threats to animal, plant and ecosystem health. *Nature* 484, 186–194.
Flannigan, B., McCabe, E.M. and McGarry, F. (1991) Allergenic and toxigenic micro-organisms in houses. *Journal of Applied Bacteriology Symposium Supplement* 20, 61S–73S.
Flannigan, B. and Miller, J.D. (1994) Health implications of fungi in indoor environments - an overview. In: Samson, A., Flannidan, R.B., Flannigan, M.E., Erhoeff, A.P., Adan, O.C.G. *et al.* (eds) *Health Implications of Fungi in Indoor Environments*. Elsevier, Amsterdam, pp. 3–28.
Fraser, J.A., Giles, S.S., Wenink, E.C., Geunes-Boyer, S.G., Wright, J.R. *et al.* (2005) Same-sex mating and the origin of the Vancouver island *Cryptococcus gattii* outbreak. *Nature* 437, 1360–1364.
Garrett, M.H., Rayment, P.R., Hooper, M.A., Abramson, M.J. and Hooper, B.M. (1998) Indoor airborne fungal spores, house dampness and associations with environmental factors and respiratory health in children. *Clinical and Experimental Allergy* 28, 459–467.
Gąska-Jedruch, U. and Dudzinska, M. (2009) Microbial contaminants in indoor air. In: *Conference Materials of Third National Congress of Environmental Engineering*, Lublin, pp. 31–40.
Gatwiri, M., Sirma, A.J., Ouko, E.O., Mburugu-Musoti, C.K., Kitala, P.M. *et al.* (2017) Exposure of Kenyan population to aflatoxins in foods with special reference to Nandi and Makueni counties. *Food Quality and Safety* 1, 131–137.
Giraud, T., Gladieux, P. and Gavrilets, S. (2010) Linking the emergence of fungal plant diseases with ecological speciation. *Trends in Ecology and Evolution* 25, 387–395.
Gottschalk, C., Bauer, J. and Meyer, K. (2008) Detection of satratoxin G and H in indoor air from a water-damaged building. *Mycopathologia* 166, 103–107.
Gugnani, H.C., Mitchell, T.G., Litvintseva, A.P., Lengeler, K.B., Heitman, J. *et al.* (2005) Isolation of *Cryptococcus gattii* and *Cryptococcus neoformans var. grubii* from the flowers and bark of Eucalyptus trees in India. *Medical Mycology* 43, 565–569.
Halo, B.A., Al-Yahyai, R.A. and Al-Sadi, A.M. (2018) *Aspergillus terreus* inhibits growth and induces morphological abnormalities in *Pythium aphanidermatum* and suppresses *Pythium*-induced damping-off of cucumber. *Frontiers in Microbiology* 9, 95.
He, Y., Zhu, M., Huang, J., Hsiang, T. and Zheng, L. (2019) Biocontrol potential of a *Bacillus subtilis* strain BJ-1 against the rice blast fungus *Magnaporthe* oryzae. *Canadian Journal of Plant Pathology* 41, 47–59.
Hendrickse, R.G. and Maxwell, S.M. (1989) Aflatoxins and child health in the tropics. *Toxin Reviews* 8, 31–41.
Hendrickse, R.G., Coulter, J.B.S., Lamplugh, S.M., Macfarlane, S.B., Williams, T.E. *et al.* (1982) Aflatoxins and kwashiorkor: A study in Sudanese children. *British Medical Journal* 285, 843–846.
Hoffman, D. (1984) Mould allergens. In: Al-Doory, Y. and Domson, J. (eds) *Mould Allergy*. Lea and Febiger, Philadelphia, pp. 104–116.
Hogan, G., Ryan, N. and Wallace Hayes, A. (1978) Aflatoxin B1 and reye's syndrome. *The Lancet* 311, 561.

Holdich, D.M., Reynolds, J.D., Souty-Grosset, C. and Sibley, P.J. (2009) A review of the ever increasing threat to European crayfish from non-indigenous crayfish species. *Knowledge and Management of Aquatic Ecosystems* 11, 394–395.

James Downer, A., Uchida, J.Y., Hodel, D.R. and Elliott, M.L. (2009) Lethal palm diseases common in the United States. *HortTechnology* 19, 710–716.

Jia, H., Wu, W.D., Lu, X., Zhang, J., He, C.H. *et al.* (2017) Role of glucagon-like peptide-1 and gastric inhibitory peptide in anorexia induction following oral exposure to the trichothecene mycotoxin deoxynivalenol (vomitoxin). *Toxicological Sciences* 159, 16–24.

Johanning, E., Morey, P.R. and Jarvis, B.B. (1993) Clinical-epidemiological investigation of health effects caused by *Stachybotrys atra* building contamination. In: *Indoor Air" 93, Proceedings of the Sixth International Conference on Indoor Air Quality and Climate*, Espoo, Finland: Helsinki University of Technology, pp. 225–230.

Karunasena, E., Larrañaga, M.D., Simoni, J.S., Douglas, D.R. and Straus, D.C. (2010) Building-associated neurological damage modeled in human cells: A mechanism of neurotoxic effects by exposure to mycotoxins in the indoor environment. *Mycopathologia* 170, 377–390.

Kashyap, P.L., Rai, P., Srivastava, A.K. and Kumar, S. (2017) Trichoderma for climate resilient agriculture. *World Journal of Microbiology and Biotechnology* 33, 155.

Kazerooni, E.A., Maharachchikumbura, S.S.N., Rethinasamy, V., Al-Mahrouqi, H. and Al-Sadi, A.M. (2017) Fungal diversity in tomato rhizosphere soil under conventional and desert farming systems. *Frontiers in Microbiology* 8, 1462.

Kendrick, B. (2000) *The fifth kingdom*. Newburyport (MA): Focus Publication, Pullins Company.

Kern, M.E. and Uecker, F.A. (1986) Maxillary sinus infection caused by the homobasidiomycetous fungus *Schizophyllum commune*. *Journal of Clinical Microbiology* 23, 1001–1005.

Kidd, S.E., Guo, H., Bartlett, K.H., Xu, J. and Kronstad, J.W. (2005) Comparative gene genealogies indicate that two clonal lineages of *Cryptococcus gattii* in British Columbia resemble strains from other geographical areas. *Eukaryotic Cell* 4, 1629–1638.

Kilburn, K.H. (2004) Role of molds and mycotoxins in being sick in buildings: Neurobehavioral and pulmonary impairment. *Advances in Applied Microbiology* 55, 339–359.

Klich, M.A. and Pitt, J.I. (1988) *A laboratory guide to the common Aspergillus species and their teleomorphs*. CSIRO, North Ryde, Australia.

Knutsen, A.P., Bush, R.K., Demain, J.G., Denning, D.W., Dixit, A. *et al.* (2012) Fungi and allergic lower respiratory tract diseases. *Journal of Allergy and Clinical Immunology* 129, 280–291.

Koiso, Y., Morisaki, N., Yamashita, Y., Mitsui, Y., Shirai, R. *et al.* (1998) Isolation and structure of an antimitotic cyclic peptide, ustiloxin F: Chemical interrelation with a homologous peptide, ustiloxin B. *Journal of Antibiotics* 51, 418–422.

Kommendahl, T. and Windels, C. (1981) Root, stalk and ear-infecting fusarium 263 species on corn in the USA. In: Nelson, P., Toussoun, T. and Cook, R. (eds) *Fusarium: Diseases, Biology and Taxonomy*. The Pennsylvania State University Press, University Park (PA), p. 265.

Kotilínek, M., Hiiesalu, I., Košnar, J., Šmilauerová, M., Šmilauer, P. *et al.* (2017) Fungal root symbionts of high-altitude vascular plants in the Himalayas. *Scientific Reports* 7, 6562.

Kreja, L. and Seidel, H.J. (2002) On the cytotoxicity of some microbial volatile organic compounds as studied in the human lung cell line A549. *Chemosphere* 49, 105–110.

Krishnamachari, K., Nagarajan, V., Bhat, R. and Tilak, T.B.G. (1975) Hepatitis due to *Aflatoxicosis*: An outbreak in Western India. *The Lancet* 305, 1061–1063.

Krzysztofik, B. (1992) *Microbiology of air*. Politechniki Warszawskiej, Warsaw, Poland, pp. 1–198.

Lacey, J. Hawksworth, D.L. (ed.). (1991) *Aerobiology and health*. CABI, UK, pp. 157–185.

Larsen, T.O. and Frisvad, J.C. (1995) Characterization of volatile metabolites from 47 *Penicillium taxa*. *Mycological Research* 99, 1153–1166.

Launay, M., Zurfluh, O., Huard, F., Buis, S., Bourgeois, G. *et al.* (2020) Robustness of crop disease response to climate change signal under modeling uncertainties. *Agricultural Systems* 178, 102733.

Levetin, E. (1995) Fungi. In: Burge, H.A. (ed.) *Bioaerosols*. Lewis, Boca Raton (FL), p. 108.

Li, D.W. and Yang, C.S. (2004) Fungal contamination as a major contributor to sick building syndrome. *Advances in Applied Microbiology* 55, 31–112.

Li, F.Q., Yoshizawa, T., Kawamura, O., Luo, X.Y. and Li, Y.W. (2001) Aflatoxins and fumonisins in corn from the high-incidence area for human hepatocellular carcinoma in Guangxi, China. *Journal of Agricultural and Food Chemistry* 49, 4122–4126.

Logrieco, A., Mule, G., Moretti, A. and Bottalico, A. (2002) Toxigenic fusarium species and mycotoxins associated with maize ear rot in Europe. *European Journal of Plant Pathology* 108, 597–609.
Lopez, D., Ribeiro, S., Label, P., Fumanal, B., Venisse, J.S. *et al.* (2018) Genome-wide analysis of *Corynespora cassiicola* leaf fall disease putative effectors. *Frontiers in Microbiology* 9, 276.
Magan, N. and Evans, P. (2000) Volatiles as an indicator of fungal activity and differentiation between species, and the potential use of electronic nose technology for early detection of grain spoilage. *Journal of Stored Products Research* 36, 319–340.
Mallet, J. (2007) Hybrid speciation. *Nature* 446, 279–283.
Malling, H.J. (1990) Diagnosis and immunotherapy of mould allergy. With special reference to *Cladosporium harbarum*. *Danish Medical Bulletin* 37, 12–22.
Marco, A., Diéguez-Uribeondo, J., Abella, E., Martín, M., Tellería, M. *et al.* (2006) Natural colonization of loggerhead turtle eggs by the pathogenic fungus *Fusarium oxysporum*. In: *Sea Turtle International Congress, Seaturtle, Greece*. Seaturtle, Greece: National Marine Fisheries Service.
Matossian, M.K. (1989) *Poisons of the past: molds, epidemics, and history*. Yale University Press, New Haven.
Maxwell, S.M., Apeagyei, F., Vries, H.R., Mwanmut, D.D. and Hendrickse, R.G. (1989) Aflatoxins in breast milk, neonatal cord blood and sera of pregnant women. *Toxin Reviews* 8, 19–29.
McBeath, J.H. and McBeath, J. (2010) *Environmental change and food security in China*. Springer Dordrecht Heidelberg, London, New York.
Miller, J.D. (1992) Fungi as contaminants in indoor air. *Atmospheric Environment. Part A. General Topics* 26, 2163–2172.
Miller, W.G., Padhye, A.A., Bonn, W., Jensen, E., Brandt, M.E. *et al.* (2002) Cryptococcosis in a bottlenose dolphin (*Tursiops truncatus*) caused by *Cryptococcus neoformans var gattii*. *Journal of Clinical Microbiology* 40, 721–724.
Mitchell, K.M., Churcher, T.S., Garner, T.W.J. and Fisher, M.C. (2008) Persistence of the emerging pathogen *Batrachochytrium dendrobatidis* outside the amphibian host greatly increases the probability of host extinction. *Proceedings of the Royal Society B: Biological Sciences* 275, 329–334.
Moularat, S., Robine, E., Ramalho, O. and Oturan, M.A. (2008) Detection of fungal development in closed spaces through the determination of specific chemical targets. *Chemosphere* 72, 224–232.
Müller, T., Thißen, R., Braun, S., Dott, W. and Fischer, G. (2004) (M)VOC and composting facilities: Part 1: (M)VOC emissions from municipal biowaste and plant refuse. *Environmental Science and Pollution Research* 11, 91–97.
Munn Sann, L., Ghazali, A.A., Mohan, J., Alwin, N. and Nair, R.C. (1995) An outbreak of acute hepatic encephalopathy due to severe aflatoxicosis in Malaysia. *The American Journal of Tropical Medicine and Hygiene* 53, 68–72.
Nakazawa, T. and Tochigi, T. (1989) Hypersensitivity pneumonitis due to mushroom (*Pholiota nameko*) spores. *Chest* 95, 1149–1151.
Naseri, B. and Ansari Hamadani, S. (2017) Characteristic agro-ecological features of soil populations of bean root rot pathogens. *Rhizosphere* 3, 203–208.
Nielsen, K.F. (2003) Mycotoxin production by indoor molds. *Fungal Genetics and Biology* 39, 103–117.
Nilsson, A., Kihlström, E., Lagesson, V., Wessén, B., Szponar, B. *et al.* (2004) Microorganisms and volatile organic compounds in airborne dust from damp residences. *Indoor Air* 14, 74–82.
Nonzom, S. and Sumbali, G. (2017) Camouflaged mycotoxins in some field crops and forages: A review. In: Satyanarayana, T., Deshmukh, S.K. and Johri, B.N. (eds) *Developments in Fungal Biology and Applied Mycology*. Springer Singapore, Singapore, pp. 563–600.
O'Hollaren, M.T., Yunginger, J.W., Offord, K.P., Ballard, D.J., Yunginger, J.W. *et al.* (1991) Exposure to an aeroallergen as a possible precipitating factor in respiratory arrest in young patients with Asthma. *New England Journal of Medicine* 324, 359–363.
Olsen, J.H., Dragsted, L. and Autrup, H. (1988) Cancer risk and occupational exposure to aflatoxins in Denmark. *British Journal of Cancer* 58, 392–396.
Ortoneda, M., Guarro, J., Madrid, M.P., Caracuel, Z., Roncero, M.I.G. *et al.* (2004) *Fusarium oxysporum* as a multihost model for the genetic dissection of fungal virulence in plants and mammals. *Infection and Immunity* 72, 1760–1766.
Oyelami, O.A., Maxwell, S.M., Adelusola, K.A., Aladekoma, T.A. and Oyelese, A.O. (1997) Aflatoxins in the lungs of children with kwashiorkor and children with miscellaneous diseases in Nigeria. *Journal of Toxicology and Environmental Health* 51, 623–628.

Park, J., Choi, S., Hwang, H. and Kim, Y. (2005) Fungal mycoflora and mycotoxins in Korean polished rice destined for humans. *International Journal of Food Microbiology* 103, 305–314.

Pei-Sheng, Y., Cui-Juan, S., Chun-Chun, H. and Guang-Feng, K. (2011) Inhibition of vomitoxin-producing *Fusarium graminearum* by marine actinomycetes and the extracellular metabolites. In: *Proceedings of the International Conference on Human Health and Biomedical Engineering*, Jilin, pp. 454–456.

Peraica, M., Radić, B., Lucić, A. and Pavlović, M. (1999) Toxic effects of mycotoxins in humans. *Bulletin of the World Health Organization* 77, 754–766.

Perera, R.H., Maharachchikumbura, S.S.N., Jones, E.B.G., Bahkali, A.H., Elgorban, A.M. *et al.* (2017) *Delonicicola siamense* gen. & sp. nov. (*Delonicicolaceae* fam. nov., *Delonicicolales* ord. nov.), a saprobic species from *Delonix regia* seed pods. *Cryptogamie Mycologie* 38, 321–340.

Phillott, A.D. and Parmenter, C.J. (2001) The distribution of failed eggs and the appearance of fungi in artificial nests of green (*Chelonia mydas*) and loggerhead (*Caretta caretta*) sea turtles. *Australian Journal of Zoology* 49, 713–718.

Pitt, J.I. (1979) *The genus Penicillium and its teleomorphic states Eupenicillium and Talaromyces*. Academic Press Inc. Ltd, London, UK.

Prom, L., Horsley, R., Steffenson, B. and Schwarz, P. (1999) Development of *Fusarium* head blight and accumulation of deoxynivalenol in barley sampled at different growth stages. *Journal of the American Society of Brewing Chemists* 57, 60–63.

Rainer, J. and Hoog, G.S. (2006) Molecular taxonomy and ecology of *Pseudallescheria*, *Petriella* and *Scedosporium prolificans* (Microascaceae) containing opportunistic agents on humans. *Mycological Research* 110, 151–160.

Rajaram, S. and Dubin, H.J. (2019) Plant diseases, global food security and the role of R. Glenn Anderson. *Canadian Journal of Plant Pathology* 41, 311–317.

Rani, R. and Sharma, V.K. (2018) Diversity analysis of northern Indian isolates of *Ustilaginoidea* virens. *Indian Phytopathology* 71, 33–42.

Rebell, G. (1981) Fusarium infections in human and veterinary medicine. In: Nelson, P., Toussoun, T. and Cook, R. (eds) *Fusarium Diseases, Biology and Taxonomy*. The Pennsylvania State University Press, University Park, pp. 210–220.

Reddy, M.K. and Srinivas, T. (2017) Mold allergens in indoor play school environment. *Energy Procedia* 109, 27–33.

Reed, C.E. (1985) What we do and do not know about mold allergy and asthma. *The Journal of Allergy and Clinical Immunology* 76, 773–775.

Richards, T.A., Soanes, D.M., Jones, M.D.M., Vasieva, O., Leonard, G. *et al.* (2011) Horizontal gene transfer facilitated the evolution of plant parasitic mechanisms in the Oomycetes. In: *Proceedings of the National Academy of Sciences of the United States of America*, Vol. 46. pp. 75–100.

Rodríguez-Gálvez, E., Guerrero, P., Barradas, C., Crous, P.W. and Alves, A. (2017) Phylogeny and pathogenicity of *Lasiodiplodia* species associated with dieback of mango in Peru. *Fungal Biology* 121, 452–465.

Ryan, N.J., Hogan, G.R. and Hayes, A.W. (1979) Aflatoxin B1: Its role in the etiology of reye's syndrome. *Pediatrics* 64, 71–75.

Rypien, K.L., Andras, J.P. and Harvell, C.D. (2008) Globally panmictic population structure in the opportunistic fungal pathogen *Aspergillus sydowii*. *Molecular Ecology* 17, 4068–4078.

Sakamoto, T., Ito, K., Yamada, M., Iguchi, H., Ueda, M. *et al.* (1990) Allergenicity of the Osmophilic fungus *Aspergillus restrictus* evaluated by skin prick test and radioallergosorbent test. *Japanese Journal of Allergology* 39, 1492–1498.

Santilli, J. and Rockwell, W. (2003) Fungal contamination of elementary schools: A new environmental hazard. *Annals of Allergy, Asthma and Immunology* 90, 203–208.

Sarma, U.P., Bhetaria, P.J., Devi, P. and Varma, A. (2017) Aflatoxins: Implications on health. *Indian Journal of Clinical Biochemistry* 32, 124–133.

Sarmiento-Ramírez, J.M., Abella, E., Martín, M.P., Tellería, M.T., López-Jurado, L.F. *et al.* (2010) *Fusarium solaniis* responsible for mass mortalities in nests of loggerhead sea turtle, Caretta caretta, in Boavista, Cape Verde. *FEMS Microbiology Letters* 312, 192–200.

Savilahti, E., Kolho, K.L., Westerholm-Ormio, M. and Verkasalo, M. (2010) Clinics of coeliac disease in children in the 2000s. *Acta Paediatrica, International Journal of Paediatrics* 99, 1026–1030.

Scauflaire, J., Mahieu, O., Louveaux, J., Foucart, G., Renard, F. *et al.* (2011) Biodiversity of *Fusarium* species in ears and stalks of maize plants in Belgium. *European Journal of Plant Pathology* 131, 59–66.

Schiefer, H.B. (1990) Mycotoxins in indoor air: A critical toxicological viewpoint. In: *Indoor Air" 90, Proceedings of the 5th International Conference on Indoor Air Quality and Climate*, Toronto, Japan, pp. 167–172.

Schumann, G.L. and D'Arcy, C.J. (2006) *Essential plant pathology*. St. Paul, Minnesota, USA.

Shank, R.C., Bourgeois, C.H., Keschamras, N. and Chandavimol, P. (1971) Aflatoxins in autopsy specimens from Thai children with an acute disease of unknown aetiology. *Food and Cosmetics Toxicology* 9, 501–504.

Sharon, A. and Shlezinger, N. (2013) Fungi infecting plants and animals: Killers, non-killers, and cell death. *PLoS Pathogens* 9, e1003517.

Singh, J. (1994) Nature and extent of deterioration in buildings due to fungi. In: Singh, J. (ed.) *Building Mycology*. Chapman and Hall, London, pp. 34–53.

Smoragiewicz, W., Cossette, B., Boutard, A. and Krzystyniak, K. (1993) Trichothecene mycotoxins in the dust of ventilation systems in office buildings. *International Archives of Occupational and Environmental Health* 65, 113–117.

Stukenbrock, E.H. and McDonald, B.A. (2008) The origins of plant pathogens in agro-ecosystems. *Annual Review of Phytopathology* 46, 75–100.

Suman, A., Nath Yadav, A. and Verma, P. (2016) Endophytic microbes in crops: Diversity and beneficial impact for sustainable agriculture. In: Singh, D.P., Singh, H.B. and Prabha, R. (eds) *Microbial Inoculants in Sustainable Agricultural Productivity*, Vol. 1. Springer India, India.

Summerbell, R. (2003) *Aspergillus*, *Fusarium*, *Sporothrix*, *Piedraia*, and their relatives. In: Howard, D. (ed.) *Pathogenic Fungi in Humans and Animals*. Marcel Dekker Inc, New York, pp. 237–498.

Tang, C., Xu, Q., Zhao, M., Wang, X. and Kang, Z. (2018) Understanding the lifestyles and pathogenicity mechanisms of obligate biotrophic fungi in wheat: The emerging genomics era. *The Crop Journal* 6, 60–67.

Thacker, P.D. (2004) Airborne mycotoxins discovered in moldy buildings. *Environmental Science and Technology* 38, 281A–282A.

Váry, Z., Mullins, E., McElwain, J.C. and Doohan, F.M. (2015) The severity of wheat diseases increases when plants and pathogens are acclimatized to elevated carbon dioxide. *Global Change Biology* 21, 2661–2669.

Weinhold, B. (2007) A spreading concern: Inhalational health effects of mold. *Environmental Health Perspectives* 115, A300–A305.

Wilkins, K., Nielsen, K.F. and Din, S.U. (2003) Patterns of volatile metabolites and nonvolatile trichothecenes produced by isolates of *Stachybotrys*, *Fusarium*, *Trichoderma*, *Trichothecium* and *Memnoniella*. *Environmental Science and Pollution Research* 10, 162–166.

Wilson, R.A. and Talbot, N.J. (2009) Under pressure: Investigating the biology of plant infection by *Magnaporthe oryzae*. *Nature Reviews Microbiology* 7, 185–195.

Windels, C. (2000) Economic and social impacts of *Fusarium* head blight: Changing farms and rural communities in the Northern great plains. *Phytopathology* 90, 17–21.

Wulff, E., Sorensen, J., Lubeck, M., Nielsen, K., Thrane, U. *et al.* (2010) *Fusarium* spp. associated with rice Bakanae: Ecology, genetic diversity, pathogenicity and toxigenicity. *Environmental Microbiology* 12, 649–657.

Xu, X. and Berrie, A. (2005) Epidemiology of mycotoxigenic fungi associated with *Fusarium* earblight and apple blue mould: A review. *Food Additives and Contaminants* 22, 290–301.

Yao, Q., Liu, J., Yu, Z., Li, Y., Jin, J. *et al.* (2017) Three years of biochar amendment alters soil physiochemical properties and fungal community composition in a black soil of northeast China. *Soil Biology and Biochemistry* 110, 56–67.

Yong, M., Deng, Q., Fan, L., Miao, J., Lai, C. *et al.* (2018) The role of *Ustilaginoidea virens* sclerotia in increasing incidence of rice false smut disease in the subtropical zone in China. *European Journal of Plant Pathology* 150, 669–677.

Yuan, Y., Feng, H., Wang, L., Li, Z., Shi, Y. *et al.* (2017) Potential of endophytic fungi isolated from cotton roots for biological control against verticillium wilt disease. *PLoS One* 12, e0170557.

Zain, M.E. (2011) Impact of mycotoxins on humans and animals. *Journal of Saudi Chemical Society* 15, 129–144.

Żukiewicz-Sobczak, W.A., Sobczak, P.T., Imbor, K., Krasowska, E., Horoch, A. *et al.* (2012) Zagrożenia grzybowe w budynkach i w mieszkaniach – wpływ na organizm człowieka. *Medycyna Ogólna i Nauki o Zdrowiu* 18, 141–146.

Zukiewicz-Sobczak, W.A. (2013) The role of fungi in allergic diseases. *Postepy Dermatologii i Alergologii* 30, 42–45.

22 *Toxocara* and its Species

Molly A. Ziegler and Calum N. L. Macpherson*

School of Graduate Studies, St. George's University, Windward Islands Research and Education Foundation, True Blue Campus, Grenada, West Indies

Abstract

This systematic review focuses on the nematode genus *Toxocara* and its zoonotic and non-zoonotic species and provides an update to that published by Warren almost half a century ago. Currently, 26 species of *Toxocara* have been described morphologically and four differentiated by molecular techniques. The most frequently reported and wide spread zoonotic species is *Toxocara canis*. Zoonotic infection with *T. cati* remains controversial and only a few infections, mostly in children with ocular larval migrans (OLM), have been reported. To date, none have been confirmed using molecular techniques. Only a single-suspected case of human infection with *T. pteropodis* has been reported and this species has yet to be confirmed as zoonotic. Of the non-zoonotic species *T. vitulorum* is of major economic importance and there are 13 minor species: *T. alienata, T. apodemi, T. genettae, T. indica, T. leonine, T. mackerrasae, T. malaysiensis, T. paradoxura, T. pearsei, T. sprenti, T. suricattae, T. tanuki* and *T. vajrasthirae*. Nine species have been reported only once: *T. canarisi, T. cynonycteridis, T. elephantis, T. herpestum, T. hippopotami, T. lyncis, T. manzadiensis, T. vincenti* and *T. warreni*. *Toxocara* occurs in many definitive host species: canids, felids, civets, mongoose, cattle, raccoons, bats and rodents. In humans, *T. canis* infections can result in four distinct syndromes: visceral larval migrans, OLM, neuro-toxocariasis and covert toxocariasis. Serological tests supplemented by molecular and imaging techniques provide the basis of diagnosis and may also add to the longitudinal monitoring of treatment. Seroprevalence in humans in developed countries ranges from 3 to 22% and in developing countries from 10 to 92%. Vertical transmission of the parasite in definitive hosts facilitates the earliest potential production of eggs from young animals and provides challenging yet important control opportunities. Climate change and increasing human and companion animal populations have facilitated an expansion in the geographical range of this zoonosis. Behavioural changes coupled with increased urbanization enhance potential transmission, as people and dogs become increasingly crowded together facilitating opportunities for *T. canis* transmission, and a greater understanding of these factors should be examined to facilitate appropriate and cost-effective control programmes. Anthelminthics used in the elimination of adult parasites from dog or cat intestines can provide an effective control with toxocariasis. Control measures using a one health approach coordinating the expertise of physicians, veterinarians, public health workers, dog owners and aided by legislation facilitates a best practice approach to control.

Keywords: *Toxocara*, Toxocariasis, *Toxocara canis*, Zoonosis

Review Methodology

To facilitate this review, all published articles and reviews using the keywords *Toxocara*, toxocariasis, *Toxocara canis* and *Toxocara* species were searched for in a variety of databases which included ScienceDirect, Scopus, National Center for Biotechnology Information and Google

*Corresponding author: cmacpherson@sgu.edu

Scholar. References from these articles were also reviewed.

Introduction

The roundworm *Toxocara* was originally described by Werner in 1782, who recovered the nematode from a domestic dog and named it *Lumbricus canis* (Werner, 1782; Warren, 1970). The evolution of the nomenclature for this organism continued in 1793 when it was renamed *Ascaris wernei*, then *Ascaris marginata* in 1802 by Rudolphi. There was a permutation of these genera by Leiper in 1902 who implemented a genus for the nematodes specific to canine hosts *Toxascaris* and another for feline hosts *Belascaris*. Stiles and Hassall did not develop the genus we know today, Warren (1970), renaming *L. canis* to *Toxocara canis*. Over the history of the genus *Toxocara* there have been as few as 11 species as stated by Warren in 1970 and as many as 30 when relevant literature is combined (Sprent, 1956; Warren, 1970; Borecka, 2010). This review considers the 26 recognized species of the genus *Toxocara*. The *species inquiraedae* are not included.

Characteristics of the species within this genus include a white-yellow to light brown long cylindrical body, and arrow-shaped anterior (Warren, 1970). Males are small and have a ventrally curved posterior spike (Radwan *et al.*, 2009). Adult *Toxocara* live in the small intestine of their definitive hosts. Females release up to 200,000 eggs daily into the environment via host faeces (Glickman and Schantz, 1981). The eggs can embryonate over a period of 2–6 weeks, depending on temperature, humidity, light, substrate, pH and vegetation cover. During this time, the larvae inside the protective egg can mature developing from L_1 to L_2, and eventually to the infective L_3 stage (Araujo, 1972). There are a wide variety of definitive host species, which live in a diversity of habitats over a wide geographical region. Transmission to the definitive host is achieved either by horizontal or vertical means. Horizontal transmission occurs through ingestion of L_3-infective larvae either in eggs from the environment or infected paratenic hosts such as soil-dwelling invertebrates, birds, rodents, rabbits and pigs (Overgaauw and Van Knapen, 2000; Mizgajska, 2001; Despommier, 2003; Sommerfelt *et al.*, 2004; Okulewicz *et al.*, 2012). Vertical transmission has been demonstrated in some hosts, either through transplacental or transmammary routes (Overgaauw and Van Knapen, 2000). Paratenic hosts, vertical transmission and resilience of the eggs in the environment are important contributors to the maintenance of transmission in endemic areas.

In humans, infection with *Toxocara* is thought to mainly occur through the accidental ingestion of microscopic-infective eggs. The economic and public health importance of toxocariasis are greatest in the tropics and subtropics, where it is estimated that more than 1 billion people are infected with parasitic helminths (Hotez *et al.*, 2007; Hotez *et al.*, 2009). The overall contribution of toxocariasis to the burden of human disease is not well defined owing to a lack of prioritization, difficulty of diagnosis and the heterogeneity of clinical symptoms from asymptomatic through non-specific symptoms, such as asthma to severe neuro- and ocular toxocariasis (Smith *et al.*, 2009).

Speciation of *Toxocara* species is based on morphology or molecular characterization. Morphological characteristics between the species consist of comparing the shape and size of the anterior body, spicule length, oesophageal gland, cervical alae and length of the nematode. For example, *T. malaysiensis* was identified as a separate species molecularly based on mitochondrial DNA (21). Molecular techniques were later used to confirm *T. canis*, *T. cati* and *T. vitulorum* as separate species (Chen *et al.*, 2012). Some may classify these species differently, but morphology and molecular techniques were the criteria used for categorization in this review.

Species are listed as zoonotic in this review only when a case of human infection was reported in the published literature. Although a few cases of human infections with *T. felis* and only a single case of *T. pteropodis* has been reported in the literature. These infections have yet remained unconfirmed by molecular techniques and their zoonotic potential for humans is unclear. Only *T. canis* infections have been clearly established as zoonotic. To date, no *T. vitulorum* cases have been reported in humans.

Non-Zoonotic Species of *Toxocara*

Of the 23 non-zoonotic *Toxocara* species, one *T. vitulorum* has a widespread distribution and is of economic importance. In addition, 13 out of the 23 non-zoonotic *Toxocara* species are of minor importance whilst nine species have only been reported once in the literature.

Toxocara vitulorum (Goeze 1782)

The Asian water buffalo (*Bubalus bubalis*), domestic cattle (*Bos taurus*), zebu (*Bos taurus indicus*) and wood bison (*Bison bison athabascae*) serve as definitive hosts of *T. vitulorum*. *T. vitulorum* has been reported in many countries (see Table 22.1) (El-Moukdad, 1979; Rekwot and Ogunsusi, 1985; Wen *et al.*, 1986; Holland *et al.*, 2000; Knopf *et al.*, 2004; Aydin *et al.*, 2006; Wymann *et al.*, 2007; Mahieu and Naves, 2008; Davila *et al.*, 2010; Avcioğlu and Balkaya, 2011; Mirani *et al.*, 2012; Kulišić *et al.*, 2012; Jyoti *et al.*, 2012; Rast *et al.*, 2013; Raza *et al.*, 2013). Until recently, *T. vitulorum* was regarded as a nematode infection of cattle mainly in the tropics and subtropics, but is a common cause of toxocariasis in cattle, water

Table 22.1. *T. vitulorum* infection in cattle and buffalo worldwide

Region/Country	% Infected	No. of samples/host	References
Central America and Caribbean			
Guadeloupe	77	247 cattle	(Sommerfelt *et al.*, 2004)
Sub-Saharan Africa			
Ivory Coast	12.3	144 cattle	(Aydin *et al.*, 2006)
Mali	7.6	790 cattle	(Vicente *et al.*, 1997)
Nigeria	54.4		(Rast *et al.*, 2013)
Asia			
China	40		(Holland *et al.*, 2000)
South and Southeast Asia			
India	8.5	1582 buffalo	(Raza *et al.*, 2013)
Laos	20.9 cattle	566 cattle	(Mirani *et al.*, 2012)
	25.5 water buffalo	333 water buffalo	
Vietnam	36	74 cattle	(Mia *et al.*, 1975)
West and Central Asia			
Pakistan	37.5 cattle	144 cattle	(Roberts, 1990)
	63.8 water buffalo	282 water buffalo	
Pakistan	8	1000 buffalo	(Roberts *et al.*, 1990)
Serbia	35	600 cattle	(Avcioğlu and Balkaya, 2011)
Syria	2.94	34 cattle	(Davila *et al.*, 2010)
Turkey	29	718 cattle	(Wymann *et al.*, 2007)
	17.7	231 cattle	
	22.2	508 cattle	(Rekwot and Ogunsusi, 1985)
North America			
US-Florida	17.6	105 cattle	(Wen *et al.*, 1986)

buffalo and bison worldwide. The morphological description of *T. vitulorum* is, 'Cervical alae present as short lateral ridge, cervical V-shaped rod extending beyond the excretory pore. Adults up to 300 mm long. Dorsal oesophageal gland nucleus asymmetrical. Parasites of ruminants' (Warren, 1970). Infection is by ingestion of eggs from the environment. Lactogenic transmission is subsequently the most widely observed route of transmission (Warren and Needham, 1969; Warren, 1971; Mia *et al.*, 1975; Roberts *et al.*, 1990; Roberts, 1990). Molecular knowledge on *T. vitulorum* consists of partial sequencing of the mitochondrial DNA, ITS-1 and ITS-2 of the ribosomal DNA (Zhu *et al.*, 2000; Li *et al.*, 2008a; Wickramasinghe *et al.*, 2009).

Adult cattle, water buffalo and bison ingest infective eggs from their environment, which hatch in their gastro-intestinal tract, then larvae migrate to the somatic tissue. In breeding female adults, it is suspected that reproductive hormones during pregnancy cause reactivation of L_3 larvae, which migrate from somatic tissue to the mammary glands 1–8 days before parturition, leading to lactogenic transmission in suckling calves (Warren, 1970; Prociv, 1987; Woodbury *et al.*, 2014). Studies in sheep have shown that lactation increases an ewe's susceptibility to intestinal helminths. This may help explain how somatic larvae in pregnant cows are re-activated and passed to calves (Lloyd *et al.*, 1983). The first week after birth, milk produced by the cow will have the highest concentration of larvae, larval output in milk will continue for up to 18 days post-partum (Goossens *et al.*, 2007). During this time, calves are infected and the prepatent period of *T. vitulorum* is 21–28 days, after which calves will shed eggs in their faeces for up to 6 months but usually stop by 4 months (Starke-Buzetti *et al.*, 2001; Davila *et al.*, 2010; Woodbury *et al.*, 2014). Males and non-breeding female cattle are dead-end hosts. Larvae mature in the small intestines to reach the adult stage in lactogenically infected calves that then shed eggs in their faeces. Eggs released into the environment require 7–12 days at 28–30°C to moult and become infective L_3, eggs can remain viable for up to 2 years outside of a host (Roberts, 1989). Transplacental infection has not been observed in cattle in the field or reported in published studies, but some suggest it is a secondary mode of transmission for *T. vitulorum* to account for adult *T. vitulorum* found in calves soon after birth (Warren, 1971; Hubbert *et al.*, 1975; Roberts, 1990; Aydin *et al.*, 2006; Starke-Buzetti, 2006). At 6 months of age, calves expel the parasites into the environment effectively ending their role as definitive hosts.

Treatment of infected cattle consisted of albendazole orally, which was 85% effective (Borgsteede *et al.*, 2012). Those still infected after administration of albendazole were given doramectin by subcutaneous injection, eliminating *T. vitulorum* from all cattle. Other studies have found treatment with fenbendazole or pyrantel and levamisole in calves to be effective. Treatment methods for cattle include: piperazine, pyrantel, febantel, and oxfendazole, ivermectin, doramectin, moxidectin, fenbendazole and eprinomectin (Roberts, 1989; Starke-Buzetti, 2006; Avcioglu and Balkaya, 2011). The most effective way to control and prevent the spread of infection in a herd is to treat the calves and improve farming conditions to discourage re-infection. *T. vitulorum* exhibits seasonal prevalence with its height in the summer; this should be considered for treatment regimens.

A high mortality rate has been reported in 15–50 day-old calves, in which masses of worms in the lumen can cause occlusions (Woodbury *et al.*, 2012). Signs of infection include: diarrhoea, inappetence, intermittent colic, tympanism or distension of the abdomen due to gas in the intestines or peritoneal cavity, dysentery, anorexia, constipation, dehydration, steatorrhoea, abdominal pain, eczema, decreased plasma proteins, leucocytosis, neutrophilia, eosinophilia, basophilia, lymphopenia, increased histamine, hepatic toxins and haemorrhagic enteritis. High mortality in a herd can lead to severe economic loss and food shortages in some areas, depending on the composition of food sources for the local human population. The economic loss has not yet been calculated for loss in cattle production and interruption of breeding programmes associated with *T. vitulorum*.

Water buffalo are farmed in 40 countries, mainly for their milk and meat, and they are also considered by many to be productive domestic animals. The countries with the highest buffalo populations are: India 53%, China 14.8%, Pakistan 12.9% and Brazil's buffalo population is increasing at a rapid pace (Starke-Buzetti, 2006). As with other species of *Toxocara*, *T. vitulorum* eggs are resilient and pose a challenge to elimination efforts. In India, *T. vitulorum* has been shown to survive in dung heaps for 17 months, over 2 years in more forgiving climates and 5 months in cattle tissue (Roberts, 1989; Starke-Buzetti, 2006). Four important key points presented by Roberts (Roberts, 1993), that remain important in understanding the tough enduring nature of this parasite are: long survival of eggs in the environment, long survival of larvae in tissues of maternal hosts, transmission through mothers and high egg output by calves over a short period of time. *T. vitulorum* has been shown difficult to eliminate from a herd once it becomes endemic, even in the Northern United States and Canada with frigid temperatures during the winter as the larvae overwinter in the tissue of female cattle.

Minor Non-Zoonotic *Toxocara* Species

Toxocara alienata (Rudolphi 1819)

Members of the procyonidae family, including the South American coati (*Nasua nasua*), ring-tailed coati (*Nasua rufa*), crab-eating raccoon (*Procyon cancrivorus*) and the collared peccary (*Pecari tajacu*) are the hosts of *T. alienata* (Vicente *et al.*, 1997). *T. alienata* has been found in Brazil and Peru (Sprent, 1982; Gomez-Puerta, 2014). The morphological description of *T. alienata is* 'Spicules 0.6 mm long, parasitic in the ring-tailed coati (*Nasua rufa*)' (Warren, 1970).

Toxocara apodemi (Olsen 1957)

The striped field (*Apodemus agrarius*) and Korean field mice (*Apodemus peninsulae*) are the hosts of *T. apodemi*, parasitic in rodents (Asakawa *et al.*, 1994). *T. apodemi* has been found in China and South Korea (Warren, 1970; Asakawa *et al.*, 1994). The morphological description of *T. apodemi* is, 'External prolongations of labial pulp asymmetrical, rounded at anterior border. Female with small terminal spike on tail. Spicules 0.55 mm long in males 35.0 mm long. Parasitic in *Apodemus peninsulae*' (Warren, 1970).

Toxocara cynonycteridis (Parona 1889)

Leschenault's rousette (*Pteropus leschenaultii*) is the host of *T. cynonycteridis*. *T. cynonycteridis* has a wide distribution having been reported from Australia, Africa and Asia including Burma (Puylaert, 1967; Sprent, 1968; Warren, 1970; Prociv, 1989; Borecka, 2010). The morphological description of *T. cynonycteridis* is: females 60–65 mm in length with males at 50 mm, two papillae on the lip, two anterior-pointed protuberances, spicules 0.042 mm in length and four pairs of pre-cloacal papillae (Prociv, 1989).

Toxocara genettae (Warren 1972)

The South African small-spotted genet (*Genetta felina*) and common genet (*Genetta genetta*) are the hosts of *T. genettae* (Alvarez *et al.*, 1990). *T. genettae* was found in South Africa and more recently in Spain (Warren, 1972; Alvarez *et al.*, 1990). The morphological description of *T. genettae* (Warren, 1972) notes the absence of cervical alae that are replaced by lateral crests supported by V-shaped cuticular bars the entire body length and a mucron on the end of the tail in males only (Sanmartín *et al.*, 1992).

Toxocara herpestum (Vuylsteke 1956)

The Egyptian mongoose (*Herpestes ichneumon*) is the host of *T. herpestum* (Vuylsteke, 1956). There have been reports from Asia and Africa (Vuylsteke, 1956; Borecka, 2010). The morphological description of *T. herpestum* is, 'slightly trilobed lips and lacking intermediate lips' (Vuylsteke, 1956).

Toxocara leonine (Rudolphi 1819)

The Margarita capuchins (*Cebus apella margaritae*), tayra (*Eira barbara*), jaguars (*Panthera onca*) and cougars (*Puma concolor*) are the hosts of *T. leonine*. *T. leonine* has been found in Venezuela (Ceballos-Mago *et al.*, 2010).

Toxocara mackerrasae (Sprent 1957)

The water rat (*Hydromys chrysogaster*) and bush rat (*Rattus fuscipes*) are hosts of *T. mackerrasae* (Naidu, 1981). *T. mackerrasae* has been found in Asia, Australia and Papua New Guinea (Sprent, 1982; Smales, 2005). The morphological description of *T. mackerrasae* (Sprent, 1957) is, 'External prolongations of labial pulp symmetrical, subdivided at anterior border. Female without small terminal spike on tail. Spicules 0.65 mm long in males 35 to 36 mm long' (Warren, 1970).

Toxocara malaysiensis (Gibbons, Jacobs, Sani 2001)

The domestic cat (*Felis catus*) is the host of *T. malaysiensis* (Gibbons *et al.*, 2001). This species is a relatively new discovery and has only been found in Vietnam, Malaysia and China (Gibbons *et al.*, 2001; Li *et al.*, 2006; Le *et al.*, 2016). There has been an increase in the number of reported cases of toxocariasis in the human population of Vietnam, but due to serological testing limitations the exact species of *Toxocara* cannot be determined. *T. malaysiensis* has not been proven to be zoonotic. The mitochondrial DNA, ITS-1 and ITS-2 from ribosomal DNA have been sequenced for this species of *Toxocara* (Jacobs *et al.*, 1997; Zhu *et al.*, 1998; Li *et al.*, 2006; Li *et al.*, 2008b). The ITS-1 and 2 were significant in distinguishing this organism for *T. canis* and provided evidence for a new species of *Toxocara* to be named. Based on molecular analysis, *T. malaysiensis* is genetically closer to *T. cati* than *T. canis* (Le *et al.*, 2016).

Toxocara paradoxura (Kou 1958)

The Viverrids including the Asian palm civet (*Paradoxurus hermaphrodites*) are the hosts of *T. paradoxura*. *T. paradoxura* has been reported in China and Taiwan (Su *et al.*, 2013). Although comparable to *T. tanuki*, this species was added to the genus *Toxocara* based on morphological differences. The morphological description of *T. paradoxura* (Kou, 1958) is, 'Spicules always greater than 2.5 mm long, adults always less than 20.0 mm long. Males and females with small terminal hooks on the tip of the tail' (Warren, 1970).

Toxocara pearsei (Chitwood 1935)

The Trinidadian funnel-eared bat (*Natalus tumidirostris*) and lesser dog-like bat (*Peropteryx macrotis*) are hosts of *T. pearsei*. *T. pearsei* has been found in the South America, Central America and the USA (Chitwood, 1935; Warren, 1970; Gibbons *et al.*, 2001). An adult of *T. pearsei* was reportedly found in the digestive tract in the crustacean snapping shrimp (*Synalpheus brooksi*) as well (Chitwood, 1935). The morphological description of *T. pearsei* from a male is: caudal alae absent, spicules subequal at 1.2 and 1.32 mm long, cervical alae 1.28 mm long and is 21 mm long (Chitwood, 1935). When the original parasite was examined by Warren, it was found to be poorly preserved and no additional information could be gained (Warren, 1970).

Toxocara sprenti (Warren 1972)

The small Indian civet (*Viverricula indica*) is the host of *T. sprenti* and it is thought that more viverrid species may be definitive hosts (Warren, 1972). *T. sprenti* was originally discovered in Australia and has been found in Thailand (Warren, 1972).

Toxocara suricattae (Ortlepp 1940)

The banded mongoose (*Mungos mungo*), black-footed mongoose (*Bdeogale nigripes*) and slender-tailed meerkat (*Suricata suricatta*) are the hosts of *T. suricattae* (Warren, 1972). *T. suricattae* has been reported in South Africa (Leclaire and Faulkner, 2014). The morphological description of *T. suricattae* is, 'Cervical alae not present. Cervical V-shaped rod extending only 50 to 60 μm from the base of the lips and not reaching the level of excretory pore. Adults never longer than 100 mm. Dorsal oesophageal gland nucleus symmetrical' (Warren, 1970).

Toxocara tanuki (Yamaguti 1941)

Raccoon dogs (*Nyctereutes procyonoides viverrinus*) and raccoons (*Procyonoides viverrinus*) are the hosts of *T. tanuki*. *T. tanuki* is found in Japan. A study conducted on the Japanese mainland revealed an infection rate of 80% in raccoons and 43% in raccoon dogs on Yakushima Island, Japan (Sato *et al.*, 1999; Sato *et al.*, 2006). As raccoon dogs are omnivores, it is suspected by the authors of the study that infection could be occurring through raccoon dogs ingesting infected rodents and birds, also found on the island. The morphological description for *T. tanuki* is 'Spicule lengths more than 3.0 mm in males 37.0 to 42.0 mm long; cervical alae approximately 0.25 mm wide' (Warren, 1970).

Non-Zoonotic *Toxocara* Species Reported Once

Toxocara canarisi (Puylaert 1967)

African servals (*Leptailurus serval*) are the host of *T. canarisi*. *T. canarisi* has been reported once from Kenya. Further studies are required on this species to provide a morphological description and other hosts (Puylaert, 1967; Warren, 1972).

Toxocara elephantis (Rudolphi 1819)

T. elephantis has only been reported in the Asian elephant (*Elephas maximus*), the infected animal was from a zoo in Switzerland (Fowler and Mikota, 2008). This species of *Toxocara* has never been reported in the wild.

Toxocara hippopotami (Canavan 1931)

The common hippopotamus (*Hippopotamus amphibious*) is the host of *T. hippopotami* (Maung, 1975). There is one record of *T. hippopotami* found in Uganda and one of a captive hippopotamus in the USA (Round, 1968; Maung, 1975). According to Warren who attempted to verify this species classification, the original parasite collected could not be located (Warren, 1970).

Toxocara indica (Naidu 1981)

The greater bandicoot rat (*Bandicota indica*) is the host of *T. indica*. This species of *Toxocara* was found in India. The morphological description for *T. indica* (Naidu, 1981) is a thick yellow brown coloured nematode with, 'Cervical alae absent, female with terminal spike on tail, spicules subequal, left 0.46–0.48 mm and right 0.51–0.62 mm long' (Naidu, 1981).

Toxocara lyncis (Macchiono 1999)

The caracals (*Caracal caracal*) and Eurasian lynx (*Lynx lynx*) are the hosts of *T. lyncis*. *T. lyncis* was reported in Somalia and this seems to be the only record in the literature. The morphological description of *T. lyncis* (Macchioni, 2000) is similar to that of *T. cati* except for the length of the spicules, oesophagus and the shape of the cervical alae are the same width for their entire length (Macchioni, 2000).

Toxocara manzadiensis (Vuylsteke 1956)

The Cape buffalo (*Syncerus caffer*) is the host of *T. manzadiensis*. *T. manzadiensis* (Vuylsteke, 1956) was found in the Congo, and no other reports were found in the literature. Warren reports that when he looked at parasites labelled *T. manzadiensis*, the morphology did not match that which was described by Vuylsteke (Warren, 1970).

Toxocara vajrasthirae (Sprent 1972)

The hog badger (*Arctonyx collaris*) is the host of *T. vajrasthirae*. *T. vajrasthirae* has only been recorded in Thailand. The morphological description of *T. vajrasthirae* (Sprent, 1972) is: eggs exhibit a coarse reticulate pattern. The adult females are 175–190 mm in length with adult males at 80–118 mm. The adults of this species look similar to those of *T. canis* but are differentiated by long spicules and the eggs display a coarse reticulate pattern (Sprent, 1972).

Toxocara vincenti (Puylaert 1967)

The Servaline genet (*Genetta servalina*) is the host of *T. vincenti* (Kingdon *et al.*, 2013). *T. vincenti* was found in the Congo. The morphological description for *T. vincenti* is, 'Interlabial cuticular projections present, small papillae anterior and posterior to each pair of double post-cloacal papillae' (Warren, 1970).

Toxocara warreni (Durette-Duset and Chabaud 1974)

The water chevrotain (*Hyemoschus aquaticus*) is the host of *T. warren* (Durette-Desset and Chabaud, 1974). *T. warreni* has been found in Gabon. No other records of this species were found in the literature.

Zoonotic Species of *Toxocara*

Toxocara cati (Schrank 1788)

T. cati was first described in a captive tiger (*Leopardus tigrinus*), then later in the wild in Pampas cats (*Leopardus colocolo*) by Molina in 1782. There are 24 known definitive host species (Table 22.2) in which *T. cati* has been reported, the most common being domestic cats. *T. cati* is now found globally. Description of *T. cati* is female adults up to 120 mm long with males much smaller at 30–70 mm long, 'Spicule lengths 1.7–2.0 mm in males 30.0 to 70.0 mm long. Cervical alae reaching their maximum width posteriorly. Horseshoe-shaped dorsal oesophageal gland nucleus' (Warren, 1970). Molecular knowledge on *T. cati* consists of the mitochondrial DNA genome, ITS-1 and ITS-2 of the ribosomal DNA having been sequenced (Zhu *et al.*, 2000; Li *et al.*, 2008b). This species of *Toxocara* was at one time referred to as *T. mystax*, but was later found to be the same species and combined with *T. cati*.

The modes of transmission for *T. cati* are ingestion of embryonated eggs, infected paratenic host and transmammary or lactogenic transmission. This species has not been found to cross the placenta and cause prenatal infection (Swerczek *et al.*, 1971). Lactogenic transmission of *T. cati* in cats follows the same life cycle as *T. canis* in dogs. There is no hepatotracheal migration in young cats infected by transmammary transmission. Larvae are released in the queen's milk for around 5 weeks after birth and eggs do not appear in the environment from kitten faeces until 47 days post birth (Overgaauw and Knapen, 2013). In older cats, infection by ingestion of embryonated eggs from the environment followed by hepato-tracheal migration is common. Migration and morphological developments of *T. cati* within kittens was studied in those that ingested infected embryonated eggs (Sprent, 1956). The distribution of larvae found in examined tissue from cats was as follows

Table 22.2. Currently accepted *Toxocara* species and their definitive domestic and feral hosts and their geographic distribution

Toxocara species	Definitive host(s)	Location(s) (Reference)	Molecular speciation (Reference)
T. canis (Z) (Werner, 1782)	*Canids*, *Canis aureus*, *Canis dingo*, *Canis familiaris*, *Canis latrans*, *Canis lupus*, *Canis mexicanus*, *Canis occidentalis*, *Crocuta crocuta*, *Fennecus zerda*, *Ichneumia albicauda*, *Lycaon pictus*, *Megalotis zerda*, *Meles anakuma*, *Nyctereutes procyonoides*, *Procyon lotor*, *Urocyon cinereoargenteus scotti*, *Vulpes fulva pennsylvanicus*, *Vulpes bengalensis*, *Vulpes fulva regalis*, *Vulpes japonica*, *Vulpes lagopus*, *Vulpes vulpes*	Argentina (Bugg *et al.*, 1999) Australia (Merigueti *et al.*, 2017) Brazil (Agudelo *et al.*, 1990; da Amaral *et al.*, 2010) Columbia (Dumenigo and Galvez, 1995) Cuba (Hernández *et al.*, 2007; Dubná *et al.*, 2007) Czech Republic (Moks *et al.*, 2006) Egypt (Hotez *et al.*, 2007) Estonia (Tavassoli *et al.*, 2012) Iran (Roddie *et al.*, 2008) Ireland (Habluetzel *et al.*, 2003; Keegan and Holland, 2010) Italy (Lee *et al.*, 1993) Japan (Sato *et al.*, 2006) Malaysia (Eguía-Aguilar *et al.*, 2005) Mexico (Overgaauw *et al.*, 2009) Netherlands (Luty, 2001) Poland (Luty, 2001) Switzerland (Reperant *et al.*, 2007) Turkey (Aydenizöz-Özkayhan *et al.*, 2008) UK (Jacobs *et al.*, 1977; Wolfe and Wright, 2003) United States (Parsons, 1987; Lucio-Forster *et al.*, 2016) Vietnam (Le *et al.*, 2016)	– Mitochondrial DNA genome sequenced (Li *et al.*, 2008a; Li *et al.*, 2008b) – ITS-1 and ITS-2 (Zhu and Gasser, 1988; (Jacobs *et al.*, 1997); (Zhu *et al.*, 2000); (Zhu *et al.*, 2001) – SSCP analysis (Zhu and Gasser, 1988)
T. cati (Z) (Sprent, 1956) (previously *T. mystax*)	*Actinomyx jubatus*, *Civettictis civetta*, *Felis catus*, *Felis Leopardus geoffroyi*, *Puma concolor*	Australia (O'Callaghan and Beveridge, 1996) Argentina (Beldomenico *et al.*, 2005) Argentina (Vega *et al.*, 2018)	– Mitochondrial DNA genome sequenced (Li *et al.*, 2008a; Li *et al.*, 2008b) – ITS-1 and ITS2 (Zhu and Gasser, 1988; Jacobs *et al.*, 1997; Zhu *et al.*, 2000; Zhu *et al.*, 2001)

Continued

Table 22.2. Continued

Toxocara species	Definitive host(s)	Location(s) (Reference)	Molecular speciation (Reference)
	Chaus, *Felis serval*, *Felis silvestris*, *Genetta*, *Helogale parvula*, *Leopardus colocolo*, *Leopardus geoffroyi*, *Leopardus pardalis*, *Leopardus tigrinus*, *Lynx baileyi*, *Lynx canadensis*, *Lynx lynx*, *Lynx pardinus*, *Lynx rufus texensis*, *Martes americana*, *Panthera leo*, *Panther pardus saxicolor*, *Panthera tigris*, *Prionailurus bengalensis euptilura*, *Prionailurus bengalensis iriomotensis*, *Puma yagouaroundi*	Belgium (Vanparijs and Thienpont, 1973; Vanparijs *et al*., 1991) Bolivia (Robbins *et al*., 2006) Brazil (Gallas and Silveira, 2013) Denmark (Engbaek *et al*., 1984; Fisher, 2003) Egypt (Khalafalla, 2011) France (Petithory *et al*., 1996) Germany (Beelitz and Göbel, 1992) Japan (Itoh, 2000) Mexico (Martínez-Barbabosa *et al*., 2003) Netherlands (Overgaauw and Nederland, 1997) Scotland (McColm and Hutchison, 1980) Spain (Calvete *et al*., 1998) Somalia (Gadale *et al*., 1988) South Africa (Baker *et al*., 1989) Taiwan (Fei and Mo, 1997) Tasmania (Milstein and Goldsmid, 1997) UK (Niak, 1972; Nichol *et al*., 1981; Gethings *et al*., 1987; Yamaguchi *et al*., 1996) USA (Kirkpatrick, 1988; Nolan and Smith, 1995)	– ITS-1 (Vega *et al*., 2018) – SSCP analysis (Zhu and Gasser, 1988)
T. pteropodis (Z) (Prociv, 1987)	*Pteropus conspicullatus*, *Pteropus hypomelanus*, *Pteropus tonganus*, *Pteropus poliocephalus*	Australia (Prociv, 1983; Prociv, 1990) India (Prociv, 1987) Indonesia (Prociv, 1987) New Guinea (Prociv, 1987) Vanuatu (Baylis, 1936)	

Continued

Table 22.2. Continued

Toxocara species	Definitive host(s)	Location(s) (Reference)	Molecular speciation (Reference)
T. vitulorum (Lamina, 1971)	*B. bison athabascae*, *Bos indicus*, *B. taurus*, *B. bubalis*	Australia (Doughty, 1972; Roberts, 1993) Belgium (Goossens *et al*., 2007) Canada (Woodbury *et al*., 2012; Woodbury *et al*., 2014) Egypt (Sultan *et al*., 2015) France (Dorchies, 2010) Germany (Lamina, 1971; Venjakob *et al*., 2017) Greece (Diakou and Papadopoulos, 2002) Guadeloupe (Mahieu and Naves, 2008) India (Jyoti *et al*., 2012) Italy (Scala *et al*., 2001) Ivory Coast (Knopf *et al*., 2004) Japan (Taira, 1991) Laos (Rast *et al*., 2013) Mali (Wymann *et al*., 2008) Netherlands (Borgsteede et al., 2012) Pakistan (Mirani *et al*., 2012; Raza *et al*., 2013) Serbia (Kulišić et al., 2012) Sri Lanka (Roberts, 1990; Roberts, 1993) Turkey (Aydin *et al*., 2006; Avcioğlu and Balkaya, 2011) UK (Jones *et al*., 2009) USA (Davila *et al*., 2010; Chelladurai *et al*., 2015) Vietnam (Holland *et al*., 2000) Yugoslavia (Surkovic-Zuko, 1997)	– Partial Mitochondrial DNA genome sequenced (Li *et al*., 2008b; Wickramasinghe *et al*., 2009) – ITS-1, ITS-2, and 28S (Zhu and Gasser, 1988; Jacobs *et al*., 1997; Zhu *et al*., 2000) – SSCP analysis (Zhu and Gasser, 1988)

Z = zoonoses, proven case of infection in human.

chronologically: stomach wall, intestinal wall, lungs, muscle, stomach wall, stomach contents and intestinal contents. When the kittens were fed mice that had been infected with *T. cati*, few larvae were found in the muscle or lungs of the definitive host, skipping hepato-tracheal migration and going directly from the stomach to the intestine in a 42-day period even though all were stage L_3 (Sprent, 1956). Earthworms, cockroaches, chickens, dogs, sheep and mice serve as paratenic hosts (Sprent, 1956; Mizgajska, 2001).

A complete description of larval morphology and the life cycle of *T. cati* has been published

(Sprent, 1956). L_4 larvae are found within the mucosal or sub-mucosal layers of the stomach; significant growth occurs here. Structural changes can be observed in the oral region where ventral lips develop, number of cells in the intestines, tail and oesophagus increase. At a length of 0.99–1.2 mm the next moult takes place, where the cuticle lining of the oesophagus is shed and the lips become more prominent. During L_4 white nodules, granulomas, appear in the stomach and intestines of hosts with high larval burdens.

Morphological changes in L_5 take place in the host's stomach contents and intestinal wall, the main developments during this stage are the lips and sexual differentiation begins. The larvae take on a more ascarid-like appearance, oesophageal ventricles become globular, the lumen is well defined, rectum thickly lined by cuticle with both the dorsal and ventral rectal glands differentiated. Once L_5 reaches the intestines, sexual differentiation begins. At the adult stage, the buccal region continues to change, forming three lips from digitiform extensions of palp, each lip has one or more papilla. In female adult worms, the vulva is open and the tail has two phasmids, while males have spicules present and changing on their tail. The tail changes present in males are that both pre-anal and post-anal papillae are present in the adult stage. Recently moulted adults of both sexes have lateral alae that extend the length of their body but the alae disappear from the posterior and widen and become shorter and assume the arrow shape at the cervical region. Adults usually reach 60 mm in length (Sprent, 1956).

Symptoms of *T. cati* infection are rarely seen in cats. When they occur, symptoms include: distended abdomen, rough coat, diarrhoea and dehydration (Overgaauw and Nederland, 1997). Treatment for infected cats can begins at 3 weeks; anthelmintics should be given every 2 weeks to both the kittens and nursing queen. Then treatment monthly until the kittens reach 6 months of age (European Scientific Counsel Companion Animal Parasites, 2019).

The zoonotic potential of *T. cati* remains controversial as to date, no molecular characterization of this species has been made in humans and only a few clinical cases in humans attributed to infection with *T. cati* have been reported (Shimokawa *et al.*, 1982; Fisher, 2003). The majority of suspected *T. cati* cases in humans have involved cases of ocular larval migrans (OLM) diagnosed by the Ouchterlony test (Fillaux and Magnaval, 2013) and a single case by enzyme linked immunosorbent assay (ELISA) (Sakai *et al.*, 1998). A single case of suspected visceral larval migrans (VLM) diagnosed by the Ouchterlony test has also been reported (Shimokawa *et al.*, 1982). Children vomiting adult worms have also been reported, but whether these represent zoonotic infections remains controversial (Eberhard and Alfano, 1998; Fisher, 2003; Macpherson, 2013).

Toxocara pteropodis (Baylis 1936)

The black flying fox (*Pteropus alecto*), spectacled flying fox (*Pteropus conspicillatus*), island fox (*Pteropus hypomelanus*), grey headed flying fox (*Pteropus poliocephalus*), little red flying fox (*Pteropus scapulatus*), Pacific flying fox (*Pteropus tonganus*) and Indian flying fox (*Pteropus medius*) are the hosts of *T. pteropodis*. *T. pteropodis* was first reported in the Pacific flying fox in Vanuatu and has been found in Australia, India, Indonesia and New Guinea (Bayils, 1936; Prociv, 1983; Prociv, 1987; Prociv, 1990). The eggs of *T. pteropodis* are thick-shelled and the morphological description of the adults is: spicule length less than 1.0 mm in males; 65.0–81.0 mm long; cervical alae 0.06–0.13 mm wide (Warren, 1970). When *T. pteropodis* eggs are fed in large numbers to juvenile bats of the genus *Pteropus*, they hatched in the intestines and reach the liver via the portal vein and do not become patent. Subsequent migration, if any, depends on the age and gender of the bat. In males the larvae accumulate in the liver, while in females the larvae also reside in the liver but migrate during parturition to the mammary glands (Prociv, 1983; Prociv, 1989). Larvae ingested during suckling by juveniles develop into patent adults which produce a daily output of around 25 000 eggs. The adult worms are spontaneously expelled at weaning which occurs at approximately 5 months (Prociv, 1989). There has been no evidence of transplacental infection from mother to young prior to parturition in bats. In studies with infected bats, more female worms were recovered in each infected bat than male worms, mother and young pairs had a higher rate of infection at 90% than adult males (Prociv, 1987).

There was a suspected zoonotic transmission of *T. pteropodis* on Palm Island, Australia in November of 1979 among the local population. It was suspected that *T. pteropodis* was the cause of hepatitis/allergic gastroenteritis which was contracted from ingesting eggs from bats deposited on mangoes subsequently ingested by humans (Moorhouse, 1982). The symptoms of those infected included: electrolyte and acid/ base disturbances, hypokalaemic acidosis, diarrhoea, glycosuria, ketonuria, proteinuria and haematuria (Byth, 1980). An alternative theory by those who challenged the classification of *T. pteropodis* as zoonotic proposed that the outbreak was caused by algal intoxication or by the algicide, copper sulphate, which was used to treat the water (Bourke *et al.*, 1983). If the outbreak was caused by *T. pteropodis*, then it would constitute the only zoonotic account for this species. This finding remains unsubstantiated.

Toxocara canis (Werner 1782)

Of the 22 recorded definitive hosts of *T. canis* (Table 22.2), the domestic dog is the most important and widely distributed geographically. Paratenic hosts, those in which *T. canis* is unable to complete its life cycle include: birds, rodents, rabbits, sheep, pigs and humans. *T. canis* has been reported from a large number of countries on all inhabited continents.

T. canis has been morphologically described as 'Spicule lengths 0.9 to 1.0 mm in males 9 to 13 cm long. Cervical alae reaching their maximum width in the middle, tapering posteriorly. Rod-shaped dorsal oesophageal gland nucleus' (Warren, 1970). Adult females are 120–180 mm in length and male worms 100–120 mm in length. Eggs of *T. canis* are approximately 75 μm, opaque yellow/brown with black/ brown granular contents, spherical in shape with a corrugated or pitted looking thick shell formed by a protein layer (Webster, 1958). Molecular knowledge on *T. canis* consists of the mitochondrial DNA genome, ITS-1 and ITS-2 of the ribosomal DNA having been sequenced (Jacobs *et al.*, 1997; Zhu *et al.*, 2000; Li *et al.*, 2008b).

In the definitive host, the start of the *T. canis* life cycle depends on how old the host is and the transmission method. There are various ways the host may be infected and the route the larvae take inside the host. This parasite can be transmitted in canids horizontally: ingestion of embryonated eggs, ingestion of larvae from infected paratenic host, or vertically: transplacental, or lactogenic/ transmammary transmission (Overgaauw and Van Knapen, 2000; Macpherson, 2013).

The complexities of *T. canis*' lifecycle have been researched. Here, a comprehensive overview is discussed including larval development and modes of infection, definitive hosts, survival of eggs in the environment, syndromes of infections in domestic dogs, studies in animal models and human toxocariasis.

Larval Development and Modes of Infection

Oral infection via egg

T. canis eggs are excreted into the environment via host faeces. Eggs require between 2 and 6 weeks (16) to embryonate to reach the L_3-infective stage. The development time depends upon the environmental conditions of temperature, humidity, substrate, light, pH and vegetation cover (Macpherson, 2013). Under optimal conditions of 25–30°C, high humidity, light but not direct sunlight and soil substrate eggs may become infective in 5–9 days (Levine, 1980; Mizgajska and Luty, 1998; Mizgajska, 2001; Maya *et al.*, 2010).

Under specific conditions, the unembryonated egg remains dormant in the environment for months to years, or if conditions become favourable, can mature (Despommier, 2003; Azam *et al.*, 2012). Once infective *T. canis* eggs are ingested by the definitive host the initial migration phase begins. The L_3 larva 'hatch' losing its shell in the duodenum 2–4 hour post infection (PI). The larvae then migrate to the small intestine and penetrate the mucosal wall, and enter the lymphatic vessels, and use the vessels as transport to the mesenteric lymph nodes, where the host's portal circulation system is used to reach the liver 24 hour PI (Webster, 1958). The L_3 remain in the liver normally for less than 12 hour before continuing to the vena cava and heart, but some larvae can become trapped in the liver, ending their migration. From the heart, they exit the pulmonary artery and then enter the lungs 24–96 hour PI. At this point the majority of infections take two different routes depending on the age of the host: under 3 months old tracheal migration begins, over 3 months old somatic migration begins.

Tracheal migrations for younger hosts, larvae exit the lungs via the alveoli wall and enter the bronchioles. In the stomach 7–15 days PI, the L_3 is thought to moult into the L_4 (Schacher, 1957; Sprent, 1958). The pre-adult stage L_5 reaches the small intestine where they develop into the adult. Worms are dioecious and following mating eggs are produced 4–5 weeks PI.

In hosts over 3 months old, larvae migrate to the alveoli wall through the lungs to the circulatory system. Here they become trapped in capillaries where they penetrate the capillary wall and migrate through tissue, causing haemorrhaging (Manhardt, 1980). After somatic migration most L_3 are found in the skeletal muscles, kidneys and liver and rarely in the central nervous system (Webster, 1958; Manhardt, 1980; Bosse *et al.*, 1980; Strube *et al.*, 2013). At these locations larval development is arrested and granulomas form around the L_3, which will eventually die or become hypobiotic.

Somatic migration rather than tracheal migration is thought to be due to age resistance. Age resistance results in acquired immunity, which is stage-specific to L_3 (Ferreira *et al.*, 1976; Barriga, 1988). In bitches infected by L_3 from their puppies' faeces, commonly ingested while cleaning and feeding their offspring, they go to the small intestines where they develop into adults producing eggs (Sprent, 1961). This only happens with ingestion of L_3 to which age resistance has not occurred. Unembryonated eggs ingested by the bitch from her puppies can pass through the bitch without development (Schnieder *et al.*, 2011). This is considered a spurious infection.

Oral infection via paratenic host

After ingestion of the L_3 from paratenic host the larvae are released during digestion of the tissue, where they are able to continue their migration to adults in the definitive host. Depending on the host, tracheal migration may be bypassed and the larvae go to the small intestines directly (Sprent, 1958). Infection via a paratenic host has been shown to take direct and tracheal migration routes (Herschel, 1981). Paratenic hosts include: birds, rodents, rabbits, pigs and earthworms (Mizgajska, 2001; Despommier, 2003; Sommerfelt *et al.*, 2004; Okulewicz *et al.*, 2012).

Prenatal infection

Prenatal infection also called transplacental and intrauterine transmission allows a bitch to infect their unborn pups. This is the most common form of transmission in canids and the least understood with no clear beneficial treatment option available to prevent it. Transplacental infection occurs when larvae in a previously infected bitch are reactivated or a bitch is newly infected during pregnancy. What signals the reactivation of the somatic larvae is a matter of debate (Yutuc, 1949; Webster, 1958; Koutz *et al.*, 1966). Multiple hypotheses exist including a hormonal signal such as prolactin, oestrogen, progesterone or TGF-β (Schneider *et al.*, 1996; Jin *et al.*, 2008;

Schnieder *et al.*, 2011). A study supporting reactivation by hormones found progesterone is highest in the second stage of gestation followed by prolactin. It is proposed that reactivation occurs during the second stage of gestation where these hormones promote the growth and development of *T. canis* larvae in bitches (Muñoz-Guzmán and Alba-Hurtado, 2018).

The L_3 larvae are transmitted from the bitch to the unborn pups via the umbilical cord during pregnancy (Koutz *et al.*, 1966). It is generally accepted that larvae transplacentally infect pups on day 42 and after (Douglas and Baker, 1959; Scothorn *et al.*, 1965; Lloyd *et al.*, 1983; Overgaauw and Nederland, 1997). Most of the parasites are expelled before the pup reaches 6 months of age (Woodbury *et al.*, 2014).

Lactogenic infection

While a much less common method of transmission in canids, lactogenic infection has been observed. As in prenatal infection, larvae are reactivated in the bitch's tissue and migrate to the mammary glands, where pups ingest L_3 via milk (Strube *et al.*, 2013). If a puppy ingests L_3 lactogenically, hepatotracheal migration does not occur, instead the L_3 go to the small intestines after ingestion where they mature into adults. Lactogenic transmission is rare in dogs and much more frequent in cats (Swerczek *et al.*, 1971; Overgaauw and Nederland, 1997). Post-partum larvae in milk increase until a maximum is reached within 7–14 days, most pups are infected within 2–3 weeks post-partum (Stoye, 1976; Schnieder *et al.*, 2011). Many studies have been conducted to examine the migratory route larvae take, when larvae reach the mammary glands, and how close to parturition a bitch can be infected and still transmit *T. canis* larvae to pups via lactogenic transmission (Stoye, 1976; Manhardt, 1980; Löwenstein, 1981; Burke and Roberson, 1985; Burke and Roberson, 1985).

Infection of paratenic host

Upon ingestion of L_3 from the environment by a paratenic host, the larvae migrate to the stomach where the egg shell is shed by the L_3. The larvae then enter the small intestine where they pass through the intestinal wall and begin somatic migration. Larvae undergo somatic migration to organs within the host, most commonly the liver, lungs, muscles, heart, eyes and brain. The larvae can be encysted and die after a period, which depends on the paratenic host species, could be years.

Definitive Hosts of *Toxocara canis*

Domestic dog (*Canis familiaris*)

Domestic dogs are found globally, as pets in many households and as strays or even feral animals living on the penumbra of human society. Dogs, mainly puppies under 1 year of age, represent the main source of infection to humans (Table 22.3).

Red fox (*Vulpes vulpes*)

Since the 1980s, with the successful control of rabies through vaccination control programmes, the population of foxes in Europe has steadily increased and the prevalence of *T. canis* in these hosts is high in most countries where studies have been conducted in Europe and in Canada. The range of *T. canis* has increased in Europe with the expansion and number of the fox population. Age-prevalence and age-intensity profiles show that *T. canis* worm burdens are usually higher in cubs than in adult foxes. Seasonal variations in worm burdens occur in red foxes and are related to the reproductive cycles of the fox. The highest prevalences and intensities occur during the spring, which coincides with the birth of cubs (Ross and Fairley, 1969; Loos-Frank and Zeyhle, 1982; Borgsteede, 1984; Richards *et al.*, 1995; Willingham *et al.*, 1996;

Table 22.3. *T. canis* infection in domestic and feral hosts

Definitive host	Country	% Infected	No. of samples/ type	References
Domestic dog	Grenada	48	306 faecal	(Schwartz, 2017)
	USA	2	2.5 million faecal	(Lucio-Forster *et al.*, 2016)
	Brazil	5.5	271 faecal	(Oliveira-Sequeira *et al.*, 2002)
	Belgium	17.4	2324 faecal	(Vanparijs *et al.*, 1991)
	Germany	6.9	3329 faecal	(Epe *et al.*, 1993)
	Italy	33.6	295 faecal	(Habluetzel *et al.*, 2003)
	Poland	32	445 faecal	(Luty, 2001)
	Nigeria	34.6	474 faecal	(Akeredolu and Sowemimo, 2014)
	Nigeria	31.8	1000 faecal	(Kutdang *et al.*, 2010)
	Ethiopia	25.8	334 faecal	(Degefu *et al.*, 2010)
	Tanzania	13.7	241 faecal	(Swai *et al.*, 2010)
Red fox	Denmark	23.5	68 faecal and intestines	(Willingham *et al.*, 1996)
	Denmark	59.4 (68.5 male, 49.4 female)	1040 intestines	(Saeed *et al.*, 2006)
	Germany	32	3573 intestines	(Loos-Frank and Zeyhle, 1982)
	Great Britain	61.6	588 small intestine	(Smith *et al.*, 2003)
	Ireland	20	91 faecal	(Stuart *et al.*, 2013)
	Ireland	35	72 intestines	(Ross and Fairley, 1969)
	Italy	9.1	129 intestine and faecal	(Magi *et al.*, 2009)
	Italy	54.4	645 small intestine	(Cerbo *et al.*, 2008)
	Poland	6.9	144 faecal	(Borecka *et al.*, 2013)
	Poland	19.1	639 small intestine	(Borecka *et al.*, 2009)
	Spain	4.4	67 small intestine and faeces	(Criado-Fornelio *et al.*, 2000)
	UK	55.9	843 small intestine	(Richards *et al.*, 1995)
	Slovak Republic	12.5	1198 faecal	(Miterpáková *et al.*, 2009)
	Netherlands	73.3	139 intestines	(Borgsteede, 1984)
	Iran	4.5	22 small intestine	(Dalimi *et al.*, 2006)
	Kyrgyzstan	30.4	151 intestines	(Ziadinov *et al.*, 2010)

Continued

Table 22.3. Continued

Definitive host	Country	% Infected	No. of samples/ type	References
	Lithuania	40.5	310 intestines	(Bružinskaitė-Schmidhalter *et al.*, 2012)
	Canada	25.1 (25.4 male, 21.7 female)	271 faecal	(Wapenaar *et al.*, 2013)
Arctic fox	Iceland	2	50 faecal	(Skirnisson *et al.*, 1993)
	Sweden	7, 30	29 and 23 dens, faecal	(Meijer *et al.*, 2011)
Japanese red fox	Japan	71	seven intestines	(Sato *et al.*, 1999)
Wolves	Belorussian Polesie	21.2	52 necropsy	(Shimalov and Shimalov, 2000)
	Estonia	8	26 intestines and faecal	(Moks *et al.*, 2006)
	Latvia	5.8	34 necropsy	(Bagrade *et al.*, 2009)
	Poland	5.6	89 faecal	(Popiołek *et al.*, 2007)
	Poland	13.5	52 faecal	(Kloch *et al.*, 2005)
	Spain	6.4	47 necropsy	(Segovia *et al.*, 2001)
Coyotes	Canada	2.2	185 faecal	(Wapenaar *et al.*, 2013)
	Canada	19	69 small intestine	(Bridger *et al.*, 2009)
Golden jackals	Hungary	20	20 internal organs and faecal	(Takács *et al.*, 2013)
	Serbia	1.6	447 intestines	(Ćirović *et al.*, 2015)
	Iran	10	ten small intestine	(Dalimi *et al.*, 2006)
Raccoon dogs	Belorussian Polesie	20.5	78 necropsy, 179 faecal	(Shimalov and Shimalov, 2002)
	Lithuania	17.6	99 intestines	(Bružinskaitė-Schmidhalter *et al.*, 2012)

Criado-Fornelio *et al.*, 2000; Smith *et al.*, 2003; Dalimi *et al.*, 2006; Saeed *et al.*, 2006; Cerbo *et al.*, 2008; Miterpáková *et al.*, 2009; Borecka *et al.*, 2009; Magi *et al.*, 2009; Ziadinov *et al.*, 2010; Bružinskaitė-Schmidhalter *et al.*, 2012; Wapenaar *et al.*, 2013; Borecka *et al.*, 2013).

Arctic fox (*Alopex lagopus*)

Arctic foxes have been found infected with *T. canis* in Iceland and Sweden (Skirnisson *et al.*, 1993; Meijer *et al.*, 2011). Prevalence rates in Sweden were reported to increase during a 2-year study in the year where rodent populations were highest (Meijer *et al.*, 2011).

Japanese red fox (*Vulpes japonica*)

In the Japanese red fox, a limited number of older foxes (seven) were found to be heavily infected with adult *T. canis* (Sato *et al.*, 1999). This is in contrast to other definitive host species where young animals have higher prevalences and intensities of *T. canis* infection. This finding in the Japanese red fox may be because of the small number of animals examined (Martínez *et al.*, 1978; Kapel and Nansen, 1996).

Wolves (*Canis lupus*)

Wolves have been found to be commonly infected with *T. canis* in a number of countries in Northern Europe. Because they have little interaction with humans and do not encroach on urban areas they pose an insignificant threat to human infection (Shimalov and Shimalov, 2000; Segovia *et al.*, 2001; Kloch *et al.*, 2005; Moks *et al.*, 2006; Popiołek *et al.*, 2007; Bagrade *et al.*, 2009).

Coyote (*Canis latrans*)

Coyotes which mostly occur in rural areas have also adapted to urban areas and their public health importance in the epidemiology of *T. canis* will increase with this trend. Infected coyotes have been reported in Costa Rica (Niehaus *et al.*, 2012) Iowa, USA (Redman *et al.*, 2016) and in Canada (Bridger *et al.*, 2009; Wapenaar *et al.*, 2013).

Golden jackal (*Canis aureus*)

A few studies in Europe have shown that golden jackals can serve as definitive hosts for *T. canis* (Dalimi *et al.*, 2006; Takács *et al.*, 2013; Ćirović *et al.*, 2015). Their importance as sources of zoonotic infection is likely to be minimal, as these animals have not become adapted to urban centres.

Raccoon dog (*Nyctereutes procyonoides*)

Racoon dogs have been reported to be definitive hosts of *T. canis* in Germany, Belorussian Polesie, Lithuania and Russia (Shimalov and Shimalov, 2002; Bružinskaitė-Schmidhalter *et al.*, 2012).

Survival of *Toxocara canis* Eggs in the Environment

Environmental conditions influence larval development inside the egg and play an important role in the geographical distribution of the parasite. Optimal egg development conditions of 25–30°C and 85–95% humidity cause eggs to mature to the L_3-infective stage in 9–15 days (Schacher, 1957; Okoshi and Usui, 1968; Smith *et al.*, 1981; Schnieder *et al.*, 2011). Factors that negatively affect the egg development are temperatures of 37°C and above, low humidity, sandy substrate and direct sunlight. Soil substrate is more favourable than sand for development and therefore favours transmission opportunities as in sand the eggs sink far below the surface where the conditions are not favourable for their development. In soil, eggs tend to remain in the top 2 cm of substrate and soil maintains a higher water content than sand, vegetation cover favours egg survival. Eggs will perish in temperatures below −15°C in the open, but can survive if under the soil surface or covered in snow up to −29°C (Levine, 1980; Overgaauw and Nederland, 1997; Azam *et al.*, 2012). *T. canis* can survive in a wide variety of environmental conditions and can also arrest development until appropriate environmental conditions arise, enabling parasite survival in most areas inhabited by humans and their dogs. Studies examining egg development, survival and availability in the environment have demonstrated that puppies under 6 months of age are the most important contributors to egg deposition (Nijsse *et al.*, 2015). Other studies have investigated host density and over dispersion of *T. canis* infection to estimate environmental contamination (Morgan *et al.*, 2013; Nijsse et al., 2015). In countries where they occur foxes and racoons play a lesser role in environmental contamination (Morgan *et al.*, 2013). In the Netherlands host egg output decreased from domestic dogs, to stray cats, to domestic cats and foxes (Nijsse *et al.*, 2015). As human populations grow and become more concentrated in urban areas with limited green spaces shared with a large number of definitive hosts the public health importance of *T. canis* is likely to increase.

Syndromes of *Toxocara canis* Infections in Dogs

Pathological changes in dogs

Pathological changes that take place during a *T. canis* infection start with eosinophilia around 7 days PI. Eosinophilia does not decrease until eggs are shed via host faeces (Zimmermann, 1983). Enzymatic changes occur during liver migration causing liver enzymes glutamate dehydrogenase and alaine transaminase to increase (Zimmermann, 1983). Larvae reach the liver 72 hour PI and leucocytes such as eosinophils, monocytes and polymorphonuclear leucocytes increase steadily for the next 24–48 hour as a part of the host's immune response to infection (Webster, 1958). The white blood cells, cause the formation of white nodules or spots as they surround larvae and form granulomas, often seen in the liver, kidneys and lungs. Granulomas may also cause tissue necrosis, haemorrhaging and fibrous tissue proliferation, resulting in scar tissue (Schnieder *et al.*, 2011). Fibrous tissue begins to form 3 weeks PI and can cause a multitude of clinical affects depending on the location.

Another pathological change caused by *T. canis* is a decreasing number of erythrocytes in puppies, which are born with low erythrocyte levels that increase until levelling off at adulthood. Infection of this parasite always results in anaemia. This is caused by the host's immune response with inflammation producing cytokines which inhibit erythrocyte production and cause internal bleeding as a result of larval migrations (Zimmermann, 1983; Schnieder *et al.*, 2011). Adults usually only exhibit increased activity of liver enzymes from migrating larvae (Overgaauw and Nederland, 1997; Macpherson, 2013).

Clinical syndromes in dogs

In definitive hosts *T. canis* infection does not typically cause clinical symptoms in adults, but in puppies symptoms can be as severe as still births or early death. Although larval migrans may not cause overt symptoms they have the potential to do damage. As *T. canis* larvae migrate through the body they leave behind a trail of internal damage including: tissue damage, bloody mucous enteritis, low to moderate enteritis, lesions in the intestinal tract, peritonitis, cachexia, spots on the liver, lesions in kidneys, obstruction and rupture of intestine, fatty degeneration of liver cells and petechial haemorrhages in lungs (Webster, 1958; Fernando, 1968; Dade and Williams, 1975; Bosse *et al.*, 1980; Herschel, 1981; Overgaauw and Nederland, 1997). Symptoms in puppies include: coughing, dyspnoea, pneumonia, distention of abdomen, diarrhoea, constipation, nasal discharge and failure to thrive (Webster, 1958). White spots, which appear on the liver are a result of L_3 larva being encapsulated by leucocytes, monocytes and eosinophils, giving the liver a mottled appearance. Granulomas appear in other places throughout the body such as the kidney and lungs. In the lungs eosinophils form white nodules and may lead to tissue necrosis and haemorrhage (Webster, 1958; Hayden and Kruiningen, 1975).

Clinical syndromes exhibited by the host are based on three variables; larval burden, host's immune response, and which organs are implicated by the larva migration route. A low larval burden may lead to pneumonia, vascular congestion, and digestive disturbances while a high larval burden can cause severe anaemia, eosinophilia, obstruction or rupture of intestines, moderate enteritis and the most severe cases death (Webster, 1958). Migration of larvae through the intestinal wall commonly causes internal bleeding, which can lead to anaemia especially in puppies (Zimmermann, 1983; Vossmann and Stoye, 1986). Involvement of the liver has been shown to cause fatty degeneration of liver cells and peritonitis when the bile ducts are affected by allowing the larvae to enter the abdominal cavity (Webster, 1958; Schnieder *et al.*, 2011). Effects of larvae entering the lungs are coughing, dyspnoea, lobular pneumonia and vascular congestion (Webster, 1958; Overgaauw and Nederland, 1997). The interaction of the host's immune system with *T. canis* excretory secretory (ES) antigen molecules released by the larvae also play an important role in the development of symptoms manifested by infected host, but their role is not well understood (Maizels *et al.*, 1984; Page *et al.*, 1992).

Diagnosis and Treatment of *Toxocara canis* in Domestic Dogs

Diagnosis in dogs consists of clinical presentation, faecal flotation or smears and spontaneous passage of worms in faeces (Macpherson, 2013).

Faecal flotation utilizes flotation solutions with a high specific gravity (1.2–1.3) and the subsequent microscopic identification of the characteristic eggs. Such techniques are sensitive for diagnosis in young puppies which usually shed large numbers of eggs, but lack sensitivity in older animals which shed eggs intermittently and/or in low numbers. Thus, samples should be taken at regular intervals if an infection is to be correctly ruled in or out using this technique. Recently, ultrasound (US) has been used to examine pre-patent infections in puppies and was shown to have a 100% specificity with an 85% sensitively in puppies 15 days post-partum (Corda *et al.*, 2019). Such a diagnosis would significantly help in the early treatment of infected puppies prior to excretion of eggs and potentially substantially reduce contamination of the environment with *T. canis* eggs.

Treatment guidelines suggest anthelmintics for puppies which should begin at 2 weeks and repeated at 4, 6 and 8 weeks then monthly until 6 months of age (Sloss *et al.*, 1994; Overgaauw and Nederland, 1997; Macpherson, 2013). High risk groups such as puppies in pet shops, dog-breeding kennels etc. should especially adhere to this treated regimen to avoid potential zoonotic transmission. Re-infection in puppies occurs through ingestion of *T. canis* larva in milk from the bitch or eggs from the environment. Treatment of a bitch during pregnancy is not recommended as anthelmintics can have negative side effects on the unborn pups such as palatoschisis and low birth rates (Bosse *et al.*, 1980; Overgaauw and Boersema, 1998). Another reason for not treating while pregnant is that it is unknown exactly when the larvae emerge from their state of stasis and migrate to the uterus and mammary glands, making treatment times a guess and anthelmintic have shown to be ineffective against somatic larvae (Overgaauw and Nederland, 1997). The time of reactivation has been cited as the last third of pregnancy, but that still leaves much room for error (Epe, 2009). It should be noted that anthelmintics have proven ineffective against somatic larvae in adult dogs, but treatment for bitches that have recently given birth is important as the larvae are active during this time (Epe, 2006; Macpherson, 2013).

Multiple studies have shown that infection is more likely when a relatively small number of embryonated eggs are ingested (Overgaauw and Knapen, 2013). This has been demonstrated when 2000 eggs were fed to 1-year-old dogs and two of four dogs developed patent infections (Greve, 1971). Another study infected puppies 2 months old with 10 000 embryonated eggs and none of the puppies developed patent infections (Dubey, 1978).

For adult dogs, faecal examinations should take place multiple times a year to assess if there is an active *T. canis* infection. Positive cases should be treated accordingly with anthelmintics (Table 22.4).

Toxocara canis Studies in Animal Models

Animal models have been used to trace the migratory route of larva, immune response from the host and how larvae evade the immune system's attacks. These studies have been conducted on mice, rats, gerbils, pigs, poultry, quail, pigeons, macaques and early on even humans (Beaver, 1956; Galvin, 1964; Glickman and Summers, 1983; Kayes *et al.*, 1985; Nagakura *et al.*, 1989; Pahari and Sasmal, 1990; Havasiová-Reiterová *et al.*, 1995; Cox and Holland, 1998; Helwigh *et al.*, 1999; Cox and Holland, 2001; Akao *et al.*, 2003; Lescano *et al.*, 2004; Akao, 2006; Merigueti *et al.*, 2018).

Table 22.4. Treatment of *T. canis* infections in dogs

Drug	mg/kg × days	Application	References
Fenbendazole	50 × 3	PO	(Penn Veterinary Medicine, n.d.; Manual, n.d.)
Febantel	25	PO	(Penn Veterinary Medicine, n.d.)
Flubendazole	22 × 5	PO	(Epe, 2006)
Mebendazole	22 × 3	PO	(Penn Veterinary Medicine, n.d.)
Pyrantel	5.0–10.0 × 1	PO	(Epe, 2006)
Pyrantel pamoate	5	PO	(Manual, n.d.)
Praziquantel + Pyrantel pamoate	5/5	PO	(Manual, n.d.)
Praziquantel + Pyrantel pamoate + Ivermectin	5/5/0.006	PO	(Manual, n.d.)
Praziquantel + Pyrantel pamoate + Febantel	5/5/25	PO	(Manual, n.d.)
Nitroscanat	50 × 1	PO	(Epe, 2006)
Ivermectin	0.2–0.4 repeat as needed	PO	(Penn Veterinary Medicine, n.d.)
Milbemycin	0.5	PO	(Penn Veterinary Medicine, n.d.; Manual, n.d.)
Milbemycin oxime	0.5/1.0 × 1	PO	(Epe, 2006)
Milbemycin oxime + lufenuron	0.5/1.0 × 1	PO	(Manual, n.d.)
Selamectin	6.0 × 1	Topical	(Epe, 2006)
Moxidectin	2.5–6.5 × 1	Topical	(Epe, 2006)
Moxidectin + imidacloprid	2.5/10	Topical	(Manual, n.d.)

[a]Adverse effects were reported in certain sheepdog breeds (Collies).

Mice have shown that early in the infection larvae are found in the liver and lungs but then later accumulate in the muscle and brain (Cox and Holland, 1998; Holland and Cox, 2001; Cox and Holland, 2001). These changes all increase a mouse's susceptibility to predators and a decrease in self-preservation. A decrease in learning capacity and memory with an increase in abnormal behaviour was also seen during this study in mice with high numbers of larvae residing in the brain (Janecek *et al.*, 2017). Mice have also been used to examine the immune response elicited by *T. canis*, showing a polarized TH2 immune response and systematic cytokine patterns (Resende *et al.*, 2015). Vertical transmission has been shown to take place in mice, the only paratenic host shown to pass on *T. canis* infection to their offspring lactogenically (Oshima, 1961). Neurotoxocariasis (NT) in mice altered myelin gene expression causing nerve fibre demyelination in the cerebrum and cerebellum (Heuer *et al.*, 2015).

Macaques (*Macaca fascicularis*) have been a valuable animal model in observing VLM commonly found in children. Symptoms of VLM include granulomatous hepatitis and encephalomyelitis for this species, while neurological changes include ataxia, nystagmus and paralysis. OLM has not been shown to occur in macaques (Tomimura *et al.*, 1976; Glickman and Summers, 1983). In other primate models, larvae have been shown to live for extended periods of time, 15 months in the eye and up to 10 years in other tissues (Beaver, 1969); raising the question of how long the larvae can survive in human tissue, a question that has yet to be answered.

Mongolian gerbils (*Meriones unguiculatus*) are prone to OLM, up to 90% of those infected present with OLM making them an important animal model for research in understanding this clinical manifestation (Takayanagi *et al.*, 1999; Alba-Hurtado *et al.*, 2000; Akao *et al.*, 2003; Flecher *et al.*, 2016). Oral infection in gerbils has shown larvae appear in the liver and lungs in 12–24 hour PI, remain in the lungs 3–5 days PI, and are found in the eye from day 5 PI until day 60 when the study ended (Alba-Hurtado *et al.*, 2009). Pathological changes seen in this animal model include: vitreous and retinal haemorrhages, circulatory system fluid build-up in lesions, granulomas and inflammation of blood vessels, all of which are comparable to changes in infected humans. Neurological symptoms are urinary incontinence, coma, difficulty with gait, ataxia and paralysis of the lower body (Strube *et al.*, 2013).

Pigs, whose immune systems are similar to humans, are an animal model used for VLM and covert toxocariasis (CT) due to their immune response and the long migrations larvae undertake (Helwigh *et al.*, 1999; Taira *et al.*, 2004; Strube *et al.*, 2013; Sommerfelt *et al.*, 2014). Pigs rarely exhibit symptoms but pathological changes are common with the liver, kidneys, lungs and lymph nodes affected. Both the liver and kidneys exhibit white spots on their exterior and granulomas can be found in the lungs of infected subjects with VLM. Changes in pigs with CT mainly take place in the brain and include: oedema, necrosis, abnormal clustering of cells, nerve cell shrinkage or destruction and damage to glial cells (Sasmal *et al.*, 2008). Toxocariasis appears to be a self-limiting parasite in pigs as after 126 days PI, no larvae were recovered from infected animals (Sommerfelt *et al.*, 2004).

Rats (*Rattus norvegicus*) have been included in a few studies showing that *T. canis* larvae follow the hepatopulmonary and myotropic–neurotrophic phases, as have been demonstrated in mice models (Strube *et al.*, 2013; dos Santos *et al.*, 2017). After oral infection larvae appear in the liver 3–5 days PI, then the lungs 5–8 days PI and are found in the brain from day 5 PI (Lescano *et al.*, 2004). Larvae in the brain lead to a decreased ability to navigate complex mazes (Olson and Rose, 1966). Similar behaviour modification seen in mice were also seen in rats, particularly with regards to spending more time in open space, where predation is more likely, making the rats easier prey (Chieffi *et al.*, 2010; Santos *et al.*, 2015). Studies on the effect of the hormone prolactin on the immune response from a host has also been explored in the rat model, providing insight into the role hormones play in reactivation of larvae in bitches (Del Rio-Araiza *et al.*, 2018).

Chickens have been used as animal models as they present a real zoonotic source for human infection via the ingestion of a paratenic host route (Taira *et al.*, 2011; Strube *et al.*, 2013; Merigueti *et al.*, 2018). In studies where chickens were orally infected, larvae have been shown to live in the liver for up to 3 months and over 3 years in other tissue (Maruyama *et al.*, 1994). In chicken meat, larvae can remain viable for extended periods of time and survive low temperatures, such as those used for freezing meat (Sprent, 1953; Zibaei *et al.*, 2017). Nematophagous fungi, *Pochonia chlamydosporia* and *Duddingtonia flagrans* showed predatory and ovicidal effects on L2 exposed to the fungi in one study. This study showed a reduction in viability of 53–87%, depending on the length of exposure and fungus (Hiura *et al.*, 2015).

Human Toxocariasis

Humans are infected with *T. canis* mainly through the ingestion of infective eggs, facilitated by behaviour which increases the opportunity for ingestion of eggs. Our understanding of the incidence of infection in humans is relatively undefined. Many seroprevalence studies have been conducted in numerous countries reviewed most recently by Ma *et al.* (Ma *et al.*, 2018), but these only provide an indication of human exposure and are usually limited through small sample sizes. One exception was the study by Farmer *et al.* (Farmer *et al.*, 2017) where over 13 000 people were studied using ELISA, which showed that infection increases with age. This is to be expected given the accidental nature of human infection. The incidence of infection is most likely highest amongst children because of their behaviour as discussed below.

Risk Factors for Transmission of *Toxocara* spp. to Humans

The incidence of *T. canis* infection is highest among children as many of their behaviours expose them to the risk of accidentally ingesting infective eggs. Such behaviour includes pica, geophagia and poor hygiene practices, including putting unwashed hands, vegetables and other objects in their mouths. Children also usually have a closer association with puppies, whose fur and their sleeping environment may be contaminated by infective eggs (Magnaval *et al.*, 2001; Strube *et al.*, 2013; Macpherson, 2013; Ma *et al.*, 2018). Other potentially highly contaminated areas include public parks, especially in urban areas where people and their pets are concentrated.

The most important route of transmission of *T. canis* to humans is from the accidental ingestion of eggs containing L_3 from the environment. Humans can also become infected by eating raw chicken liver and meat from duck, pig, cattle and rabbits all of whom serve as paratenic hosts (Salem and Schantz, 1992; Yoshikawa *et al.*, 2008; Antolová *et al.*, 2013; Fillaux and Magnaval, 2013). The consumption of smoked, pickled or cured foods from paratenic hosts may also be a source of infection.

Risk factors other than age and hygiene include gender, profession, geographic location, socioeconomic status, education level, pet ownership and the increasing proclivity of eating uncooked or preserved foods which might have a cultural or popular trend basis, which are difficult to quantify (Carvalho and Rocha, 2011; Macpherson, 2013; Lee et al., 2014). Raw cow's liver is often eaten in parts of South East Asia and has been shown in South Korea to be an important source of human exposure to *T. canis* infection (Won *et al.*, 2015).

Clinical manifestations of *T. canis* infections in humans

It is likely that the majority of patients infected with *T. canis* remains asymptomatic or develop clinical symptoms that have yet to be routinely associated with the parasite. Seroprevalence studies conducted in many parts of the world show that a large percentage of people may be exposed to this parasite yet few are reported with overt clinical manifestations. Further studies are required to link infection with this parasite and its range of clinical manifestations in people.

Clinical manifestations are due primarily to mechanical damage and the immune response to the excretory secretions (ES) by the L_3. The ES antigens are produced by the oesophageal gland and excretory column of the L_3 (Page *et al.*, 1992). A component of ES is TBA-1, which results in the allergenic reaction seen (Sugane and Oshima, 1983; Glickman *et al.*, 1987; Yahiro *et al.*, 1998). There are other glycoproteins produced by the epicuticular layer that have not yet been identified. Four clinical syndromes of toxocariasis have been described and include: VLM, OLM, CT and NT.

Visceral Larval Migrans (VLM)

This is the most commonly diagnosed syndrome and often present in children. VLM is associated with a heavy infection load and clinically presents as fever, hepatomegaly, abdominal pain, vomiting, diarrhoea, asthma, weight loss, headache, fatigue, pneumonitis, pulmonary infiltrates, pleural effusion, pericarditis, eosinophilic myocarditis, endomyocardial fibrosis, anaemia, hepatitis, respiratory symptoms, leucocytosis, hypergammaglobulinaemia, myalgia, splenomegaly, nephritis, arthritis, eczema, pruritus, urticaria, vasculitis and eosinophilia (Beaver *et al.*, 1952; Smith *et al.*, 2009; Hotez and Wilkins, 2009; Stoicescu *et al.*, 2011; Nicoletti, 2013; Fan *et al.*, 2013; Strube *et al.*, 2013; Macpherson, 2013; Zibaei, 2017; Ain Tiewsoh *et al.*, 2018; Ma *et al.*, 2018). It is also associated with allergy related manifestations including chronic urticaria, prurigo, reactive arthritis and angioedema (Magnaval and Glickman, 2006). Long-term effects of VLM have been associated with asthma and pulmonary fibrosis (Ma *et al.*, 2018).

Ocular Larval Migrans (OLM)

OLM is caused when L_3 migrate or become entrapped in the eye, and may result in a variety of symptoms depending on the activity and location of the larvae in the choroid. Clinical symptoms include: visual distortion, heterotopia, detachment of the macula or retina, cystoid macular oedema, strabismus, leucocoria, eosinophilic abscesses, vitreous haze, cataracts, papillitis, endophthalmitis, uveitis, granulomatous lesions, granulomatous larval tracks in retina, diffuse endophthalmitis, and in extreme cases can result in blindness, which is usually uniocular (Shields, 1984; Gillespie *et al.*, 1993; Stewart *et al.*, 2005; De Visser *et al.*, 2008; Woodhall *et al.*, 2012; Macpherson, 2013). These symptoms occur rapidly and evolve over days or weeks.

Covert Toxocariasis (CT)

CT, sometimes called common toxocariasis, is a *Toxocara* infection that displays non-specific mild clinical symptoms. It is the toxocariasis syndrome that is mostly observed in children. However, CT occurs in children and adults manifesting with different symptoms. In children: fever, anorexia, headache, abdominal pain, nausea, vomiting, lethargy, sleep and behavioural disorders, limb pain, cervical lymphadenitis, pharyngitis, pneumonia, cough, pulmonary symptoms and hepatomegaly have been reported (Nicoletti, 2013; Fillaux and Magnaval, 2013; Strube *et al.*, 2013; Macpherson, 2013; Ma *et al.*, 2018). In adults: weakness, pruritus, urticaria, pulmonary dysfunction, abdominal pain, with or without eosinophilia may occur (Fan *et al.*, 2013; Macpherson, 2013; Nicoletti, 2013; Ma *et al.*, 2018).

Neurotoxocariasis (NT)

NT is thought to be rare and occurs when L_3 enter the brain or spinal cord. Symptoms for NT include: meningitis, encephalitis, myelitis, cerebral vasculitis, seizures, motor impairment, headache, fever, photophobia, weakness, dorsalgia, confusion, depression, fatigue, optic neuritis, eosinophilic meningitis, cerebral lesions, astrocyte apoptosis, meningoencephalitis, meningoradiculitis and transverse myelitis (Xinou *et al.*, 2003; Vidal *et al.*, 2003; Eberhardt *et al.*, 2005; Hotez and Wilkins, 2009; Strube *et al.*, 2013; Caldera *et al.*, 2013; Nicoletti, 2013; Fillaux and Magnaval, 2013; Jabbour *et al.*, 2014; Chou and Fan, 2018). NT is considered by some authorities to be a contributing factor to neuro-degenerative disorders such as dementia, epilepsy, Parkinson's, schizophrenia, seizures and developmental delays (Nicoletti *et al.*, 2007; Quattrocchi *et al.*, 2012; Fan *et al.*, 2015; Ma *et al.*, 2018). The behavioural effects observed in other paratenic hosts, such as mice, including reduction of aggression, less tendency towards exploration, increase in immobility and favouring open areas have thus far not been described in humans and this requires further investigation (Cox and Holland, 2001; Janecek *et al.*, 2017).

Diagnosis and treatment of *Toxocara canis* infection in humans

Diagnosis of toxocariasis consists of multiple methods, as some patients do not present with overt symptoms. Until recently, it was recommended for many cases that serological testing with an ELISA to detect the antigen immunoglobulin E (IgE) or IgG followed by a western blot (WB) to confirm was the best diagnostic practice (De Savigny *et al.*, 1979;

Alcântara-Neves *et al.*, 2008; Mohamad *et al.*, 2009; Fillaux and Magnaval, 2013). The reliability of the ELISA depends on the antigens and type of antibody used for the test, there have been some issues with cross reactivity to other parasites such as *Strongyloides stercoralis* and *Trichinella spiralis* that may be co-infecting the patient (Jacquier et al., 1991; Fillaux and Magnaval, 2013). Although there are many serological tests, the distinction of *T. canis* infection from *T. cati* infection has not been achieved yet in serological studies. Despite this, the sensitivity and specificity of the ELISA tests are high and given the high prevalence of the infection in most endemic countries, the positive predictive value is also high. Polymerase chain reaction (PCR) of tissue or body fluids was recommended as the most reliable as PCR testing can provide a definitive *Toxocara* species identification (Ma *et al.*, 2018). A comprehensive review of the serological tests available has recently been published (Ma *et al.*, 2018). Along with serological and immunologic tests other methods of detection include medical imaging techniques using US, computed tomography and magnetic resonance imaging (MRI) (Vidal *et al.*, 2003; Eberhardt *et al.*, 2005; Macpherson, 2013; Fillaux and Magnaval, 2013). Histopathological exams and morphologic assessment of larvae are rare because the larvae's location within the body is not usually known.

Diagnosis of OLM consists of serological testing of the vitreous or aqueous humour with imaging techniques, especially ocular US used to assist (Macpherson, 2013; Martinez-Pulgarin *et al.*, 2015; Ma *et al.*, 2018). NT diagnosis consists of eosinophils in the cerebral spinal fluid (CSF), antigens found during serology, in addition to imaging techniques such as MRI, rarely larvae may be detected in the CSF of patients with NT (Macpherson, 2013; Caldera *et al.*, 2013; Ma *et al.*, 2018). Diagnosis for CT consists of clinical presentation, patient history, ELISA, followed by confirmation with WB (Hotez and Wilkins, 2009). Diagnosis for VLM is serological and immunologic testing used in conjunction with imaging techniques, mainly US (Macpherson, 2013; Ma *et al.*, 2018). Diagnostic methods for the four clinical syndromes are not agreed upon by all and would benefit from improvement in diagnosis protocols.

Treatment of *Toxocara canis* syndromes in humans

Recommended treatment depends on the syndrome and severity of symptoms. VLM, NT or CT treatment usually consists of anthelmintics, such as mebendazole or albendazole, which are administered alone or in conjunction with corticosteroids (Magnaval and Glickman, 2006). Treatment with diethylcarbamazine is administered alone and not with corticosteroids, as they inhibit the function of this anthelmintic (Maizels and Denham, 1992).

Albendazole appears to be the treatment of choice with a reported cure rate of 47% (Stürchler *et al.*, 1989). Diethylcarbamazine has the highest success rate at 70%, but is associated with a high rate of neurological side effects (Magnaval, 1995). Thiabendazole is not recommended for treatment of toxocariasis as it has a 50–53% success rate and 50–60% of patients had side effects (Magnaval and Charlet, 1987; Stürchler *et al.*, 1989).

Because OLM is a rare diagnosis there is little consolidated evidence on the best treatment protocols for this condition, linking ophthalmological clinics would be a useful development in generating sufficient information to guide the best evidence-based treatment protocol. Currently treatment is using surgical techniques, such as laser, to ablate the larva and there is increasing evidence that use of albendazole and corticosteroids would be more preferable in some cases (Magnaval and Glickman, 2006; Ma *et al.*, 2018).

Control of *Toxocara canis*

The high prevalence of *T. canis* in dogs and their ubiquitous distribution coupled to the high seroprevalence in humans and the poor understanding of the true public health implications of infection suggests that control of this parasite should be given a greater priority than is presently the case. Climate change and population growth is facilitating the expansion of the geographical range of both the parasite and its definitive host species (Jenkins *et al.*, 2013). The rapid urbanization of populations concentrates people and definitive hosts into greater proximities.

Control of *T. canis* has to focus on the production of eggs from definitive hosts. Once in the environment eggs are extremely resistant to environmental conditions and are almost impossible to kill being resistant to chemicals and disinfectants. Eggs remain viable after 8 days in 40% formalin or Lysol, 1 month in 10% hydrochloric acid or 10% formalin, and 18 days in 5.25% sodium hypochlorite solution (Levine, 1980; von Dohlen *et al.*, 2017). Eggs can also survive conventional sewer treatments or being composted (Pegg and Donald, 1978; Strauch, 1991). Direct sunlight, drying and temperatures above 37°C kill eggs (Levine, 1980; Mizgajska, 2001; Tiyo *et al.*, 2008). Nematophagous fungi including *Mucor circinelloides* and *D. flagrans* have recently been shown to have predatory activity on *T. canis* eggs passed by puppies, reducing their viability up to 57% (Hernández *et al.*, 2018).

Today, most developed countries have instituted poop and scoop laws mandating that owners pick up their dog's faeces from public areas or face a fine. Such laws were first introduced in 1935 in London and were adopted widely: New York instituted the law in 1978 with a $250 fine for noncompliance (Brulliard, 2016). In Madrid, dog owners can be fined up to $1700. Other cities including Mexico City, Paris and Taipei have instituted incentives, such as free Wi-Fi and lottery tickets, instead of fines (Brulliard, 2016).

Wild definitive hosts, stray and feral dogs present a separate challenge for control. Trap, treat and relocation programmes have been introduced with the Animal Birth Control method (Glickman and Schantz, 1981; Rubel *et al.*, 2003; Totton *et al.*, 2010; Fan *et al.*, 2013; Akeredolu and Sowemimo, 2014; Yoak *et al.*, 2014).

Although there are 26 species of *Toxocara* nine have only been reported once, and most of the other species are restricted to a few older records. The zoonotic *T. canis* and *T. cati* require control programmes. Their importance in causing human toxocariasis requires further study to determine the public health and economic impact. The lack of knowledge by many medical physicians and veterinarians is of concern (Overgaauw, 1998; Smith *et al.*, 2009). Zoonotic *Toxocara* is a neglected tropical disease with an expanding global distribution and whose public health importance is still unclear. As pet ownership increases and more people live in urban areas with increasing numbers of domestic and wild definitive hosts *Toxocara* should no longer be ignored.

References

Agudelo, C., Villareal, E., Caceres, E., Lopez, C., Eljach, J. *et al.* (1990) Human and dogs *Toxocara canis* infection in a poor neighborhood in Bogota. *Memórias Do Instituto Oswaldo Cruz* 85(1), 75–78.

Ain Tiewsoh, J.B., Khurana, S., Mewara, A., Sehgal, R. and Singh, A. (2018) Clinical and laboratory characteristics of patients with toxocariasis encountered at a tertiary care centre in North India. *Indian Journal of Medical Microbiology* 36(3), 432–434.

Akao, N., Tomoda, M., Hayashi, E., Suzuki, R., Shimizu-Suganuma, M. *et al.* (2003) *Cerebellar ataxia* due to *Toxocara* infection in *Mongolian gerbils, Meriones Unguiculatus*. *Veterinary Parasitology* 113(3–4), 229–237.

Akao, N. (2006) Critical assessment of existing and novel model systems of toxocariasis. In: Holland, C.V. and Smith, H.V. (eds) *Toxocara: The Enigmatic Parasite*. CABI Publishing, Wallingford, pp. 74–85.

Akeredolu, A.B. and Sowemimo, O.A. (2014) Prevalence, intensity and associated risk factors for *Toxocara canis* infection in Nigerian dogs. *Journal of Parasitology and Vector Biology* 6(8), 111–116.

Alba-Hurtado, F., Tórtora, P.J., Tsutsumi, V. and Ortega-Pierres, M. (2000) Histopathological investigation of experimental ocular toxocariasis in *Gerbils*. *International Journal for Parasitology* 30(2), 143–147.

Alba-Hurtado, F., Muñoz-Guzmán, M.A., Valdivia-Anda, G., Tórtora, J.L. and Ortega-Pierres, M.G. (2009) *Toxocara canis*: Larval migration dynamics, detection of antibody reactivity to larval excretory–secretory antigens and clinical findings during experimental infection of gerbils (*Meriones unguiculatus*). *Experimental Parasitology* 122(1), 1–5.

Alcântara-Neves, N.M., Santos, A.B., Mendonça, L.R., Figueiredo, C.A.V. and Pontes-de-Carvalho, L. (2008) An improved method to obtain antigen-excreting *Toxocara canis* larvae. *Experimental Parasitology* 119(3), 349–351.

Alvarez, F., Iglesias, R., Bos, J., Tojo, J. and Sanmartin, M.L. (1990) New findings on the helminth fauna of the common European genet (*Genetta genetta L.*): First record of *Toxocara genettae* Warren, 1972 (*Ascarididae*) in Europe. *Annales de Parasitologie Humaine et Comparee* 65(5–6), 244–248.

Antolová, D., Reiterová, K., Stanko, M., Zalesny, G., Fričová, J. *et al.* (2013) Small mammals: Paratenic hosts for species of *Toxocara* in eastern Slovakia. *Journal of Helminthology* 87(1), 52–58.

Araujo, P. (1972) Observations on the early ecdyses of larvae of *Ascaris lumbricoides*, *A. suum* and *Toxocara canis*. *Revista Do Instituto de Medicina Tropical de São Paulo* 14(2), 83–90.

Asakawa, M., Li, J.-F., Guo, A.H., Yang, X.-Y., Liu, Z.L. *et al.* (1994) A new host and locality record for *Toxocara apodemi* (Olsen, 1957) (Nematoda: Ascarididae) from striped field mice, *Apodemus agrarius* (Pallas) (Rodentia: Murinae) in Changsha, China. *Journal of Rakuno Gakuen University, Natural Science* 19(1), 193–196.

Avcioglu, H. and Balkaya, I. (2011) A comparison of the efficacy of subcutaneously administered ivermectin, doramectin, and moxidectin against naturally infected *Toxocara vitulorum* in calves. *Tropical Animal Health and Production* 43(6), 1097–1099.

Avcioğlu, H. and Balkaya, İ. (2011) Prevalence of *Toxocara vitulorum* in calves in Erzurum, Turkey. *Kafkas Universitesi Veteriner Fakultesi Dergisi* 17(3), 345–347.

Aydenizöz-Özkayhan, M., Yağcı, B.B. and Erat, S. (2008) The investigation of *Toxocara canis* eggs in coats of different dog breeds as a potential transmission route in human toxocariasis. *Veterinary Parasitology* 152(1–2), 94–100.

Aydin, A., Goz, Y., Yuksek, N. and Ayaz, E. (2006) Prevalence of *Toxocara vitulorum* in Hakkari eastern region of Turkey. *Bulletin-Veterinary Institute in Pulawy* 50(1), 51–54.

Azam, D., Ukpai, O.M., Said, A., Abd-Allah, G.A. and Morgan, E.R. (2012) Temperature and the development and survival of infective *Toxocara canis* larvae. *Parasitology Research* 110(2), 649–656.

Bagrade, G., Kirjušina, M., Vismanis, K. and Ozoliņš, J. (2009) Helminth parasites of the wolf *Canis lupus* from Latvia. *Journal of Helminthology* 83(1), 63–68.

Baker, M.K., Lange, L. and Verster, A. (1989) A survey of helminths in domestic cats in the Pretoria area of Transvaal, republic of South Africa. Part 1: The prevalence and comparison of burdens of helminths in adult and juvenile cats. *Journal of the South African Veterinary Association* 60(3), 139–142.

Barriga, O.O. (1988) A critical look at the importance, prevalence and control of toxocariasis and the possibilities of immunological control. *Veterinary Parasitology* 29(2–3), 195–234.

Baylis, H.A. (1936) A new *Ascarid* from a bat. *Journal of Natural History* 17(99), 360–365.

Beaver, P.C. (1956) Larva migrans. *Experimental Parasitology* 5(6), 587–621.

Beaver, P.C. (1969) The nature of visceral larva migrans. *Journal of Parasitology* 55(1), 2–12.

Beaver, P.C., Snyder, C.H., Carrera, G.M., Dent, J.H. and Lafferty, J.W. (1952) Chronic eosinophilia due to visceral larva migrans: Report of three cases. *Pediatrics* 9(1), 7–19.

Beelitz, P. and Göbel, E. (1992) Fauna and incidence of endoparasites in kittens and their mothers from different husbandry situations in south Germany. *Tierarztl Prax* 20(3), 297–300.

Beldomenico, P.M., Kinsella, J.M., Uhart, M.M., Gutierrez, G.L. and Pereira, J. (2005) Helminths of Geoffroy's cat, *oncifelis geoffroyi* (Carnivora, Felidae) from the Monte desert, central Argentina. *Acta Parasitologica* 50(3), 263–266.

Borecka, A. (2010) Rozprzestrzenienie nicieni z rodzaju *Toxocara* na świecie The spread of nematodes from Toxocara genus in the world. *Wiadomości Parazytologiczne* 56(2), 117–124.

Borecka, A., Gawor, J., Malczewska, M. and Malczewski, A. (2009) Prevalence of zoonotic helminth parasites of the small intestine in red foxes from central Poland. *Medycyna Weterynaryjna* 65(1), 33–35.

Borecka, A., Gawor, J. and Zieba, F. (2013) A survey of intestinal helminths in wild carnivores from the Tatra National Park, southern Poland. *Annals of Parasitology* 59(4), 169–172.

Borgsteede, F.H.M. (1984) Helminth parasites of wild foxes (*Vulpes vulpes* L.) in The Netherlands. *Zeitschrift Für Parasitenkunde* 70(3), 281–285.

Borgsteede, F.H.M., Holzhauer, M., Herder, F.L., Veldhuis-Wolterbeek, E.G. and Hegeman, C. (2012) *Toxocara vitulorum* in suckling calves in the Netherlands. *Research in Veterinary Science* 92(2), 254–256.

Bosse, M., Manhardt, J. and Stoye, M. (1980) Epizootiology and control of neonatal helminth infections in dogs. *Fortschritte Der Veterinarmedizin* (30), 247–256.

Bourke, A.T.C., Hawes, R.B., Neilson, A. and Stallman, N.D. (1983) An outbreak of hepato-enteritis (the Palm Island mystery disease) possibly caused by algal intoxication. *Toxicon* 21, 45–48.

Bridger, K.E., Baggs, E.M. and Finney-Crawley, J. (2009) Endoparasites of the coyote (*Canis latrans*), a recent migrant to insular Newfoundland. *Journal of Wildlife Diseases* 45(4), 1221–1226.

Brulliard, K. (2016) Cities go to extreme lengths to tackle a dog poop epidemic. Internet. The Washington Post. Available at: https://www.washingtonpost.com/news/animalia/wp/2016/04/27/madrid-is-the-latest-city-to-fight-a-dog-poop-epidemic-that (accessed 28 July 2018).

Bružinskaitė-Schmidhalter, R., Šarkūnas, M., Malakauskas, A., Mathis, A., Torgerson, P.R. *et al.* (2012) Helminths of red foxes (*Vulpes vulpes*) and raccoon dogs (*Nyctereutes procyonoides*) in Lithuania. *Parasitology* 139(1), 120–127.

Bugg, R.J., Robertson, I.D., Elliot, A.D. and Thompson, R.C.A. (1999) Gastrointestinal parasites of urban dogs in Perth, Western Australia. *Veterinary Journal* 157(3), 295–301.

Burke, T.M. and Roberson, E.L. (1985) Prenatal and lactational transmission of *Toxocara canis* and *Ancylostoma caninum*: Experimental infection of the bitch at midpregnancy and at parturition. *International Journal for Parasitology* 15(5), 485–490.

Byth, S. (1980) Palm Island mystery disease. *Medical Journal of Australia* 2(1), 40–42.

Caldera, F., Burlone, M.E., Genchi, C., Pirisi, M. and Bartoli, E. (2013) *Toxocara* encephalitis presenting with autonomous nervous system involvement. *Infection* 41(3), 691–694.

Calvete, C., Lucientes, J., Castillo, J.A., Estrada, R., Gracia, M.J. *et al.* (1998) Gastrointestinal helminth parasites in stray cats from the mid-Ebro Valley, Spain. *Veterinary Parasitology* 75(2–3), 235–240.

Carvalho, E.A.A. and Rocha, R.L. (2011) Toxocariasis: Visceral larva migrans in children. *Jornal de Pediatria (Rio J)* 87(2), 100–110.

Ceballos-Mago, N., González, C.E. and Chivers, D.J. (2010) Impact of the pet trade on the Margarita capuchin monkey *Cebus apella margaritae*. *Endangered Species Research* 12(1), 57–68.

Cerbo, A., Manfredi, M., Trevisiol, K., Bregoli, M., Ferrari, N. *et al.* (2008) Intestinal helminth communities of the red fox (*Vulpes vulpes L.*) in the Italian Alps. *Acta Parasitologica* 53(3), 302–311.

Chelladurai, J.J., Bader, C., Snobl, T., Magstadt, D., Cooper, V. *et al.* (2015) *Toxocara vitulorum* infection in a cohort of beef calves in Iowa. *Veterinary Parasitology* 214(1–2), 96–99.

Chen, J., Zhou, D.-H., Nisbet, A.J., Xu, M.-J., Huang, S.-Y. *et al.* (2012) Advances in molecular identification, taxonomy, genetic variation and diagnosis of *Toxocara spp*. *Infection, Genetics and Evolution* 12(7), 1344–1348.

Chieffi, P.P., Aquino, R.T.R., Pasqualotti, M.A., Ribeiro, M. and Nasello, A.G. (2010) Behavioral changes in *Rattus norvegicus* experimentally infected by *Toxocara canis* larvae. *Revista Do Instituto de Medicina Tropical de São Paulo* 52(5), 243–246.

Chitwood, B.G. (1935) Nematodes parasitic in, and associated with, Crustacea, and descriptions of some new species and a new variety. *Proceedings of the Helminthological Society of Washington* 2(2), 93–96.

Chou, C.-M. and Fan, C.-K. (2018) Significant apoptosis rather autophagy predominates in astrocytes caused by *Toxocara canis* larval excretory-secretory antigens. *Journal of Microbiology, Immunology and Infection* 18, 3022–3028.

Ćirović, D., Pavlović, I., Penezić, A., Kulišić, Z. and Selaković, S. (2015) Levels of infection of intestinal helminth species in the golden jackal *Canis aureus* from Serbia. *Journal of Helminthology* 89(1), 28–33.

Corda, A., Tamponi, C., Meloni, R., Varcasia, A., Parpaglia, M.L.P. *et al.* (2019) Ultrasonography for early diagnosis of *Toxocara canis* infection in puppies. *Parasitology Research* 118(3), 873–880.

Cox, D.M. and Holland, C.V. (1998) The relationship between numbers of larvae recovered from the brain of *Toxocara canis*-infected mice and social behaviour and anxiety in the host. *Parasitology* 116(6), 579–594.

Cox, D.M. and Holland, C.V. (2001) Influence of mouse strain, infective dose and larval burden in the brain on activity in *Toxocara*-infected mice. *Journal of Helminthology* 75(1), 23–32.

Criado-Fornelio, A., Gutierrez-Garcia, L., Rodriguez-Caabeiro, F., Reus-Garcia, E., Roldan-Soriano, M.A. *et al.* (2000) A parasitological survey of wild red foxes (*Vulpes vulpes*) from the province of Guadalajara, Spain. *Veterinary Parasitology* 92(4), 245–251.

da Amaral, H.L.C., Rassier, G.L., Pepe, M.S., Gallina, T., Villela, M.M. *et al.* (2010) Presence of *Toxocara canis* eggs on the hair of dogs: A risk factor for visceral larva migrans. *Veterinary Parasitology* 174(1–2), 115–118.

Dade, A.W. and Williams, J.F. (1975) Hepattic and peritoneal invasion by adult ascarids (*Toxocara canis*) in a dog. Veterinary Medicine, Small Animal Clinician.

Dalimi, A., Sattari, A. and Motamedi, G.H. (2006) A study on intestinal helminths of dogs, foxes and jackals in the western part of Iran. *Veterinary Parasitology* 142(1–2), 129–133.

Davila, G., Irsik, M. and Greiner, E.C. (2010) *Toxocara vitulorum* in beef calves in North Central Florida. *Veterinary Parasitology* 168(3–4), 261–263.

De Savigny, D.H., Voller, A. and Woodruff, A.W. (1979) Toxocariasis: Serological diagnosis by enzyme immunoassay. *Journal of Clinical Pathology* 32(3), 284–288.

De Visser, L., Rothova, A., De Boer, J.H., Van Loon, A.M., Kerkhoff, F.T. *et al*. (2008) Diagnosis of ocular toxocariasis by establishing intraocular antibody production. *American Journal of Ophthalmology* 145(2), 369–374.

Degefu, H., Tefera, A. and Yohannes, M. (2010) Zoonotic helminth parasites in fecal samples of households in Jimma Town, Ethiopia. *Journal of Public Health and Epidemiology* 3(4), 138–143.

Del Rio-Araiza, V.H., Nava-Castro, K.E., Alba-Hurtado, F., Quintanar-Stephano, A., Aguilar-Díaz, H. *et al*. (2018) Prolactin as immune cell regulator in *Toxocara canis* somatic larvae chronic infection. *Bioscience Reports* 38(4). DOI: 10.1042/BSR20180305.

Despommier, D. (2003) Toxocariasis: Clinical aspects, epidemiology, medical ecology, and molecular aspects. *Clinical Microbiology Reviews* 16(2), 265–272.

Diakou, A. and Papadopoulos, E. (2002) Prevalence of gastrointestinal parasites of cattle in Greece. *Journal of the Hellenic Veterinary Medical Society* 53(4), 304–309.

Dorchies, P. (2010) *Toxocara vitulorum* and *Strongyloides papillosus*: The enemies of very young calves. *Bulletin Des GTV* (52), 55–56.

dos Santos, S.V., Santos, F.H.Y., Lescano, S.A.Z., Santos, D.M., Tiago, E.S. *et al*. (2017) Migration pattern of *Toxocara canis* larvae in experimentally infected male and female *Rattus norvegicus*. *Revista Da Sociedade Brasileira de Medicina Tropical* 50(5), 698–700.

Doughty, F.R. (1972) *Toxocara vitulorum*. *Australian Veterinary Journal* 48(2), 62–63.

Douglas, J.R. and Baker, N.F. (1959) The chronology of experimental intrauterine infections with *Toxocara canis* (Werner, 1782) in the dog. *Journal of Parasitology* 43–44.

Dubey, J.P. (1978) Patent *Toxocara canis* infection in ascarid-naive dogs. *Journal of Parasitology* 64(6), 1021–1023.

Dubná, S., Langrová, I., Nápravník, J., Jankovská, I., Vadlejch, J. *et al*. (2007) The prevalence of intestinal parasites in dogs from Prague, rural areas, and shelters of the Czech republic. *Veterinary Parasitology* 145(1–2), 120–128.

Dumenigo, B. and Galvez, D. (1995) Soil contamination in Ciudad de La Habana province with *Toxocara canis* eggs. *Revista Cubana de Medicina Tropical* 47(3), 178–180.

Durette-Desset, M.-C. and Chabaud, A.G. (1974) Trois nouveaux nématodes parasites du chevrotain aquatique: *Hyemoschus aquaticus* au Gabon (collection G. Dubost). *Bulletin Du Muséum National d'histoire Naturelle* 105, 75–87.

Eberhard, M.L. and Alfano, E. (1998) Adult *Toxocara cati* infections in US children: Report of four cases. *American Journal of Tropical Medicine and Hygiene* 59(3), 404–406.

Eberhardt, O., Bialek, R., Nägele, T. and Dichgans, J. (2005) *Eosinophilic meningomyelitis* in toxocariasis: Case report and review of the literature. *Clinical Neurology and Neurosurgery* 107(5), 432–438.

Eguía-Aguilar, P., Cruz-Reyes, A. and Martínez-Maya, J.J. (2005) Ecological analysis and description of the intestinal helminths present in dogs in Mexico City. *Veterinary Parasitology* 127(2), 139–146.

El-Moukdad, A.R. (1979) Helminth fauna of Syrian cattle. *Angewandte Parasitologie* 20(1), 11–16.

Engbaek, K., Madsen, H. and Larsen, S.O. (1984) A survey of helminths in stray cats from Copenhagen with ecological aspects. *Zeitschrift Für Parasitenkunde* 70(1), 87–94.

Epe, C. (2009) Intestinal nematodes: Biology and control. *Veterinary Clinics of North America: Small Animal Practice* 39(6), 1091–1107.

Epe, C., Ising-Volmer, S. and Stoye, M. (1993) Parasitological fecal studies of equids, dogs, cats and hedgehogs during the years 1984–1991. *Deutsche Tierärztliche Wochenschrift* 100(11), 426–428.

Epe, C. (2006) *16 current and future options for the prevention and treatment of canids*. In: Holland, C.V. and Smith, H.V. (eds) *Toxocara: The Enigmatic Parasite*. CABI, Wallingford, UK, pp. 239–252.

European Scientific Counsel Companion Animal Parasites (2019) *MG1: Worm Control in Dogs and Cats*. ESCCAP, Malvern, Worcestershire, UK.

Fan, C.-K., Liao, C.-W. and Cheng, Y.-C. (2013) Factors affecting disease manifestation of Toxocarosis in humans: Genetics and environment. *Veterinary Parasitology* 193(4), 342–352.
Fan, C.-K., Loxton, K. and Barghouth, U. (2015) Cerebral toxocariasis: Silent progression to neurodegenerative disorders? *Clinical Microbiology Reviews* 28(3), 663–686.
Farmer, A., Beltran, T. and Choi, Y.S. (2017) Prevalence of *Toxocara* species infection in the U.S.: Results from the National Health and Nutrition Examination Survey, 2011–2014. *PLoS Neglected Tropical Diseases* 11(7), e0005818.
Fei, A.-Y. and Mo, K.-M. (1997) A survey of endoparasitic zoonoses of stray dogs and cats in Taipei city. *Journal of the Chinese Society of Veterinary Science* 23, 26–33.
Fernando, S.T. (1968) Immunological response of rabbits to *Toxocara canis* infection. *Parasitology* 58(1), 91–103.
Ferreira, L.F., Oliveira, E.L. and Camillo-Coura, L. (1976) Sobre a presença de ovos de *Toxocara* em praças da cidade do Rio de Janeiro. *Revista Da Sociedade Brasileira de Medicina Tropical* 10(2), 51–54.
Fillaux, J. and Magnaval, J.-F. (2013) Laboratory diagnosis of human toxocariasis. *Veterinary Parasitology* 193(4), 327–336.
Fisher, M. (2003) *Toxocara cati*: An underestimated zoonotic agent. *Trends in Parasitology* 19(4), 167–170.
Flecher, M.C., Musso, C., Martins, I.V.F. and Pereira, F.E.L. (2016) Larval migration of the ascarid nematode *Toxocara canis* following infection and re-infection in the gerbil *Meriones unguiculatus*. *Journal of Helminthology* 90(5), 569–576.
Fowler, M.E. and Mikota, S.K. (2008) *Biology, Medicine, and Surgery of Elephants*. John Wiley & Sons, USA, p. 596.
Gadale, O.I., Capelli, G., Ali, A.A. and Poglayen, G. (1988) Intestinal helminths of cats. First reports in Somalia. Boletinol Scientifico Della Facolta Di Zootecnia e Veterinaria. Universita Nazionale.
Gallas, M. and Silveira, E.F. (2013) *Toxocara cati* (Nematoda, Ascarididae) in different wild feline species in Brazil: New host records. *Biotemas* 26(3), 117–125.
Galvin, T.J. (1964) Experimental toxocara canis infections in chickens and pigeons. *Journal of Parasitology* 50(1), 124–127.
Gethings, P.M., Stephens, G.L., Wills, J.M., Howard, P., Balfour, A.H. *et al.* (1987) Prevalence of *Chlamydia, Toxoplasma, Toxocara* and ringworm in farm cats in south-west England. *Veterinary Record* 121(10), 213–216.
Gibbons, L.M., Jacobs, D.E. and Sani, R.A. (2001) *Toxocara malaysiensis* n. sp (Nematoda: Ascaridoidea) from the domestic cat (*Felis catus* Linnaeus, 1758). *Journal of Parasitology* 87(3), 660–665.
Gillespie, S.H., Dinning, W.J., Voller, A. and Crowcroft, N.S. (1993) The spectrum of ocular toxocariasis. *Eye* 7(3), 415–418.
Glickman, L.T. and Schantz, P.M. (1981) Epidemiology and pathogenesis of zoonotic toxocariasis. *Epidemiologic Reviews* 3, 230–250.
Glickman, L.T. and Summers, B.A. (1983) Experimental toxocara canis infection in Cynomolgus macaques (*Macaca fascicularis*). *American Journal of Veterinary Research* 44(12), 2347–2354.
Glickman, L.T., Magnaval, J.-F., Domanski, L.M., Shofer, F.S., Lauria, S.S. *et al.* (1987) Visceral larva migrans in French adults: A new disease syndrome? *American Journal of Epidemiology* 125(6), 1019–1034.
Gomez-Puerta, L.A. (2014) Primeros registros de *Hysterothylacium pelagicum* (Anisakidae) y *Toxocara alienata* (Toxocaridae) en el Perú. *Revista Peruana de Biología* 21(2), 171–174.
Goossens, E., Dorny, P., Vervaecke, H., Roden, C., Vercammen, F. *et al.* (2007) *Toxocara vitulorum* in American bison (*Bison bison*) calves. *Veterinary Record* 160(16), 556.
Greve, J.H. (1971) Age resistance to toxocara canis in ascarid-free dogs. *American Journal of Veterinary Research* 32(8), 1185–1192.
Habluetzel, A., Traldi, G., Ruggieri, S., Attili, A.R., Scuppa, P. *et al.* (2003) An estimation of *Toxocara canis* prevalence in dogs, environmental egg contamination and risk of human infection in the Marche region of Italy. *Veterinary Parasitology* 113(3–4), 243–252.
Havasiová-Reiterová, K., Tomašovicová, O. and Dubinský, P. (1995) Effect of various doses of infective *Toxocara canis* and *Toxocara cati* eggs on the humoral response and distribution of larvae in mice. *Parasitology Research* 81(1), 13–17.
Hayden, D.W. and Kruiningen, H.J. (1975) Experimentally induced canine toxocariasis: Laboratory examinations and pathologic changes, with emphasis on the gastrointestinal tract. *American Journal of Veterinary Research* 36(11), 1605–1614.

Helwigh, A.B., Lind, P. and Nansen, P. (1999) Visceral larva migrans: Migratory pattern of *Toxocara canis* in pigs. *International Journal for Parasitology* 29(4), 559–565.

Hernández, J.Á., Cazapal-Monteiro, C.F., Sanchís, J., Sánchez-Andrade, R., Paz-Silva, A. *et al.* (2018) Potential usefulness of filamentous fungi to prevent zoonotic soil-transmitted helminths. *Vector-Borne and Zoonotic Diseases* 12, 690–696.

Hernández, R.M., Fidel, A.N. and Pelayo, L.D. (2007) Zoonotic potential of intestinal helminth infections in stray dogs from City of Havana. *Revista Cubana de Medicina Tropical* 59(3), 234–240.

Herschel, A.-M. (1981) Zum Verhalten der Larven von *Toxocara canis* WERNER 1782 (Anisakidae) aus paratenischen Wirten im Hund (Beagle). *Tieraerztliche Hochschule Hannover.*

Heuer, L., Beyerbach, M., Lühder, F., Beineke, A. and Strube, C. (2015) Neurotoxocarosis alters myelin protein gene transcription and expression. *Parasitology Research* 114(6), 2175–2186.

Hiura, E., del Carmen Garcia Lopes, A., da Paz, J.S., Gava, M.G., Flecher, M.C. *et al.* (2015) Fungi predatory activity on embryonated *Toxocara canis* eggs inoculated in domestic chickens (*Gallus gallus domesticus*) and destruction of second stage larvae. *Parasitology Research* 114(9), 3301–3308.

Holland, C.V. and Cox, D.M. (2001) Toxocara in the mouse: A model for parasite-altered host behaviour? *Journal of Helminthology* 75(2), 125.

Holland, W.G., Luong, T.T., Nguyen, L.A., Do, T.T. and Vercruysse, J. (2000) The epidemiology of nematode and fluke infections in cattle in the Red River Delta in Vietnam. *Veterinary Parasitology* 93(2), 141–147.

Hotez, P.J. and Wilkins, P.P. (2009) Toxocariasis: America's most common neglected infection of poverty and a helminthiasis of global importance? *PLoS Neglected Tropical Diseases* 3(3), e400.

Hotez, P.J., Molyneux, D.H., Fenwick, A., Kumaresan, J., Sachs, S.E. *et al.* (2007) Control of neglected tropical diseases. *New England Journal of Medicine* 357(10), 1018–1027.

Hotez, P.J., Fenwick, A., Savioli, L. and Molyneux, D.H. (2009) Rescuing the bottom billion through control of neglected tropical diseases. *Lancet* 373(9674), 1570–1575.

Hubbert, W.T., Bryner, J.H., Foley, J.W. and Estes, P.C. (1975) Parasitic infection of the bovine perinate: A review. *Theriogenology* 3(2), 43–63.

Itoh, N. (2000) Survey on *Toxocara cati* in domestic cats. *Journal of the Japanese Association for Infectious Diseases* 74(10), 824–827.

Jabbour, R., Sawaya, R., Yamout, B., Kanj-Sharara, S. and Atweh, S. (2014) A large series of *Toxocara canis* myelitis. *Multiple Sclerosis and Related Disorders* 3(6), 742.

Jacobs, D.E., Pegg, E.J. and Stevenson, P. (1977) Helminths of british dogs: *Toxocara canis* – A veterinary perspective. *Journal of Small Animal Practice* 18(2), 79–92.

Jacobs, D.E., Zhu, X., Gasser, R.B. and Chilton, N.B. (1997) PCR-basedmethods for identification of potentially zoonotic ascaridoidparasites of the dog, fox and cat. *Acta Tropica* 68(2), 191–200.

Jacquier, P., Gottstein, B., Stingelin, Y. and Eckert, J. (1991) Immunodiagnosis of Toxocarosis in humans: Evaluation of a new enzyme-linked immunosorbent assay kit. *Journal of Clinical Microbiology* 29(9), 1831–1835.

Janecek, E., Waindok, P., Bankstahl, M. and Strube, C. (2017) Abnormal neurobehaviour and impaired memory function as a consequence of *Toxocara canis*-as well as *Toxocara cati*-induced neurotoxocarosis. *PLoS Neglected Tropical Diseases* 11(5), e0005594.

Jenkins, E.J., Castrodale, L.J., de Rosemond, S.J.C., Dixon, B.R., Elmore, S.A. *et al.* (2013) Tradition and transition: Parasitic zoonoses of people and animals in Alaska, Northern Canada, and Greenland. In: *Advances in Parasitology*. Academic Press, pp. 33–204.

Jin, Z., Akao, N. and Ohta, N. (2008) Prolactin evokes lactational transmission of larvae in mice infected with *Toxocara canis*. *Parasitology International* 57(4), 495–498.

Jones, J.R., Mitchell, E.S.E., Redman, E. and Gilleard, J.S. (2009) *Toxocara vitulorum* infection in a cattle herd in the UK. *Veterinary Record* 164(6), 171–172.

Jyoti, N.K., Singh, P.O. and Juyal, M.H. (2012) Epidemiology of gastrointestinal parasites in buffalo calves of Punjab state. *Journal of Veterinary Parasitology* 26, 19–22.

Kapel, C.M.O. and Nansen, P. (1996) Gastrointestinal helminths of arctic foxes (*Alopex lagopus*) from different bioclimatological regions in Greenland. *Journal of Parasitology* 82(1), 17–24.

Kayes, S.G., Omholt, P.E. and Grieve, R.B. (1985) Immune responses of CBA/J mice to graded infections with *Toxocara canis*. *Infection and Immunity* 48(3), 697–703.

Keegan, J.D. and Holland, C.V. (2010) Contamination of the hair of owned dogs with the eggs of *Toxocara* spp. *Veterinary Parasitology* 173(1–2), 161–164.

Khalafalla, R.E. (2011) A survey study on gastrointestinal parasites of stray cats in Northern Region of Nile Delta, Egypt. *PLoS One* 6(7), e20283.

Kingdon, J., Happold, D., Butynski, T., Hoffmann, M., Happold, M. *et al.* (2013) *Mammals of Africa*. Bloomsbury Publishing, UK, pp. 243–245.

Kirkpatrick, C.E. (1988) Epizootiology of endoparasitic infections in pet dogs and cats presented to a veterinary teaching hospital. *Veterinary Parasitology* 30(2), 113–124.

Kloch, A., Bednarska, M. and Bajer, A. (2005) Intestinal macro-and microparasites of wolves (*Canis lupus* L.) from north-eastern Poland recovered by coprological study. *Annals of Agricultural and Environmental Medicine* 12(2), 237–247.

Knopf, L., Komoin Oka, C., Betschart, B., Gottstein, B. and Zinsstag, J. (2004) Paramètres de production et de santé en relation avec le parasitisme chez les bovins N'Dama villageois en savane guinéenne de la Côte d'Ivoire. *Revue d'élevage et de Médecine Vétérinaire Des Pays Tropicaux* 57(1–2), 95.

Kou, C.C. (1958) Studies on parasitic nematodes of mammals from canton. I. Some new species from *Paradoxurus minor exitus* Schwarz, *Paguma larvata larvata* (Hamilton Smith), and *Manís pentadactyla aurita* Hodgson. *Acta Zoologica Sinica* 10(1), 60–72.

Koutz, F.R., Groves, H.F. and Scothorn, M.W. (1966) The prenatal migration of toxocara canis larvae and their relationship to infection in pregnant bitches and in pups. *American Journal of Veterinary Research* 27(118), 789–795.

Kulišić, Z., Aleksić, N., Đorđević, M., Gajić, B., Tambur, Z. *et al.* (2012) Prevalence of gastrointestinal helminths in calves in Western Serbia. *Acta Veterinaria Brunensis* 62(5–6), 665–673.

Kutdang, E.T., Bukbuk, D.N. and Ajayi, J.A. (2010) The prevalence of intestinal helminths of dogs (*Canis familiaris*) in Jos, Plateau State, Nigeria. *Researcher* 2(8), 51–56.

Lamina, J. (1971) New findings on the calf ascarid *Toxocara vitulorum* (syn. *Neoascaris Vitulorum*, Goeze, 1782). *Deutsche Tierärztliche Wochenschrift* 78(6), 181–182.

Le, T.H., Anh, N.T.L., Nguyen, K.T., Nguyen, N.T.B. and Gasser, R.B. (2016) *Toxocara malaysiensis* infection in domestic cats in Vietnam – an emerging zoonotic issue? *Infection, Genetics and Evolution* 37, 94–98.

Leclaire, S. and Faulkner, C.T. (2014) Gastrointestinal parasites in relation to host traits and group factors in wild meerkats *Suricata suricatta*. *Parasitology* 141(7), 925–933.

Lee, C.C., Cheng, N. and Bohari, Y. (1993) *Toxocara canis* From Domestic Cats in Kuala Lumpur, Vol. 10. Tropical Biomedicine. International Book Service, USA, pp. 79–80.

Lee, R.M., Moore, L.B., Bottazzi, M.E. and Hotez, P.J. (2014) Toxocariasis in North America: A systematic review. *PLoS Neglected Tropical Diseases* 8(8), e3116.

Lescano, S.Z., Queiroz, M.L. and Chieffi, P.P. (2004) Larval recovery of *Toxocara canis* in organs and tissues of experimentally infected *Rattus norvegicus*. *Memórias Do Instituto Oswaldo Cruz* 99(6), 627–628.

Levine, N.D. (1980) *Nematode Parasites of Domestic Animals and Man*, 2nd ed. Burgess Publishing Co, Minneapolis, MN, USA, pp. 317–372.

Li, M., Lin, R., Song, H., Sani, R.A., Wu, X. *et al.* (2008a) Electrophoretic analysis of sequence variability in three mitochondrial DNA regions for ascaridoid parasites of human and animal health significance. *Electrophoresis* 29(13), 2912–2917.

Li, M.-W., Zhu, X.-Q., Gasser, R.B., Lin, R.-Q., Sani, R.A. *et al.* (2006) The occurrence of *Toxocara malaysiensis* in cats in China, confirmed by sequence-based analyses of ribosomal DNA. *Parasitology Research* 99(5), 554–557.

Li, M.-W., Lin, R.-Q., Song, H.-Q., Wu, X.-Y. and Zhu, X.-Q. (2008b) The complete mitochondrial genomes for three *Toxocara* species of human and animal health significance. *BMC Genomics* 9(1), 224.

Lloyd, S., Amerasinghe, P.H. and Soulsby, E.J.L. (1983) Periparturient immunosuppression in the bitch and its influence on infection with *Toxocara canis*. *Journal of Small Animal Practice* 24(4), 237–247.

Loos-Frank, B. and Zeyhle, E. (1982) The intestinal helminths of the red fox and some other carnivores in Southwest Germany. *Zeitschrift Für Parasitenkunde* 67(1), 99–113.

Löwenstein, M.D. (1981) *Quantitative Untersuchungen über die Wanderung der Larven von Toxocara canis WERNER 1782 (Anisakidae) im definitiven Wirt (Beagle) nach einmaliger Reinfektion*. University of Veterinary Medicine Hannover, Hannover, Germany.

Lucio-Forster, A., Mizhquiri Barbecho, J.S., Mohammed, H.O., Kornreich, B.G. and Bowman, D.D. (2016) Comparison of the prevalence of *Toxocara* egg shedding by pet cats and dogs in the U.S.A., 2011–2014. *Veterinary Parasitology: Regional Studies and Reports* 5, 1–13.

Luty, T. (2001) Prevalence of species of *Toxocara* in dogs, cats and red foxes from the Poznan region, Poland. *Journal of Helminthology* 75(2), 153–156.

Ma, G., Wang, T., Hofmann, A., Fan, C.-K., Maizels, R.M. *et al.* (2018) Human toxocariasis. *Lancet Infectious Diseases* 18(1), e14–e24.

Macchioni, G. (2000) A new species, *Toxocara lyncis*, in the caracal (*Lynx caracal*). *Parassitologia* 41(4), 529–532.

Macpherson, C.N.L. (2013) The epidemiology and public health importance of toxocariasis: A zoonosis of global importance. *International Journal for Parasitology* 43(12–13), 999–1008.

Magi, M., Macchioni, F., Dell'Omodarme, M., Prati, M.C., Calderini, P. *et al.* (2009) Endoparasites of red fox (*Vulpes vulpes*) in central Italy. *Journal of Wildlife Diseases* 45(3), 881–885.

Magnaval, J.F. (1995) Comparative efficacy of diethylcarbamazine and mebendazole for the treatment of human toxocariasis. *Parasitology* 110(5), 529–533.

Magnaval, J.F. and Charlet, J.P. (1987) Efficacité comparée du thiabendazole et du mébendazole dans le traitement de la toxocarose. *Therapie* 42(6), 541–544.

Magnaval, J., Berry, A., Fabre, R. and Morassin, B. (2001) Eosinophil cationic protein as a possible marker of active human *Toxocara* infection. *Allergy* 56(11), 1096–1099.

Magnaval, J. and Glickman, L. (2006) Management and treatment options for human toxocariasis. In: Holland, C. and Smith, H.V. (eds) *Toxocara: The Enigmatic Parasite*. CABI, pp. 113–126.

Mahieu, M. and Naves, M. (2008) Incidence of *Toxocara vitulorum* in Creole calves of Guadeloupe. *Tropical Animal Health and Production* 40(4), 243–248.

Maizels, R.M. and Denham, D.A. (1992) Diethylcarbamazine (DEC): Immunopharmacological interactions of an anti-filarial drug. *Parasitology* 105(S1), S49–60.

Maizels, R.M., Savigny, D.D. and Ogilvie, B.M. (1984) Characterization of surface and excretory-secretory antigens of *Toxocara canis* infective larvae. *Parasite Immunology* 6(1), 23–37.

Manhardt, J. (1980) *The Behavior of the Larvae of Toxocara canis WERNER 1782 (Anisakidae) During and After Migration Through the Lungs of a Definitive Host (Beagle)*. University of Veterinary Medicine Hannover, Germany.

Merck Manual (n.d.) *Roundworms in Small Animals – Digestive System*. Merck Veterinary Manual. Merck Publishing, Rahway, NJ, USA.

Martinez-Pulgarin, D.F., Muñoz-Urbano, M., Gomez-Suta, L.D., Delgado, O.M. and Rodriguez-Morales, A.J. (2015) Ocular toxocariasis: New diagnostic and therapeutic perspectives. *Recent Patents on Anti-Infective Drug Discovery* 10(1), 35–41.

Martínez, F., Hernández, S., Calero, R. and Moreno, T. (1978) Contribución al conocimiento de los parásitos del zorro (*Vulpes vulpes*). *Revista Ibérica de Parasitología* 38, 207–211.

Martínez-Barbabosa, I., Tsuji, O.V., Cabello, R.R., Cárdenas, E.M.G. and Chasin, O.A. (2003) The prevalence of *Toxocara cati* in domestic cats in Mexico City. *Veterinary Parasitology* 114(1), 43–49.

Maruyama, S., Nino, T., Yamamoto, K. and Katsube, Y. (1994) Parasitism of *Toxocara canis* larvae in chickens inoculated with the ascarid eggs. *Journal of Veterinary Medical Science* 56(1), 139–141.

Maung, M. (1975) An ascaridoid nematode from a hippopotamus. *International Journal for Parasitology* 5(4), 431–439.

Maya, C., Ortiz, M. and Jiménez, B. (2010) Viability of ascaris and other helminth genera non larval eggs in different conditions of temperature, lime (pH) and humidity. *Water Science & Technology* 62(11), 2616–2624.

McColm, A.A. and Hutchison, W.M. (1980) The prevalence of intestinal helminths in stray cats in central Scotland. *Journal of Helminthology* 54(4), 255–257.

Meijer, T., Mattsson, R., Angerbjörn, A., Osterman-Lind, E., Fernández-Aguilar, X. *et al.* (2011) Endoparasites in the endangered fennoscandian population of arctic foxes (*Vulpes lagopus*). *European Journal of Wildlife Research* 57(4), 923–927.

Merigueti, Y., Santarém, V.A., Ramires, L.M., Silveira Batista, A., Costa Beserra, L.V. *et al.* (2017) Protective and risk factors associated with the presence of *Toxocara* spp. eggs in dog hair. *Veterinary Parasitology* 244, 39–43.

Merigueti, Y., Silva Raposo, R., Zampieri, B.P., Lima Cerazo, L.M., Pereira, L. *et al.* (2018) Dispersion and infectivity of *Toxocara canis* eggs after passage through chicken intestine. *Parasitology Research* 117(11), 3481–3486.

Mia, S., Dewan, M.L., Uddin, M. and Chowdhury, M.U.A. (1975) The route of infection of buffalo calves by, *Toxocara (neoascaris) vitulorum*. *Tropical Animal Health and Production* 7, 153–156.

Milstein, T.C. and Goldsmid, J.M. (1997) Parasites of feral cats from southern Tasmania and their potential significance. *Australian Veterinary Journal* 75(3), 218–219.
Mirani, A.H., Mirbahar, K.B., Khan, M.S., Lochi, G.M., Khan, I.U. *et al.* (2012) Prevalence of coccidiosis and other gastrointestinal nematode species in buffalo calves at Hyderabad, Sindh, Pakistan. *African Journal of Microbiology Research* 6(33), 6291–6294.
Miterpáková, M., Hurníková, Z., Antolová, D. and Dubinský, P. (2009) Endoparasites of red fox (*Vulpes vulpes*) in the Slovak Republic with the emphasis on zoonotic species *Echinococcus multilocularis* and *Trichinella* spp. *Helminthologia* 46(2), 73–79.
Mizgajska, H. (2001) Eggs of *Toxocara* spp. in the environment and their public health implications. *Journal of Helminthology* 75(2), 147–151.
Mizgajska, H. and Luty, T. (1998) Toxocariasis in dogs and contamination of soil with *Toxocara* spp. eggs in the Poznań region. *Przegląd Epidemiologiczny* 52(4), 441–446.
Mohamad, S., Azmi, N.C. and Noordin, R. (2009) Development and evaluation of a sensitive and specific assay for diagnosis of human toxocariasis by use of three recombinant antigens (TES-26, TES-30USM, and TES-120). *Journal of Clinical Microbiology* 47(6), 1712–1717.
Moks, E., Jõgisalu, I., Saarma, U., Talvik, H., Järvis, T. *et al.* (2006) Helminthologic survey of the wolf (*Canis lupus*) in Estonia, with an emphasis on *Echinococcus granulosus*. *Journal of Wildlife Diseases* 42(2), 359–365.
Moorhouse, D.E. (1982) *Toxocariasis*. A possible cause of the Palm Island mystery disease. *Medical Journal of Australia* 1(4), 172–173.
Morgan, E.R., Azam, D. and Pegler, K. (2013) Quantifying sources of environmental contamination with *Toxocara* spp. eggs. *Veterinary Parasitology* 193(4), 390–397.
Muñoz-Guzmán, M.A. and Alba-Hurtado, F. (2018) Progesterone and prolactin: Hormones important for the reactivation of *Toxocara canis* larvae in bitches. *Advances in Neuroimmune Biology* 7(1), 77–88.
Nagakura, K., Tachibana, H., Kaneda, Y. and Kato, Y. (1989) Toxocariasis possibly caused by ingesting raw chicken. *Journal of Infectious Diseases* 160(4), 735–736.
Naidu, T.S.V. (1981) Two new ascarid nematodes from vertebrate hosts from India. *Folia Parasitologica (Praha)* 28(4), 327–334.
Niak, A. (1972) The prevalence of *Toxocara cati* and other parasites in Liverpool cats. *Veterinary Record* 91(22), 534–536.
Nichol, S., Ball, S.J. and Snow, K.R. (1981) Prevalence of intestinal parasites in feral cats in some urban areas of England. *Veterinary Parasitology* 9(2), 107–110.
Nicoletti, A., Bartoloni, A., Sofia, V., Mantella, A., Nsengiyumva, G. *et al.* (2007) Epilepsy and toxocariasis: A Case-Control Study in Burundi. *Epilepsia* 48(5), 894–899.
Nicoletti, A. (2013) Toxocariasis. In: Garcia, H.H., Tanowitz, H.B. and Del Brutto, O.H. (eds) *Handbook of Clinical Neurology*. Elsevier, the Netherlands, pp. 217–228.
Niehaus, C., Valerio, I., Blanco, K. and Chinchilla, M. (2012) [Parasitic infections of coyote, *Canis latrans* (Carnivora: Canidae) in a Costa Rican National Park and a surrounding agricultural area]. *Revista De Biologia Tropical* 60(2), 799–808.
Nijsse, R., Mughini-Gras, L., Wagenaar, J.A., Franssen, F. and Ploeger, H.W. (2015) Environmental contamination with *Toxocara* eggs: A quantitative approach to estimate the relative contributions of dogs, cats and foxes, and to assess the efficacy of advised interventions in dogs. *Parasites and Vectors* 8(1), 397.
Nolan, T.J. and Smith, G. (1995) Time series analysis of the prevalence of endoparasitic infections in cats and dogs presented to a veterinary teaching hospital. *Veterinary Parasitology* 59(2), 87–96.
O'Callaghan, M.G. and Beveridge, I. (1996) Gastro-intestinal parasites of feral cats in the Northern Territory. *Transactions of the Royal Society of South Australia* 120(3/4), 175–176.
Okoshi, S. and Usui, M. (1968) Experimental studies on *Toxascaris leonina*. IV. Development of eggs of three ascarids, *T. leonina*, *Toxocara canis* and *Toxocara cati*, in dogs and cats. *Japanese Journal of Veterinary Science* 30(1), 29–38.
Okulewicz, A., Perec-Matysiak, A., Buńkowska, K. and Hildebrand, J. (2012) *Toxocara canis*, *Toxocara cati* and *Toxascaris leonina* in wild and domestic carnivores. *Helminthologia* 49(1), 3–10.
Oliveira-Sequeira, T.C.G., Amarante, A.F.T., Ferrari, T.B. and Nunes, L.C. (2002) Prevalence of intestinal parasites in dogs from São Paulo State, Brazil. *Veterinary Parasitology* 103(1–2), 19–27.
Olson, L.J. and Rose, J.E. (1966) Effect of *Toxocara canis* infection on the ability of white rats to solve maze problems. *Experimental Parasitology* 19(1), 77–84.

Oshima, T. (1961) Standardization of techniques for infecting mice with *Toxocara canis* and observations on the normal migration routes of the larvae. *Journal of Parasitology* 47(4), 652–656.

Overgaauw, P.A.M. (1998) *Toxocara* infections in dogs and cats and public health implications. *Veterinary Quarterly* 20(Suppl.1), 97–98.

Overgaauw, P.A.M. and Nederland, V. (1997) Aspects of *Toxocara* epidemiology: Toxocarosis in dogs and cats. *Critical Reviews in Microbiology* 23(3), 233–251.

Overgaauw, P.A.M. and Boersema, J.H. (1998) Nematode infections in dog breeding kennels in the Netherlands, with special reference to *Toxocara*. *Veterinary Quarterly* 20(1), 12–15.

Overgaauw, P.A.M. and Knapen, F. (2013) Veterinary and public health aspects of *Toxocara* spp. *Veterinary Parasitology* 193(4), 398–403.

Overgaauw, P.A.M. and Van Knapen, F. (2000) Dogs and nematode zoonoses. In: Macpherson, C.N.L., Meslin, F.X. and Wandeler, A.I. (eds) *Dogs, Zoonoses and Public Health*. CABI Publishing, Wallingford, UK, pp. 213–256.

Overgaauw, P.A.M., Zutphen, L., Hoek, D., Yaya, F.O., Roelfsema, J. *et al.* (2009) Zoonotic parasites in fecal samples and fur from dogs and cats in the Netherlands. *Veterinary Parasitology* 163(1–2), 115–122.

Page, A.P., Rudin, W., Fluri, E., Blaxter, M.L. and Maizels, R.M. (1992) *Toxocara canis*: A labile antigenic surface coat overlying the epicuticle of infective larvae. *Experimental Parasitology* 75(1), 72–86.

Pahari, T.K. and Sasmal, N.K. (1990) Infection of Japanese quail with *Toxocara canis* larvae and establishment of patent infection in pups. *Veterinary Parasitology* 35(4), 357–364.

Parsons, J.C. (1987) Ascarid infections of cats and dogs. *Veterinary Clinics of North America: Small Animal Practice* 17(6), 1307–1339.

Pegg, E.J. and Donald, C.R. (1978) The effects of composting on the eggs of *Toxocara canis* and *Toxascaris leonina*. *Journal of Institute of Animal Technology* 29, 29–30.

Penn Veterinary Medicine (n.d.) *Diagnosis of Veterinary Endoparasitic Infections*. *Toxocara canis*.

Petithory, J.C., Vandemeulebroucke, E., Jousserand, P. and Bisognani, A.C. (1996) Prevalence of *Toxocara cati* in cats in France. *Bulletin de La Societe Francaise de Parasitologie* 14, 79–84.

Popiołek, M., Szczęsna, J., Nowak, S. and Mysłajek, R.W. (2007) Helminth infections in faecal samples of wolves *Canis lupus* L. from the western Beskidy Mountains in southern Poland. *Journal of Helminthology* 81(4), 339–344.

Prociv, P. (1983) Observations on the transmission and development of *Toxocara pteropodis* (Ascaridoidea: Nematoda) in the Australian grey-headed flying-fox, *Pteropus poliocephalus* (Pteropodidae: Megachiroptera). *Zeitschrift Für Parasitenkunde* 69(6), 773–781.

Prociv, P. (1987) *Toxocara pteropodis Baylis, 1936: life-cycle, epizootiology and zoonotic potential*. The University of Queensland.

Prociv, P. (1989) Toxocara pteropodis and visceral larva migrans. *Parasitology Today* 5(4), 106–109.

Prociv, P. (1989) Some comments on the validity of *Toxocara cynonycteridis* (Parona, 1889). *International Journal for Parasitology* 19(4), 445–446.

Prociv, P. (1989) Larval migration in oral and parenteral *Toxocara pteropodis* infections and a comparison with *T. canis* dispersal in the flying fox, *Pteropus poliocephalus*. *International Journal for Parasitology* 19(8), 891–896.

Prociv, P. (1989) Observations on egg production by *Toxocara pteropodis*. *International Journal for Parasitology* 19(4), 441–443.

Prociv, P. (1990) Aberrant migration by *Toxocara pteropodis* in flying-foxes – two case reports. *Journal of Wildlife Diseases* 26(4), 532–534.

Puylaert, F.A. (1967) Un nouvel ascaride, *Toxocara canarisi* sp. n. parasite de Felis (Leptailurus) seerval Schreber (Vermes-Nematoda). *Revue de Zoologie et de Botanique Africaines* 76(3/4), 235–243.

Quattrocchi, G., Nicoletti, A., Marin, B., Bruno, E., Druet-Cabanac, M. *et al.* (2012) Toxocariasis and epilepsy: Systematic review and meta-analysis. *PLoS Neglected Tropical Diseases* 6(8), e1775.

Radwan, N.A., Khalil, A.I. and El Mahi, R.A. (2009) Morphology and occurrence of species of *Toxocara* in wild mammal populations from Egypt. *Comparative Parasitology* 76(2), 273–282.

Rast, L., Lee, S., Nampanya, S., Toribio, J.-A., Khounsy, S. *et al.* (2013) Prevalence and clinical impact of *Toxocara vitulorum* in cattle and buffalo calves in northern Lao PDR. *Tropical Animal Health and Production* 45(2), 539–546.

Raza, M.A., Murtaza, S., Ayaz, M.M., Akhtar, S., Arshad, H. *et al.* (2013) *Toxocara vitulorum* infestation and associated risk factors in cattle and buffalo at Multan district, Pakistan. *Science International* 25(2), 291–294.

Redman, W.K., Bryant, J.E. and Ahmad, G. (2016) Gastrointestinal helminths of Coyotes (*Canis latrans*) from Southeast Nebraska and Shenandoah area of Iowa. *Veterinary World* 9(9), 970–975.

Rekwot, P.I. and Ogunsusi, R.A. (1985) Prevalence of *Toxocara (neoascaris) vitulorum* infection in cattle around Zaria, Nigeria. *Journal of Animal Production Research* 5, 201–207.

Reperant, L.A., Hegglin, D., Fischer, C., Kohler, L., Weber, J.-M. *et al.* (2007) Influence of urbanization on the epidemiology of intestinal helminths of the red fox (*Vulpes vulpes*) in Geneva, Switzerland. *Parasitology Research* 101(3), 605–611.

Resende, N.M., Gazzinelli-Guimarães, P.H., Barbosa, F.S., Oliveira, L.M., Nogueira, D.S. *et al.* (2015) New insights into the immunopathology of early *Toxocara canis* infection in mice. *Parasites and Vectors* 8(1), 354.

Richards, D.T., Harris, S. and Lewis, J.W. (1995) Epidemiological studies on intestinal helminth parasites of rural and urban red foxes (*Vulpes vulpes*) in the United Kingdom. *Veterinary Parasitology* 59(1), 39–51.

Robbins, R.G., Maffei, L. and Wade, S.E. (2006) Parasites of free-ranging small canids and felids in the Bolivian Chaco. *Journal of Zoo and Wildlife Medicine* 37(2), 130–134.

Roberts, J.A. (1989) The extraparasitic life cycle of *Toxocara vitulorum* in the village environment of Sri Lanka. *Veterinary Research Communications* 13(5), 377–388.

Roberts, J.A. (1989) Toxocara vitulorum: Treatment based on the duration of the infectivity of buffalo cows (*Bubalus bubalis*) for their calves. *Journal of Veterinary Pharmacology and Therapeutics* 12(1), 5–13.

Roberts, J.A. (1990) The egg production of *Toxocara vitulorum* in Asian buffalo (*Bubalus bubalis*). *Veterinary Parasitology* 37(2), 113–120.

Roberts, J.A. (1990) The life cycle of *Toxocara vitulorum* in Asian buffalo (*Bubalus bubalis*). *International Journal for Parasitology* 20(7), 833–840.

Roberts, J.A. (1993) *Toxocara vitulorum* in ruminants. *Helminthology Abstracts* 62(4), 151–174.

Roberts, J.A., Fernando, S.T. and Sivanathan, S. (1990) *Toxocara vitulorum* in the milk of buffalo (*Bubalus bubalis*) cows. *Research in Veterinary Science* 49(3), 289–291.

Roddie, G., Holland, C., Stafford, P. and Wolfe, A. (2008) Contamination of fox hair with eggs of *Toxocara canis*. *Journal of Helminthology* 82(4), 293–296.

Ross, J.G. and Fairley, J.S. (1969) Studies of disease in the red fox (*Vulpes vulpes*) in Northern Ireland. *Journal of Zoology* 157(3), 375–381.

Round, M.C. (1968) *Check list of the helminth parasites of african mammals of the orders carnivora, tubulidentata, proboscidea, hyra-coidea, artiodactyla and perissodactyla*. Commonwealth Agricultural Bureaux, Farnham Royal.

Rubel, D., Zunino, G., Santillán, G. and Wisnivesky, C. (2003) Epidemiology of *Toxocara canis* in the dog population from two areas of different socioeconomic status, Greater Buenos Aires, Argentina. *Veterinary Parasitology* 115(3), 275–286.

Saeed, I., Maddox-Hyttel, C., Monrad, J. and Kapel, C.M.O. (2006) Helminths of red foxes (*Vulpes vulpes*) in Denmark. *Veterinary Parasitology* 139(1–3), 168–179.

Sakai, R., Kawashima, H., Shibui, H., Kamata, K., Kambara, C. *et al.* (1998) *Toxocara cati*-induced ocular toxocariasis. *Archives of Ophthalmology* 116(12), 1686–1687.

Salem, G. and Schantz, P. (1992) Toxocaral visceral larva migrans after ingestion of raw lamb liver. *Clinical Infectious Diseases* 15(4), 743–744.

Sanmartín, M.L., Alvarez, F., Gijón Botella, H., Iglesias, R., Estévez, J. *et al.* (1992) A scanning electron microscope study of *Toxocara genettae* Warren, 1972 (Ascaridae), with data on morphometric variation. *Folia Parasitologica* 39, 355–367.

Santos, S.V., Moura, J.V.L., Lescano, S.A.Z., Castro, J.M., Ribeiro, M. *et al.* (2015) Behavioural changes and muscle strength in rattus norvegicus experimentally infected with *Toxocara cati* and *T. canis*. *Journal of Helminthology* 89(4), 465–470.

Sasmal, N.K., Acharya, S. and Laha, R. (2008) Larval migration of *Toxocara canis* in piglets and transfer of larvae from infected porcine tissue to mice. *Journal of Helminthology* 82(3), 245–249.

Sato, H., Inaba, T., Ihama, Y. and Kamiya, H. (1999) Parasitological survey on wild Carnivora in North-Western Tohoku, Japan. *Journal of Veterinary Medical Science* 61(9), 1023–1026.

Sato, H., Suzuki, K. and Aoki, M. (2006) Nematodes from raccoon dogs (*Nyctereutes procyonoides viverrinus*) introduced recently on Yakushima Island, Japan. *Journal of Veterinary Medical Science* 68(7), 693–700.

Scala, A., Carfagna, G., Uras, P., Poglayen, G., Giannetto, S. *et al.* (2001) Parasitological survey about cattle reared in Gallura (Sardinia). *Atti Della Societa' Italiana Di Buiatria*.

Schacher, J.F. (1957) A contribution to the life history and larval morphology of *Toxocara canis*. *Journal of Parasitology* 43(6), 599–612.

Schneider, S.L., Gollnick, S.O., Grande, C., Pazik, J.E. and Tomasi, T.B. (1996) Differential regulation of TGF-β2 by hormones in rat uterus and mammary gland. *Journal of Reproductive Immunology* 32(2), 125–144.

Schnieder, T., Laabs, E.-M. and Welz, C. (2011) Larval development of *Toxocara canis* in dogs. *Veterinary Parasitology* 175(3–4), 193–206.

Schwartz, R. (2017) *Toxocara canis in Puppies and Their Public Health Importance in Grenada. St.* George's University, Grenada, West Indies.

Scothorn, M.W., Koutz, F.R. and Groves, H.F. (1965) Prenatal toxocara canis infection in pups. *Journal of the American Veterinary Medical Association* 146(1), 45–48.

Segovia, J.M., Torres, J., Miquel, J., Llaneza, L. and Feliu, C. (2001) Helminths in the wolf, *Canis lupus* from north-western Spain. *Journal of Helminthology* 75(2), 183–192.

Shields, J.A. (1984) *Ocular toxocariasis*. A review. *Survey of Ophthalmology* 28(5), 361–381.

Shimalov, V. and Shimalov, V. (2002) Helminth fauna of the racoon dog (*Nyctereutes procyonoides* Gray, 1834) in Belorussian Polesie. *Parasitology Research* 88(10), 944–945.

Shimalov, V.V. and Shimalov, V.T. (2000) Helminth fauna of the wolf (*Canis lupus* Linnaeus, 1758) in Belorussian Polesie. *Parasitology Research* 86(2), 163–164.

Shimokawa, H., Nakashima, T., Akagi, K., Omae, T. and Tsuji, M. (1982) Visceral larva migrans by *Toxocara cati*. *Fukuoka Igaku Zasshi* 73, 64–69.

Skirnisson, K., Eydal, M., Gunnarsson, E. and Hersteinsson, P. (1993) Parasites of the Arctic fox (*Alopex lagopus*) in Iceland. *Journal of Wildlife Diseases* 29(3), 440–446.

Sloss, M.W., Kemp, R. and Zajac, A. (1994) Veterinary Clinical Parasitology. American Association of Veterinary Parasitologists. Iowa State University Press, Ames, Iowa.

Smales, L.R. (2005) Helminth parasites of the grassland melomys (Muridae: Hydromyinae) from Australia and Papua New Guinea. *Australian Journal of Zoology* 53(6), 369.

Smith, G.C., Gangadharan, B., Taylor, Z., Laurenson, M.K., Bradshaw, H. *et al.* (2003) Prevalence of zoonotic important parasites in the red fox (*Vulpes vulpes*) in Great Britain. *Veterinary Parasitology* 118(1–2), 133–142.

Smith, H., Holland, C., Taylor, M., Magnaval, J.-F., Schantz, P. *et al.* (2009) How common is human toxocariasis? Towards standardizing our knowledge. *Trends in Parasitology* 25(4), 182–188.

Smith, H.V., Quinn, R., Kusel, J.R. and Girdwood, R.W.A. (1981) The effect of temperature and antimetabolites on antibody binding to the outer surface of second stage *Toxocara canis* larvae. *Molecular and Biochemical Parasitology* 4(3–4), 183–193.

Sommerfelt, I.E., Duchene, A., Daprato, B., Lopez, C.M., Cardillo, N. *et al.* (2014) Experimental infection with *Toxocara cati* in pigs: Migratory pattern and pathological response in early phase. *Revista Do Instituto de Medicina Tropical de São Paulo* 56(4), 347–352.

Sommerfelt, I.E.E., Rosa, A., Duchene, A., Degregorio, O., López, C. *et al.* (2004) *Toxocara canis* in experimentally infected pigs: Migratory pattern and tissue lesions. *Veterinary Parasitology* 125(3–4), 323–334.

Sprent, J.F. (1972) *Toxocara vajrasthirae* sp. nov. from the hog-badger (*Arctonyx collaris*) of Thailand. *Parasitology* 65(3), 491–498.

Sprent, J.F.A. (1953) On the migratory behavior of the larvae of various *Ascaris* species in white mice: II. Longevity. *Journal of Infectious Diseases* 92(2), 114–117.

Sprent, J.F.A. (1956) The life history and development of *Toxocara cati* (Schrank 1788) in the domestic cat. *Parasitology* 46(1–2), 54–78.

Sprent, J.F.A. (1957) A new species of Neoascaris from *Rattus assimilis*, with a redefinition of the genus. *Parasitology* 47(3–4), 350–360.

Sprent, J.F.A. (1958) Observations on the development of *Toxocara canis* (Werner, 1782) in the dog. *Parasitology* 48(1–2), 184–209.

Sprent, J.F.A. (1961) Post-parturient infection of the bitch with *Toxocara canis*. *Journal of Parasitology* 47(2), 284.

Sprent, J.F.A. (1968) Notes on *Ascaris* and *Toxascaris*, with a definition of *Baylisascaris* gen. nov. *Parasitology* 58(1), 185–198.

Sprent, J.F.A. (1982) Ascaridoid nematodes of South American mammals, with a definition of a new genus. *Journal of Helminthology* 56(3), 275–295.

Starke-Buzetti, W.A., Machado, R.Z. and Zocoller-Seno, M.C. (2001) An enzyme-linked immunosorbent assay (ELISA) for detection of antibodies against *Toxocara vitulorum* in water buffaloes. *Veterinary Parasitology* 97(1), 55–64.

Starke-Buzetti, W.A. (2006) 18 *Toxocara vitulorum* in livestock. In: Holland, C.V. and Smith, H.V. (eds) *Toxocara: The Enigmatic Parasite*. CABI, Wallingford, UK, pp. 260–277.

Stewart, J.M., Cubillan, L.D. and Cunningham, J.R.E.T. (2005) Prevalence, clinical features, and causes of vision loss among patients with ocular toxocariasis. *Retina* 25(8), 1005–1013.

Stoicescu, R.M., Mihai, C.M. and Giannakopoulou, A.D. (2011) Marked hypereosinophilia in a toddler: A case report. *Journal of Medicine and Life* 4(1), 105–108.

Stoye, M. (1976) Galaktogene und pranatale infektionen mit *Toxocara canis* beim Hund (Beagle). *Deutsche Tierärztliche Wochenschrift* 83, 107–108.

Strauch, D. (1991) Survival of pathogenic micro-organisms and parasites in excreta, manure and sewage sludge. *Scientific and Technical Review of the Office International Des Epizooties (Paris)* 10(3), 813–846.

Strube, C., Heuer, L. and Janecek, E. (2013) *Toxocara* spp. Infections in paratenic hosts. *Veterinary Parasitology* 193(4), 375–389.

Stuart, P., Golden, O., Zintl, A., Waal, T., Mulcahy, G. *et al.* (2013) A coprological survey of parasites of wild carnivores in Ireland. *Parasitology Research* 112(10), 3587–3593.

Stürchler, D., Schubarth, P., Gualzata, M., Gottstein, B. and Oettli, A. (1989) Thiabendazole vs. albendazole in treatment of toxocariasis: A clinical trial. *Annals of Tropical Medicine and Parasitology* 83(5), 473–478.

Su, H., Su, Y. and Huffman, M.A. (2013) Leaf swallowing and parasitic infection of the Chinese lesser civet *Viverricula indica* in northeastern Taiwan. *Zoological Studies* 52(1), 22.

Sugane, K. and Oshima, T. (1983) Purification and characterization of excretory and secretory antigen of *Toxocara canis* larvae. *Immunology* 50(1), 113–120.

Sultan, K., Omar, M., Desouky, A.Y. and El-Seify, M.A. (2015) Molecular and phylogenetic study on *Toxocara vitulorum* from cattle in the mid-Delta of Egypt. *Journal of Parasitic Diseases* 39(3), 584–587.

Surkovic-Zuko, A. (1997) Endoparasites in cattle in the Travnik region. *Veterinaria Sarajevo* 46, 107–119.

Swai, E.S., Kaaya, E.J., Mshanga, D.A. and Mbise, E.W. (2010) A survey on gastro-intestinal parasites of non-descript dogs in and around Arusha Municipality, Tanzania. *Journal of Animal and Veterinary Advances* 3(2), 63–67.

Swerczek, T.W., Nielsen, S.W. and Helmboldt, C.J. (1971) Transmammary passage of *Toxocara cati* in the cat. *American Journal of Veterinary Research* 32(1), 89–92.

Taira, N.F.J. (1991) Morphological observation of *Toxocara vitulorum* found in Japanese calves. *Journal of Veterinary Medical Science* 53(3), 409–413.

Taira, K., Saeed, I., Permin, A. and Kapel, C.M.O. (2004) Zoonotic risk of *Toxocara canis* infection through consumption of pig or poultry viscera. *Veterinary Parasitology* 121(1–2), 115–124.

Taira, K., Saitoh, Y. and Kapel, C.M.O. (2011) *Toxocara cati* larvae persist and retain high infectivity in muscles of experimentally infected chickens. *Veterinary Parasitology* 180(3–4), 287–291.

Takács, A., Szabó, L., Juhász, L., Lanszki, J., Takács, P. *et al.* (2013) Data on the parasitological status of golden jackal (*Canis aureus* L., 1758) in Hungary. *Acta Veterinaria Hungarica* 62(1), 33–41.

Takayanagi, T.H., Akao, N., Suzuki, R., Tomoda, M., Tsukidate, S. *et al.* (1999) New animal model for human ocular toxocariasis: Ophthalmoscopic observation. *British Journal of Ophthalmology* 83(8), 967–972.

Tavassoli, M., Javadi, S., Firozi, R., Rezaei, F., Khezri, A.R. *et al.* (2012) Hair contamination of sheepdog and pet dogs with *Toxocara canis* eggs. *Iranian Journal of Parasitology* 7(4), 110–115.

Tiyo, R., Guedes, T.A., Falavigna, D.L.M. and Falavigna-Guilherme, A.L. (2008) Seasonal contamination of public squares and lawns by parasites with zoonotic potential in southern Brazil. *Journal of Helminthology* 82(1), 1–6.

Tomimura, T., Yokota, M. and Takiguchi, H. (1976) Experimental visceral larva migrans in monkeys. I. Clinical, hematological, biochemical and gross pathological observations on monkeys inoculated with embryonated eggs of the dog ascarid, *Toxocara canis*. *Japanese Journal of Veterinary Science* 38(6), 533–548.

Totton, S.C., Wandeler, A.I., Zinsstag, J., Bauch, C.T., Ribble, C.S. *et al.* (2010) Stray dog population demographics in Jodhpur, India following a population control/rabies vaccination program. *Preventive Veterinary Medicine* 97(1), 51–57.

Vanparijs, O.F.J. and Thienpont, D.C. (1973) Canine and feline helminth and protozoan infections in Belgium. *Journal of Parasitology* 59(2), 327–330.

Vega, R.M., González Prous, C., Krivokapich, S., Gatti, G., Brugni, N.L. *et al.* (2018) Toxocariasis in Carnivora from Argentinean patagonia: Species molecular identification, hosts, and geographical distribution. *International Journal for Parasitology: Parasites and Wildlife* 7(1), 106–110.

Vanparijs, O., Hermans, L. and Van Der Flaes, L. (1991) Helminth and protozoan parasites in dogs and cats in Belgium. *Veterinary Parasitology* 38(1), 67–73.

Venjakob, P.L., Thiele, G., Clausen, P.-H. and Nijhof, A.M. (2017) *Toxocara vitulorum* infection in German beef cattle. *Parasitology Research* 116(3), 1085–1088.

Vicente, J.J., Oliveira Rodrigues, H. and Gomes, D.C. (1997) Nematóides do Brasil. Parte V; nematóides de mamíferos. Brazillan nematodes. Part V; nematodes of mammals. *Revista Brasileira de Zoologia* 14(1), 1–452.

Vidal, J., Sztajnbok, J. and Seguro, A. (2003) Eosinophilic meningoencephalitis due to *Toxocara canis*: Case report and review of the literature. *American Journal of Tropical Medicine and Hygiene* 69(3), 341–343.

von Dohlen, A.R., Houk-Miles, A.E., Zajac, A.M. and Lindsay, D.S. (2017) Flotation of *Toxocara canis* eggs in commercial bleach and effects of bleach treatment times on larval development in these eggs. *Journal of Parasitology* 103(2), 183–186.

Vossmann, T. and Stoye, M. (1986) Klinische, hämatologische und serologische Befunde bei Welpen nach pränataler infektion mit *Toxocara canis* WERNER 1782 (Anisakidae). *Journal of Veterinary Medicine Series B* 33(1–10), 574–585.

Vuylsteke, C. (1956) Note sur quelques nématodes parasites avec description de neuf espèces nouvelles. *Revue de Zoologie et de Botanique Africaines* 53(3/4), 441–477.

Wapenaar, W., Barkema, H.W. and O'Handley, R. (2013) Fecal shedding of *Toxocara canis* and other parasites in foxes and coyotes on Prince Edward Island, Canada. *Journal of Wildlife Diseases* 49(2), 394–397.

Warren, E.G. (1971) Observations on the migration and development of *Toxocara vitulorum* in natural and experimental hosts. *International Journal for Parasitology* 1(1), 85–99.

Warren, E.G. (1972) Some hosts of ascaridoid nematodes in Africa. *Annales de Parasitologie Humaine et Comparee* 47(5), 763–764.

Warren, E.G. (1972) Two new species of *Toxocara* from viverrid hosts. *Parasitology* 65(2), 179–187.

Warren, G. (1970) Studies on the morphology and taxonomy of the genera *Toxocara* stiles, 1905 and *Neoascaris* Travassos, 1927. *Zoologischer Anzeiger* 185(5/6), 393–441.

Warren, E.G. and Needham, D.J. (1969) On the presence of *Neoascaris vitulorum* in calves from New South Wales. *Australian Veterinary Journal* 45(1), 22–23.

Webster, G.A. (1958) A report on *Toxocara canis* Werner, 1782. *Canadian Journal of Comparative Medicine and Veterinary Science* 22(8), 272–279.

Wen, Y.L., Zhvang, Z.L., Lin, B.M., Pan, Y.D., Gao, B.Z. *et al.* (1986) An epidemiologic survey of *Neoascaris* in calves. *Chinese Journal of Veterinary Science and Technology* 8, 18–20.

Werner, P.C.F. (1782) *Vermium Intestinalium Praesertim Taeniae Humanae Brevis Expositio*, Vol. 1. Apud Siegfried Lebrecht Crusium.

Wickramasinghe, S., Yatawara, L., Rajapakse, R. and Agatsuma, T. (2009) *Toxocara vitulorum* (Ascaridida: Nematoda): Mitochondrial gene content, arrangement and composition compared with other *Toxocara* species. *Molecular and Biochemical Parasitology* 166(1), 89–92.

Willingham, A.L., Ockens, N.W., Kapel, C.M.O. and Monrad, J. (1996) A helminthological survey of wild red foxes (*Vulpes vulpes*) from the metropolitan area of Copenhagen. *Journal of Helminthology* 70(3), 259–263.

Wolfe, A. and Wright, I.P. (2003) Human toxocariasis and direct contact with dogs. *Veterinary Record* 152(14), 419–421.

Won, E.J., Kim, J., Shin, M.-G., Shin, J.H., Suh, S.P. *et al.* (2015) Seroepidemiology of toxocariasis and its clinical implications in Gwangju and Jeonnam-province, Korea. *Annals of Laboratory Medicine* 35(4), 449.

Woodbury, M.R., Copeland, S., Wagner, B., Fernando, C., Hill, J.E. *et al.* (2012) *Toxocara vitulorum* in a bison (*Bison bison*) herd from western Canada. *Canadian Veterinary Journal* 53(7), 791–794.
Woodbury, M.R., Wagner, B., Ben-Ezra, E., Douma, D. and Wilkins, W. (2014) A survey to detect *Toxocara vitulorum* and other gastrointestinal parasites in bison (*Bison bison*) herds from Manitoba and Saskatchewan. *Canadian Veterinary Journal* 55(9), 870–874.
Woodhall, D., Starr, M.C., Montgomery, S.P., Jones, J.L., Lum, F. *et al.* (2012) *Ocular toxocariasis*: Epidemiologic, anatomic, and therapeutic variations based on a survey of ophthalmic subspecialists. *Ophthalmology* 119(6), 1211–1217.
Wymann, M.N., Bonfoh, B., Traore, K., Tembely, S. and Zinsstag, J. (2007) Species diversity and acquisition of gastrointestinal parasites in calves aged 0–13 months in periurban livestock production in Mali. *Veterinary Parasitology* 143(1), 67–73.
Wymann, M.N., Traore, K., Bonfoh, B., Tembely, S., Tembely, S. *et al.* (2008) Gastrointestinal parasite egg excretion in young calves in periurban livestock production in Mali. *Research in Veterinary Science* 84(2), 225–231.
Xinou, E., Lefkopoulos, A., Gelagoti, M., Drevelegas, A., Diakou, A. *et al.* (2003) CT and MR imaging findings in cerebral toxocaral disease. *American Journal of Neuroradiology* 24(4), 714–718.
Yahiro, S., Cain, G. and Butler, J.E. (1998) Identification, characterization and expression of *Toxocara canis* nematode polyprotein allergen TBA-1. *Parasite Immunology* 20(8), 351–357.
Yamaguchi, N., Macdonald, D.W., Passanisi, W.C., Harbour, D.A. and Hopper, C.D. (1996) Parasite prevalence in free-ranging farm cats, *Felis silvestris catus*. *Epidemiology and Infection* 116(2), 217–223.
Yoak, A.J., Reece, J.F., Gehrt, S.D. and Hamilton, I.M. (2014) Disease control through fertility control: Secondary benefits of animal birth control in indian street dogs. *Preventive Veterinary Medicine* 113(1), 152–156.
Yoshikawa, M., Nishiofuku, M., Moriya, K., Ouji, Y., Ishizaka, S. *et al.* (2008) A familial case of visceral toxocariasis due to consumption of raw bovine liver. *Parasitology International* 57(4), 525–529.
Yutuc, L.M. (1949) Prenatal infection of dogs with ascarids, *Toxocara canis* and hookworms. *Ancylostoma Caninum*. *Journal of Parasitology* 35(4), 358–360.
Zhu, X., Gasser, R.B., Jacobs, D.E., Hung, G.-C. and Chilton, N.B. (2000) Relationships among some ascaridoid nematodes based on ribosomal DNA sequence data. *Parasitology Research* 86(9), 738–744.
Zhu, X.Q. and Gasser, R.B. (1988) Single-strand conformation polymorphism (SSCP)-based mutation scanning approaches to fingerprint sequence variation in ribosomal DNA of ascaridoid nematodes. *Electrophoresis* 19(8–9), 1366–1373.
Zhu, X.Q., Gasser, R.B., Chilton, N.B. and Jacobs, D.E. (2001) Molecular approaches for studying ascaridoid nematodes with zoonotic potential, with an emphasis on *Toxocara* species. *Journal of Helminthology* 75(2), 101–108.
Zhu, X.Q., Jacobs, D.E., Chilton, N.B., Sani, R.A., Cheng, N. *et al.* (1998) Molecular characterization of a *Toxocara variant* from cats in Kuala Lumpur, Malaysia. *Parasitology* 117(2), 155–164.
Ziadinov, I., Deplazes, P., Mathis, A., Mutunova, B., Abdykerimov, K. *et al.* (2010) Frequency distribution of *Echinococcus multilocularis* and other helminths of foxes in Kyrgyzstan. *Veterinary Parasitology* 171(3–4), 286–292.
Zibaei, M. (2017) Helminth infections and cardiovascular diseases: *Toxocara* species is contributing to the disease. *Current Cardiology Reviews* 13(1), 56–62.
Zibaei, M., Sadjjadi, S.M. and Maraghi, S. (2017) The occurrence of *Toxocara* species in naturally infected broiler chickens revealed by molecular approaches. *Journal of Helminthology* 91(5), 633–636.
Zimmermann, U. (1983) *Quantitative Untersuchungen über die Wanderung und Streuung der Larven von Toxocara canis WERNER 1782 (Anisakidae) im definitiven Wirt (Beagle) nach fraktionierter Erst-und Reinfektion*. University of Veterinary Medicine Hannover, Germany.

23 Feline Obesity and Diabetes: A One Health Perspective

Moira S. Lewitt*

School of Health and Life Sciences, University of the West of Scotland, PA1 2BE, UK

Abstract

There is increasing awareness of obesity and diabetes mellitus in cats that parallels the 'epidemic' of obesity and type 2 diabetes in humans. Likewise, understanding of the pathophysiology and management of feline obesity and diabetes has developed alongside and draws from human medicine. As in human medicine, overweight and obesity are associated with the development with diabetes; however, there are other genetic and environmental influences that contribute to this risk, some of which are shared. In cats, the body condition score appears to be a good diagnostic tool. It is reliable in the hands of owners and is likely to reflect visceral adiposity. However, the diagnostic label of feline obesity should be considered against the rate of success of any intervention, owner perspectives and impact on cat quality of life, as well as risk of future disease. The classification of human diabetes is evolving towards one that is more closely linked to disease outcome and therefore management. Consideration could be given to classifying the diabetes of hypersomatotropism and that associated with exogenous glucocorticoid administration in cats, separately in veterinary medicine. Rather regarding feline obesity and diabetes as models of human disease, a closer interdisciplinary 'One Health' approach between veterinary and human medicine is warranted to advance research and clinical care in this field.

Keywords: Feline, Diabetes, Obesity, Metabolic syndrome, One Health

Introduction

There is increasing awareness of obesity and diabetes mellitus in cats that parallels the 'epidemic' of obesity and type two diabetes in humans. Most knowledge of the pathophysiology of obesity derives from clinical and experimental studies in humans and rodent models which are used as the basis for understanding feline obesity and its management (Loftus and Wakshlag, 2015). Conversely, feline obesity and diabetes are often regarded as models of human obesity and type two diabetes (Hoenig, 2006; Van de Velde *et al.*, 2013; Osto and Lutz, 2015). The aim of this review is to compare and contrast the definition, diagnosis, aetiology, pathogenesis and management of feline obesity and diabetes mellitus with the conditions in humans. The terms 'feline' and 'obesity' or 'diabetes' were used to search the PubMed and ScienceDirect databases. The title and abstracts of the items retrieved were searched manually for English language papers that focussed primarily on obesity or diabetes in cats, resulting in 702

*Corresponding author: Moira.Lewitt@uws.ac.uk

relevant papers dating from 1946 being identified. The growth of the literature was found to fit an exponential curve ($r^2 = 0.996$), with a doubling time of 9.2 years (95% confidence interval 9.0–9.4 years). Two hundred were reviews or commentaries (28%), a proportion that has remained stable over time. Emerging themes guided the incorporation of relevant literature from human medicine.

Definitions and Diagnosis

Overweight and obesity

Weight can be used to track changes in body mass in individuals both human and feline. According to the World Health Organisation, overweight is '*a condition characterised by excess weight relative to height*' (World Health Organization, 2018) and recommends use of the body mass index (BMI) to define overweight (25.00–29.99 kg/m^2) and obesity (≥30.00 kg/m^2). While these definitions are useful in adult populations, age, gender and pubertal status must also be taken into account in defining overweight and obesity in children. Furthermore, the BMI does not reflect adipose tissue distribution. Waist measurement is a significant predictor of health risk (Janssen *et al.*, 2004) and is a good marker of visceral adiposity (Engin, 2017). Adult cats vary considerably in body mass, and the diagnosis of overweight and obesity in feline medicine rests to a large extent on observations of body shape. Using line drawings (Laflamme, 1997), owners are able to identify a body condition score (BCS) and make judgements that closely agree with experienced veterinarians (Peron *et al.*, 2016). However, using a nine-point visual scale, where 6–9 is overweight or obese, owners perceive a BCS of 7 as indicating ideal body weight (Rowe *et al.*, 2017; Ohlund *et al.*, 2018). Thus, while scoring might be considered reliable, owner education is needed if these are to have an influence on feline care. It has been suggested that a feline BMI score that utilizes the length from the top of the patella to the end of the calcaneous might be more sensitive and useful than the BCS (Kawasumi *et al.*, 2016). However, as for waist measurement in human, feline BCS which assesses fat covering the ribs, abdomen and lumbar area might be a better marker of visceral adiposity than the feline BMI score.

Metabolic syndrome

The metabolic syndrome has emerged as a useful clinical concept in humans. The risk of cardiovascular disease is increased when abdominal adiposity is associated with evidence of glucose intolerance, dyslipidaemia or hypertension (Engin, 2017). In cats, atherosclerosis does not present as a clinical problem. Nevertheless, since an elevated BCS is associated with insulin resistance (Hoenig *et al.*, 2007), it has been suggested that an additional classification of feline metabolic syndrome, using BCS associated with increased blood glucose, dyslipidaemia and low adiponectin (Okada *et al.*, 2017). However, whether such a classification has practical clinical value is yet to be determined.

Diabetes mellitus

There is no agreed definition of diabetes mellitus in cats and this is considered a limitation in systematic reviews of this area (Gostelow *et al.*, 2014). In human health, there is a global consensus on the diagnostic criteria for diabetes (World Health Organization, 2006), and there is also consensus on the definition of cure (Buse *et al.*, 2009). In feline clinical practice, the presence of signs (polyuria, polydipsia, polyphagia and weight loss), along with persistent hyperglycaemia or glycosuria, is used to make a diagnosis of diabetes mellitus, and treatment is commenced on that basis (Nelson and Reusch, 2014). It would be useful to have a marker of pre-diabetes to use, for example, in cats with a high BCS score. In humans, the 75g oral glucose tolerance test is used as a standard to screen for impaired glucose tolerance. It is preferred to intravenous glucose tolerance testing where there is no incretin response. In cats, administration of oral glucose requires careful handling techniques to minimize struggling and stress hyperglycaemia (Rand *et al.*, 2002) and therefore intravenous glucose is used. Selection of a glucose concentration based on body weight, however, may lead to an overestimation in obese cats, and thereby an overdiagnosis of impaired glucose tolerance (Reeve-Johnson *et al.*, 2016). The lack of glucokinase in cats may account for a prolonged elevation of blood glucose after a meal (Hewson-Hughes *et al.*, 2011) and needs to be considered in tests of glucose clearance.

Glucose is ubiquitously present in the urine of euglycaemic cats (Zeugswetter *et al.*, 2018) and therefore cannot be relied on in the diagnosis or monitoring of feline diabetes. In the absence of stress, fasting blood glucose values do not exceed 7 mmol/L in cats and it has been proposed that 'persistent values above this are diagnostic, if supported by documentation of elevated fructosamine or glycosylated haemoglobin, regardless of clinical signs' (Gilor *et al.*, 2016). Cut-off points of fasting blood glucose for the diagnosis of prediabetes in otherwise healthy older cats (>8 years) have been proposed (Reeve-Johnson *et al.*, 2016). In clinically healthy cats, fructosamine concentrations are positively associated with body weight and are higher in male cats than in female cats matched for age, weight and BCS (Gilor *et al.*, 2010). While the use of fructosamine as a screening test for prediabetes is yet to be evaluated, it is well established as a measure of glycaemic control in cats with a diagnosis of diabetes (Reusch *et al.*, 1993).

Risk Factors for Overweight and Obesity

Genetic predisposition

In humans, there is an interaction between genes and environment in determining predisposition to obesity across childhood and adolescence (Dubois *et al.*, 2012). Research using cat colonies indicates that obesity is also determined early in life (Cave *et al.*, 2018) and there is likely to be a genetic component in its development (Haring *et al.*, 2011). Healthy weight intact male cats in a population genetically predisposed to overweight (Haring *et al.*, 2011) have similar metabolic responses to a high carbohydrate to genetically lean cats, but lower fasting insulin levels (Keller *et al.*, 2017) might indicate relative insulin sensitivity. A population study of cats in metropolitan Sydney, Australia, identified that mixed breed and British shorthair were more likely to be overweight than other purebred cats (Teng *et al.*, 2017).

Nutrition and physical activity

It is well known that cats are obligate carnivores, which means evolutionary pressures have resulted in requirements for nutrients, including amino acids and vitamins, that are met by consuming prey (Verbrugghe and Hesta, 2017). There are adaptions in feline carbohydrate metabolism which have been interpreted as indicting that high carbohydrate diets are a risk factor for the development of feline obesity. Consistent with this, feline overweight and obesity is associated with dry food consumption (Ohlund *et al.*, 2018), as early as 1 year of age (Rowe *et al.*, 2015). Commercial dry foods contain more carbohydrate than wet diets (Villaverde and Fascetti, 2014). However, high wet food consumption at a young age and owners giving cat 'treats' are also associated with overweight (Rowe *et al.*, 2017) and it is likely that consumption of excess calories through overfeeding is the key risk factor (Verbrugghe and Hesta, 2017). Compared with veterinary physicians, owners are less likely to perceive that their cat is obese (Rowe *et al.*, 2017) and owner characteristics, such as age and income, are potential risk factors for feline obesity (Larsen and Villaverde, 2016). There is an interaction between food consumption and energy expenditure in determining predisposition to weight gain. Evidence shows that lean cats are more active than overweight cats, have a greater anticipatory physical activity prior to feeding and greater social interaction with humans (De Godoy and Shoveller, 2017). Another study has shown a stronger diurnal activity pattern of cats when water is added to a dry food diet, compared with a wet canned diet of similar moisture content, the mechanism for which is unexplained (Thomas *et al.*, 2017).

Endocrine disruptors and hormonal influences

Perfluoroalkyl substances (PFAS) have endocrine disrupting effects and are associated with increased risk of childhood obesity (Braun,

2017). In adult humans, higher plasma PFAS concentrations are associated with greater weight regain after a weight loss programme, particularly in women (Liu *et al.*, 2018). Since indoor cats have elevated PFAS levels that are similar to those in human sera (Bost *et al.*, 2016), this environmental influence on obesity predisposition may be shared with humans and is worthy of further collaborative research.

In many countries, surgical neutering is a common procedure and considered a likely factor influencing obesity in cats (Larsen, 2017). Neutering in urban free-roaming cats is associated with an increased prevalence of feline obesity (Gunther *et al.*, 2018). After neutering, male cats still have decreased insulin tolerance compared with female cats, and lower adiponectin levels (Bjornvad *et al.*, 2014).

Adipose tissue is an endocrine organ. Feline obesity is associated with increased adipocyte size and altered adipokine gene expression, with similar patterns to human obesity, with higher leptin and lower adiponectin levels in the circulation, and an increase in expression pro-inflammatory cytokines and chemokines (Van de Velde *et al.*, 2013; Takashima *et al.*, 2016; Zapata *et al.*, 2017). In healthy cats, nearly 40% of the variance in final body weight after 8 weeks of *ad libitum* feeding is explained by initial body weight, energy requirements for maintenance and fasting leptin (Coradini *et al.*, 2014). Adiponectin has been used in a classification of feline metabolic syndrome (Okada *et al.*, 2017). The role of other adipokines in prediction and pathogenesis of overweight and obesity requires further study.

Is Obesity a Disease?

If feline obesity is a disease, it is one of the most prevalent. Prevalence of overweight and obesity in cats of 35% (Lund, 2005) and 39% (Courcier *et al.*, 2010) have been reported using a five-point BCS and as high as 45% (Ohlund *et al.*, 2018) and 65% (Vandendriessche *et al.*, 2017) using a nine-point scale. Despite suggestions that feline overweight and obesity might be increasing in prevalence in parallel with human obesity, a cross-sectional study in New Zealand found no evidence for an increase between 1993 and 2007 (Cave *et al.*, 2012).

In humans, while obesity is increasing in prevalence, the level of risk appears to be decreasing. The lowest all-cause mortality in Denmark has increased from a BMI of 24 kg/m^2 in 1976–1978 to 27 kg/m^2 three decades later (Afzal and Nordestgaard, 2016). In a US study, while the risk of diabetes among obese individuals is the same, cardiovascular risk has declined over this time period (Gregg *et al.*, 2005). Human obesity is classified as a nutritional disorder in the WHO International Classification of Disease (World Health Organization, 2018). However, there are calls to improve that definition based on aetiology, degree of adiposity and health risk (Hebebrand *et al.*, 2017). The American Medical Association has classified obesity as a disease; however, this has generated debate around diagnostic criteria, classification and risk (Stoner and Cornwall, 2014). Recent studies in humans suggest that some individuals with obesity are in fact 'metabolically healthy'. However, the risk of mortality and morbidity remains greater than in metabolically healthy normal weight individuals, and this difference is largely explained by cardiorespiratory fitness (Ortega *et al.*, 2018).

In cats, obesity is associated with reduced insulin sensitivity of glucose and fat metabolism (Hoenig *et al.*, 2007) and a low or absent first phase insulin response following intravenous glucose (Nelson *et al.*, 1990; Appleton et al., 2001). There are clear links between obesity and the development of diabetes and hepatic lipidosis in cats (Clark and Hoenig, 2016). However, not all obese cats develop disease and it is not clear that all cats with obesity would have improved quality of life with weight loss. Useful predictive markers of disease in obese cats are yet to be identified. As in humans, prevention of obesity development and relapse is of key importance in reducing prevalence of this condition (German, 2016).

Management of Obesity

It has been emphasized that, rather than focussing on the achievement of an 'ideal weight', the goal of weight loss should be established and a robust management approach designed in collaboration with the owner (German,

2016). Restricted feeding of a moderate protein high-fibre diet is regarded as safe and effective for weight loss in cats (Pallotto *et al.*, 2018). Restricted high-protein diets might be beneficial for minimizing decreases in energy expenditure during weight loss (Des Courtis *et al.*, 2015). In clinical practice the effectiveness is modest, with an average weight loss of 0.8% starting body weight per week and a 41% non-completion rate during a 3-month programme (Flanagan *et al.*, 2018). Regain in weight is common, particularly in younger cats (Deagle *et al.*, 2014). Strategies that increase physical activity, such as increased feeding frequency (Deng *et al.*, 2014; De Godoy *et al.*, 2015), running wheels (Detweiler *et al.*, 2017) and social interaction with humans (De Godoy and Shoveller, 2017) may help in the prevention and management of overweight and obesity. It seems that, similar to humans, there is a stigma attached to a diagnosis of obesity in pets. Veterinarians are observed to use humour to cope with the discomfort surrounding the topic when talking to owners and the discussion is often avoided, suggesting the need for training towards history-taking and information-giving around nutritional intake (Phillips *et al.*, 2017) including communication skills (Churchill and Ward, 2016).

Feline Diabetes Mellitus

There is a prevalence of feline diabetes mellitus of 0.58% in veterinary primary care clinics in England today (O'Neill *et al.*, 2016). In North America, the prevalence of feline diabetes presenting to a veterinary teaching hospital has increased, which may reflect changes in the willingness of owners to present or for veterinary physicians to refer, as well as increasing prevalence of risk factors (Prahl *et al.*, 2007). Studies indicate an increased incidence in some cat breeds. An increased risk of diabetes has been observed in Burmese cats in England (O'Neill *et al.*, 2016), Australia (Lederer *et al.*, 2009) and Sweden (Ohlund *et al.*, 2015), which interestingly has not been reported in the USA, where breeding programmes have been kept separate (Alhaddad *et al.*, 2013). An increased prevalence has been documented in Norwegian Forest cats (Ohlund *et al.*, 2015; O'Neill *et al.*, 2016), Tonkinese (O'Neill *et al.*, 2016) and in Russian Blue and Abyssinian (Ohlund *et al.*, 2015), compared with other breeds. There is a higher prevalence of obesity in cats with diabetes (Panciera *et al.*, 1990). As in humans, a polymorphism in the melanocortin four receptor gene is associated with diabetes in overweight cats (Forcada *et al.*, 2014). In normal weight cats, there is an association between dry food intake and an increased risk of diabetes (Öhlund *et al.*, 2017). Since dry food is widely used by pet owners, it is important that this observation is further investigated.

In addition to the genetic predisposition and obesity, some of the factors associated with feline diabetes are also associated with type two diabetes risk in humans. Physical inactivity (and indoor confinement) (Slingerland *et al.*, 2009) and advancing age (O'Neill *et al.*, 2016) are associated with increased risk of feline diabetes. Male cats have lower total adiponectin and decreased insulin tolerance compared with female cats (Bjornvad *et al.*, 2014) and the risk of diabetes is higher (Prahl *et al.*, 2007; Lederer *et al.*, 2009; Ohlund *et al.*, 2015; O'Neill *et al.*, 2016). In cats, it has long been recognized that exogenous glucocorticoid administration is associated with diabetes onset (Buse *et al.*, 1957) and under these conditions, the pancreatic islets may be protected by insulin (Lukens *et al.*, 1961). There is a greater chance of remission if cats have a history of corticosteroid treatment in the 6 months prior to diabetes diagnosis (Hewson-Hughes *et al.*, 2011). In cats with endogenous hyperadrenocorticism, it is reported that the incidence of diabetes is 80% (Niessen *et al.*, 2013).

Growth hormone has important lipolytic effects, and in humans with growth hormone excess (acromegaly), total body fat is reduced (Berryman and List, 2017). However, growth hormone has anti-insulin activities and acromegaly is associated with a high prevalence of glucose intolerance and diabetes, the severity of which is predicted by age, BMI and IGF-I concentrations (Dreval *et al.*, 2014). Growth hormone-secreting pituitary tumours are well described in association with diabetes in cats (Lichtensteiger *et al.*, 1986), although cases of feline acromegaly without diabetes have also been reported (Fletcher *et al.*, 2016). Report of a prevalence of 25% of hypersomatotropism in feline diabetes in primary care settings in the UK (Niessen *et al.*, 2015) has led to a conclusion that screening for the disease should be undertaken in all cats presenting with diabetes (Gilor *et al.*, 2016). However, many of these cats lack any other clinical features of acromegaly. Furthermore, while treatment that is directed at the tumour is likely to improve glucose tolerance, it is costly and invasive. In a series of 12 cases managed surgically, seven of the ten surviving cats achieved insulin independence (Kenny *et al.*, 2015). A wide reference interval of 90–1207 ng/ml in a population of healthy cats (Strage *et al.*, 2015) indicates that the current use of IGF-I concentration of >1000 ng/ml in screening might be set too high. Furthermore, IGF-I concentrations have been observed to increase in cats with diabetes in the weeks following the commencement of insulin (Strage *et al.*, 2018). Since abnormalities seen in pituitary imaging may be incidental, it would be prudent to continue to exercise caution in the diagnosis of feline acromegaly until further research is undertaken.

Veterinary medicine has adopted the nomenclature of human medicine, and currently uses the terms type 1 (T1DM) and type two diabetes (T2DM). Although there are reports of lymphocytic infiltration of the endocrine pancreas, T1DM is likely to be rare in cats (Nelson and Reusch, 2014). Extensive pancreatic inflammation and destruction can, theoretically, cause insulin-deficient diabetes in any species. However, the converse may also be true. T2DM is associated with an increased risk of pancreatitis in humans (Yang *et al.*, 2013). Experimental hyperglycaemia in cats is associated with increased pancreatic neutrophils (Zini *et al.*, 2010) and elevated serum pancreatic lipase activity and ultrasound findings consistent with pancreatitis have been documented in cats with diabetes, in the absence of clinical signs (Zini *et al.*, 2015).

Historically, most feline diabetes was classified as insulin-dependent diabetes or type 1 (Stogdale, 1986), however it is now clear that it resembles human T2DM, with a combination of insulin resistance, amyloid deposition in pancreatic islets and abnormal β-cell function (Lutz and Rand, 1993; Nelson and Reusch, 2014). However, recently in human medicine it has been recognized that diabetes mellitus is a more heterogeneous disorder and a new substratification, based on disease progression and risk of complications, has been proposed (Ahlqvist *et al.*, 2018). The value of such an approach is to help in targeting management approaches. It is emphasized that protocols for diagnosis and treatment of diabetes are not appropriate for animals (Niaz *et al.*, 2018). Thus there are limitations in using human aetiology-based classification systems for companion animals, and development of alternative approaches may be of more practical use for prognosis and management (Gilor *et al.*, 2016).

Management of Diabetes

In diabetic cats, circulating insulin concentrations are reduced (Finn *et al.*, 1970; Lutz and Rand, 1996). Very early experimental work demonstrated that pancreatic islet lesions could be induced by administration of glucose (Dohan and Lukens, 1947) and glucotoxicity is now regarded as the key factor for declining β-cell function (Nelson and Reusch, 2014). Recently, the mechanisms underlying the effect on β-cell function are the subject of intensive study using rodent models (Rorsman and Ashcroft, 2018). In humans, intensive insulin therapy in newly diagnosed patients with T2DM is associated with long-term restoration of insulin sensitivity and partial restoration of β-cell function (Hu *et al.*, 2011). Despite this observation, early intensive insulin regimens remain an unconventional approach to management in human medicine. In veterinary care, on the other hand, it is widely recognized that intensive management with insulin, along with a low carbohydrate diet and home blood glucose monitoring, which aims for near-euglycaemia, is associated with diabetes remission (Nack and DeClue, 2014). This success contrasts to earlier reports of high morbidity and mortality associated with the disease (Goossens *et al.*, 1998). However, overall, the published evidence is moderate in quality at best (Gostelow *et al.*, 2014) and, apart from a history of steroid administration (Roomp and Rand, 2009) and the IGF-I response to insulin (Strage *et al.*, 2018) being associated with an increased rate of remission, no single factor predicts successful independence from insulin therapy (Gostelow *et al.*, 2014). Intensive treatment regimens for feline diabetes impact on quality of life, with the risk of hypoglycaemia perceived by owners as one of the biggest concerns (Niessen *et al.*, 2010), despite the fact that it is uncommon in glargine-treated cats (Roomp and Rand, 2015) and symptomatic hypoglycaemia is usually explained by vomiting after a meal or accidental double-dosing of insulin (Viebrock and Dennis, 2018). This highlights the importance of good communication between veterinary physicians and owners, in a collaborative approach that allows individualized care (Lewitt *et al.*, 2016). This requires that owners be provided with evidence and choice, as in the human domain, where the International Diabetes Federation recommends that diabetes self-management education is critical in laying the foundation for effective care in T2DM (International Diabetes Federation, 2012). It has been reported that, amongst owners willing to take on the task of home blood glucose monitoring, there is a positive impact on quality of life for pet and owner, even in the absence of an impact on glycaemic control (Hazuchova *et al.*, 2018). Continuous glucose monitoring systems have been tested in cats and would provide an alternative that reduces the number of venepunctures and therefore potentia stress to the animal (Ristic *et al.*, 2005).

While insulin remains the mainstay of treatment of feline diabetes, a response to the oral hypoglycaemic agent glipizide is observed in approximately 50% of animals where there is residual β-cell function (Miller *et al.*, 1992; Nelson *et al.*, 1993). Pioglitazone improves insulin sensitivity and improves lipid metabolism in obese cats (Clark *et al.*, 2014) and therefore shows promise. Use of the α-glucosidase inhibitor, acarbose, along with a low carbohydrate diet, is associated with reduced insulin requirements, particularly in obese cats (Mazzaferro *et al.*, 2003). Alternative approaches are emerging that parallel the developments in human medicine. Glucagon-like peptide-1 (GLP-1) is an incretin, secreted in response to food intake and increasing insulin secretion and sensitivity. It is lower in obese, compared with lean cats, in the fasting state and following oral glucose (Hoenig *et al.*, 2010) and increased in cats with diabetes compared with lean and obese animals (McMillan *et al.*, 2016). GLP-1 receptor agonists reduce appetite and body weight, and increase insulin and decrease glucagon concentrations in healthy cats (Hall *et al.*, 2015) and, when added to the insulin regimen in diabetic cats, are associated with weight loss and decreased insulin requirements (Scuderi *et al.*, 2018). A better understanding of the normal feline incretin response to dietary macronutrients (McCool *et al.*, 2018) will contribute to understanding the role these agonists might play. The sodium-glucose cotransporter two inhibitor, velaglifiozin, increases urinary glucose excretion in obese cats (Hoenig *et al.*, 2018), and may be useful in the future management of hyperglycaemia.

One Health Approach to Obesity and Diabetes

One Health has been a long history of rediscovery (Evans and Leighton, 2014), and has expanded even further since the American Veterinary Medical Association and American Medical Association resolved to increase collaboration between their communities (Gibbs, 2014). Although there is no standard definition, the concept of how to improve animal and human health through interdisciplinary approaches is a useful one. The One Health concept thus implies that feline conditions should not be seen as simply models of human disease. In the context of obesity and diabetes, it is clear that a sharing of knowledge and clinical practice is helpful to feline and human medicine. There are shared lifestyle and environmental factors underpinning obesity that can be addressed concurrently and in interdisciplinary ways (Sandoe *et al.*, 2014;

Bomberg *et al.*, 2017; Chandler *et al.*, 2017). In diabetes care, human medicine could learn from the emphasis on intensive management while veterinary medicine could learn from the shift to precision medicine based on better disease classification.

Human–animal social interaction is important in the management of obesity in pets (Linder and Mueller, 2014; De Godoy and Shoveller, 2017) and there is evidence that managing diabetes in pets pivots on their recognition as 'sentient selves' (Rock and Babinec, 2008). It is imperative to involve the owner closely in environment and behaviour modification (Murphy, 2016) and in the complexities of diabetes management (Lewitt *et al.*, 2016). While there is evidence of a closer relationship between overweight cats and their owners, playing with the cat is more important to the owners of normal weight cats (Kienzle and Bergler, 2006). It has been suggested that styles of pet ownership might mirror parenting styles and provide comparative insights into the links to childhood obesity (German, 2015). Behavioural addiction treatment methods are recommended for both overweight children and overweight pets, and studies of outcomes of these approaches are likely to be of value to both disciplines (Pretlow and Corbee, 2016).

Summary and Recommendations

Our understanding of the pathophysiology and management of feline obesity and diabetes has developed in parallel to human medicine. The definition of human overweight and obesity, and the classification of human diabetes is being challenged. In the light of this, it is timely to reconsider feline obesity and diabetes. In particular, a reclassification of diabetes that is management-focussed would seem appropriate. The diabetes of hypersomatotropism and that associated with exogenous glucocorticoid administration, for example, might be classified separately. The BCS appears to be a good diagnostic tool. It is reliable in the hands of owners and is likely to reflect visceral adiposity. Therefore, given the limitations in the use of BMI that have been identified in human medicine, efforts to develop a similar index for cats would seem unnecessary. As in human medicine, overweight and obesity are associated with the development of diabetes; however, there are other genetic and environmental influences that contribute to this risk, some of which are shared. Rather regarding feline obesity and diabetes as models of human disease, a closer interdisciplinary 'One Health' approach between veterinary and human medicine is warranted to advance research and clinical care in this field.

Acknowledgement

The author is grateful to Marisa Stevenson for helpful comments on manuscript drafts.

References

Afzal, S. and Nordestgaard, B.G. (2016) Body mass index and all-cause mortality-reply. *JAMA* 316(9), 992.

Ahlqvist, E., Storm, P., Karajamaki, A., Martinell, M., Dorkhan, M. *et al.* (2018) Novel subgroups of adult-onset diabetes and their association with outcomes: A data-driven cluster analysis of six variables. *The Lancet. Diabetes & Endocrinology* 6(5), 361–369.

Alhaddad, H., Khan, R., Grahn, R.A., Gandolfi, B., Mullikin, J.C. *et al.* (2013) Extent of linkage disequilibrium in the domestic cat, *Felis silvestris catus*, and its breeds. *PLoS ONE* 8(1), e53537.

Appleton, D.J., Rand, J.S. and Sunvold, G.D. (2001) Insulin sensitivity decreases with obesity, and lean cats with low insulin sensitivity are at greatest risk of glucose intolerance with weight gain. *Journal of Feline Medicine and Surgery* 3(4), 211–228.

Berryman, D.E. and List, E.O. (2017) Growth hormone's effect on adipose tissue: Quality versus quantity. *International Journal of Molecular Sciences* 18(8), E1621. DOI: 10.3390/ijms18081621.

Bjornvad, C.R., Rand, J.S., Tan, H.Y., Jensen, K.S., Rose, F.J. *et al.* (2014) Obesity and sex influence insulin resistance and total and multimer adiponectin levels in adult neutered domestic shorthair client-owned cats. *Domestic Animal Endocrinology* 47, 55–64.

Bomberg, E., Birch, L., Endenburg, N., German, A.J., Neilson, J. *et al.* (2017) The financial costs, behaviour and psychology of obesity: A one health analysis. *Journal of Comparative Pathology* 156(4), 310–325.

Bost, P.C., Strynar, M.J., Reiner, J.L., Zweigenbaum, J.A., Secoura, P.L. *et al.* (2016) Domestic cats as sentinels for perfluoroalkyl substances: Possible linkages with housing, obesity, and disease. *Environmental Research* 151, 145–153.

Braun, J.M. (2017) Early-life exposure to EDCs: Role in childhood obesity and neurodevelopment. *Nature Reviews. Endocrinology* 13(3), 161–173.

Buse, J., Gundersen, K. and Lukens, F.D. (1957) Steroid diabetes in the cat. *Diabetes* 6(5), 428–432.

Buse, J.B., Caprio, S., Cefalu, W.T., Ceriello, A., Del Prato, S. *et al.* (2009) How do we define cure of diabetes? *Diabetes Care* 32(11), 2133–2135.

Cave N.J., Allan F.J., Schokkenbroek S.L., Metekohy C.A., Pfeiffer D.U. A cross-sectional study to compare changes in the prevalence and risk factors for feline obesity between 1993 and 2007 in New Zealand. Preventive Veterinary Medicine 2012;107(1–2):121–133.

Cave, N.J., Bridges, J.P., Weidgraaf, K. and Thomas, D.G. (2018) Nonlinear mixed models of growth curves from domestic shorthair cats in a breeding colony, housed in a seasonal facility to predict obesity. *Journal of Animal Physiology and Animal Nutrition* 102(5), 1390–1400.

Chandler, M., Cunningham, S., Lund, E.M., Khanna, C., Naramore, R. *et al.* (2017) Obesity and associated comorbidities in people and companion animals: A one health perspective. *Journal of Comparative Pathology* 156(4), 296–309.

Churchill, J. and Ward, E. (2016) Communicating with pet owners about obesity: Roles of the veterinary health care team. *The Veterinary Clinics of North America. Small Animal Practice* 46(5), 899–911.

Clark, M. and Hoenig, M. (2016) Metabolic effects of obesity and its interaction with endocrine diseases. *The Veterinary Clinics of North America. Small Animal Practice* 46(5), 797–815.

Clark, M., Thomaseth, K., Dirikolu, L., Ferguson, D.C., Hoenig, M. Effects of pioglitazone on insulin sensitivity and serum lipids in obese cats. Journal of Veterinary Internal Medicine 2014;28(1):166–174.

Coradini, M., Rand, J.S., Morton, J.M., Rawlings, J.M. Metabolic determinants of body weight after cats were fed a low-carbohydrate high-protein diet or a high-carbohydrate low-protein diet ad libitum for 8 wk. Domestic Animal Endocrinology 2014;49:70–79.

Courcier, E.A., O'Higgins, R., Mellor, D.J., Yam, P.S. Prevalence and risk factors for feline obesity in a first opinion practice in Glasgow, Scotland. Journal of Feline Medicine and Surgery 2010;12(10):746–753.

De Godoy, M.R., Ochi, K., De Oliveira Mateus, L.F., De Justino, A.C. and Swanson, K.S. (2015) Feeding frequency, but not dietary water content, affects voluntary physical activity in young lean adult female cats. *Journal of Animal Science* 93(5), 2597–2601.

De Godoy, M.R., Shoveller, A.K. (2017) Overweight adult cats have significantly lower voluntary physical activity than adult lean cats. *Journal of Feline Medicine and Surgery* 19(12), 1267–1273.

Deagle, G., Holden, S.L., Biourge, V., Morris, P.J. and German, A.J. (2014) Long-term follow-up after weight management in obese cats. *Journal of Nutritional Science* 3, e25.

Deng, P., Iwazaki, E., Suchy, S.A., Pallotto, M.R. and Swanson, K.S. (2014) Effects of feeding frequency and dietary water content on voluntary physical activity in healthy adult cats. *Journal of Animal Science* 92(3), 1271–1277.

Des Courtis, X., Wei, A., Kass, P.H., Fascetti, A.J., Graham, J.L. *et al.* (2015) Influence of dietary protein level on body composition and energy expenditure in calorically restricted overweight cats. *Journal of Animal Physiology and Animal Nutrition* 99(3), 474–482.

Detweiler, K.B., Rawal, S., Swanson, K.S. and Godoy, M.R.C. (2017) Physical activity level of female and male adult cats before and after running wheel habituation. *Journal of Nutritional Science* 6, e17.

Dohan, F.C. and Lukens, F.D. (1947) Lesions of the pancreatic islets produced in cats by administration of glucose. *Science* 105(2720), 183.

Dreval, A.V., Trigolosova, I.V., Misnikova, I.V., Kovalyova, Y.A., Tishenina, R.S. *et al.* (2014) Prevalence of diabetes mellitus in patients with acromegaly. *Endocrine Connections* 3(2), 93–98.

Dubois, L., Ohm Kyvik, K., Girard, M., Tatone-Tokuda, F., Perusse, D. *et al.* (2012) Genetic and environmental contributions to weight, height, and BMI from birth to 19 years of age: An international study of over 12,000 twin pairs. *PLoS ONE* 7(2), e30153.

Engin, A. (2017) The definition and prevalence of obesity and metabolic syndrome. *Advances in Experimental Medicine and Biology* 960, 1–17.

Evans, B.R. and Leighton, F.A. (2014) A history of one health. *Revue Scientifique et Technique* 33(2), 413–420.

Finn, J.P., Martin, C.L. and Manns, J.G. (1970) Feline pancreatic islet cell hyalinosis associated with diabetes mellitus and lowered serum-insulin concentrations. *Journal of Small Animal Practice* 11(9), 607–619.

Flanagan, J., Bissot, T., Hours, M.A., Moreno, B. and German, A.J. (2018) An international multi-centre cohort study of weight loss in overweight cats: Differences in outcome in different geographical locations. *PLoS ONE* 13(7), e0200414.

Fletcher, J.M., Scudder, C.J., Kiupel, M., Pipe-Martin, H.N., Kenny, P.J. *et al.* (2016) Hypersomatotropism in 3 cats without concurrent diabetes mellitus. *Journal of Veterinary Internal Medicine* 30(4), 1216–1221.

Forcada, Y., Holder, A., Church, D.B. and Catchpole, B. (2014) A polymorphism in the melanocortin 4 receptor gene (MC4R: c.92C>T) is associated with diabetes mellitus in overweight domestic short-haired cats. *Journal of Veterinary Internal Medicine* 28(2), 458–464.

German, A.J. (2015) Style over substance: What can parenting styles tell us about ownership styles and obesity in companion animals? *British Journal of Nutrition* 113(Suppl), S72–S77.

German, A.J. (2016) Obesity prevention and weight maintenance after loss. *The Veterinary Clinics of North America. Small Animal Practice* 46(5), 913–929.

German, A.J. (2016) Weight management in obese pets: The tailoring concept and how it can improve results. *Acta Veterinaria Scandinavica* 58, 57.

Gibbs, E.P. (2014) The evolution of one health: A decade of progress and challenges for the future. *The Veterinary Record* 174(4), 85–91.

Gilor, C., Graves, T.K., Lascelles, B.D., Thomson, A.E., Simpson, W. *et al.* (2010) The effects of body weight, body condition score, sex, and age on serum fructosamine concentrations in clinically healthy cats. *Veterinary Clinical Pathology* 39(3), 322–328.

Gilor, C., Niessen, S.J., Furrow, E. and DiBartola, S.P. (2016) What's in a name? Classification of diabetes mellitus in veterinary medicine and why it matters. *Journal of Veterinary Internal Medicine* 30(4), 927–940.

Goossens, M.M., Nelson, R.W., Feldman, E.C. and Griffey, S.M. (1998) Response to insulin treatment and survival in 104 cats with diabetes mellitus (1985–1995). *Journal of Veterinary Internal Medicine* 12(1), 1–6.

Gostelow, R., Forcada, Y., Graves, T., Church, D. and Niessen, S. (2014) Systematic review of feline diabetic remission: Separating fact from opinion. *Veterinary Journal* 202(2), 208–221.

Gregg, E.W., Cheng, Y.J., Cadwell, B.L., Imperatore, G., Williams, D.E. *et al.* (2005) Secular trends in cardiovascular disease risk factors according to body mass index in US adults. *JAMA* 293(15), 1868–1874.

Gunther, I., Raz, T. and Klement, E. (2018) Association of neutering with health and welfare of urban free-roaming cat population in Israel, during 2012–2014. *Preventive Veterinary Medicine* 157, 26–33.

Hall, M.J., Adin, C.A., Borin-Crivellenti, S., Rudinsky, A.J., Rajala-Schultz, P. *et al.* (2015) Pharmacokinetics and pharmacodynamics of the glucagon-like peptide-1 analog liraglutide in healthy cats. *Domestic Animal Endocrinology* 51, 114–121.

Haring, T., Wichert, B., Dolf, G. and Haase, B. (2011) Segregation analysis of overweight body condition in an experimental cat population. *Journal of Heredity* 102, S28–S31.

Hazuchova, K., Gostelow, R., Scudder, C., Forcada, Y., Church, D.B. *et al.* (2018) Acceptance of home blood glucose monitoring by owners of recently diagnosed diabetic cats and impact on quality of life changes in cat and owner. *Journal of Feline Medicine and Surgery* 20(8), 711–720.

Hebebrand, J., Holm, J.C., Woodward, E., Baker, J.L., Blaak, E. *et al.* (2017) A proposal of the European association for the study of obesity to improve the ICD-11 diagnostic criteria for obesity based on the three dimensions etiology, degree of adiposity and health risk. *Obesity Facts* 10(4), 284–307.

Hewson-Hughes, A.K., Gilham, M.S., Upton, S., Colyer, A., Butterwick, R. *et al.* (2011) The effect of dietary starch level on postprandial glucose and insulin concentrations in cats and dogs. *British Journal of Nutrition* S105–S109.

Hoenig, M. (2006) The cat as a model for human nutrition and disease. *Current Opinion in Clinical Nutrition and Metabolic Care* 9(5), 584–588.

Hoenig, M., Thomaseth, K., Waldron, M. and Ferguson, D.C. (2007) Insulin sensitivity, fat distribution, and adipocytokine response to different diets in lean and obese cats before and after weight loss. *American Journal of Physiology. Regulatory, Integrative and Comparative Physiology* 292(1), R227–R234.

Hoenig, M., Jordan, E.T., Ferguson, D.C. and Vries, F. (2010) Oral glucose leads to a differential response in glucose, insulin, and GLP-1 in lean versus obese cats. *Domestic Animal Endocrinology* 38(2), 95–102.

Hoenig, M., Clark, M., Schaeffer, D.J. and Reiche, D. (2018) Effects of the sodium-glucose cotransporter 2 (SGLT2) inhibitor velagliflozin, a new drug with therapeutic potential to treat diabetes in cats. *Journal of Veterinary Pharmacology and Therapeutics* 41(2), 266–273.

Hu, Y., Li, L., Xu, Y., Yu, T., Tong, G. *et al.* (2011) Short-term intensive therapy in newly diagnosed type 2 diabetes partially restores both insulin sensitivity and beta-cell function in subjects with long-term remission. *Diabetes Care* 34(8), 1848–1853.

International Diabetes Federation (2012) *Global guideline for type 2 diabetes*. ISBN 2-930229-43-8

Janssen, I., Katzmarzyk, P.T. and Ross, R. (2004) Waist circumference and not body mass index explains obesity-related health risk. *American Journal of Clinical Nutrition* 79(3), 379–384.

Kawasumi, K., Iwazaki, E., Okada, Y. and Arai, T. (2016) Effectiveness of feline body mass index (fBMI) as new diagnostic tool for obesity. *Japanese Journal of Veterinary Research* 64(1), 51–56.

Keller, C., Liesegang, A., Frey, D. and Wichert, B. (2017) Metabolic response to three different diets in lean cats and cats predisposed to overweight. *BMC Veterinary Research* 13(1), 184.

Kenny, P.J., Scudder, C., Keyte, S.V., Swann, J.W., Fowkes, R.C. *et al.* (2015) Experiences of a newly established hypophysectomy clinic for treatment of feline hypersomatotropism. *Journal of Veterinary Internal Medicine* 29, 319–350.

Kienzle, E. and Bergler, R. (2006) Human-animal relationship of owners of normal and overweight cats. *Journal of Nutrition* 136, 1947S–1950S.

Laflamme, D. (1997) Development and validation of a body condition score system for cats: A clinical tool. *Feline Practice* 25(5–6), 13–18.

Larsen, J.A. (2017) Risk of obesity in the neutered cat. *Journal of Feline Medicine and Surgery* 19(8), 779–783.

Larsen, J.A. and Villaverde, C. (2016) Scope of the problem and perception by owners and veterinarians. *The Veterinary Clinics of North America. Small Animal Practice* 46(5), 761–772.

Lederer, R., Rand, J.S., Jonsson, N.N., Hughes, I.P. and Morton, J.M. (2009) Frequency of feline diabetes mellitus and breed predisposition in domestic cats in Australia. *Veterinary Journal* 179(2), 254–258.

Lewitt, M.S., Strage, E. and Church, D. (2016) An individual approach to feline diabetes care: A case report and literature review. *Acta Veterinaria Scandinavica* 58, 63.

Lichtensteiger, C.A., Wortman, J.A. and Eigenmann, J.E. (1986) Functional pituitary acidophil adenoma in a cat with diabetes mellitus and acromegalic features. *Veterinary Pathology* 23(4), 518–521.

Linder, D. and Mueller, M. (2014) Pet obesity management: Beyond nutrition. *The Veterinary Clinics of North America. Small Animal Practice* 44(4), 789–806.

Liu, G., Dhana, K., Furtado, J.D., Rood, J., Zong, G. *et al.* (2018) Perfluoroalkyl substances and changes in body weight and resting metabolic rate in response to weight-loss diets: A prospective study. *PLoS Medicine* 15(2), e1002502.

Loftus, J.P. and Wakshlag, J.J. (2015) Canine and feline obesity: A review of pathophysiology, epidemiology, and clinical management. *Veterinary Medicine* 6, 49–60.

Lukens, F.D., Cohen, S.N. and Goto, Y. (1961) Steroid diabetes in the cat. protection of the islets by insulin or phlorhizin. *Diabetes* 10, 182–189.

Lund E.M. Prevalence and risk factors for obesity in adult cats from private US veterinary practices. *International Journal of Applied Research in Veterinary Medicine* 2005;3(2):88–96.

Lutz, T.A. and Rand, J.S. (1993) A review of new developments in type 2 diabetes in human beings and cats. *The British Veterinary Journal* 149(6), 527–536.

Lutz, T.A. and Rand, J.S. (1996) Plasma amylin and insulin concentrations in normoglycemic and hyperglycemic cats. *The Canadian Veterinary Journal* 37(1), 27–34.

Mazzaferro, E.M., Greco, D.S., Turner, A.S., Fettman, M.J. (2003) Treatment of feline diabetes mellitus using an α-glucosidase inhibitor and a low-carbohydrate diet. *Journal of Feline Medicine & Surgery* 5(3), 183–189.

McCool, K.E., Rudinsky, A.J., Parker, V.J., Herbert, C.O. and Gilor, C. (2018) The effect of diet, adiposity, and weight loss on the secretion of incretin hormones in cats. *Domestic Animal Endocrinology* 62, 67–75.

McMillan, C.J., Zapata, R.C., Chelikani, P.K., Snead, E.C. and Cosford, K. (2016) Circulating concentrations of glucagon-like peptide 1, glucose-dependent insulinotropic peptide, peptide YY, and insulin in client-owned lean, overweight, and diabetic cats. *Domestic Animal Endocrinology* 54, 85–94.

Miller A.B., Nelson R.W., Kirk C.A., Neal L., Feldman E.C. Effect of glipizide on serum insulin and glucose concentrations in healthy cats. Research in Veterinary Science 1992;52(2):177–181.

Murphy, M. (2016) Obesity treatment: Environment and behavior modification. *The Veterinary Clinics of North America. Small Animal Practice* 46(5), 883–898.

Nack, R. and DeClue, A.E. (2014) In cats with newly diagnosed diabetes mellitus, use of a near-euglycemic management paradigm improves remission rate over a traditional paradigm. *Veterinary Quarterly* 34(3), 132–136.

Nelson, R.W. and Reusch, C.E. (2014) Animal models of disease: classification and etiology of diabetes in dogs and cats. *Journal of Endocrinology* 222(3), T1–T9.

Nelson, R.W., Himsel, C.A., Feldman, E.C. and Bottoms, G.D. (1990) Glucose tolerance and insulin response in normal-weight and obese cats. *American Journal of Veterinary Research* 51(9), 1357–1362.

Nelson, R.W., Feldman, E.C., Ford, S.L., Roemer, O.P. (1993) Effect of an orally administered sulfonylurea, glipizide, for treatment of diabetes mellitus in cats. *Journal of the American Veterinary Medical Association* 203(6), 821–827.

Niaz, K., Maqbool, F., Khan, F., Hassan, F.I., Momtaz, S. *et al.* (2018) Comparative occurrence of diabetes in canine, feline, and few wild animals and their association with pancreatic diseases and ketoacidosis with therapeutic approach. *Veterinary World* 11(4), 410–422.

Niessen, S.J., Powney, S., Guitian, J., Niessen, A.P., Pion, P.D. *et al.* (2010) Evaluation of a quality-of-life tool for cats with diabetes mellitus. *Journal of Veterinary Internal Medicine* 24(5), 1098–1105.

Niessen, S.J., Church, D.B. and Forcada, Y. (2013) Hypersomatotropism, acromegaly, and hyperadrenocorticism and feline diabetes mellitus. *The Veterinary Clinics of North America. Small Animal Practice* 43(2), 319–350.

Niessen, S.J., Forcada, Y., Mantis, P., Lamb, C.R., Harrington, N. *et al.* (2015) Studying cat (*Felis catus*) diabetes: Beware of the acromegalic imposter. *PLoS ONE* 10(5), e0127794.

Ohlund, M., Fall, T., Strom Holst, B., Hansson-Hamlin, H., Bonnett, B. *et al.* (2015) Incidence of diabetes mellitus in insured Swedish cats in relation to age, breed and sex. *Journal of Veterinary Internal Medicine* 29(5), 1342–1347.

Öhlund, M., Egenvall, A., Fall, T., Hansson-Hamlin, H., Röcklinsberg, H. *et al.* (2017) Environmental risk factors for diabetes mellitus in cats. *Journal of Veterinary Internal Medicine* 31(1), 29–35.

Ohlund, M., Palmgren, M. and Holst, B.S. (2018) Overweight in adult cats: A cross-sectional study. *Acta Veterinaria Scandinavica* 60(1), 5.

Okada, Y., Kobayashi, M., Sawamura, M. and Arai, T. (2017) Comparison of visceral fat accumulation and metabolome markers among cats of varying BCS and novel classification of feline obesity and metabolic syndrome. *Frontiers in Veterinary Science* 4, 17.

O'Neill, D.G., Gostelow, R., Orme, C., Church, D.B., Niessen, S.J. *et al.* (2016) Epidemiology of diabetes mellitus among 193,435 cats attending primary-care veterinary practices in England. *Journal of Veterinary Internal Medicine* 30(4), 964–972.

Ortega, F.B., Cadenas-Sanchez, C., Migueles, J.H., Labayen, I., Ruiz, J.R. *et al.* (2018) Role of physical activity and fitness in the characterization and prognosis of the metabolically healthy obesity phenotype: A systematic review and meta-analysis. *Progress in Cardiovascular Diseases* 61(2), 190–205.

Osto, M. and Lutz, T.A. (2015) Translational value of animal models of obesity-focus on dogs and cats. *European Journal of Pharmacology* 759, 240–252.

Pallotto, M.R., Godoy, M.R.C., Holscher, H.D., Buff, P.R. and Swanson, K.S. (2018) Effects of weight loss with a moderate-protein, high-fiber diet on body composition, voluntary physical activity, and fecal microbiota of obese cats. *American Journal of Veterinary Research* 79(2), 181–190.

Panciera, D.L., Thomas, C.B., Eicker, S.W. and Atkins, C.E. (1990) Epizootiologic patterns of diabetes mellitus in cats: 333 cases (1980–1986). *Journal of the American Veterinary Medical Association* 197(11), 1504–1508.

Peron, L., Rahal, S.C., Castilho, M.S., Melchert, A., Vassalo, F.G. *et al.* (2016) Owners perception for detecting feline body condition based on questionnaire and scores. *Topics in Companion Animal Medicine* 31(3), 122–124.

Phillips, A.M., Coe, J.B., Rock, M.J. and Adams, C.L. (2017) Feline obesity in veterinary medicine: Insights from a thematic analysis of communication in practice. *Frontiers in Veterinary Science* (4), 117.

Prahl, A., Guptill, L., Glickman, N.W., Tetrick, M. and Glickman, L.T. (2007) Time trends and risk factors for diabetes mellitus in cats presented to veterinary teaching hospitals. *Journal of Feline Medicine and Surgery* 9(5), 351–358.

Pretlow, R.A. and Corbee, R.J. (2016) Similarities between obesity in pets and children: The addiction model. *British Journal of Nutrition* 116(5), 944–949.

Rand, J.S., Kinnaird, E., Baglioni, A., Blackshaw, J. and Priest, J. (2002) Acute stress hyperglycemia in cats is associated with struggling and increased concentrations of lactate and norepinephrine. *Journal of Veterinary Internal Medicine* 16(2), 123–132.

Reeve-Johnson, M.K., Rand, J.S., Anderson, S.T., Appleton, D.J., Morton, J.M. *et al.* (2016) Dosing obese cats based on body weight spuriously affects some measures of glucose tolerance. *Domestic Animal Endocrinology* 57, 133–142.

Reeve-Johnson, M.K., Rand, J.S., Vankan, D., Anderson, S.T., Marshall, R. *et al.* (2016) Diagnosis of prediabetes in cats: Glucose concentration cut points for impaired fasting glucose and impaired glucose tolerance. *Domestic Animal Endocrinology* 57, 55–62.

Reusch, C.E., Liehs, M.R., Hoyer, M. and Fructosamine, V.R. (1993) A new parameter for diagnosis and metabolic control in diabetic dogs and cats. *Journal of Veterinary Internal Medicine* 7(3), 177–182.

Ristic, J.M.E., Herrtage, M.E., Walti-Lauger, S.M.M., Slater, L.A., Church, D.B., Davison, L.J. *et al.* (2005) Evaluation of a continuous glucose monitoring system in cats with diabetes mellitus. *Journal of Feline Medicine and Surgery* 7(3), 153–162.

Rock, M. and Babinec, P. (2008) Diabetes in people, cats, and dogs: Biomedicine and manifold ontologies. *Medical Anthropology* 27(4), 324–352.

Roomp, K. and Rand, J. (2009) Intensive blood glucose control is safe and effective in diabetic cats using home monitoring and treatment with glargine. *Journal of Feline Medicine and Surgery* 11(8), 668–682.

Roomp, K. and Rand, J. (2015) Rebound hyperglycaemia in diabetic cats. *Journal of Feline Medicine and Surgery* 18(8), 587–596.

Rorsman, P. and Ashcroft, F.M. (2018) Pancreatic beta-cell electrical activity and insulin secretion: Of mice and men. *Physiological Reviews* 98(1), 117–214.

Rowe, E., Browne, W., Casey, R., Gruffydd-Jones, T. and Murray, J. (2015) Risk factors identified for owner-reported feline obesity at around one year of age: Dry diet and indoor lifestyle. *Preventive Veterinary Medicine* 121(3–4), 273–281.

Rowe, E.C., Browne, W.J., Casey, R.A., Gruffydd-Jones, T.J. and Murray, J.K. (2017) Early-life risk factors identified for owner-reported feline overweight and obesity at around two years of age. *Preventive Veterinary Medicine* 143, 39–48.

Sandoe, P., Palmer, C., Corr, S., Astrup, A. and Bjornvad, C.R. (2014) Canine and feline obesity: A one health perspective. *The Veterinary Record* 175(24), 610–616.

Scuderi, M.A., Ribeiro Petito, M., Unniappan, S., Waldner, C., Mehain, S. *et al.* (2018) Safety and efficacy assessment of a GLP-1 mimetic: Insulin glargine combination for treatment of feline diabetes mellitus. *Domestic Animal Endocrinology* 65, 80–89.

Slingerland, L.I., Fazilova, V.V., Plantinga, E.A., Kooistra, H.S. and Beynen, A.C. (2009) Indoor confinement and physical inactivity rather than the proportion of dry food are risk factors in the development of feline type 2 diabetes mellitus. *Veterinary Journal* 179(2), 247–253.

Stogdale, L. (1986) Definition of diabetes mellitus. *The Cornell Veterinarian* 76(2), 156–174.

Stoner, L. and Cornwall, J. (2014) Did the american medical association make the correct decision classifying obesity as a disease? *The Australasian Medical Journal* 7(11), 462–464.

Strage, E.M., Theodorsson, E., Strom Holst, B., Lilliehook, I. and Lewitt, M.S. (2015) Insulin-like growth factor I in cats: Validation of an enzyme-linked immunosorbent assay and determination of biologic variation. *Veterinary Clinical Pathology* 44(4), 542–551.

Strage, E.M., Sundberg, M., Holst, B.S., Andersson Franko, M., Ramstrom, M. *et al.* (2018) Effect of insulin treatment on circulating insulin-like growth factor i and IGF-binding proteins in cats with diabetes mellitus. *Journal of Veterinary Internal Medicine*.

Takashima, S., Nishii, N., Kato, A., Matsubara, T., Shibata, S. *et al.* (2016) Molecular cloning of feline resistin and the expression of resistin, leptin and adiponectin in the adipose tissue of normal and obese cats. *Journal of Veterinary Medical Science* 78(1), 23–28.

Teng, K.T., McGreevy, P.D., Toribio, J., Raubenheimer, D., Kendall, K. *et al.* (2017) Risk factors for underweight and overweight in cats in metropolitan Sydney, Australia. *Preventive Veterinary Medicine* 144, 102–111.

Thomas, D.G., Post, M. and Bosch, G. (2017) The effect of changing the moisture levels of dry extruded and wet canned diets on physical activity in cats. *Journal of Nutritional Science* 6, e9.

Van de Velde, H., Janssens, G.P., De Rooster, H., Polis, I., Peters, I. *et al.* (2013) The cat as a model for human obesity: Insights into depot-specific inflammation associated with feline obesity. *British Journal of Nutrition* 110(7), 1326–1335.

Vandendriessche, V.L., Picavet, P. and Hesta, M. (2017) First detailed nutritional survey in a referral companion animal population. *Journal of Animal Physiology and Animal Nutrition* 101, 4–14.

Verbrugghe, A. and Hesta, M. (2017) Cats and carbohydrates: The carnivore fantasy? *Veterinary Science* 4(4), E55.

Viebrock, K.A. and Dennis, J. (2018) Hypoglycemic episodes in cats with diabetes mellitus: 30 cases (2013–2015). *Journal of Feline Medicine and Surgery* 20(6), 563–570.

Villaverde, C. and Fascetti, A.J. (2014) Macronutrients in feline health. *The Veterinary Clinics of North America. Small Animal Practice* 44(4), v–vi.

World Health Organisation (2006) Definition and diagnosis of diabetes mellitus and intermediate hyperglycemia: Report of a WHO/IDF consultation. ISBN 92 4 159493 4

World Health Organisation (2018) *International Classification of Diseases ICD-11*. Available at: http://www.who.int/classifications/icd/en

Yang, L., He, Z., Tang, X. and Liu, J. (2013) Type 2 diabetes mellitus and the risk of acute pancreatitis: A meta-analysis. *European Journal of Gastroenterology & Hepatology* 25(2), 225–231.

Zapata, R.C., Meachem, M.D., Cardoso, N.C., Mehain, S.O., McMillan, C.J. *et al.* (2017) Differential circulating concentrations of adipokines, glucagon and adropin in a clinical population of lean, overweight and diabetic cats. *BMC Veterinary Research* 13(1), 85.

Zeugswetter, F.K., Polsterer, T., Krempl, H. and Schwendenwein, I. (2018) Basal glucosuria in cats. *Journal of Animal Physiology and Animal Nutrition (Berl)* 103(1), 324–330.

Zini, E., Osto, M., Moretti, S., Franchini, M., Kook, P.H. *et al.* (2010) Hyperglycaemia but not hyperlipidaemia decreases serum amylase and increases neutrophils in the exocrine pancreas of cats. *Research in Veterinary Science* 89(1), 20–26.

Zini, E., Hafner, M., Kook, P., Lutz, T.A., Ohlerth, S. *et al.* (2015) Longitudinal evaluation of serum pancreatic enzymes and ultrasonographic findings in diabetic cats without clinically relevant pancreatitis at diagnosis. *Journal of Veterinary Internal Medicine* 29(2), 589–596.

24 Integrative View of Diseases in Ruminants: Towards a Holistic Model

Ricardo Piña-Martínez[1], Cintli Martínez-Ortiz-de-Montellano[1]*, Claudia Cecilia Márquez-Mota[2] and Edgar Dantán-González[3]

[1]Departamento de Parasitología, Facultad de Medicina Veterinaria y Zootecnia, Universidad Nacional Autónoma de México, Colonia UNAM, CU, Delegación Coyoacán, C.P. 04510, Ciudad de México, México; [2]Departamento de Nutrición Animal y Bioquímica, Facultad de Medicina Veterinaria y Zootecnia, Universidad Nacional Autónoma de México, Colonia UNAM, CU, Delegación Coyoacán, C.P. 04510, Ciudad de México, México; [3]Centro de Investigación en Biotecnología, Universidad Autónoma del Estado de Morelos, Av. Universidad 1001, Colonia Chamilpa, Cuernavaca, Morelos, 62209, México

Abstract

The holobiontic approach in ruminants presents an integrative vision of the organism, where both the microbiota and macrobiota are considered distinct entities that influence animal welfare. The early establishment of these communities in the ruminant holobiont is crucial for regulating digestive, immunological, and metabolic processes. Not only do they facilitate fiber breakdown in the rumen, but they also play a key role in disease prevention, helping the animal resist pathological imbalances. The gastrointestinal ecosystem is significantly influenced by both biotic factors, such as nutrition, and abiotic factors, like drug use. The resistance of the microbiota and macrobiota in ruminants is essential, as it affects the success of conventional treatments and parasite management and can disrupt the balance within these populations. In this context, the veterinarian plays a critical role in preserving these ecological niches, ensuring equilibrium and functionality through effective therapeutic interventions and continuous monitoring. Holistic strategies, including integrated parasite management and omics sciences, allow for more comprehensive analyses and a deeper understanding of infectious diseases in ruminants. These approaches promote sustainability in animal health and ensure a holistic view that supports the welfare of animals and the ecosystems they inhabit, aligning with the One Welfare concept.

Keywords: holobiont, ruminants, macrobiota, microbiota, animal welfare, One Welfare

Introduction

Animal welfare is a critical component of the health and productivity of ruminants. As conceptualized by the OIE (2024), animal welfare is rooted in the five fundamental freedoms: freedom from hunger, thirst, and malnutrition; freedom from fear and *distress*; freedom from physical and thermal discomfort; freedom from pain, injury, and disease; and freedom to express natural behavior. It is important to recognize that both biotic and abiotic factors significantly

*Corresponding author: cintli@unam.mx

impact the well-being of the ruminant *holobiont*. Various factors can induce stress, either *eustress* (positive) or *distress* (negative), which directly affect homeostasis (Muñoz-Vargas *et al.*, 2023). In ruminant production, the goal of the food security system is to ensure that all individuals have physical and economic access to sufficient, safe, and nutritious food that meets their dietary needs (FAO, 2011). However, the relationship between animal welfare and food security has largely been approached from a commercial standpoint, resulting in a limited understanding. This narrow perspective presents several challenges, including the tendency to view the relationship as a misunderstood trend and to equate animal welfare with quality consumption. Furthermore, these concepts are often used in marketing and sales strategies, distorting their true meaning. Nevertheless, the need to increase productivity and reduce food safety risks remains essential, all while preserving public health and, above all, consumer confidence (Muñoz-Vargas *et al.*, 2023).

Within the context of *One Welfare*, which recognizes the interconnections between animal–human welfare, and the physical and social environment (García-Pinillos, 2017), it is essential to develop holistic preventive veterinary programs that prioritize the overall health of ruminants. The holobiontic approach to these animals, which considers both the *microbiota* and *macrobiota*, is crucial for their welfare and health. Recent studies have shown that helminths, especially nematodes, which are part of the macrobiota, play a vital role in shaping the composition and *diversity* of the gastrointestinal microbiota in ruminants. These organisms, far from being mere parasites, contribute as beneficial symbionts to the *host* animal (Limborg *et al.*, 2024). Understanding the interactions between *ecological niches*, such as the microbiota and macrobiota, is key to maintaining a healthy *gastrointestinal ecosystem*. Therefore, it is important to promote the use of cutting-edge feeding technologies, including *prebiotics*, *probiotics*, *postbiotics*, and *eubiotics*, in animal nutrition. These strategies should be supported by omics sciences and not only optimize animal health but also reduce the reliance on chemicals like antibiotics and antiparasitics. This, in turn, reduces the chemical and critical load on ecosystems and enhances the sustainability of animal production systems. The aim of this article is to dynamically incorporate the concepts of a holobiont perspective for a *holistic approach* to infectious diseases in ruminants, utilizing strategies such as integrated parasite management and omics sciences, in alignment with One Welfare principles (Box 24.1).

Review Methodology

The literature consulted for the development of this bibliographic review was obtained from various databases with access to scientific research articles available in high impact factor journals and books related to veterinary parasitology, bacteriology and dynamics studies of the gastrointestinal microbiota in ruminants, as well as articles related to the basics of omics sciences and their application. The main databases consulted were Google Scholar, Science Direct, NCBI-PubMed, Wiley, Frontiers. The search strategy was based on the combination of keywords such as 'microbiota', 'macrobiota', 'holobiont', 'ruminant', 'animal welfare', 'one welfare'. Multiple combinations of these terms were made to obtain an integrative view of the perspective of different authors on the interaction between macrobiota and microbiota in the context of ruminant health and welfare. The search was not limited by country or geographical region, but only recent studies, not older than 10 years, were included. The above search dynamics and selection of articles allow us to have a wide and updated variety of studies from different regions of the world, enriching the study of the interaction between macrobiota and microbiota in ruminants. Mendeley software was used to manage, organize and cite bibliographic references, facilitating the follow-up of the literature reviewed and the correct insertion of citations in the document.

Ruminant Holobiontic Vision

The One Welfare concept (García-Pinillos, 2017) permits the visualization of animal health as

Box 24.1. Glossary.

- **Holistic approach**: Perceiving diseases from an integrative aspect where the properties and components nents of biological systems must be analysed as a whole and not only through their component parts.
- **Abundance**: Refers to the distribution of the bacterial group and the degree of dominance.
- **Animal welfare**: The physical and mental state of an animal in relation to the conditions in which it lives and dies considering the five freedoms: freedom from hunger, thirst and malnutrition, freedom from fear and distress, freedom from physical and thermal discomfort, freedom from pain, injury and disease, and freedom to exhibit natural behavior.
- **Distress**: Chronic and persistent conditions, where pathological alterations can be observed that trigger hormonal and metabolic changes that are difficult to overcome.
- **Dysbiosis**: Imbalance in the composition and taxonomic diversity of the gut ecosystem leading to possibly lethal effects on the holobiont.
- **Diversity**: Species richness or number of species involved in a given microbiota.
- **Gastrointestinal ecosystem**: Biological system composed of bacteria, protozoa, fungi, viruses, archaea and non-living elements interacting with each other in the gastrointestinal lumen.
- **Eubiosis**: Refers to the stability of the intestinal ecosystem in which beneficial species belonging mainly to the phylum Firmicutes and Bacteroidetes predominate.
- **Eubiotic**: Orally administered natural strains of intestinal bacteria that colonise the gastrointestinal tract, thereby preventing the overgrowth of pathogenic micro-organisms and ensuring better digestion and optimal nutrient utilisation.
- **Eustress**: An optimal and adaptive level of stress associated with positive situations and a healthy physiological state.
- **Holobiont**: From the Greek holos (all) and bios (life), it refers to individuals in which there is a huge consortium of interactions in which a large number of species from different taxonomic kingdoms coexist.
- **Host:** Organism component of parasitism that harbours another taxonomically distinct organism that benefits from it and, depending on biotic and abiotic factors, may or may not cause harm to it.
- **Macrobiome:** Diversity of genetic material of the metazoan species that make up the holobiont.
- **Macrobiota:** Population of metazoans interacting with the holobiont and its microbiota.
- **Microbiome:** Diversity of genetic material of the species of micro-organisms residing in the holobiont.
- **Microbiota:** A complex set of interactions between different organisms that make up a biological microsystem in which bacteria, protozoa, fungi, viruses and archaea coexist with another taxonomically superior organism.
- **Ecological niche:** Environmental, biotic and abiotic conditions that interact to enable the existence and coexistence of an individual.
- **Evolutionary niche:** Refers to the sum of disturbing selection factors affecting a population.
- **One Welfare:** Interconnection between animal welfare, human welfare, physical and social environment.
- **Parasitiasis:** The term 'parasitism' refers to a variety of parasitism where the host is able to cope with the presence of parasitic organisms by establishing a balanced relationship that preserves homeostasis.
- **Parasitism:** A symbiotic relationship established between two organisms of different taxonomic origin in which one benefits metabolically while the other may be affected depending on its ability to resist.
- **Parasitosis:** Variety of parasitism where the presence of the parasite overwhelms the host's ability to establish a positive symbiotic relationship leading to homeostatic imbalance and subsequent disease.
- **Pathobiome:** Diversity of genetic material from pathobionts.
- **Pathobiont:** Commensal or opportunistic micro-organisms that under certain conditions are potentially capable of causing homeostatic imbalance leading to the development of disease or death.
- **Perturbation:** Causal event that changes the immediate environment or directly the community and can vary in magnitude, rhythmicity and context.
- **Postbiotic:** Inactivated microbial cells and bioactive cellular components or metabolites generated from fermentation by cultures of active probiotic microorganisms.
- **Prebiotics:** Fructooligosaccharides and galactooligosaccharides derived from non-digestible carbohydrates of the yeast cell wall useful as health promoters of the microbiota.
- **Probiotic:** Live bacteria or yeasts beneficial to intestinal homeostasis.

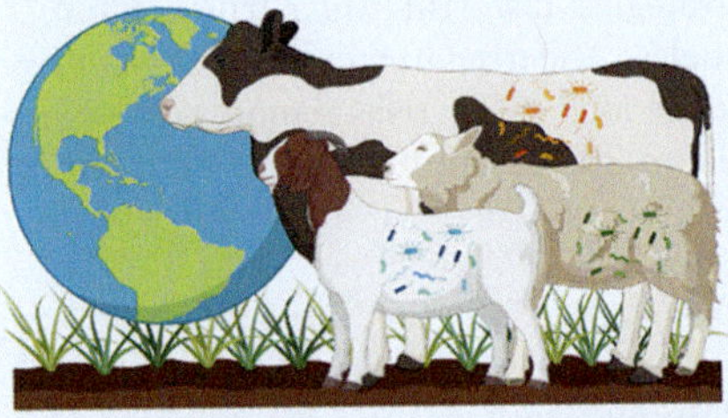

a constituent element of a complex system, designated as the 'planet,' wherein each organism is deemed to play a pivotal role in ensuring optimal functionality. In this context, it can be posited that a holobiont ruminant functions in a similar manner, comprising the ecological niche of millions of microorganisms that constitute a system of dynamic interactions. These interactions are key to the maintenance of a balance that enables the ruminant to enjoy good health and, thus, animal welfare (OIE, 2024). The equilibrium that enables the well-being of ruminants is reinforced by three essential components: the microbiota, the macrobiota, and the gastrointestinal ecosystem. The latter provides most of the factors necessary for the interaction between these groups of organisms to maintain a state of *eubiosis*, which favors the health of the host. The maintenance of homeostasis in this system is contingent upon the presence of not only the macrobiota and microbiota, but also the entirety of the *microbiome* and *macrobiome*. The coexistence of related and unrelated species within this ecosystem is vital for the stability and health of the ruminant, as it promotes biological and functional diversity. The concept of animal welfare cannot be considered in isolation; rather, it must be viewed through a holistic lens. This is because every eukaryotic organism exists within a complex microbial ecosystem. The symbiotic relationship between prokaryotes and eukaryotes is particularly crucial for ruminants within a specific ecosystem. Although this interaction is essential for eukaryotes, prokaryotes do not depend on this coexistence, as they thrived long before eukaryotes emerged (Limborg *et al.*, 2024). Prokaryotes have been inhabitants of Earth for billions of years and have been able to adapt and evolve in multiple environments, which have allowed them to form independent or dependent relationships with eukaryotic organisms.

Establishment of the Microbiota and Macrobiota in the Ruminant Holobiont

Understanding the benefits ruminants derive from their gastrointestinal ecosystem requires examining how newborns acquire the diverse microorganisms that colonize their digestive tract, skin, mucous membranes, and body cavities. In the case of the microbiota, this process is influenced by several factors, including genetics, maternal health, the conditions of parturition, and the choice between artificial or natural lactation. Notably, even if a newborn ruminant is fed exclusively on milk during its initial days or weeks, its gastrointestinal tract is colonized by a diverse microbiota shortly after birth (Cherbuy, 2016; Dunière *et al.*, 2023). The various components of the microbiota are introduced at birth and throughout the early years of life from multiple sources, including the maternal vaginal and vulvar canal, udder mucosa, skin, colostrum, as well as the surrounding environment, bedding feces, and maternal saliva. The presence of the dam or other adult ruminants is critical for the neonate's colonization by bacteria, fungi, and protozoa. For instance, studies have shown that neonates separated from their mothers after parturition exhibit poor establishment of the cellulolytic bacterium *Fibrobacter succinogenes* and protozoa from the genus *Entodinium*, both of which are crucial for digestion and fermentation in the rumen (Chaucheyras-Durand *et al.*, 2019; Dunière *et al.*, 2023; Yu *et al.*, 2024). Weaning represents a focal period in ruminant development, during which the digestive system transitions from monogastric to fermentative, accompanied by the development of the rumen and other compartments. The mature rumen, now exposed to a new fiber-rich diet typical of conventional herbivorous diets, harbors a dense and diverse microbiota (Chiu and Gilbert, 2020). This microbiota is continuously subjected to both biotic and abiotic *perturbations* (Box 24.2). Among the microbiota established in these early stages, certain protozoa can be considered *pathobionts*, such as *Cryptosporidium* species and various *Eimeria* species (Peek *et al.*, 2018; Bowman, 2022), as well as fungi from the genus *Aspergillus* (Peek *et al.*, 2018). Additionally, the gastric compartments harbor complex and still poorly understood interactions involving free viruses and bacteriophages that play a role in the ruminant's life cycle. These interactions encompass not only pathobionts but also *pathobiomes*, which enhance the gastrointestinal ecosystem's diversity by facilitating gene distribution through horizontal gene transfer mechanisms (Gilbert *et al.*, 2020). The establishment of the macrobiota is similarly influenced by the factors mentioned earlier, but it is especially dependent on host characteristics such as age and metabolic state, as well as the nature of the parasites present in the ecological niche. The establishment of *evolutionary niches* between species and the ecological zone in which the ruminants reside are also critical factors (Box 24.2). Through maternal interactions, ruminants can encounter larvae and eggs of helminths, particularly gastrointestinal nematodes, which are abundant and diverse. Notable genera include *Gongylonema, Haemonchus, Teladorsagia, Ostertagia, Toxocara, Trichostrongylus, Cooperia, Strongyloides, Bunostomum, Nematodirus, Oesophagostomum, Chabertia*, and *Trichuris*, as

Box 24.2. Key factors that enable the coexistence of microbiota and macrobiota within the ruminal holobiont (Taken and modified from Martínez Ortiz de Montellano *et al.*, 2022a).

Abiotic environmental factors

- Time of the year.
- Meteorological conditions (Temperature, humidity)
- Radiation
- Global warming, contamination.
- Antibiotic and antiparasitic treatments.

Biotic environmental factors

- Population density
- Eustress (birth, weaning, grazing)
- Distress (malnutrition, bad housing, sickness)
- Interspecific and intraspecific reservoirs

Pathobiont characteristics

- Dose
- Infectivity
- Virulence
- Intergroup competition
- Order of infection time
- Coevolution history

Host characteristics

- Innate and acquired immunity
- Corporal condition
- Age
- Type of housing
- Zootechnical purpose/ physiological stage

well as flatworms from genera such as *Fasciola*, *Paramphistomum*, *Thysanosoma*, and cestodes as *Moniezia* and multiple metacestodes; not to mention numerous arthropods that act as ectoparasites, such as lice, mites, flies, and those responsible for cavitary myiasis (Peek *et al.*, 2018; Bowman, 2022).

The Importance of Microbiota and Macrobiota in the Ruminant Holobiont

Understanding the interaction among various agents such as bacteria, viruses, fungi, protozoa, and metazoa with the host in veterinary medicine is often framed in terms of health compromise or infectious disease. However, many components of the gastrointestinal microbiota and macrobiota in ruminants are either harmless or even beneficial to the host (Cherbuy, 2016). The symbionts residing within the holobiont protect it from enteropathogens, enhance nutrient metabolism, and contribute to optimal immune function (Dunière *et al.*, 2023). It is important to note that not all instances of *parasitism* result in disease or death. A clear example is found in the distinction between the terms *parasitiasis* and *parasitosis*, where the former indicates a state of eustress while the latter is associated with distress (Muñoz-Vargas *et al.*, 2023). Metazoans, particularly helminths, provoke immune responses that incorporate powerful regulatory components capable of controlling inflammation, safeguarding barrier function, and mitigating tissue damage (Medzhitov *et al.*, 2012). Additionally, these organisms secrete products that can influence microbiota composition, potentially affecting its proper functioning (Hewitson *et al.*, 2009). Conversely, alterations in microbiota can influence susceptibility to infections by the macrobiota (Mumcuoglu, 2019). For instance, a study on alpine goats conducted under experimental conditions demonstrated that infection with *Haemonchus contortus* not only impaired weight gain but also resulted in an increase in abomasal pH (Liu *et al.*, 2020). This condition led to significant alterations in the microbial composition of the abomasum by disrupting the balance between archaea and bacteria. Another investigation showed an increase in the *abundance* of bacteria from the Pasteurellaceae family in goats primoinfected with *H. contortus*, alongside a 19% change in the abundance of 432 resident bacterial species within the gastrointestinal microbiome (Li *et al.*, 2016). In contrast, Rooney *et al.* (2024) reported that some helminths can produce antimicrobial peptides consisting of fewer than 100 amino acids, which possess chemical properties enabling them to function as broad-spectrum antibiotics against both eukaryotes and prokaryotes. Research in pigs has suggested a beneficial role for *Ascaris suum*, demonstrating a high bactericidal potential against bacteria such as *Escherichia coli*, *Staphylococcus aureus*, and *Salmonella typhimurium*. The excretory and secretory products of these nematodes can disrupt bacterial membrane formation, leading to lysis or lethal agglutination of cells (Midha *et al.*, 2018). Similarly, *in vitro* experiments have indicated that the parasite *Teladorsagia circumcincta*, an abomasal parasite of small ruminants, can significantly reduce *E. coli* colony-forming units within 3 hours (Rooney *et al.*, 2022). This diaphony between these two distinct groups represents a constant crosstalk that, when in equilibrium, plays a crucial role in promoting eubiosis and host eustress (Gause and Maizels, 2016). This dynamic presents a challenge for scientific inquiry, as further research is needed to elucidate many underlying mechanisms, as highlighted by Limborg *et al.* (2024). A key aspect of this interaction is the molecular dialogue established to maintain balance in this crosstalk, which can be explored through various fields of omics science.

What is known to date is that a gastrointestinal ecosystem can respond to any perturbation under four possible scenarios (Fig. 24.1) previously described by Moya and Ferrer (2016), Sommer *et al.* (2017), and Martínez-Ortiz-de-Montellano *et al.* (2023):

1. *Resistance* is defined as the property of an ecosystem that remains unchanged in the face of a perturbation. In the context of the microbiota, this means that its composition does not vary despite external disturbances, thereby ensuring that the bacterial communities inhabiting the holobiont remain balanced.

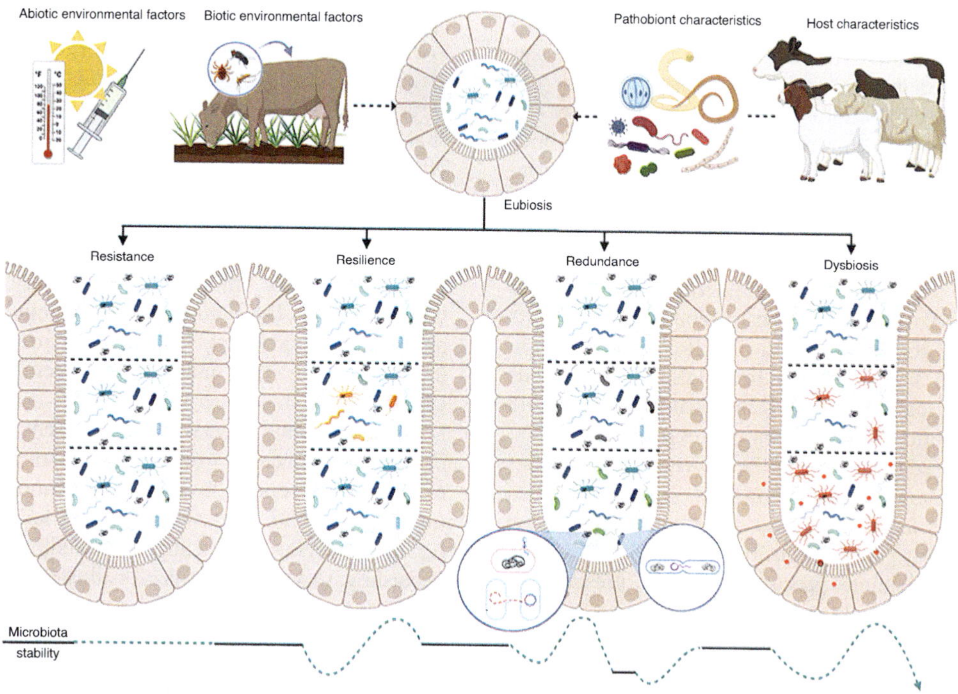

Fig. 24.1. The four microbiota scenarios against perturbation. The holobiont is constantly exposed to a series of factors that represent changes for the microbiota to which they must adapt if they are to survive as part of the organism that hosts them. Initially, the animal is in eubiosis, but any environmental disturbance, abiotic or biotic, characteristic of a pathobiont or of the holobiont itself, will lead to the development of one of four scenarios: resistance, resilience, redundancy and dysbiosis. Among these adaptation mechanisms, there is a high genetic diversity, which is as dynamic as the microbiota organisms and is constantly changing thanks to the mechanisms of horizontal gene transfer, giving the bacteria, above all, the ability to adapt or acquire skills that allow them to maintain equilibrium. Otherwise, the proliferation of pathobionts is inevitable, leading to colonization and invasion, with an unfortunate outcome for the holobiont. The stability of the microbiota is represented by a straight line, and in the presence of perturbations the line becomes distorted, and the ability of the microbiota to recover will determine whether the line continues or leads to dysbiosis (Moya and Ferrer, 2016; Sommer *et al.*, 2017; Martínez-Ortiz-de-Montellano *et al.*, 2023). Created in BioRender.com.

2. *Resilience* describes the extent of stress a system can withstand before its homeostatic state shifts to a new equilibrium, which may exhibit different functional characteristics. In the case of the microbiota, while changes may occur following a perturbation, this does not affect key bacterial groups responsible for critical functions such as metabolic regulation.
3. *Redundancy* is exemplified by alterations that modify the original composition of the microbiota without affecting its metabolic functions, due to the repopulation by newly established commensal groups. This principle is significant as it introduces the concept that species within a given microbiota can be somewhat interchangeable in terms of their functional roles. Indeed, two holobionts with distinct microbiota compositions may exhibit similar behaviors. Functions conferred by multiple bacteria may be shared among both related and unrelated species, reflecting the evolutionary convergence of unrelated taxa. As a result, variable combinations of species from different phyla may fulfill partial functional redundancy, allowing different metabolically active bacteria to perform analogous functions in diverse individuals.

These three principles, resilience, resistance, and redundancy, characterize the so-called 'robust' microbiota, which possess the ability to restore a phenotype beneficial to the holobiont. However, a fourth principle defines a disruption in the robustness of the bacterial population.

Dysbiosis is interpreted as an imbalance in the robustness and taxonomic composition of the gastrointestinal microbiota, potentially leading to severe consequences in ruminants due to alterations in population composition and function. The investigation of various microbiota scenarios in relation to biotic and abiotic factors remains relatively underexplored in ruminants. However, studies in other species, including humans, have established that factors such as diet—considering type, quality, and quantity—alongside age, sex, management practices, and the presence of disease, influence the perturbation of the metacommunity and its capacity to respond.

Similarly, dysbiosis can lead to three potential scenarios associated with the emergence of bacterial diseases (Moreno-Calderón, 2022). This, in turn, can cause alterations in macrobiota populations, manifesting as *parasitosis* (Gause and Maizels, 2016).

a. Increase of pathobionts: These are members of the gastro-intestinal microbiota that typically act as natural colonizers and commensals but can proliferate significantly when disruptions occur in the gastrointestinal ecosystem (Moreno-Calderón, 2022). An example of this phenomenon in ruminants is enterotoxemia, which is caused by *Clostridium perfringens*. As a normal inhabitant of the intestine, *C. perfringens* proliferates excessively and produces a wide range of toxins when there are abrupt dietary changes or other factors that remain poorly understood. These toxins may be absorbed into the systemic circulation and/or exert local effects in the intestine, leading to disease (Ortega *et al.*, 2019). The proliferation of pathobionts can result in detrimental modifications to the gastrointestinal environment, potentially reducing the proliferation of or even killing other microorganisms participating in the microbiota. Subacute ruminal acidosis is an alteration of the ruminal microbiota caused by an increase in volatile fatty acids, resulting in a moderate decrease in pH (Silberberg *et al.*, 2013). An increase in highly fermentable carbohydrates has been shown to induce changes in the integrity of the microbiota. These conditions facilitate the growth, death, and lysis of certain Gram-negative bacteria, which release endotoxins such as bacterial lipopolysaccharides. This not only elicits a systemic inflammatory response but also alters the composition of Gram-positive bacteria, yeasts, and other natural inhabitants of the holobiont (Moreno-Calderón, 2022).
b. Loss of microbial diversity: The presence of dysbiosis typically results in a reduction of initial microbial diversity. This inter- and intraspecific consortium is initially highly diverse but can be modified according to host patterns. As illustrated in the preceding paragraph, sudden and unanticipated changes in dietary patterns – such as an increase in highly fermentable carbohydrates or the introduction of weaned lambs to leafy pastures – can act as catalysts for the loss of microbial integrity, leading to a decline or surge in specific bacterial genera (Alsaab *et al.*, 2021; Moreno-Calderón, 2022).
c. Alterations in macrobiota populations: Dysbiosis can also lead to significant changes in the composition and function of macrobiota populations (Gause and Maizels, 2016; Mumcuoglu, 2019; Rooney *et al.*, 2022), which may result in the manifestation of parasitosis. The interplay between dysbiosis and macrobiota alterations highlights the importance of maintaining microbial balance to prevent the onset of bacterial diseases in ruminants.

Global Scope of Antibiotic and Antiparasitic Resistance in the Context of One Welfare

The global scope of antibiotic and antiparasitic resistance, as a concern within the One Welfare agenda, is extensive and represents a challenge that surpasses current control and treatment strategies. Since the inception of the use of these molecules, the management of parasitic and bacterial diseases has primarily focused on their application, often overlooking the fact that diseases arise from a complex interplay of factors rather than a single causal agent. Issues related to chemical resistance stem from a negative human perception of the presence of bacteria or parasites in organisms, leading to a focus on eradication and associating these microorganisms with disease, while neglecting essential components of the ecological dynamics within the gastrointestinal ecosystem of the holobiont. In particular, the management of metazoans or macrobiota has traditionally involved the routine or continuous deworming of all animals in a herd or flock, often without any diagnostic evidence, solely aiming to eradicate populations of insects, ticks, nematodes, or trematodes. Reports of increasing resistance to these drugs have emerged in several countries, raising concerns about the potential consequences of antiparasitic-resistant parasite populations on global ruminant production (OIE, 2022; Martínez Ortiz de *et al.*, 2022b). The impact of anthelmintics extends beyond their role in developing resistance mechanisms; it also encompasses the detrimental effects on the ecosystems in which these animals reside. According to García Pinillos and Huertas Canén (2023), field contamination with antiparasitic and antimicrobial residues poses a significant risk to human and animal health, food safety, and the overall ecosystem. A substantial proportion of these residues is excreted in feces or urine, spreading through the environment alongside resistant populations. The resistance genes associated with these newly resistant species are released into the soil and water, facilitating the emergence of new generations of previously susceptible species that have become resistant to treatments. The circulation of these emerging generations further exacerbates resistance through the repeated infection of hosts. Additionally, ecological toxicity represents another form of contamination that adversely affects the activity and composition of soil microbial communities and the diverse fauna, particularly arthropods (García Pinillos and Huertas Canén, 2023). For the treatment of parasitosis in ruminants, various chemical molecules are utilized, classified into three main families: benzimidazoles, macrocyclic lactones, and imidazothiazoles. The efficacy of these drugs is influenced by the evolutionary and ecological characteristics of nematodes, including their short life cycles, high reproductive rates, rapid evolutionary rates, and extremely large population sizes, which contribute to generational genetic mutations. The gradual emergence of resistance can be attributed to the selective pressure exerted by each molecule, which eliminates the most susceptible nematodes while allowing those with resistance traits to survive. As previously mentioned, the scope of anthelmintic resistance is extensive, with causes that extend beyond the biology of the macrobiota. Factors such as increased reliance on a single drug family, under- and overdosing, inadequate governmental regulation regarding the sale of these drugs, and inappropriate veterinary practices lacking diagnostic evidence and strategic deworming analysis have intensified the issue in both national and international production units (Sargison, 2016; WOAH, 2020). Table 24.1 summarizes the primary families of anthelmintics used in ruminant production and how nematodes develop resistance genes in response. Over the years, deworming strategies for metazoan populations have become homogenized across domestic ruminant species. In other words, bovine medicine has often been applied uniformly to small ruminants, without considering the physiological differences between sheep, goats, and cattle. There have even been attempts to apply identical doses of anthelmintics to sheep and goats, disregarding the fact that parasitism manifests differently within each holobiont (Martínez Ortiz de *et al.*, 2022b).

Antimicrobials are regarded as one of the most significant inventions of the last century for both human and animal medicine. However, their excessive use as growth promoters in ruminants, often in the absence of any semiological evidence of disease, has led to a substantial increase in consumption. This, in turn, has resulted in the accumulation of these residues and fostered the emergence of antibiotic-resistant bacteria within the gastrointestinal microbiota. The overuse of these drugs not only promotes the selection of bacterial species resistant to the mechanisms of

Table 24.1. Overview of the mechanisms of action, resistance, doses and presentation of antiparasitic drugs commonly used in ruminants.

Drug families	Benzimidazoles	Macrocyclic lactones	Imidazothiazoles
Mechanism of action	The attack on the cellular metabolism of nematodes deprives them of usable energy. This is achieved by binding to a target receptor (β-tubulin) present on tubulin protein, which alters the balance of microtubules. This results in depolymerization, immobilization, and death of the nematode.	High-affinity agonists on glutamate receptors, associated with chloride channels and GABA (γ-aminobutyric acid) receptors, have been demonstrated to cause an increase in chloride ion concentration and hyperpolarization of the nematode neuron, leading to spastic paralysis. These agonists have exhibited high potency at low doses.	They function as cholinergic agonists at the neuromuscular junctions, acting on nicotinic acetylcholine receptors to exert both muscarinic and nicotinic effects. This results in depolarization and spastic paralysis in the parasite.
Resistance mechanism	The high gene flow between nematode populations, a consequence of their high prolificacy, gives rise to a high diversity of β-tubulin resistance mutations. Several studies have identified three amino acid codons that may be involved in the development of polymorphisms that determine resistance to benzimidazoles.	Two mechanisms associated with resistance have been identified. The initial mechanism pertains to the occurrence of mutations in two subunits of the chloride channel of the parasite that has developed resistance. Conversely, various researchers have indicated that the GluCl receptor plays a part in the emergence of resistance.	The mutations associated with the acquisition of resistance are related to the disappearance of acetylcholine receptors. Other studies have indicated that channel dynamics in resistant strains are altered, with a reduction in the opening time and a decrease in depolarization.
Presentation	Suspension	Suspension	Suspension
Common name	Febendazole, Albendazole, Thiabendazole, Mebendazole, Ricobendazole, Febantel, Oxfendazole	Ivermectin, Doramectin, Moxidectin	Levamisole
Dose mg/kg BB			
Cattle	7.5–10	0.2	4.5
Sheep	5–20	0.2	8–12
Goat	5–20	0.2	8–12

Pugh and Baird (2012); Lambertz *et al.* (2019); Yanuartono *et al.* (2019); Pivoto *et al.* (2020).
[a]It is advised that the cited bibliographies be consulted for specific values according to the anthelmintic of interest.

action of chemotherapeutics but also leads to residual contamination in food of animal origin consumed by humans, directly affecting the ecosystem and the resident microbiota of various holobionts, including domestic ruminants (Jian *et al.*, 2021). To develop resistance to antibiotics, bacteria can employ two mechanisms: intrinsic and acquired (Baran *et al.*, 2023). The distinction between these two lies in their origin; intrinsic resistance occurs naturally due to the functional or structural characteristics of bacteria that inhibit drug action. Physical mechanisms such as efflux through porins or the inability of antibiotics to penetrate the membrane due to their molecular structure exemplify intrinsic resistance. Another intrinsic mechanism involves the differences in phospholipid ratios between Gram-positive and Gram-negative bacteria; the lower presence of anionic phospholipids in Gram-positive membranes reduces the efficiency of daptomycin insertion mediated by calcium. Lastly, the production of enzymes that modify antibiotics to inhibit their mechanisms of action showcases the functional properties of bacteria that confer resistance to traditional methods for treating bacterial infections (Jian *et al.*, 2021; Baran *et al.*, 2023). The second mechanism is linked to the abundant microbiome within the gastrointestinal ecosystem. Among the genes present in this ecological niche are antibiotic-resistance genes responsible for developing traits that enable bacteria to counteract the effects of these drugs. Pathogenic bacteria can acquire these and other resistance genes through horizontal gene transfer, which can occur via plasmid exchange with other bacteria, *conjugation*; by taking up genes from lysed bacteria that expose their genetic material, *transformation*; and through the transfer of resistance genes by phages, *transduction* (Jian *et al.*, 2021; Moura de Sousa *et al.*, 2023). As discussed, the effects of chemotherapeutic treatments aimed at controlling bacterial and parasitic diseases are not always entirely beneficial. Additionally, the perception among producers and veterinarians that parasites are the primary cause of production losses may lead to a misguided focus on eradicating helminths in animals that, with appropriate diagnostics, may not require treatment. This approach can promote irresponsible and inappropriate use of these molecules, contributing to the development of resistance mechanisms in both the microbiota and the macrobiota (Moon *et al.*, 2021). Another negative effect that has received limited attention is the potential for anthelmintic molecules to harm bacterial populations within the gastrointestinal ecosystem. The molecular composition of drugs such as benzimidazoles and macrocyclic lactones affects not only helminth populations but also bacteria and even fungi (Bansal and Silakari, 2012). The macrocyclic ring structure of drugs like abamectin or moxidectin is a structural component associated with antimicrobial activity, leading to the hypothesis that the use of broad-spectrum anthelmintics could induce changes in the microbiota. Such disruptions may result in distress for the animals and pose a threat to their welfare (Moon *et al.*, 2021). Another important consideration is that treating lambs, kids, or calves assumed to have diarrhea without a prior coproparasitological diagnosis, particularly if coccidiosis is suspected, with coccidicides such as gentamicin, sulfas, or toltrazuril can disrupt the microbiota. Treatments do not solely target protozoa like *Eimeria*; they can also affect bacteria, fungi, and other microbial populations within the gastrointestinal ecosystem.

Holistic Approach of the Veterinarian as a Conservationist of the Microbiota and Macrobiota of Ruminants

It is essential for veterinarians to adopt a holistic perspective, avoiding a reductionist view that focuses solely on isolated pathological causes. Instead, they should consider the pathophysiological processes that can trigger dysbiosis, anaphylaxis, disseminated intravascular coagulation, hemoconcentration, hypovolemic shock, respiratory arrest, cardiac arrest, and ultimately, death. A clear example of this comprehensive approach is enterotoxemia, a disease caused by *C. perfringens*, a Gram-positive, aerotolerant bacterium capable of producing more than 20 toxins with devastating effects on the host. Although *C. perfringens* is a normal inhabitant of the intestine, it can proliferate uncontrollably when exposed to external factors, such as sudden dietary changes or the presence of other pathogens. For instance, *Trichostrongylus colubriformis*, a strongylid nematode that resides in the duodenum, causes local hyperemia, mucus production, and inflammation due to the abrasion of parietal cells. These effects alter intestinal pH and promote dysbiosis, allowing the proliferation of pathogens such as *C. perfringens*. Furthermore, hormonal imbalances in cholecystokinin can lead to loss of appetite, decreased voluntary intake, and anorexia, contributing to the clinical deterioration of the animal, which may ultimately culminate in death. The massive proliferation of *C. perfringens* results in toxin production that invades the systemic circulation or acts locally in the intestine, causing severe clinical manifestations (Ortega *et al.*, 2019). Among the toxins secreted by this bacterium are sialidases, hyaluronidases, fibronectin-binding proteins, and toxins alpha, beta, delta, and perfringolysin. These toxins catalyze the degradation of extracellular matrix proteins and cell membrane components, such as phosphatidylcholine and sphingomyelin. Additionally, they can form protein complexes that create pores in cell membranes. In synergy with the rapid multiplication of the bacteria, these toxins cross the epithelial barrier and disseminate to various organs, including the central nervous system, potentially leading to the animal's death (Mehdizadeh Gohari *et al.*, 2021). The uncertainty remains regarding which agent initiated colonization, highlighting the complex crosstalk that is difficult to elucidate. The holistic approach of the veterinarian entails the application of these concepts aimed at enhancing welfare within the One Welfare background (García-Pinillos, 2017). This model advocates for the integration of various management aspects, including parasite control, as part of an integrative and holistic view of disease management (Esteve-Gasent *et al.*, 2020; Martínez Ortiz de Montellano *et al.*, 2022a).

Holistic Strategies for the Management of Infectious Diseases in Ruminants

The term Integrated Parasite Management (IPM) refers to a system that proposes multiple control strategies to address parasitosis in an integrated manner, considering economic and epidemiological aspects, the status of resistance to anthelmintics, the dynamics of the production system, and its structured management (Box 24.3). The primary objective is to utilize treatment and control alternatives from various products with different mechanisms of action, allowing for the reduction of nematodes in pastures and animals while completely abandoning the idea of total eradication.

Box 24.3. Principles of Integrated Parasite Management in ruminants (Taken and modified from Martínez Ortiz de *et al.*, 2022b).

1. <u>Enhance host response against parasites</u>
   - Nutrition
   - Microbiota care
   - Genetic selection
   - Vaccines

2. <u>Mitigate the population of parasites within the host</u>
   - Rational use of anthelmintic molecules
   - Target Selective Treatment
   - Bioactive compounds of plants
   - Nutraceutical plants
   - Cooper needles

3. <u>Deplete source of environmental contamination from parasites</u>
   - Shelter management
   - Pasture and grazing management
   - Biological control

This approach aims to gradually decrease dependence on conventional anthelmintics and significantly reduce the incidence of gastrointestinal nematodes (Maqbool *et al.*, 2017). Integrated parasite management is built upon three fundamental pillars:

1. optimizing the host response to nematodes,
2. reducing or eliminating environmental contamination by parasites, and
3. decreasing the parasite burden within the host (Martínez Ortiz de *et al.*, 2022b) (Box 24.3).

The significance of animal nutrition and microbiota management is crucial to the first pillar of IPM, which focuses on optimizing the host response to parasites. While the microbiota has been extensively studied for its role in rumen metabolism, its interaction with metazoans is still emerging. In ruminants, the rumen microbiota is well documented for its involvement in feed metabolism, particularly in the production of volatile fatty acids and the absorption of essential nutrients for energy and protein synthesis (Wang *et al.*, 2021). The intestines, both large and small, are home to a diverse array of microorganisms that contribute to numerous functions necessary for animal homeostasis. Studies have demonstrated that the intestinal microbiota not only aids in the breakdown of dietary carbohydrates but also plays a pivotal role in balancing the immune response and stabilizing the gastrointestinal ecosystem (Wang *et al.*, 2021). Maintaining the integrity of the ruminant's gastrointestinal microbiota is critical for achieving balance within the holobiont. A state of eubiosis allows the individual to sustain beneficial functions derived from symbiosis with commensal microorganisms. From a therapeutic perspective, regulating the integrity of the microbiota has focused on implementing preventive treatments that enrich and shape its composition (Castañeda-Guillot, 2019). The use of eubiotics, probiotics, prebiotics, and postbiotics in ruminant production presents a promising alternative for dietary supplementation, especially as traditional practices of using antibiotics as additives and growth promoters have been restricted (Kiczorowska *et al.*, 2017). These new tools, derived from natural sources, offer options that enhance productive performance while ensuring welfare, as they support various links in the animal product production chain, guaranteeing food safety and animal welfare while providing more environmentally friendly solutions (Estrada-Angulo *et al.*, 2021). Eubiotics are among the most widely used supplements in cattle, recognized as natural feed additives with minimal reports of adverse effects on environmental, human, or animal health. Their mechanisms of action promote intestinal homeostasis by balancing the microbiota and enhancing enzymatic activity in the gastrointestinal tract, leading to improved animal growth, development, and productivity. For instance, the addition of eubiotics to the diets of dairy cows not only enhances productivity and health but has also been proposed to modify the nutritional profile of milk, particularly in its fatty acid composition (Kiczorowska *et al.*, 2017). Probiotics and prebiotics offer natural alternatives to replace antibiotics as dietary additives for ruminants. Although these 'symbiotics' may not share identical mechanisms of action, they often exhibit synergistic effects under specific conditions. The combination of these two supplements has been shown to reduce morbidity and mortality rates in dairy cattle compared to those that have not been supplemented (Kiczorowska *et al.*, 2017). Other studies indicate that symbiotic supplementation in lambs contributes to increased weight gain and improved adaptation to subtropical climatic conditions, particularly in terms of dietary energy utilization (Estrada-Angulo *et al.*, 2021). Like previous supplementation alternatives that enrich the gastrointestinal ecosystem, postbiotics, when consumed in adequate quantities, provide a wide range of biological benefits for maintaining digestive homeostasis. Moreover, the ingestion of postbiotics may influence physiological mechanisms and regulatory processes associated with microbiota function. Investigations into these components have revealed that many postbiotics, including short-chain fatty acids, linoleic acid, glycoproteins, peptidoglycans, proteins, peptides, lactic acid, and exopolysaccharides, exhibit significant antioxidant and antibacterial potential (Abbasi *et al.*, 2023). On the other hand, the tools provided by omics sciences enable in-depth studies of microbiota composition and its interactions with the macrobiota. Through disciplines such as transcriptomics, proteomics, metabolomics, and others, advanced food technology has been developed, highlighting the significance of prebiotics, probiotics, postbiotics, and eubiotics in nutrition and integrated parasite management for ruminants. When combined with preventive medicine strategies, these tools are essential for optimizing the health and welfare of ruminants (Fig. 24.2).

Conclusion

Only through a revolution and paradigm shift can we fully grasp that veterinary medicine must evolve, particularly in recognizing the so-called pathobionts. Complete eradication of diseases is not feasible within sustainable systems under the One Welfare basis. A holistic perspective on parasitism encourages us to address disease by enhancing nutrition within the gastrointestinal ecosystem of the ruminant holobiont, while

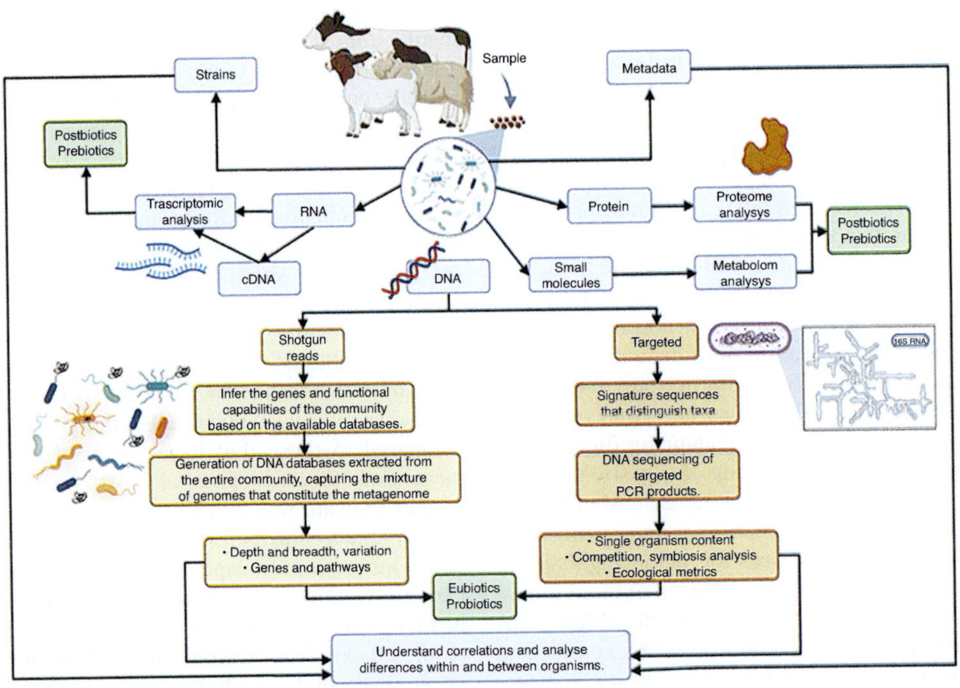

Fig. 24.2. The omics sciences and their impact on understanding the interaction of microbiota and how to enrich their coexistence. The omics sciences offer the possibility of knowing the diversity of the population that constitutes the microbiota, its genetic diversity, and the knowledge of genes and their functional capacity by building databases through shotgun readings. It is also possible to know the characteristics of specific genera, allowing us to know the individual genetic content, ecological metrics, and symbiotic interactions between species. These new technologies not only allow us to know the composition of the microbiota but also promise the possibility of producing compounds that benefit the health of the microbiota, for example, eubiotics, prebiotics, postbiotics and probiotics, through its different branches of study such as transcriptomics, metabolomics, and proteomics (Weinstock, 2012). Created in BioRender.com.

considering the complex molecular interactions that remain largely misunderstood and unknown to humans. Integrated parasite management encompasses a range of tools that, when applied effectively, can not only enhance animal welfare but also promote the balance and health of our ruminant holobionts. In conclusion, advancing toward a more integrative approach to veterinary medicine that fosters coexistence and balance among the organisms comprising the holobiont is essential for ensuring sustainable production systems aligned with the principles of global animal welfare and public health.

Acknowledgment

This work was made possible thanks to the support of the Dirección General del Personal Académico (DGAPA) at UNAM, through the Program for the Support of Research and Technological Innovation Projects (PAPIIT), under Project number IT202024, which funded the master's thesis of Ricardo Piña Martínez, the first author of this work. The first author also received a scholarship from CONAHCYT to support his master's degree studies.

Funding

The study was funded by the Dirección General de Asuntos del Personal Académico, Universidad Nacional Autónoma de México with the project number PAPIIT IT202024.

Author Contributions

CMOM conceptualized the data, contributed in funding acquisition and project administration, and supervised the study; CMOM and EDG visualized the study; RPM contributed in writing – original draft; CMOM, CCMM, and EDG contributed in writing – review and editing.

References

Abbasi, A., Sabahi, S., Bazzaz, S., Tajani, A.G., Lahouty, M. *et al.* (2023) An edible coating utilizing *Malva sylvestris* seed polysaccharide mucilage and postbiotic from *Saccharomyces cerevisiae* var. *boulardii* for the preservation of lamb meat. *International Journal of Biological Macromolecules* 246, 125660. DOI: 10.1016/j.ijbiomac.2023.125660.

Alsaab, F., Wahdan, A. and Saeed, E.M.A. (2021) Phenotypic detection and genotyping of *Clostridium perfringens* associated with enterotoxemia in sheep in the Qassim Region of Saudi Arabia. *Veterinary World* 14(3), 578–584.

Bansal, Y. and Silakari, O. (2012) The therapeutic journey of benzimidazoles: A review. *Bioorganic & Medicinal Chemistry* 20(21), 6208–6236. DOI: 10.1016/j.bmc.2012.09.013.

Baran, A., Kwiatkowska, A. and Potocki, L. (2023) Antibiotics and bacterial resistance—A short story of an endless arms race. *International Journal of Molecular Sciences* 24(6), 5777. DOI: 10.3390/ijms24065777.

Bowman, D.D. (2022) *Georgi. Parasitología para Veterinarios*. Elsevier Health Sciences.
Castañeda-Guillot, C. (2019) Probióticos de nueva generación. *Belize Journal of Medicine*. Available at: https://Bjomed.Org/Index.Php/Bjm/Article
Chaucheyras-Durand, F., Ameilbonne, A., Auffret, P., Bernard, M., Mialon, M.-M. *et al.* (2019) Supplementation of live yeast based feed additive in early life promotes rumen microbial colonization and fibrolytic potential in lambs. *Scientific Reports* 9(1), 19216. DOI: 10.1038/s41598-019-55825-0.
Cherbuy, C. (2016) Gut microbiota and host health: From infancy to adulthood. In: *Taste, Nutrition and Health of the Horse*.
Chiu, L. and Gilbert, S.F. (2020) Niche construction and the transition to herbivory: phenotype switching and the organization of new nutritional modes. In: *Phenotypic Switching*. Elsevier, Chennai, India, pp. 459–482. DOI: 10.1016/B978-0-12-817996-3.00015-3.
Dunière, L., Ruiz, P., Lebbaoui, Y., Guillot, L., Bernard, M. *et al.* (2023) Effects of rearing mode on gastro-intestinal microbiota and development, immunocompetence, sanitary status and growth performance of lambs from birth to two months of age. *Animal Microbiome* 5(1), 34. DOI: 10.1186/s42523-023-00255-7.
Esteve-Gasent, M.D., Rodríguez-Vivas, R.I., Medina, R.F., Ellis, D., Schwartz, A. *et al.* (2020) Research on integrated management for cattle fever ticks and bovine babesiosis in the United States and Mexico: Current status and opportunities for binational coordination. *Pathogens* 9(11), 871. DOI: 10.3390/pathogens9110871.
Estrada-Angulo, A., Zapata-Ramírez, O., Castro-Pérez, B.I., Urías-Estrada, J.D., Gaxiola-Camacho, S. *et al.* (2021) The effects of single or combined supplementation of probiotics and prebiotics on growth performance, dietary energetics, carcass traits, and visceral mass in lambs finished under subtropical climate conditions. *Biology* 10(11), 1137. DOI: 10.3390/biology10111137.
FAO (2011) *Programa Especial para la Seguridad Alimentaria (PESA) Centroamérica. Conceptos básicos*.
García Pinillos, R. and Huertas Canén, S.M. (2023) *One Welfare Animal Health and Welfare, Food Security and Sustainability*. CABI Wallingford, UK. DOI: 10.1079/9781789249507.0000.
García-Pinillos, R. (2017) Un solo bienestar. marco de trabajo para a apoyar la implementacion de las normas de bienestar animal de la OIE. *OIE* 1, 1–8. DOI: 10.20506/bull.issue.2017.1.2586.
Gause, W.C. and Maizels, R.M. (2016) Macrobiota – helminths as active participants and partners of the microbiota in host intestinal homeostasis. *Current Opinion in Microbiology* 32, 14–18. DOI: 10.1016/j.mib.2016.04.004.
Gilbert, R.A., Townsend, E.M., Crew, K.S., Hitch, T.C.A., Friedersdorff, J.C.A. *et al.* (2020) Rumen virus populations: Technological advances enhancing current understanding. *Frontiers in Microbiology* 1, 11–14. DOI: 10.3389/fmicb.2020.00450.
Hewitson, J.P., Grainger, J.R. and Maizels, R.M. (2009) Helminth immunoregulation: The role of parasitc secreted proteins in modulating host immunity. *Molecular and Biochemical Parasitology* 167(1), 1–11. DOI: 10.1016/j.molbiopara.2009.04.008.
Jian, Z., Zeng, L., Xu, T., Sun, S., Yan, S. *et al.* (2021) Antibiotic resistance genes in bacteria: occurrence, spread, and control. *Journal of Basic Microbiology* 61(12), 1049–1070. DOI: 10.1002/jobm.202100201.
Kiczorowska, B., Samolińska, W., Marczuk, J., Winiarska-Mieczan, A., Klebaniuk, R. *et al.* (2017) Comparative effects of organic, traditional, and intensive production with probiotics on the fatty acid profile of cow's milk. *Journal of Food Composition and Analysis* 63, 157–163. DOI: 10.1016/j.jfca.2017.08.002.
Lambertz, C., Poulopoulou, I., Wuthijaree, K. and Gauly, M. (2019) Anthelmintic efficacy against gastrointestinal nematodes in goats raised under mountain farming conditions in northern Italy. *BMC Veterinary Research* 15(1), 216. DOI: 10.1186/s12917-019-1968-8.
Li, R.W., Li, W., Sun, J., Yu, P., Baldwin, R.L. *et al.* (2016) The effect of helminth infection on the microbial composition and structure of the caprine abomasal microbiome. *Scientific Reports* 6(1), 20606. DOI: 10.1038/srep20606.
Limborg, M.T., Winther-Have, C.S., Morueta-Holme, N., Gilbert, M.T.P. and Rasmussen, J.A. (2024) The overlooked biodiversity loss. *Trends in Ecology & Evolution* 39(10), 889–890. DOI: 10.1016/j.tree.2024.08.001.
Liu, F., Xie, Y., Zajac, A.M., Hu, Y., Aroian, R.V. *et al.* (2020) Gut microbial signatures associated with moxidectin treatment efficacy of *Haemonchus contortus* in infected goats. *Veterinary Microbiology* 242, 108607. DOI: 10.1016/j.vetmic.2020.108607.

Maqbool, I., Wani, Z.A., Shahardar, R.A., Allaie, I.M. and Shah, M.M. (2017) Integrated parasite management with special reference to gastro-intestinal nematodes. *Journal of Parasitic Diseases* 41(1), 1–8. DOI: 10.1007/s12639-016-0765-6.

Martínez Ortiz de, C., Torres-Avosta, J.F.J., Ojeda-Robertos, N.F., González-Reyes, L. and Muñoz-Marín, S.A. (2022b) Manejo integrado de parásitos en pequeños rumiantes. *Bioagrociencias* 15(2), 1–10.

Martínez Ortiz de Montellano, C., Quiroz-Castañeda, R.E., Dantán-González, E., Aguilar-Díaz, H., Márquez-Mota, C.C. *et al.* (2022a) Concepción integrativa del parasitismo: Redefiniendo nuevos conceptos. *Bioagrociencias* 48–59.

Martínez-Ortiz-de-Montellano, C., Márquez-Mota, C.C., Montes-Carreto, L.M., Quiroz-Catañeda, R.E., Dantán-González, E. *et al.* (2023) Caracterización de la microbiota fecal en caballos con ciatostomosis en México. *Tropical and Subtropical Agroecosystems* 26(1), 10–13. DOI: 10.56369/tsaes.4546.

Medzhitov, R., Schneider, D.S. and Soares, M.P. (2012) Disease tolerance as a defense strategy. *Science* 335(6071), 936–941. DOI: 10.1126/science.1214935.

Mehdizadeh Gohari, I., Navarro, M.A., Li, J., Shrestha, A., Uzal, F. *et al.* (2021) Pathogenicity and virulence of *Clostridium perfringens*. *Virulence* 12(1), 723–753. DOI: 10.1080/21505594.2021.1886777.

Midha, A., Janek, K., Niewienda, A., Henklein, P., Guenther, S. *et al.* (2018) The intestinal roundworm *Ascaris suum* releases antimicrobial factors which interfere with bacterial growth and biofilm formation. *Frontiers in Cellular and Infection Microbiology* 8, 5–10. DOI: 10.3389/fcimb.2018.00271.

Moon, C.D., Carvalho, L., Kirk, M.R., McCulloch, A.F., Kittelmann, S. *et al.* (2021) Effects of long-acting, broad spectra anthelmintic treatments on the rumen microbial community compositions of grazing sheep. *Scientific Reports* 11(1), 3836. DOI: 10.1038/s41598-021-82815-y.

Moreno-Calderón, X. (2022) Disbiosis en la microbiota intestinal. *GEN* 76(1), 17–23.

Moura de Sousa, J., Lourenço, M. and Gordo, I. (2023) Horizontal gene transfer among host-associated microbes. *Cell Host & Microbe* 31(4), 513–527. DOI: 10.1016/j.chom.2023.03.017.

Moya, A. and Ferrer, M. (2016) Functional redundancy-induced stability of gut microbiota subjected to disturbance. *Trends in Microbiology* 24(5), 402–413. DOI: 10.1016/j.tim.2016.02.002.

Mumcuoglu, I. (2019) Interactions between parasites and human microbiota. *European Journal of Therapeutics* 25(1), 6–11. DOI: 10.5152/EurJTher.2019.18080.

Muñoz-Vargas, L., Zamora-Sanabria, R. and Hidalgo-Jara, W. (2023) Animal welfare, stress and food safety. In: *One Welfare Animal Health and Welfare, Food Security and Sustainability*. CABI, Wallingford, UK, pp. 62–88.

OIE (2024) *Código Sanitario para los Animales Terrestres*. Available at: https://www.woah.org/fileadmin/Home/esp/Health_standards/tahc/current/es_preface.htm (accessed 28 May 2025).

Organización Mundial de Sanidad Animal (OIE) (2022) *Uso responsable y prudente de los fármacos antihelmínticos para contribuir al control de la resistencia a antihelmínticos en las especies ganaderas herbívoras*. OIE.

Ortega, J., Verdes, J.M., Morrell, E.L., Finnie, J.W., Manavis, J. *et al.* (2019) Intramural vascular edema in the brain of goats with *Clostridium perfringens* Type D enterotoxemia. *Veterinary Pathology* 56(3), 452–459. DOI: 10.1177/0300985818817071.

Peek, S.F., Mcguirk, S.M., Sweeney, R.W. and Cummings, K.J. (2018) Infectious diseases of the gastrointestinal tract. In: *Rebhun's Diseases of Dairy Cattle*. Elsevier, St, Louis, MO, pp. 249–356. DOI: 10.1016/B978-0-323-39055-2.00006-1.

Pivoto, F.L., Cezar, A.S., Vogel, F.S.F. and do Rego Leal, M.L. (2020) Effects of long-term indiscriminate use of macrocyclic lactones in cattle: Parasite resistance, clinical helminthosis, and production losses. *Veterinary Parasitology: Regional Studies and Reports* 20, 100381. DOI: 10.1016/j.vprsr.2020.100381.

Pugh, D.G. and Baird, A.N. (2012) *Sheep and Goat Medicine*, 2nd edn. Elsevier, London.

Rooney, J., Williams, T.L., Northcote, H.M., Frankl, F.E.K., Price, D.R.G. *et al.* (2022) Excretory-secretory products from the brown stomach worm, *Teladorsagia circumcincta*, exert antimicrobial activity in in vitro growth assays. *Parasites & Vectors* 15(1), 354. DOI: 10.1186/s13071-022-05443-z.

Rooney, J., Rivera-de-Torre, E., Li, R., Mclean, K., Price, D.R.G. *et al.* (2024) Structural and functional analyses of nematode-derived antimicrobial peptides support the occurrence of direct mechanisms of worm-microbiota interactions. *Computational and Structural Biotechnology Journal* 23, 1522–1533. DOI: 10.1016/j.csbj.2024.04.019.

Sargison, N.D. (2016) Keys to solving health problems in small ruminants: Anthelmintic resistance as a threat to sustainable nematode control. *Small Ruminant Research* 142, 11–15. DOI: 10.1016/j.smallrumres.2016.02.021.

Silberberg, M., Chaucheyras-Durand, F., Commun, L., Mialon, M.M., Monteils, V. *et al.* (2013) Repeated acidosis challenges and live yeast supplementation shape rumen microbiota and fermentations and modulate inflammatory status in sheep. *Animal* 7(12), 1910–1920. DOI: 10.1017/S1751731113001705.

Sommer, F., Anderson, J.M., Bharti, R., Raes, J. and Rosenstiel, P. (2017) The resilience of the intestinal microbiota influences health and disease. *Nature Reviews. Microbiology* 15(10), 630–638. DOI: 10.1038/NRMICRO.2017.58.

Wang, X., Hu, L., Liu, H., Xu, T., Zhao, N. *et al.* (2021) Characterization of the bacterial microbiota across the different intestinal segments of the Qinghai semi-fine wool sheep on the Qinghai-Tibetan Plateau. *Animal Bioscience* 34(12), 1921–1929. DOI: 10.5713/ab.20.0809.

Weinstock, G.M. (2012) Genomic approaches to studying the human microbiota. *Nature* 489(7415), 250–256. DOI: 10.1038/nature11553.

WOAH (2020) *Uso responsable y prudente de los fármacos antihelmínticos para contribuir al control de la resistencia a antihelmínticos en las especies ganaderas herbívoras*. Organización Mundial de Sanidad Animal. Available at: es-oie-anthelmintics-prudent-and-responsible-use-v4-web (accessed 28 May 2025).

Yanuartono, Y., Indarjulianto, S., Nururrozi, A. and Purnamaningsih, H. (2019) Nematodes resistance on anthelmintics group of benzimidazole in ruminants. *Journal of Livestock Science and Production* 3(1), 164–178. DOI: 10.31002/jalspro.v3i1.1464.

Yu, Z., Yan, M. and Somasundaram, S. (2024) Rumen protozoa and viruses: The predators within and their functions – A mini-review. *JDS Communications* 5(3), 236–240. DOI: 10.3168/jdsc.2023-0433.

Index

Printed and bound by CPI Group (UK) Ltd, Croydon, CR0 4YY

13/09/2026

14961085-0008